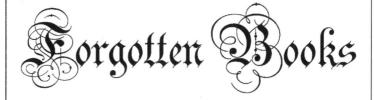

ISBN 978-1-330-49211-6
PIBN 10069110

1 MONTH OF
FREE
READING

at

www.ForgottenBooks.com

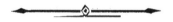

By purchasing this book you are eligible for one month membership to ForgottenBooks.com, giving you unlimited access to our entire collection of over 1,000,000 titles via our web site and mobile apps.

To claim your free month visit: www.forgottenbooks.com/free69110

English
Français
Deutsche
Italiano
Español
Português

www.forgottenbooks.com

Mythology Photography **Fiction**
Fishing Christianity **Art** Cooking
Essays Buddhism Freemasonry
Medicine **Biology** Music **Ancient
Egypt** Evolution Carpentry Physics
Dance Geology **Mathematics** Fitness
Shakespeare **Folklore** Yoga Marketing
Confidence Immortality Biographies
Poetry **Psychology** Witchcraft
Electronics Chemistry History **Law**
Accounting **Philosophy** Anthropology
Alchemy Drama Quantum Mechanics
Atheism Sexual Health **Ancient History**
Entrepreneurship Languages Sport
Paleontology Needlework Islam
Metaphysics Investment Archaeology
Parenting Statistics Criminology
Motivational

THE

STUDY OF MEDICINE.

BY JOHN MASON GOOD,
M.D. F.R.S. F.R.S.L.
MEM. AM. PHIL. SOC. AND F.L.S. OF PHILADELPHIA.

IMPROVED FROM THE AUTHOR'S MANUSCRIPTS,

AND BY REFERENCE TO THE LATEST ADVANCES IN

𝔓𝔥𝔶𝔰𝔦𝔬𝔩𝔬𝔤𝔶, 𝔓𝔞𝔱𝔥𝔬𝔩𝔬𝔤𝔶, 𝔞𝔫𝔡 𝔓𝔯𝔞𝔠𝔱𝔦𝔠𝔢.

BY SAMUEL COOPER,
PROFESSOR OF SURGERY IN THE UNIVERSITY OF LONDON, ETC.

SIXTH AMERICAN, FROM THE LAST ENGLISH EDITION.

WITH NOTES,

BY A. SIDNEY DOANE, A.M. M.D.

TO WHICH IS PREFIXED,

A SKETCH OF THE HISTORY OF MEDICINE,
FROM ITS ORIGIN TO THE COMMENCEMENT OF THE NINETEENTH CENTURY.

BY J. BOSTOCK, M.D. F.R.S.

IN TWO VOLUMES.
VOL. II.

NEW-YORK:

PUBLISHED BY HARPER & BROTHERS,
NO. 82 CLIFF-STREET.

1835.

HÆMATICA.

DISEASES OF THE SANGUINEOUS FUNCTION.

ORDER IV.

DYSTHETICA.

CACHEXIES.

ORDER IV.

DYSTHETICA.

CACHEXIES.

MORBID STATE OF THE BLOOD OR BLOODVES-
SELS; ALONE, OR CONNECTED WITH A MOR-
BID STATE OF THE FLUIDS, PRODUCING A
DISEASED HABIT.

THE words ordinarily used to import the diseases meant to be comprehended under the
present order, are CACHEXIA and IMPETIGO, or,
as the Greeks expressed it, λύης, LUES, or LYES.
None of these, however, exactly answer, and
that on two accounts: first, because the order
is limited to those depravities which seem to
originate or manifest themselves chiefly in vessels or fluids of the sanguineous function; and,
secondly, because no very definite sense has
hitherto been assigned to either of these terms,
and they have in consequence been used in
very different meanings by different writers,
from the time of Celsus to our own day.

· Upon this subject the author has dwelt at
large in his volume of Nosology, and it is not
necessary to add to the remarks there offered.
The word DYSTHETICA has hence been adopted
for the purpose of avoiding confusion, and is
justified by the EUSTHESIA and EUSTHETICA
(ΕΥΣΘΕΣΙΑ) and (ΕΥΣΘΕΤΙΚΑ) of Hippocrates
and Galen, importing a "well-conditioned habit
of body," as their opposite, DYSTHETICA, from
the same root, imports "an ill-conditioned habit,"
but a habit, as just observed, originating in, or
dependant upon, the organized parts or fluids
of the sanguineous function. Thus explained,
it will be found to embrace the following
genera:—

I.	Plethora.	Plethora.
II.	Hæmorrhagia.	Hemorrhage.
III.	Marasmus.	Emaciation.
IV.	Melanosis.	Melanose.
V.	Struma.	Scrofula. King's Evil.
VI.	Carcinus.	Cancer.
VII.	Lues.	Venereal Disease.
VIII.	Elephantiasis.	Elephant-skin.
IX.	Catacausis.	Spontaneous Ignescence.
X.	Porphyra.	Scurvy.
XI.	Exangia.	Vascular Divarication.
XII.	Gangræna.	Gangrene.
XIII.	Ulcus.	Ulcers.

A 2

GENUS I.

PLETHORA.

PLETHORA.

COMPLEXION FLORID; VEINS DISTENDED; UNDUE
SENSE OF HEAT AND FULNESS; OPPRESSION
OF THE HEAD, CHEST, OR OTHER INTERNAL
ORGANS.

PLETHORA is seldom ranked as a disease, and
hence seldom treated of in a course of medical
instruction. From what cause this omission
proceeds I know not, nor is it worth while to
inquire. That it is an important omission, will
be obvious to every student before he has been
six months in practice; for there will probably
be few affections on which he will be sooner or
more frequently consulted. Yet, the subject
has not always been neglected by nosologists;
for plethora, as a genus, occurs in the classifi-
cations both of Linnæus and Sagar.

In a state of health, the quantity of blood
produced from the substances that constitute
our common diet, bears an exact proportion to
the quantity demanded by the vascular system
in its ordinary diameter and the various secretions which are perpetually taking place in every
part of the body. But the quantity of blood
produced within a given period of time may
vary; and the diameter of the bloodvessels,
or the call of the different secernent organs,
may vary; yet, so long as a due balance is
maintained, and the proportion of new-formed
blood is answerable to the demand, the general
health continues perfect, or is little interfered
with. Thus, a man exhausted and worn down
by shipwreck, or by having lost his way in a
desert, or who is just recovering from a fever,
will devour double the food and elaborate double
the quantity of chyle, in the course of four-
and-twenty hours, to what he would have done
in the ordinary wear of life; but the whole
system demands this double exertion; the double supply is made use of, and the general harmony of the frame is as accurately maintained
as at any former period; there is no accumulation or plethora.

It should also be observed, that in this case,
the same remedial or instinctive power that
stimulates the sanguific organs to the formation
of a larger proportion of blood, stimulates also
the bloodvessels to a diminution of their ordi-

nary capacity, and lessens the activity of the secernents ; and hence the difficulty to which the animal machine is reduced is also met-another way, and a balance between the contained fluid and the containing tubes is often preserved as completely during the utmost degree of exhaustion as in the fullest flow of healthy plenitude.

We sometimes, however, meet with cases in which an increased supply of blood is furnished when no such increase is wanted, and the vessels remain of their ordinary capacity. And we also sometimes meet with cases in which, from a peculiar diathesis, the capacity of the vessels is unduly contracted, while no change takes place in the ordinary supply of blood. It is evident that in both these contingences, there must be an equal disturbance of the balance between the substance contained and the substance containing, and that the measure of the former must be too large for the measure of the latter. In other words, there must be in both cases an excess of fluid, or a plethora, though from very different, and are usually regarded as opposite, causes : and hence it has been distinguished by different names; that proceeding from an actual surplus of blood being denominated a plethora ad molem, or a plethora in respect to its general mass or absolute quantity ; and that proceeding from a diminished capacity of the vessels being denominated a plethora ad spatium, or a plethora in respect to the space to be occupied.

It is possible, however, for both these causes of plethora to exist at the same time, and for the vessels to evince a contractile habit or diathesis, while the blood is produced in an inordinate proportion. And this, in truth, is by no means an uncommon state of the animal frame ; for, where the excess of blood is the result of a highly vigorous action or eutony of the organs of sanguification, we often see proof of the same entony or highly vigorous action through the whole range of the vascular system, and, indeed, of every other part of the machine ; the pulse is full, strong, and rebounding ; the muscular fibres firm and energetic, the complexion florid, the whole figure strongly marked. We have here the sanguine temperament ; and this kind of plethora has hence been called the SANGUINE PLETHORA.

But we often meet with an inordinate formation of blood in a constitution where the vascular action is peculiarly weak, instead of being peculiarly vigorous ; the muscular fibres are relaxed, instead of being firm ; and the coats of the vessels readily give way, and become enlarged, instead of being diminished in their diameter ; and where, instead of entony, or excess of strength, there is considerable irritability, or deficiency of strength in the organs of sanguification.

Yet though the cause is different, the result is the same ; the vessels, notwithstanding their facility of dilatation, at length become distended, and a plethora is produced which has been denominated a plethora ad vires ; or a plethora as it respects the actual strength of the system.

The pulse is here indeed full, but frequent and feeble ; the vital actions are languid ; the skin smooth and soft, the figure plump, but inexpressive ; all which are symptoms of debility of the living power, or rather of that peculiar diathesis which has been distinguished by the name of the serous, phlegmatic, or pituitary temperament ; and hence this sort of plethora has been commonly denominated SEROUS PLETHORA.

We have hence a foundation for the two following very distinct species of this affection, the names of which are derived from their proximate causes.

1. Plethora Entonica.   Sanguine Plethora.
2. ——— Atonica.   Serous Plethora.*

SPECIES I.
PLETHORA ENTONICA.
SANGUINE PLETHORA.

PULSE FULL, STRONG, REBOUNDING : MUSCULAR FIBRES FIRM AND VIGOROUS.

SANGUINE plethora is more common to men ; serous to women. It is the disease of manhood, of the robust and athletic. Plethora of this kind must be distinguished from obesity ; in effect, they are rarely found in conjunction, for the entony, or excess of vigorous action, is common to every part of the animal frame ; and hence, though it is probable that a larger portion of animal oil is secreted than in many other conditions of the body, yet it is carried off by the activity of the absorbents, and there is no leisure for its accumulation in the cellular membrane. And hence, persons, labouring under sanguine plethora, are rather muscular than fat, and their distended veins lie superficially, and appear to peep through the skin.

In this state of the bloodvessels, slight excitements produce congestion in the larger vessels or organs. The head feels heavy and comatose ; the sleep is disturbed by tumultuous dreams ; the lungs labour in respiration ; and the muscles feel a want of freedom or elasticity in exercise. If fever arise, it will assume the inflammatory type ; and a slight excess in feasting or conviviality will endanger an apoplexy.†

The cure, however, is not in general accom-

---

* Dr. Barlow distinguishes plethora into *absolute* and *relative* (Cycl. of Pract. Med., art. PLETHORA); the former term implying that the redundance of blood exceeds what the healthy state of the individual constitution would require or bear ; the latter, that its quantity, without being absolutely excessive, is so in relation to the deficient powers of the constitution to dispose of it. But as these varieties of plethora do not comprise the whole subject, he notices a third condition of the blood, which takes place when, under moderate nutrition, there is defective excretion. In this state the system is oppressed, not so much by the quantity of nutriment, or the labour of disposing of it, as by the load of excrementitious matter with which the blood is overcharged.—ED.

† Instead of saying that plethora is " the parent of pure inflammation" (Cyclop. of Pract. Med.), it would be more correct to regard it as creating a predisposition to inflammatory disorders.—ED.

panied with much difficulty; and far more easily effected in this species than in the ensuing: for the entonic power may readily be lowered by venesection and purgatives; and its disposition to return may commonly be prevented by the use of refrigerants, as nitrate of potash, or other neutral salts, and an adherence to a reduced diet and liberal exercise; at the same time it should be observed, that, where the plethora depends upon a sanguineous temperament or phlogistic diathesis, venesection, though rightly employed at first, should be repeated with great caution, as it will tend to generate in the system a periodical necessity for the same kind of depletion, and consequently promote the disease it is designed to cure.* ...

SPECIES II.
PLETHORA ATONICA.
SEROUS PLETHORA.

PULSE FULL, FREQUENT, FEEBLE: VITAL ACTIONS LANGUID; SKIN SMOOTH AND SOFT; FIGURE PLUMP, BUT INEXPRESSIVE.

THE general pathology we have already treated of: and the reasons given under the last species for the usual appearance of sanguine plethora in persons of a spare and slender make, will explain the plumpness of figure and glossiness of skin which so peculiarly mark the species before us. In the first, there is great and universal vigour and rapidity of action; the secretions are all hurried forward in their elaborations, and carried off as soon as produced. In the second, there is little vigour or activity of any kind, and whatever is eliminated is suffered to accumulate. Hence costiveness is a common symptom; the ankles are cold and pituitous; and the animal oil, when once separated and deposited in the chambers of the cellular membrane, remains there, becomes augmented, and produces corpulency and sleekness. The inertness of the body is communicated to the mind; every exertion is a fatigue; and the mind thus participating in the inertness of the body, the countenance, though fair and rounded, is without expression, and often vacant.

Debility is always a source of irritability;

* An increase of bulk and a florid complexion, as Dr. Barlow observes, in which so many exult as evincing sound health, and which they endeavour by all the aids of good living to promote, should not be a source of unmixed congratulation; because they predispose to consequences by which both health and life may be forfeited. "Up to this period, however, disease cannot be said to have commenced, however it may have approached; and reduction of diet, with free bowels, and increase of active exercise, would suffice for getting back to sounder health, without any need of medical interference. When abatement of healthful energies becomes evinced by a low and oppressed pulse, diseased actions may be said to commence; and when the stage of irregular action ensues, sensible progress may be considered as made towards the establishment of febrile action and inflammatory disease." Medical aid and active discipline now become indispensable.—See Cyclop. of Pract. Med., art. PLETHORA.—ED.

and hence there is great irregularity, and a seeming fickleness in many of the symptoms by which this species of plethora is characterized, and the results to which it leads. The bowels, though usually quiescent and costive, are sometimes all of a sudden attacked with flatulent spasms, or a troublesome looseness. The appetite is languid and capricious; the heart teased with palpitations, the chest with dyspnœa and wheezing; the head is heavy and somnolent; the urine pale, small in quantity, and discharged frequently.

In this species, as in the last, we are compelled to begin with cupping or the use of the lancet. But though the distended and overflowing vessels demand an abstraction of blood, it should never be forgotten, that the relief hereby afforded is only temporary; and that, as the disease is, in this case, an effect of debility, we are directly adding to the cause as often as we have recourse to the lancet. Our leading object should be to give tone to the relaxed fibres; and to take off the morbid tendency to the production of a surplus of blood by counteracting the irritability which gives rise to it. Our attack must be made upon the entire habit, which, as far as possible, should undergo a total change. The diet should be nutritious, but perfectly simple, and the meals less frequent, or less abundant, than usual; the sedentary life should give way to exercise, at first easy and gentle, but by degrees more active, and of longer extent or duration. Tonics, as bitters, astringents, and sea-bathing, may now be employed with advantage; and the muscular fibres will become firmer as the cellular substance loses its bulk.

The whole, however, must be the work of time; for although in morals it is a wholesome principle, that bad habits cannot too speedily be thrown off, it is a mischievous doctrine in medicine. Health being the middle term between excess and deficiency, every day is giving us a proof, that where either of these extremes has become habitual, the system can only be let up or let down by slow degrees, so as to reach and rest at the middle point with certainty and without inconvenience. Professor Monro has furnished us with several very striking examples of this fact: and particularly among those who had acquired a habit of drinking very large quantities of spirituous potation. A man of this description, who had broken both bones of one leg, and was put, for a more speedy recovery, upon a diet of milk and water and water-gruel, was hereby thrown into a low fever with an intermitting pulse, twitching tendons, and delirium; during which he got out of bed and kicked away the box in which his leg was confined. A by-stander and friend of the patient's, of the same irregular habit, ventured to tell the professor, that he would certainly kill him if he did not allow him ale and brandy; since, for several years antecedently, he had been accustomed to both these as his common drink: a little of each was, in consequence, permitted him, but the patient's friends did not tie him down to this little; for, extending the grant of an inch to an ell, they instantly gave the man a Scots quart of ale and a gill of brandy, which was his usual allowance for the evening: he slept well and sound; the next morning was free from delirium and fever; and, by a perseverance in the same regimen, obtained a speedy cure without the least accident.

GENUS II.
HÆMORRHAGIA.
HEMORRHAGE.
FLUX OF BLOOD WITHOUT EXTERNAL VIOLENCE.

THE term hæmorrhagia, or hemorrhage, is derived from the Greek αἷμα, "sanguis," and ῥήγνυμι, ",rumpo." Dr. Cullen has adopted the same name for an order of diseases; but few parts of his arrangement are more open to animadversion, and in fact have been more animadverted upon, than the present. The order of hemorrhages, or fluxes of blood, ranks in Dr. Cullen's system under the class pyrexiæ, or febrile diseases. Pyrexy, however, is only an accidental symptom in idiopathic hemorrhages of any kind, and has hence been omitted by all, or nearly all, other nosologists in their definitions: while Dr. Cullen himself has found it impossible to apply it to many hemorrhages, among which are all those that are called passive; and he has hence been obliged to transfer the whole of these to another part of his system, notwithstanding their natural connexion with the active, and to distinguish them by the feeble name of *profusions*, instead of by their own proper denomination.

Blood, from whatever organ it flows, may have two causes for its issue. The vessels may be ruptured by a morbid distention and impetus; or they may give way from debility and relaxation, their tunics breaking without any peculiar force urged against them, or their exhalants admitting the flow of red blood, instead of the more attenuate serum.† To the former de-

scription of hemorrhages, Dr. Cullen has given the name of active; to the latter that of passive.† The distinction is sufficiently clear; and, under the names already employed in the preceding genus of this system, will lay a foundation for the two following species:—

1. Hæmorrhagia Ento- Entonic Hemorrhage.
   nica.
2. ————— Atonica. Atonic Hemorrhage.

SPECIES I.
HÆMORRHAGIA ENTONICA.
ENTONIC HEMORRHAGE.
ACCOMPANIED WITH INCREASED VASCULAR ACTION; THE BLOOD FLORID AND TENACIOUS.

As the outlets of the body are but few, and all of them communicate with numerous organs, we cannot always determine with strict accuracy from what particular part the discharge flows. We have, however, sufficient reason for the following varieties:—

α Narium.	Entonic bleeding at the nose.
β Hæmoptysis.	——— spitting of blood.
γ Hæmatemesis.	——— vomiting of blood.
δ Hæmaturia.	——— bloody urine.
ε Uterina.	——— uterine hemorrhage.
ζ Proctica.	——— anal hemorrhage.

The great predisponent cause of active hemorrhage, wherever it makes its appearance, is plethora or congestion. A plethoric diathesis will, however, only predispose to a hemorrhage *somewhere* or *other*; and hence there must be a distinct local cause that fixes it upon one particular organ rather than upon another.*

---

* Edin. Med. Ess., vol. v., part II., art. XLVI. With regard to the treatment of plethora from inadequate excretion, Dr. Barlow has remarked, that a constitution naturally feeble, especially if insufficient exercise be taken, sends the blood to the surface too languidly for proper exhalation from the skin to take place. The best preventive of this diseased condition seems, to him, to be exercise, slighter degrees of which would also be the most effectual cure. Dr. Barlow is likewise an advocate for warm bathing, combined with frictions, and other means of softening and detaching hardened cuticle. The Russian vapour-bath, so accurately described by the late Dr. Clarke, appears well calculated for establishing a healthy state of the cutaneous functions.—ED.

† On this subject some judicious observations are made by M. Andral (Anat. Pathol., tom. i., p. 338), who cautions the practitioner not to confound discharges of blood from mucous membranes with other affections, of which a degree of inflammation is necessarily a part. In hemorrhage, there may, indeed, be determination of blood to the part; but it seems as if the fluid, instead of accumulating in the vessels of the mucous membrane, escaped as soon as it reached them, owing to some unknown modification of them. There may also be a passive fulness of them, as in obstruction of the venous circulation.

But an unusual flow of blood to, or fulness of the vessels, is not essentially concerned in every kind of hemorrhage; for the qualities of the blood may be so altered, that the natural cohesion of its particles may one another may be weakened, and then it may readily escape from the vessels, producing hemorrhage, quite independent of irritation, in several parts of the system at the same time. This is what is observed in scurvy and typhoid fevers, and in every case where attention to causes, and the look of the blood itself, afford a conviction that this fluid is materially altered.—ED.

* The reader will find many valuable observations on internal hemorrhages in the Lumleian Lectures, delivered at the College of Physicians in May, 1832, by Dr. Watson, and published in the Medical Gazette, vol. x. He espouses the doctrine that, in a great majority of instances, the escape of the blood is not dependant upon rupture of the vessels, but is effused through those pores or outlets which afford a passage to the natural fluids of the part, and to which we apply the name of exhalants. These hemorrhages by exhalation he divides into the *idiopathic*, or such as are independent of any discoverable change of texture in any part of the body; and the *symptomatic*, or those which are connected with organic disease; and this latter class is subdivided into two species; the first including cases in which the hemorrhage is dependant upon disease in the part from which the blood proceeds; and the second, those examples in which the disease is situated in some other part, capable of influencing the circulation in the

The chief local cause is a greater degree of debility in the vessels of such organ, than belongs to the vascular system generally. But there are other and more extensive causes that operate upon some organs, and which consist in an unequal distribution of the blood, and its peculiar accumulation in some vessels rather than in others. Thus, some organs acquire development and perfection sooner than others, of which the head, peculiarly large, even in infancy, furnishes us with a striking example; and, in the promotion of such development, the flow of the blood is directed with greater force and in greater abundance. And hence while the coats of the bloodvessels in this organ are yet tender, and destitute of that firmness which they derive from age, we have reason to expect hemorrhage as a frequent occurrence, and particularly from the vessels of the nostrils; because there is in the nose, for the use of the olfactory sense, a considerable network of bloodvessels expanded on the internal surface of the nostrils, and covered only by thin and weak integuments. And on this account, we see why young persons are so much more subject to bleedings from this organ, than those in mature life. Hæmoptysis, or spitting of blood, takes place more commonly a few years later, and when the animal frame has acquired its full growth, and, consequently, the vascular system its full extent or longitude. Antecedently to this, the impetus and determination of blood are greater in the aorta and its extreme ramifications than in the pulmonary artery, because more of the vital fluid is demanded for the progressive elongation of the very numerous arteries that issue from the former: and consequently, a greater tendency to plethora exists in this direction till the age of about fifteen or eighteen, than in the direction of the lungs. Till this period of life, therefore, we have no reason to expect hemorrhage from the respiratory organs. When this term, however, has arrived, the bias is thrown on the other side: and, the vessels of the corporeal and of the pulmonary circulation being equally perfected, the tendency to accumulation will be in the latter, in consequence of their shorter extent. This tendency will continue till about the age of thirty-five; which is exactly correspondent with the observation of Hippocrates, who has remarked, that hæmoptysis commonly occurs between the age of fifteen and that of five-and-thirty. We have explained why it does not often occur before fifteen; but what is the rea-

son of its seldom occurring after the latter period? Dr. Cullen has ingeniously explained it in the following manner. The experiments of Sir Clifton Wintringham, he observes, have shown, that the density of the coats of the veins, compared with that of the arteries, is greater in young than in old animals; from which it may be presumed, that the resistance to the passage of the blood from the arteries into the veins is greater in young animals than in old; and while this resistance continues, the plethoric state of the arteries must be perpetually kept up. The very action, however, of an increased pressure against the coats of the arteries gradually thickens and strengthens them, and renders them more capable of resistance; whence in time they come not only to be on a balance with those of the veins, but to prevail over them; a fact which is also established by the experiments just adverted to.

After thirty-five, therefore, the constitutional balance becomes completely changed, and the veins, instead of the arteries, are chiefly subject to accumulation. The greatest congestion will usually, perhaps, be found in the vena portarum, in which the motion of the venous blood is slower than elsewhere; and such congestion alone will frequently act upon the neighbouring arteries, and induce what may be called a reflex plethora upon them, in consequence of their inability of unloading themselves: and hence the chief origin of hæmatemesis, anal hemorrhage, and various other hemorrhages from the abdominal and pelvic organs.*

All these organs, however, are exposed to hemorrhage from incidental causes, as well as

* The following conditions are specified by Andral, as liable to bring on hemorrhage from the mucous membrane of the digestive tube (Anat. Pathol., tom. ii., p. 150):— 1. A mechanical obstruction of the circulation in the vena portæ. 2. Irritation of the mucous coat of the stomach and bowels. Thus, certain corrosive poisons, taken into the stomach, will be followed by hæmatemesis, and strong drastic medicines will occasion hemorrhage from the bowels. 3. Sanguineous congestion, neither of a mechanical kind, as in the first case, nor the result of irritation, as in the second. The blood simply accumulates at a certain point, and makes its escape, and that is all that can be ascertained. 4. Certain states of the blood itself, making it disposed to quit its proper channels, as exemplified where particular poisons are absorbed; in typhus, and also in yellow fever, with black vomit. 5. Lastly, blood in the cavity of the stomach and bowels may have got there by being swallowed, as happens when an aneurism of the aorta bursts into the œsophagus.

In hæmatemesis, the blood is usually poured out by a kind of exhalation; the bleeding from ulceration of any considerable artery, or vein, being comparatively rare. Three examples of the latter occurrence are quoted by Dr. Watson (Med. Gazette, vol. x., p. 434); one from the Journ. Hebdomadaire for May, 1830; a second from Dr. Latham's patients in St. Bartholomew's Hospital; and a third from the practice of Dr. Clark. In all these cases, there had been marked symptoms of gastric disorder for some time previously to the hemorrhage, and two of the subjects had been habitual drunkards.—ED.

former, by reason of some intelligible connexion between them, either of structure, or function, or mutual relation. Dr. Watson adverts to the fact, that hemorrhage by exhalation occurs much more frequently from the mucous membranes, than from any other tissues of the body; and also to the remarkable circumstance, that hemorrhage from the brain differs from most other internal bleedings, in not taking place by exhalation, but from actual rupture of a bloodvessel. This is attempted to be accounted for, partly by a reference to the structure and arrangement of the cerebral arteries, but chiefly by the consideration of their great liability to disease.—ED.

that constitutional change which has a tendency to produce the disease vicariously.

Thus, hemorrhage in all of them is occasionally produced by violent exertion, as great muscular force, vehement anger, or other passions or emotions of the mind ; severe vomiting, or coughing ; suppressed evacuations of various kinds, especially hemorrhoids of long standing, catamenia, habitual ulcers, issues, or chronic eruptions of the skin :* as also by the wound of a leech swallowed accidentally.† But in this last case it is probable, that the living principle of the stomach is in a state of weakness, as in all other cases in which exotic worms are found to continue alive under its action : since we know that this action, when in full vigour, is sufficient to destroy oysters, frogs, slugs, leeches, and various other cold-blooded animals in a short time. Hæmoptysis is also said by many writers to have been produced by leeches accidentally taken into the stomach by a draught of water.‡ But it is probable, that in this case there is a deception ; and that the blood, discharged by coughing from the trachea, has first passed into it from the stomach and mouth.

Local stimulants are also an occasional cause. Thus the vessels both of the kidneys and rectum have been excited to hemorrhage by an injudicious use of aloes, terebinthinate preparations, and pungent alliaceous sauces. And the former by cantharides, whether applied externally or internally : for Schenck and other writers have given examples of hæmaturia excited in irritable constitutions by vesicatories alone §

Occasionally, however, all the various kinds of hemorrhages before us have assumed a different character, and proved salutary and critical. Thus, cephalitis has often ceased suddenly on a free and sudden discharge of blood from the nostrils ; pneumonitis, from what has been deemed an alarming hæmoptysis : visceral infarctions, from a liberal evacuation of the hemorrhoidal vessels ; a jaundice has been carried off by a profuse hæmaturia,‖ and fevers of various kinds have instantly yielded to a spontaneous appearance of any of them.

Such hemorrhages, however, though salutary in their onset, must be cautiously watched ; since, if not checked when they have accomplished their object, they are apt to pass into a chronic or periodic form. Hence, many persons have monthly discharges from the rectum ; others from the nostrils ; others, again, occasioual or periodic, from the lungs ; and a few from the stomach.¶ Tulpius gives a case of chronic hæmoptysis that continued for thirty years ;** and there are other instances of much longer duration.††

There is also another reason for an early attention to spontaneous hemorrhages, and that is, the profuseness of the discharge which sometimes takes place, and the alarming exhaustion which follows. Dr. Bauyer* gives a case of this sort, in which the discharge was from the bladder : Büchner, another case from the same organ, in which it amounted to not less than four pounds :† and other writers bring examples of its having proved fatal.

The largest quantities, however, are usually lost from the nostrils. Ten, twelve, and upwards of twenty pounds have been known to flow away before the hemorrhage has ceased. Bartholin mentions a case of forty-eight pounds ;‡ Rhodius another of eighteen pounds lost within thirty-six hours ;§ and a respectable writer, in the Leipsic Acta Erudita, a third, of not less than seventy-five pounds within ten days ;‖ which is most probably nearly three times as much as the patient possessed in his entire body at the time the hemorrhage commenced. In the Ephemera of Natural Curiosities is a case in which the quantity indeed is not given, probably from the difficulty of taking an account of it, but which continued without cessation for six weeks.¶

In ACTIVE HEMORRHAGES FROM THE NOSTRILS, the epistaxis of many writers, the discharge is usually preceded by some degree of local heat and itching ; and occasionally by a flushing of the face, a throbbing of the temporal arteries, a ringing in the ears, or a pain or sense of weight and fulness in the head. Yet, not unfrequently, the blood issues suddenly without any of these precursories ; for, as we have already observed, the arteries, distributed over the Schneiderian membrane, are very numerous and superficial, and a very slight irritation is often sufficient to rupture them. That insolation, or exposure to the direct rays of the sun, a cold in the head, cold applied to the feet or hands, coughing, or sneezing, especially upon the use of sternutatories, an accidental blow upon the upper part of the nose or forehead, or a jar of the entire frame, as on stumbling, should be sufficient to produce this effect, can easily be conceived ; and these, in truth, are the common occasional causes : but it is singular that it should follow, in some highly irritable idiosyncrasies, upon such very trivial excitements as have been noticed by many pathologists. Thus, Bruyerin** gives an example in which the nostrils flowed with blood upon smelling at an apple ; Rhodius,†† upon the smell of a rose ; and Blancard,‡‡ upon the ringing of bells : and when we find the same effect produced by various emotions of the mind, as terror, anger, and even a simple excitement of the imagination,§§ we may readily trace by

* Percival's Essays, ii., p. 181.
† Galen, De Loc. Affect., lib., iv., cap. v. Riverius, Observ. Med., cent. iv., obs. 26.
‡ Galen, De Loc. Affect., lib. iv., cap. v. Borelli, cent. i., obs. 24.
§ Schenck, lib. vii., obs. 124, ex Langio. Hist. Mort. Uratislav., p. 58.
‖ Schenck, obs., lib. iii., serm. ii., n. 258.
¶ Rhodius, cent. ii., obs. 94.
** Lib. ii., cap. ii.
†† N. Act. Nat. Cur., vol. i., obs. 1.

* Phil. Trans., vol. xlii.
† Miscell. 1728, p. 1496.
‡ Anat. Renov., lib. ii., cap. vi.
§ Cent. i., obs. 90.   ‖ Lib. 1688, p. 205.
¶ Dec. i., ann. iii., obs. 243.
** De Re Cibariâ, lib. i., cap. 24.
†† Cent. iii., obs. 99.
‡‡ Collect. Med. Phys., cent. vi., obs. 74.
§§ Rhodius, cent. i., obs. 89.

by what means the philosophers and poets of the eastern world, and even some of those of the western, were led to regard the nose as the seat of mental irritation, the peculiar organ of heat, wrath, and anger ; and may discover how the same term אף (ap or aph) came to be employed among the Hebrews to signify both the organ and its effect, the nose and the passion of anger to which it was supposed to give rise.

We have already observed, that the quantity of blood discharged by a spontaneous hemorrhage from the nostrils, is sometimes enormous. This, however, is a more common result of passive than of active hemorrhage ; and is more usually found in advanced than in early life : the two stages in which nasal hemorrhage chiefly shows itself. And where it frequently returns, it is apt, like the hemorrhoids, to form a habit of recurrence that cannot be broken through without danger, except by an employment of evacuants, or some other drain.*

If it be evidently connected with entonic plethora, or accompanied with the local symptoms just enumerated, it will afford a more effectual relief than bleeding in any other way, and should not be restrained till it has answered its purpose. Even a small portion of blood, not amounting to more than a table-spoonful or two, when thus locally and spontaneously evacuated, has afforded, on some occasions, a wonderful freedom and elasticity to an oppressed and heavy head : and, when more copious, has probably prevented an apoplectic fit, as it has often formed a salutary crisis in inflammation of the brain, or fevers in which the brain has been much affected.

But when these reasons do not exist, the bleeding should be checked by astringent applications. Cold is the ordinary application for this purpose, and it commonly succeeds without much trouble. Cold water may be sniffed up the nostrils, or thrown up with a syringe ; but the exertion of sniffing, or even the impetus of the water alone, where a syringe is employed, sometimes proves an excitement that more than counterbalances the frigoric effect. Independently of which, there is an advantage in leaving the blood to coagulate on the ruptured orifice of the vessel, which these methods do not allow. By means of a syringe, however, we can throw up, when necessary, astringents of more power than cold water, as vinegar, or the sulphuric acid properly diluted, or a solution of sulphate of zinc, copper, iron, or lead ; after which we should force up tents of lint moistened with the same, and particularly with extract of lead diluted with only an equal quantity of water, as high as we are able, with a probe or small forceps, so as to form a tight compress : the styptic agarics can be rarely used to advantage. The face may, at the same time, be frequently immersed in ice-water, or water artificially chilled to the freezing point ; and the temples, or even the whole of the head, be surrounded with a band or napkin moistened

with the same, and changed as soon as it acquires the warmth of the skin. When tents are used, they have sometimes been dipped in moistened powder of charcoal, which, of itself, has proved an excellent styptic. Cold applied to the back sometimes succeeds, but often fails ; it is more certain of success when applied to the genitals.

Emetics have occasionally been of service, and are recommended by Stoll.* The principle upon which they may be presumed to act will be noticed under hæmoptysis. The bleeding has sometimes been checked by a sudden fright,† probably from the cold sweat that so often attends such an emotion : and Reidlin gives a case in which it was cured by sneezing ;‡ but this was probably a case of atonic hemorrhage, in which the spasmodic action might assist in corrugating the mouths of the bleeding vessels.

It is rarely necessary, or even proper, in this variety of hemorrhage, to employ any internal astringent or other tonic ; but if this discharge should be excessive, and produce debility, the same plan may be resorted to as will be recommended under the ensuing species.

In ʜᴀ̨ᴍᴏᴘᴛʏsɪs, or sᴘɪᴛᴛɪɴɢ ᴏғ ʙʟᴏᴏᴅ, it is not always easy to determine from what vessel, or even from what organ, the bleeding proceeds : for the blood may issue from the posterior cavity of the nostrils, or from the fauces, as well as from the lungs. If, however, from the first, it will cease upon bending the head forward, or lying procumbent, and will probably flow from the nose : if from the second, we shall commonly be able to satisfy ourselves by inspection. Blood from the stomach is of a darker colour, thrown up by vomiting, and betrays an intermixture of food.

If the hæmoptysis be from the lungs, and belong strictly to the present species, and more especially if it be a result of entonic plethora, the blood will be chiefly thrown up by coughing ; and the discharge will be preceded by flushed cheeks, dyspnœa, and pain in the chest. There is usually, also, a sense of tickling about the fauces, which often descends considerably lower : Salmuth asserts, that he has known it extend to the scrobiculus cordis.◊ These symptoms, moreover, indicate that the blood flows from a branch of the pulmonary, rather than of the bronchial artery. The blood is here of a florid hue, and the hemorrhage sudden and often copious. If a branch of the bronchial artery give way, the flow of blood is usually much slower, and smaller in quantity ; there are no precursive symptoms, the blood is rather hawked or spit up intermixed with saliva, and, from being longer in its ascent, is of a darker colour. From its lodgment, however, in the air-vesicles, it becomes a cause of irritation, and a frothy cough ensues, sometimes accompanied with a little increase of the pulse and other febrile

---

* J. P. Frank, De Cur. Hom. Morb. Epit., tom. vi., lib. vi., part iii. 8vo. Viennæ, 1821.

* Rat. Med., part iii., p. 21.
† Panarol. Pentecost., v., obs. 27.
‡ Linn. Med., ann. i., obs. 24.
◊ Cent. iii., obs.

symptoms, as a feeling of heat and some degree of pain in the breast, which subsides after the ejection, and returns if there be a fresh issue.

If the structure of the lungs be sound, we have no reason to prognosticate danger. On the contrary, it often affords great relief to a gorged liver, and has proved critical in obstructed menstruation.* Excreted with the sputum, it is frequently serviceable, as we have already observed, in cases of asthma, pleurisy, and peripneumony. But if it have been preceded by symptoms of phthisis, or a strumous diathesis, there is a great reason for alarm; for we can have little hope that the ruptured vessel will heal kindly and speedily, and have much to fear from the fresh jets by which the extravasated blood becomes deposited, and forms a perpetual stimulus in an irritable organ.

The general pathology has been already laid down. The incidental causes are, misformation of the chest; undue exertion of the respiratory muscles, whether in running, wrestling, singing, or blowing wind instruments; excess in eating and drinking; or a violent cough. As a symptom or sequel, it occurs in wounds, phthisis, or the suppression of some accustomed discharge.

In active hemorrhage from the lungs, venesection is one of the most important steps towards a cure; and the blood should be drawn freely at once, rather than sparingly and repeatedly; though a second and even a third copious use of the lancet will often be found expedient. Emetics have been recommended, but they are of doubtful effect. They augment the vascular volume by relaxing the capillaries; but they stimulate locally by the act of rejection. Drastic purgatives are avoided, because of the straining; but the straining in vomition is greater and more direct.

Dr. Brian Robinson of Dublin, who was one of the most strenuous promoters of this mode of practice in his day, accounted for the benefit of emetics by the constriction which he conceived they produce upon the extreme vessels everywhere; but, to act thus, they should rather nauseate than vomit; for in nausea we have great vascular depression, and a cold and general collapse on the surface; while vomiting is known to rouse the system generally and determine towards the surface. Upon the recommendation of Dr. Robinson, Dr. Cullen followed the plan in several cases: "but in one instance the vomiting," says he, "increased the hemorrhage to a great and dangerous degree; and the possibility of such an accident again happening

* In the Lumleian Lectures for 1832, Dr. Watson related some striking examples, in which the menstruation, as one might say, took place for several years through the lungs, without any apparent injury of the general health. Among the patients of the celebrated Hoffman was a woman, who, for eight years, remained subject to a bleeding from the nose, which came on regularly every month, a few days before the menstrual period, and ceased upon the flowing of the catamenia. Then the direction of this periodical discharge was changed; and, for six years more, instead of epistaxis, she suffered hæmoptysis, and afterward this was exchanged for hæmatemesis.—ED.

has prevented all my further trials of such a remedy."* Nauseating has on this account been preferred on the continent to full vomiting in hemorrhage from the stomach, and indeed various other organs, as well as from the lungs; and ipecacuanha in small doses has been generally preferred to the metallic salts, as more manageable; half a grain, or even a quarter of a grain, being given every quarter of an hour, for many hours in succession.†

In general, however, we shall find it as successful and far less distressing to employ mild aperients and sedatives. The first, and particularly neutral salts, are alone of great benefit, and their action should be steadily maintained. Sedatives are of still higher importance, and especially those that reduce the tone of the circulation, as nitre and digitalis. The first, in about ten grains to a dose, should be given in iced water, and swallowed while dissolving; the dose being repeated every hour or two, according to the urgency of the case. If there be much cough, it must be allayed by opium and blisters. Local astringents we cannot use, and general astringents are here manifestly counter-indicated, however useful in passive hemorrhage: though it should be recollected that, when an active hemorrhage from the lungs is profuse and obstinate, the vessels lose their tone, and fall into a passive state.

In HÆMATEMESIS, the blood is evacuated from the alimentary canal at either extremity, whether that of the mouth or of the anus; for the term is used thus extensively by the Greek writers. In both cases it is discharged in active hemorrhage with a considerable expulsive effort; and the discharge is preceded by tensive pain about the stomach; and accompanied with anxiety and faintness.

The quantity discharged from the stomach is in most cases larger than what is discharged from the lungs, and of a deeper hue: it is also thrown up by the act of vomiting, and usually intermixed with some of the contents of the stomach. And hence there is no great difficulty in determining as to the source of the hemorrhage.‡ Hæmatemesis, however, is far more frequently a disease of atony than of eutony, and hence, chiefly belongs to the next species. Its usual exciting causes, when it occurs under an entonic character, are concussion or other external violence, as a shock of electricity,§ some strong emotion of the mind, as rage or terror, vomiting, or pregnancy. It has also occasionally been found to afford relief in suppressed catamenia, or been vicarious of it.

The pathology we have already given: the blood may proceed from the spleen, the liver,

* Mat. Med., part ii., ch. xix., p. 470.
† Keck, Abhand. und Beobach. Med. Wochen. blatt, 1783. No. xlix.
‡ The blood, which comes from the lungs, is commonly florid, and mixed with bubbles of air, *frothy*; that which proceeds from the stomach is usually dark-coloured, coagulated, or grumous, and mingled with fragments of the food, with mucus, or bile.—Dr. Watson in Lumleian Lectures for 1832.—ED.
§ Percival's Essays, vol. ii., p. 181.

the pancreas,* the stomach itself, or the smaller intestines ; and the mode of treatment should be as already advised for hæmoptysis. [From the effects of that insidious disease, chronic inflammation of the stomach, an hæmatemesis is sometimes produced, that rapidly cuts off the patient.—(*Dr. Abercrombie, in Edin. Med. Journ.,* No. lxxviii., p. 2.) Hæmatemesis is also one of the earliest symptoms of scirrhus or cancer of that organ ; taking place long before the commencement of ulceration, as well as in the ultimate stages of the disease. Then, as Dr. Watson conceives (*Med. Gaz.*, vol. x., p. 436), it may be owing to a breach in some vessel of magnitude, though he represents it as being more commonly a general oozing or exhalation from the ulcerated surface.]

In ʜᴀᴍᴀᴛᴜʀɪᴀ, the blood is evacuated at the urethra, and the evacuation is preceded by pain in the region of the bladder or kidneys, and accompanied with faintness. The blood is sometimes intermixed with urine, but occasionally flows pure and uncombined : and, in this last state, the disease is called by Vogel stymatosis, and the bleeding is supposed to proceed from the bladder rather than from the kidneys ; that from the latter being smaller in quantity, and remaining a longer time in the passages, and consequently of a darker colour. There is some ground for this opinion ; for, when the bladder is the seat affected, there is far more local pain and faintness than when the affection is in the kidneys. Hippocrates, indeed, has observed, that when the blood flows pure, copiously, and suddenly, and without pain, it proceeds from the kidneys, but, when it is small in quantity, and of a blackish colour, and accompanied with much heat or pain, or both, its source is the bladder. But this remark, instead of opposing, tends rather to corroborate, the preceding ; for, according to both views, the seat of disease is distinguished by the greater or less degree of uneasiness that attends the discharge ; and this whether the quantity discharged be larger or smaller.

It is not often, though sometimes, an entonic disease, or an active hemorrhage. Its exciting

* The statement with respect to the blood proceeding from the spleen, liver, or pancreas, is not correct. Disease of these organs may lead to hæmatemesis, or exist simultaneously with it ; but the source of the blood is in the vessels of the mucous coat of the stomach itself. As Dr. Watson has observed, a great majority of cases of hemorrhage from the stomach are symptomatic. That which depends upon incipient cancer of the stomach, while it is by no means of rare occurrence, is also more frequently obscure than other instances. In general, an attention to symptoms, and the past history of the patient, will readily elucidate hæmatemesis from the action of corrosive poisons ; from the rupture of an aneurism ; from the influence of scurvy, or purpura ; from cancer of the stomach in its advanced stages; from organic diseases of the liver, spleen, or heart ; from an attack of yellow fever ; from suppressed or imperfect menstruation ; or from the pressure of the gravid uterus.—See Dr. Watson's Observations, as published in Med. Gaz., vol. x., p. 439.—Eᴅ.

cause is frequently a stone in the bladder, or a violent blow on the kidneys, or on the bladder, especially when the latter is full. It is also said by Schenck (Lib. vii., obs. i., 24), and other writers, to be occasionally produced by cantharides, whether employed externally or internally.*

In connexion with the general course of treatment already recommended in the preceding varieties, the compound powder of ipecacuanha may here be employed with great advantage : for the pain and irritation are often intolerably distressing, and, on this account, demulcent drinks are frequently found to produce considerable relief.

In ᴜᴛᴇʀɪɴᴇ ʜᴇᴍᴏʀʀʜᴀɢᴇ, the blood is discharged from the womb with a sense of weight in the loins, and of pressure upon the vagina. This is the menorrhagia of most of the nosologists, and is often, but very erroneously, described as an excess of the menstrual flux. It is, in truth, a real hemorrhage or issue of blood, instead of menstrual secretion, which is often entirely suppressed, though sometimes a small but inadequate portion is intermixed with the uterine bleeding : and hence Hoffman has properly denominated it uteri hemorrhagia. It occurs both in an entonic and an atonic state of the vessels, and especially of the general system : and, from the remarks offered under Pʟᴇᴛʜᴏʀᴀ, it is not at all to be wondered at that

* Hist. Mort. Uratislav., p. 58. The editor has known hæmaturia occur in several cases in which cancerous disease of the neck of the uterus had extended by ulceration into the bladder. In one woman, whom he lately attended in Boswell-Court, Devonshire-street, the bladder would sometimes become so full of coagulated blood, that a retention of urine used to be induced, in which the catheter had little effect, unless introduced much further than usual. He has also known profuse hæmaturia arise from a cancerous disease of the bladder ; a case that was remarkable as having been attended with a spontaneous fracture of the left thigh bone and one rib. The particulars have been published in the Trans. of Med. Chir. Society, vol. xvii. M. Andral mentions a very curious example of hæmaturia.—(Anat. Pathol., tom. i., p. 339.) It took place in an old woman who had a cancer of the stomach. A fortnight before her death, numerous purple spots appeared on her skin, and a remarkable quantity of blood was daily voided with her urine. Red spots occurred on the conjunctiva, and one of them, rendered very prominent by the blood under it, formed a purple ring round the cornea, like what is observed in chemosis. On opening the body, numerous ecchymoses were found in the cellular texture on the outside of the peritonæum and the pleura, on the inside of the cavities of the heart, and in different parts of the alimentary canal. The urinary passages contained a bloody fluid, which might also be pressed out of the mamillæ or the tubular substance of the kidneys. No blood was anywhere found, except what was of a purple colour, and quite liquid, without any appearance of coagulum. A similar case is recorded by M. Stoltz.—(Archives de Méd., tom. xv.) The patient, in the latter instance, was a pregnant woman, and it is curious that ecchymoses, resembling those noticed in most textures of her body, were also found in the lungs, pericardium, heart, and vessels of the fœtus.—Eᴅ.

hemorrhage should in both conditions take place from the uterus very frequently, and, perhaps, more so than from any other organ.

For reasons we shall have occasion to explain in a subsequent part of this work, the uterus, from the period of the completion of the female form, is stimulated, once in every lunation, to the secretion and elimination of a peculiar fluid, which exhibits the colour, though it is deficient in many of the properties, of blood ; and for this purpose the uterine arteries are, at such seasons, peculiarly turgid and irritable. There is hence always a tendency on such occasions to a hemorrhage in this quarter in females of a firm and robust texture, and of a plethoric habit. But if, from cold or any other cause, the uterine secernents do not at these seasons fulfil their office, and throw forth the proper fluid, the uterine arteries will be inordinately gorged ; the regular stimulus will be greatly augmented ; pain, tension, and spasm will extend over the loins, and the extremities of the vessels be ruptured, or their mouths give way by anastomosis, and a considerable hemorrhage the consequence.

. This is the ordinary period in which uterine hemorrhage takes place, though it may occur during any part of the interval between the catamenial terms, upon any of the occasional causes that operate upon other organs, and form the preceding varieties ; as it is well known to occur at times, with great violence, during pregnancy and in childbed.

When we come to treat of diseases appertaining to the sexual organs, we shall have to notice some singular cases of precocity in female infants, and especially that of a regular menstruation. It is upon this principle alone that we can account for uterine hemorrhage in new-born infants, of which the medical records give several examples, and especially the Ephemerides of Natural Curiosities.

In suppressed menstruation, uterine hemorrhage affords relief to the spasms and pains that harass the loins, and the headache and difficulty of breathing which have usually preceded the lumbar distress. But the discharge may be immoderate, and become habitual. And it is hence best to be upon our guard, and to use venesection as a substitute, and to prevent or diminish the spasmodic action by gentle aperients and the sedatives already recommended in hæmoptysis, after which the case will become a disease of suppressed menstruation alone, and must be treated according to the method recommended under that malady ; for a restoration of the catamenial secretion is its natural cure. I may observe, however, that, when the suppression of this secretion has been of some standing, and a uterine hemorrhage has periodically taken its place, accompanied with distressing pains in the whole circle of the pelvic region, we can sometimes suddenly restore a healthy action to the organ by a plan of anticipation. For this purpose, I have prescribed venesection about ten days before the return of the monthly paroxysms, and having thus taken off plethoric impetus, I have, a few days afterward, recommended the hip-bath to be used in a tepid state

every night, and persevered in till the period of relapse ; when I have often found that there has been neither tension nor spasms, that the loins have continued easy, and the hemorrhage has yielded to the natural secretion.

In HEMORRHAGE STRICTLY ANAL, the flux of blood issues chiefly from the hemorrhoidal vessels, and, as these are large, and but little supported by any surrounding organization, they readily give way both in an entonic and atonic state of the frame, and particularly in case of plethora upon very slight excitements, as in straining to expel hardened fæces, taking cold in the feet, or walking a little too far. Irritants introduced by the mouth have also proved a frequent cause of this variety of hemorrhage ; as an injudicious use of aloes, terebinthinate preparations, or even pungent alliaceous sauces. The irritation of piles is also a very common cause, and hence by some writers anal hemorrhage is only treated of as a symptom of that variety of this last disease, which is known by the name of bleeding piles. But this is highly incorrect, as anal hemorrhage often occurs, and very profusely, where no piles have ever been experienced. This power of hemorrhage, when active, as it is called, or in an entonic habit, is usually preceded by a sense of weight and pain within the rectum, and sometimes by a load in the head. And it has often, as already observed, proved critical and salutary, and carried off congestions from the abdominal viscera. It is, however, peculiarly apt to become profuse, and to establish an order of recurrence, and hence must be overpowered by the reducent and sedative plan, recommended in most of the preceding varieties, and particularly in that of hæmoptysis. The aperients employed, however, should here be peculiarly mild and alterant ; and sulphur, which does not readily dissolve in the course of the intestinal canal, and often reaches the rectum in an unmixed state, is one of the best, and is often found strikingly serviceable. All stimulant foods, moreover, must be especially avoided ; and the ordinary drink should be water, soda-water, or lemonade.

Here also we are able, as in the case of hemorrhage from the nose, to employ local astringents, though it would be improper to use those that act generally, so long as plethora or an entonic habit continues. The patient may sit in a bidet of ice-water, or water cooled artificially to the freezing point, or may use a cold hip-bath, and have injections of cold water, or astringent lotions, as of alum, zinc, or even lead, thrown up the rectum ; the latter of which should be in such proportions as to remain there for half an hour or an hour.

————

SPECIES II.

HÆMORRHAGIA ATONICA.

ATONIC HEMORRHAGE.

ACCOMPANIED WITH GENERAL LAXITY OR DEBILITY, AND WEAK VASCULAR ACTION ; BLOOD ATTENUATE, AND OF A DILUTED RED.

THOUGH the effect in this species is the same as in the preceding, the proximate cause, as well as the more obvious signs, are directly opposite. The general pathology has been given in the introductory remarks to the genus, and the more common organs from which the hemorrhage proceeds are the same as already noticed under the preceding species ; and hence the varieties of that may be regarded as those of the species before us.

When plethora is the remote cause, which it often is, it is atonic plethora, or plethora of debility ; but whatever has a tendency to loosen or enervate the tone of the solidum vivum, or living fibre, will lay a foundation for this kind of hemorrhage. It is hence a characteristic disease of advanced age, as entonic plethora is of youth and adult life ; and often takes place in those whose vigour is reduced by meager or innutritious food, close confinement, without exercise, in a foul and stagnant atmosphere, or immoderate indulgence in the pleasures of wine or sexual intercourse. Hence, too, its frequent occurrence, as a symptom, in tabes, atrophy, struma, scurvy, and low fevers.*

The CHARACTERS of the several varieties of this species, as distinguished from those of the preceding, are as follow ; for it is not necessary to put the varieties themselves into a tabular form :—

In HEMORRHAGE FROM THE NOSTRILS, the blood flows without heat or headache.

In that from the RESPIRATORY ORGAN, it is usually produced without even the exertion of coughing, and is often accompanied with a scirrhous or calculous affection of the lungs ; the countenance is pale and emaciated.

In HEMORRHAGE FROM THE ALIMENTARY CANAL, the blood is discharged without tensive pain : though there must necessarily be an expulsive effort ; and, from the inanition hereby produced, some degree of nausea and faintness.

When evacuated by the URETHRA, there is, for the same reason, faintness, but little or no previous pain. The most singular and severe examples of hemorrhages from the urethra are those that have occurred during coition ; sometimes intermixed with semen, sometimes instead of it, and sometimes immediately after emission. The individuals have been generally persons of highly irritable and delicate habits ; and who have weakened themselves by too free an indulgence in pleasures of this kind. Numerous instances of this sort of hemorrhage are given in the Collections of Medical Curiosities, and especially in several of the German Ephemerides.†

* The more correct principles, on which the fact is accounted for by Andral, are adverted to in some of the notes in the preceding pages.—Ed.

† The employment of caustic bougies, or the rough introduction of instruments into the urethra, occasionally causes profuse hemorrhage. The editor is attending a man at this time (Nov., 1830), who was cut for the stone in Guy's Hospital about twenty years ago, and who is voiding a considerable quantity of blood from the urethra, in consequence, as he states, of slipping down with his thighs widely and very forcibly separated. Hæmaturia atonica may attend typhus fever, smallpox, and purpura hæmorrhagica. When entirely passive and unaccompanied by inflamma-

There is little pain in ATONIC HEMORRHAGE FROM THE UTERUS : and it generally occurs at the natural cessation of the menstrual flux, or within a few years afterward. As a concomitant, hemorrhage from this quarter is also frequently found in a scirrhous, cancerous, or other morbid states of the uterus, in whatever period of life these may occur ; which, however, they do most usually after the age of forty or fifty.

ATONIC HEMORRHAGE FROM THE ANUS ordinarily takes place spontaneously, with little or no pain ; but commonly with varices or congestions of the hemorrhoidal vessels, and is very apt to produce a habit of recurrence.

In all these varieties, venesection must be had recourse to sparingly, and never, unless where we have satisfactory evidence of atonic plethora or congestion. It may sometimes be requisite to use the lancet in nasal hemorrhage, for the head may feel oppressed and drowsy : and it will still more frequently be necessary in hemorrhage from the uterus ; but the blood extracted should rarely exceed seven or eight ounces ; and, in all other varieties, as a general rule, it will be better to withhold our hand, and to proceed at once with a tonic plan of treatment.

Into this plan we may, in the present species, freely admit the use of general astringents, in conjunction with their local application, however objectionable in the preceding ; for a laxity and inelasticity of the fibrous structure are among the chief symptoms we have to oppose : and hence the mineral acids and metallic salts may be had recourse to with great advantage, along with bitters ; and, with a few exceptions, we cannot well err in the selection. The preparations of iron may be rather too heating in hæmoptysis, and perhaps in all atonic hemorrhages accompanied with much irritability. One of its mildest and best forms is that of a subcarbonate ; and perhaps the best mode of obtaining it in this form is by the celebrated compositiou of Dr. Griffiths. The myrrh is also in his preparation a useful article for the present purpose, and we shall rarely do better than employ it. In the London Pharmacopœia, it is given under the name of mistura ferri composita.

From the manifest power of opium to restrain most evacuations, it has often been employed in hemorrhages. It does not appear, however, to have any direct effect in checking the discharge ; and in entonic hemorrhages, and especially when employed early, has been highly mischievous. But where, in hæmoptysis, there is a perpetual cough from irritation, or in uterine hemorrhages a frequent recurrence of spasmodic pains, it has been tried with considerable success. And the same remark will apply to hyoscyamus, and various other narcotics, which seem to be only useful on the same account.

Cinchona, which is peculiarly objectionable in the preceding species, may here be had recourse to, the exhibition of turpentine in small doses, from twenty to twenty-five drops, every six hours, should be adopted, and the system supported.—See Elliotson's Lects., delivered at Lond. Univ., in Med. Gaz. for Aug., 1833.—Ed.

course to with considerable promise. It seems, however, to be chiefly serviceable in uterine hemorrhage, where the disease depends upon a laxity of the extremities of the vessels, which are therefore readily opened by every irritation, applied to the system or to the diseased part. Whether in this case it acts altogether as a bitter, as supposed by Dr. Cullen, or partly also as an astringent, it may be difficult to determine ; but the question is not of importance.

For other general roborants to which it may be necessary to have recourse, the reader may turn to the treatment of LIMOSIS *dyspepsia*, or indigestion (Class I., Ord. I., vol. i., p. 98) ; and he may govern the patient's diet and regimen by the general plan there laid down.

The local astringents and refrigerants already recommended under the former species, may be here employed with even less reserve : and where the bleeding has become chronic, which it is far more likely to do than in entonic hemorrhage, or has been so profuse as very considerably to exhaust the system, a little wine or some other cordial should be administered as soon as we are consulted : for, however small the vessel that is ruptured, its orifice is incapable of contracting from a total loss of tone ; and hence a diffusible stimulus gives it the irritation it stands in need of, and forms a salutary constringent. A striking case of this kind has already been given in treating of accidental hemorrhages from extracting teeth ; and it is not long since, that the author was requested to attend in a similar hemorrhage from the nose. The patient was a lady of about fifty years of age, of slender and delicate frame, who had for some years ceased to menstruate. The bleeding had continued incessantly for three or four days, during which she had been restrained to a very low diet, and allowed nothing but toast and water for her common drink. She was faint, felt sick, and had a feeble pulse, and must have lost many pounds of blood, though no exact measure had been taken. I gave her instantly a free draught of negus made with port wine, and camphire mixture with the aromatic spirit of ammonia, had the nostrils syringed with equal parts of tincture of catechu and water, and applied a neckerchief wetted with cold water round the temples, directing it to be renewed every ten minutes. In half an hour the hemorrhage ceased, and, on the ensuing day, I found no other symptom than weakness, for which a nutritious but inirritant regimen was prescribed. A few days afterward the hemorrhage returned from sneezing or some other incidental stimulus, and was restrained, as I was told, for I did not see her, by a recurrence to the same plan. I recommended, however, carriage-exercise, and an excursion to the seacoast, which was immediately complied with, and there was no recurrence of the disease.

To effect the same intention, I have occasionally advised cardiacs combined with astringents in hæmatemesis, where the discharge of blood has been profuse, and has continued for some days, and the patient has become considerably exhausted : and I do not recollect an instance in which the plan has proved unfriendly. In like manner, in very great faintness or deliquium produced by a copious and protracted hemorrhage from the uterus, I have had the vagina injected with equal parts of port wine and water acidulated with sulphuric acid, and have found it equally successful.

The acetate of lead is also a preparation which, in all such cases, ought to be tried internally. It was at one time greatly out of favour, from the writings of Sir George Baker, and the concurrent opinion of Dr. Heberden. Of the mischievous effects of various preparations of this metal when employed internally, the former has given numerous examples, and concludes with the following corollary : "that lead taken into the stomach is a poison . I do not say ex proprietate naturæ et totâ substantiâ ; but which is capable of doing much more hurt than good to the generality of men in all the known ways of using it ; and, consequently, that it cannot be avoided with too much caution."— (*Med. Transact.*, vol. i., p. 311.) In corroboration of which Dr. Heberden tells us, that its good effects are by no means so certain as its mischief ; and, in most cases, would be far overbalanced by it. In the form of an acetate, however, all its evils seem to be subdued by a combination with opium ; for the first distinct knowledge of which the medical world is indebted to the penetration and judgment of Dr. Reynolds, who tried it, in this state of union, in various cases, with the most perfect success, and without the least unfavourable symptom whatever, whether of pain or even costiveness. He also employed with equal benefit the old tinctura saturnia, and the sugar of lead : of the former, giving eighteen drops with three drops of laudanum to a dose, and repeating the dose every four hours in a little barley-water ; of the latter, giving one grain with three drops of laudanum mixed into a pill with conserve of roses ; to he repeated every six hours. And, under both forms, he employed these materials with great and unalloyed advantages in hemorrhages of most sorts, especially uterine, pulmonary, and nasal.—(*Med. Transact.*, vol. iii., art. xiii.)

Dr. Latham (vol. v., art. xxi.) has since confirmed this practice of Dr. Reynolds in its fullest degree, and even extended its range ; and so little inconvenience has he found from the use of the acetate, that he has employed it "in doses of a grain three times a day for six, eight, and ten weeks successively ; usually, but not always, combining it with opium or conium ; without any other precaution than desiring the patients to obviate any costiveness by oleum ricini or confectio sennæ." He has occasionally given two grains of the acetate as an evening dose ; once, in consultation with Dr. Reynolds, five grains ; and mentions another case in which he was concerned, where ten grains a day were taken without any inconvenience. By a mistake for sugar, a young woman, respecting whom he was consulted, swallowed at one time about two drachms of it, yet without any serious evil : the fauces and œsophagus were considerably constringed, and this seems to have been the chief mischief; for the bowels were opened by oleum ricini and other purgatives in the course of the day, and the patient was not at all worse for the accident on the ensuing morning.

Imboldened by these facts, Dr. Latham has employed the same medicine in other diseases in which irritant astringents and tonics seem requisite, as in colliquative diarrhœas and hectic perspirations, and more especially in that semi-purulent expectoration which too often terminates in pulmonary ulceration and consumption : and, as he confidently assures us, with great advantage. And he hence concludes, that whatever deleterious properties may appertain to lead in some of its salts and oxydes, nothing pernicious exists in its acetate ; in the process for which, he conceives it either to be more completely freed from arsenical or other poisonous minerals than in its other forms, or rendered innocuous by the addition of the acetic acid.

It only remains to be added, that where entonic hemorrhage has occurred so profusely, or has continued so long, as to reduce the system to an atonic state, it then becomes a disease of debility, and is to be treated as though originating under the present species.

GENUS III.

MARASMUS.

EMACIATION.

GENERAL EXTENUATION, OF THE BODY, WITH DEBILITY.

MARASMUS is a Greek term, derived from μαραίνω, "marcesco," "marcescere reddo." It was long ago used collectively to comprehend atrophy, tabes, and phthisis ; and in employing it therefore in the present system as a generic name, we only restore it to its earlier sense. The generic character is common to all these subdivisions ; for each is distinguished by a general emaciation of the frame, accompanied with debility, and consequently forms a species to marasmus as a genus.

With these species the reader, however, will now find two others united ; M. ANHÆMIA, to which I shall advert presently, and M. CLIMAC-TERICUS : the last from a high authority, with which I fully coincide ; and which is intended to imbody that extraordinary decline of all the corporeal powers, which, before the system falls a prey to confirmed old age, sometimes makes its appearance in advanced life without any sufficiently ostensible cause, and is occasionally succeeded by a renovation of health and vigour, though it more generally precipitates the patient into the grave.

Extenuation or leanness is not necessarily a disease ; for many persons who are peculiarly lean are peculiarly healthy, while some take pains to fall away in flesh, that they may increase in health and become stronger. But if an individual grow weaker as he grows leaner, it affords a full proof that he is under a morbid influence ; and it is this influence, this conjunction of extenuation with debility, as noticed

in the definition, that is imported by the term MARASMUS, and its synonyme EMACIATION.

It is curious to observe how much more easily the body wastes under a disease of some organs than of others ; and it would be a subjcet of no small moment to inquire into the cuuse of this, and to draw up a scale of organs effecting this change, from the lowest to the highest degree. Dr. Pemberton, in a work of considerable merit, published many years ago, threw out some valuable hints upon this subject, which it is to be lamented that he did not afterward follow up to a fuller extent. The following passage is well worthy of notice, and aptly illustrative of what is here intended. "Let us take," says he, "the two cases of a diseased state of the mesenteric glands, and a diseased or scrofulous affection of the breast. In the former, we shall find there is a great emaciation ; in the latter, none at all. In an ulceration of the small intestines, great emaciation takes place : in scirrhus of the rectum, none. In a disease of the gall-bladder, which is subservient to the liver, the bulk of the body is diminished ; but in a disease of the urinary bladder, which is subservient to the kidneys, scarcely any diminution of bulk is to be perceived. In an abscess of the liver, the body becomes much emaciated ; but in an abscess of the kidneys, the bulk is not diminished.

"If we examine into the function of those parts, the diseases of which do or do not occasion emaciation, we may perhaps be led to the true cause of this difference of their effect on the bulk. In order, however, to understand more clearly how the functions of these parts bear relation to each other, it may be necessary to premise, that the glands of the body are divided into those which secrete a fluid from the blood for the use of the system, and those which secrete a fluid to be discharged from it. The former may be termed glands of supply ; the latter, glands of waste.

"The smaller intestines, in consideration of the great number of absorbents with which they are provided for the repair of the system, may be considered as performing the office of glands of supply. The large intestines, on the contrary, may be considered as performing the office of glands of waste ; insomuch as they are furnished very scantily with absorbents, and abundantly with a set of glands which secrete or withdraw from the system a fluid which serves to lubricate the canal for the passage of the feces, and which itself, together with the feces, is destined to be discharged from the system. The glands which secrete a fluid to be employed in the system, as well as the glands of direct supply, may be considered the liver, the pancreas, the mesenteric glands, perhaps the stomach, and the small intestines ; and the glands of waste are the kidneys, breasts, exhalant arteries, and the larger intestines."

The first set are, in fact, the general assemblage of the chylific organs ; and it is upon their direct or indirect inability to carry into execution their proper function, that the first of the species we are now about to enter upon, that of ATRO-

PHY, is founded in all its varieties. How far these remarks will apply to the other species of the present genus is not quite so clear. The seat of the third and fourth may be doubtful, perhaps variable ; that of PHTHISIS, or the fifth, admits of no debate. Are the lungs to be regarded as an organ of waste or of supply? The question may be answered in opposite ways, according to the hypothesis adopted respecting the doctrine of respiration. They throw off carbonic acid gas. Do they introduce oxygen or any other vital gas into the circulating system? As an organ of waste, we cannot, upon the principle here laid down, account for the emaciation which flows from a diseased condition of them. If it can be substantiated that they are an organ of supply, they confirm and extend the principle. Will this principle, moreover, apply in dropsy, in which there is even more emaciation than in phthisis? The subject is worth enucleating; but we have not space for it, and must proceed to arrange the five species that appertain to the genus before us :—

1. Marasmus Atrophia. Atrophy.
2. ——— Anhæmia. Exsanguinity.
3. ——— Climactericus. Decay of Nature.
4. ——— Tabes. Decline.
5. ——— Phthisis. Consumption.

Most of these follow in regular order, as genera or species in most of the nosological arrangements, and are set down as subdivisions of macies or marasmus. By Dr. Cullen, phthisis is regarded as a mere sequel of hæmoptysis, upon which we shall have to observe in its proper place ; while atrophia and tabes are given as distinct diseases under the ordinary head, only that, for macies or marasmus he employs marcores as an ordinal term. The common distinguishing marks are, that atrophy is emaciation without hectic fever ; tabes, emaciation with hectic fever ; and phthisis, emaciation and hectic fever coupled with pulmonary disease. And such, with the exception of phthisis, is the distinction continued by Dr. Cullen in his Synopsis. But, in his Practice of Physic, he informs us that his views upon this subject had undergone a change, not only in respect to the subdivisions or varieties of these two diseases, but as to the diseases themselves. "I doubt," says he, "if ever the distinction of TABES and ATROPHIA, attempted in the Nosology, will properly apply ; as I think there are certain diseases of the same nature, which sometimes appear with and sometimes without fever."—(Vol. iv., part iii., book i., sect. 1618.) This is written in the spirit of candour that so peculiarly characterizes this great man. But I cannot thus readily consent to relinquish a distinction which has received the sanction of so many observant pathologists, and which appears to me to have a sufficient foundation. It is difficult, undoubtedly, to assign a proper place to all the varieties or subdivisions of these species ; but this is a difficulty common to many other diseases equally ; for we perceive fevers, nervous affections, and those of the digestive organs perpetually running into each other in different varieties, yet

we find it convenient to arrange and describe them as distinct diseases. And, with the caution attempted to be exercised in respect to the species before us, I trust that the reader will not discern a greater transgression of boundary in the present, than in various other cases of general allowance.

SPECIES I.

MARASMUS ATROPHIA.

ATROPHY.

COMPLEXION PALE, OFTEN SQUALID ; SKIN DRY AND WRINKLED ; MUSCLES SHRUNK AND INELASTIC ; LITTLE OR NO FEVER.

THE specific is a Greek term deduced from α privative, and τρέφω, "nutrio," and is literally, therefore, INNUTRITION ; a designation peculiarly significant, as the disease, in all its forms or varieties, seems to be dependant on a defect in the quantity, quality, or application of the nutrient part of the blood ; and thus lays a foundation for the three following varieties :—

α Inopiæ. Blood innutritious from scarcity or pravity of food.
Atrophy of want.
β Profusionis. Blood deprived of nutrition by profuse evacuations.
Atrophy of waste.
γ Debilitatis. Nutrition not sufficiently introduced into the blood by the chylific organs, or not sufficiently separated from it by the assimilating.
Atrophy of debility.

In order that the body should maintain its proper strength and plumpness, it is necessary that the digestive organs should be supplied with a proportion of food adequate to the perpetual wear of its respective parts : for this wear, as we all know, produces a waste ; and hence the emaciation sustained by those who suffer from famine, in which there is no food introduced into the stomach, or from a meager or unwholesome diet, in which the quantity introduced is below the ordinary demand. It is this condition that forms the first of the subdivisions or varieties, the ATROPHY OF WANT, under which the species before us is contemplated in the present arrangement.

But the ordinary demand may not be sufficient for the body, or some part of it may be in a state of inordinate wear and waste, as in very severe and protracted labour, in which the supply is rapidly carried off by profuse perspiration, or in rupturing or puncturing a large artery, in which the same effect is produced by a profuse hemorrhage. Any other extreme or chronic evacuation may prove equally mischievous, as an excessive secretion from the bowels, from the vagina, from the salivary glands, from the breasts ; as where a delicate wet-nurse suckles two strong infants. And hence the origin of the second of the above varieties, or the ATROPHY OF WASTE.

Now, in all these cases, wherever the system is in possession of an ordinary portion of health, there is a strong effort made by the digestive powers to recruit the excessive expenditure by an additional elaboration of nutriment; and the instinctive effort runs through the entire chain of action to the utmost reach of the assimilating powers, or those secernents with which every organ is furnished, to supply itself with a succession of like matter from the common pabulum of the blood. Hence, the stomach is always in a state of hunger, as in the case of famine, profuse loss of blood, or recovery from fever.; all the chylific organs secrete an unusual quantity of resolvent juices, an almost incredible quantity of food is demanded, and is chymified, chylified, and absorbed almost as soon as it enters the stomach; the heart beats quicker, the circulation is increased, and the new and unripe blood is hurried forward to the lungs, which more rapidly expand themselves for the purpose, to be completed by the process of ventilation: in which state it is as rapidly laid hold of by the assimilating powers of every organ it seems to fly to, and almost instantly converted into its own substance. Such is the wonderful sympathy that pervades the entire frame; and that runs more particularly through that extensive chain of action which commences with the digestive and reaches to the assimilating organs, constituting its two extremities.

So long as the surplus of supply is equal to the surplus of expenditure, no perceptible degree of waste ensues; but the greater the demand the greater the labour, and the turmoil is too violent to be long persevered in. The excited organs must have rest, or their action will by degrees become feeble and inefficient. And if this take place while the waste is still continuing, emaciation will be a necessary consequence, even in the midst of the greatest abundance; and hence, an explanation of the variety of emaciation before us, constituting the second.

Thus far we have contemplated the animal frame in a firm and healthy constitution: and have supposed a general harmony of action pervading every link of the extensive chain of nutrition, from the digestive organs to the assimilating powers. But we do not always find it in this condition; and occasionally perceive, or think we perceive, that this necessary harmony is intercepted in some part or other of its tenour: that the digestive powers, or some of them, do not perform their trust as they should do, or, that the assimilating powers, or some of them, exhibit a like default; or, that the blood is not sufficiently elaborated in its course, or becomes loaded with some peculiar acrimony. And hence another cause, or rather an assemblage of other causes, competent to the disease before us.

It is from the one or the other of these sources that we are in most, perhaps in all cases, to derive the third modification of this disease, which is here distinguished, for want of a better term, by that of ᴀᴛʀᴏᴘʜʏ ᴏғ ᴅᴇʙɪʟɪᴛʏ. The disease under this form is often very complex, and it is difficult to trace out what link in the great chain of action has first given way. Most probably, indeed, it is sometimes one link, and sometimes another. But, from the sympathy

which so strikingly pervades the whole, we see at once how easy it is for unsoundness in one quarter to extend its influence to another, till the disease becomes general to the system. Yet I am much disposed to think that the atrophy so conspicuous in feeble habits, and the feeblest periods of life, as infancy and old age, commences most usually at the one or the other end of the chain, and immediately operates by sympathy on its opposite. This remark is in consonance with a very common law of life, by which impressions are more powerfully and more readily communicated from one extreme of an organ to another, than they are to any of the intermediate points. It is hence the will operates instantly on the fingers, the stomach on the capillaries of the skin; and that the irritation produced by a stone in the bladder is felt chiefly in the glans penis. And hence the close correspondence which we have already seen to prevail between these two extremities of the nutritive function in the case of want and hunger.

Where atrophy is connected with a morbid state of the digestive organs, we have a little light thrown on the nature of the disease, but not much. For first, indigestion does not necessarily produce this effect, since it is no uncommon thing for dyspeptic patients to become plethoric, and gain, instead of lose, in bulk of body. And next, the morbid state of these organs may be a secondary, instead of a primary affection, and be dependant upon a general hebetude, or some other unsound condition of the assimilating powers, constituting the other end of the chain; and hence exercising a stronger sympathy over them than over any intermediate organs whatever: as the digestive organs themselves, if the disease should have originated in them, may exercise a like sympathy over the assimilating powers, and hence produce that general extenuation which, as we have just observed, is not a necessary consequence of dyspepsy. It is at least put, I think, beyond a doubt, that more than one set of organs are connected in the atrophy of debility.

Where this atrophy takes place in infants at the breast, or young children, it is ushered in by a flaccidity of the flesh, a paleness of the countenance, sometimes alternating with flushes, bloated prominence of the belly, irregularity of the bowels, pendulousness of the lower limbs, general sluggishness and debility, and, where walking has been acquired, a disinclination to motion, with fretfulness in the day, and restlessness at night.

There is at first no perceptible fever, no cough, nor difficulty of breathing: but if the disease continue, all these will appear as the result of general irritation, and the skin will become dry and heated, and be covered over with ecthyma, impetigo, or some other squalid eruption. The breath is generally offensive; the urine varies in colour and quantity; and, in infants at the breast, the stools are often ash-coloured or lienteric, or greenish, loose, and griping. The appetite varies; in some cases it fails, in others it is insatiable.

Where these symptoms or the greater part of them occur to an infant at the breast, it becomes us, in the first place, to be particularly attentive to the manner in which it has been nursed, in respect to cleanliness, purity of air, warmth, and exercise ; we have next to turn our attention to the nurse's milk ; and afterward to an examination whether the infant is breeding teeth, or has worms, or there be any scrofulous taint in the blood. For the last we have no immediate remedy ; the rest we must correct as we find occasion. And if we have no reason to be satisfied upon any of these points, it may still be advisable to change the milk. It is not easy to detect all the peculiarities of milk that may render it incapable of affording full nutrition : and there is reason to believe, that one infant may pine away on what proves a healthy breast to another. I have given this advice in some dilemmas, and have often found a wonderful improvement on its being followed.

In children on their feet, who are confined in the filth and suffocating air of a narrow cell, the common habitation of a crowded family from Sunday morning to Saturday night ; or who are pressed into the service of a manufactory, and have learned to become a part of its machinery before they have learned their mother-tongue ; there is no difficulty in accounting for the atrophy that so often prevails among them. The appetite does not here so much fail as the general strength ; their meals are, perhaps, doled out at the allotted hours by weight and measure : but still they are falling victims to emaciation ; and are affording proof, that air and exercise are of as much importance as food itself ; that there are other organs than those of digestion, upon which the emaciation must depend : and that, unless the supply furnished by the food to the bloodvessels be sufficiently oxygenized by ventilation, and coagulated by exercise, the blood itself, however pure from all incidental defect or hereditary taint, will never stimulate the secernents of the various organs to which it travels to a proper separation of its constituent principles, and a conversion to their own substance.

In all these cases, therefore, the proximate cause seems to be lodged principally in the assimilating powers of the system ; and whenever the digestive organs grow infirm also, it is rather by sympathy with the former than by any primary affection of their own.

There is a singular case of atrophy quoted by Sauvages, to which he has given the name of *lateralis*, and which unquestionably belongs to this variety. It occurred in a young child, and took possession of just one half the body ; the left side, from the axilla to the heel, being so completely wasted, that the bones seemed only to be covered with skin, while the right side was fat. Under the influence of topical antispasmodics, and sudorifics continued *for seven years*, the writer of the account tells us that he *began* to get better—" meliùs habere cæpit."—(*Nos. Med.*, cl. x., ord. i. ; *Ex. Collect. Acad.*, tom. iii., p. 693.)

In the atrophy of debility, common to old age,

the cellular membrane, that is, the part containing, as well as the parts contained, seems rather to shrivel away, in many cases to be carried away, by absorption, and the muscular fibres to become dried up and rigid, rather than loose and flabby. In this case, the assimilating powers seem to have done their duty to the last, and, like an empty stomach when loaded with gastric juice in a moment of sudden death, to have preyed upon and devoured themselves : since it is probable, that nearly all the animal oil, and more than half the bulk of the muscles and of the parenchyma of many of the organs, is carried off in the same manner ; for, that all these are capable of being converted into a like substance is clear, since all of them are transformable into adipocire by a chymical action after death, and into a steatomatous material by a morbid action of the living power, while every other organ continues in good health ; and there are many facts that lead to the conclusion that all, under the circumstances before us, are capable of yielding a common substitute for the natural food of the system. Here, therefore, we are to look for the proximate cause of the disease towards the other end of the chain, or among the chylific viscera. And we shall not in general look in vain. Not, indeed, that we shall always, or even commonly, find it in the stomach or in the liver, for the appetite may not fail, though its demand is but small and is easily satisfied ; and it probably digests what is introduced into it. Yet here the greater part of the food rests ; or rather, most of it passes through the intestines, and very little goes into the lacteals ; insomuch that many of our most celebrated anatomists have thought, as I have had occasion to observe (vol. i., p. 228, Parabysma Mesentericum), that the mesenteric glands of old people become obliterated ; while Ruysch contended, that mankind pass the latter part of their lives without lacteals, and that he himself was doing so at the time of writing.

The mode of treatment needs not detain us. Where the disease depends upon a want of wholesome food, or of food of any kind, the cure is obvious : where upon profuse evacuations, it falls within the precincts of some other disease, and is to be governed by its remedies. And where the cause is an infirm condition of any part of the chain of nutritive functions, from the chylific to the assimilating organs, the same tonic course of medicine that may be advisable in the one case, will be equally advisable in the other. The bowels should be kept in a state of regularity ; mercurial alterants may sometimes be required, though less frequently than under one or two varieties of tabes ; the different preparations of iodine will often exercise a healthful stimulus, and prove the deobstruent that is stood in need of ; the bitters and astringents enumerated under DYSPEPSY may also be had recourse to, according to the peculiarity of the case ; and cleanliness, fresh air, exercise, and cold-bathing will complete the rest. The atrophy of old age is to be met by the richest foods, wine, and the warmth of another person sleeping in the same bed.

SPECIES II.
MARASMUS ANHÆMIA.
EXSANGUINITY.

FACE, LIPS, AND GENERAL SURFACE GHASTLY PALE; PULSE QUICK AND FEEBLE; APPETITE IMPAIRED; ALVINE EVACUATIONS IRREGULAR, BLACK, AND FETID, OCCASIONALLY WITH SEVERE GRIPINGS; LANGUOR AND EMACIATION EXTREME.

THE specific name. for this disease is sometimes written ANÆMIA, but incorrectly; for the aspirate ought to be retained, and is so, indeed, in common usage, as in *anhæmous*, vulnerary or styptic, from the same root; *enharmonic; errhine; cachexy; amphemera; anthelmintic*. The most striking peculiarity of the affection is, that the bloodlessness of the exterior precisely corresponds with that of the interior; since dissections show that the largest and deepest vessels are nearly as destitute of blood as those on the surface.* It is in this ghastly pallor of the whole exterior, as directly expressive of the same condition within, that this disease chiefly differs from the atrophy of want, of waste, and of debility, which constitute the different modifications of the preceding species.

The disease itself has often been referred to, and at times described by the old writers, as Becher (*Diss. Resolutio casûs practici Anæmiæ, Sanguinis miros fructus repræsentantis*, Leid., 1663), Albert (*Diss. De Anæmiâ*, Hall., 1732), and Janson (*Diss. De Morbis ex Defectu Liquidi vitalis*, Lugd. Bat., 1748); and still more lately by Hoffman, De Haen, and Isenflamm. Several of their cases, however, are confounded with the different forms of the preceding species, and consist of nothing more than an exhausted state of the bloodvessels, from hemorrhage or other profuse evacuations, in one case, indeed, from hemorrhoids.—(*Robin, Journ. de Médecine*, tom. xxxii., p. 48.) And hence Lieutaud and Isenflamm undertook, in the middle of the last century, to distinguish the real disease from those which were thus confounded with it; tracing out the separate causes and symptoms, and marking them by different names; as *anæmia chlorosis*, and *anæmia consecutiva*, which were the appellations of Lieutaud (*Précis de la Médecine Pratique*, 1761); and a. *vera*, and a. *spuria*, which were those of Isenflamm. These distinctions, however, seem to have made less impression on the world of medicine than they ought to have done: for we find M. de Sauvages, in the first edition of his Nosologia Methodica, published subsequently to Lieutaud's Summary,

following Strach and Ramazzini in describing anæmia, if, indeed, he has described it at all, as a modification of spurious chlorosis, or pallor, under the name of *chlorosis rhachialgica*.—(*Nos. Med.*, cl. x.; *Cachexiæ*, ord. vi.; *Icteritiæ*, gen. xxxv.; *Ramazzini De Morbis Artific.*, cl. i., ii.)

Of late years, however, something more of light and far more of correct description have been thrown upon this very extraordinary malady by the contributions of several writers, and particularly of Professor Halle, of Paris, and Dr. Combe, of Edinburgh.* Nothing can be more different than the occupations, habits, and modes of life, of two distinct classes of individuals, who are hereby brought forward as the subjects of anhæmia. And yet the close resemblance, and, allowance being made for incidental circumstances, we may say the identity of the symptoms exhibited in situations so perfectly unlike, furnish an adequate proof of an identity of disease.†

The most strictly idiopathic example, and the one most free from influential incidents, is that of Dr. Combe.—(*Case of Anæmia; Transact. of Med. Chir. Soc. of Edin.*, vol. i., p. 194.) The patient was forty-seven years of age, was born in the country, and for the most part had been occupied in agricultural employments: he was married, but without a family; was leading a regular and temperate life; had enjoyed perfect health ever since childhood, and had never been blooded. At the time of his applying to Dr. Combe for advice, he had been unwell for about two months, or something more; his chief complaint having been loss of strength, uneasiness in the head, and a sickly complexion. "I was much struck," says Dr. Combe, "by his peculiar appearance. He exactly resembled a person just recovering from an attack of syncope. His face, lips, and the whole extent of the surface, were of a deadly pale colour: the albuginea of his eye bluish. his motions and speech were languid: he complained much of weakness; his respiration, free when at rest, became

* Professor Samuel Jackson, of Philadelphia, considers anhæmia under four divisions: complete and incomplete; general and local or partial; under each division he has made some very pertinent remarks:—When anhæmia becomes a complication superadded to other affections, an epiphenomenon, as it was formerly expressed, the treatment of the original disease must be modified by this circumstance.—See Hays's Cyclop. of Med., art. ANEMIA.—D.

† A general anhæmia may come on without any discoverable cause. Andral noticed its existence in the bodies of several individuals who died dropsical, and in whom no alteration whatever of the solids could be traced.—(Clinique Méd., tom. iii., p. 558, et suiv.) The restriction to a diet not sufficiently nutritious, the habitual respiration of impure, damp air, deprived of the sun's influence, and which prevents the elaborating functions of the skin and lungs from being duly performed, a disease that affects the direct or indirect organs of hæmatosis, are the circumstances adverted to by Andral as capable of producing a more or less complete general anhæmia.—See Anat. Pathol., tom. i., p. 81.—ED.

* The blood may be so diminished in quantity, that it seems, during life, to forsake the surface, which is only pervaded (to use Andral's expression) by a kind of serosity; and, after death, no blood is found, not only in the arterial trunks, great veins, and right cavities of the heart, but in the several capillary networks, all of which seem remarkably pale. In this state, completely destitute of blood, are found all the membranous and parenchymatous tissues, as the brain, the lungs, the liver, the kidneys, the alimentary canal, and the texture of the heart and muscles.—See Andral, Anat. Pathol., tom. i., p. 80.—ED.

hurried on the slightest exertion : pulse eighty, and feeble : tongue covered with a dry fur; the inner part of the lips and fauces nearly as colourless as the surface." His bowels were very irregular, though generally relaxed : the stools very dark and fetid; urine copious and pale : appetite impaired, and latterly a rejection of almost every kind of food; constant thirst; no pain referable to any part, nor any determinable derangement of structure.

These symptoms continued with little variation for about three months, with the exception that, for a short time, he appeared to be improving. Yet, upon the whole, the disorder gained ground; the feeble pulse was easily excited; a copious perspiration followed any exertion; the veins on the arms and neck could be felt on making pressure, but the colour of the blood did not appear through the skin. At one time, an affection of the liver was suspected; at another, from the thirst and great flow of urine, *paruria mellita;* but none of these indications were stationary. Tonics did no service, nor a sea-voyage, which was tried, nor the use of a chalybeate spring. He grew gradually weaker, continued to lose flesh; but, with a strong resemblance to the delusive confidence of phthisis, his spirits remained for the most part undepressed, and he still looked forward to a speedy recovery. Meanwhile all the symptoms were deteriorating, and the constitution was evidently sinking under their pressure. In about six months from the period of his application for relief, the œdema extended over his face and upper extremities, evident marks presented themselves of effusion into the chest, and he died with all the symptoms of hydrothorax.

The body was examined thirty-six hours after death. The waxy pallor of the surface remained unchanged : the subcutaneous fat was scanty, of a pale yellow, and semi-fluid. Not a drop of blood escaped on dividing the scalp : the dura mater was pale, presented few vessels, and those empty. The pia mater was equally pale, its bloodvessels contained a pale serum and a considerable quantity of air. The lateral sinuses were moderately filled with a pale fluid blood; the arteries at the basis were empty. The substance of the brain was very soft and pultaceous, mapped with very few vessels. The lungs were of a pale gray, without any marks of gravitated blood. The heart, when cut into, was of a pale colour, and did not tinge the linen when rubbed upon it; it appeared like flesh macerated many days in water. The right ventricle contained a pale coagulum. The left side was wholly empty. The coronary arteries were sound. The inner coat of the aorta was of a fine red colour for some inches, without any turgescence or ossification. All the valves were sound. A considerable moisture bedewed the viscera of the abdomen. The liver was of its proper size and structure, but of a light brown colour; there was no exudation of blood on cutting into its substance. The spleen was the only viscus of its usual colour : it was very soft, and its contents, when pressed, turned out as from a sac. The kidneys were nearly bloodless : the pancreas of a pale reddish hue. The stomach and intestines were perfectly sound, thin, showing no vessels, and transparent. The muscular substance throughout the body was, like that of the heart, very pale, and exuded no blood, but only a pale serum when cut into. The arteries were universally empty, as were also the jugular, humeral, and femoral veins. The lower cava alone, about the bifurcation, with the exception of the lateral sinuses, contained any appreciable quantity of blood.

Besides these appearances, about three pounds of a lemon-coloured serum was found effused in the thorax, and a considerable ossification, about an inch long, rough and irregular, was traced imbedded in the plicæ of the dura mater near the vertex, being almost the only morbid deviations, with the exception of those that relate to the sanguineous system; the first of which Dr. Combe justly regards as a mere consequence of the disease; while he thinks it may admit of a doubt whether the second had any connexion with the bloodless state of the system. In truth, it seems to have been an incidental concomitant.

It is impossible to conceive a more total exhaustion of the vital fluid from the entire system, than this singular case presents to us ; and instead of wondering at the deadly waxiness of the complexion, the feebleness of the pulse, the utter debility and emaciation which this incarnate ghost must have presented, the greater and almost the only wonder is, how the living principle could so long have remained attached to so exhausted a receiver, and the sensorial power have derived its means of recruit ; at a time, too, when all the functions, in the midst of their feebleness, were urged on by the force of the morbid excitement to the performance of double duty : the pulse was quickened; the animal spirits were maintained above the standard of sober health ; the peristaltic action, though irregular, for the most part accelerated, the perspiration redundant, and the urine often profuse.

The post-obit examination, while it unveils little or nothing of the proximate cause of the disease, discloses to us most manifestly the inroad that had been made upon the general substance of the frame for the want of a due supply of nourishment, and how completely every organ had been living upon itself, and the whole had been living upon the remnant of the blood almost to its last drop. The fault does not, therefore, so much seem to have been in the secernent system, or assimilating powers, as in the lacteals, or digestive function : in the commencement, rather than in the termination of the chain.

It was the opinion of Ruysch, as we have lately had occasion to observe, that this commencing part of the catenated organ of supply gradually loses its power with the advance of years, and that, in old age, it entirely ceases to act : so that being himself, at the time of writing, in this very season of life, he conceived he was then living, and had been living for a long period, upon himself : upon such nourishment as the fat, blood, flesh, parenchyma, and even brain, can produce when melted down by the action of the absorbents. And he further conceived that, from the little wear and tear which usually takes place in old age, the flame of life might be kept burning for a considerable term by the fuel hereby supplied ; the growing emaciation being a pretty correct measure of the material consumed.

How far such may have been the fact with Ruysch himself, or with any other person in the ordinary advance of life, we need not at present examine : but something very like it appears to have occurred in the extraordinary malady before us. We have seen that the digestive function was habitually impaired, and that at length food of all kinds was rejected from the stomach ; and we shall find by other instances presently, that the stomach, under the influence of this disease, seems to be always, even at the best estate, capricious or fastidious.* But the lacteals seem to have participated in the same infirmity ; and to have laboured under an atony or paresis so considerable, though invisible to the eye of the anatomist, as to have transmitted whatever aliment might have been subacted very imperfectly, or not at all, into the course of the circulation. And hence, while the blood actually in existence was perpetually drained off in support of the different organs and their respective functions, a small quantity only of an unelaborated fluid was able to reach the heart and larger arteries, which were, in consequence, pale and empty, or only partially supplied with a thin, watery, and scarcely tinged liquid. And, in confirmation of this idea, we shall find in the sequel of our examination, that the mesentery, in various instances, gives proof of disturbance, and appears enlarged, even to an external examination, while the hypochondria are free from such affection.

Such then seems to have been the proximate cause, though undeveloped by dissection, if we may be allowed to hazard a conjecture upon a subject involved in so much obscurity. Yet the exciting cause seems still more effectually to elude our penetration : for the constitution of the individual seems to have been strong and hearty, and every thing in his situation, occupation, and habits of life, apparently concurred in promising him a long continuance of health.

In various cases of the disease, however, that have occurred, we have some degree of insight into the occasional, as well as into the proximate cause. And I now particularly allude to the endemic appearance of this complaint at Auzain near Valenciennes, as described by Professor Halle.†

At Anzain is a large coal-mine, reaching to two or three adjoining villages. It was in one of the galleries of this mine that the complaint made its appearance, and to this it was confined, though no difference had hitherto been detected between the contaminated gallery and the rest. It is of the same depth, being a hundred and twenty fathoms from the level ground, and excavated in the same manner, but is longer, and hence does not so readily admit of an efflux of pure air. Its temperature is 64° Fahrenheit : it exhales an odour of sulphuretted hydrogen gas, which renders respiration difficult. Some caustic mineral, perhaps some metallic salt, appears to be dissolved in the water that drips from the mine, as it produces blains or blisters on any part of the body to which it is applied. Yet the water has been occasionally drunk to allay thirst, and the mine had been worked for eleven years without any such complaint as that before us : and it is hence obvious, that some new combination of vapour, incapable of detection by the senses, had found vent into the atmosphere of the gallery ; or some new mineral substance had become dissolved in its percolating water, which had a direct power of loosening and destroying the tone of the restorative system, at the commencement of its chain.

The symptoms, in their general features, were strikingly similar to those we have just described ; and seem only to have been modified by the peculiarity of the exciting cause, being often, though by no means always, accompanied from the first with severe gripings, and more violent affection of the abdominal viscera, and hence more rapid in their progress. Dr. Combe is inclined to think from these symptoms, that this disease was not a strict idiopathic anhæmia, but a modification of rhachialgia, the colic of lead or arsenic, and that it is hence more nearly allied to the *chlorosis rhachialgica* of Sauvages, than to the *anhæmia chlorosis* of Lieutaud. But in no instance do I find the back-bone ache, or spine-ache, from which rhachialgia derives its name, and by which, together with an extension of this aching over the upper and sometimes the lower extremities, with a strong tendency to paralysis, it is specifically distinguished. Neither indeed is the colicky pain itself to be regarded as a pathognomonic sign, or necessary attendant : for of the four patients who were sent for examination and treatment from Auzain to Paris, while two suffered from it, the other two were without any such symptom. Nor did the treatment usually found most serviceable in rhachialgia, prove of much, if indeed of any, benefit in the anhæmia of Auzain ; so that the medical superintendents, who had at first embraced this idea, found themselves obliged to abandon such a course, and the view of the disease on which it was founded, and to regard it as a direct exemplification of idiopathic anhæmia.

At the time of opening their correspondence

---

* After sp a g of the effects of a scanty quantity of blood on the system, upon the nervous system, respiratory organs, &c., Andral observes, that digestion is likewise disturbed, because, after the stomach has received food, the regular performance of that important function requires that the stomach shall become the seat of sanguineous congestion, which, in persons labouring under anhæmia, cannot take place.—See Anat. Pathol., tom. i., p. 82.—Eo.

† Journ. de Médecine, Chirurg. Pharm., &c. Par M M. Corvisart, Leroux, et Boyer, tom. ix., p.

3, Paris, An xiii.—See a translation of this in the Edin. Journ., vol. iii., p. 170.

with the School of Medicine at Paris, fifty patients, all belonging to the same gallery, had been attacked with the disorder, three of whom had died, and the number of patients was almost daily increasing, notwithstanding that the gallery was at this time shut up. Some of the sufferers had been ill for fifteen, others for twelve, others for eight months; and many were recent cases. It was obvious, however, that those were the most unfortunate subjects, and exhibited the highest degree of severity, who had been attacked while actually employed in the gallery: while those who did not complain till it was closed, passed through it, not indeed with speed, but in a more favourable way. So that the disorder seemed capable of being divided into two distinct states or varieties, an acute and a chronic.

The general symptoms under the former, independently of those of colic, were pallor of skin, great emaciation, weak, feeble, quick, contracted pulse palpitations of the heart, anhelation, extreme debility, so as to render walking difficult; bloated countenance, habitual perspiration, especially at night; stools black or greenish. These symptoms often continued without much change for many months, sometimes for upwards of a year; when they were united, manifestly from augmented weakness, with headache, frequent faintings, intolerance of light and sound.

Where colic was an accompaniment, there was much griping pain in the stomach and intestines, inflation of the abdomen, and at times, towards the close, purulent stools.

Four patients were selected out of the aggregate body to be sent to the School of Medicine at Paris for examination and advice. They were all young; their ages being from sixteen to twenty-one: one of them had worked in the mine for six years, the others for ten or eleven; and as they had all been ill for nearly a twelvemonth, it is obvious that they had been attacked while labouring in the gallery; and were hence regarded as having received the complaint in its acute state.

We have already observed, that, of these four, two had experienced colicky pains from the first, and two had not been troubled with them. The pulse varied from seventy to a hundred and four strokes in a minute, but the stroke was extremely feeble and scarcely perceptible; the least excitement, moreover, would accelerate it almost beyond the power of counting.

The stomach appears to have been generally capricious; they could relish food if allowed to exercise a choice; but one of them was subject to frequent vomiting; and in all the digestion was manifestly imperfect, as the food was partially discharged with little change, intermixed with black or greenish feces. The mesentery, as we have already observed, seemed considerably enlarged to the touch, but was destitute of pain on pressure: nor did the enlargement extend to any other region.

So extreme was the weakness, that none of these patients were able to walk more than a few steps without palpitation of the heart, and being compelled to sit down, and especially on mounting a staircase. Yet the same delusive hope, the same eparsis, or mental elation, that often accompanies consumption, and appeared, as we have already observed, in Dr. Combe's patient, was generally conspicuous in the cases before us. Even the death of one of them did not seem to destroy this enviable feeling. "We were afraid," says Professor Halle, "lest the melancholy fate of the first patient should have had an influence on the minds of his companions; but we had here no difficulty to encounter. The hope that the opening of his body would put us upon a more successful mode of treatment predominated in their minds, without taking away their regret for his loss." It is thus that we sometimes meet with a few cordial drops intermixed with the bitterest cup of suffering, and enabling the patient to support his trial, not only with composure, but with an elevated spirit.

The individual who thus fell a sacrifice, seems to have been attacked with more than ordinary severity at the very onset of the disease: and was one of those who had to contend with the pains of colic in addition to the specific symptoms. Mercurial inunction was early tried, but abandoned in a few days, from its being found to augment the pulse and increase the tendency to fever. When he reached Paris he had been ill for eleven months, having previously been employed in the mine for a period of eight years. He at length gave manifest proofs of hectic fever, the remissions of which became gradually shorter, till at length the fever assumed a continued type. But, though the skin was burning hot, it did not lose its paleness, nor was the slightest blush discernible on the tongue, the lips, or the conjunctiva: a remark which is indeed equally applicable to all the rest. He seems to have sunk under the pressure of debility alone; his most prominent symptoms at last being those of great difficulty of breathing, a feeble and intermitting pulse, and cold extremities.

The appearances on dissection were, as nearly as may be, those of Dr. Combe's patient, as we have already described them. The parenchymatous viscera were all pale, diminished, and shrivelled, with the exception of the heart, which preserved its natural size. Even the spleen, which, in the preceding case, retained its proper colour, and does not seem to have had its size much interfered with, was here of a reduced magnitude, and of the same spongy softness which the preceding case disclosed.

The almost utter bloodlessness of all the vessels, however, formed the predominant feature. "In the three cavities all the vessels, as well arteries as veins, were destitute of coloured blood, and contained only a small quantity of serous fluid. No blood was found in the aorta, as far as its crural subdivisions, nor in the accompanying veins, nor in the system of the hepatic vessels, nor in any of the sinuses of the brain. Upon making a deep incision into the flesh of the thighs, a small quantity of liquid and black blood flowed out; but none issued from a cut in any other part whatever. The flesh of the muscles which cover the thorax was exceedingly red, but that of the extremities much less so. And we are told that the same destitution of blood which distinguished this case, occurred also in all the other dissections that were made at any time; so that the want of colour in the interior precisely corresponded with that of the surface, and of the whole capillary system. "This condition, therefore," observes M. Halle, "may be regarded as peculiarly dependant on the disease; as exhibiting itself by manifest signs during its entire progress; and as reaching its height when it is on the point of terminating, and has reached its last stage."

From the extensive spread of the malady, there was a pretty ample opportunity of putting various plans of treatment to an effective test; and the opportunity was not neglected.

Mercury, as we have already observed, did not seem to answer. Two cases recovered under its use; but, in general, it produced febrile excitement, and hence no credit was given to it even in the instances of restoration. Emetics, sudorifics, acids, sedatives, tonics, and stimulants were all tried simultaneously, or in succession. But by far the most successful, as, indeed, the most rational plan, and that most corresponding with the nature of the proximate cause we have endeavoured to illustrate, consisted in a combined employment of the two last of these classes, stimulant and tonic medicines, with a free use of opium where the tormina required it, and the employment of gentle laxatives on the return of constipation. The best stimulants appear to have been camphire and ether; the best tonics, bark and iron.* While this plan was continued the patients generally improved in strength, lost their palpitation on walking, and evinced a slight return of colour; and in every instance in which this process was discontinued at too early a period, they appear to have relapsed; and only to have renewed their advantage upon a return to the same treatment. The diet was generous and nutritious, and altogether harmonized with the pharmaceutic intention.

SPECIES III.
MARASMUS CLIMACTERICUS.
DECAY OF NATURE: CLIMACTERIC DISEASE.

GENERAL DECLINE OF BULK AND STRENGTH, WITH OCCASIONAL RENOVATION, AT THE AGE OF SENESCENCE, WITHOUT ANY MANIFEST CAUSE.

For the groundwork of this species of marásmus, I am entirely indebted to Sir Henry Halford's elegant and perspicuous description of

---

* The subcarbonate, in doses of one or two drachms, three times a day. In the anhæmia connected with enlarged spleen, preparations of iron are extremely beneficial. This fact is mentioned by Tomassini, in his Clinical Reports.—ED.

---

it in the Medical Transactions. The disease has hitherto never appeared in any nosological arrangement, but it has characters sufficiently distinct and striking for a separate species. In several of its features, it bears a strong resemblance to the marasmus or atrophy of old age, described under the first species : but it differs essentially in the instance which it affords of a complete rally and recovery : and, if the train of reasoning about to be employed in developing its physiology proves correct it will be found to differ also in its chief seat and proximate cause.

The ordinary duration of life seems to have undergone little or no change from the Mosaic age, in which, as in the present day, it varied from threescore and ten to fourscore years. In passing through this term, however, we meet with particular epochs at which the body is peculiarly affected, and suffers a considerable alteration. These epochs the Greek physiologists contemplated as five. And, from the word climax (κλίμαξ), which signifies a gradation, they denominated them climacterics. They begin with the seventh year, which forms the first climacteric; and are afterward regulated by a multiplication of the figures three, seven, and nine, into each other; as, the twenty-first year being the result of three times seven; the forty-ninth, produced by seven times seven; the sixty-third, or nine times seven; and the eighty-first, or nine times nine. A more perfect scale might perhaps have been laid down; but the general principle is well founded and it is not worth while to correct it. The two last were called grand climacterics, or climacterics emphatically so denominated, as being those in which the life of man was supposed to have consummated itself; and beyond which nothing is to be accomplished but a preparation for the grave.

With the changes that occur on or about the first three of these periods we have no concern at present, and shall hence proceed to that which frequently strikes our attention as taking place about the fourth, or in the interval between the fourth and fifth. This change is of two distinct and opposite kinds, and it is necessary to notice each.

We sometimes find the system, at the period before us, exhibiting all of a sudden a very extraordinary renovation of powers. The author has seen persons who had been deaf for twenty years abruptly recover their hearing, so as in some cases to hear very acutely : he has seen others as abruptly recover their sight, and throw away their spectacles, which had been in habitual employment for as long a period; and he has seen others return to the process of dentition, and reproduce a smaller or larger number of teeth to supply vacuities progressively produced in earlier life. Under the genus ODONTIA, in the first class and first order of the present system, several of these singular facts have been already noticed, and examples given of entire sets of teeth cut at this period. That the hair should evince a similar regeneration, of which instances are also adduced in the same place, and of which Forestus affords other examples (Lib. xxxi., obs. 6), is, perhaps, less surprising, since this has been known to grow again, and even to change its colour, after death.* But I have occasionally seen several of these singularities, and especially the renewal of the sight and hearing, or of the sight and teeth, occur simultaneously. And hence Glanville spoke correctly when he affirmed that "the restoration of gray hairs to juvenility, and renewing exhausted marrow, may be effected without a miracle."

On the other hand, instead of a renovation of powers at the period before us, we sometimes perceive as sudden and extraordinary a decline. We behold a man apparently in good health, without any perceptible cause abruptly sinking into a general decay, His strength, his spirits, his appetite, his sleep, fail equally, his flesh falls away, and his constitution appears to be breaking up. In many instances this is, perhaps, the real fact, and no human wisdom or vigilance can save him from the tomb. But, in many examples also, it is an actual disease in which medical aid and kindly attention may be of essential service, and upon an application of which we behold the powers of life, as in other diseases, rally; the general strength return; the flesh grow fuller and firmer; the complexion brighten; the muscles become, once more, broad and elastic; and the whole occasionally succeeded by some of those extraordinary renovations of lost powers, or even lost organs, to which I have just adverted.

The subject is obscure, and it is as difficult, perhaps, to account for either of these extremes—for the sudden and unexpected decline as for the sudden and singular restoration. That the decline, however, is a real malady, and not a natural or constitutional decay, is perfectly obvious from the recovery. And hence Sir Henry Halford, in reference to the period in which it occurs, and by which, no doubt, it is influenced, has emphatically denominated it the CLIMACTERIC DISEASE.

Under the first species the author observed, that the great chain of the organs of nutrition extends from the chylific viscera to the assimilating secernents; that these form the ends of the chain; that a powerful sympathetic action runs through the whole: but that this action is more powerful between the one end of the chain and the other, than between any of its intermediate links. He observed farther, that, in the atrophy of old age, the failure of action seems to commence and to be chiefly seated at the chylific or chyliferous end, and that the assimilating secernents exhibit the same failure only afterward and by sympathy: that the lacteals become generally, and sometimes altogether obliterated, while the assimilating process is supported by an absorption, first of the animal oil deposited in the cellular membrane, then of this membrane itself, and, lastly, of much of the

muscular and parenchymatous structure of the general frame. In the disease before us, the reverse of all this seems to take place; and for its origin we must look to the assimilating powers constituting the other end of the chain. The patient falls away in flesh and strength before he complains of any loss of appetite, or has any dyspeptic symptoms; which only appear to take place afterward by sympathy. And that the mesentery and lacteals are not paralyzed and obliterated, as in the atrophy of old age, is incontrovertible, from the renovation of power and reproduction of bulk that form an occasional termination of the disease.

In watching carefully the symptoms of this malady when totally unconnected with any concomitant source of irritation, either mental or bodily, we shall often perceive that it creeps on so gradually and insensibly, that the patient himself is hardly aware of its commencement. "He perceives," to adopt the language of Sir Henry Halford, "that he is tired sooner than usual, and that he is thinner than he was; but yet he has nothing material to complain of. In process of time, his appetite becomes seriously impaired; his nights are sleepless, or, if he gets sleep, he is not refreshed by it. His face becomes visibly extenuated, or perhaps acquires a bloated look: His tongue is white, and he suspects that he has fever. If he ask advice, his pulse is found quicker than it should be, and he acknowledges that he has felt pains in his head and chest, and that his legs are disposed to swell; yet there is no deficiency in the quantity of his urine, nor any other sensible failure in the action of the abdominal viscera, except that the bowels are more sluggish than they used to be."

Sometimes he feels pains shooting over different parts of the body, conceived to be rheumatic, but without the proper character of rheumatism; and sometimes the headache is accompanied with vertigo. Towards the close of the disease, when it terminates fatally, the stomach seems to lose all its powers; the frame becomes more and more emaciated; the cellular membrane in the lower limbs is laden with fluid; there is an insurmountable restlessness by day, and a total want of sleep at night; the mind grows torpid and indifferent to what formerly interested it; and the patient sinks at last; seeming rather to cease to live than to die of a mortal distemper.

Such is the ordinary course of this disorder in its simplest form, when it proves fatal, and the powers of the constitution are incapable of coping with its influence. Yet it is seldom that we can have an opportunity of observing it in the simple form, and never perhaps, but in a patient whose previous life has been entirely healthy, and whose mind is unruffled by anxiety. For if this complaint, whatever be its cause, should show itself in a person who is already a prey to grief, or care, or mental distress of any kind, or in whom some one or more of the larger and more important organs of the body, as the liver, the lungs, or the heart, has been weakened or otherwise injured by accident or irreg-

---

* Eph. Nat. Cur., passim. The growth of the hair after death is a manifest impossibility, unless it be assumed that vascular action, circulation, deposition, and secretion, can continue after the extinction of life.—ED.

ularity, or is influenced by a gouty or other morbid diathesis, the symptoms will assume a mixed character, and the disease be greatly aggravated. It is these accidents, indeed, that for the most part constitute the exciting cause, as well as the most fearful auxiliary, of the disease; for, without such, it is highly probable that the predisposition might remain dormant; and that many a patient who falls a sacrifice to it, would be enabled to glide quietly through the sequestered vale of age to the remotest limit of natural life, and at length quit the scene around him without any violent struggle or protracted suffering, with a euthanasia sometimes, though rarely attained, but ardently desired by us all.

Sir Henry Halford has remarked, that the disease, according to his experience, is less common to women than to men. The author's own experience coincides with this observation. And we can be at no loss to account for the difference, when we reflect on the greater exposure of the latter than of the former, to those contingencies which so frequently become occasional causes or auxiliaries, and which, at the period now alluded to, strike more deeply and produce a much more lasting effect, than in the heyday and ebulliency of life.

There are some events, however, that apply equally to both sexes, and which very frequently lead to this affection; as, for instance, the loss of a long-tried and confidential friend; of a beloved or only child; or of a wife or husband assimilated to each other in habits, disposition, general views, and sentiments, by an intercourse of perhaps thirty or forty years' standing. This last, as it has occurred to me, is a more marked and more frequent cause of excitement than any other. I have seen it in some instances operate very rapidly: and have my eye at this moment directed to the melancholy fate of a very excellent clergyman; between fifty and sixty years of age, the father of ten children, who were all dependant upon him, and whose benefice would have enabled him, in all probability, to provide for them respectably had he lived; but who, having lost the beloved mother of his family while lying-in of her tenth living child, was never able to recover from the blow, and followed her to the grave in less than three months.

I have at other times seen the same effect produced as clearly and decidedly, though with a much tardier step, and unaccompanied with any sudden shock. I attended not long since a lady in Edgeware Road, who died of a consumption at the age of fifty-four. Her husband, though not a man of keen sensibility, had attentively nursed her through the whole of her lingering illness, and had lived happily with her from an early period of life. He was aware of her approaching end, and prepared for it: and, in a few weeks after her decease, seemed to have recovered his usual serenity. Not long afterward, however, he applied to me on his own account. I found him dispirited, and losing flesh; his appetite was diminishing, and his nights restless, with little fever, and alto-

gether without any manifest local disorder. The emaciation with its accompanying evils nevertheless increased, the general disease became confirmed, and, in about five months, he fell a sacrifice to it.

Occasionally, however, where the climacteric temperament, if I may so express myself, is lurking, a very trivial accidental excitement proves sufficient to rouse it into action. "I have known," says Sir Henry Halford, "an act of intemperance, where intemperance was not habitual, the first apparent cause of it. A fall, which did not appear of consequence at the moment, and which would not have been so at any other time, has sometimes jarred the frame into this disordered action. A marriage, contracted late in life, has also afforded the first occasion to this change."

It has in some instances followed a cutaneous eruption, of which the ensuing case will afford a very striking example, and show in the clearest colours the general want of tone, which, under this morbid influence, prevails throughout the system.

Most of my readers of this metropolis have heard of, and many of them have perhaps had the pleasure of being personally acquainted with, the late James Cobb, Esq., Secretary to the East India Company, the history of whose life, from his intimate and extensive connexion and correspondence with the most brilliant and distinguished characters of the age that have figured either in political or fashionable life, and more especially from his own fine taste and commanding talents, and his unwearied efforts to patronise merit in whatever rank it was to be found, ought not to have been withheld from the world. In November, 1816, this gentleman, then in his sixty-first year, and blessed with one of the firmest and most vigorous constitutions that I have ever known, applied to me for an erysipelatous affection of the face. It was troublesome, and for nearly a fortnight accompanied with a slight fever, and a good deal of irritation. It subsided at length, but left a degree of debility which called for a change of air, and relaxation from public duty. He made a short excursion to France, and returned much improved, but evidently not quite restored to all the strength and elasticity he formerly enjoyed. Insensibly, and without any ostensible cause, he became emaciated, walked from Russell Square to the East India House with less freedom than usual, and found his carriage a relief to him in returning home. His appetite diminished, his nights were less quiet, and his pulse a little quickened. At one time he complained of an inextinguishable thirst, and voided an unusual quantity of urine, so as to excite some apprehension of *paruria mellita*. But the urine evinced no sweetness, and both these symptoms rapidly disappeared under the medical treatment laid down for him. The general waste and debility, however, continued to increase; his natural cheerfulness began to flag occasionally, and exertion was a weariness. At this period an inflammation commenced suddenly on the left side of the nates, which soon produced a tumour somewhat larger than a goose's egg, and suppurated very kindly. Sir Gilbert Blane and Sir Walter Farquhar were now engaged in consultation with myself, as was Dr. Hooper afterward. It was a doubtful question, what would be the result of this abscess? It might be regarded as an effort of nature to re-invigorate the system by a critical excitement; and, in this view of the case, there was reason for congratulation. But it was at the same time obvious, that if the strength of the system should not be found equal to this new source of exhaustion, and could not be stimulated to meet it, the abscess might prove highly unfavourable. The tumour was opened, and about a quarter of a pint of well-formed pus discharged: but the morbid symptoms remained without alteration, and the cavity seemed rather disposed to run into a sinus along the perinæum than to fill up. The opening was enlarged, but no advantage followed: it was evident there was too little vigour in the system to excite healthy action. The abscess was alternately stimulated with tincture of myrrh, a solution of nitrate of silver, and red precipitate; but the surface continued glassy, with a display of pale and flabby granulations, that vanished soon after they made their appearance. Mr. Cline was now united in consultation, and concurred in opinion, that the wound was of subordinate importance, and would follow the fortune of the general frame. The issue was still doubtful, for the constitution resisted pertinaciously, though upon the whole the disorder was gaining ground. Yet, even at this time, there was not a single organ we could pitch upon, with the exception of the abscess, that gave indication of the slightest structural disease. The lungs were perfectly sound and unaffected; the heart without palpitation; the mind in the fullest possession of all its powers; the head at all times free from pain or stupor, even after very large doses of opium and other narcotics: the bile was duly secreted; the urine in sufficient abundance; and the bladder capable of retaining it without inconvenience through the whole night. The pulse, however, was quick, the stomach fastidious, and the bowels irregular, sometimes costive, and at others suddenly attacked with a diarrhœa that required instant and active attention to prevent a fatal deliquium. The wound continued on a balance: there was energy enough to prevent gangrene, but too little for incarnation.

A clearer example of the disease before us cannot be wished for or conceived. Unfortunately, its progress, though retarded by the arms of medicines, was retarded alone. One of the last recommendations was a removal into the country; but Mr. Cobb was now become so debilitated and infirm that this was found a work of some difficulty, and required contrivance. His Royal Highness the Duke of Sussex, however, being kind enough to accommodate our patient with the use of his easy and convenient sofa-carriage, for as long a period as he might choose, he proceeded without

much fatigue to a house provided for him on the borders of Windsor Forest. The distance was now become too considerable for me to attend him statedly, and I visited him but once or twice afterward. He continued, however, to decline gradually, and, in about a month from the time of his going to Windsor, sunk suddenly under a return of the diarrhœa.

In the progress of this disease, medicine will generally be found to accomplish but little. The constitutional debility must be met by tonics, cordials, and a generous diet: and a scrupulous attention should be paid to such contingencies of body or mind as may form an exciting cause, or aggravate the morbid diathesis if already in a state of activity. Congestions must be removed where they exist, and every organ have room for the little play that the rigidity of advanced life allows to it: and where aperients are necessary, they should consist principally of the warm and bitter roots or resins, as rhubarb, guaiacum, and spikealoes. In many instances the Bath water, and in a few that of Cheltenham, will be also found of collateral use; and especially where we have reason to hope that a beneficial impression has been made on the disease, and that the system is about to recover itself.

The last remark I shall beg leave to offer, I must give in the words of Sir Henry Halford himself. If not strictly medical, it is of more than medical importance; and I have very great pleasure in seeing it put forth from so high an authority, and finding its way into a professional volume. "For the rest," says he, "the patient must minister to himself. To be able to contemplate with complacency either issue of a disorder which the great Author of our being may, in his kindness, have intended as a warning to us to prepare for a better existence, is of prodigious advantage to recovery, as well as to comfort; and the retrospect of a well-spent life is a cordial of infinitely more efficacy than all the resources of the medical art."*

SPECIES IV.
MARASMUS TABES.
DECLINE.

GENERAL LANGUOR; DEPRESSION OF STRENGTH, AND, MOSTLY, OF SPIRITS; HECTIC FEVER.

TABES is a Latin term, of doubtful origin. The lexicographers derive it from the Greek τήκω, "macero," varied in the Doric dialect to τάκω,—whence Scaliger makes a compound of τακόβιος, "macerans vita," "a consuming life, or life of consumption;" and supposes that such a word existed formerly, and that tabes is

* In the medical writings of Dr. Rush may be seen a paper of peculiar interest, entitled, "An account of the state of the Body and Mind in Old Age, with Observations on its Diseases and their Remedies." Many of the remarks of Dr. Rush are particularly applicable to this species of marasmus. Dr. Rush puts much stress upon circumstances connected with hereditary predisposition.—D.

a derivative from it. This is ingenious, but nothing more. *Tab-eo* or *tab-es*, is most probably derived from the Hebrew אב (tab), literally " to pine away or consume ;" which is the exact meaning of the Latin terms.

Tabes is sufficiently distinguished from atrophy by the presence of hectic fever ; from climacteric decay, by the tendency to depressed spirits, as well as its appearing at any age ; and from consumption, by the local symptoms of the latter.

Its ordinary causes are commonly supposed to be an absorption of pus into the blood, or the introduction of some poisonous substance, as quicksilver or arsenic ; or a scrofulous taint ; or an irritation produced by excess in libidinous indulgences ; thus laying a groundwork for the four following varieties :—

a Purulenta.	Purulent decline.
β Venenata.	Decline from poison.
γ Strumosa.	Scrofulous decline.
δ Dorsalis.	Decline of intemperance.

In the FIRST OF THESE VARIETIES, the absorbed pus may be contemplated as acting the part of a foreign and irritating substance,[*] and as acting upon a peculiarity of constitution : but, unless the latter be present, pus will rarely, if ever, be found to produce a tabid frame : for, as already observed under hectic fever, if absorbed pus be capable, independently of idiosyncrasy, of inducing a decline in one instance, it ought to do so in every instance ; yet this we know is not the case, since buboes, empyemas, and other apostemes and abscesses of large extent, have been removed by absorption, and yet no tabes has accompanied the process. It is said to occur more frequently where an abscess or a vomica is open ; in consequence of pus becoming more acrimonious by the action of the air. But this supposition is altogether gratuitous : and where hectic fever accompanies a sore or open abscess, it is more probably from increased irritation on the edges or internal surface of the cavity, as already observed when treating on psoas abscess.

In TABES VENENATA, Dr. Cullen conceives that one cause of emaciation is produced by an absorption of oil from the cells of the cellular membrane into the blood, for the purpose of inviscating the acrimonious spiculæ of the poisonous substance. This, however, is mere hypothesis, without a shadow of proof ; and by far the greater number of poisons that enter the blood, whether by deglutition or inhalation, act by a chymical rather than by a mechanical

---

[*] Armstrong, Diss. de Tabe Purulentâ, Edin., 1732. Pus, when absorbed into the circulation from common abscesses, is thought by Cruveilhier (Anat. Pathol.) to undergo some change by the action of the absorbing vessels on it, which change prevents it from having hurtful effects on the constitution ; whereas, if pus be introduced directly into the circulation, without being acted upon by the absorbents, it causes capillary venous phlebitis, visceral abscesses, and severe and fatal consequences ; but no disorder resembling what Dr. Good calls tabes purulenta.—Ed.

power. Let them, however, act as they may, the hypothesis is not necessary to account for the emaciation ; for the offensive matter with which the blood is hereby contaminated, is alone sufficient to excite and maintain the hectic ; as the hectic is alone sufficient to wear away the strength and substance of the system, and produces the waste. It is a disease, as Scheffler has observed, chiefly common to miners and mineralogists (*Von der Gesundheit der Bergleute*, Chemnitz, 1770) ; and, next to these, is to be found, perhaps, most frequently, among the labourers in chymical laboratories.

There are other poisonous irritants which are altogether ingenerate or hereditary, that, by their perpetual stimulation, ultimately produce the same effect ; as those of chronic syphilis, cancer and scurvy.

A more common cause, however, than any of these, is to be found in a state of the system which has apparently a very near relation to that of scrofula, though it is difficult precisely to identify them. The VARIETY FROM THIS CAUSE is hence frequently treated of under the head of scrofula or struma ; but as it is peculiarly connected with a morbid condition of one or more of the organs of nutrition, including those of digestion and assimilation, and is uniformly accompanied with emaciation, irritation, and some degree of hectic fever, it more properly falls within the range of the genus MARASMUS than that of STRUMA, and constitutes a peculiar variety of DECLINE.

Of all the contaminations that lurk in the blood, and are propagable in a dormant state, that of scrofula shows itself sooner than any of the rest. It is curious, indeed, to observe the different periods of time that hereditary diatheses of a morbid kind demand for their maturity, unless quickened into development by some incidental cause. Scrofula very generally shows itself in infancy ; phthisis, rarely till the age of puberty ; gout, in mature life ; mania, some years later ; and cancer still later than mania. Scrofula runs its course first, and becomes dormant, though rarely extinct ; phthisis travels through a term of fifteen or twenty years, and if it do not destroy its victim by the age of thirty-eight, generally consents to a truce, and is sometimes completely subjugated. All the rest persevere throughout the journey of life ; they may indeed hide their heads for a longer or shorter interval, but they commonly continue their harassings till the close of the scene.

When the strumous taint is excited into action in infant life, it generally fixes itself upon the chylific or chyliferous glands, especially when they are in a weakly state ; most commonly upon the mesentery, and to this quarter it often confines itself ; insomuch that " I have frequently," says Dr. Cullen, " found the case occurring in persons who did not show any external appearance of scrofula ; but in whom the mesenteric obstruction was afterward discovered by dissection."—(*Practice of Physic*, part iii., book i.; § 1606.) It is supposed by Dr. Cullen, and by most pathologists, that the emaciation is, in this case, produced invariably by an obstruction of the conglobate or lymphatic glands of the mesentery, through which the chyle must necessarily pass to the thoracic duct. That an obstruction thus total may occur is not to be altogether disputed, because the lymph has been found stagnated in its course by such an obstruction of lymphatic glands in other parts; but I have already observed that it is an interruption of very rare occurrence (Vol. i., p. 228, Cl. I., Ord. II.,·Parabysma Mesentericum); so rare that Mr. Cruickshank affirms he never saw such a stagnation on the dissection of any mesenteric case whatever. And that scrofulous enlargement of the glands of the mesentery does not necessarily produce a total obstruction is certain, because children in whom mesenteric enlargement can be felt in the form of knots protuberating in the abdomen, have lived for a considerable number of years, sometimes ten or twelve, and have at last died of some other disease. And hence it is perhaps more frequently the hectic fever, kept up by the local irritation of the mesentery, and the scrofulous taint in the blood, that produces the emaciation in this case, than the pressure of a scrofulous infarction.

"The mesenteric decline," says Dr. Young, "is generally preceded by more or less of a headache, languor, and want of appetite. It is more immediately distinguished by acute pain in the back and loins, by fulness, and, as the disease advances, pain and tenderness of the abdomen. These symptoms are accompanied or succeeded by a chalky appearance, and want of consistency in the alvine evacuations, as if the chyle were rejected by the absorbents, and left in the form of a milky fluid in the intestines; and the functions of the liver were at the same time impaired, the natural tinge of the bile being wanting. The evacuations are also sometimes mixed with mucus and blood; and are attended by pain, irritation, and tenesmus, somewhat resembling those that occur in a true dysentery. Occasionally, also, there are symptoms of dropsy, and especially of ascites; as if the absorption of the fluid, poured into the cavity of the abdomen, were prevented by local obstacles: the absorbent glands, which are enlarged, being rendered impervious, and pressing also on the lacteals and lymphatics which enter them and pass by them." The appetite is generally good, and often ravenous; probably produced by some remote irritation acting sympathetically on the stomach: as that of the mesentery, or more likely that of the assimilating powers that constitute the opposite end of the chain of nutrient organs, and which, from their morbid excitement, produce a morbid waste, and demand a larger supply than they receive. As worms are easily generated, and multiply in the digestive organs when in a state of debility, they have often been found in a considerable number in this disease, and have sometimes been mistaken for the cause of the malady instead of the effect.—(*Chesneau*, lib. v., obs. 27.) Balme gives a case in which they were equally discharged by the mouth and anus.—(*Journ. de Méd.*, 1790, Sept.,

No. i.) In the strumous enlargements are occasionally found calcareous concretions; and similar concretions are sometimes discovered in the lacteals and the liver.—(*Histoire de l'Acad. des Sciences*, &c., 1684.) Where the irritation or inflammation is considerable, the intestinal canal is peculiarly apt to unite in the morbid action, producing, with many of the symptoms we have just noticed, hectic fever, and forming what has often been called the FEBRIS INFANTUM REMITTENS.

The decline from an intemperate indulgence in libidinous pleasures has been denominated TABES DORSALIS, from the weakness which it introduces into the back, or rather into the loins. It is a disease of considerable antiquity; for we find traces of it in the oldest historical records that have reached our own day; and it is particularly described by Hippocrates under the name of 'ΦΘΙΣΙΣ ΝΩΤΙΑΣ (Περὶ τῶν ἔθνος Παθῶν, Opp., p. 539, as also Περὶ Νουσῶν ii., Opp., p. 479), literally "HUMID TABES," from the frequent and involuntary secretion of a gleety matter, or rather of a dilute and imperfect seminal fluid. He explains it to be a disorder of the spinal marrow, incident to persons of a salacious disposition, or who are newly married, and have too largely indulged in conjugal pleasures. He represents the patient as complaining of a sense of formication, or a feeling like that of ants creeping from the upper part of his body, as his head, into the spine of his back; and tells us, that when he discharges his urine or excrements, there is at the same time a copious evacuation of semen, in consequence of which he is incapable of propagating his species, or answering the purpose of marriage. He is generally shortbreathed and weak, especially after exercise; he is sensible of a weight in his head, his memory is inconstant, and he is affected with a failure of sight, and a ringing in his ears. Though without fever at first, he at length becomes severely feverish, and dies of that variety of remittent which the Greeks called leipyria, a sort of causus or ardent fever, attended with great coldness of the extremities, but with a burning fire and intolerable heat within, an insupportable anxiety and unconquerable dryness of the tongue. This description is fully confirmed by Professor Frank in his history of the miserable condition of two young men who had induced the same disease by a habit of self-pollution, one of whom, together with extreme emaciation, suffered excruciating pains in every limb from head to foot, was incapable of standing, and subject to epileptic fits; while the other, after a long career of acute suffering in various ways, was at length seized with a hemiplegia.—(*De Cur. Hom. Morb. Epit.*, tom. v., p. 259.)

From this sketch it is obvious that the disease is one of great danger, though it is occasionally combated with success. In the Hôpital des Enfans Malades at Paris, the fatal cases are calculated by M. Guersent, one of the physicians to the establishment, at from five to six in every hundred of boys, and from seven to eight in every hundred of girls, whose names enter in the tables of mortality.—(*Dict. de Méd.*, art. Carreau.) Upon the treatment, we shall offer a few remarks towards the close of the species.

Dr. Cullen does not think that the quantity of seminal fluid discharged by undue indulgence can ever be so considerable as to account for this general deficiency of fluids in the body, and the debility that accompanies it, and adds, that we must therefore seek for another explanation of these evils. " And whether," says he, " the effects of this evacuation may be accounted for either from the quality of the. fluid evacuated, or from the singularly enervating pleasure attending the evacuation, or from the evacuation's taking off the tension of parts, the tension of which has a singular power in supporting the tension and vigour of the whole body, I cannot positively determine ; but I apprehend that upon one or other of these suppositions, the emaciation attending the tabes dorsalis must be accounted for."—(*Pract. of Physic.*, part iii., b. i., § 690.)

It is not difficult to trace this result in a less doubtful and more direct way. The sexual organs, both in males and females, have a close and striking sympathy with the brain. Morbid salacity is no uncommon cause of madness, as we shall have occasion to observe hereafter. Irritation of the uterus shortly after childbirth, is a still more frequent cause of the same mental affection. The testes are not capable of secreting their proper fluid till the sensorial organ has acquired, or is on the point of acquiring, maturity, so that both become perfect nearly at the same time ; the mere apprehension of failure, when in the act of embracing, has at once, in a variety of instances, unnerved the orgasm, and prevented the seminal flow so effectually, that the unhappy individual has often required many weeks, or even months, before he could recover a sufficient confidence to render the operation complete ; while, as Dr. Cullen has correctly observed, the evacuation itself, even when conducted naturally, produces a pleasure of a singularly enervating kind. It is in truth. a shock that thrills through all the senses ; and hence, in persons of an epileptic temperament, has been known, as we shall have occasion to observe more fully hereafter, to bring on a paroxysm while in the act of interunion.

It is hence easy to see, that an immoderate excitement of the generic organs, and secretion of seminal fluid, must weaken the sensorial powers even at their fountain ; and consequently that the nervous and muscular fibres throughout the entire frame, and even the mind itself, must be influenced by the debility of the sensorium. This we might suppose if there were no chronic flux from the seminal vessels. But when we consider the effect often produced on the general frame by the discharge, or rather the irritation, of a single blister ; or, which is perhaps more to the purpose, of a small seton or issue, we can be at no loss to account for all the evils that haunt the worn-out debauchee, and especially the self-abuser, from involuntary emissions of a seminal fluid, however dilute and spiritless, in connexion with the dreadful debility we have just noticed, and which is the cause of this emission. The nervous irritation which results from this debility, is the source of the hectic by which the miserable victim is devoured ; and hence the heavy terrors and insupportable anxiety, corporeal as well as mental, the sense of formication and other phantasms, the flaccidity of the back and loins, the withering of the entire body, the constant desire of erection, with an utter inability of accomplishing it, which haunt him by day and by night, and throw him into a state of despondency. A fearful picture, which cannot be too often before the eyes of a young man in this licentious metropolis, in order to deter him from plunging into evils to which he is so often exposed.[*]

Even where sexual inability has not taken place, the system, by an habitual excess of libidinous indulgence, is not unfrequently roused and kept up to such a state of excitement as to produce hectic fever and great debility, or other derangement of the spinal cord. Of this we shall hereafter have to give a most appalling example (when treating of paraplegia) in a young debauchee, who, at the age of forty-five fell a sacrifice chiefly to this enervating propensity, after refusing to take the warning that a constitution naturally feeble and rachetic was well calculated to offer ; but which might, by care and prudent nursing, have held out to the ordinary term of old age. The upper limbs were, for years before his death, motionless and rigid ; and the spinal marrow, through a considerable portion of its length, was found disorganized and liquescent.

Much of the medical treatment it may be proper to pursue, has been anticipated in several of the preceding species.

The first variety, in which the decline is dependant on the stimulus of an abscess or sore, or the introduction of pus into the circulation, can only be cured by a cure of the local affection. The strength may in the meanwhile be supported by a course of inirritant tonics, as cinchona and the mineral acids, nutritious diet, gentle exercise, and pure air. And, if stimulants be at any time employed with a view of acting more directly on the morbid irritation, and changing its nature, they should be limited to the milder resins, as myrrh, or the milder terebinthinates, as camphire, and balsam of copayva.

In decline from the inhalation of metallic or other deleterious vapours, if Dr. Cullen's hypothesis were established, that the emaciation is the mere result of the vis medicatrix naturæ, and produced by an absorption of oil from the cellular membrane for the purpose of sheathing the minute goads of the poison, it would be our duty to follow up this indication, and employ inviscating demulcents, both oils and mucilages. But this practice has rarely been productive of any success ; and we have much more reason

<hr/>

[*] Lewis's Essay upon the Tabes Dorsalis, Lond., 1758. Brendal, Diss. de Tabe Dorsali, Goett., 1748. Swediaur, vol. i., p. 251. Spermacrasia Asthenica.

to expect benefit from a use of the alkalis, which, by uniting with the metallic salts, if they still exist in the circulation, may disengage their acid principle, reduce the metallic base to a harmless regulus, and, by the new combination hereby produced, form a cooling, perhaps a sedative neutral. The first step, however, is to remove the patient from the deleterious scene to an atmosphere of fresh air, then to purify the blood, whether we employ the alkalis or not, with alterant diluents, as the decoction of sarsaparilla, and afterward to have recourse to bitters, astringents, and the chalybeate mineral waters.

In strumous decline, the mode of treatment should run precisely parallel with that for most of the species of PARABYSMA, or VISCERAL TURGESCENCE, already laid down under their respective heads, and particularly with that for mesenteric parabysma, to which the reader may turn.

In the treatment of *tabes dorsalis*, or decline from intemperate indulgence, our attention must be directed to the mind as well as to the body: for it is a mixed complaint, and each suffers equally. A summer's excursion with a cheerful and steady friend, into some untried and picturesque country, where the beauty and novelty of the surrounding scenery may by degrees attract the eye, and afford food for conversation, will be the most effectual step to be pursued if the symptoms be not very severe. The hours should be regular, with early rising in the morning; the diet light, nutritive, and invigorating, and a little wine may be allowed after dinner; since it will almost always be found that the patient has too freely indulged in wine formerly; and he must be let down to the proper point of abstinence by degrees.* The metallic tonics will commonly be found of more use than the vegetable, with the exception of iron, which is generally too heating: though the chalybeate waters may be drunk, if sufficiently combined with neutral salts. The local cold bath of a bidet should be used from the first, and afterward bathing in the open sea.

If the disease have made such an inroad on the constitution that travelling cannot be accomplished; if the mind be overwhelmed, the back perpetually harassed with pain and feebleness, and the nights sleepless with hectic sweats and a frequent involuntary discharge, two grains of opium, or more if needful, should be taken constantly on going to bed; diluted acids, vegetable or mineral, should form the usual beverage, and a caustic be applied to the loins on each side. Hippocrates recommends the actual cautery, and that it should descend on each side of the back, from the neck to the sacrum. Sayin bougies have been prescribed by some writers as a topical stimulus; but a bidet of cold water is preferable; with injections of zinc or copper, at first not rendered very astringent, but gradually increased in power.

* See Wichmann, De Pollutione Diurnâ, frequentiori, sed rarius observatâ, Tabescentiæ causâ, Goett., 1782.

SPECIES V.
MARASMUS PHTHISIS.
CONSUMPTION.

COUGH : PAIN OR UNEASINESS IN THE CHEST, CHIEFLY ON DECUMBITURE : HECTIC FEVER : DELUSIVE HOPE OF RECOVERY.

CONSUMPTION, or PHTHISIS, as it is sometimes called by old medical writers, is by Dr. Cullen contemplated as nothing more than a sequel of hæmoptysis, instead of being regarded as an idiopathic affection; and his species, which are two, can only be viewed, and so appear to have been by Dr. Cullen himself, as separate stages in the progress of the complaint; his first species being denominated *phthisis incipiens*, and characterized by an absence of purulent expectoration; and his second *phthisis confirmata*, distinguished by the presence of this last symptom.

This, however, is a very unsatisfactory as well as a very unscientific view of the subject, and evidently betrays the trammels of Dr. Cullen's classification; since he seems only to have placed the disease in this position because he could find no other to receive it: for he admits, in his First Lines, that "phthisis arises also from other causes besides hæmoptysis."— (Part i., book iv., ch. i., sect. 852.) No man of experience can doubt that phthisis occurs, or at least commences, more frequently without hemorrhage from the lungs than with it, and consequently that hæmoptysis ought much rather to be regarded as a symptom or sequel of phthisis, than phthisis of hæmoptysis.

"Hæmoptysis," observes Dr. Young, in a work that has the rare advantage of combining great research and learning, comprehensive judgment, and a study of the present disease in his own person, "is usually enumerated among the exciting, or even among the more remote causes of consumption; but, in a healthy constitution, hæmoptysis is not materially formidable; and it is conjectured that, when it appears to produce consumption, it has itself been occasioned by an incipient obstruction of a different kind."—(*Treatise on Consumptive Diseases*, p. 45.) So that, on a concurrence of the two, we may commonly adopt the opinion of Desault, and call it an hæmoptysis from consumption, rather than a consumption from hæmoptysis.—(*Sur les Mal. Vén., la Rage, Phthisie*, &c., Bord., 1733.)

Of the three varieties we, are about to describe, we shall find hæmoptysis a frequent cause of the second, but rarely of either of the others. These varieties I have taken from Dr. Duncan's valuable "Observations" on consumption: they are evidently drawn from a close and practical attention to the disease, and are as follow :—

a Catarrhalis.   Catarrhal consumption.
β Apostematosa.   Apostematous consumption.
γ Tubercularis.   Tubercular consumption.*

* The editor prefers considering no case as true phthisis that is not accompanied with tubercles. If once this criterion be deviated from, the pathologist is obliged to confound diseases which have not the slightest analogy to one another. Chronic

In the FIRST VARIETY the cough is requent and violent, with a copious excretion of a thin, offensive, purulent mucus, rarely mixed with blood ; generally soreness in the chest, and transitory pains shifting from side to side. It is chiefly produced by catching cold, or the neglect of a common catarrh.*

In the APOSTEMATOUS VARIETY the cough returns in fits, but is dry : there is a fixed, obtuse, circumscribed pain in the chest, sometimes pulsatory ; with a strikingly difficult decumbiture on one side ; the dry cough at length terminates in a sudden and copious discharge of purulent matter, occasionally threatening suffocation ; the other symptoms being temporarily, in a few rare instances, perhaps, permanently relieved.

In the TUBERCULAR VARIETY the cough is short and tickling ; and there is an excretion of the watery whey-like sanies, sometimes tinged with blood ; the pain in the chest is slight ; and there is mostly an habitual elevation of spirits. Usually the result of a scrofulous diathesis.

In Dr. Duncan's observations, consumption or phthisis is introduced as a genus, and consequently the varieties now offered are reckoned as so many species ; yet as the tubercular may run into the apostematous variety, and the catarrhal into both, according to the peculiarity of the constitution and other concurrent circumstances, and more especially as a common cause may produce all of them in different idiosyncrasies, the present subdivision will perhaps be found the most correct.

Dr. Wilson Philip has formed another variety (with him species) of consumption, to which he has given the name of *Dyspeptic Phthisis*, and which he supposes to be produced by a previously diseased state of the digestive organs, in which the lungs ultimately participate. "Drunkards," says he, "at that time of life which disposes to phthisis, frequently fall a sacrifice to this form of the disease ; and those who have been long subject to severe attacks of dyspepsy, and what are called bilious complaints, are liable to it. What is the nature of the relation observed between the affection of the lungs and that of the digestive organs, in this species of phthisis ? Is the one a consequence of the other, or are they simultaneous

affections, arising from a common cause ? They are not simultaneous affections, for the one always precedes the other. In by far the majority of cases in which both the lungs and digestive organs are affected, the affection of the digestive organs precedes that of the lungs. In some instances, we find the affection of the lungs the primary disease ; but, in these, the case does not assume the form above described, but that of simple phthisis ; and the hepatic affection, which is always the most prominent feature of this derangement in the digestive organs, does not show itself till a late period of the disease, and then little, if at all, influences the essential symptoms."—(*Trans. of Medico-Chirurg. Soc.*, vol. vii., p. 499.)

These remarks show clearly that dyspeptic phthisis is a sequel of a prior disorder, rather than an idiopathic affection ; and, as such, needs not be pursued further in describing the present species. If it outlast the primary malady, or this disease, as is sometimes the case, is converted into it, the digestive organs recovering health, and the lungs appearing to concentrate the morbid action in themselves, it is then reduced to a case of simple or idiopathic phthisis of the one or the other of the varieties now offered.

It would, however, be tedious, and of no practical use, to notice the different ramifications into which consumption has been followed up by many pathologists. Among modern writers more especially, it has been very unnecessarily subdivided : thus Bayle gives us six species, derived from supposed organic causes (*Recherches sur la Phthisie Pulmonaire*, Paris, 1810), of most of which we can know nothing till the death of the patient ; Portal fourteen (*Obs. sur la Nat. et le Traite. de la Phthisie Pulm.*, 2 tom., 8vo., Paris, 1809), the first two of which, the scrofulous and plethoric, are peculiarly entitled to attention, while the rest are drawn from other diseases with which it is often complicated, or of which it is a sequel. In Morton and Sauvages, the divisions and subdivisions are almost innumerable. The Greek pathologists are not chargeable with the same error ; for in general they treat of the disease under two branches alone, phthisis and phthoe : the first importing abscess of the lungs, or the apostematous variety of the present classification ; and the second, ulceration of the lungs, embracing perhaps the greater part of the other two. The terms are those of Hippocrates, and they are thus interpreted by Aretæus.—(*Morb. Chron.*, i., 10.)

Of the varieties here noticed, by far the most frequent is the TUBERCULAR ; concerning which it is necessary to offer an explanation, as the term TUBERCLE has been used in very different senses by different writers, and as the morbid change it imports has been derived from very different sources.

The term, considered etymologically, is a diminutive of *tuber*, a bump or knot of any kind ; in the present work PHYMA ; and has hence been conveniently applied to minute prominences generally : though, when accompanied with in-

---

catarrh may partially resemble phthisis in symptoms ; but its nature is totally different, and this, notwithstanding it may sometimes even lead to the production of tubercles, or real consumption, where the constitution is so disposed. As for apostematous consumption, it is only a particular stage of the tubercular. With respect to the species described by Bayle, under the name of *granular, ulcerous, calculous, cancerous*, and *with melanosis*, Laennec observes, that the first is a mere variety of the tubercular ; the third is a partial gangrene of the lungs ; and the three others are affections which have nothing in common with tubercular phthisis, except that they have their seat in the same organ.—See Laennec on Diseases of the Chest, &c., 2d edit., p. 272, tr. by Forbes.—ED.

* Broussais's History of Chronic Phlegmasiæ, or Inflammations, translated from the French by Drs. Hays & Griffith, vol. i., Philad., 1832.

flammation, they are usually called *papulæ* or pimples, and when filled with a limpid fluid, vesicles: and if the vesicles, or rather the vesicular cysts, be supposed to possess an independent or animalcular life, hydatids.

There is not an organ of the body but is capable, as well in its substance as its parenchyma, of producing tubercles* of some kind or other; and occasionally of almost every kind at the same time; for Bonet, Boerhaave, and De Haen, as well as innumerable writers in our own day, have given striking examples of clusters of cystic tubers, or enlarged tubercles, of every diversity of size, existing both in the abdomen and in the thorax, formed in the interior of their respective viscera, or issuing from the surface of their serous membranes, some of which are filled with a limpid fluid, others with a gelatinous, a mucous, or a puriform, and others again with a cheesy, pulpy, or steatomatous mass.

It is not improbable, that even a certain degree of inflammation itself is often favourable to the growth and general spread of tubercles. In their origin they seem to be single cysts, or often perhaps single follicles, but as they enlarge, the interior is at times divided by reticulations of vessels, or membranous bands, or distinct

---

* In whatever organ the formation of tuberculous matter takes place, " the mucous system, if constituting a part of that organ, is, in general, either the exclusive seat of this morbid product, or is far more extensively affected with it than any of the other systems or tissues of the same organ."—(See Carswell's Illustrations of the Elementary Forms of Disease, fasc. i.) In the lungs he exhibits the tuberculous matter formed on the secreting surface, and collected within the air-cells and bronchi; in the intestines, within the isolated and aggregated follicles; in the liver, within the biliary ducts and their extremities; in the kidneys, within the infundibula, pelvis, and ureters: in the uterus, within the cavity of that organ and Fallopian tubes; and, in the testicle, within the tubuli seminifen, epididimis, and vas deferens. The formation and subsequent diffusion of tuberculous matter are also described, by Dr. Carswell, as taking place likewise on the secreting surface of serous membranes, particularly the pleura and peritoneum, and in the numerous minute cavities of the cellular tissue. The accumulation of it in the lacteals and lymphatics, both before and after they unite to form their respective glands, he finds to be often very considerable. Dr. Carswell has also given representations of tuberculous matter in the substance of the brain and cerebellum, in accidental cellular tissue, and in the blood; and adverts to its occasional formation in accidental products.—ED.

† Some of the opinions here delivered are not universally admitted; the productions to which several pathologists now restrict the name of tubercle, being, in fact, less diversified than those described in the text. Thus Andral defines those of the lungs to be of a pale yellow colour, mostly of a globular form, and of infinitely various sizes; at their commencement firm, but brittle; afterward softening; and, in a later stage, changing into a substance which is not homogeneous, but consists of whitish friable masses, suspended in a sero-purulent fluid.—(Anat. Pathol., tom. i., p. 408.) The round form of the tubercular substance is consid-

cells, thus exhibiting almost every variety of the animal structure; while the external tunic usually becomes stouter, sometimes duplicate, and at times cartilaginous.†

---

ered by Professor Carswell as quite an accidental circumstance. The tubercle assumes the form of a shut or open globular sac, if confined to the secreting surface, and of a solid globular tumour of various sizes, if it fills completely the cavity of the air-cells; and, for similar reasons, it presents in the bronchi a tubular or cylindrical form, having a ramiform distribution, terminated by a cauliflower arrangement of the air-cells. In the mucous follicles, its shape is similar to that which it receives from the air-cells. The granular arrangement of tuberculous matter in the lungs, is ascribed by Dr. Carswell to its accumulation in contiguous cells; and the lobular character, to its being confined to the air-cells of a single lobule.—(See illustrations of the Elementary Forms of Disease, fasc. i.) Their derivation from obstructed follicles and inflammation, is a doctrine which Andral, as well as Laennec, rejects, as a general proposition, which, indeed, in relation to inflammation as a cause, it is right to say, the words of Dr. Good would by no means countenance. The sequel of the text will show that, on this point, he inclined to the opinion of Bichat. In the text, however, cysts of nearly every kind, simple and complicated, with fluid, fatty, or fleshy contents, and contents of various other sorts, are all comprised under the term; a view not adopted at the present time, when so much light has been thrown upon the subject by the researches of MM. Lombard, Laennec, Andral, Armstrong, Cruveilhier, Carswell, and other distinguished cultivators of morbid anatomy. Although a tubercle assumes different appearances in its different stages, its transformations are less numerous than Dr. Baron and M. Dupuy (Traité de l'Affection Tuberculeuse, 8vo., 1817) imply in the hypothesis which they maintain, that a tubercle is at first a transparent vesicle, or hydatid. The following is Dr. Carswell's definition of tubercle, or rather of the tuberculous matter, which constitutes the essential anatomical character of those diseases to which the term tubercular is now *exclusively* restricted. Tuberculous matter, says he, is a pale yellow, or yellowish-gray, opaque, unorganized substance, the form, consistence, and composition of which vary with the nature of the part in which it is formed, and the period at which it is examined. He describes it as an unorganized secretion, or as a cheesy-looking material without any trace of organization. When the process of softening takes place in tubercular matter, it is clear, as Dr. Carswell observes, that the change cannot originate in the inorganic substance itself. " After having become firm, it may be converted into a granular-looking pulp, or pale grumous fluid of various colours, from the admixture of serosity, pus, blood, &c., which have been effused or secreted by the tissues subject to its irritating influence. The pus and serosity pervade the substance of the tuberculous matter, loosen and detach it. These changes are further promoted by atrophy, ulceration, or mortification of the surrounding or enclosed tissues, the bloodvessels of which have been compressed or obliterated by the tuberculous matter." Dr. Carswell considers the doctrine, that the softening of tubercles always begins in their centre, as extremely incorrect. According to his researches, when tuberculous matter is formed in the lungs, it is generally contained in the air-cells and bronchi. " If, therefore, this morbid product is confined to the surface of either, or has accumulated to such a degree as to

In many cases the cysts or niduses of tubercles possess so little energy of action,[*] as never to exceed the size of small shot, or to consist of more than an insipid fluid, rendered glairy or caseous by an absorption of the finer particles of the material effused or secreted ;[†] but which, by being united with a few corpuscles of red blood, or of carbonaceous matter, become not unfrequently of a black or chocolate hue, the melanosis of Bayle, but not that of Breschet and Laennec ; and which, by other unions or other changes, produced, perhaps, by the anomalous operation of the still inherent principle of life, furnish us with all those appearances which dissections bring to light on the surface or in the substance of the lungs, or whatever other organ may chance to be affected.

Many writers conceive that, for the growth of tubercles, it is absolutely necessary that inflammation should take place, and that the whole of the new matter must be supplied from the sanguiferous system immediately : a doctrine rather upheld by Mr. Hunter's followers than by himself, and directly opposed, as Bichat has justly observed (*Anat. Gén.*, tom. iv., p. 517), by the absence of all the signs of inflammation in by far the greater number of passing cases, at least till the morbid growth has fully established itself, and operates by mechanical pressure or some other excitement. While other physiolo-

gists have limited such morbid growths to the operation of the absorbent system, or to minute bladders containing a limpid fluid which they have called hydatids ; the term being sometimes employed as a mere synonyme of bladders or turgid vesicles of serum, in the language of Boerhaave, "hydatids, sive vesiculæ sero turgentes" (*Epist. Anat. ad Fred. Ruysch*, p. 82) ; and at other times importing a parasitic animalcule forming a subdivision under the genus tænia of Linnéus, and of which we have already spoken under turgescence of the liver.—(Vol. i., Cl. 1., Ord. III., Gen. IV., Spe. 1.)

[With regard to the important question, whether tubercles of the lungs are the product of inflammation, the subject is one concerning which some of the greatest men in the profession are yet divided. "If," says Laennec, "we question any practitioner, ignorant of morbid anatomy, but who is a man of observation and free from prejudices, he will give it as his opinion, that the symptoms of phthisis very rarely supervene to acute pneumonia. Even in the cases where this sequence is observed, it is impossible to say whether the pneumonia has given rise to the tubercles, or whether these, acting as irritating bodies, have not excited the pneumonia." The latter view was adopted by a late eminent physician of this country ; for, he distinctly observes, that the number and the increase of the size of tubercles frequently create irritation in their vicinity, so that a *consequent* inflammation of the surrounding texture is not an uncommon circumstance.—(*Armstrong's Morbid Anat. of the Bowels*, &c., p. 16, Lond., 1828, 4to.) The solution of the question by a reference to pathological anatomy, Laennec deems far more simple, since it is certain, that we very rarely find tubercles in the lungs of those who die of pneumonia, and that the greater number of consumptive subjects exhibit no symptom of this disease during the progress of their fatal malady, nor any trace of it after death. Many of these have even never been affected with it during the whole course of their lives. If tubercles were merely a product of acute peripneumony, we should be able to ascertain the different steps of the transition of the one into the other, which is not the case. It is said that chymical analysis discovers no difference between the softened matter of tubercles and true pus :[*] in

---

leave only a limited central portion of their cavities unoccupied, it is obvious that, when they are divided transversely, the following appearances will be observed—1. A bronchial tube will resemble a tubercle having a central depression, or soft central point, on account of the centre of the tube not being, or never having been occupied by tuberculous matter, and of its containing a small quantity of mucus or other secreted fluids. 2. The air-cells will exhibit a number of similar appearances, or rings of tuberculous matter grouped together, and containing in their centre a quantity of similar fluids. When the bronchi or air-cells are completely filled, the tuberculous matter presents no such appearances."—(Professor Carswell's Illustrations of the Elementary Forms of Disease, fasc. i.) Softening, he says, most frequently begins at the circumference of firm tuberculous matter, where its presence, as a foreign body, is most felt by the surrounding tissues.—Ed.

[*] In the lungs, the idea of encysted tubercle appears to Dr. Carswell erroneous, the distended walls of the air-cells being commonly mistaken for cysts. He admits, however, that tuberculous matter is sometimes encysted, but not until it has undergone changes preparatory to its ultimate removal from the organ in which it is formed.—Ed.

[†] The common pulmonary tubercle is most indurated in its early stages, and the change which it afterward undergoes is a softening or dissolution, which Andral refers to the effect of the pus secreted around it. An increased hardness of the tubercular matter, after its first secretion, has not yet been proved, with the exception of a few instances, in which a large proportion of phosphate and carbonate of lime is deposited in the substance of the tubercles. According to M. Andral, this happens chiefly in cases where these bodies have for a long time ceased to have any serious effect upon the constitution. In this respect, the earthy transformation is quite the converse of the process by which a tubercle is softened.—Ed.

---

[*] As already observed, the softening of tubercles is ascribed by Laennec, Andral, and Carswell, to the effect of suppuration around them; in other words, the tubercular matter dissolves in the pus. If this explanation be correct, though disagreeing with the admission of Andral, that the softening of tubercles often begins in their centre, it is not surprising that the analysis of suppurated tubercles should resemble that of purulent matter. But the analysis of a solid tubercle is different, being, according to M. Thénard, animal matter, 98.15 ; muriate of soda, phosphate of lime, carbonate of lime, 1.85; with some traces of oxyde of iron. There are tubercles, however, the analysis of which is still more different from that of pus ; viz., those which contain a very large proportion of phosphate and carbonate of lime, and which are generally such as have existed a long while, with-

like manner, Laennec replies, it discovers none between the albumen of the egg and the secretion of certain cancers. These facts only prove the imperfection of chymistry, and not the identity of the matters in question. In almost all their physical characters, tubercles differ from pus. After the complete evacuation of a softened tubercle, its contents are never renewed; while the sides of an abscess, after it is opened, are well known to continue to secrete pus. Laennec admits that acute pneumonia and tubercles occasionally coexist; but the complication is rare, when the great frequency of both diseases is taken into consideration. In nineteen twentieths of the cases of this complication, the tubercular affection evidently precedes the other; and we may therefore infer, either that the tubercles are the occasion of pneumonia, or that the diseases, although co-existing, have no etiological relation to each other. Laennec concedes, however, as a matter of no evil consequence in practice, and of no importance in theory (although he thinks it supported neither by direct experiment nor positive observation), that in the small number of cases where phthisis is seen to arise during the convalescence from acute peripneumony, the inflammation may sometimes accelerate the development of tubercles, to which the patient was disposed from some other cause, of the nature of which we are ignorant, but which is assuredly different from inflammation.—(Op. cit., p. 291.) According to M. Andral, if the *disposition to tubercles be very strong*, the slightest local congestion of blood will give rise to them; wherever such congestion takes place, the same product appears, or the *tubercular diathesis* is produced. If this disposition be less strong, it is requisite for the formation of a tubercle, that the congestion of blood should be so considerable and permanent, as to amount to inflammation. But, *when there exists no such predisposition, the most intense and the longest inflammation will not produce a tubercle.*—(*Andral, Clinique Méd.,* tom. iii., p. 13.)

The latter admission is virtually an acknowledgment, that the formation of tubercles depends essentially upon a peculiar diathesis. Against the idea of tubercles being simply the

---

out any serious effect on the system. They consist of animal matter, 3; saline matter, 96. These are the only kind of pulmonary tubercles which can be said to become more indurated with time. Professor Carswell observes, that the chymical composition of tuberculous matter varies not only at the different periods at which it is examined, but in different animals, and probably in different organs. In man, he says, it is chiefly composed of albumen, with various proportions of gelatin and fibrin. The most important fact relating to this part of the subject is, " that either from the nature of its constituent parts, the mode in which they are combined, or the condition in which they are placed, they are not susceptible of organization, and consequently give rise to a morbid compound, capable of undergoing no change that is not induced in it by the influence of external agents."— See Professor Carswell's Illustrations of the Elementary Forms of Disease, fasc. i.—ED.

effect of inflammation, Dr. Armstrong instances the following fact: in many cases, where tubercular points are scattered over the pleura or peritoneum, the serous membrane is transparent up to these points, and only becomes reddened or opaque when the tumour has enlarged so as to produce local irritation. The tubercle, he admits, is probably connected with effusion of fibrin, but, according to his observations, such effusion is not necessarily connected with inflammation.—(*Armstrong's Morbid Anatomy of the Bowels,* &c., p. 17, 4to., Lond., 1828.)*

The ancients ascribed to inflammation all kinds of scirrhi, tumours, and tubercles. In the course of the eighteenth century, this doctrine encountered opposition; but it was not till M. Bayle directed his powerful mind to the subject, that many positive facts were collected in formidable array against the hypothesis. On the other hand, the celebrated Broussais (*Exam. des Doctr. Méd.,* 1816) has continued to be an active defender of the ancient opinion; and, as far as tubercles of the lungs are concerned, he can still boast of distinguished partisans, among whom be it sufficient to mention the name of Alison. The cases which this gentleman has seen, and which seemed to him to furnish the best evidence on this point, have occurred, he says, in young children. From them he has been led to think, that when the constitutional *tendency to them prevails,* tubercles may form in very different circumstances, and probably with various rapidity. He has little doubt, that *they do often form without being preceded by inflammation of such a character as to be detected by symptoms* during life; and that, in the lungs at least, *the inflammation,* of which the undeniable marks are so often found along with them after death, *has really often been posterior to them in date.* But he has also been led to believe that *it is not merely,* as Laennec states, *a possibility, but a real and frequent occurrence, that inflammation, acute or chronic* (to which he would add *febrile action*), however produced, *becomes, in certain constitutions, the occasion of the development of tubercles.*—(*Edin. Med. Chir. Trans.,* vol. i., p. 407.)

The cases which seem to Dr. Alison to confirm the doctrine, that tubercles sometimes form in consequence of inflammation, he arranges under two heads:—

1. The first consists of cases in which the tubercles did not cause death, and were found on dissection in an incipient state, but so imme-

---

* A late American writer, Dr. Morton, adduces much able reasoning to prove, " 1st. That tubercles are an altered secretion of the albuminous halitus, proper to the cellular tissue forming the parenchyma of organs. 2d. That inflammation is not necessary to their development. 3d. That the cellular tissue which envelops and intersects tubercles, sooner or later takes on inflammation and secretes pus, by which process the tubercular matter is eliminated and an abscess is formed."— See Illustrations of Pulmonary Consumption, its anatomical characters, causes, symptoms, and treatment, with 12 plates, drawn and coloured from nature; by Samuel George Morton, M. D., Philadelphia, 1834.—D.

diately succeeding to the symptom, and *so closely connected with*, or *even passing by insensible degrees into, the undeniable effects of inflammation*, that it was impossible to suppose their formation independent of it.

2. The second consists of examples in which children, previously in good health, or at least unaffected with any pulmonary complaint, have been seized with well-marked inflammatory symptoms, generally from a known cause, certainly adequate to that effect. These symptoms have lasted some time, and been manifestly dangerous to life,—have subsided very imperfectly,—the children have passed into the state of phthisis, and died within a few months; and, on dissection, tubercles have been found in various stages of progress, but with little or no other appearance which could be considered either as the effect of the inflammation *known to have existed*, or as the cause of death.

In a paper of later date,* Dr. Alison strength-

* Edin. Med. Chir. Trans., vol. iii., p. 274. The expression, "*in certain constitutions*," employed by Dr. Alison, is an important limit to the doctrine. With this understanding, there is no material difference between his views and those of Laennec and Andral. The latter pathologist distinctly affirms, that irritation alone will not necessarily give rise to tubercles, which are frequently formed without any irritation that can be perceived. Without the concurrence of other causes, mere irritation will not account for their production.—(Anat. Pathol., tom. i., p. 438.) Like many other writers, he ascribes much to peculiarity of constitution. Tubercles, he says, are particularly apt to form in individuals whose skin is very white, and, as it were, shrivelled, without any traces of colouring matter in its capillary network; and whose cheeks exhibit a red patch, making a singular contrast to the dead white of the rest of the face. The colouring matter is also deficient in the eyes, which retain the blue colour of infancy; and the hair is of a light hue, and its quantity small. The muscles are slender and flabby, with little strength of contraction. The blood is serous, and poor in fibrin and colouring matter; and the mucous secretions predominate. In persons of this diathesis, sanguineous congestions readily take place in the skin and mucous membranes; and, when once produced, do not terminate, but continue in a chronic form, and are frequently followed by ulcerations, and various disorganizations very difficult of cure, and often needing remedies of an opposite nature to such as are termed antiphlogistic. These individuals seem to retain in adult age several traits which appertain to infancy, considered both in its healthy and diseased state; and the development of their organization is impeded. This kind of constitution may be formed without the influence of any manifest external cause. In other instances it appears to be acquired: a residence in an impure air, or such as is not renewed often enough; the crowding of many persons together; absence of the sun's rays; an habitually damp atmosphere; food of a quality inadequate to repair the strength of the system; and various excesses, which exhaust the strength and nervous influence, and injure nutrition, are enumerated by Andral as so many causes which, at the same time that they render the blood so poor as to account for the state of the skin and muscles externally, give a chronic character to every inflammatory complaint, and a

ens; by additional facts and observations, the proposition that, *in certain constitutions*, inflammation, acute or chronic, but most generally chronic, does frequently and directly lead to the deposition of tubercles.

The first fact to which he adverts is, that tubercles are very seldom found in the bodies of children who are stillborn, or die very shortly after birth.—(*Denis, Recherches d'Anat. et de Physiologie Pathologiques sur plusieurs Maladies des Enfans nouveau-nés.*) Velpeau and Breschet had frequently sought for tubercles in the fœtus, but could never find them; and though Orfila and West have seen them, it was only in small number.* Dr. Alison therefore infers, that in most of the numerous cases where tubercles are found in the bodies of young children, the diseased actions by which they are formed originate after birth, parents transmitting to their offspring only the tendency to this kind of diseased action, and very seldom the actual disease.

Dr. Alison next quotes the observation of Magendie, that in those cases where he had detected tubercles of the smallest size, and apparently in the earliest stages of the bodies of young children, they were surrounded by circumscribed vascularity. This Dr. Alison has also observed, not uniformly, but in many cases. Lastly, Dr. Alison, in support of his views, adverts to the frequency of phthisis in masons, as is supposed from the irritation of the particles of sand inhaled; and to certain experiments by Dr. J. P. Kay, in which the introduction of a globule of mercury into the tracheæ of rabbits led to the production of clusters of tubercles in the lungs, each tubercle containing in its centre a small particle of mercury. As for these experiments, and others recorded by Cruveilhier (*Anat.- Pathol.*), the editor thinks that they merely show that the particles of mercury, like other extraneous bodies, led to the effusion of lymph around them, by which they became encysted, just as a leaden shot or bullet has frequently been observed to be, when it has been lodged in the lungs for some time previously to death. The same process happens in all other parts, so as to circumscribe extraneous bodies.

tendency in every organ to the tubercular secretion. It is not to be supposed, however, that tubercles form only in these constitutions; and Andral admits that it is not uncommon for phthisis to destroy persons of dark complexion, very black hair, and a muscular system strongly developed. We know, indeed, that so far is a dark complexion from being a certain protection from phthisis, that the blacks of Africa, when brought to this climate, are particularly liable to the disease; though here the disposition to it may be set down as acquired. At this present time (Dec., 1830), the editor has a patient with phthisis, in the King's Bench, whose complexion is remarkably dark, and his hair black. However, he believes with M. Andral, that the natural disposition to tubercles is most frequent in the above description of subjects, and especially the tendency to their simultaneous production in several organs.—Op. cit.) p. 434.—Ed.

* One or two additional cases of this kind are recorded in Lloyd's work on Scrofula. The preparations are in Mr. Langstaff's museum.—Ed.

The analogy between these cases and others in which tubercles are produced extensively throughout the lungs, by a process in which frequently the presence of no extraneous body can be suspected, certainly does not seem very evident.]

A few years ago, Dr. Baron brought forward an hypothesis, founded upon the hydatid basis. Waving the question of the animalcular origin of the hydatid, as contended for by Dr. Jenner and others, and resigning the critical meaning of the term tubercle as a diminutive substantive, he employs tubercle, vesicle, and hydatid as nearly synonymes. Tubercles in their incipient state being with him "small vesicular bodies with fluid contents" (Inquiry illustrating the Nature of Tuberculated Accretion, &c., p. 214), the hydatids of his friend Dr. Jenner, and vesicles being parallel with both, and distinguished from tumour as follows :—" I would employ the word tubercle to denote those disorganizations that are composed of one cyst, whatever may be its magnitude or the nature of its contents ; and by tumour I would understand those morbid structures that appear to be composed of more than one tubercle."

From this source Dr. Baron derives tumours of almost every kind, varied merely by the peculiarity of the constitution, or the concomitant circumstances of the organ in which their vesicular or hydatid form first makes its appearance ; and hence ramifying into encysted tumours, however diversified in their contents,—whether limpid, gelatinous, cheesy, pultaceous, medullary, or steatomatous,—sarcomatous tumours, scirrhous tumours, cartilaginous tumours, cancer, and the fungus hæmatodes. He limits their formation to the absorbent system alone, conceiving the sanguiferous to have little or nothing to do with the morbid productions ; and upon this point it is that he is chiefly in a state of challenge with the ablest supporters of the Hunterian doctrines.

According to Dr. Baron, the tubercle "may be pendulous, or imbedded in any soft part, or it may be found between the layers of membranes, and wherever the textures are of such a nature as to admit of its growth. It may be so small as to be scarcely visible, or it may acquire a very great magnitude. Single tubercles are often seen in a viscus, while all the rest of the organ is free from disease, and its functions are performed in an uninterrupted manner. But it is evident that the same state of the system, whatever that may be, which calls one tubercle into existence, may generate an indefinite number : that they may be diffused through the whole of a viscus, leaving nothing of its original texture ; or they may occupy any portion of it, or extend to the contiguous parts, and involve them in the same form of disease."—(P. 216.)

If the organ or the general constitution be not much predisposed to a generation of tubercles, a few may remain for a long time inert, and without any multiplication whatever ; but there is often a particular diathesis that favours such a complaint, and facilitates its being called from a latent state into an active manifestation by a thousand little accidents ; and which, when once excited, encourages the growth of tubercles in great abundance, and finds a rich and ready soil for them, not in one organ only, but in every one. A case, strikingly illustrative of this form of the disease, is recorded by Mr. Langstaff.—(Med. Chir. Trans., vol. ix.)

[Some valuable observations, lately published by Dr. Abercrombie (Edin. Med. Chir. Trans., vol. i., p. 682), are very unfavourable to the hypothesis that tubercles consist of hydatids. A chymical examination of the mesenteric glands affected with tubercular disease, he found to present some curious results. When a gland, having a soft fleshy appearance, is plunged into boiling water, it instantly contracts considerably in its dimensions, its textures become much firmer, and its colour changes from that of flesh to an opaque white or ash-colour. By boiling for a short time, it loses a great part of its weight ; but a residuum is left, which has increased much in firmness during the boiling, has lost entirely the flesh colour, and exhibits the appearance, consistence, and properties of coagulated albumen. The part that is lost seems to consist partly of water, but chiefly of the muco-extractive matter ; sometimes, but not always, there is a mixture of gelatin ; and, in some specimens, the coagulated part gave traces of fibrin, but in small quantity.

According to Dr. Abercrombie's report, the proportions of these ingredients varied exceedingly in different specimens, and apparently in different periods of the disease. In the softest state, glands which were considerably enlarged, lost by boiling about five sixths of their weight ; the remaining one sixth being a firm mass, with the appearance of the firm white tubercle, and the properties of coagulated albumen. Glands, examined in a more advanced stage of the disease, lost by boiling perhaps from two thirds to one half. Portions in the semi-transparent, cartilaginous state, lost about one fourth, leaving three fourths of their weight in the same state of firm, opaque, albuminous coagulum. The white, opaque, tubercular matter lost a still smaller proportion, and what was left was a firm white substance, resembling coagulated albumen. The same results were obtained from an examination of the white tuberele of the lungs, the tubercular disease of the bronchial glands, tubercles of the liver, certain tumours of the brain, and of similar masses in other situations.

As the mesenteric and lymphatic glands, approaching the healthy state, do not exhibit any traces of albumen, Dr. Abercrombie infers, that the deposition of this substance in them is a morbid process, and that there is good ground for conjecture that this deposition of albumen is the origin of tubercular disease.

The tuberculated disease of the peritoneum, on which so much of Dr. Baron's hypothesis is founded, presented, in Dr. Abercrombie's experiments, characters considerably different from those of tubercles of the lungs, or of the tubercular disease of the lymphatic glands. The specimens presented an irregular surface, elevated into variously-shaped nodules of a semi-pellucid appearance and firm texture. By boiling in water, these nodules were nearly dissolved, leaving only a small central part, to which they seemed to have been attached, and which had undergone little or no change during this first boiling. The part that was dissolved seemed to consist entirely of the muco-extractive matter, and the part that remained was the same substance in a more concrete state, with a small trace of albumen. In all Dr. Abercrombie's examinations, this substance seemed remarkably different from what is observed in the proper tubercle. They both differ, however, from the contents of a hydatid, which consist of water, holding in solution about one hundredth part of saline matter, and one fortieth part of muco-extractive animal matter ; a fact weighing heavily against Dr. Baron's hypothesis.*

The researches of Dr. Armstrong taught him that the vesicular appearance of a tubercle is an accidental occurrence, dependant on the texture of the part in which it is placed ; a fact agreeing with Dr. Carswell's investigations. Thus, tubercles in their origin may have the vesicular appearance in the lungs ; but if minutely examined, he says they will be found to be the extremities of the bronchial tubes, or air-cells, into which the peculiar deposite constituting tubercle often takes place. He has frequently examined them in a strong light, and never found them to be, strictly speaking, vesicles, though the tubercular points have been in many cases extremely minute.†

Dr. Baron attempts to prove that tubercles are essentially hydatids, and that the progress of tubercular disease is precisely the reverse of Laennec's description ; and that, instead of passing from an indurated to a softened and fluid state, they are first simple vesicles of fluid ;‡ and that they generally pass through a

process of inspissation, until they become quite hard, in which state, he says, there is the strongest reason for believing that they do not subsequently soften ! This theory seems to Dr. Forbes incompatible with the best established facts, and susceptible of ready refutation by any person versed in modern pathology. Dr. Baron, as a critic has remarked, has betrayed not only a singular misapprehension of the pathology of the diseases of which he treats, but actually not a due acquaintance with the natural history of hydatids themselves, on which all his opinions repose. He reproaches Laennec with indulging in unnecessary minuteness in his description of tubercles ; forgetting, in his zeal for the hydatid doctrine of disease, that nature's forms may be very diversified, and that it is the privilege of theory only to be just as simple as the theorist could desire. Real instances of hydatids in the lungs are extremely rare, Andral having met with only four or five cases among six thousand subjects.*

---

* Dr. Carswell has always found tuberculous matter in scrofulous glands ; and, when the cutis is pale, and they happen to lie directly under it, they are almost completely filled with this morbid product. " When, therefore, enlarged glands, in a scrofulous patient, ultimately disappear, we may conclude, almost with certainty, that we have witnessed the cure of a tubercular disease."—See Illustrations of the Elementary Forms of Disease, fasc. i.—Ed.

† See Morbid Anatomy of the Bowels, &c., p. 16 Dr. Armstrong's belief that tubercles are originally the extremities of the bronchial tubes, or air-cells, may have been derived from the fact, that tubercles are sometimes situated in the substance of the parietes of the air-cells, and of the minute ramifications of the bronchiæ. Matter, like that of tubercles, has been found, however, in cavities lined by mucous membrane, after ulceration has taken place. Mucous follicles and lymphatic vessels have been occasionally remarked to contain a similar substance.—(Andral, Anat. Pathol., tom. i., p. 419.) The cellular tissue is, then, not the only nidus for tubercles.—Ed.

‡ According to Professor Carswell, tuberculous matter does not acqnire its maximum of consistence until an indefinite period after its formation : and he states that it is frequently found in

its primitive state, in the bronchi, air-cells, and other situations, resembling a mixture of soft cheese and water.—(See Illustrations of the Elementary Forms of Disease, fasc. i.) M. Cruveilhier believes, that previously to the period when a tubercle presents itself as a firm substance, it has a less advanced stage, in which it exists in a fluid form. In his experiments to produce tubercles artificially in animals, on an examination of their bodies at the very commencement of the disease, he found, close to the white bodies, which were already indurated, other productions, which differed from them only in having less consistence, and being in a state of fluidity. In the human lungs, filled with tubercles, M. Andral has also seen dispersed, throughout the interior of those viscera, white points, consisting of a liquid matter, like a small drop of pus. Yet he is of opinion, that the doctrine of M. Cruveilhier has not been sufficiently proved ; and that the above appearances are only accidental, and not constant ; and that, however minute a tubercle may be, it is mostly met with in a solid shape. At all events, there is one great difference between M. Cruveilhier and Dr. Baron, inasmuch as the former does not suppose that hardened tubercles cannot soften.—Ed.

* Laennec on Diseases of the Chest, note by Dr. Forbes, 2d edit., p. 298. Andral, Clinique Méd.; tom. iii., p. 93. In another publication (Anat. Pathol., tom. i., p. 408), the latter author mentions, that he has seen only a single instance of transparent vesicles in the human lungs, accompanied by tubercles ; but he has met with this association more than once in phthisical horses, and, in some of these examples, the fluid of the vesicle became turbid, and surrounded by a white opaque cyst. His inferences are, that the transparent vesicles observed in a few uncommon cases, in the vicinity of tubercles, are an accidental complication. If they were the original form of tubercles, they would be more frequently noticed. They may sometimes secrete, instead of their usual contents, a peculiar matter, the physical qualities of which may have more or less resemblance to those of a tubercle ; but this is no proof of the latter having been always preceded by a serous cyst, and secreted from it. As well might it be argued, that a tubercle is always secreted by a mucous follicle, or lymphatic vessel, because a substance like that of tubercle has been occasionally observed within

When the morbid action commences in the abdominal organs, it far more readily passes into those of the chest, than when it commences in the chest, into those of the abdomen ; instances of which have been sufficiently noticed under the complicated species of Parabysma.—(Vol. i., Cl. I., Ord. II., Gen. IV., Spe. 7.) These, however, are extreme examples ; for, in most cases of tubercular phthisis, the disease has made far less progress at the time of its proving fatal, and is often confined to the seat of the lungs alone, and even to an evolution of tubercles of minute size and uniform simplicity of contents, mostly consisting of a whey-like or cheesy material. A certain but low degree of inflammatory action, however, seems to favour a more rapid formation of fresh tumours, and an enlargement of those already in existence ; and the same may be observed of the accompanying hectic fever. If this be decided and considerable, the disease may run its course in four or five months, and sometimes sooner. If the hectic be undecided and only occasional, the disease may play about the system for some years, and at length prove equally fatal. If the inflammatory action exceed the low degree we have just adverted to, ulceration and suppuration usually follow, and the tubercular form passes into, or is united with, the apostematous.

M. Louis, like his friend M. Laennec, refers every case of phthisis to a tubercular origin ; and where the predisposition to the formation of such growths is very predominant, he has traced them, in post-obit dissections, to a still wider range than the example furnished by Mr. Langstaff : in various instances, indeed, over almost every viscus of the abdominal, as well as of the thoracic cavity. In one or two of these, he has even found the tubercular structure to have been far more manifest and elaborated than in the lungs, and especially in the stomach, the mesenteric glands, the ileum or jejunum, but rarely in the duodenum. But he positively asserts that he has never traced these morbid appearances in other parts, without some kind of manifestation of them in the lungs : and he hence concludes, that a development of tubercles in this last organ is essential to their formation elsewhere. So far as he has examined, however,— and his field of observation has been very extensive, as well as closely followed up, in the Hôpital de la Charité,—phthisis has seldom limited its structural ravages to the region of the lungs. Tubercles, or ulcerations, have usually been detected elsewhere on dissection ; often, indeed, in the trachea, larynx, and epiglottis, and occasionally in the pharynx and œsophagus, as well as in the stomach. And when the hectic has been active, there is scarcely an organ but what he

has found at times entering more or less into the general circle of action ; as the large intestines, the liver, the spleen, the peritoneum, the lymphatic glands, the aorta, and even the brain. The heart, and the urinary organs, have usually escaped with less structural injury than any others.—(Recherches Anatomico-Pathologiques sur la Phthisie, par P. Ch. A. Louis, Paris, 8vo., 1825.)

With one exception out of 350 dissections, whenever M. Louis found tubercles in the lungs, he always found them in other organs.* In a few instances, however, Laennec found tubercles to commence in other parts, especially in the mucous membrane of the intestines, and in the lymphatic glands, their formation in the lungs having been secondary.—(Laennec, op. cit., p. 285.) The occurrence of tubercles in various organs without the presence of any in the lungs, has been noticed by M. Andral more frequently than by M. Louis. Such cases are more common in children than adults. In the former, there is a disposition to tubercles in a larger number of parts at once ; and the organs most frequently affected in them are not the same as in the adult subject. The parts which are most frequently the seat of them in the adults are, first, the lungs, and then the small intestines : in children, first, the bronchial glands ; secondly, the mesenteric glands ; thirdly, the spleen ; fourthly, the kidneys ; and fifthly, the intestines, &c. In children under fifteen, tubercles are least frequent between the first and second years of their age ; and most common from the end of the fourth until the commencement of the fifth. —(Anat. Pathol., tom. i., p. 424.)]

Phthisis, as already observed, is a disease of high antiquity, as well as of most alarming frequeney and fatality. So frequent, indeed, is it, as to carry off prematurely, according to Dr. Young's estimate, and the calculation is by no means overcharged, one fourth part of the inhabitants of Europe (On Consumptive Diseases, ch. iii., p. 20) : and so fatal, that M. Bayle will not allow it possible for any one to recover who suffers from it in its genuine form.—(Recherches sur la Phthisie Pulmonaire, Paris, 1810.) I can distinctly aver, however, that I have seen it terminate favourably in one or two instances, where the patient has appeared to be in the last stage of disease, with a pint and a half of pus and purulent mucus expectorated daily, exhausting night-sweats, and anasarca ; but whether from the treatment pursued, or a remedial exertion of nature, I will not undertake

* Recherches sur la Phthisic, &c., p. 179. In the 350 post-mortem examinations mentioned in the text, M. Louis found tubercles in various organs besides the lungs, in the following proportions :—In 2-3 of subjects, small intestines ; in 1-9, large intestines ; in 1-4, mesenteric glands ; in 1-10, the cervical glands ; in 1-11, the lumbar glands ; in 1-13, the prostate ; in 1-14, the spleen ; in 1-20, the ovaries ; in 1-40, the kidneys ; 1-350, the womb ; 1-350, the brain ; 1-350, the cerebellum ; 1-350, the ureter. M. Louis makes no mention of tubercles in the testis, which are common ; nor does he say any thing about their occasional formation in the bones.—Ed.

such parts. Transparent cysts are very common in the diseased lungs of pigs, where they even exceed tubercles in number ; and it seems to M. Andral, that this fact is the chief ground of the opinion that tubercles commence in the shape of hydatids. He also warns us not to mistake the deposition of tubercular matter around hydatids (an instance of which he met with in a rabbit) for the conversion of vesicles into tubercles.—Ed.

to say. Dr. Parr affirms that he has witnessed six cases of decided phthisis recover spontaneously.

[Previously to the knowledge of the true nature of tubercles, and while consumption was considered simply as a consequence of chronic inflammation and suppuration of the pulmonary tissue, phthisis was deemed curable, at least, when properly treated before it had made too much progress. But, says Laennec, it is now the general opinion of all well-informed pathologists, that *the tubercular affection*, like cancer, *is absolutely incurable.* The observations contained in the treatise of M. Bayle, as well as Laennec's remarks on the development of tubercles, prove how illusive the idea is of curing consumption in its early stage. Crude tubercles tend essentially to increase in size, and to become soft. Nature and art may retard, or even arrest their progress, but neither can reverse it. But, while Laennec admits the incurability of consumption in the early stages, he is convinced, from a great number of facts, that, *in some cases, the disease is curable in the latter stages,* that is, *after the softening of the tubercles, and the formation of an ulcerous excavation.**

---

* Laennec on Diseases of the Chest, 2d edit., p. 299. In Dr. Carswell's Illustrations of the Elementary Forms of Disease, fasc. i., the reader will find some particularly interesting facts, confirming Laennec's views of this part of the subject; for he has traced the several steps of the curative process in the bronchial glands, in individuals who had recovered from scrofula and phthisis, but died some time afterward of other diseases. He has found in these glands a greater or less quantity of a substance resembling putty, or dry mortar, the consistence of which was sometimes equal to that of sandstone or bone, and presented spiculæ, which had excited inflammation, ulceration, and perforation of the lining of the bronchi or trachea with which they were in contact. A direct communication was thus formed between the cavity of the air-tubes and the diseased glands, through which the cretaceous bodies passed; and they were rejected along with the expectorated fluids. Dr. Carswell has seen several examples of cure of tubercular disease of the bronchial glands in the manner just described. When these glands have discharged the whole of their contents, they are found atrophiated, and converted into a fibrous tissue, which fills up the external orifice of the perforated tube. The accidental opening now contracts, becomes obliterated, and leaves in its place a puckered depression or cicatrix, seen on the internal surface of the air-tube. Dr. Carswell adds, that similar appearances, indicating the removal of the serous and albuminous parts of the tuberculous matter, and the condensation of its earthy salts, have frequently been observed in the lungs of persons whose history left no doubt of their having been affected, at some period of their lives, with tubercular phthisis. For a particular description of the changes referred to, as leading to this fortunate amendment, the reader is advised to consult Carswell's Illustrations of the Elementary Forms of Disease, fasc. i. It appears, that if the bronchi remain pervious, the tubercular matter is gradually removed by expectoration; and, if they are closed, it is removed by absorption.—ED.

Eight or ten cases of cicatrization of the lungs after tubercles are recorded by Andral.—(*Clinique Méd.*, tom. iii., p. 382.) The learned translator of Laennec's work is of opinion, however, that this author has exaggerated the frequency of recoveries in this way; and that he has considered certain appearances as signs of cicatrization, which were probably owing to other causes. Dr. Forbes considers it likely, that simple pneumonia, or pleuro-pneumonia, may give rise to many of the slighter deviations from the natural structure, considered by Laennec as tubercular cicatrices.—(See *note in translation of Laennec*, p. 311; also, *Louis, Recherches*, &c., p. 36.) Notwithstanding what has here been advanced, many experienced practitioners still incline to Bayle's opinion, that tubercular consumption is incurable; the disease, however, may be retarded, and patients may live with it sometimes thirty or forty years.]

The ordinary period of the consumptive diathesis has been stated to be from the age of eighteen to that of thirty-five, occasionally anticipating the first, and overpassing the second of these limits: the mean term of its proving fatal has been fixed at about thirty; and the annual victims to its ravages in Great Britain, Dr. Woolcombe has calculated at fifty-five thousand.—(*Remarks on the Frequency and Fatality of different Diseases*, &c., 8vo., Lond., 1808.)

During the last half century, it is said to have been considerably on the increase; but this is, perhaps, chiefly owing to the greater number of infants of delicate health who are saved from an early grave by the introduction of a better system of nursing than was formerly practised; yet who only escape from a disease of infant life to fall before one of adolescence or adult years. And, for the same reason, savages rarely suffer from consumption, as they only rear a healthy race, and lose the sickly soon after birth.

The question, however, concerning the actual range of the consumptive diathesis, or in other words, at what period of life consumption is most frequent, is still open to inquiry. It was a common doctrine among the Greek physicians, and it has very generally descended to our own day, that phthisis rarely occurs before fifteen or after thirty-five years of age; and Dr. Cullen has entered into an ingenious argument to show why it should be so. Yet the tables that have been kept in most parts of the world seem to indicate the contrary; or that, at least, as many die of this disease, and even originate it, after thirty-five or forty years of age, as antecedently to this period. One of the first pathologists who appears to have called the public attention to this general concurrence of the tables and bills of mortality, is Dr. Woolcombe; and he particularly adverts to the proportions observed in the Dispensary of Plymouth, as being the chief source from which he drew his calculations. He tells us, that of seventy-five deaths from consumption, which occurred within the range of this establishment, ten took place before the age of fifteen, sixteen between fifteen and thirty, and forty-nine above the age of thirty; twenty-three of these forty-nine, moreover, being above the age of forty.—(Op. cit., &c., p. 75.)

Dr. Alison (On the Pathology of Scrofulous Diseases ; Transact. of the Medico- Chir. Soc. Edin., vol. i.) has given the result of various other tables, most of which are in consonance with Dr. Woolcombe's. Thus Bayle, in his Treatise on Consumption, notices a hundred cases above fifteen years of age, all of which terminated fatally in the hospital of La Charité at Paris, and after the following proportions : thirty-three below the age of thirty, and sixty-seven above it, of whom forty-four were upwards of forty.* So Haygarth, in his account of the deaths from phthisis in the course of two years at Chester, makes the total a hundred and thirty-five ; of which twenty-five occurred before the age of fifteen, forty-two between fifteen and thirty, and sixty-eight above thirty ; forty-four of these last being above forty.—(Phil. Transact., lxiv., lxv.) "In the practice of the New Town Dispensary at Edinburgh, Dr. Alison tells us, there have been fifty-five deaths from phthisis in the last two years ; of these, eight occurred before fifteen years of age, thirteen between fifteen and thirty ; thirty-four after thirty ; and of these last, twenty-four after forty."

So in Sussmilah's table of deaths at Berlin in 1746, out of six hundred deaths from phthisis, two hundred and fifty-one are stated to have occurred before fifteen years of age, seventy-three between fifteen and thirty, and two hundred and ninety-six above the age of thirty ; two hundred and thirty of which occurred after the age of thirty. In this last table, a greater number of deaths took place within the first fifteen years than in any fifteen years afterward. And a like surplus occurs in the calculations at Warrington recorded by Dr. Aikin : the proportions being twenty-four below the age of fourteen, thirty-six between fourteen and fifteen, and the same number above the age of forty-five.—(Phil. Trans., vol. liv.) While at Carlisle, as we learn from Dr. Heysham, out of two hundred and fourteen deaths, fifty-nine anticipated the age of fifteen, sixty took place between this period and thirty, and ninety-five above the age of thirty ; sixty-one of these being above that of forty.†

The general result, therefore, seems, at first sight, to oppose in a very striking degree the doc-

trine of the Greek schools, and those who have followed them ; and to show that the age from fifteen to thirty is most exempt from consumption, while that above thirty, or even forty, to the close of life, is most distinguished by fatality from this disease, though the period below fifteen is also seriously invaded by it.

But the doctrine of the Greek schools relates to idiopathic consumption as the product of a phthisical diathesis ; or, in other words, affirms that this diathesis, when not called into action by accidental excitements, is most disposed to show itself between the ages of fifteen and thirty-five. And, thus modified· it is probable that the doctrine holds good to the present day, notwithstanding the apparent contradiction of the tables now adverted to. For, with respect to the cases of consumption that anticipate the age of fifteen, by far the greater part of them are secondary, instead of primary or idiopathic affections, and follow as sequels of a strumous habit that has previously shown itself in a morbid condition of the mesentery or some other organ, with which the lungs at length associate in action ; though, but for such an incidental excitement, they would probably have remained quiescent for several years longer. In many instances, indeed, they are to the last rather tabes strumosa, strumous or mesenteric decline, than phthisis or consumption properly so called, though included in the bills of mortality or other tables under this last name. And as we have already observed, that variolous and vaccine inoculation carry various sickly infants through the period of infancy, who would otherwise have fallen victims to the smallpox, yet who, a few years afterward, from the same sickliness of constitution, sink beneath the assault of decline or phthisis, we see sufficient reason for the greater number of early deaths in our own day from what is ordinarily called consumption, and what often is strictly so, though of a secondary or catenating, instead of a primary or idiopathic kind, than was known to the Greek authorities, whose doctrine relating to idiopathic phthisis alone is not hereby interfered with. The observations of M. Louis, to which we have just adverted, and which seem to have been made and persevered in with great accuracy, are directly coincident with these remarks, and support the calculation of the Greek school. "The number of individuals who die of phthisis," says this attentive pathologist, "is more considerable between the ages of twenty and forty than between forty and sixty, although the general mortality is less in the first than in the second of these periods." And, in support of this assertion, he subjoins the following table as the result under his own eye :—

Age.	No. of Deaths.	Age.	No. of Deaths.
From 15 to 20	11	From 40 to 50	23
20 - 30	39	50 - 60	12
30 - 40	33	60 - 70	5

scrofula is more likely to occur in the lungs between the ages of 18 and 30, than at any other time of life.—See Lect. at Lond. Univ., as published in Med. Gaz. for 1833, p. 231.—Ed.

* Bayle, p. 42. Of 223 deaths from phthisis, recorded by Bayle and Louis, 21 occurred between the ages of 15 and 20, 62 between the ages of 20 and 30, 56 between those of 30 and 40, 44 between those of 40 and 50, 27 between those of 50 and 60, 13 between those of 60 and 70.—See Laennec, tr. by Forbes, note, p. 352.—Ed.

† Milne, on Annuities, vol. ii., p. 464. After puberty, Andral has calculated that tubercles are most common in men between the age of 21 and 28 ; but that females are most liable to the disease ere they attain their 21st year.—(Anat. Pathol., tom. i., p. 429.) These estimates, it is to be observed, refer only to the periods of the existence of the disease, and not to the time of life in which the greater or lesser number of deaths takes place from it. The latter is a very different question ; because numerous consumptive patients linger many years. Dr. Elliotson observes, that in this country

And in effect the proportions, as arranged by M. Bayle, do not essentially vary when given in his own tabular form, instead of being generalized, as they are by Dr. Alison, in the reference just quoted. In this form they occur as follows :—

Age.	No. of Deaths.	Age.	No. of Deaths.
From 15 to 20	- 10	From 40 to 50	- 21
20 - 30	- 23	50 - 60	- 15
30 - 40	- 23	60 - 70	- 8

In respect to the exuberant cases that occur in later life than thirty, they are, for the most part, far less a result of a phthisical diathesis than of an accidental exposure to causes peculiarly operating upon the lungs, and exciting them to a morbid action, so as to produce the disease, whether there be any hereditary taint or predisposition to consumption, or whether there be none.

These causes are chiefly the habitual influence of a higher degree of heat or of cold, and especially the latter, than is consistent with that euthesy or perfection of constitution on which sound health depends; and particularly the mischievous influence of a temperature perpetually varying from high degrees of heat to those of cold; and a like mischievous exposure to irritating gases, or spicular dust, perpetually inhaled in various chymical or handicraft occupations. Above thirty years of age, the stations of mankind are usually fixed, and whether healthy or unhealthy, they cannot easily be abandoned.

If, then, we examine the kind of consumption which takes place above this age, we shall find it, in by far the greater number of cases, confined to the lower classes—to those engaged in the occupations just noticed, or who have injured themselves by intemperance; while the classes above them, who have passed safely through the period of from fifteen to thirty or forty years of age, and are free from the incidental excitements alluded to, rarely add to the number of deaths from consumption; and may be regarded as having, in a considerable degree, lost whatever predisposition they had to the disease in an anterior stage of life. Thus again confirming the correctness of the earlier and more common doctrine upon this subject, which refers chiefly to consumption as issuing from a phthisical diathesis.

Hence a material difference is very generally discernible in the nature of the disease as occuring in earlier life, or during the natural range of the predisposition, and as occurring from incidental excitements afterward. The first is usually, though not always, of the tubercular variety; the last, as usually of the catarrhal or apostematous, most commonly of the catarrhal modification, originating from habitual irritation and repeated and neglected inflammation, not at first of an unhealthy character, for the most part more active than tubercular inflammation; and, where suppuration does not take place freely, leading to a dark-hued or hepatized induration.

The causes of phthisis, then, are of two kinds; the predisponent, and those that excite the predisposition into action, or operate even where there is no predisposition whatever.

Of the nature of the predisponent cause, we know little more than that it appertains to a peculiarity of constitution, which will be noticed presently.* The exciting or occasional causes are very numerous, as mechanical irritation of the lungs from swallowing a piece of bone; the dust of metallic or other hard substances perpetually inhaled; frequent and sudden changes of temperature, or exposure of the body to cold when in a heated state and unprepared for it; overaction in speaking, singing, or playing on a wind instrument; the irritation of various other diseases, as worms, scrofula,† syphilis, or measles; too rapid a growth of the body; and various passions perpetually preying upon the individual, as mortified ambition, disappointed love, home-longing (R. Hamilton, in Duncan's Med. Comm., xi., p. 343), when at a remote distance from one's friends and country. .

Examples of consumption from a mechanical irritation of the lungs are peculiarly numerous, and they furnish cases of every variety of the disease, according to the habit or idiosyncrasy, though the apostematous is less frequent than the rest. So common is this complaint among persons employed in dry grinding, or pointing needles in needle-manufactories, that Dr. Johnstone, of Worcester, informs us they seldom live to be forty, from the accumulation of the dust of the grindstones in the air-cells of the lungs, and the irritation and suppuration which follow.—(Mem. Med. Soc., v., 1799, p. 89.) It appears to be little less common among knife and scythe-grinders, whence, according to Dr. Simmons, the disease thus originating is called the grinder's rot (Pract. Observ. on the Treat. of Consumptions, 8vo., 1780); and Wepfer gives an account of its proving endemic at Waldshut, on the Rhine, where there is a cavern in which mill-stones are dug and wrought : the air is always hot, even in the winter, and a very fine dust floats in it, which penetrates leathern bags, and discolours money contained in them. "All the workmen," says he, "become consumptive if they remain there for a year, and some even in a shorter time; and they all die unless they apply early for assistance."—(Observationes de Affect. Capitis, 4to., Schaff., 1727-8, quoted by Young on Consumptive Diseases, p. 206.) And hence, Dr. Fordyce had much reason for regarding the dust of the streets of London as a se-

---

* Many would escape the disease were it not for their being exposed to wet and cold, for want of proper lodging and clothing. These circumstances, together with unwholesome food, are well known to create a tendency to, and even to excite, scrofulous diseases in general, among which must undoubtedly be placed tubercular phthisis. It is alleged, says Dr. Elliotson, that formerly in Scotland the people were all dressed in woollen, and phthisis was rare among them; but that since they have changed it for cotton, the disease has become very prevalent in that country.—ED.

† Tubercular phthisis is considered, by the most accurate pathologists of the present day, as a scrofulous disease itself.—ED.

rious cause of pulmonic disorders (*Trans. of Soc. for the Impr. of Med. and Chir. Knowledge*, vol. i., p. 252), though it is a cause that has been much diminished since the introduction of paving and watering.* As there are causes that operate at all ages, consumption among such persons occurs at all ages also ; in patients, however, beyond forty, it may for the most part be regarded as a strictly original disease, the consumptive diathesis having by this time, as already observed, gradually lost its influence. And it is on this account that Dr. Alison regards the tubercular or strumous form as rarely taking place after the age of thirty-five or forty (*Edin. Medico-Chir. Transact.*, vol. i., 1824), thus confirming the ancient, and indeed the common opinion, how much soever opposed by the tables we have already referred to.

A lodgment of some fragment of a bone even in the œsophagus has, in like manner, been a frequent cause of phthisis, which has often been protracted through a long period of time. Thus Claubry gives a case of this kind which had continued for fourteen years, and the patient seemed to be in the last stage of a consumption, when he was fortunate enough to bring up the piece of bone spontaneously, in consequence of which he recovered, though for the preceding four years he had laboured under an hæmoptysis.—(*Sedill. Journ. Gen. Med.*, xxxiv., p. 13, 1809.) Mr. Holman describes a similar case that had run on for fifteen years, accompanied with cough, hæmoptysis, and hectic diarrhœa ; and which was also speedily relieved in consequence of the bony fragment, three quarters of an inch in length, and apparently carious, being suddenly coughed up after the discharge of a pint of blood.—(*Lond. Med. Journ.*, vii., p. 120.)

A moderate use of the vocal organs, as of any other, tends to strengthen them, and to enable public speakers, singers, and performers on wind-instruments to go through great exertion without inconvenience, which would be extremely fatiguing to those who are but little practised in any of these branches ; but the labour is often carried too far, and the lungs become habitually irritated, and hæmoptysis succeeds. I have known this terminate fatally among clergymen ; who have lamented, when too late, that in the earlier part of life they spent their strength unsparingly in the duties of the pulpit.† Hence,

Dr. Young observes from Rammazini (*On Consumptive Diseases*, p. 264), that public speakers, readers, and singers are most liable to pulmonary diseases, and that Morgagni and Valsalva have confirmed the observation. Cicero himself felt it necessary, as he tells us in his book on orators, to retire from the forum for two years, during which he travelled into Asia, and afterward returned with renewed vigour to the duties of his profession ; and Molière died of hæmoptysis, immediately after performing, for the fourth time, his Malade Imaginaire.—(*Van Swieten*, Aph. iv., § 1201, p. 49.)

Many diseases have a peculiar tendency to excite phthisis, from their close connexion with the lungs, or affinity to hectic fever, which is one of its most prominent symptoms. Thus, neglected catarrhs form a frequent foundation, and measles for the same reason.

[This hypothesis of the origin of consumption from catarrh is very ancient, but not at present universally admitted. In most phthisical cases, as Laennec allows, the first symptoms are catarrhal ; but, as he also acknowledges, we find very large and very numerous tubercles in subjects who exhibit no signs of catarrh. If it be said that the tubercles are the product of former catarrhs, Laennec replies, that they exist in persons who have not had catarrh for years, or even at all. Pulmonary catarrh is, indeed, often the first symptom of tubercular phthisis : this, however, may have existed long in a latent state ; since we find, on examining the chest of such persons, all the physical signs of tubercles, and sometimes even of tubercles already excavated. On the other hand, thousands of persons have catarrh several times every year, and yet very few of them become phthisical.—(*Op. cit.*, p. 293.) Some arguments and facts against the doctrine of tubercles being a consequence of pleurisy, peripneumony, and catarrh, are noticed by M. Louis. Of eighty phthisical subjects, into whose previous history he had particularly inquired, only seven had ever been affected with pneumonia, and four of these had been perfectly free from any pectoral affection for several years before the invasion of phthisis. He notices the fact, mentioned by Laennec, of tubercles being most frequent in the upper lobes, while peripneumony most commonly occupies the lower. He adds, that pneumonia rarely af-

---

* The diminution of the supposed cause, and the undiminished frequency of consumption, seem to contradict Fordyce's hypothesis.—ED.

† On this subject Dr. John Ware, of Boston, very justly remarks (Med. Dissertations, Boston, 1820), " The most obvious cause of this liability to pulmonary disease in clergymen is the great and long-continued exercise of the lungs, required in the performance of public worship. To this, as the peculiar duty of the profession, our attention is apt to be principally and almost exclusively devoted ; we are too ready to consider it as a sufficient cause in itself ; and to avoid examining the influence of other circumstances. It is not found that members of other professions who are in the habit of exerting their lungs, are more liable than the average of mankind to pulmonary disease. We do not hear of any extraordinary proportion of deaths from consumption among lawyers, public

actors, public singers," &c.—" The reason I believe to be this, that the duties of the profession are only occasional, and occur at too great intervals to allow the formation of a habit ; while at the same time they are sufficiently difficult to overexercise, fatigue, and exhaust the organ. They are from the first as long and laborious as they ever will be, and there is no opportunity for that slow and gradual increase which enables one to acquire strength and facility of exertion."—" Occasional extraordinary exertion, carried to the point of fatigue, and then omitted until the fatigue is entirely removed, can only have the most injurious effect, and it is exactly in this way that the lungs are exercised in preaching. They are wearied by the services of the Sabbath, and are then suffered to remain perfectly at rest through the interval of the week."—D.

fects both lungs, while phthisis almost always does so; and that the former is most common in men, while the latter is so in women. The same remarks, he says, apply to pleurisy and catarrh, with this addition, that in cases of chronic pleurisy, he has found as many tubercles in the lung of the sound as in that of the diseased side. Out of the eighty cases of phthisis above alluded to, only twenty-three had been particularly subject to catarrh.—(*Louis, Recherches*, &c., p. 503, et seq.; also, *Forbes, in note to transl. of Laennec*, p. 323, 2d edit.)]

Whether the tubercles found in the substance of the lungs, in the tubercular variety of consumption, be, in every instance, strictly scrofulous, may admit of a doubt; that they are so in many cases is unquestionable; and hence scrofula becomes very generally an exciting, and not unfrequently, perhaps, a primary cause of this disease.*

The tendency of the syphilitic poison to pro-

---

* In Great Britain, where strumous habits are admitted to exist much more extensively than in the United States, the connexion between scrofula and consumption ought not to be questioned. In this country scrofula is rare when compared with Great Britain, and yet the mortality by consumption is nearly the same as there. To what circumstances is this to be attributed? To the extraordinary vicissitudes in the climate, " to the mischievous influence of a temperature perpetually varying from high degrees of heat to those of cold." Consumption too is evidently increasing among us, and within the city of New-York the weekly number of deaths from this disease within the last five years, has risen from 18 to 36; a ratio of one hundred per cent., while the increase in population is not more than ten per cent.; thus, notwithstanding the improvements in medicine, our treatment is not much more successful than it was formerly: this increase may be ascribed partly to the modified habits and manners of our people, especially in the larger cities, where greater errors of life prevail; to imprudence in dress, improprieties in diet, and the excesses and indiscretions which mark the extremes of society, the rich and the poor. The truth of this remark will be readily seen by comparing the mortality by consumption at the present time with that which prevailed about a century ago. Dr. Colden, speaking of the climate of New-York some ninety years since, remarks, " the air of the country being almost always clear, and its spring strong, we have few consumptions or diseases of the lungs. Persons inclined to be consumptive in England, are often perfectly cured by our fine air." —(Am. Med. and Phil. Reg., vol. i., p. 309.) If these premises be allowed as correct, we have strong reason to think that inflammation is the more common cause of consumption, and to regard with more favour than many eminent writers abroad, the principle of the entonic or acute character of the disease. Dr. Rush was unguardedly led into an error in stating that the Indians are exempt from pulmonary disease; an acute observer, one who resided long among those " sons of the forest," remarks, that consumption is one of the common causes of death among them.—(See Hunter on Diseases of the Indians, in the N. York Med. and Phys. Journal, vol. i.) Nine deaths from the same cause have occurred in the family of the celebrated Indian chief Red-Jacket.—(See Francis on the Mineral Waters of Avon.) The liability of blacks to consumption is well known.—D.

---

duce phthisis has been noticed by almost every writer from the time of Bennet, who particularly dwells upon it (*Vestibulum Tabidorum*, 8vo., 1654, Leyd.); but whether this would be adequate to such a purpose without an hereditary predisposition is uncertain.* And the same remark may be made respecting worms, which Morgagni has stated to be a very common cause.—(*De Morb. Thoracis*, lib. ij., Ep. Anat. xxi., 43.) Indeed, any habitual irritation in any part of the alimentary canal, seems capable of exciting a sympathetic action in the lungs: and hence Wilson, in Dr. Duncan's Annals, gives a case of hectic in a child produced by swallowing a nail two inches long, which remained in the stomach fifteen months, and was then thrown up, and succeeded by a recovery of health.†

Rapid growth is always attended with debility; and, where there is a predisposition to consumption, it often becomes its harbinger. Richerand relates a case of this kind that terminated fatally, the individual having grown more than an English foot in a year.—(*Sedill. Journ. Gen. Med.*, xx., p. 255.) I have known a still more rapid growth, without any other inconvenience than that of languor; but, in this case, there was no phthisical predisposition.

Where the chest labours under any misformation, we can readily trace another cause of excitement, and are prepared to meet the examples that from this source so frequently occur to us in practice. But it is less easy to explain by what means persons otherwise deformed, and particularly those who have had limbs amputated, should be more liable to consumption than others; yet this also is a remark that has been made by Bennet.‡

Of all the occasional or accidental causes of phthisis, however, frequent and sudden vicissitudes of temperature are probably the most common (*Broussais*, ut sup.; *Hastings, Essay on Bronchial Inflammation*); so common, indeed, and at the same time so active, as often to be a cause of consumption in constitutions where we cannot trace any peculiar taint or predisposition whatever. Several hundred cases of phthisis from this cause, among which were many fatal ones, occurred in the channel fleet that blockaded the port of Brest in April, 1800. The summer was hot and dry, the duty severe,

---

* " The varieties termed scorbutic, venereal, &c. are all essentially tuberculous, differing only from the common species by the cause (perhaps gratuitous) to which the development of the tubercles is attributed."—(Laennec, p. 272.) No modern practitioner of any judgment now believes in the existence of a form of phthisis depending upon and kept up by the syphilitic poison.—Eo.

† Vol. i., 1796. Our author here, and in some other places, seems not to have made an adequate distinction between phthisis and hectic fever.—Ed.

‡ Tabid. Theatr., p. 99. Perhaps some explanation of the circumstance, if true, might be deduced from the consideration that most amputations, in this country at least, are done for scrofulous diseases of joints, and consequently on individuals of strumous diathesis; in whom alone, probably, tubercles of the lungs ever form.—Ed.

the sailors, wet with sweat, were frequently exposed to currents of air at the port-holes; and little time was allowed for refitting.*

Hence, the most frequent examples of consumption are to be found in countries which are most subject to changes of temperature. In Great Britain it is calculated that this disease carries off usually about one fourth of the inhabitants; at Paris, about one fifth; and at Vienna, one sixth: while it is by no means common in Russia, and still less so in the West Indies; † for it is checked in both regions by the greater uniformity of the atmosphere, whether hotter or colder.‡ It is a singular fact, and not well accounted for, that of all places which have hitherto been compared, the proportional mortality from consumption appears to have been the greatest at Bristol; and this, not among its occasional visiters, but its permanent inhabitants; and yet, as though in defiance of expericuce, this very place has been chosen as the great resort of consumptive persons.—(*Young, ut suprà,* p. 42.) Nor does its mineral water seem entitled to any higher compliment than its atmosphere. Dr. Beddoes affirms, in direct terms, that it is of no manner of use.—(*Manual of Health, &c.,* 12mo., Lond., 1806.)

Heat, when above the range of health and entony, is often found a cause as well as cold, though it does not act so manifestly or so rapidly. But of its power of action, we have a clear proof in the greater frequency and fatality of consumption among the native troops of hot climates during the fatigues of war, than among

---

* Trotter's Medicina Nautica, vol. iii., p. 325. While Laennec partly admits the truth of the statement respecting the effects of vicissitudes of temperature, he observes, that too light clothing, and the impression of cold, when the body is heated, much more frequently give rise to catarrhs, peripneumonies, and pleurisies, which are not followed by the tubercular disease; so that he concludes that phthisis, when it follows these complaints, has been merely accelerated by them, the tubercles having previously existed. In opposition to Dr. Trotter's account, Laennec says, that most naval surgeons whom he has conversed with, inform him that they had scarcely ever known a man become phthisical in the course of a long voyage, and that they had frequently seen sailors who had pulmonary complaints at the time of putting to sea, return benefited or cured.—Op. cit., p. 352.—ED.

† If we examine the official records of mortality, we shall find that consumption annually destroys its thousands in the United States also. The statistical tables of Dr. Emerson, of Philadelphia, present the following as the relative number of deaths by consumption in the principal cities of the union. Deaths by consumption in proportion to the whole mortality—New-York, 1-5,23; Boston, 1-5,54; Baltimore, 1-6,21; Philadelphia, 1-6,38. Number of deaths in proportion to the population—New-York, 1-39,36; Baltimore, 1-39,17; Boston, 1,44-93; Philadelphia, 1-47,86. The number of deaths by consumption in the city of New-York during the last seven years, is nearly eight thousand.—D.

‡ Woolcombe (Dr. W.), remarks on the Frequency and Fatality of Diseases, 8vo., London, 1808. Southey (Dr. H. H.), Observations on Pulmonary Consumption, 8vo., Lond., 1814.

Europeans who have just been inured to the climate, and have for a less period of time been under the influence of its relaxing agency. "We know at least," observes Dr. Alison, "that a great majority of the inhabitants of these climates, both negroes and Hindoos, are unusually prone to scrofula when they come to temperate climates, and even suffer from it, in some instances, in their own, where Europeans are nearly free from it. I was favoured by Dr. Fergusson, lately inspector of hospitals in the Windward and Leeward Islands, with a perusal of the report of the deaths and chief diseases occurring in the army in these colonies, in each quarter, from March, 1816, till March, 1817, distinguishing the deaths among the white and black troops."—(*Trans. Medico-Chir. Society Edin.,* vol. i., p. 397.) According to these reports, the average strength of the army, for the entire year, consisted of seven thousand three hundred and thirty-seven whites, and five thousand seven hundred and seventy-two blacks: out of which there died of fever, whites, one in 15.3; blacks, one in 151.8: of dysentery, whites, one in 21.4; blacks, one in 58.9: but of pulmonic disease, whites, one in 89.1; blacks, one in 45. "Fever, therefore," remarks Dr. Alison, "caused ten times as great a mortality among the white troops as among the blacks, and dysentery nearly three times as great; but pulmonary complaints caused twice as great a mortality among the blacks as among the whites. The deaths from this cause were one in 10.9 of the whole mortality among the whites; and one in 2.06 of the whole mortality among the blacks. The pulmonic disease among the black troops was almost exclusively phthisis, which attacked them chiefly in the more elevated situations of the interior of the islands, where the heat is least oppressive, and where the Europeans were most free from the diseases which, to them, are in that climate most fatal."—(*Trans. Med.-Chir. Soc. Edin.,* vol. i., p. 398.)

On this account we can readily see whence, in numerous instances, a residence in the warmer regions of Europe proves remedial to occasional visiters from colder and less genial countries, although the tables of mortality do not show a much greater immunity from consumption among the natives than exists in higher latitudes. Negroes and Hindoos are by no means exempt from this disease; and we shall presently have to notice, that the southern borders of the Mediterranean give proofs of a frequency and fatality that would be sufficient to deter strangers from trying those coasts as a cure, did not daily observation justify our recommending them to patients of a more northerly origin.*

---

* An exact comparative view of the degree in which consumption prevails in different parts of the world, has not yet been satisfactorily obtained. According to Laennec, the complaint is very rare among the natives of high mountainous countries, particularly the Alps. Dr. Forbes thinks it tolerably well made out, that, in the most northern parts of Europe, particularly Russia, and still more conspicuously between the tropics, the disease is

Where a consumptive diathesis has once originated, it is often very evidently transmitted to succeeding generations; and there is great reason to believe that the disease is in a certain degree contagious. M. Portal, and a few other pathologists of distinction, have doubted or denied that it possesses any such property; but the apparent instances of communication among near relations and close attentive nurses, and especially between husbands and wives, who have fallen victims to it in succession, are so frequent, that its contagious power has been admitted by most practitioners, and in most ages. Aristotle appeals to it as a matter of general belief among the Greeks in his day (*Problem,* sect. i., 7); and it has since been assented to in succession by Galen, Morton, Hoffmann, Vogel, Desault, Morgagni, Darwin, and most modern writers.*

I have myself been witness to various cases which could not be ascribed to any other cause; and Dr. Rush has given an account of a consumption manifestly contagious, which spread from the proprietors of an estate among the negroes, who were neither related to the first victims, nor had been subjected to fatigue or anxiety on their account, and among whom it scarcely ever makes its appearance.—(*Medical Inquiries and Obs.*, &c., vol. i., 8vo., Phila., 1789.) The disease, however, is but slightly contagious, admitting it to be so at all; and seems to demand a long and intimate communion, as, for instance, that of sleeping or constantly living in the same room, to render the miasm effective.

[Respecting the contagious nature of phthisis, the editor must take this opportunity of observing, that a belief in it is not entertained in this country: Laennec distinctly affirms, that the disease does not appear to be contagious in France. When the great frequency of consumption, and other pulmonary complaints confounded with it, is fairly considered, the extensive co-existence of such cases, or their continual succession, or seeming transmissions from one individual to another, can be very well accounted for, without unnecessarily resorting to the doctrine of contagion. If one fourth or one fifth of the population die phthisical, such events

considerably less prevalent than in more temperate climates. It is extremely prevalent in every part of Great Britain, Germany, France, Italy, Spain, and in the islands and on all the coasts of the Mediterranean sea. Laennec believed the inhabitants of maritime situations to be less liable to consumption than those who reside away from the sea; but in England this is not found to be the fact.—See note by Dr. Forbes, in Laennec's Treatise, p. 324.—Ed.

* In Languedoc, Spain, Portugal, Italy, and Malta, phthisis is yet regarded as contagious. When the editor was in the latter island, many years ago, a consumptive person could hardly procure a lodging for money; and in Spain and Portugal, the clothes of persons who die with consumption are burned by the civil authorities. Morgagni was so frightened about its contagiousness, that he would not open the bodies of those who died of it.—Ed.

must of course be frequent. Is it meant to insinuate that all phthisical diseases are contagious, notwithstanding the wide difference in their nature, even as viewed by the author of the present work? Or is it intended to limit the doctrine exclusively to tubercular consumption?]

The diathesis strictly consumptive is usually associated, in the language of Hippocrates (*Epidem.*, v., p. 1142) and Aretæus (*Chron.*, Diss. i., 10, 12), with a smooth, fair, and ruddy complexion, light or reddish hair, blue eyes, a long neck, a narrow chest, slender form, and high shoulders, or, in the words of Hippocrates, shoulders projecting like wings, and a sanguine disposition. In some instances, however, the skin is dark, and the hair almost black.* According to Dr. Withering and Dr. Darwin, the most constant mark of a consumptive habit is an unusual magnitude of the pupil, to which some have added long and dark eyelashes; but this last character seems loose and unestablished. It is a remark far better supported, that the teeth are peculiarly clear, and the eyes exceedingly bright; and that both become more so when the disease has once commenced its inroad; the former assuming a milky whiteness, and the latter a pearly lustre.

Professor Camper, and most physicians with him, affirm that this appearance accompanies all the varieties of the disease; but Dr. Foart Simmons limits it to the tubercular alone, and conceives it to be a distinguishing characteristic of this form of the disease, or of a predisposition to it. And he remarks further, that, of those who are carried off by tubercular phthisis, the greater number will be found never to have had a carious tooth.—(*Practical Obs. on Consumption,* 8vo., London, 1779.)

The earliest symptoms of phthisis, in whatever manner excited, are insidious, and show themselves obscurely. The patient is, perhaps, sensible of an unusual languor, and breathes with less freedom than formerly, so that his respirations are shorter and increased in number. He coughs occasionally, but does not complain of its being troublesome, and rarely expectorates at the same time; yet, if he make a deep inspiration, he is sensible of some degree of uneasiness in a particular part of the chest. These symptoms gradually increase, and at length the pulse is found quicker than usual, particularly towards the evening; a more than ordinary perspiration takes place in the course of the night; and if the sleep be not disturbed by coughing, a considerable paroxysm of coughing takes place in the morning, and the patient feels relaxed and enfeebled. This may be said to form the first stage of the disease; and it is the only hopeful season for the interposition of medical aid.

The malady is now decidedly established;

* Nearly two thirds of the consumptive patients seen by Dr. S. G. Morton, have had dark eyes and hair, and sallow or dark complexions, and many of the remainder had reddish hair and a sandy complexion.—(See his Illustrations of Pulmonary Consumption, &c., Philadelphia, 1834.)—D.

the cough increases in frequency, and from being dry is accompanied with a purulent mucus, varying, according to the peculiar modification of the disease, from a watery whey-like sanies, occasionally tinged with blood, to a sputum of nearly genuine pus : which, as Aretæus has well observed, may be livid, deep black, light brown, or light green ; flattened or round ; hard or soft ; fetid or without smell.* In many cases it is very scanty ; and we may also add, with Aretæus, that, in some consumptions, there is no expectoration at all : for in the apostematous variety, the sufferer has sometimes died before the vomica has broken. The uneasiness in the chest, only perceived at first on making a deep inspiration, is now permanent, and attended with a sense of weight ;† the hectic fever has assumed its full character ; the patient can only lie with comfort on one side, which is usually the side affected ; and the breathing, as Bennet has remarked, is frequently accompanied by a sound like the ticking of a watch. The strength now fails apace ; the pulse varies from about a hundred to a hundred and twenty or thirty ; the teeth increase in transparency, and the sclerotica of the eye is pearly-white ; "the fingers," to continue the elegant description of Aretæus, as given by Dr. Young, "are shrunk, except at

---

* In the earliest stage of the disease, according to Dr. Forbes's valuable description, the cough is either quite dry, or attended by a mere watery, or slightly viscid, frothy, and colourless fluid. This, on the approach of the second stage, gradually changes into an opaque, greenish, thicker fluid, intermixed with fine streaks of a yellow colour. At this period, also, the sputa are sometimes intermixed with small specks of a dead white, or slightly yellow colour, varying from the size of a pin's head to that of a grain of rice. After the complete evacuation of the tubercles, the expectoration puts on various forms of purulency ; but frequently assumes one particular character, which has always appeared to Dr. Forbes pathognomonic of phthisis, although he says it has been noticed by other pathologists in simple catarrh. This expectoration consists of a series of globular masses, of a whitish yellow colour, with a rugged woolly surface, and somewhat like little balls of cotton or wool. They commonly, but not always, sink in water. They are most common in young scrofulous subjects, in whom the disease is hereditary. At other times, in cases where these globular masses are observed, and also in those in which they have not appeared, the expectoration assumes the common characters of the pus of an abscess, with an occasional tinge of red, and sometimes more or less fetor.—See Laennec, by Forbes, note, p. 352, 2d edit.

† The researches of M. Louis tend to support the opinion, that the pain in phthisis depends upon slight chronic pleurisies, which occasion the adhesions found after death, and not upon the tubercles.—(Recherches, &c., p. 205.) As, however, one direct effect of tubercles in the lungs is to lessen the capacity of these organs for the air of respiration, and to diminish that surface by which the purposes of breathing are accomplished, it is difficult to conceive this approach to suffocation, slow as it is, unattended with more or less uneasiness and pain. The tubercular matter itself, being unorganized, cannot, of course, be susceptible of pain.—Ed.

---

the joints, which become prominent : the nails are bent for want of support, and become painful ; the nose is sharp, the cheeks are red, the eyes sunk, but bright, the countenance as if smiling ; the whole body is shrivelled ; the spine projects, instead of sinking, from the decay of the muscles ; and the shoulder-blades stand out like the wings of birds."

The third stage is melancholy and distressing, but usually of short duration. It commences with a depressing and colliquative diarrhœa ; but, till this period, and occasionally indeed through it, the patient supports his spirits, and flatters himself with ultimate success, while all his friends about him are in despondency, and find it difficult to suppress their feelings. The voice becomes hoarse, the fauces aphthous, or the throat ulcerated, with a difficulty of swallowing. Dropsy, in various forms, now makes its approach ; the limbs are anasarcous, the belly tumid, or the chest fluctuating ; and the oppression is only relieved by an augmentation of the night-sweats or of the diarrhœa ; for it is generally to be found, that the one set of symptoms is less as the other is greater. "A few days before the patient's death, he is frequently unable to expectorate from apparent weakness, and sometimes dies absolutely suffocated : but much more commonly the secretion of pus, as well as the expectoration, has ceased : as if the capillary arteries had lost their power, or the fluids of the system were exhausted. There is also sometimes a degree of languid delirium for some days, and occasionally a total imbecility for a week or two : though, in general, the faculties are entire, and the senses acute, the patient being perfectly alive to the danger and distress of his situation, and retaining, even when his extremities are becoming cold, a considerable quickness of hearing and feeling. The closing scene is often painful, but it sometimes consists in the gradual and almost imperceptible approach of a sleep which is the actual commencement of death."—(*Young on Consumptive Diseases*, p. 28.)

[One very frequent symptom is not noticed in the preceding account : the editor alludes to a sore oppressive sensation in the throat, attended with a feeling as if an extraneous mass were lodged in the larynx, and generally accompanied by more or less difficulty of swallowing. In numerous cases seen by him, this symptom occurred a few days before death : it depends upon ulceration within the larynx, which is often noticed on dissection.

In the dissections performed by M. Louis, the mucous membrane of the trachea was found either red, or somewhat thickened and softened, in one fifth of the cases, and ulcerated in rather less than one third, while the larynx and epiglottis were ulcerated in one fifth. According to Bayle, the proportion is one sixth, and to Andral, three fourths. The ulceration of the larynx, and more particularly of the trachea and epiglottis, is deemed by M. Louis peculiar to phthisis. Dr. Bright says, it is generally betrayed by the hoarseness of the voice, and the clanging sound which accompanies the cough. The most usual seat of it, he observes, is immediately below the rima glottidis, where it begins with one or two very small round ulcers, which soon extend, and become irregular in form, assuming the appearance of superficial abrasion. The situation and extent, however, vary a little : sometimes the epiglottis itself is ulcerated, and, occasionally, small independent ulcers take place in the mucous membrane of the trachea, two or three inches below the larynx. When the ulceration in the larynx has taken place early, it has not unfrequently, according to Dr. Bright, drawn the attention both of the patient and the practitioner from the more important seat of disease ; for the irritation and uneasiness occasioned by it is more forced upon the attention than the inconvenience and dyspnœa, seldom amounting to pain, which accompany the tubercular deposite in the lungs.—(See *Bright's Reports of Medical Cases*, p. 149, 4to., Lond., 1827.)]

Such is the common progress and termination of the disease ; but it varies considerably in the character and combination of its symptoms, and particularly in the tardiness or rapidity of its march, according to the habit or idiosyncrasy of the individual, or the variety of the disease itself. Where the constitution is firm, and the hereditary predisposition striking, it commonly assumes the apostematous form, and runs on to the fatal goal with prodigious speed, constituting what among the vulgar is called, with great force of expression, a galloping consumption. In this case, the activity of the lymphatic, and, indeed, of every other part of the general system, is wonderful : the whole frame is in a state of estuation, and greedily preying upon itself. The animal spirits are more than ordinarily recruited, and all is hope and ardent imagination ; the secernents play with equal vigour, and the skin is drenched with moisture ; the bronchial vessels are overloaded with mucus, vomica after vomica becomes distended with pus, and the bowels are a mere channel of looseness. The absorbents drink greedily ; and animal oil, cellular membrane, parenchyma, and muscle, are all swallowed up and carried away, till every organ* is rapidly reduced to half its proper

---

* This statement should be qualified : it is true, as Laennec explains, that the greater number of phthisical subjects, before they die, fall into that extreme degree of emaciation, from which the Greeks derived the name of the disease. This emaciation is strongly marked in the adipose cellular membrane and muscles, but, with the exception of the heart, *not at all in the internal organs.* The intestines may appear contracted, but this is chiefly owing to their containing very little air. The brain, nerves, genital organs, spleen, pancreas, and other glands, present no marks of emaciation. The bloodvessels usually seem dwindled, owing to the quantity of the circulating fluid having been reduced by copious evacuations and low regimen. The bones are not at all shortened ; but Laennec thought that he had frequently noticed, in protracted cases, a diminution of their diameter, and their specific gravity is certainly lessened. The narrowness and contraction of the chest are known to everybody.—(See Laennec, by Forbes, p. 286, 2d edit.) With regard to the heart, the statement of Andral is different from that above given ; for

weight and bulk, and the entire figure becomes a shrivelled skeleton. So swift was the progress of the disease in the case of the Dutchess de Pienne, that M. Portal informs us she died in ten or twelve days from the first alarm.

If, before this, an extensive vomica burst suddenly and with a wide opening into the trachea, or larger bronchial tubes, suffocation follows instantly. If its aperture be small, a purulent matter, often diversicoloured, is expectorated in the course of a violent fit of coughing : the expuition then ceases for a few days, and, at times, with an apparent relief to the patient ; but it returns in a short time, and is always ushered by an increase of the febrile state for the preceding four-and-twenty hours. The breath now becomes tainted, and is offensive to by-standers ; the appetite is lost, and the lightest foods and most desirable dainties produce a sense of increased languor and anxiety. The patient becomes daily more emaciated : all the symptoms just noticed are exacerbated, till, at length, a supervening colliquative diarrhœa first diminishes, and then totally suppresses the expectoration, and the sufferer turns himself unexpectedly on his back, and, in a very few days afterward, draws up his legs, and, in this position, usually expires suddenly.

[A tuberculous cavity sometimes opens into the pleura. In the cases recorded by M. Louis, the rupture was indicated by an instantaneous acute pain at one point of the chest, with dyspnœa and extreme anxiety, followed by the common symptoms of acute pleurisy, and death within a period varying from one to thirty-six days. "In every case of this kind," says Dr. Forbes, "the diagnosis derives unerring certainty from auscultation and percussion." In five of the cases described by M. Louis, the perforation took place opposite the angle of the third and fourth ribs of the left side, and it did the same in a case attended by Dr. Forbes.—(See *Laennec, by Forbes*, p. 341 ; and *Louis sur la Phthisie*, ch. vii., p. 446.)]*

On other occasions the march of the consumption is remarkable for its tardiness. This is particularly the case with the tubercular variety, when not quickened in its pace by returns of hæmoptysis. Hoffmann gives instances of two or three who lived under the disease for

---

he observes, that although, in several diseases which carry off the patients in a very emaciated condition, the heart partakes of the atrophy of the rest of the muscular system, this is not constantly the case, and the hearts of many consumptive persons, who die in the extreme of marasmus, are quite free from atrophy. If, in such a case, the heart should appear diminished in size, it is because, being empty of blood, it has contracted ; its cavities are small, but its parietes are of their natural thickness.—Andral, Anat. Pathol., tom. ii., p. 288.—ED.

* Dr. Morton, in his valuable Illustrations of Pulmonary Consumption already cited, has figured a case (Pl. vii., ix.), in which pus passed between two ribs, infiltrated into the muscles of the back where a large abscess formed, by which the spinous processes of several vertebræ were exposed.—D.

thirty years:* and in the Edinburgh Communications is the case of an individual, who passed nearly the whole of a long life under its influence, who was consumptive from eighteen to seventy-two, and died of the complaint at last. Of two hundred cases, however, selected by M. Bayle, a hundred and four died within nine months, which may hence be regarded as the mean term.

Dissections concur in showing, in almost every instance, an indurated and ulcerated state of the lungs, while the changes thus exhibited vary greatly in the morbid structure they develop; the more obvious of which, though perhaps constituting the two extremes of these changes, are the white and the dark-coloured or hepatized knobs. The first seems to move forward to a state of inflammation with a slow and pausing step, and forms the basis of the tubercular variety before us. The second is more rapid and uniform in its action, and constitutes the catarrhal or purulent modifications. While, not unfrequently, we meet with both these appearances intermixed in every possible proportion. Yet we perceive, concurrently with the diagnostics of the disease, that its most frequent form is the tubercular; so much so, indeed, that M. Laennec has confined his attention to this variety alone, and will hardly admit of any other.—(*De l'Auscultation Médiate; ou Traité du Diagnostic des Maladies des Poumons*, &c., 2 tomes, Paris, 1819.) The tubercles are found indiscriminately in all parts of the cellular texture of the lungs, but more abundantly at the upper and posterior parts. As already observed, they exhibit every diversity of size; are often very minute, but more generally consist of those circumscribed nodules or indurations which Wesser has called grandines. They are whitish and opaque, like small absorbent glands, but sometimes more transparent, like cartilage, with black dots in their substance. They augment by degrees, till they are half an inch or more in diameter; but in general, when they have acquired the size of large peas, they begin to soften in the centre, and then open by one or more small apertures into the neighbouring bronchiæ, or remain for a longer time closed, and constitute small vomicæ, containing a curdy half-formed pus. Occasionally, as we have stated, they are found to unite into large abscesses.† [Whatever be the form under which the tubercular matter is developed, it presents at first, according to Laennec,‡ the

appearance of a gray, semi-transparent granulation, which gradually becomes yellow, opaque, and very dense. Afterward it softens, and gradually acquires a fluidity nearly equal to that of pus. It is then expelled through the bronchiæ, and cavities are left, vulgarly called *ulcers of the lungs*, but which Laennec designated *tubercular excavations*.] Now as we have before observed from Dr. Baillie, that nothing like a gland is to be found in the cellular membrane of the lungs in a sound state, constituting the seat of these tubercles,* and as scrofula selects for its abode a glandular structure, tubercular consumption cannot perhaps with strict propriety be called a scrofulous disease; yet as the untempered fluid contained in the tubercles resembles that of scrofula, and, more especially, as this variety of consumption is very generally found in constitutions distinctly scrofulous, the analogy between the two is extremely close, and has often led to a similar mode of treatment. M. Portal, indeed, contends that glands exist in great numbers through the whole structure of the lungs, but rather from analogy than from demonstration. And to the same effect M. Laennec; "The

noticed in lymphatic glands, in which a tubercle can be examined in every stage of its progress? Have they ever been seen in the brain, liver, spleen, or the cellular tissue under mucous or serous membranes, or between the muscles? The small, grayish, irregularly globular bodies, dispersed sometimes over the free surface of serous membranes, he contends, are as different as possible from ordinary granulations of the lungs. As for the grayish granulations, sometimes noticed on the surface of mucous membranes, they seem to Andral to be merely enlarged follicles. At the same time, he admits that tubercular matter may be formed within granulations of the lungs. —Anat. Pathol., tom. i., p. 411.—ED.

* This doctrine does not coincide with Andral's observations, whose researches lead him to consider tubercles as a secretion, which may take place indifferently, either in the ultimate bronchial tubes and air-cells, in the cellular tissue interposed between these, or in the interlobular cellular texture. He inclines to the opinion, adopted also by Professor Carswell, that the tubercular matter is at first liquid, and afterward becomes solid; and that a congestion, and even inflammation, are often concerned in giving rise to their production. "Observation proves," says he, "that the tubercular matter may be deposited on the surface of the mucous lining of the bronchiæ or air-cells, or in the cellular tissue uniting together the different parts of the lung." M. Magendie, and subsequently M. Cruveilhier, promulgated the opinion, that tubercular matter might be formed in the ultimate ramifications of the bronchiæ; and Andral confirms its truth by various facts, and, among others, by the appearances found in the lungs of a glandered horse. Andral also proves, by dissection, that tubercles may sometimes occur primarily in the lymphatic glands within the lungs; and he relates two rare instances, in which the tubercular matter filled the superficial lymphatic vessels of the lungs, and, in one of the cases, the lymphatics of other parts, and likewise the thoracic duct.— (See Clinique Méd., tom. iii., p. 13–20.) The corroboration of Andral's views by Professor Carswell's observations, as given in his Illustrations of the Elementary Forms of Disease, fasc. i., has been noticed in the foregoing pages.—ED.

---

* In 1828, a person named Robert Jeffries, aged 56, died in the Fleet prison, who had had a cough and shortness of breath for thirty years, and whose lungs were found, after death, filled with tubercles and abscesses.—ED.

† Young, ut suprà. Portal, Observations sur la Nature et le Traitement de la Phthisie. Bayle, Recherches sur la Phthisie Pulmonaire, Paris, 1810.

‡ On Diseases of the Chest, by Forbes, 2d edit., p. 272. Andral objects to Laennec's view, that if a tubercle necessarily began as a grayish semi-transparent granulation, this would be found in every situation where tubercles are met with. But, he asks, have such granulations ever been

tubercles in the lungs," says he, "differ in no respect from those situated in the glands; and which, under the name of scrofula, after being softened and evacuated, are often followed by a perfect cure." Here, however, the hollows are not incarned or filled up with a new material, but have their surfaces covered with a semi-cartilaginous membrane, which, as they thus heal, leave as many sound fistulæ as there were formerly tubercles.

In some cases, proper abscesses or larger vomicæ are found without any trace of tubercles: and especially when the disease has rapidly followed peripneumony, or taken place in persons of robust or plethoric habits. And when the catarrhal symptoms have been striking, and, in the increasing hoarseness and free discharge of muculent pus, have evinced extensive inflammation on the surface of the trachea, M. Portal has found the whole extent of the tube lined by a crust resembling bone. In some instances, the lungs, from the accretion of new matter, have weighed not less than five or six pounds, which is nearly four times their ordinary weight; but, in others, they have been so reduced as, in the language of the same writer, to leave "a vacant space" in the chest; or, in that of M. Bayle, "to be shrivelled into leather." On this account, breathing would be impossible, if it were not that the lungs in a state of health are capable of containing ten times as much air as is received by an ordinary act of inspiration; and hence are capable of losing a very large portion of their capacity without suffocation. In some cases, one lung has been entirely destroyed, and the office of respiration maintained by the remaining lung alone for many years.—(*Boneti Sepulchr.*, lib. i., sect. ii., obs. 167; *Parotti, Raccolti d' Opuscoli Scientifici*, xlvi., p. 275.) In other cases, blood, and even pins have been thrown up from time to time in considerable quantities without the least trace of ulceration, or breach of continuity in the membrane, or any part of the structure of the lungs.—(*De Haen, Ratio Med.*, i., xi., p 60; *Willan's Reports*, 1796, March 20.)

[Laennec has particularly invited the attention of practitioners to the successive development of tubercles in different parts of the lungs, as very important in a therapeutical point of view. Tubercles, he says, begin to show themselves in the first place, almost always in the top of the upper lobes, more particularly the right; and it is in these points that tubercular excavations of large size are most commonly met with. M. Louis coincides with Stark in stating, that such excavations are nearer the posterior than the anterior part of the lungs. According to Laennec, it is by no means unfrequent here to meet with cavities of this kind, when the rest of the lungs is quite sound, and does not contain a single tubercle; but, in this class of cases, the symptoms have only been equivocal, and the patient has died of some other disease. It is much more usual, however, to find one single excavation and several crude tubercles, in a pretty advanced state, in the upper part of the lungs; and the remainder of

these organs, though still crepitous, and in other respects sound, crowded with innumerable tubercles of the miliary kind, extremely small, semi-transparent, and hardly any of them with the yellow speck in the centre. This secondary crop of tubercles Laennec represents as being produced about the time when the first set begin to be softened. A third, still later crop, composed of crude miliary tubercles, with some yellow points in their centre, is situated still lower, and, finally, the basis and inferior edge exhibit the most recent formation of all.—(Op. cit., p. 282.)

The preceding account, given by Laennec, of the greater frequency of tubercles in the right than the left lung, does not agree with the statements of other distinguished pathologists. Of thirty-eight cases, in which M. Louis found one upper lobe wholly disorganized, twenty-eight were on the left side; of eight cases of perforation, seven were on the left side; and of the seven cases in which the tubercles were confined to one lung, five were on the left side.—(*Recherches sur la Phthisie Pulmon.*, p. 7, et seq.) According to Stark, the left lungs are more frequently affected than the right; an observation agreeing with the researches of Dr. C. Smyth.—(See *note by Forbes in Laennec*, p. 283.) The secondary production of tubercles is not confined to the lungs; and, at the period when the first crop is being softened, others make their appearance in various other organs. In fact, it is observed by Laennec that it is very rare in phthisical subjects to find these bodies only in the lungs; they almost always exist at the same time in the coats of the intestines, where they give rise to ulcers, which become the cause of the colliquative diarrhœa so often accompanying phthisis.—(Op. cit., p. 284.) With respect to the origin of intestinal ulcers, as described by Laennec and Dr. Bright, Andral admits that it may be the case in some instances but he contends that it is not so in all; for he has examined the bodies of several phthisical subjects, where the intestines presented an infinite number of ulcers, yet without any appearance countenancing the idea that they had originated in tubercles under the mucous membrane.—(*G. Andral, Anat. Pathol.*, tom. ii., p. 95.) In five sixths of the cases adverted to by M. Louis, the small intestines were more or less ulcerated. The ulcers were also nearly as frequent in the large intestines, the whole, or a great portion of the mucous membrane of which, in one half of the cases, although often red and thickened, was as soft as mucus. In only three cases did M. Louis find the large intestines universally healthy.—(*Louis, Recherches Anat. Pathol. sur la Phthisie*, p. 175, Paris, 1825.) In sixty-seven cases out of a hundred, Bayle also found the intestines in a state of ulceration; while Andral's dissections* con-

---

* Andral, Clinique Méd., tom. iii., p. 306. In his latter publication he remarks, that in phthisis the digestive canal is so commonly unsound, that this state may be considered, in some measure, as one of the elements of phthisis, and almost a constitu

firm all these reports by the fact, recorded in his most valuable work, that the intestines were perfectly sound in only one fifth of all the numerous cases under M. Lerminier in La Charité. The morbid changes in the mucous membrane of the intestines in phthisis are particularly noticed by Dr. Bright. They are denoted, he says, by unequivocal symptoms during life, and are traced in two different forms after death; "sometimes giving proof of a diffused irritation along the whole membrane from the pylorus to the termination of the rectum, evinced by increased vascularity, or by the appearance of innumerable minute black specks, which give a general gray colour to all the parts where they are most frequent; and sometimes affording evidence of a more severe affection, by the formation of numerous ulcers, which are found sometimes in the upper part of the duodenum, frequently dispersed along the whole course of the small intestines, but usually most abundant about the valve, and through the whole extent of the colon. These ulcers, as found in the small intestines, are usually, in the first place, very small and circular, and appear to originate from round, opaque, white bodies, about the size of half a sweet pea; but, whether these are altogether morbid tubercles, or are only enlarged mucous glands, it is no easy matter to decide. Certain it is, that they are most generally placed in that part of the circumference of the intestines which is most distant from the mesentery, and where the mucous follicular structure is most developed."—The ulceration of the large intestines is, according to Dr. Bright, most conspicuous about the cœcum and valve of the colon, where it also begins, as in the small intestines, by opaque deposites; but the disease proceeds to a much greater extent, sometimes involving the cœcum in one continued ulcer, and occasionally, though rarely, affecting the lining of the vermiform process itself. In the colon, the ulcers are generally oval, with elevated edges, and more or less distributed along the sides of the longitudinal bands. They are frequently found as low as the sigmoid flexure, and sometimes even in the rectum. They appear to Dr. Bright occasionally to undergo a healing process, their tubercular edges becoming softened down, and their flattened edges adhering

ent part of it. In about four fifths of consumptive patients who die in an advanced stage of this disease, the intestines are found seriously affected. Ulcerations are the most common change in them, and ordinarily situated at the end of the small intestines, and in the cœcum. Varying in number, shape, and size, and occupying (though not constantly) the follicles of Peyer, they are produced most frequently without pain, and occasion merely a more or less copious looseness. Even in the very commencement of phthisis, it is not uncommon to observe slight marks of intestinal irritation, alternations of constipation and diarrhœa, the latter gradually becoming permanent, like the lesion on which it depends.—(Anat. Pathol., tom. ii., p. 222.) The great opportunities which I have had of observing the progress of phthisis in the branches of the public service with which I am connected, lead me to recognise fully the truth of these valuable observations.—ED.

to the parts denuded by ulceration; but he states that this is not a frequent occurrence, because the more usual course of phthisis is to go on from worse to worse till it terminates in death; and little attempt is made by practitioners to change the condition of the intestines, while they consider the more urgent disease to be in another organ.—(Reports of Medical Cases, p. 151, 4to., Lond., 1827.) Sometimes, when phthisis is accompanied by numerous ulcerations of the intestinal canal, one of them makes its way completely through the bowel, and the immediate cause of the patient's death is peritonitis. —(G. Andral, Anat. Pathol., tom. ii., p. 106.) The inflammation thus excited in the peritoneum is generally acute and rapidly fatal; but sometimes of a chronic character, with symptoms of slower progress. Thus, Andral says, he can never forget the case of a consumptive young man, from whose navel, one day, an ascaris lumbricoides was discharged. He lived several weeks after the occurrence, the fistulous opening daily emitting a small quantity of matter resembling what the intestines usually contain. Examination of the body after death disclosed the existence of chronic peritonitis, with numerous pseudo-membranes, between which were formed several worms of the above kind, floating in the extravasated matter, some of which issued from the navel every day.—(Op. cit., vol. cit., p. 114.)

Besides the morbid appearances already mentioned as often complicating phthisis, are to be enumerated a softening of the mucous coat of the stomach, and frequently a general attenuation of all its coats; but, according to Andral, it is not usual to meet with ulcerations or tubercles in it (Andral, Anat. Pathol., tom. ii., p. 222), an increased vascularity and softened state of the brain, and disease of the absorbent glands of the bronchiæ and mesentery. In phthisical persons, the cartilages of the ribs and larynx are observed to become prematurely ossified.—(Andral, Anat. Pathol., tom. i., p. 300.)

Many ingenious experiments have been invented to distinguish between pus and mucus, in order to determine the actual nature of the disease. Such trials may gratify the curiosity of the pathologists, but from the variable and frequently complicated nature of the expectoration, as well in the most dangerous as in the earlier stages of the complaint, we can derive little assistance from this distinction. Mr. Hunter, as a test, employed muriate of ammonia, having observed that a drop of pus, united with a drop of this fluid, is rendered soapy, while neither blood nor mucus is affected by it.—(See Apostema Commune, vol. i., 503.) Mr. Charles Darwin—

"Heu miserande puer! si quâ fata aspera rumpas.
Tu Marcellus eris"—

proposed a double test of sulphuric acid and a solution of pure potass. If, on the addition of water to pus dissolved in each of these separately, there be a powerful precipitation, the matter made use of is determined to be pus; if there be no precipitation in either, it is mucus. But the simplest and truest character of pus, as was first observed and described by Sir Everard

Home, is, that it is a whitish fluid composed of globules contained in a transparent liquid ; that it does not coagulate by heat ; and is only condensed by alcohol. The presence of the globules, as remarked by Dr. Young, may be easily determined by putting a small quantity of the liquid between two pieces of plate-glass. If it be pus, we shall perceive, on looking through it towards a candle placed a little way off, the appearance, even in the daytime, of a bright circular corona of colours, of which the candle will be the centre ; a red area surrounded by a circle of green, and this again by another of red ; the colours being so much the brighter, as the globules are more numerous and more equable. If the substance be simply mucus, there will be no rings of colours ; though a confused coloured halo may sometimes be perceived by the mixture of mucus with blood or some other material.

As, however, consumption is by far more frequently a tubercular than a strictly purulent disease, and, perhaps, more generally fatal under the former than under the latter modification, the distinction here sought for is of less importance. It is of more consequence to ascertain whether morbid excavations from any cause, ulcerative or tubercular, have taken place at all ; and to this point the attention of physicians has been peculiarly directed, for the purpose, if possible, of obtaining a criterion.

It is now well known that M. Avenbrügger of Vienna suggested, more than half a century ago, the possibility of determining whether there were such morbid hollows, or other diseased condition of the chest, by the means of percussion by the hand (*Inventum Novum ex Percussione Thoracis Humani,* Vienna, 8vo., 1761): and that M. Corvisart was so much impressed with the importance of the suggestion, that he not only translated Avenbrugger's work on the subject from the German into the French tongue, but recommended his method warmly in his Clinical Lectures, and employed it so generally in his practice as to obtain for it a considerable degree of reputation. There is no doubt of its giving us a correct information at times : but the whole process is accompanied with difficulties which we shall notice presently, and its application is also of limited use. To remedy these evils, M. Laennec, from an early period of his life, conceived it possible to attain the same end, and with much greater exactness, by an acoustic instrument.* His mind was directed

to the fact, that if the ear be applied to one end of a beam of wood, we may distinctly hear the scratch of a pin when made at the other end : and, taking advantage of this hint, he first made a roll of a sheet of paper, wound up close, and well tied, when "applying," says he, "one end of it to the region of the præcordia, and placing the ear at the other end, I was as much surprised as gratified on hearing the heart beat more clearly and distinctly than I had ever done by a direct application of the ear itself." And hence he foresaw that the same instrument might also be employed to ascertain a variety of modifications in the pulsation of the heart and the larger arteries.

Having experimented upon a series of substances, he found that bodies of such a density as folded paper, wood, or cane, were best calculated for the purpose ; and he at length fixed upon a cylinder of wood of a foot long, and an inch and a half in diameter, with a bore or canal in the centre three lines in diameter. To render this instrument more portable, he made it divisible in the middle, like a German flute, the parts, however, being united by a screw.

When this cylinder, to which he gives the name of a STETHOSCOPE, is applied to the chest of a healthy person in the act of speaking or singing, nothing is heard but a kind of low murmuring, more distinct in some parts of the chest than in others : yet where an ulcer or other morbid excavation exists in the lungs, a very singular change takes place ; for the voice of the invalid is no longer heard by the disengaged ear, but comes entire to the observant ear that is applied to the end of the cylinder opposite to that affixed to the chest. This phenomenon M. Laennec ascribes to the greater degree of strength which the vocal sound exercises in a cavity of wider calibre than the bronchiæ themselves. And the opinion is rendered probable as the same phenomenon occurs when the cylinder is applied to the trachea or larynx. To this apparent transfer of the voice to the chest, the experimenter has given the awkward name of *pectoriloquism,* or *mediate auscultation of the voice.* And as the same instrument, or with slight variations, is capable of determining the morbid changes that take place in the breathing or contraction of the heart, he hence employs it in like manner to obtain a *mediate auscultation of the respiration,* or of the *pulsation of the heart,* or *the aorta.* For the first of these two purposes, however, the canal should be

---

* De l'Auscultation Médiate, ou Traité du Diagnostique des Maladies des Poumons et du Cœur, 2 tom., 8vo., Paris, 1819. Two years previously, M. Double had brought out his Semeiologie Générale, in which he mentions auscultation as a method peculiar to himself.—(See tom. ii., p. 31.) In the history of auscultation is a curious passage in Hook's Posthumous Works, p. 39, who, though not of the medical profession, actually foretold, as Dr. Elliotson has observed, the invention and uses of the stethoscope. The following short biographical notice of Avenbrugger is from the pen of Dr. Forbes :—Avenbrugger was born at Graets in Styria, in 1722. He graduated at Vienna, and afterward became physician in ordinary of the Spanish nation, in the Imperial

Hospital in that city. In Ersh and Puchelt's Literatur der Medicin, he is recorded as the author of two other works, relating to madness, one in Latin, published in 1776, and the other in German, in 1783. In the same record, Avenbrügger is stated to have died so late as the year 1809, in the 87th year of his age. The Inventum Novum was first translated into French in 1770, by Rozière ; but the subject attracted little attention till a second translation was published by Corvisart in 1808. The only English translation came out in 1824, with a selection of Corvisart's Commentaries, and additional notes.—See Original Cases, &c., by John Forbes, M. D., 1824 ; and art. Auscultation, in Cyclopædia of Pract. Med.—Ed.

graduall widened at the end applied to the chest, iny a funnel-form, to an ascent of about an inch, and then suffered to return suddenly to it general calibre. For the second purpose, the canal should be entirely obliterated, which may be easily done by a plug of the same kind of wood; the pulses being propagated through the cylinder by vibratory chords.[*]

PERCUSSION and AUSCULTATION are used simultaneously by many physicians in France; they were so by Laennec himself; and their comparative pretensions have been ably estimated in the same country by Dr. Colin (*Des Diverses Méthodes d'Exploration de la Poitrine,* Paris, 1824), as they have in our own by Dr. Forbes.—(*Original Cases,* &c., 8vo., London, 1824.)

The diseases in which the former method is chiefly employed, are phthisis, dropsy of the chest, chronic pleurisy, chronic peripneumony, emphysema of the lungs, pneumo-thorax, or a morbid communication of the interior of the lungs with the thoracic cavity, and hypertrophy of the heart, or a morbid enlargement of its substance.

In the use of this kind of exploration, the patient should be in a sitting posture, the points of the fingers brought close together may be employed, or the flat of the hand, and either upon the naked chest or with the body linen drawn tight over it. The action of percussion is applied, as circumstances may direct, to the forepart of the chest, the sides, or the back. In the first of which cases, the patient is to hold his head erect, and throw back his shoulders, that the chest may be protruded, and the skin and muscles drawn tight over its bones, by which the sound is rendered most distinct. In striking the lateral parts of the chest, the patient is to hold his arms across his head, so that the walls of the thorax may become tense, and the sounds rise distinct, as in the former instance. If the back be operated upon, the patient is for the same reason to bend forward, and draw his shoulders towards the anterior part of the chest, hereby rounding the dorsal region. The degree of percussion is to be varied according to the subject and the place; so that a more powerful impulse is to be employed in a fat or robust, than in a slender and emaciated subject; for the stroke that is sufficient to educe a clear sound in the latter case, may draw forth none in the former.

The amount of the sound must depend upon the general sum of the hollow contained in the chest, as in striking a cask, to which M. Avenbrugger very forcibly compares it. And hence, to determine whether this amount be more or less than it ought, it is necessary we should become first acquainted with its character in a healthy state, and accustom ourselves to the

* De l'Auscultation Médiate, &c., par R. T. H. Laennec, 1818. For a particular description of the construction of the stethoscope, consult Dr. Williams's Rational Exposition of Physical Signs, ed. 2, 1833. The best maker of stethoscopes that he has been able to meet with, is Grumbridge, turner, 42 Poland-street, Oxford-street.—ED.

percussion of those who are well. Its changes from this standard are of three kinds: it may be greater or stronger than natural; dull or obscure; or totally wanting. The first takes place where the cavity or hollow is enlarged, as in emphysema of the lungs, which, so to speak, resembles a cask comparatively empty, or rather containing a large volume of air: the second in œdema of the lungs, severe catarrh, or the earlier stage of peripneumony; in which the interior is more than usually occupied with dense matter: and the third in a tuberculated or hepatized state of the lungs, or when they are crowded with any other morbid secretion or induration, so as to be choked up, and leave no room for resonance.

The chief difficulties attending the diagnostic of percussion, are the long habit required for its use before it can be employed with any advantage, and the peculiar tact or address with which the stroke must be applied to produce its proper effect: the limited power of our having recourse to it in many cases of females, on the score of delicacy; and its occasional uselessness, perhaps deception, in other cases. Thus it is altogether unavailing in patients possessing much corpulence; and, although it affords a pretty clear indication in hydrothorax, when the chest is but partially loaded, and in peripneumony, before suppuration has taken place, yet as no sound is yielded when the chest is quite full of fluid, and a very different sound to what was at first elicited when a vomica has burst, both these diseases may be mistaken in their most important stage. In nervous coughs, asthmas, dyspnœas, and polypous concretions about the heart in young subjects, M. Avenbrugger himself admits the total inefficiency of his method.

The diagnostic of AUSCULTATION has some advantage in most of these respects. It is employed, as we have already observed, for three distinct purposes; as a test of the VOICE, of the RESPIRATION, and of the ACTION OF THE HEART AND AORTA.

When employed for the first purpose, or that of determining the state of the voice, it affords, under different circumstances, four different kinds of measure: as that of its degree of intensity, which M. Laennec has denominated *resonance*; its articulation, to which, as above stated, he has given the name of *pectoriloquism*; its suppression, or under-tone, which, from its supposed resemblance to the voice of goats, he has called *ægophonism*; and its vibratory clink, distinguished by the name of *metallic tinkling*. The first of these tests, when existing in a higher tone than natural, is supposed, for the most part, to indicate a certain degree of induration in the substance of the lungs. The second, or that of pectoriloquism, we have already noticed: it is a measurer of tubercular excavations communicating with the bronchia. The third indicates, in the opinion of M. Laennec, a flattening of the bronchial tubes. And the fourth a morbid communication of the interior of the lungs with the cavity of the chest.

Where the stethoscope, or chest-sound, is

employed as a measure of the RESPIRATION, it runs parallel with the modifications of percussion; and determines its intensity, its atony, and its absence; and detects also its combination with foreign sounds. Under the first modification it strikes the ear like the strong and sonorous breathing of children, into which the action of the trachea greatly enters; and on this account, the present modification is distinguished by M. Laennec by the name of *puerile*, or *tracheal*. It occurs especially in cases in which an entire lung, or a considerable portion of both, is rendered impervious to air, and particularly in acute diseases. The modifications of a *weak* or *absent* respiration upon the use of the cylinder indicate a general obstruction in the respiratory organ, and only vary in the degree or extent of such morbid change; and hence, as in the parallel modifications of percussion, they become tests of certain different stages of hydrothorax and peripneumony. The *foreign sounds* with which the cylinder detects the respiration to be occasionally combined, are various kinds of *râle* or *rattle*, to which the inventor of the present method has given the name of *crepitous*, and *subcrepitous, mucous, sonorous, sibilous*. The first, or *crepitous rattle*, is denominated from its resembling in sound the crepitation of salt in a heated vessel, or that emitted by frying butter. It is supposed to be a pathognomonic sign in peripneumony on its first attack, and occurs sometimes in hæmoptysis. The *subcrepitous* is an under-sound of the same kind, and indicates an œdematous state of the lungs. The *mucous rattle* is that peculiar kind of stertor called "the dead rattles" by the vulgar of our own country, though in a less degree of intensity. It is produced by a transmission of the breath through fluids accumulated in the trachea or bronchiæ, and measures the extent of such accumulation in catarrhal phthisis, hæmoptysis, and other important diseases. The *sonorous* and *sibilous* rattle are of less importance as diagnostics, and exhibit considerable ramifications in their character. The former gives sometimes a loud, and sometimes a deep snore, and sometimes the cooing of a wood-pigeon; the latter consists of a whizzing, or whispering tone, or of chirping like that of birds, often alternately ceasing and renewing its murmur. Both descriptions indicate some partial obstruction of the bronchial tubes; the latter perhaps of the smaller cells.

But the method of mediate auscultation is also employed to determine the degree of the STRENGTH AND ACTION OF THE HEART. And it is supposed to do this in four distinct ways: by measuring the extent of the pulsation; its shock or impulse; its sound; and its rhythm.

In a healthy person, of moderate stoutness, and well-proportioned heart, the action of this last organ, upon an application of the stethoscope, is not found to EXTEND beyond the range of the cardiac region, or the space comprised between the cartilages of the fifth and seventh ribs, and under the lower end of the sternum. It is, however, often traced, in a state of disease, through the whole of the left or the right side of the chest, as well as in the region posterior to them: which is generally owing to the feebleness of the heart, and the extenuation of its walls. It may therefore be taken as a general rule, according to M. Laennec, that a perceptible extent of the heart's action is in the direct ratio of its thinness and weakness, or inversely to its substance and power. A wide range of sound is often, indeed, traced when the heart is enlarged; but in this case its walls are often morbidly slender; and the enlargement consists in a mere dilatation of its ventricles. And hence this diseased extent of action is often traced in particular kinds of a hypertrophy of the organ.

The heart is also frequently found to be hereby affected in the SHOCK or IMPULSE of its stroke. The stouter and thicker the walls of the heart, the more violent is the impulse, insomuch that, as we have already had occasion to observe, the bed-clothes have sometimes been seen to be hereby elevated. This impulse is peculiarly caught hold of by the stethoscope: and is in some cases so energetic as even to lift up the observer's head, and to give an unpleasant shock to his ear. In proper hypertrophies, therefore, or such enlargements of the heart as are opposed to the preceding, in which the natural cavities are not much interfered with, and the augment consists altogether in a thickening of the parietes, we have reason to expect the present effect; which, in like manner, becomes a pathognomonic sign of such a disorder, and indicates its existence.

The stethoscope, also, measures the SOUND of the heart's pulsation. When the action of the heart is peculiarly violent, as in vehement palpitations, the individual himself becomes sensible of a peculiar sound, as well as of an increased impulse; and it has, indeed, in a few rare cases, been heard at a distance from the patient's person. Now, the application of the stethoscope heightens the sound of the pulsation considerably at all times, insomuch that, in its ordinary tenour of health, it communicates a certain degree of sonorous vibration, which cannot be perceived otherwise; the sound, however, produced by the contract on of the ventricles, and which is accompanied by the stroke of the pulse, being much clearer than that produced by the contraction or systole of the auricles, so that there is at all times to the ear of the experimenter a double or alternate sound, consisting of a louder volume succeeded by a lower. The seat of this double sound, in a state of health, is the cardiac region, to which it is limited; but in a state of disease it spreads much wider, and is heard distinctly in other places. The sound, moreover, varies from the standard of health both in intensity and in hebetude. Where the diameter of the heart is enlarged by a dilatation of its cavities, while its walls are weakened and rendered thinner, the sound is loud and distinct; but where, on the contrary, its walls are considerably thickened and enlarged, the cavities remaining but little disturbed, the sound is morbidly dull or obscure; and where the same organic thickening exists in considerable excess, the contraction of the ventricles produces a mere shock or impulse without any sound whatever.

The sound, moreover, is not only varied in its intensity, but in its vibration from a natural state. It is sometimes accompanied with a peculiar hissing, like that of a pair of bellows, and is in this state either continuous or intermittent, indicating, according to M. Laennec, a spasm or some other temporary and partial obstruction of the first organs of the circulating system. At other times, the accompanying noise is like that of a rasp or file ; which is always permanent, and evinces a permanent obstruction in some of the orifices of the heart. And in one or two instances, Dr. Colin has observed it combined with a crackling like that of new leather, which he supposes to be a pathognomonic indication of an inflammation of the pericardium, from his having traced this affection in a person who died during its existence.

The stethoscope is also supposed to detect in a peculiar degree the RHYTHM or relative duration and succession of the ventricular and auricular contractions. These are sometimes alternated with considerable but irregular intermissions, and sometimes far too rapid in their succession: both which changes from the rhythm of health indicate that kind of organic affection which is dependant upon delicacy of constitution, and is often congenital. They do not, however, augur the existence of any dangerous or even very serious malady.

It appears from this general outline, that the method of MEDIATE AUSCULTATION may be advantageously applied in one or all its forms to a detection of various important diseases of the chest, and especially to the different varieties of phthisis ; that it may be more generally employed than that of percussion, since corpulescency will seldom prove a bar to its use ; and that it is often more definite in its results.*

Notwithstanding, however, all the ingenuity that it evinces, it must often be found an imperfect guide in deciding on the actual state of a disease, or even indicating the disease itself, to say nothing of the long and repeated experience which is absolutely necessary to its being employed with precision. For, first, it

---

* For an extensive practical application of this method, see Andral's Clinique Médicale, ou Choix d'Observations Recueillies à la Clinique de M. Lerminier; Médecin de l'Hôpital de la Charité, Deuxième Partie, Maladies de Poitrine, 8vo., Paris, 1824 ; also Colin, des Diverses Méthodes d'Exploration de la Poitrine, &c., 8vo., Paris, 1824. John Forbes, M. D., Original Cases, with Dissections and Observations, illustrating the Use of the Stethoscope and Percussion in the Diagnosis of Diseases of the Chest, &c., 8vo., 1824. P. A. Piorry, de la Percussion Médiate, et des Signes Obtenus à l'aide de ce Nouveau Moyen d'Exploration dans les Maladies des Organes Thoraciques et Abdominaux, 8vo., 1828. Lisfranc, Mém. sur des Nouvelles Applications du Stéthoscope, 8vo., Paris, 1824. J. Hope, M. D., on the Diseases of the Heart and Great Vessels, Lond., 1832. John Elliotson, M. D., on Diseases of the Heart, fol.—Ed.

gives us a very doubtful kind of information concerning the existence of tubercles or vomicæ till they have actually broken, and produced numerous excavations, and consequently is of little use in the earlier stages of the disease.* Next, as it has been observed by M. Laennec himself, that some persons have an habitually relaxed state of some of the bronchial vessels, from hooping-cough or chronic catarrh, or a few

---

* The following information is derived from Professor Elliotson's Lectures :—It is only when the tubercles increase to a certain size, and approximate so as to form a mass, that you can expect any symptoms that are discernible by the ear. You will easily see that this must be the case, when you consider that, in the first instance, the tubercles which constitute this disease are exceedingly small and few, leaving a large portion of pulmonary structure perfectly healthy. The parts in which the symptoms cognizable by the ear are first noticed, are those below the clavicle, and this even before the tubercles have softened ; but, when they have become sufficiently large and numerous to occupy some space, you will not find, on striking the part under which such deposite is situated, the hollow sound of health, but a degree of dulness. In proportion to the size of the tubercular deposite, is the dulness of the sound. Then, if you listen with the stethoscope, and make the patient speak, you will find the voice resounds there in an unnatural way, because the solid substance of the tubercles is a much better medium for the conveyance of sound than the loose structure of the healthy lung. The sound, therefore, where the tubercles exist, is louder than elsewhere. You will likewise perceive what is termed *bronchophony ;* the same sound you hear on putting the stethoscope over the large bronchiæ. But it is to be remembered, that the voice naturally sounds louder under the clavicle than elsewhere, on account of the large tubes being there, and consequently you should not depend on this symptom alone ; but, to justify a decided inference that the bronchophony depends upon tubercular deposition, it should be united with the dead sound on percussion. Dr. Elliotson very properly also advises a careful comparison of the sounds perceptible on each side of the chest. When the tubercular mass softens, and a portion is discharged, so that the cavity is emptied, or nearly so, a new symptom presents itself, viz., *pectoriloquy,* or *pectoriloquism ;* for, as the bronchial tubes enter this cavity, you hear with the stethoscope the same sound as is heard on putting it over the trachea. If you make the patient cough, you hear a mucous rattle ; and, in proportion as more and more of the tubercular matter is spit up, and mere mucus remains in the cavity, the gurgling sound becomes louder and more distinct. In thin persons, pectoriloquy under the clavicles is natural, though no tubercles may exist : it should be heard decidedly in other parts of the chest to be sufficient evidence of the disease. When pectoriloquy is established, the dull sound on percussion ceases: The tubercular solid mass, which gave the dull sound, no longer exists ; and the part being now excavated, yields the same hollow sound as in health. It is to be remembered, says Dr. Elliotson, that though you have pectoriloquy, and a large space which ought not to be there, yet, the Ph· nomenon does not show the nature of the cavity, and it is only from the general symptoms that you are satisfied it is the cavity of the phthisis. A part of the lungs is sometimes separated by gan-

minute excavations in the organ of the lungs, without any serious deviation from a state of ordinary health; as also that patients occasionally recover from the tubercular species of consumption, and have the interior of the hollows or fistulæ hereby produced not filled up, but lined with a semicartilaginous membrane, thus effecting a natural cure,—the phenomenon of pectoriloquism will here be as distinct as in a morbid state of the pulmonary organ, and consequently may often lead the practitioner astray. And, lastly, as the stethoscope is limited, or nearly so, to the ulcerative forms of phthisis, the disease may exist in the catarrhal variety, and still elude its power. For these and other reasons, little dependance is placed on this instrument by M. Rostan, and still less by M. Foderé ; nor is it likely to obtain a very extensive use in our own country.* [It has

grene, and a cavity will remain ; so that you may here have pectoriloquy ; but the nature of the case is denoted by the fetor of expectoration, sudden extreme debility, &c. In chronic bronchitis the bronchial tubes may be very much enlarged at one spot ; and here, also, there may be pectoriloquy ; but the general symptoms of phthisis will be absent. No reliance is to be placed on the ear alone ; the symptoms which are audible, are only to be taken in conjunction with those which are general. Certainly, a very wrong view is taken of auscultation, when it is regarded as superseding the necessity of attending to the whole of the symptoms. As Dr. Elliotson further explains, a person may be labouring under ulceration of the lungs, and yet he may not afford the sign of pectoriloquy. If the cavity be near the surface of the chest, and the walls of the cavity be very thin, and if the bronchial tubes that open into the cavity have mouths so small as to bear no proportion to the cavity itself, you may have a large cavity, and yet no pectoriloquy at all. Here is another instance of the fallacy of observations made by the ear alone, to the exclusion of the other symptoms. The walls of the cavity must be of a certain thickness for pectoriloquy to be produced, and the bronchial tubes, opening into the cavity, must bear a certain proportion to it; but, when the cavity is near the surface of the lung, and only covered by pleura, there will be no pectoriloquy. If, however, you had seen the patient before the cavity became so large as to be out of proportion to the bronchial tubes opening into it, and before the sides of the cavity had become so thin, you would have had pectoriloquy. When the excavation is very large indeed, you will sometimes hear the metallic tinkling, a silvery-ringing sound, when the patient coughs, speaks, or breathes. The metallic tinkling, however, as Laennec observed, is heard also whenever a communication is formed between the air-cells and the cavity of the pleura. In the first stage of phthisis, nothing is to be learned from the ear ; and as the case proceeds, the case is generally clear enough without the information to be derived from this source ; but, when it is questionable whether the disease be bronchitis or phthisis, the existence of pectoriloquy in the latter affection, previously to the excavation becoming too large, will prove the true character of the complaint, and serve for the discrimination of one case from the other.—See Professor Elliotson's Lectures at the Lond. Univ., as published in Med. Gaz. for 1833, p. 227.—Ed.

* The editor does not coincide in this remark ; but he beheves, that, for the elucidation of many

also been employed to ascertain the existence of pregnancy, by catching the sounds of the pulsations of the fœtal heart, and of the movement of the blood in the utero-placental arteries.]

Such is the general history of phthisis. The pathology and practice are in a most unsatisfactory and unsettled state : nor can any thing be conceived more contradictory than the writings upon both these subjects. Boerhaave regarded consumption as a local disease, or conversion of all the blood and chyle into pus by means of an erosive ulcer seated in the lungs : Stahl as a general disease, unaffected by pus or any other acrimony. The latter ascribed consumption to the very abundant use of bark which was then prevailing in Europe ; while Morton regarded bark as his sheet-anchor in effecting a cure. Consumption, according to Brillouet and many other writers, is identic with scrofula, and is only to be cured by tonics, alkalis, corrosive sublimate, or other mercurial alterants employed for the cure of scrofulous affections.—(*Journ. de Méd.*, 1777.) According to Cullen, though it has an apparent connexion with scrofula, the analogy affords us no assistance in the treatment, and the remedies for the one are of no avail in the other.

Dr. Rush contemplated it for the most part as an entonic or inflammatory disease, and particularly in its first stage, though it is sometimes accompanied with a hectic, or even a typhus fever. And hence his principal remedies were, salivation, or bleeding, which he sometimes prescribed fifteen times in six weeks ; emetics, nitre in large doses, a milk and vegetable diet, walking in cold air even during an hæmoptysis, and afterward severe exercise. The hardships of a military life, says he, have effected cures in a multitude of cases of confirmed consumption ; and a riding postman has been relieved more than once by the pursuit of his occupation.—(*Med. Inquir. and Observ.*, i., 8vo., Phil., 1789 ; ii., 1793 ; v., 1802.) This bold practice excited many followers, and was tried with variable success upon a large scale. But a practice of an opposite kind, equally bold, and which soon became equally popular, was proposed at the same time by M. Salvadori, of Trent.—(*Del. Morbo-Tisico*, 2 vols., 8vo., Trent, 1787.) Consumption, in the view of this pathologist, is an atonic, instead of an entonic disorder from the beginning—a disease of direct debility, and not of inflammation ; and hence is only to be cured by an active plan of stimulants and roborants from the first. The patient's diet is to consist of copious meals of meat and wine, and his chief regimen to be that of climbing

ambiguous cases in the practice both of physic and surgery, the stethoscope will always be a valuable instrument. Its use in the examination of tumours, suspected to be of the aneurismal kind, but attended with obscurity, is generally recognised. For ascertaining doubtful fractures, and sometimes the presence of a calculus in the bladder, the stethoscope has also been recommended. —See Lisfranc, Mém. sur les Nouvelles Applications du Stéthoscope ; or Alcock's Translation ; and Dr. Ferguson's Obs. in Dublin Trans., vol. i.— Editor.

hills, or precipitous steeps, in the morning, as quickly as he is able, till he is out of breath and bathed in sweat, and then augmenting the perspiration by placing himself near a large fire. Mr. May, who adopted the same general principle, seems to have postponed the gymnastic part of the process till the symptoms were alleviated, and to have called in the aid of medicines which Salvadori regarded as superfluous. May's medicinal means were emetics, bark, and laudanum night and morning ; and for diet, he prescribed soup, meat, wine, porter, brandy and water, eggs, oysters, with proper condiments. Swinging was interposed twice a day, and horse-exercise was to complete the cure.—(*Lond. Med. Journ.*, ix., 1788.)

Many later writers believe consumption to be very generally produced by a habit of drinking vinegar daily to improve the figure : and Desault relates a case in which this effect was produced in the course of a month:—(*Sur les Maladies Vénériennes, la Rage, et la Phthisie*, 12mo., Bord., 1739.) Galen recommends vinegar as the best refrigerant we can employ : and Dr. Gregory, in 1794, gave the case of a patient, who recovered by using three dozen lemons daily. Dr. Beddoes felt justified in declaring fox-glove a cure for consumption as certain as bark for agues (*Essay on the Causes, Early Signs, and Prevention of Pulmonary Consumption*, 1799); Dr. Barton, of Philadelphia, has never known but one case cured by it, though others may have been palliated (*Collections for a Materia Medica*, 8vo., Philadelphia, 1798) ; and Dr. Parr asserts roundly, that it is more injurious than beneficial.—(*Med. Dict. in verb., Phthisis*, vol. ii., p. 410.)

Contradictory, however, as are these statements with each other, they are chiefly so, as being either too highly coloured or too indiscriminate. We have already considered phthisis under three varieties - or modifications, chiefly in respect to its being deep-seated or superficial ; the apostematous lying lowermost, the tubercular somewhat higher, and the catarrhal on the surface. But each of these, as it occurs in different constitutions, or under different circumstances, may exhibit very different symptoms, and demand a very different, and perhaps an opposite mode of treatment. And hence, most of the principles on which the preceding opinions and modes of practice are founded, may derive authority from particular examples of success ; and are so far correct, though, perhaps, none of them will apply to the whole. So considerable, indeed, are the shades of distinction from this multiplicity of causes, that every separate case of consumption should be allowed to speak for itself, and must call for much deviation from the widest line of treatment we can ever propose to ourselves under the form of general rules.

[Whether tubercular phthisis be ever really curable, is yet a contested point. It is certain, however, that the progress of the disease may be checked, and that some patients will live thirty years or more, without sinking under its effects. From various cases which Laennec

has reported, this distinguished pathologist concludes that tubercular phthisis is not beyond the powers of nature, though he admits that art possesses no certain means of accomplishing a cure. We may be well assured, he says, that a disease is irremediable, when we find employed in its treatment almost every known medicament, however different, or even opposite in effect ; when we see new remedies proposed every day, and old ones revived, after having lain long in merited oblivion ; when, in short, we find no plan constant but that of giving palliatives, and no means persevered in but such as are proper for fulfilling indications purely symptomatic.

With respect to what our author denominates *catarrhal phthisis*, if it be unattended with tubercles, the frequency of its cure is as undoubted as its total difference from a case of tuberculated lungs. But the apostematous phthisis, spoken of in the preceding pages, seems to imply either an abscess in the lungs from some cause not essentially connected with tubercles, or else the effect of that process by which pulmonary tubercles become more or less dissolved, and converted into a fluid exhibiting many of the qualities of pus. Apostematous phthisis, in the first of these meanings, must often admit of cure ; but, in the second, the frequency and even the possibility of cure are matters of dispute. After a careful perusal of the facts recorded by Laennec, in illustration of the mode in which nature sometimes cures phthisis, or repairs tubercular excavations, and after an impartial consideration of Professor Carswell's observations (*Illustrations of the Elementary Forms of Disease*, fasc. i., 4to., 1833), the editor conceives that the absolute incurability of apostematous phthisis must not be positively asserted, though the extreme rarity of a cure is as certain as any fact whatsoever in the whole mass of medical knowledge.[*]

According to Laennec, and with reference to the ascertained progress of tubercles, as detailed in the foregoing pages, the following are the most rational indications :—

1. As soon as we have ascertained the existence of the disease, our aim should be to prevent the formation of the second set of tubercles ; as, in this case, says Laennec, if the primary tubercular masses be not extremely large or numerous, which they very seldom are, a cure will necessarily take place after they are softened and evacuated.

* The following is Professor Elliotson's opinion on the important question of the curability of tubercular phthisis :—"I am quite sure, on account of the succession of tubercles, that persons *rarely* recover ; and I doubt whether the cavities heal so often as Laennec thought they did." The puckering and subjacent induration, noticed by Laennec as proofs of cicatrization of the lungs, are not considered by Dr. Elliotson to furnish unequivocal evidence of the fact, because similar appearances are commonly observed in the liver, under circumstances where there could have been no suppuration and ulceration.—(See Lect. at Lond. Univ., as published in Med. Gaz. for 1833, p. 230.) Andral has arrived at the same conclusion.—Ed.

2. The second indication should be to promote the softening and evacuation, or the absorption of the existing tubercles. These indications being comprised in the following ones, considered by the author of the present work, though expressed in different language, the editor does not find it necessary to deviate from the arrangement preferred by Dr. Good.]

The general intentions by which practitioners seem to have been guided in the midst of all the above contrarieties of practice, are the ensuing:—

I. To take off the inflammatory action.
II. To correct the specific cause, or phthisical diathesis.
III. To support under debility.
IV. To subdue the local irritation, and improve the expectoration.
V. To excite a change of action.

I. If the patient be of a robust habit, and in the prime and vigour of life, and if the symptoms indicate considerable inflammation, whether in the lungs or bronchiæ, such as, in the former case, fixed pain and weight in the chest, increased by lying on one side, with a dry but troublesome cough; and in the latter, a general soreness rather than pain in the chest, frequent and violent cough, with a copious excretion of a thin, offensive, and purulent mucus; and, in both cases, with a full and strong pulse, the fever, though remissive, making an approach towards a cauma, constituting the plethoric species of Portal, and the inflammatory of Dr. Rush, our object in both these cases should be to diminish vascular action by every means in our power. Venesection should be had recourse to with all speed: and though we shall seldom be called upon so closely to follow the steps of Dr. Dover as to repeat the operation fifty times in succession (*Ancient Physician's Legacy to his Country*, 8vo., Lond.) before we desist, it may be necessary to follow it up rapidly to the third, fourth, or fifth time. Portal, in the catarrhal variety, bled a man, seventy-eight years old, three times, with the happiest effect.*

[With regard to bleeding, Laennec does not consider it as a means of curing, or even preventing phthisis, but only as calculated to allay the inflammatory affections with which it is sometimes complicated. Laennec, as we have already explained, conceived that inflammation had little share in the production of tubercular phthisis, and he positively asserts that bleeding can neither prevent the formation of tubercles, nor cure them when formed.—(*On Diseases of the Chest*, p. 362, 2d edit. by Forbes.) The

* The patient may occasionally have attacks of inflammation, and suffer violent stitches in the side, with aggravation of the cough. Under these circumstances a few ounces of blood may be taken away, or the chest may be cupped and blistered. You have then, as Dr. Elliotson observes, to treat the case as one of inflammation of the chest, in a constitution of little power.—(See his Med. Lect. at Lond. Univ., as published in Med. Gaz. for 1833, p. 235.) If the patients be seized with hemorrhage, it is often necessary to treat them in the same way, and keep them on low diet.—ED.

latter part of the proposition is more generally admitted than the former; and the celebrated Broussais declares, that, in putting a stop to catarrh, a mild peripneumony, and pleurisy, by very active treatment at their onset, the occurrence of phthisis may be rendered very rare, whatever be the constitutional predisposition of the patient.—(*Doct. Med.*, p. 686.)]

Immediately after the use of the lancet, we should employ small doses of ipecacuanha or antimonial powder, so as to maintain a nausea till the pulse is lowered. Where the symptoms approach to peripneumony, the latter is to be preferred; where they lean to an inflammation of the mucous membrane of the bronchiæ, the former, of which three or four grains may be given three or four times a day, and will often prove expectorant, and unload the mucous follicles of the air-cells. The bowels should, in the meantime, be thoroughly opened by neutral salts, or uniting three or four grains of calomel with the nauseating powder: and after this, the fox-glove may be prescribed. Van Helmont first employed this last medicine as a specific for scrofula; but the only specific influence we know it to possess is on the kidneys, and on the action of the heart and arteries. It is for this last effect that we look to it in the present instance; the only effect, in all probability, that renders it of any advantage in consumption. In catarrhal phthisis, it seems sometimes, however, to improve the character of the exspuition: but this is, perhaps, a collateral result of the diminished action of the arterial system.

When a sufficient inroad has thus been made upon the inflammatory diathesis, we may content ourselves with an administration of the cooling neutrals, of which the nitrate of potash is one of the best. It may be given in almond emulsion in the proportion of a scruple to half a pint; and, if the cough be still troublesome, may be conveniently united with some light narcotic, as the extract of hyoscyamus or white poppy. The diet and general regimen are points of great importance; but upon these we shall have to speak presently.

It is not often, however, that phthisis commences with the inflammatory action we have been contemplating. Its ordinary march is unostentatious and insidious; and it takes possession of the fair and delicate, rather than of the firm and athletic frame, and chiefly in those possessing this figure who can trace the disease in their ancestors.

II. Of the proximate cause of this predisponent diathesis we know nothing: it is generally supposed to have a near analogy to that of scrofula; and when called into action, it commonly shows itself in the form of the tubercular variety; the tubercles themselves, though not occurring in a structure strictly glandular, bearing a considerable resemblance to scrofulous indurations. And on this account, as there are various medicines and a particular regimen that seem to have a beneficial effect upon a scrofulous habit, the same have often been resorted to for the cure of consumption. Thus; sea-water, the alkalis, almost all the metallic salts, and especially those of mercury, have been repeatedly tried, but apparently with very doubtful success. Mr. Spalding gives the case of a patient who had taken nearly two pounds of potash and soda, intermixed like common salt, with his ordinary food ; and, he states, with considerable benefit, after fox-glove, sulphuric acid, and bitters, had been successively found to disagree (*American Med. Repository*, vol. v., p. 220) ; and Dr. Trotter affirms, that among seamen in scrofulous consumption, as he calls the tubercular, salt and salt diet have proved of eminent service, but that the most effectual remedy is cinchona with sulphur.—(*Medecina Nautica*, vol. ii., p. 359.) Yet, though serviceable in particular cases of tubercular consumption, this class of medicines is far less efficacious than in strumous affections ; and the remark of Dr. Cullen, which he has confined to two or three varieties of them, may be extended to the whole. " In scrofula," says he, " the remedies that are seemingly of most power are, sea-water, and certain mineral waters ; but these have generally proved hurtful in the case of tubercles of the lungs. I have known," he adds, " several instances of mercury very fully employed in certain diseases in persons who were supposed at the time to have tubercles formed, or forming, in their lungs : but though the mercury proved a cure for those other diseases, it was of no service in preventing phthisis, and, in some cases, seemed to hurry it on."—(*Pract. of Phys.*, vol. ii., sect. 907, p. 293.) Nor have any other metallic salts been of more use than those of mercury. Dr. Roberts has had the spirit and perseverance to run through the whole range of such of them as can in any way be thought applicable to this complaint ; and has also had the candour, after a sufficient scale of trial in St. Bartholomew's (a candour how seldom to be met with l), to confess that none of them were administered with success. The experimental list consisted of silver in its nitrate ; lead in its superacetate, combined with opium, for counteracting its deleterious effects, zinc, in its sulphate and oxyde ; and the precipitate from the sulphate of potash, combined with myrrh ; arsenic in the neutral salt formed by a combination with potash ; manganese in its white oxyde, in doses of ten grains every six hours ;. cobalt in its black oxyde, in doses of from one grain to four ; ammoniated copper, and muriate of barytes. And with a like want of success, he tells us, in addition, were employed the vegetable narcotics aconite, hyoscyamus, stramonium, belladonna, as also toxicodendron.* We may hence, I think, nearly

conclude with Dr. Cullen, that " the analogy of scrofula gives no assistance in this matter." —(*Pract. of Phys.*, vol. ii., sect. 907.) And it is probably on this account, that M. Foderé has treated of tubercular and scrofulous con- sumption as two distinct forms of the disease.— (*Leçons sur les Epidémies et l'Hygiène Pub- lique*, tom. ii., Paris, 1823)

The preparations of iodine have a fair claim to attention here, as well as in scrofula, though great caution is necessary in employing them ; while it is only where the affection is pretty evidently tubercular that we have any reason to expect success from their use ; and even here, only in an incipient state of this variety. I have found a local application of the ointment re- lieve the cough and pain in the side, in some cases, more effectually than the tartar-emetic eruption. And if the erythema hereby produced should prevent a continuance of the applica- tion,* we may substitute the form of pills or of tincture ; giving half a grain of the iodine, in either mode of preparation, two or three times a day. [From the remarkable power of iodine in removing bronchocele, and reducing the size of diseased lymphatic glands on the surface of the body, the employment of it for the dispersion of pulmonary tubercles, as Dr. Forbes observes, was at once prompted and justified by the fairest analogy.† But, says he, there exists so material a difference between tuberculous diseases of the lungs and bronchocele, or enlargement of the external glands, notwithstanding their seeming analogy, as renders the efficacy of iodine in the former disease more than problematical. He considers it, however, as deserving of further trial.]

This part of our subject, however, ought not to be closed without briefly adverting to the practice of giving very small doses of tartar- emetic, dissolved in a large body of some simple menstruum, and continuing it for an almost in- definite period of time. Dr. Balfour dissolves two grains in six ounces of water, and prescribes an ounce of this mixture, that is, a third part of a grain of the tartarized antimony, to be taken every hour, and a smaller quantity where this is found to nauseate. M. Lenthois, in his Méthode Préservative, first directs a grain of tartarized antimony to be dissolved in eight tablespoonfuls of distilled water, and then six or eight pints of water, and sometimes not less than twelve, to be added. The solution, thus weakened, is em- ployed by the patient for common drink in every case and stage of consumption, either alone or with some other drink at meals, or occasionally with wine. [Tartarized antimony was strongly recommended by Dr. Jenner (*Letter to Dr. Parry*, 1822), but Dr. Forbes says that he has tried it, as well as setons, blisters, &c., without any benefit.]

III. Although in consumption we can avail

---

* Med. Trans., vol. iv., p. 129. Professor Cars- well has traced abundance of tubercular matter in scrofulous lymphatic glands : and since swellings of this kind are sometimes cured, he regards the circumstance as a consideration against the infer- ence, that tubercles of the lungs are absolutely incurable.—(See his Illustrations of the Element- ary Forms of Disease, fasc. i., 4to., Lond., 1833.) The tubercular substance being unorganized, can- not itself be affected or influenced by medicine ; and hence no doubt one principal difficulty in the attempt to cure phthisis.—ED.

* For its other troublesome effects, see Vol. II., Cl. VI., Ord. I., Gen. II., Spe. 1, Emphymá Sar- coma Bronchocele, p. 315.

† See Baron's Illustrations of the Inquiry re- specting Tuberculous Diseases, p. 220, and Gaird- ner on the Effects of Iodine, 1824.

ourselves but little of the treatment which applies to scrofula, and know nothing whatever of the nature of its specific cause, we see enough to convince us that consumption, in its general character, is, like scrofula, a disease of debility; and that wherever it exhibits an excess of vascular action, it is merely in consequence of being planted upon a plethoric or entonic temperament.* And hence another principle, conspicuous in most of the remedial plans to which it has given birth, is that of supporting the system while labouring under its influence.

This principle is well founded, but of difficult application; and, like the opposite principle of reduction, has been often carried to an extreme. During the last century, Salvadori in the Tyrol, and, in the present day, Dr. Stewart of Edinburgh, are justly chargeable with having done this by a very general allowance of nourishing diet, in conjunction with pure or diluted wine, bark, steel, and other tonics; exercise on horseback, and affusion with vinegar and cold water. In its ordinary course the disease itself is not only peculiarly prodigal of animal strength, but extremely protracted in its duration; while the fever, though remissive, rarely subsides altogether, or allows any interval of which we can avail ourselves.

In some instances, however, it does allow such interval, and especially where it has continued for a long period, and has broken down the general vigour of the frame; in which case, Moreton occasionally found the inflammatory form with which it commenced converted into a low intermittent, sometimes assuming the quotidian, but more generally the tertian type; beginning with cold fits, and succeeded by intense heat and profuse sweats, which exhausted the patient, though they left him in high spirits during the intermissions. And in such instances, it is possible that the tonic and stimulant plan of bark, wine, and even high-seasoned dishes, with cold air, cold bathing, and active exercise, so warmly eulogized by the writers just referred to, as well as by many others, may occasionally prove successful; and particularly where the disease is of the apostematous or catarrhal variety, and there is no constitutional taint to oppose at the same time. And it is here also, if anywhere, that the bustling and violent exercise, so strenuously recommended by Dr. Rush and Dr. Jackson, have a chance of proving beneficial. Dr. Chisholm tells us that, in particular cases, he found both these plans of decided service.—(*Climate and Diseases of Tropical Countries*, &c., 8vo., p. 112, Lond., 1822.)

But these are plans which cannot be brought into general practice; and, in supporting the strength of the system, we are ordinarily compelled to pursue a very different course: a doctrine, in a few rare instances, admitted even by Dr. Stewart himself.

The first means by which we are to aim at

accomplishing this is of a negative kind; and consists in saving the frame as much as possible from the profuse exhaustion it is daily sustaining, by calming the febrile irritation, and checking the colliquative sweats, which, as already observed, are never of a critical kind.

"I have sometimes succeeded very decidedly," says Dr. Young in a note to the author, while the first edition was printing, "in checking the sweats by Dover's powder; but I do not know that the progress of the disease has been much retarded by this palliation."

Bleeding, however plausible and even advantageous when the pulse is full and strong, and the pain in the side acute, can rarely be allowed when the frame is delicate and irritable, and the pulse small and weak. Where the local distress is considerable, it may be had recourse to as a palliative, but never carried beyond a few ounces, nor repeated without great hesitation.

To emetics there is less objection, but vomiting is here to be preferred to nauseating. The latter, though it lowers the pulse, produces considerable fatigue and distress. The former emulges the bronchial glands, and diminishes the local irritation by transferring it, through the means of a general glow and moisture, over the system at large. The dose may be repeated three or four times a week, and should have its power limited, as nearly as may be, to a single inversion of the stomach.

In the selection of emetics, some judgment is required; for those should be carefully avoided which, like the antimonial preparations, produce loose evacuations, and excite considerable sweating. The ipecacuanha is, perhaps, one of the simplest and the best. Dr. Simmons, however, preferred the sulphate of copper, giving first of all half a pint of water to the patient, and then the blue vitriol from two grains to twenty, according to his age and strength, dissolved in an additional cupful of water. In general he found, that the moment the emetic reached the stomach it was thrown up again, upon which the patient was ordered to swallow another half pint of water, which was sufficient to take off the nausea.—(*Practical Observations on the Treatment of Consumption*, &c.)

[Besides the use of ipecacuanha as one of the best emetics in phthisis, it is an important medicine for palliating the diarrhœa, under which many patients sink. This complaint, it is true, is often quite incurable, being connected with morbid changes in the bowels, already described in the preceding pages; but whatever benefit it does admit of will be derived from small doses of ipecacuanha. Thus, Dr. Bright says, when the disorder of the mucous membrane of the bowels is a prominent feature in phthisis, the purging may often be diminished, and the stools rendered natural in appearance, by giving the patient two grains of ipecacuanha three times a day.—(*Reports*, &c., p. 152.) The editor can add his testimony in favour of the practice, especially when the ipecacuanha is made into a pill with four or five grains of the confectio opii.]

The reason that prohibits nauseating, prohibits also the use of fox-glove: for though the

---

* Excess of vascular action sometimes depends upon phthisis being conjoined with various degrees of inflammation in the chest.—Ed.

pulse may be diminished, nothing more is obtained, and even this is obtained at too great an expense of sensorial power in the degree of debility we are now contemplating: and the remark will apply to most of the narcotics, whether of the umbellate or solanaceous order.. The neutral salts answer better, and especially nitre; and there is no modification of the disease in which this may not be given, and will not prove an excellent refrigerant as well as sedative. The general error, however, has been in administering it too freely, as in doses of fifteen grams or a scruple; in which case it becomes a direct irritant, and does much more harm than good. Seven or eight grains at a time, as already observed, is a far better proportion, and even in this quantity it will answer best if considerably diluted. It is often united with narcotics; but these are never found of use, unless they palliate the cough or local distress; for otherwise they increase the heat and quicken the pulse.

Most of the acids may also be employed for the same purpose, and with equally good effect. They may, indeed, be regarded in the joint character of sedatives, refrigerants, and astringent tonics: and have hence every claim to attention. The mineral have been most commonly in use; but, from their erosive quality, they cannot be thrown in sufficient abundance into the circulating fluids: and, on this account, the vegetable are to be preferred; and, of the vegetable, the fermented acids, which, though somewhat less grateful than the native, seem to be more effectual as tonics. The acetous acid was employed freely by Galen, diluted with water, who regarded it as the best refrigerant we can select. It is continued to the present day among the Moorish physicians at Tunis, and, according to the late M. Orban, with decided success. He observed its effects, during three months, upon one patient who appeared to be labouring under a confirmed phthisis from a neglected catarrh. The quantity of vinegar drunk in the course of every twenty-four hours, was seven fluid ounces intermixed with seven times as much rain-water, and sweetened with two ounces of refined sugar. This apozem was accompanied with astringent and tonic pills, composed chiefly of alum and sulphate of iron, of each of which two grains and a half were taken daily. The diet allowed was very slender, and consisted of nothing more than vermicelli or millet, boiled in water, and seasoned with a little oil and salt. Of this, only two meals in the four-and-twenty hours were allowed for several weeks. And, on the patient's becoming very costive under its use, the Moorish physician paid no attention to the symptom, but told M. Orban that a constipated state of the bowels was the best symptom that could occur, and that the more strikingly this prevailed, the more certain he was of a cure. M. Orban* left his patient in

a state of convalescence bordering on perfect health; and, on his return to France, pursued the same plan, with the exception of the iron, which he omitted as too stimulant, and found it, in many cases, eminently successful, though not in all. It has since been tried in our own country, and has often proved equally advantageous. Dr. Roberts has paid particular attention to its effects; and, upon a pretty extensive scale, has been satisfied with them. One of his cases was of a very unpromising aspeet, and consisted of a young gentleman, seventeen years of age, whose elder brother had died of phthisis. The cough, which in the morning was very considerable, was accompanied with expectoration sometimes streaked with blood; a confirmed hectic preyed upon him, and the night-sweat was so profuse that his hair was drenched with it. "My patient," says Dr. Roberts, "was at once relieved by the use of the acid, and in a short time so lost his complaints, that, by advice, he discontinued the remedy."—(Med. Trans., ut suprà.) The acetic and acetous acid seem to have been employed indiscriminately; over which the citric, which was also tried, did not seem to have any advantage. The acetous was usually given in half-ounce doses, with an ounce of infusion of cascarilla, and a little mucilaginous powder or sirup, the dose being repeated three or four times a day.

From these facts, as well as from a host of others of the same kind that might be adduced, the acetous acid appears to be a powerful sedative. It diminishes action generally, checks night-sweats, restrains hæmoptysis, retards the pulse, and produces costiveness. In hæmoptysis, I have carried the use of the acetous acid much farther than was prescribed by Dr. Roberts, and with manifest and unmixed advantage.

The proper astringents have also not unfrequently been employed in phthisis for the same negative purpose of producing strength by checking the exhausting discharges of sweat, pus or mucus, blood, and often diarrhœa; but they have rarely proved successful. Some degree of benefit seems occasionally to have been derived from the use of oak bark, several of the agarics (De Haen, Rat. Med., tom. ii., 567; Dufresnoy, in Corvisart, Journ. Med., cent. vii., 531, 1804) given in the form of lozenges, and the acetate of lead;* but they have far more generally been employed without success, or with more mischief than advantage.

The most direct means of supporting the system would be by those tonics that unite an astringent with a bitter principle; but we have

---

* Med. Trans., vol. v., art. xviii. This treatment with vinegar falls under the head of what is called the empirical practice. The account is altogether unsatisfactory: the case is called a confirmed phthisis; but was it of the tubercular kind?—ED.

* Ewell in Sédilot's Journ. Gén. Méd., xliv.; Hildebrand, id., xxxvi. Frequently the largest doses of opium, such as will produce great stupor, and astringents in doses that even overload the stomach, will not succeed in checking the diarrhœa. Frequently there is ulceration of the intestines, and then the sulphate of copper is recommended by Dr. Elliotson. It has a tendency to produce sickness; but this may be subdued by hydrocyanic acid. In the event of this not answering, we may try ipecacuanha in small doses joined with opium, as already mentioned.—ED.

already observed, that the system is usually, and particularly in the beginning and at the height of the disease, in too high a degree of irritation for a convenient use of any medicines of this kind; though where the complaint has lasted for many months, and appears to be rather of the tubercular or catarrhal, than of the apostematous variety, these may sometimes be employed with great success. The Angustura bark generally agrees better than the cinchona; and to this myrrh and iron may at such times be added in increasing doses, and particularly as prepared in the mistura ferri composita of the London College. In the tubercular variety, the cinchona seldom agrees in any stage: Dr. Cullen conceives never; and tells us that, even where the disease has assumed something of an intermittent character, quotidian or tertian,— and he has, on this account, been tempted to try it in free doses,—he has in no instances succeeded so as to establish a complete cure. "For in spite," says he, "of large exhibitions of the bark, the paroxysms, in less than a fortnight or three weeks after they had been stopped, always returned, and with greater violence, and proved fatal." In the latter stages of the apostematous variety, and especially where the vomicæ are small and in perpetual succession, he thinks, however, it may be of service in restoring a healthy action, and promoting a secretion of genuine pus.

In this last case, and here perhaps only, we may venture with success on the use of the cold bath. In a more irritable state or stage of the complaint, the tepid bath may occasionally prove serviceable; and, where it does so, should be repeated three or four times a week, or even oftener. Of the effect of the *baños de tierra* of the once-celebrated Solano de Luque, I cannot speak from personal knowledge. It consists in burying the patient up to the chin in fresh mould. It would be most obvious to suppose that this was designed to act as a tonic, and check the undue tendency to perspiration by a protracted chill, but that Van Swieten tells us the smell of fresh earth is serviceable, and approves of it on this account. It has since been recommended by Dr. Simmons and M. Pouteau.

Before, however, the hectic, or the general irritability of the system, has so far subsided as to render tonics advisable, our chief dependance for giving support to the system must be upon diet and regimen.

The diet should be of the lightest kinds, and in very small proportion, and with long intervals of rest; for some degree of exacerbation, in the stage of the disease we are now contemplating, is always produced by the process of digestion. Under *limosis expers* we have already seen how very small a portion of food is necessary for the support of life; when neither mental nor muscular exercise is made use of; and though hectic fever itself is a source of very great exhaustion, this exhaustion will be less in proportion as we produce less excitement, whether from eating or any other cause. And hence the most cautious physicians, from the time of the Greeks to our own day, have concurred in recommending food in small quantity; as well as of the lightest materials. It is not merely the stomach and its collatitious organs that are hereby put at rest, but the circulating system, the assimilating powers, the brain, and the intestines.

The food itself should consist principally of milk and the farinaceous parts of plants, if it be not limited entirely to these: and upon a diet of this kind, in conjunction with temperate air and exercise, the Greek physicians placed their only hopes of a cure. Whether it be necessary to pay that strict attention to the different kinds of milk which we find inculcated by many writers of established reputation, I cannot fully determine. Galen recommends woman's milk as lightest of all, then ass's, next goat's or ewe's, and lastly cow's (*Opp.*, tom. vi., 130, 131, edit. Basil., 1542); and Van Swieten adopts the recommendation of Galen.—(*Comment.*, tom. iv., sect. 1211, edit. Lugd. Bat., 1764.) Mare's milk has since been proposed as preferable to all these: but the analyses published by different chymists vary so much from each other, that it is difficult to come to a conclusion. If the experiments of Stipriaan may be depended upon, mare's milk contains most sugar, and least cream, butter, or caseous matter; and woman's milk most sugar, and least butter and caseous matter, next to mare's, with most cream, next to sheep's.—(*Crell's Chemische Annales,* sect. viii, p. 138, 1794.) Whence mare's milk should be the lightest of the whole, but less nutritive than woman's. According to Parmentier, however, ass's milk contains less proportion of caseous matter than any of the rest.

Peculiar properties may sometimes be given to milk by the food fed upon; and hence Galen endeavoured to render it more astringent, by placing the animal that was to furnish it in pasturage enriched for the purpose with agrostis, lotus, polygonum, and melyssophyllum. And as the patient became convalescent, and could bear a richer nutriment, he was allowed to sail down the Tiber and use the cow's milk of Stabiæ, which was peculiarly celebrated for its excellence.

When ass's milk cannot conveniently be obtained, its place may be supplied with what has been called artificial ass's milk; which is a mixture of cow's milk and animal mucilage, diluted in a farinaceous apozem, rendered slightly sweetish and aromatic by eryngo. The ordinary form consists in boiling eighteen contused snails with an ounce of hartshorn shavings, of eryngo-root, and pearl-barley, in six pints of water, to half its quantity, and then adding an ounce and a half of sirup of Tolu. Four ounces of this are usually taken morning and evening, with an equal quantity of fresh milk from the cow.—(*Med. Trans.*, vol. ii., p. 341.)

The chief foods which have been allowed in the general treatment of consumption in its earlier and middle stages, in conjunction with milk and the farinacea, are the vegetable and animal mucilages, but particularly the former. And of these, that obtained from the Iceland liverwort has been held, and deservedly so, in the highest degree of estimation ; for, to an aliment of sufficient nourishment, it adds a tonic power by its bitterness ; yet a power that, so far from increasing vascular action, seems rather to quiet it ; as though the bitter principle were itself in possession of something of the sedative quality of the hop, Ignatius's bean, or some other plant that decisively unites the two.

In supporting or recruiting the strength, a due attention to air and exercise is also of high importance. The advantages offered by the first are those of a mild, dry, and equable atmosphere ; and, probably, these are the whole. If the patient's own country give him these, he need not wander from home. If it do not, he must create an artificial atmosphere in his own chamber, or set of chambers, by keeping the thermometer at from 60° to 65° of Fahrenheit, and confining himself to this temperature ; or he must seek the atmosphere he stands in need of in a foreign climate. The disadvantage of the former is, that though he may support the requisite temperature, he cannot conveniently obtain a sufficient change of air, nor so well avail himself of the various exercises that might be useful to him, as if he were at liberty to go abroad.

Hence a change of abode has been recommended in all ages to those whose native soil is subject to considerable and sudden atmospherical variations, though pathologists have by no means agreed upon a meteorological standard. For the patient's residence in our own country, the southwestern boundary of the Cornish coast, and particularly Penzance, seems to offer the best asylum : and where a foreign climate is recommended, it should lie between thirty and forty degrees of latitude : if lower than this, the disease, and especially where ulceration has taken place, seems to be exacerbated instead of diminished, and, consequently, its fatal issue to be quickened (*Sir G. Blane, Observations on the Diseases of Seamen,* 8vo., 1785) ; notwithstanding that to the natives consumption is little known within the tropics.

In Great Britain, the annual mortality from this disease in 1811, when the population was calculated at 23,353,000, seems to have amounted to 55,000, being a proportion of 1 in 224. In Geneva, from a very exact register, M. Prevost Moulton estimates it at 1 in 521.— (*Chisholm, on Tropical Climates,* p. 234.)

Generally speaking, however, a change of climate or of local situation has been determined upon too late ; and hence has not been attended with all the benefit that might otherwise have been reasonably hoped for. On which account many pathologists have considered it as of little importance, if not more injurious than staying at home, though the most celebrated spots should be selected.

Thus Dr. Carmichael Smyth asserts, that Madeira is unfavourable to the consumptive when the lungs are materially injured, notwithstanding the mildness and equability of its climate.[*] Nice and Naples are said to be equally

unfriendly from the neighbourhood of mountains ; and Dr. Southey's inquiry has led him to conclude that, in Malta, Sicily, and other islands in the Mediterranean, phthisis, though a rare disease among the natives, does not appear to be retarded in those who visit them for a cure.[*] M. Portal dissuades from all such trials by affirming that there is no dependance to be placed upon them, since he has seen the disease accelerated in Englishmen, or those of other northern nations, by a visit in quest of milder air to the south of France ; while, in the natives of Languedoc or Provence, it has been restrained by a removal to Paris.—(*Obs. sur la Nature et le Traitement de la Phthisie Pulmonaire,* ii., p. 358.) Nor are the observations of M. Foderé much more encouraging to a trial of any part of France : as he expressly tells us that, in the provinces on the borders of the Mediterranean, phthisis commits the most horrible ravages ; while, out of 62,447 deaths which took place at Paris in the years 1816, 1817, and 1818, thirteen thousand eight hundred and eighteen fell victims to diseases of the chest.—(*Leçons sur les Epidémies et l'Hygiène Publique,* tom. ii., 1813.)

The whole of this, however, only shows us that very great care is necessary in ascertaining the state and stage of the disease, the patient's constitution, and the local features of the situation that may be proposed for his residence : and we have already shown how it is possible for a mild and relaxing climate to prove remedial to strangers, while it may even become a predisponent cause of phthisis to natives. Where, in the commencement of the disease, there is great irritability or an inflammatory diathesis ; or, in its advance, the strength of the constitution is greatly reduced ; and especially where an obstinate diarrhœa has supervened, the fatigues of journeying and of a sea-voyage, and the necessary relinquishment of many of those minuter, but still important conveniences, to which the patient has been accustomed at home, will more than counterbalance all the advantages he might derive from the possession of a milder and more equable atmosphere.

The topography of the situation about to be chosen is of equal importance ; for if it be strongly marked by lofty cliffs or mountains,[†] the air will seldom circulate freely, but rush in currents in some parts, and be obstructed and become stagnant in others. Such is the state of Hastings on the Sussex coast of our own country,

---

monary Consumption, &c., 8vo., 1787. In Madeira the thermometer commonly ranges from 60° to 75° ; and, in the greatest extremes, seldom exceeds these limits by more than 5°.—See Journ. of Morbid Anatomy, Ophthalmic Medicine, &c., vol i., p. 103.—ED.

[*] Obs. on Pulmonary Consumption, 8vo., 1814. Phthisis was common enough among the inhabitants of Malta and Minorca when the editor formerly visited those islands as an army surgeon. —ED.

[†] Laennec observes that, though phthisis is unfrequent in mountainous countries, it runs a very rapid course when it does occur in them.—On Diseases of the Chest, p. 368, 2d edit. by Forbes.

---

[*] Account of the Effects of Swinging in Pul-

which would otherwise form an excellent asylum for those who are subject to pulmonary affections, and cannot remove far from their native abodes. The shore is skirted by two enormous cliffs of sandstone, that rise between two and three hundred feet in perpendicular height. The old town is built in a deep ravine opening towards the northeast, that lies between them, and the new town immediately under the cliffs, fronting south and west; and hence, while the air is rushing in a perpetual current through the former, it becomes stagnant, heated, and suffocative in the latter.* On this account, it has been uniformly found that small islands, without any great boldness of feature, enjoy the most equable temperature, and, when within the range already pointed out, form the most favourable situations for consumptive cases. Madeira, in some of its positions, is one of the best foreign stations in the winter season; but from its mountainous face, and the snow, sleet, and cold winds to which it is occasionally liable, catarrhal affections, and even genuine consumption itself, are, according to Dr. Gourlay, not uncommon to the natives; and in removing to it, therefore, it will be necessary to select a spot of sufficient elevation, and equally sheltered from the meteorological evils of currents, tempests, and suffocative heat. And, however fortunate a patient may be in procuring such a residence at Madeira, he will, in all probability, succeed still better, and obtain a greater choice of desirable situations, at Nice, Pisa, or even Hières; and might be more comfortable at Villa Franca than even at any of these, if the town were now of sufficient extent and population to offer him the conveniences he will always want, and especially that of a roomy and excellent lodging-house, which, in the present decayed state of this town, is not a little difficult to be obtained. The depth of the bay, and the very abrupt elevation of the hills that rise in a most beautiful and romantic amphitheatre behind it, enable the patient to make a considerable range without exposure to sudden currents. The east is its only unsheltered quarter, and, from the evils attendant on occasional chills, he must sedulously avoid this.

But we have already shown that a high degree of heat habitually applied to the body, as in intertropical regions, as a source of debility and irritation, may itself call forth a latent consumptive predisposition into action, and become a source of phthisis, as well as a temperature of unfriendly cold. The variety in this case, as we have already observed, is almost always the tubercular, and often combined with a strumous diathesis, if it do not originate from it. The change must here, therefore, be to a cooler instead of to a warmer temperature; to an atmosphere of a more refreshing and invigorating power; to a climate still mild, but less exciting, equable in its thermometer, and tonic in its general influence.*

After all, the most equable of temperatures is that of the sea itself: and hence many patients who feel inconvenience from a residence on the seaside, are almost instantly relieved by sailing a few miles distance from it. This has often been resolved into the exercise of sailing, or the sea-sickness which in many instances is hereby excited. It is, nevertheless, a distinct advantage from either, and resolvable into the explanation just stated.

Sea-sickness, however, is of unquestionable service in many cases, and particularly in those in which a protracted nausea by other means has already been recommended. The exercise of sailing is useful on another and a very different account All motion without exertion, or with no more exertion than gives a pleasurable feeling to the system, which the Greeks expressed by the term æora, instead of exhausting, tranquillizes and proves sedative. It retards the pulse, calms the irregularities of the heart, produces sleep, and even costiveness. Hence sailing on the Tiber was a common prescription among the Roman physicians, and many consumptive patients have found great benefit from long voyages, in which they have suffered no seasickness, and have been exposed to many varieties of atmospherical temperature. Hence, too, the well-known advantage of exercise in a swing, or in a carriage, on horseback, or even on foot, as soon as these can be engaged in with comfort; the organs of respiration, like those of every other kind, deriving strength, instead of weakness, from a temperate use of them.

Gymnastic medicine, however, seems by many pathologists to have been carried to an extreme; and especially by Sydenham, who employed horse-exercise in all stages of the dis-

* For a more inviting account of Hastings, as a place of resort for invalids, see Harwood's Curative Influence of the Southern Coast: or the Journal of Morbid Anatomy, &c., by Dr. Farre, vol. i., p. 121.• Laennec considered maritime situations as exhibiting a less prevalency of consumption; but Dr. Forbes, who has resided long on the southern coast of England, deems the opinion unestablished by proof During a residence of five years at Penzance, Cornwall, a place much frequented by consumptive patients on account of the mildness and equability of its temperature, Dr. Forbes had extensive opportunities of observing the effect of change of climate on phthisis; and he says, that, in the greater number of cases, the change was not beneficial.—Transl. of Laennec, 2d edit., pp. 324 and 367.

* The following remarks by Dr. Clark deserve attention:—"A change of climate having been decided on, the particular situation to be selected becomes a question. Professor Laennec's decided preference of a maritime residence is not, perhaps, founded on very extensive experience. Certain it is, however, that as well in this country as on the continent, the places usually resorted to by consumptive invalids are on the seacoast, or at no great distance from it. In almost every case, when the removal to a milder climate can be effected by sea, this means is much preferable to a journey by land. In some cases, the good effects produced by a voyage are very remarkable."—(See Laennec, by Forbes, 2d edit., p. 368.) No doubt, as Dr. Forbes has explained, change of climate often fails, because tried too late; and some deception prevails respecting such cases as are benefited, and which are frequently only specimens of chronic catarrh, or chronic bronchitis.—ED.

ease, and roundly affirms, that neither mercury in syphilis, nor bark in intermittents, is more effectual than riding in consumptions.—(*Opp.*, P. 629.) Nor is carriage-exercise, says he, by any means to be despised, though not equal to that of the saddle. Hoffmann and Baglivi adopted the same opinion, and laid it down in terms nearly as unqualified. Where phthisis is a secondary disease, and dependant upon some obstruction of the digestive viscera, exercise of this kind may, in many instances, be employed as in important co-operation with other means, even from the beginning ; and to such cases of consumption Desault judiciously limits it. In the present day, it has been revived by Dr. Stewart under a variety of ingenious modifications, and appears in many cases to have afforded relief : but the constitutions of mankind must strangely have altered since the days of Sydenham, if the severity of horse-exercise could at that period have been employed as a specific remedy in consumptions of every kind. Stoll did not find it so in the middle of the last century ; for he tells us, that, if a consumptive patient mount his horse, he will ride to the banks of the Styx as surely as if he were in a pleurisy. —(*Rat. Med.*, i.) And Stoerck died consumptive, though in the habit of riding, killed by an hæmoptysis apparently produced by this exercise.—(*Quarin*, pp. 162, 163.)

IV. Another part of the curative process in the disease before us has consisted in endeavouring to subdue the local irritation, and improve the secretion from the lungs. This has been chiefly attempted by fumigations, medicated airs, expectorants, and sedatives.

Bennet was strongly attached to the first of these, and thought they proved peculiarly detergent, and enabled the patient to throw up a more laudable discharge with increased facility. He sometimes employed aromatic herbs immersed in hot water, over which the patient held his head, surrounded with cloths to confine the vapour, which was thus inhaled with every inspiration. But he seems to have placed more dependance on an inhalation of the fumes of various terebinthinate resins, as frankincense, styrax, and turpentine itself, mixed into a powder or troche with a few other ingredients, and burnt on coals : to which he sometimes added a considerable proportion of orpiment. And such was the success ascribed to this practice, that Willis, not many years after, resolved the greater exemption of certain parts of England and Holland from coughs and consumptions, to the turf and peat fires which the inhabitants were in the habit of using, and the arsenical principle which was intermixed with the material. In our own day, terebinthinate fumigations have been very extensively tried, in consequence of the warm recommendation of Sir Alexander Crichton,[*] who thought he had perceived great and decisive advantage from the aroma of pitch

and tar diffused through rope manufactories, ships, and other places where these articles are in perpetual use. I have tried this repeatedly by heating a tin vessel of tar over an oil or spirit-lamp, and thus impregnating the atmosphere of the chamber with the powerful vapour that arises. In doing this, however, we must be careful not to burn the tar ; for in such case the room will be filled with an empyreumatic smoke, that will greatly augment the patient's cough instead of diminishing it : and it will be also advisable, as recommended by Dr. Paris (*Pharmacologia*, vol. ii., p. 339, edit. 1822), to add about half an ounce of subcarbonate of potash to every pound of tar, for the purpose of neutralizing its pyroligneous acid, the fume of which will otherwise ascend and prove irritating.

In those states of the disease in which terebinthinates, as myrrh, benzoin, or copayva, may be taken internally with a prospect of success, this kind of fumigation will sometimes prove useful also, and it is hence far better adapted to the tubercular and catarrhal than to the apostematous variety. In a chronic state of the first two I have sometimes thought it serviceable, but I have more frequently used it without any avail. The experience of Dr. James Forbes, who has tried this remedy upon an extensive scale, very closely coincides with these remarks. Of nineteen cases of phthisis, of which he has given us an account, it neither cured nor improved any ; on eight it had no effeet ; and mischievously suppressed the secretion, injured the breathing, and increased the disease in eleven. In cases of chronic catarrh, where the secretion constitutes the disease, and tonics and astringents are useful, it often succeeded. Of thirty-two cases narrated, it had no mischievous effect on any ; no effect whatever on eighteen ; improved six, and cured eight.—(*Remarks on Tar-Vapour, by James Forbes, M. D.*, 8vo , 1822.)

Pneumatic medicine, which about thirty years ago was in the highest popularity, does not appear, when candidly examined, to have been more successful. Oxygen gas has, in almost every instance, proved so stimulant, and so much increased the signs of inflammatory action, that, though it has seemed occasionally to afford a momentary relief in a few cases, it has rarely been persevered in more than a fortnight, by which time it has often suppressed the usual expectoration, and produced an hæmoptysis.— (*Fourcroy, Annales de Chim.*, iv., p. 83, 1790.)

There was much more reason and ingenuity in recommending an inhalation of hydrogen intermixed with common air than of oxygen, since the effect of this gas in destroying the irritability of the living fibre is known to every one ; and it was hence a plausible conjecture, that, by being applied immediately to the seat of the disease, it might sufficiently subdue the inflammatory impetus, change the action of the ulcerated surface, improve the secretion, and annihilate the hectic. The experiment has been tried at home and abroad upon a pretty extensive scale, by employing different proportions of hydrogen, so that the patient has twice a day

---

[*] Practical Observations on the Treatment and Cure of several Varieties of Pulmonary Consumption ; and on the Effects of the Vapour of Boiling Tar in that Disease, Lond., 8vo., 1823.

breathed from a pint to a quart of gas at a time, diluted with from twelve to six times its measure of common air ; and, making every allowance for an exaggeration of statement in those who have most warmly engaged in the practice, it seems difficult not to concede that it has proved serviceable in various cases.

A combination of hydrogen with common air seems, indeed, to be beneficial in various other modes of application ; but whether by lowering the ordinary stimulus of common air, or by directly diminishing and exhausting the nervous influence communicated to the lungs, it is not easy to determine. In either way, however, it has an equal tendency to indispose them to inflammatory action. Thus Clapier relates a case of confirmed consumption cured by an habitual residence in a coal-mine (*Journ. Méd.*, xviii., 59), and expressly states that the matter expectorated soon began to assume a more healthy appearance, and was excreted more freely. It is, in like manner, a common remark, that the miners of Cornwall are more generally exempt from phthisis than most other persons (*Southey, Observations on Pulmonary Consumption*, 8vo., 1814), and that butchers, who are perpetually engaged in slaughter-houses, and surrounded by a vapour impregnated with hydrogen, possess an equal emancipation. It is probably to this cause, if to any, we are to ascribe the benefit which Bergius found consumptive patients derive from a residence in cow-houses (*Neue Schwed. Abhandl.*, 1782, part iii., p. 298), and which was, not long since, a fashionable mode of practice in our own country.*

Expectorants and demulcents have also very generally been employed for the same purpose —that of subduing the disease by exciting a healing action in the tubercles or ulcerations, indicated by improvement in the exspuition.

Of the general nature and mode of action of these classes of medicines, we have already spoken at large in discussing the treatment of cough and asthma : and our remarks, therefore, upon the present occasion, will be but few.

Where the irritation is considerable, and accompanied with much increase of vascular action, as in the commencement of the apostematous and catarrhal varieties, the best demulcents, and, indeed, the only medicines of this

kind we can employ as palliatives, are the vegetable mucilages, as of tragacanth, quince-seeds, or gumarabic. Where it is necessary to diminish the general action, these may be united with small doses of ipecacuanha, or of squills, which have the double power of exciting nausea, and unloading the mucous follicles of the bronchiæ as expectorants. And, where the cough is very troublesome and the pain acute, they should be united with narcotics, as opium or hyoscyamus.

In a more advanced stage of the disease, and through the entire course of the tubercular variety, except where hæmoptysis is present, the expectorants, more properly so called, have often been employed with advantage. One of the oldest of these is sulphur, and, perhaps, one of the best : from its not readily dissolving in the first passages, it is carried to the rectum, and skin sometimes, with little alteration, and hence gently stimulates both extremities, loosens the bowels, and excites a pleasing diapnoe on the surface. It is in this way it appears to be serviceable in an inflammatory or tubercular state of the lungs. It was in high repute among the Greek and Roman physicians, who, when employing it as an expectorant, usually combined it with yelk of egg ; and it has maintained its character to the present day. In the tubercular or scrofulous variety, as it is often called, it has frequently been united with some other preparation, as diaphoretic antimony, with which it was joined by Hoffmann, dulcamara by Videt (*Médecine Expectante*, tom. iii., p. 237, 8vo., Lyons, 1803), and cinchona by Dr. Trotter.— (*Medicina Nautica*, vol. iii., p. 325.)

The vulnerary balsams and resins, however, have been more generally had recourse to, but ought rarely, perhaps never, to be employed in an early stage of the disease. Their action is common, and depends upon their possession of a terebinthinate principle, and hence they might be used indiscriminately, but that some of them are less stimulant and heating than the rest. Myrrh and camphire are among the least irritant, and may often be employed when we dare not trust to any other. Copayva, though of somewhat greater balsamic pungency, has often been found essentially useful. Marryatt was peculiarly attached to it : he gave twenty drops of it night and morning upon sugar, and asserts that, when an ulcer has been formed, it ought never to be omitted (*Therapeutica*, Lond., 1758) ; and Dr. Simmonds appears to hold it in nearly as high an estimation.—(*Pract. Obs. on the Treatment of Consumption*, Lond., 1780.)

Many of the remedies already enumerated under the present head act with a sedative influence, and of opium we have already spoken. But there is a medicine which immediately belongs to the present place, not yet noticed, that has of late years been strongly urged upon the public in the warmest terms of panegyric, and by many celebrated writers been regarded as a specific in consumption ; and that is, the prussic or hydrocyanic acid. M. Magendie has been highly sanguine concerning it in France.—(*Recherches sur l'Emploi de l'Acide Prussique,* &c.,

---

* Of late years the inhalation of iodine and chlorine has been extensively tried. When iodine is employed, it is only in a minute quantity, and mixed with hydriodate of potassa. Dr. Elliotson informs us, that he has seen more *mitigation* from the chlorine than the iodine ; but *he has never seen a case cured* by either of them. He has known a single drop of tincture of iodine, put into a pint of fluid, produce great irritation ; but chlorine is borne much better : the mitigation afforded by it, however, is but temporary. The following is the mode of using it recommended by Dr. Elliotson :—Into three quarters of a pint of water, drop four or five minims of a saturated solution of chlorine ; but he considers it best to begin with one or two minims, and to increase the quantity gradually, in proportion as the patient can bear it.—See Lect. at Lond. Univ., as published in Med. Gaz. for 1833, p. 236. —ED.

par F. Magendie, D. M., &c., 8vo., Paris, 1819.) MM. Brera, Manzoni, and Borda (*Storia della Febre Petecchiale di Ginova*, &c.) in Italy, and Dr. Granville in our own country (*Observations on the Internal Use of the Hydrocyanic Acid in Pulmonary Complaints*, &c.); yet not a single case of actual cure in confirmed phthisis has hitherto been advanced by any of them. We have already noticed this powerful medicine as a most valuable subduer of nervous irritation in periodic nervous cough and hooping-cough, and there can be no question that it will often be found capable of acting in the same manner in phthisis. But, from the greater degree of debility and relaxation in this last than in the preceding diseases, we have more to fear from the mischievous effects of the prussic acid, which cannot always be guarded against, and which M. Magendie admits to have taken place occasionally with very fearful apprehensions, such as vomiting, diarrhœa, great depression of spirits, prostration of strength, and even syncope. And hence, if it be employed as a palliative at all, it should be in the earlier stages of the disease ; for, in the latter, where it is most wanted, it is altogether unsafe, and must yield to most of the forms of opium. And the same remark may be made concerning aconite, another of the famous counter-stimulants of the present Italian school of medicine, and with which M. Borda tells us he has sometimes snatched the patient from the jaws of death.

V. The last part of the general therapeutic process, which has been attempted in most ages, has consisted in endeavouring to diminish or carry off the local affection by a transfer of action.

Blisters have very generally been applied for this purpose to the back or the chest. Their service is temporary, but often very efficacious, and they ought never to be neglected. It was formerly the custom to render them perpetual by the use of savin ointment or some other escharotic. But it is less painful and more beneficial to let the skin heal, and renew them after short intervals.

Setons, issues, and caustics, however, where the constitution is not very delicate, nor the habit very irritable, have proved far more powerful revellents, on account of their more violent stimulus and greater permanency of action. The actual cautery, though much abstained from in modern practice, from its apparent, and, indeed, real severity, was in almost universal use in ancient times ; and, in the mode described by Celsus, was undoubtedly a very formidable operation. When the disease, says he, has taken a deep root, the cautery must be applied under the chin, in the throat, twice on each breast, and under the shoulder-blades ; and the ulcers must not be healed as long as the cough continues.

The obvious intention is to produce a revulsion, and hence, by transferring the morbid action to a part of less importance, to allow the lungs to return to a healthy condition. Such transfer may, by these means, in some cases be rendered total, though, in general, the morbid irritation is only partially, instead of entirely, carried off. There are other means, however, by which it seems to be removed altogether, although they are seldom put into our hands.

Thus M. Bayle's fifty-third case is that of a medical man who was fully prepared to meet his fate, and resolved to take no medicine whatever. At this time a severe rigour from an unknown cause attacked him, succeeded by a sweating-fit so profuse, that his linen was changed two-and-twenty times in a night, and even this was not sufficient. The paroxysm proved critical, and the disease was thus carried off by an ephemera.

Sir Gilbert Blane gives an account of a like singular and salutary change excited by a hurricane at Barbadoes in 1780, which produced such an effect on the air or on the nerves of the sick, that some who were labouring under incipient consumption were cured by it : while others who had reached a more advanced stage were decidedly relieved, and freed for a time from many of their symptoms.—(*Observations on the Diseases of Seamen*, 8vo., Lond., 1785.)

No affection seems to keep a consumptive diathesis in so complete a state of subjugation as pregnancy. Most practitioners have seen cases in which a female has dropped all the symptoms of phthisis upon conception, and has continued free from the disease till her delivery. Suckling does not seem to continue the truce ; but, if she conceive again shortly afterward, she renews it : and there have been instances in which, from a rapid succession of pregnancies, the suspension has been so long protracted, that the morbid diathesis has run through its course and entirely subsided, leaving the patient in possession of firm and established health.

As one disease, therefore, or state of body, is well known to have a frequent influence upon another, and consumption is found to be thus influenced by various affections, it is a question well worth inquiring into, whether there be any malady of less importance, which, like cowpox over smallpox, by forestalling an influence on the constitution, may render it insusceptible of an attack of phthisis? Dr. Wells, not many years ago, very ingeniously engaged in an inquiry of this kind, and, finding that it was common for the consumptive in Flanders to remove to the marshy parts of the country where agues were frequent, began to think, not indeed that agues might give an exemption from consumptions, but that the situation which produced the former might prove a guard against the latter. And, so far as his topographical investigations have been carried, and they have extended over some part or other of all the quarters of the globe, this opinion has been countenanced ; for he has discovered that, wherever intermittents are endemic, consumption is rarely to be met with, while the latter has become frequent in proportion as draining has been introduced.— (*Trans. Medico-Chir. Soc.*, vol. iii., p. 471.) The later inquiries of Dr. Southey do not supt port this hypothesis, but the question is yet unsettled, and well worth pursuing ; and Mr. Mansford, who practises in the interior of Somersetshire, has still more lately published a work, which, though not written as a defence of Dr. Wells's opinion, indirectly confirms it, by endeavouring to prove that a low, inland situation, like the vales of his own country, is far better calculated as a residence for consumptive patients than the air of·mountains, or of the seacoast.—(*Inquiry into the Influence of Situation on Pulmonary Consumption, by J. G. Mansford,* &c., 8vo., 1818.)*

* As the pathology of consumption is not yet fixed, so too the treatment of this disease varies with different physicians : the assumption that the forming stage of phthisis is, in many cases, of an inflammatory character, has led the profession in the U. States to a more active method of relief in early periods, than is sanctioned by the practice of Europe : phthisis has generally been considered in this country as allied to pneumonitis, bronchitis, &c., and as requiring the use of the lancet, purgatives, antimonials, &c., during the first stage, which practice is warmly advocated by Dr. Hosack (Essays, vol. ii.) : few however would imitate the extreme depletory practice of Rush ; bloodletting has its limits. In regard to purgatives, morbid anatomy has so often shown an inflammatory condition of the mucous membrane of the alimentary canal, that the milder cathartics seem more appropriate than drastic purgatives.

Antimonials, in the earlier stages of the disease, are almost universally recommended, and Dr. Balfour's practice of tartar-emetic ointment is extremely popular. Practitioners differ widely as to the remedial powers of digitalis : while it is much extolled-by some as lessening the activity of the heart and arteries, it is rejected by others as increasing the debility and irritability. Dr. Eberle's estimate of its value seems to us to be just : "that under careful management, and in conjunction with a well-regulated diet and proper attention to the cutaneous functions, much good may be derived from its employment in incipient phthisis." "Tar fumigations, employed as directed in the text, have been found highly serviceable by American practitioners. In regard to iodine, a gentleman of ample experience, Dr. Morton of Philadelphia, remarks (Illustrations of Pulmonary Consumptions), that " in a large number of instances, it has appeared, especially in incipient consumption, to arrest or suspend the tubercular secretion, and with it the hectic, marasmus, cough, dyspnœa, and other urgent symptoms ;" and again, " in a majority of cases, even in the second stage of phthisis, I have been much gratified with the results ; thus, it often relieves the dyspnœa, improves the complexion, and restores the appetite, even when the advanced progress of the disease precludes all hope of recovery." Dr. Rush urges salivation as important in treating pulmonary consumption ; we are aware that the American journals contain some interesting reports in which this plan of treatment has been successful, but there are habits of body, peculiarities of temperament, and other circumstances, which, in some cases of phthisis, would forbid it.

The respiration of cold air was proposed as a remedy in pulmonary diseases by the late Dr. C. Drake, of New-York. He states, " that its sensible effects were tolerably uniform. The most 'constant effect on the pulse was to render it fuller : when it was preternaturally frequent, it commonly rendered it slower; it very generally mitigated the cough, diminishing its frequency, and rendered the expectoration freer and easier." For a view of the

E 2

GENUS IV.
MELANOSIS.*
MELANOSE.

SECRETION OF A BLACK MATERIAL, MORE OR LESS INSPISSATED ; STAINING OR STUDDING THE VISCERAL AND OTHER ORGANS.†

THE tubercles and tubers of struma chiefly originate in the texture of the glands, especially the lymphatic, and are often confined to them. There are other tubercles, as those of mesenteric tabes, that spread rapidly into different textures, and sometimes originate in them. But there are none that seem to commence or extend over so large a field as those we are now about to describe, or so seriously to affect the constitution.‡ There is not, indeed, a single organ of the simplest or most complicated kind, from the cellular texture to the unravelled elaboration of the brain, which is not occasionally loaded with them ; while, in various parts, the black pigment, which gives them their hue, is found diffused in extensive sheets, without tubercles, or the pulpy matter that fills their cysts ; transforming the natural colour of the organs, to which it is conveyed, into its own morbid jet. [The most frequent seat of true melanosis, however, is found by Dr. Carswell to be the serous tissue, more especially where this tissue constitutes the cellular element of organs. Here the melanotic matter accumulates in the cells, and forms tumours of various sizes. Its formation, as a secretion, is still more conspicuous in the loose cellular tissue, and especially on extensive serous surfaces.]

The last change has hitherto been found chiefly in the bones, but sometimes also in the membranes, and even the parenchyma of organs, constituting, in the language of M. Breschet, a false membrane or membranous expansion on the surface of the mucous and other textures ; and it is hence possible that examples may hereafter be met with of a generally DIFFUSED, as well as a generally TUBERCULAR, form of the disease. But as the second, with a few local exceptions, is the only mode under which it has hitherto appeared,§ we have at present but one

apparatus employed by Dr. Drake, see the Am. Journ. of Med. Sc., vol. iii., p. 53.—D.

* Melanose, Laennec ; Melanoma, Dr. Carswell ; Black Cancer, Baron Dupuytren.

† " True melanosis consists in the formation of a morbid product of secretion of a deep brown or black colour, of various degrees of intensity, unorganized, the form and consistence of which present considerable variety, solely in consequence of the influence of external agents."—(Dr. Carswell, in Illustrations of Elementary Forms of Disease, fasc. iv.)—ED.

‡ If we advert to tubercular diseases of the lungs, peritoneum, spleen, and some other organs, and at the same time recognise them, with many of the best modern pathologists, as scrofulous affections, some of our author's doctrine, as here laid down, will appear incorrect.—ED.

§ Since the period when this was written melanosis has been investigated with considerable attention, and our knowledge of its nature has been

species of the genus, which we shall proceed to describe under the name of Melanosis Tubercularis. Tubercular Melanose.*

SPECIES I.

MELANOSIS TUBERCULARIS.

TUBERCULAR MELANOSE.

THE BLACK SECRETION PULTACEOUS, IN EN-CYSTED† TUBERCLES, PEA-SIZED OR WALNUT-SIZED, SCATTERED IN GROUPS OVER MOST OF THE ORGANS ; CHIEFLY BELOW THE SURFACE, SOMETIMES UPON IT : FEVER MOSTLY A HEC-TIC : GREAT DEBILITY.‡

IT is singular that this very striking disease should not have been traced, or rather, perhaps, not have attracted much of the attention of

---

much extended. We are now aware that it presents itself in various forms, which have been treated of with great ability and discrimination by Professor Carswell, in his Illustrations of the Elementary Forms of Disease, fasciculus iv., Lond., 4to., 1834. He divides melanotic formations into two kinds, the *true* and *spurious.* Thus, when these formations or products depend on a change taking place in that process of secretion, whence the natural colour of certain parts of the body is derived, or, in other words, when they constitute what is called an idiopathic disease, he considers them as belonging to the first kind ; and, when they originate in the accumulation of a carbonaceous substance, introduced into the body from without, the action of chymical agents on the blood, or the stagnation of this fluid, he includes them in the second kind.—ED.

* Four varieties, or species, are described by Professor Carswell, namely,—1. Punctiform. 2. Tuberiform. 3. Stratiform. 4. Liquiform. The tuberiform, which is by far the most common, corresponds to Dr. Good's melanosis tubercularis, or the *melanose en masse* of French pathologists. Tuberiform melanosis agrees with the " concrétions mélaniques ;" punctiform with the "mélanose infiltrée ;" stratiform with the " mélanose membraniforme ;" and liquiform with the " mélanose liquide" of Laennec, Breschet, Andral, and other writers. It was Breschet who applied the term liquid melanosis to one of the varieties.—ED.

† " Tantôt la matière est enkystée, tantôt elle n'est contenue dans aucun réservoir ; et elle paroit être exhalée à la surface des tissus, ou épanchée dans une cavité."—(Breschet.) " La mélanose en masse peut être entourée d'un kyste, ou en être dépourvue. Le premier cas est infiniment plus rare que le second."—(Andral, Précis d'Anat. Pathol., tom. i., p. 451.) Laennec's distinctions of encysted and unencysted melanosis are of much less importance than similar distinctions in relation to cancer; in fact, cysts are rarely met with, and, when they are present, consist of such a cellular loose tissue, that they have little effect as boundaries to melanotic humours.—(Blandin, Dict. de Méd. et de Chir. Pratiques, art. MELANOSE.) According to Dr. Carswell, melanosis is perhaps never found encysted in compound tissues or organs, as the brain, lungs, liver, or kidneys; whereas it is always so in the cellular and adipose tissue, and sometimes also on the surface of serous membranes.—See Illustrat. of the Elementary Forms of Disease, fasc. iv.—ED.

‡ In the majority of cases, melanosis does not produce great constitutional disturbance. We find it sometimes attaining considerable magni-

---

pathologists, till a few years back, at least in the nosology of man. For it has been long observed in many kinds of quadrupeds, as the dog, cat, hare, but especially the horse, and, among the veterinary surgeons of France, has obtained the name of charbon, or maladie charbonneuse. It is, however, to the ingenious anatomical researches of MM. Laennec and Bayle (See *Journ. de Méd. de Corvisart,* &c., tom. ix., p. 368) that we are indebted for our first knowledge of the disease as it exists in man;* and for the very appropriate generic name of MELANOSIS,† or MORBID DENIGRATION, by which it is now generally distinguished.

[The colour of melanosis varies from dark yellow to brown, deep blue approaching to black, and to complete black, which is the most common. It is readily detected by its peculiar shades of colour in any organ containing it ; more especially as the surrounding tissues are lighter coloured, and form a contrast with it. No smell proceeds from it, a circumstance distinguishing it from gangrene, which always emits a very offensive odour ; nor has it any particular taste, a character which belongs to it in common with most other morbid formations. The minute texture of melanosis is little known : if we except the cyst, no vessels nor nerves have been discerned in it ; and it seems as if it were an inorganic substance deposited in or upon various parts. The melanosis described in the definition prefixed to this article by Dr. Good, is the most common or the tubercular va-

---

tude in the liver, and in the common cellular tissue, without giving rise to any functional derangement sufficient to excite the suspicion of its existence ; it may merely occasion a degree of uneasiness by its mechanical effects on the contiguous parts.—ED.

* Breschet assigns the honour of having first described this organic affection to Dupuytren, who declared, when MM. Bayle and Laennec (Bulletins de la Soc. de l'Ecole de Méd., No. ii., 1806) published their observations, that he had for several years described the disease in his lectures. Some controversial papers on this point may be seen in Corvisart's Journ., tom. ix., p. 360 and 441, and tom. x., p. 89 and 96. An allusion to the disease, however, may be traced in the writings of Morgagni, Bonetus, and Haller. In Epist. iv., No. iv., De Sedibus et Causis Morb., Morgagni informs us, that in one body which he opened, the lungs looked as if they had been stained with ink ; and in another place, he describes the lungs as having been found indurated and black. In a dropsical patient, the liver, after death, was also black.—(Epist. vii., No. xi.) In Haller's Opuscula Pathol., obs. xvii., notice is taken of an example in which the lungs were found not filled with pus, but with a matter as black as ink ; and of another case, in which the author met with black matter in the cavity of the chest.—ED.

† Breschet says, however, " Cette désignation ne se trouve ni très-rigoureuse ni très-exacte, car on voit plus souvent ces matières être jaunes-brunes, couleur de suie ou de bistre, que véritablement noires. Cependant j'en ai rencontré, qui étoient parfaitement noires, et qui coloroient les tissus de lin et le papier, comme le fait la solution aqueuse de l'encre de la Chine."—See Journ. de Physiol., tom. i, p. 354.—ED.

riety of it, but it presents itself in other shapes.* The melanotic deposite takes place in three distinct forms: 1st, Very much divided and suspended in liquids; hence the black tinge of the serous fluid of certain cavities, and especially as frequently presented by the serosity of the peritoneum, when the liver, bowels, stomach, or uterus, are the seats of cancerous disease.† Breschet, Andral, and Cruveilhier, describe a melanotic secretion from the surface of a mucous membrane, or the cavity of the stomach; but, in doing so, it seems to Professor Carswell that they have mistaken the black discoloration of the blood, produced by the action of the gastric juice on this fluid, when effused, for true liquiform melanosis.—(Op. cit., fasc. iv.) 2dly, As a very thin layer spread over serous membranes, the stratiform or membraniform melanosis. In this case it sometimes exhibits a fine glossy black colour, resembling that of Indian-ink. The, layers are more or less extensive; and M. Mérat has seen the whole of the peritoneal coat of the intestines covered with them. The matter is adherent to the serous membranes, which are almost the only ones upon which it assumes this form; but they are not at all altered by it, being neither thickened nor otherwise affected; and it is remarked, that individuals who die with this modification of melanosis do not fall victims to it, but to other organic changes. Layers of black matter are noticed on some portions of the mucous system, as on the tongue in typhoid and other fevers; and Mérat even conceives that such appearance is a specimen of one kind of melanosis. 3dly, Melanosis most frequently assumes a globular shape, or the form of a tubercle, varying from the size of a millet-seed to that of an egg, or even a larger body. Its shape is moulded by the containing parts; and hence it is in general less symmetrically spherical in soft parts, and more regularly globular

in such as are firm. 4thly, A fourth variety is that in which the disease is diffused through certain tissues, the "mélanose infiltrée" of Laennec, the "punctiform melanosis" of Carswell.*]

The cause, progress, diagnosis, and mode of treatment of tubercular melanosis, are at present obscure and unsatisfactory. The individual labouring under it frequently exhibits, when he first applies for help, a considerable degree of febrile excitement, debility, and oppression in the thorax or abdomen; most commonly about the pleura or in the loins.

Every case of melanosis that came under the observation of Dr. Armstrong was accompanied by more or less chronic bronchitis, which, however, he admits, is not sufficient of itself to produce melanosis, as numerous examples of it take place without any traces of the latter affection.—(Morb. Anat., &c., p. 25.) [Melanosis is alleged to be more frequently combined with carcinoma than with any other disease; but, as Dr. Carswell observes, there is no similarity between these two diseases, their anatomical, physical, and chymical characters being totally different. Several varieties of the former (regarded as such in Dr. Carswell's classification) are highly organized, while melanosis itself is an unorganized substance, injurious only from its quantity, the number of organs which it affects, its situation, and mechanical operation. In Dr. Carswell's work may be seen representations of melanosis, combined with fibrous, carcinomatous, and erectile tissues.]

The above, however, are not always the introductory symptoms; for the disease sometimes commences with catarrhal or rheumatic affections after exposure to cold, succeeded by shivering fits.† The patient seems generally unwell for the first five or six weeks after this attack; but when it has once firmly established itself, and evinced the thoracic or abdominal signs just adverted to, it proceeds with a rapid

---

* This form is exemplified occasionally in most of the organs of the body, and also sometimes on serous surfaces, as the pleura and peritoneum. In compendd organs, the disease is generally a single swelling; but in the cellular and adipose tissues there is an aggregation of tumours, producing tuberculated masses. In the liver, lungs, and kidneys, according to Dr. Carswell, the tuberiform melanosis is always combined with the punctiform.—ED.

† Breschet, in Magendie's Journ., tom. i., p. 359. Laennec takes no notice of the fluid variety. Indeed, as he describes melanosis as a tissue, he could not regard a liquid as meriting the name. But other pathologists, who look upon melanosis as a simple deposite of unorganized colouring matter, have no more difficulty in conceiving its fluid than its solid state. The liquiform variety of true melanosis has in general been confined to natural or accidental serous cavities. Dr. Carswell has never seen it in man, as a product of secretion, but has met with it in consequence of the destruction of melanotic tumours, and the effusion of their contents into the serous cavities, the walls of which they had perforated. The accidental serous cavities in which it is found are those which constitute cysts, particularly in the ovaries.—ED.

* The punctiform melanosis appears in minute points or dots, grouped together in a small space, or scattered irregularly over a considerable extent of surface. Such appearances are most frequently seen in the liver, the cut surface seeming as if it had been dusted over with soot or charcoal powder. When examined with the aid of a lens, the black points sometimes present a stellated or peniciliated arrangement, which, in some cases, can be distinctly seen to originate in the ramiform expansion of a minute vein, filled with melanotic matter. At other times, this matter appears to be deposited in the molecular structure of this organ, consisting of the most minute points disseminated throughout the acini of the liver, of various depths of shade, terminating in black.—See Carswell's Illustrations of the Elementary Forms of Disease, fasc. iv.—ED.

† Melanosis often produces, at its first formation, no disturbance of the health, and the existence of the disease is frequently not suspected previously to dissection. However, several patients were cut off by the disorder who had a sallow complexion, excessive debility, and more or less œdema, being in a state very similar to the advanced stage of scurvy.—See Magendie's Journ., tom. i., p. 365.—ED.

and fatal step, and in about a fortnight, he falls a victim to the hectic fever, perspiration, emaclation, and debility by which he is jointly assaulted : the prodromi or incursive symptoms, whether affecting the loins or chest, usually giving way before the closing scene arrives, and deceiving the sufferer, and sometimes even his medical attendant, into a belief that he is improving ; when he suddenly sinks from debility alone.

If the patient be examined accurately at this time, a few tubercles or clusters of tubercles may occasionally be felt under the skin, especially that of the abdomen or of the breasts. And sometimes also a cyst, much larger than the rest, may be found projecting, and even forcing its way externally through the integuments. In a few instances this larger cyst ulcerates, of which a striking example occurred to M. Breschet in 1821, and is particularly noticed by Mr. Cullen. In the right groin of the patient, who was a female, an ulcerative surface was perceived about as large as a crown piece, the bottom of which consisted of the ordinary black material of the disease before us, jetty as China ink, of the consistence of cream above, but much more inspissated below, where it was in contact with the cellular texture. There were sufficient proofs that it was not à mere sloughing sore ; among which it may be observed that it was destitute of fetor, and that in its immediate vicinity, as well as in other parts of the body, as was afterward ascertained by opening into them, there was a crop of defined melanotic tubers of different forms and diameters.

One of the best marked instances upon record is the following, which occurred to Professor Alison in the Royal Infirmary, Edinburgh. The patient's name was Rachael Bruce, she was admitted on the third of June.—(*Trans. of the Medico-Chir. Soc. of Edin.*, vol. i., p. 275, 1824.) She complained of severe pains shooting down from the loins to the inferior extremities, and to the abdomen. She had similar pains in the right shoulder and arm, increased in the night-time, or by motion. She had become weak and emaciated since her complaints began, and was liable to shivering, followed by flushing and profuse perspiration, which increased her debility without relieving her pains. The abdomen was swelled, but did not fluctuate on percussion, and the distention varied in degree at different hours of the day. She had thirst, with scanty, high-coloured urine, not coagulating by heat. The integuments of the abdomen were flaccid ; and a hard, moveable tumour could be felt in the iliac and hypogastric regions. She was also liable to paroxysms of dyspnœa during the night. Her appetite was impaired. She had a bad taste in the mouth, with white and dry tongue. Her bowels were reported to be regular ; but she had occasional nausea.

She stated her complaints, which were of five or six weeks standing, to have commenced, after exposure to cold, with shivering and pain, and stiffness of the loins, and of the hip and knee-joints of the left side. The enlargement and induration of the abdomen had been remarked only during the last fortnight.

Up to June the 20th, being seventeen days from the time of admission, the symptoms continued with little variation. On the 21st were perceived several small painful tumours on the integuments of the abdomen, which she declared to have existed from the commencement of her illness. She was on this day examined by a skilful accoucheur, who reported the tumour felt in the hypogastric region to be unconnected with the uterus. On the 24th a copious sweating, with involuntary discharge of urine, was added to the other symptoms. From this moment there was great debility, with decided hectic fever ; and a tendency to sloughing of the sacrum. On the evening of the 7th she had vomiting of a dark-coloured matter, and soon afterward died.

The course is usually more rapid : and in the case of John Houston, à shoemaker, admitted into the same infirmary under the care of Dr. Home, extended only to thirteen days. His chief symptoms at the time of admission were those of pleurisy, with a severe cough and difficult expectoration. The bladder was also affected ; and on the eighth day he was troubled with painful hemorrhoidal tumours, probably produced by the action of repeated purgatives. The other symptoms gradually diminished, but the debility increased. On the twelfth day, as we learn from a diary of the symptoms and treatment, furnished us by Sir Andrew Halliday, his pulse was 112 ; heat 98¾ Fahrenheit ; he was allowed a beefsteak, and a quarter of a pint of sherry. On the ensuing night he made complaint of great weakness ; his pulse quickened to 140, and he died at four in the morning.—(*London Medical Repository*, vol. xix., p. 442.)*

The treatment is yet to be learned ; and the cases before us afford little instruction upon the subject. The first was resisted by little more than palliatives, as leeches, laxatives, anodynes, and Dover's powder. The second unfolds a bolder plan, though the patient still sooner reached his end. It consisted in venesection to sixteen ounces, two days in succession, and powerful purgatives, at first often repeated, of calomel, jalap, and sulphate of magnesia, &c.

---

* A case of melanosis, affecting the parotid gland, is recorded by Dr. Valentine Mott, in the Am. Journ. of Med. Sc., vol. x., p. 16. The description is accompanied with a coloured engraving of the melanotic body, which was extirpated. On dividing the tumour longitudinally, not a vestige of the original organization of the gland could be observed. The inner surfaces had the appearance of firm tar, and imparted a black colour to the fingers when touched. After the operation, the patient seemed to do well ; but in about a month several tumours appeared on the scalp, a dark spot showed itself in the integuments of the diseased side of the face, the knee swelled, and hectic supervened. The patient died fifty-three days after the operation. No examination of the body could be made, but Dr. Mott is confident that the disease was constitutional melanosis.—D.

But this was not long continued, no benefit appearing to issue from it ; and it yielded to sedative mucilages and a tonic diet.

In reasoning speculatively, we should speak with great modesty. But admitting the material which forms the tubercles to be a peculiar secretion, and that the constitutional excitement consists mainly in this new and stimulant action, perhaps it may, in future cases, be found useful to combine the two intentions of allaying the peculiar irritation, and, at the same time, urging the secernents to a renewal of their proper action ; or, in other words, to employ the conjoint force of sedatives and counter-irritants ; which may be effected by a union of opium, or Dover's powder, with the tincture of iodine. The great and beneficial influence which the latter is well known to exercise in many cases over strumous tubercles, should indicate its use on the present occasion. And it is also not improbable, from the approach which the disease seems occasionally to make to the more irritant cases of phthisis, in its excitement of the chest and its hectic fever, that the hydrocyanic acid might at times, with great advantage, take the place of all other sedatives. Such coincidences of symptoms, moreover, show us clearly the place which melanosis should occupy in a general nosological arrangement.*

Before hazarding a syllable upon the physiology of this very extraordinary disease, it is requisite to put the reader into possession of the general appearances afforded by post-obit examinations ; and the case already alluded to, as under Professor Alison's care, is admirably adapted to this purpose, if put into an abridged form.

The body evinced great and general emaciation, and various small dark-coloured tumours, perceptible during life, were still distributed over it. In the mammæ, these were largest and most numerous : they were traced in cysts, and imbedded in the cellular substance ; and when cut into were found to contain a deep black-coloured matter, of a soft and pulpy consistence. Within the abdomen, most of the cellular and adipose textures had disappeared. The peritoneum lining the parietes was of a blackish colour, and the black matter was irregularly deposited in striæ and spots upon the inner side of the membrane, which had lost much of its natural transparency. The omentum presented a similar appearance, and several globular shining tumours of a black colour were appended to it, which, when cut into, poured out a similarly coloured fluid. Spots and tubercles of a like kind were traced in the serous or outer membrane of the intestines, and between the folds of the mesentery. The ovaria were several times as large as their natural size, seated in front of the uterus, and occupying the lateral iliac regions.

* When a melanotic tumour is so situated as to admit of being removed with a knife, this is the proper practice. In the human subject such an operation has been done for the extirpation of the eye affected with this extraordinary disease. Melanotic tumours have often been successfully removed from horses.—See Archiv. Gén. de Méd., Juin, 1828, p. 180.—ED.

Their external surface had a dark, shining, lobulated appearance, with numerous ramifications of vessels upon the peritoneal covering ; beneath which black matter was irregularly deposited in spots, giving a mottled appearance to the whole. When cut into, their substance was uniformly black. The cellular texture still retained its consistence, and vessels containing red coagulated blood could be traced through it. Several distinct cysts or cavities were found in their substance, which poured out a black liquid when opened. The kidneys, liver, spleen, and the mucous or interior membrane of the stomach and intestines, were all free from black matter, although it was deposited in the cellular tissue connected with these organs. On uncovering the breast-bone and scull-cap, it was observed that the whole texture of the sternum, the anterior portion of the ribs, and a great part of the parietal and occipital bones, were black, more brittle, and of softer consistence than natural, but without enlargement or ulceration. The periosteum was nearly natural, but the whole inner table of the scull, when removed from the dura mater, was of a darker hue than natural, and in some places where the black matter was deposited in irregular patches of the bone, there were corresponding stains on the surface of the dura mater. The substance of the brain was healthy, but a few black striæ were discernible in the membranes, and the tunics of several of the vessels. A large quantity of serum was effused under the arachnoid membrane and in the ventricles. Within the thorax, the costal pleura and surface of the lungs were studded with black tubercles like those of the integuments, while some of them were larger. The substance of the lungs was dark, and some minute tubercles were imbedded in it, and like spots were noticed beneath the pericardial coverings of the heart, which contained some coagulated blood in its cavities, and was softer than usual.

It should further be observed, that in a few places in the present subject, but more generally in others, the black material varied considerably from its ordinary degree of consistence, and instead of being pulpy or nearly solid, was a fluent liquid ; and that several of the tubercles were filled with a white and brain-like substance, while those that surrounded them were of a deep jet.

The first opinion formed respecting the nature of these enlargements by MM. Bresclæt and Laennec was, that the dark material was congested blood that had escaped from the capillary vessels into the cellular substance by a rupture of their coats, or by anastomosis from relaxation. But this conjecture was soon found untenable, as it was sufficiently ascertained that the material is a distinct secretion, and is now supposed to be a secretion sui generis. Nor is another opinion of M. Laennec's much more tenable, which advances that the black material evinces different stages of elaboration ; that when first thrown forth it is pultaceous or nearly solid, and in a state of crudity, but that it gradually matures, and advances to a state of ramollissement or fluidity. For it is well observed by Dr. Cullen, that, were this true, we should expect to find the largest cysts or reservoirs in the highest state of liquefaction, and the smallest in the highest state of solidity ; the contrary of which is usually the course pursued. [Mr. Fawdington (*Case of Melanosis, with General Observations on the Pathology of this interesting Disease*, 1826), however, follows Laennec in placing the stage of fluidity posterior to that of solidity. At first it seems difficult to conceive how the melanotic matter can be originally deposited in any other than a liquid form ; and if in a solid state, how from its organic nature it can undergo the process by which it is afterward softened. Yet, that tubercles of the lungs are first solid and afterward soften, though their substance has no organization, is the general belief.*]

It is also justly remarked by Dr. Cullen of Edinburgh, that the characters of tubercular melanosis completely distinguish it from cancer and fungus hæmatodes ; since it is well known to exist without local pain,† and to propagate itself by cysts and boundary lines, while both the others are accompanied with severe lancinating pains, and burst through every bond, and extend their ravages in every direction.

[Dr. Armstrong, in noticing the opinion that melanosis, like tubercle, scirrhus, and fungus, is associated with an organized affection *sui generis* of the solids, takes the opportunity to remark, that in all the cases examined by him, the disease seemed to be nothing but a secretion, sometimes occurring in textures otherwise apparently natural, sometimes in those chronically inflamed, and sometimes co-existent with either scirrhus or fungus.—(*Armstrong's Morbid Anatomy*, &c., p. 24, 8vo., London, 1828.) It is a peculiar feature in the nature of melanosis, that the animal textures are never, strictly speaking, converted into it, unless it be proved that the oily matter of the cellular tissue undergoes this change ; and even on this supposition

---

* M. Blandin supports Laennec's view by observing that melanotic tumours may change into a softened state, particularly when they are situated near the surface ; the skin becomes thin and ulcerates, and from the surface of the sore is discharged a glutinous black matter, which is characteristic of the disease. A case exemplifying these changes was seen by M. Blandin in the Salpétrière, and the particulars of it were published by Breschet.—(See Journ. de Physiol. Expériment, tom. i., p. 354.) The old woman, the subject of it, and who is referred to in our text, had melanotic tumours in the right groin, thigh, and breasts. It seems that the part, after having ulcerated, will sometimes form granulations and heal. This fact was illustrated in a horse, from which M. Damoiseau removed a melanotic tumour, as related by M. Trousseau.—Archives Gén., &c., Juin, 1828, p, 180.—ED.

† "Comme elle (la mélancse) paroit être absolument insensible, les viscères où elle existe ne manifestent aucune douleur, même à la pression ; s'il y a de la douleur, on peut affirmer, que cette lésion organique n'y est pas seule. La mélanose serait entièrement sans inconvénient, si elle ne gênait pas par son volume des viscères essentiels."—Dict. des Sciences Méd., tom. xxxii., p. 185.—ED.

---

it would be the conversion of an inorganic secretion rather than of an organic issue, into melanosis. On the contrary, the new matter is deposited in the substance of the textures or organs, or between their component fibres. These circumstances, together with its appearance in several of the bones, where it seems to have occupied the situation of the marrow,* would give some countenance to the notion that melanotic matter was a diseased modification of the adipose secretion. To this idea, however, an objection is presented in the melanotic masses found occasionally in the liver, spleen, and substance of the kidneys. Its occurrence in the pancreas forms little or no valid objection ; for the quantity of adipose cellular substance with which the portions of this gland are connected, might be regarded as the primary matrix of the morbid deposition.—(*Edin. Med. Journal*, No. xc., p. 162.) All this, however, is only conjecture ; but the following observations respecting the anatomical distribution and preference to certain textures exhibited by melanosis, seem to be founded upon the careful consideration of facts.

First, The cellular tissue and adipose membrane are both most abundantly and most generally the seat of the melanotic deposition ; that is to say, of the tubercular melanosis. The subcutaneous and intermuscular cellular tissue is a common situation of it ; as well as other parts of great laxity, where the cellular membrane is abundant, as in the genital organs, around the rectum, within the pelvis, and on the forepart or at the sides of the spine.

Secondly, The delicate cellular tissue which connects the serous membrane to contiguous parts and to the enclosed organs, presents this melanotic deposite nearly in the same, if not in a greater degree, than the common cellular membrane. This was particularly noticed in the case recorded by Mr. Fawdington. In Dr. Home's patient, though the pleura was studded with melanose tubercles, no mention is made whether they were upon or under it ; but as the lungs are described as extensively occupied by melanotic masses, there is reason to infer that this is meant of the cellular tissue beneath the pleura, and connecting that membrane to the pulmonic lobules. In like manner, when, in the same case, the substance of the heart is said to be affected ; when, in the case of Rachael Bruce, spots are said to have been noticed beneath the pericardiac coverings of the heart ; and when, in Mr. Fawdington's case, the surface of the heart is described as covered with melanose spots, chiefly subjacent to the pericardium ; little doubt can be entertained that the tissue of melanotic infiltration is the subserous and intermuscular structure. Infiltration of the abdominal subserous cellular tissue is particularly remarked in the case of Rachael Bruce, related by Dr. Cullen and Dr. Carswell, and also in Mr. Fawdington's examples. Next to the cellular

---

‡ Breschet states, however, that he has never seen melanosis in the central cavities of the bones, in the synovial membranes, nor in cartilages.—See Magendie's Journ., tom. i., p. 364.

and adipose tissue, several of the internal organs, termed parenchymatous, are most frequently the seat of the disease. Thus, not only the lungs (which, indeed, by the French writers are deemed the most common situation*), but the liver, the spleen, and the kidneys, are stated, in the case of Houston, to have been occupied with melanotic masses. In Mr. Fawdington's case, the liver, pancreas, spleen, and kidneys, were extensively affected; while in Dr. Alison's case, though the substance of both mammæ and of both ovaries was completely melanosed, the liver, spleen, and kidneys were exempt from the disease. When melanotic tubercles take place in the liver, they are frequently of considerable size, and sometimes as large as an egg...

Lastly, It is to be observed, that, in the case of Houston, one of the ribs and a part of the clavicle were melanosed. In that of Rachael Bruce, a part of the inner table of the scull was darker than natural, and the surface of the bone was stained with particles of black matter. A great part of the parietal and occipital bones was black, less consistent and more brittle than natural; and similar changes were observed in the sternum and sternal ends of the ribs. According to Breschet, the parts of bones connected with the muscles are most commonly affected. Some textures seem either quite exempt from melanosis, or only to be very slightly affected by it. Thus the nerves, the proper arterial tissue,† and muscular fibre, are scarcely ever the seat of it; and it is doubtful whether the serous and mucous membranes ever become penetrated by the melanotic deposition.‡ The above critic errs, however, in setting down the skin as rarely or never affected. In the cutaneous texture, says Breschet, melanoses are common; and he has found an infinite number of small black tumours, resembling grains of cassia, situated in the skin, and appearing to originate from the rete mucosum. An example of this kind, which was seen by Breschet, is recorded by Alibert, who denominates it *cancer mélané.—(Magendie's Journ.*, tom. i., p. 361; and *Alibert, Nosologic,* &c.) It ought to have been mentioned, that melanosis often attacks the lymphatic glands, the eye, and fat of the orbit; and that traces of it are frequently met with, as Dr. Armstrong confirms, in various diseased structures.]

We have reason to conclude that the disease before us is at first local, or commences in a particular organ; and that, from the general sympathy of the secernent system with the part where it first appears, it ramifies in every direction, over the most solid and compact, as well as over the most loose and yielding tex-

tures; accumulating and forming reservoirs where there are cells or other hollows for its reception, and spreading as a jet, die, or sheath on the surface, or through the parenchyma, where these are not.

[The doctrine of the disease being at first local, is liable to several objections: first, the great disorder of the health frequently preceding the melanotic formation;* secondly, the great extent of the affection, and the many internal organs found after death studded with melanotic tubercles; thirdly, some peculiarity of constitution appears requisite, from the curious circumstance that the disease, when it occurs in horses, is chiefly observed in such as have a white or gray-coat.†]

What is the nature of the black die or pigment, and by what means is it produced? Much more attention to the subject is necessary, before any satisfactory reply can be given to this question. The material to which it seems most nearly to make an approach, in temperate climates, is the black pigment of the choroid membrane, and perhaps that which is supplied from the rete mucosum as a colouring matter for black hair. Both these are evidently productions of the secernent system. They are indeed small in quantity; but if we turn our eyes to the intertropical climates, we shall find the same, or a like jet pigment, thrown forth over the entire surface, and continued by a permanent supply, as the die antecedently furnished is carried off. And if we attend to the curious economy which takes place in this subject respecting the children of negroes, we shall also find this material produced in very large abundance in a short time: for the infants

---

* This is not, however, a constant circumstance: many patients with melanosis have not suffered at first much constitutional disturbance; and Dr. Carswell, we know, ascribes the injurious effects of melanotic formations principally to their mechanical pressure on the neighbouring parts; they are not themselves organized.—Ed.

† See G. Breschet, in Magendie's Journ. Expér. de Physiologie, tom. i., p. 355. "The much greater frequency of melanosis in the gray and white than in the bay, brown, or black horse, is a circumstance which may be noticed here as favourable to the theory which ascribes the origin of this disease to the accumulation in the blood of the carbon which is naturally employed to colour different parts of the body, as the hair, rete mucosum, choroid, and other parts."—(See Carswell's Illustrations of the Elementary Forms of Disease, fasc. iv.) Remarkable examples of melanosis in the horse are recorded by MM. Goyer and Rodet (Journ. de Méd. Vétérinaire, tom. ii., p. 273); and MM. Trousseau and Le Blanc relate other interesting facts of the same kind.—(Archiv. Gén. de Méd., Juin, 1828.) Speaking of the melanosis being principally seen only in white or gray horses, M. Blandin observes:—"On dirait que chez eux la matière colorante s'est, pour ainsi dire, refugiée dans ces tumeurs."—(Dict. de Méd. et Chir. Pratiques, art. Melanose.) Occasionally, however, melanosis is met with in horses of other colours, and both Rodet and Andral have noticed it in those of a bay colour. In the horse, melanotic tumours are most liable to form under the tail, whence they extend into the pelvis.—Ed

---

* "Le poumon est, de tous les viscères, celui où on les voit le plus fréquemment."—Dict. des Sciences Méd., tom. xxxii., p. 185.

† This is true, notwithstanding, as Breschet remarks, "les vaisseaux sanguins sont parfois entourés de ces tumeurs, et le vaisseau est caché au milieu de la matière mélanique."

‡ See Edin. Med. Journ., No. xc., p. 157; also Dr. Cullen and Dr. Carswell, in Edin. Med. Chir. Trans., vol. i.; and Fawdington's Case of Melanosis, 1826.

of negroes, as we shall have occasion to observe more at large when treating of EPICHROSIS or MACULAR-SKIN,* are nearly fair when first born, and only become coloured with the black effusion a few weeks afterward; which at first gives little more than a tawny hue, but gradually advances to a jet.

We shall also have occasion to notice, in the same place, that this black die, like the pigment in melanosis, is on some occasions secreted in the form of a finer and more fluent liquid, and in others in a more inspissated state, and united with a coarser material, constituting the rete mucosum of Malpighi; who, moreover, gave it the name of rete from a belief that he was able to trace in it something of a fibrous structure; an idea that has not been realized by Cruickshank or any later anatomist. And it is not a little singular, that as in melanosis we sometimes meet with a few patches or tubercles of the preternatural secretion destitute of its colouring die, and presenting a variegated appearance of black and white mosaic, so, in the distribution of the natural pigment of the negro over the surface, we sometimes meet with the same casual obstruction to the flow of the black die, producing that marbled skin which gives the individuals the name of piebald negroes.

[According to the researches of Breschet and Cruveilhier, when the black matter of melanosis is not concrete, but liquid, or when it is deposited in layers on the surface of a serous or mucous membrane, the minute bloodvessels are filled with a black of precisely the same kind as that exhaled.†

Dr. Armstrong suggests, that as melanosis is frequently combined with chronic bronchitis, the venous character imparted to the whole mass of blood by this last disease may facilitate the dark and peculiar secretion of the first disorder. He observes, that the secretion peculiar to melanosis varies in colour from á dark brown to a deep blue or green black. It is sometimes spread, like so much paint, under the serous membrane of the intestines, for instance, or diffused through the substance of the spleen; while, in other cases, it is circumscribed in distinct patches, as in the parenchyma of the lungs, liver, or kidneys; in short, being occasionally found thus diffused or limited in most organs.—(*Morbid Anatomy of the Bowels,* &c., p. 24.)]

The chymical analyses of MM. Barruel and Lassaigne show that melanotic tumours consist, first, of coloured fibrin; secondly, of a blackish colouring matter, soluble in weak sulphuric acid, and in a solution of subcarbonate of soda, which become reddish; thirdly, of a small quantity of albumen; and, fourthly, of a chloruret of sodium, subcarbonate of soda, phosphate of lime, and oxyde of iron. The principles of melanosis, therefore, nearly resemble the constituent elements of the blood.* It is homogeneous, opaque, and destitute of any particular smell or taste. Thénard ascertained that it contains a very large proportion of carbon. When exposed to the air, it putrefies slowly.†

GENUS V.
STRUMA
SCROFULA.

INDOLENT, GLANDULAR TUMOURS, FREQUENTLY IN THE NECK; SUPPURATING SLOWLY AND IMPERFECTLY, AND HEALING WITH DIFFICULTY; UPPER LIP THICKENED; SKIN SMOOTH; COUNTENANCE USUALLY FLORID.

THE Greeks denominated this disease ΧΟΙΡΑΣ, the nosologists of recent times SCROFULA, thus literally translating the Greek, and importing *swine-evil, swine-swellings*, or morbid tumours to which swine are subject. Celsus employs STRUMA, which was common in his own day, and has well described the complaint under this name, which is therefore selected on the present occasion. It is probably derived from στρῶμα, "congestion," or "coacervation," as of straw in a litter, feathers in a bed, or tumours in a body; in which last sense Cicero elegantly employs the metaphor in the phrase "struma civitatis," "the scrofula or king's evil of the state." The medical dictionaries and glossaries concur in deriving struma from the Latin *struo*, but the terminating syllable of the noun should rather prove it to issue from a Greek source.

Other animals are subject to this disease besides man. It is, as already observed, from the frequency of its appearance among swine, that the Greek name, as well as the more recent one of scrofula, is derived. Among horses we meet with it at least as often, when it is called farcy; under which modification it is propagable by transfusion of blood from the diseased horse, not only to other horses, but to asses also, as

---

* Dr. Foy instituted a comparative analysis of medullary, scirrhous, and melanotic substances, and found them to contain albumen, fibrin, and salts, having for their basis soda, potash, and lime; also oxyde of iron, which was in rather greater proportion in the first two diseases than in melanosis; and in this latter alone he detected a highly carbonized principle, probably altered carbon, which constituted nearly a third of the morbid mass.—(See Archives Gén. de. Méd., Juin, 1828.) The colouring matter of melanosis is generally thought to bear a considerable analogy to the colouring matter of the blood.—ED.

† A singular appearance lately presented itself to the American editor, who, in company with Dr. Benj. Drake of New-York, examined the body of a rhinoceros to ascertain the cause of its decease, which was found to be pulmonary congestion. The small intestines, which were thirty feet in length, presented in nearly their whole course, minute black dots, resembling what is termed punctiform melanosis. Whether this appearance was natural or the result of disease, we are not prepared to say.—D.

---

* Vol. ii., Cl. VI., Ord. III., Gen. X., Spe. 2, 6, and comp. with the introductory note to Gen. IX., Trichosis.

† When melanotic matter is found in bloodvessels, it is chiefly in the venous capillaries, and "under circumstances which show that it must have been formed in these vessels."—See Professor Carswell's Illustrations of the Elementary Forms of Disease, fasc. iv.—ED

has been lately proved by Professor Coleman at the Veterinary Institution. Sauvages, who has many species under the generic character, has two for the forms now referred to. The porcine species he denominates scrofula *Chalasis,* and the equine s. *Farcimen.*

As it is not the intention of the present work to notice the diseases of other animals, otherwise than by an occasional and incidental glance, we shall proceed to a contemplation of the present genus under the single species of

1. Struma Vulgaris.　　King's Evil.

The strumous and mesenteric decline, in the present classification *atrophia strumosa,* is often introduced as a second species; but, though nearly allied to the present genus, it has so much closer a connexion with all the subdivisions of the genus MARASMUS, and especially with that of atrophia, that the former is evidently its proper place, and we have accordingly treated of it under that genus.*

SPECIES I.
STRUMA VULGARIS.
KING'S EVIL.

TUMOURS CONFINED TO THE EXTERNAL CONGLOBATE GLANDS;[†] PEA-SIZED OR CHESTNUT-SIZED; APPEARING IN INFANCY OR YOUTH; SUBSIDING ON MATURE AGE; HEREDITARY.

SCROFULA, though not a contagious disease, is unquestionably hereditary,[‡] and hence very generally dependant upon a peculiar diathesis. Yet, like many other hereditary diseases, it is also occasionally generated as a primary affection, without any hereditary taint that can be discovered. I had very lately a gentleman under my care, who has been greatly afflicted with it for many years, and is now chiefly labouring under its sequelæ; for the sores, which are in different glands and joints, and some of which have affected the bones, are healing; yet, of eight brothers and sisters who have reached the middle of life, he is the only one who has discovered any tendency to such complaint, nor is it to be traced through any part of the family lineage as far as it can be ascended.

----

* Tubercular diseases of the lungs, spleen, and peritoneum, are regarded by many pathologists of the present day as scrofulous affections: so are particular diseases of the eyes, bones, and joints, and likewise some chronic abscesses, of which one of the most remarkable examples is the psoas, or lumbar abscess. A tendency to the formation of abscesses in a very slow and sometimes hardly perceptible manner, unpreceded by any very obvious exciting cause, is a common occurrence in scrofulous individuals. We see, then, how imperfect is Dr. Good's definition of scrofula, and how much more comprehensive it might have been made.—ED.

† The editor is at a loss to understand why the deep-seated lymphatic glands, which are often the seat of scrofulous disease, should be excepted.

‡ Kirkland, On the Present State of Surgery, vol. ii. Kortum, Comment. de Vitio Scrofuloso, Lemgoviæ, 1789. Baumes, sur le Virus Scrofuleux, &c.

When it occurs as a primary or ingenerated affection, it is by no means always limited to any particular temperament or habit of body. The individual just noticed is of moderate stature, brown complexion, dark brown hair, and ruddy face: and I am still occasionally attending a lady who has long been subject to the same complaint, without any trace of hereditary predisposition, of a sallow countenance, dark eyes and hair, and of rather tall and slender make. But, where scrofula appears hereditary, and especially where it does not show itself very early, it is often accompanied with a peculiar constitution.* "It most commonly," says Dr. Cullen, "affects children of soft and flaccid flesh, of fair hair and blue eyes, smooth skins and rosy cheeks: and such children have frequently a tumid upper lip, with a chop in the middle of it; and this tumour is often considerable, and extended, to the columna nasi and lower part of the nostrils." And it is a further remark of Dr. Cullen, but which I have not found to hold very generally, that, where it takes place in children whose parents have given no signs of it, the latter have nevertheless evinced much of the habit and constitution by which the disease is ordinarily characterized.

From all this we have a clear proof that king's evil is a disease of debility, operating by a specific influence on the circulation, and particularly on the lymphatic system.—(*Garn, Kranken geschichten,* p. 121.) Whether this influence be the result of a specific matter is by no means so clear, however common the opinion. It is also a general belief that this specific matter is, from the first, a specific irritant or acrimony. But this, at least, is a mistake; for the disease is accompanied throughout with diminished, instead of with increased irritability (*Richter, Chir. Bibl.,* band viii., p. 501); and hence the power producing it must be of a sedative, rather than of an exciting or acuating quality. And it is in this diminution of irritability that scrofula differs from all other atonic diseases, since the debility and irritability generally augment in like proportion, and maintain an equal march.

Early life is peculiarly characterized by an abundance of albumen, as its maturity is by an abundance of fibrin. Dr. Parr ascribes the scrofulous diathesis to a redundance of albumen at this period, together with an excess of oxygen and a deficiency of azote, evidenced by the florid hue of the countenance. By this hypothesis he obtains a sort of lentor in the circulating system, and accounts for the origin of scrofulous tumours by arguing that, since the mobility of the lymphatic system is peculiarly affected and diminished, the viscid fluids will be most disposed to stagnate there, and particularly in the lymphatic

----

* The numerous disordered conditions of the function of nutrition evinced in scrofulous persons, are certainly independent of one another: all of them proceed from a cause that is manifested to us by the existence of those modifications of nutrition and secretion, the assemblage of which makes what is termed a scrofulous constitution. —See Andral, Anat. Pathol., tom. i., p. 5, 8vo., Paris, 1829.—ED.

glands, as they must necessarily stagnate most where the impelling power is least.*

It is here, indeed, rather than in any other modification of tubers or tubercles, that we find most to oppose to the opinion of those physiologists, as M. Broussais and Dr. Alison, who ascribe the origin of all tubercles to the existence of a higher or lower degree of inflammation. Yet it is singular that, at the same time, we here meet with proofs of the most advanced state of a living action in the morbid growths themselves, the most perfect specimens of vascularity and sensation, and particularly where they originate in a glandular texture, which is their proper seat. This living property, however, they do not seem capable of retaining long; for they soon run through their career of vitality, and become decomposed. Such was the short-lived date, according to the first physiological poet of Rome, of those monster-growths which sprang in the infancy of the world, but were soon cut off by Nature, as incongruous with her laws and hateful to her survey.

" Cætera de genere hoc monstra, ac portenta, creabat :
Nequidquam ; quoniam Natura absterruit auctum ;
Nec potuere cupitum ætatis tangere florem,
Nec reperire cibum, nec jungi per Veneris res."†

These sprang at first, and things alike uncouth:
Yet vainly ; for abhorrent Nature quick
Check'd their vile growth ; so life's consummate flower
Ne'er reach'd they, foods appropriate never cropp'd,
Nor tasted joys venereal.

As occurring in early life, when, as we have already observed, there is a peculiar abundance of albumen, with a comparatively less portion of fibrin or coagulable lymph, it is highly probable that a morbid deposition of albumen forms the commencement of the strumous tuber. And such, indeed, seems to be proved by the chymical tests to which Dr. Abercrombie has put them.—(*Trans. Medico-Chir. Soc. Edin.*, vol. i., p. 686.) It is at first, perhaps, deposited in a soft state, and involved in the structure of the gland, the part being in other respects vascular and organized, and probably capable of performing its functions. As the disease advances the proportion of albumen seems to increase, while, at the same time, it assumes a more concrete and structural figure, and evinces a vascular and sensitive character. "In this first state of enlargement," says Dr. Abercrombie, "these glands

present, when cut into, a pale flesh-colour, and a uniform, soft, fleshy texture. As the disease advances, the texture becomes firmer and the colour rather paler. In what may be regarded as the next stage, we observe portions that have lost the flesh-colour and have acquired a kind of transparency, and a texture approaching to that of soft cartilage. While these changes are going on, we generally observe, in other specimens, the commencement of the opaque white structure, which seems to be the last step in these morbid changes, and is strictly analogous, in its appearance and properties, to the white tubercle of the lungs.* In a mass of considerable size we can sometimes observe all these structures, often in alternate strata ; some of the strata being composed of the opaque white matter ; others presenting the semi-pellucid appearance ; while in other parts of the same mass, we find portions which retain the fleshy appearance. In the most advanced stage, the opaque, white, or ash-coloured tubercular matter is the most abundant, and this afterward appears to be gradually softened, until it degenerates into the soft cheesy matter or ill-conditioned suppuration so familiar to us in affections of this nature." The morbid growth, therefore, as it recedes from its more vascular and vital elaboration, gradually subsides into the simple pretension of coagulated albumen, of which it consisted at first. In the second stage, the part is probably susceptible of active inflammation and healthy suppuration, or suppuration making a near approach to that of a healthy character. In its closing stage it seems incapable of healthy action, and only passes into that peculiar state of softening which arises from a simple decomposition of the tubercular organization.

We have already described at some length the probable origin of tubercles in other textures, chiefly in the serous and mucous membranes of organs, and in the structure of the lungs. The remarks now offered will enable us in some degree to judge in what respect the tubercles of proper glands, as those of the lymphatics and the mesentery, are assimilated to these, and in what respects they differ from them. The subject, however, is still open to inquiry, and

---

* The doctrine of Andral is exactly the reverse of this : a morbid state of the lymphatic glands is most frequent at the period of life when the nutrition of these organs is most active. This, says he, affords a confirmation of the general law, in virtue of which the frequency of the disease of every organ is in a direct ratio to the development of its structure and action.—(Anat. Pathol., tom. ii., p. 449, 8vo., Paris, 1829.) Then, what are we to think of the hypothesis of stagnation in the lymphatic glands, when we find, from the experiments of Becker, that when they are diseased, quicksilver pervades them in the freest manner ?—ED.

† Lucret., De Rer. Nat., v., 845.

* In the section on tubercular phthisis, reference bas been made to Dr. Carswell's observation that the same kind of substance as constitutes tubercles in the lungs has been traced in scrofulous lymphatic glands. According to Andral, the latter organs rank as parts of the body in which tubercular matter is most commonly detected. At present this deposite is supposed to take place in the substance of these organs ; but Andral conceives it probable that future researches may trace its seat to be within the lymphatic vessels which communicate together in these organs. In fact, cases have come under his notice, where tubercular matter was found in the thoracic duct, and in several of the absorbent vessels.—(Anat. Pathol., tom. i., p. 451.) This view seems, however, to disagree with the assertion, that mercury will readily pass through the vessels of diseased lymphatic glands. We are yet in want of precise information respecting the state of the absorbent vessels in the glands, when these latter are in various conditions of disease.—ED.

much remains to be accomplished before a full and satisfactory result is likely to be obtained.

Be the proximate cause of scrofula, however, what it may, as the remōte cause is of a debilitating kind, we can readily see what are likely to prove occasional and co-operative causes, or those calculated to call the remote cause into a state of activity. They must consist of every thing that directly lowers and reduces the tone of the living fibre, and puts the system out of that state of firm and vigorous elasticity which is the best prophylactic against the disease, and keeps the scrofulous diathesis most effectually in a state of subjection. And hence we find the common debilitating powers of cold, damp, meager or unwholesome food, want of cleanliness, and a close and suffocating atmosphere, the most usual incidental sources of strumous affections.—(*E. A. Lloyd's Treatise on Scrofula,* &c., 8vo., Lond., 1821.)

But for these, a scrofulous predisposition might remain dormant in the constitution through the whole of life; and descend to and disorder the next generation, without having in the least disturbed the present. But the moment any of these occasional causes become adjuncts with the scrofulous diathesis, scrofula, rather than any other disease they are also calculated to promote, will make its appearance and commence its ravage. And hence the frequency of this disease in large manufacturing towns, and in higher and colder latitudes than 45°.

Heat, as a relaxing and debilitating power, tending to produce languid action, is also a frequent cause whenever applied in excess and habitually; and particularly where, like cold, it is combined with sudden variations of temperature. Scrofula is known to be particularly frequent in Hindoos, Hottentots, and negroes, when they come to temperate climates; and especially in the children of settlers in intertropical regions, upon their quitting such regions for countries of a milder temperature.

[The unusual frequency of phthisis among negroes and Hindoos, and even among mulattoes and half-caste people, in this climate, is, as Dr. Alison observes (*Edin. Med. Chir. Trans.,* vol. i., p. 399), generally admitted. At the same time he grants, that, as the black population of tropical countries have other peculiarities besides that of being brought up in hot climates, we are not entitled to ascribe their scrofulous tendency exclusively to this circumstance. Yet, says he, when we connect the facts above stated with the enervating influence produced by long residence in hot climates on European constitutions, so strikingly shown in the different forms assumed by fever and by hepatitis in the old settlers and the newly-arrived Europeans; and this, again, with the facts already adduced to show the connexion of general debility with scrofula; it seems to Dr. Alison extremely probable, that this part of the constitution of negroes and Hindoos is very much owing to the long-continued application of heat in early life, and particularly to this cause acting on many generations in succession.]

The influence of excessive cold, however, is much more rapid than that of excessive heat, and far more obvious to the sense. Yet it is often sustained with impunity where the constitution is firm, and the cold rarely subject to vicissitudes; and especially where there is no other debilitating cause to contend with, as the depressing passions, a sedentary occupation, scanty and innutritive diet, damp and impure air, or any kind of personal neglect or uncleanliness. And it is on this account, we meet with a far smaller proportion of scrofula in early life among the peasantry of higher latitudes and mountain scenery, as that of Scotland and Switzerland, than among the mechanics of crowded and warmer cities. "I was told," says Dr. Alison, "by one of the physicians of the Hôpital des Enfans Malades, at Paris, where upwards of five hundred children die annually, whose bodies are almost uniformly opened, that he believed nearly one half of the bodies he saw opened had scrofulous tubercles in some part or other." This is indeed a higher aggregate than is to be found in the metropolis of our own country, and obviously includes mesenteric or strumous tubers, of which we have treated already, as well as every other modification of scrofula. But the same writer calculates, from data furnished by Dr. Perceval, that the proportion of scrofulous fatal cases among children at Manchester, at the time Dr. Perceval wrote, generalizing them as above, could not be less than a third of the whole infantine mortality; while at Waverton, a country parish near Chester, it appears from the same documents that the deaths from scrofula in children under five years of age, did not amount to a fourth part of this proportion. In the bordering village of Reyton, the difference appears to have been still greater; for the whole mortality of children under five years of age in this last parish, compared with the same period of parallel mortality at Manchester, was only as two, to seven; not more than one seventh part of the children born in this village appearing to die before they had attained their fifth year. "I examined lately," says Dr. Alison, "a register, which I know to have been kept with great accuracy for nearly four years, of the deaths of a country parish in Scotland, that of Rafford, near Forres, the population of which parish is almost exactly a thousand persons. Of forty-two deaths that had occurred in that time, two only, or one in twenty-one, were below the age of two; and three only, or one in fourteen, below that of five years;" while in the town of Manchester, to which we have just referred, Dr. Perceval assures us, on an average of twenty years, that the proportion of deaths under two years to the whole deaths was 1 to 2.9.—(*Perceval's Works,* vol. iii., p. 107.)

To add any thing further is unnecessary. Scrofula is manifestly a disease of weak vascular action, and is sure to be found in abundance with other diseases, issuing from the same soil, consociate, to whose fatality it largely adds. Extreme heat and cold, though powerful predisponents, are far more injurious when flowing in irregular vicissitudes, than when in a uniform tenour; and the mischievous effect of the latter is often counteracted where combined with the tonic powers of a pure and dry atmosphere, a regular plan of diet and exercise, the salubrious exhalations from growing vegetables, and the grateful stimulus of their odours in village scenery.

[And, as Dr. Alison has judiciously remarked, those who suffer most from the agency of cold, as a cause of disease in general, are by no means those who are most frequently exposed to it; but those whose previous condition is such as to favour its operation on the body, and particularly those in whom the circulation, either from the state of the constitution or accidental circumstances, is feeble and easily depressed. The same well-informed physician elsewhere observes, that what is true of the production of disease in general by exposure to cold, seems to be true of the production of scrofulous diseases in particular; but with these limitations:— 1. That scrofulous action appears to be excited almost solely in the earlier periods of life. 2. That, for the production of this kind of diseased action, there appears to be required, besides other conditions, a certain peculiarity of habit, not understood, but, manifestly, in Dr. Alison's opinion hereditary. 3. That the constitutional debility which disposes to scrofulous disease from cold, appears to be more permanent and habitual than that which disposes to other diseases resulting from this cause.] .

For the reasons just urged, scrofula has at times been called into activity by local injuries, the depressing influence of severe grief, or a sudden reverse of worldly prosperity. It is also sometimes joined with or follows rickets; and is frequently a sequel of severe febrile disease, smallpox, yaws, measles, syphilis, scarlatina, several obstinate cutaneous affections, and the long use of mercury.

But though scrofula usually commences in the lymphatic glands, it often extends beyond them: as gout, that ordinarily shows itself at first in the small joints, and rheumatism, that begins in the large joints, spread not unfrequently to the membranes and the muscles. I have said that, under the influence of the scrofulous diathesis, the circulating system is weakened generally; and hence also we frequently find the eyes, the mucous glands of the nose, the tonsils, and even the joints and bones, successively yielding to its influence.*

The disease for the most part shows itself early in life, though rarely before the second,† and commonly not till the third year of infancy; from which period it continues to prey on the system till the seventh, when, in ordinary cases, it gradually subsides and disappears. If the predisposition be not considerable, the attack is sometimes postponed till after the seventh year, and has occasionally been retarded till the age of puberty, after which, however, we have very seldom any first manifestation of the disease.

. The first tumours we meet with are usually upon the sides of the neck, below the ears, or under the chin; and confined to the lymphatic glands in these parts. The tumours are, perhaps, two or three in number, moveable, soft, and slightly elastic, of a globular or oval figure, without pain or discoloration of the skin. In this state they continue for a year or two; after which they grow larger and become more fixed, and acquire a purplish redness. They then give that feeling of greater softness, and at length of fluctuation, to which we have just adverted; after which the skin, in one or more of them, becomes paler, and a peculiar liquid is poured forth at several small apertures, apparently like immature pus, but growing daily less purulent, and at length assuming a cheesy or curd-like form.* The tumour, or cluster of tumours, then subsides, but others rise in the neighbourhood; and in this manner the disease proceeds, fresh tumours forming, chiefly in the course of the spring, as the older disappear, and the same process is continued for several years; after which the ulcers heal spontaneously, with puckered and indelible indentations, provided the disease terminates favourably; but if not, other parts of the system, as we have already observed, become tainted with the morbid influence, and add to the sum of distress. If the attack fall upon the eyelids, they become inflamed, are swollen and red, and pour forth from their minute glands an erosive but viscid secretion, which glues them together at night, so that in the morning they are opened with difficulty. The adnata partakes of the irritation, which is at length communicated to the whole globe of the eye, and not unfrequently to the cheek, from the acrid discharge that flows down. An unsightly lippitude, and eversion of the lower eye-

---

* Sometimes the disease commences in the eyes, joints, spleen, lungs, peritoneum, or other organs, and the lymphatic glands may either escape, or be affected only secondarily. For this and other reasons, the editor regards the definition at the head of the present section as liable to objections.—Ed.

† When the mother has been scrofulous, tubercles in the lungs, and strumous disease of the kidneys, have been sometimes, though rarely, noticed in the fœtus or stillborn infant.—See Lloyd, op. cit., p. 23.—Ed.

---

* According to Mr. Wardrop, "the matter has at first a firm curdy consistence, and, as the process advances, some portions become more fluid; until, ultimately, the suppurative cavity contains a matter partly curdy, partly puriform, and partly serous. When this matter is removed by ulceration of the parietes of the cavity containing it, an irregular-shaped cavity remains in the substance of the gland. While the swelling of the part diminishes, the sides of this cavity become covered with a curdy yellow incrustation, more or less firm, and from its surface a puriform matter is secreted. This incrustation prevents the formation of granulations, and is the cause of scrofulous cavities not healing up; while it is by the separation of this crust, in consequence of laying open these abscesses, that granulations form and heal up the cavity.

"The incrustation covering the internal surface of the scrofulous abscess, when of very long standing, acquires a surface which resembles a mucous membrane, from which the puriform fluid is secreted."—Baillie's Works, by Wardrop, vol. ii Preliminary Obs., p. 33.

lid are hence a very common result of a scrofulous attack on this organ.

In like manner the disease, in this unfavourable and aggravated state, often makes its assault on the limbs, and fixes on the ligaments, cartilages, or even the bones themselves; and particularly whenever any injury occurs to a joint. An indolent tumour first shows itself, which tardily advances in magnitude with a kind of smothered inflammation, and at length opens on the surface from one or more minute ulcerations, which discharge the sanious kind of fluid we have already noticed. And it is here we perceive how nearly scrofula is related to hydarthrus, or white swelling; and how readily the former may become a cause of the latter, as already observed under that species. If the strumous diathesis be excited by the fracture of a bone, the broken ends unite with great difficulty, and sometimes not at all. A specific tumour forms in the seat of the injury, the soft parts are often affected with a weak inflammation, and ulcerate slowly, and the bone is rendered carious. If the injury occur in the middle of a cylindrical bone, an exfoliation may take place in a long course of time; but if at its extremity, it will become spongy, enlarged, and disorganized. If a cure be at length effected, the enlargement will remain and the articulation be lost; yet amputation will be of no use while the part continues under the influence of the scrofulous taint.*

[The susceptibility of scrofula, inherent in different parts, is said to be altered by age: "Thus, in children, the upper lip, eyes, glands of the neck, and those of the mesentery, are generally the parts first affected; the lungs, bones, and other parts being subsequently attacked.—(*Lloyd on Scrofula*, p. 5.)]

In the worst and severest stage of the disease, the entire system appears to be contaminated; hectic fever ensues, and sometimes tubercular phthisis, which gradually puts an end to the contest.

[The urine of scrofulous subjects is said to contain less phosphoric acid than the urine of healthy persons, and an increased quantity of phosphate of lime. This earth is also sometimes found after death in the lymphatic glands, in the thoracic duct, and in the substance of the viscera.‡]

In attending to the cure, we must not be unmindful of the principle we have endeavoured to establish, that scrofula is a disease of debility, principally affecting the lymphatic system, accompanied with diminished irritability.* And it hence follows that our chief dependance must be upon a tonic and stimulant plan, so modified as to meet the patient's age, idiosyncrasy, and manner of life.

An old hypothesis is, that scrofula depends upon an acrimony in the system, and hence sedatives and narcotics have found a place among the most celebrated of its remedies; while, as the chymical character of the acrimony has been also pretended to be developed, and has been declared to be a specific acid, another class of remedies had recourse to has been the alkalis.

That the latter are often of considerable service, ought I think freely to be admitted; but we have assuredly no proof that they become beneficial as correctors of acidity. They are gentle stimulants, admirably adapted to the debilitated and indolent condition of the vascular system they are intended to excite; and hence, in whatever form they are given, have a chance of doing good. And it is to this principle we are, perhaps, to resolve all the advantage that has been stated by different writers, and in different ages of the world, to have resulted from the use of burnt sponge, burnt cuttlefish, shells of all kinds, burnt hartshorn, and even burnt secundines, which last were at one time in high request, and are to be found as a sovereign remedy in Schroeder's Pharmacopœia.—(Lib. v., p. 288.) All these have in our own day deservedly yielded to the carbonate of soda and subcarbonate of ammonia; which, in a more elegant, and concentrated form, offer whatever virtues may be contained in the older medicines: and still more lately to iodine, not long ago detected by M. Courtois in kelp and other saltworts; for a more particular account of which medicine the reader may turn to the treatment of ʙʀᴏɴᴄʜᴏᴄᴇʟᴇ.—(Vol. ii., Cl. VI., Ord. I., Gen. II., Spe. 1, *Emphyma Sarcoma Bronchocele.*) The author has, at this moment of

---

* This is not quite correct, as no stumps generally heal more favourably than those resulting from the amputation of scrofulous joints.—Eᴅ.

† Pinel, Nosogr. Philosophique. We know from the researches of Dr. Carswell, that tubercular matter, the same kind of unorganized deposite as is found in tubercles of the lungs, is also sometimes detected in scrofulous glands; and, as these are sometimes cured, the fact has been adduced as an argument in favour of tubercular phthisis not being absolutely incurable.—See Dr. Carswell's Illustrations of the Elementary Forms of Disease.—Eᴅ.

* How contrary this theory is to that entertained by some other writers, may be seen by a reference to Crowther's work on white swelling, &c., ed. 1808. A still later author remarks:—" In scrofulous disease there is generally what is termed a delicate state of the health, great nervous irritation, greater susceptibility than natural; so that certain external agents, as cold, &c., applied to the body, produce unusual effects; and there is always more or less disorder of the digestive organs; and, upon accurate investigation, this state of the system will always be found to have existed for some time previous to the appearance of the disease in any particular part."—(Lloyd on Scrofula, p. 32.) The editor believes that we know nothing about the proximate cause of scrofula; and that the digestive organs cannot be essentially concerned in the production of the disease, is as clear as the fact pointed out by Mr. Lloyd, that scrofula sometimes affects the fœtus in utero. The disorder of these organs, in many examples, is certainly only an effect; yet it is not here intended to deny the possibility of the origin of scrofula being promoted by derangement of the functions of the digestive organs. But that something else is requisite appears certain, as these organs are frequently disordered without a single symptom of scrofula showing itself.—Eᴅ.

writing, among other patients who have been ben-efited by this plan, a lad about thirteen years of age, with weak eyes, inflamed and irritable con-junctiva, and such an enlargement of the parotid glands* as to make them nearly meet, so that the mouth opens with uneasiness. He has now applied the ointment of iodine for three weeks, and at the same time taken half a grain twice a day in the form of a pill, and is essentially im-proved in every respect. [Iodine may be said to be the medicine to which the generality of medical practitioners are turning their attention as a means of curing various forms of scrofulous disease. Its extraordinary power in.dispersing many strumous swellings cannot be doubted; but whether it possess any specific power for the correction of the scrofulous diathesis, still re-mains to be proved.†]

Lime-water and the muriate of barytes,‡ which last was thought by Dr. Adair Crawford to be nearly a specific, if they have any pretensions whatever, can only derive them from the general principle of their being stimulants, and esp-ecially of the lymphatic system. And the same may be observed of petroselinum, sarsa, meze-reon, balsam of sulphur, and calamus aromaticus.

Muriate of soda, or common sea-salt, posses-ses a like character, and has undoubtedly been found of far more use in many cases. It has hence been employed very freely, both inter-nally and externally. In the latter case gener-ally through the medium of the bibulous marine plants, which contain it in a larger proportion, and have been applied to the strumous tumours in the form of epithems, as sea-wrack (fucus vesiculosus), sea-tang (alga marina), and sea-oak (quercus marina).

The mineral waters of every description have in like manner been had recourse to, chalybeate, sulphureous, and saline ; and perhaps, as Dr. Cullen observes, with nearly a like reputation and success ; though it is by no means improbable

---

* The editor believes that this case must have been either a bronchocele, or a general enlarge-ment of the lymphatic glands on each side of the neck and behind the jaw ; for, besides the fact that the parotid gland is seldom or never the seat of scrofula, the extension of the disease under the chin seems to prove that the disease could not have consisted in the parotid.—ED.

† The strongest facts on record proving the use-fulness of iodine in scrofulous diseases, are those published by Dr. Lugol (Mém. sur l'Emploi de l'Iode dans les Maladies Scrofuleuses, 8vo., Paris, 1829), who employs this medicine, however, in a greater variety of ways and forms than we have taken the trouble to do in this country. Instead of the tincture. he prescribes an aqueous solution of iodine of different strengths, with a proportion of the hydriodate of potash in them. He also ap-plies iodine in the form of baths, lotions, and col-lyria ; sometimes also as a stimulating or rubefa-cient application ; and, in particular cases, as an escharotic. Whoever wishes to give iodine a fair trial in scrofula, should prescribe it in Lugol's manner, whose formulæ may be seen in his work. —Eo.

‡ This article is highly recommended by Dr. Williamson.—See Potter's Med. and Phil. Lyce-um, Baltimore, 1811.—D.

---

that some waters may prove a more remedial stimulant or alterant to some constitutions, and others to others. And we thus possess a more plausible reason for their being advantageous than that offered by Dr. Cullen ; namely, that, " if they are ever successful, it is the element-ary water that is the chief part of the remedy" (Practice of Physic, vol. iv., 1752) ; which, he tells us in another place, " may be of use by washing out the lymphatic system."

Stimulant external applications, besides sea-water, have also been tried, and undoubtedly been often found serviceable ; as a long con-tinued friction of the hand over the scrofulous protuberances, mercurial or ammoniacal plas-ters, or the-convenient form in the London Phar-macopœia that combines both these ingredients ; irritant ointments, especially those containing iodine, the aura of voltaism, or moderate shocks of electricity.

The means of this kind, however, to which we have recourse, whether external or internal, should always be gentle at first, however we may venture upon augmenting them afterward. If we stimulate violently, we shall do mischief rather than good, and add to the debility in-stead of diminishing it. Scrofula is a strictly chronic disease ; it never has been, and never can be cured rapidly ; and wherever any bene-ficial influence has been produced upon it, it has always been, as in the use of alkalis and of mineral waters, by lenient means and patient perseverance.

But we have to increase the power as well as to take off the irritability ; and hence tonics seem to be as much demanded as stimulants, and have in fact been as generally made use of.

It is very singular, that, of this class of med-icines, the only two which Dr. Cullen has thought it worth while to notice, are bark and coltsfoot ; of the first of these he speaks very doubtfully ; while he seems to depend more on the second than on any other remedy whatever. This opinion he expresses in his Practice of Physic, published in 1783; but in his Materia Medica, published six years afterward, he gives it the same high character, and tells us that he was induced to try it in scrofulous cases upon the testimony and recommendation of Fuller. He employed both an expressed juice of the fresh leaves, and a decoction of the dry ; but preferred the former, of which he gave " some ounces every day," and affirms that " in several in-stances it had occasioned the healing up of scrofulous sores." He admits, however, that neither of them was, in some trials, sufficiently effectual.

The metallic salts have been more generally used, and have at least acquired a higher repu-tation ; though, with the exception of calomel, I do not know of any of them that can appeal to any decided testimonies in proof of their suc-cess ; and even calomel may perhaps be regard-ed rather as an alterant or mild stimulant, than as a tonic. Salivation has always done harm ; and, on this account, mercury in every form must be given in minute doses. Combined with some preparations of antimony, and particularly with the precipitated sulphuret, as in Plummer's pills, it is said to have been chiefly serviceable. But in my own practice, I have not found this medicine of any manifest service in the present disease.

The acids have also been tried, but are of little or no avail.

Upon the whole, however, the tonic class of medicines has thus far proved considerably less decisive and important, in the treatment of scrofula, than we might fairly have conjectured. Yet a tonic regimen of sea-air, sea-bathing, liberal exercise, and a diet somewhat generous, is of the highest consequence in promoting improvement, and ought by no means to be dispensed with. The infirmary at Margate is on this account a noble institution, and cannot be too liberally supported.

Of the specific benefit of narcotics, as hemlock, henbane, foxglove, solanum, asclepias, vincetoxicum, and many others, I have yet to be persuaded. They may possibly be of some use in quieting the irritation occasionally produced by congestion and mechanical pressure where the tumours are peculiarly indurated and large, and in such cases may assist in softening and diminishing them. And they may, perhaps, operate in the same way where, in the latter and more malignant stages of the disease, the secretion is become virulent, the open ulcers irritable, and a foundation is hereby laid for hectic fever. But I can conscientiously say, with Dr. Cullen, that they have often disappointed me, and have not seemed to dispose scrofulous ulcers to heal.

The local applications, like the internal remedies, should be slightly stimulant ; and, where the tumours have broken, usually consist of digestive ointments combined with the caustic metallic salts of mercury, zinc, or copper, and of digestive lotions of a dilute solution of alum or nitrate of silver. These are well calculated to coincide with the general intention ; but we must not expect a sound cure till the morbid impression is set at rest in the constitution, or utterly extirpated from it.

[Those who espouse the hypothesis that in scrofula there always is more or less disorder of the functions of the digestive organs, and primarily of no other important function, of course renounce all faith in specifics, and consider the principal indication to be that of improving the state of those functions by attention to diet, and by keeping the bowels regular, and the hepatic secretions natural. - The editor believes that more good may be effected in scrofulous cases by endeavouring to rectify any obvious defect in the constitution, or, in other words, to improve the health in general, than by trying the effect of various medicines, supposed to have a specific power over the disease. On this very principle, however, iodine, carbonate of soda, blended with rhubarb and columbo powder, and other alteratives and tonics, will frequently be proper, as well as small doses of the blue-pill, the compound calomel pill, and the compound decoction of sarsaparilla ; with occasional mild purgatives, so much confided in by those prac-

Vol. II.—F

titioners who believe the cause of scrofula to be essentially connected with disorder of the digestive organs.]*

GENUS VI.
CARCINUS.
CANCER.†

SCIRRHOUS, LIVID TUMOUR, INTERSECTED WITH FIRM, WHITISH, DIVERGENT BANDS, FOUND CHIEFLY IN THE SECERNENT GLANDS ; PAINS ACUTE AND LANCINATING ; OFTEN PROPAGATED TO OTHER PARTS ; TERMINATING IN A FETID AND ICHOROUS ULCER.

Of this genus there is but one known species : for the division into occult and open, or

---

* Struma is comparatively of rare occurrence in the more northern portions of the United States; the official report of deaths by this disease in the city of New-York for the past five years, amounting only to sixty-five ; but in the southern country the case is far different, and there this malady proves a complete scourge to the black population, who in the northern states also appear more disposed to it than do the whites ; among the latter, it seems to affect foreigners rather than Americans, and to be often called into action by the confined air of narrow and dirty habitations, by unwholesome diet, &c.

The treatment of scrofula is conducted on the principle that the disease is often constitutional ; the popular idea that the muriate of barytes was useful, has led many to our mineral springs, and more particularly to that of Ballston in the state of New-York, inasmuch as chymical analyses had shown that this compound of barytes was a constituent part of these mineral waters. Chalybeates, more particularly the carbonates and phosphates of iron, are now commonly prescribed, attention being previously paid to the digestive organs. Iodine, also, has many firm friends with us.—D.

† One of the heterologous formations, as they are termed by Professor Carswell, in his Illustrations of the Elementary Forms of Disease. The essential character of the heterologous formations, he founds on the presence of a substance which does not enter into the original composition of the body. When the heterologous deposite is collected at numerous points, in the shape of a hard, gray, semitransparent substance, intersected by a dull-white, or pale straw-coloured, fibrous, or condensed cellular tissue, the disease is usually termed *scirrhus*. When it assumes a regular lobulated arrangement, so as to present an appearance similar to a section of the pancreas, it constitutes the *pancreatic sarcoma* of Abernethy. For other varieties, named by the French *tissue lardacé, matiére colloid*, and *cancer gélatiforme*, or *aréolaire*, consult Dr. Carswell's work. In order to trace the precise seat, origin, and mode of formation of cancer, it is necessary, as this excellent pathologist observes, "to catch the disease, as it were, at the earliest period of its formation ; that is to say, when the heterologous substance of which it consists has just been deposited, and has not effaced the particular texture or structure of the part in which it is contained. Investigated in this its first stage, we ascertain, with greater or less facility, that this substance becomes manifest to our senses, either as a production of nutrition or secretion. In the former case, it is deposited in the same manner as the nutritive element of the blood enters into the molecular structure, and assumes

indolent and ulcerative, introduced by Hippocrates, and continued to the time of Boerhaave, is unnecessary in pathology, and incorrect in a nosological arrangement; as the distinctions it contemplates are nothing more than so many stages or modifications of the same disease in different habits, or affected by different concomitants. This species is what is generally described under the name of

1. Carcinus vulgaris.   Common cancer:

and it is not necessary to alter the term.

SPECIES I.
CARCINUS VULGARIS.
COMMON CANCER.

TUMOUR BURNING, KNOTTY; WITH DARK, CANCRIFORM VARICES; ULCER, WITH THICK, LIVID, RETORTED LIPS.

THERE is a soft, fungous, and bleeding ulcer, possessing the name of fungus hæmatodes, which has by many writers of celebrity been supposed to be of a cancerous origin; and, under their authority, it has been so regarded in the author's volume on Nosology: but as it seems to differ from cancer in its constitutional influence, and in some of its local characters,* it is better to contemplate it as a malignant ULCER of a peculiar kind; and in the present work it is referred to that genus accordingly.†

The term carcinus (καρκίνος) is Greek, and imports a crab; the disease being thus call-

the form and arrangement of the tissue or organ into which it is thus introduced. In the latter, it makes its appearance on a free surface, after the manner of natural secretions, as on serous surfaces in general. Proceeding still further in our researches, we find this substance existing not only in the molecular structure, and on the free surface of organs, but also on the blood of the venous and capillary divisions of the vascular system."—Professor Carswell, op. cit.—ED.

* One fact, mentioned by Dr. Carswell, is exceedingly curious and important in relation to these malignant diseases:—"Numerous examples," says he, "might be given of scirrhus, medullary sarcoma, and fungus hæmatodes, originating in the same morbid state, and passing successively from the one into the other, in the order in which I have named them. Indeed, we often meet with all the varieties which I have enumerated of both species, not only in different organs of the same individual, but even in a single organ."—(See Illustrations of the Elementary Forms of Disease, 4to., fasc. ii., Lond., 1833.) One evening, at the London University, Sir Astley Cooper lately mentioned to Dr. Carswell and the editor, that he knew of a case in which a lady, whose breast had been removed, and was found to have the true scirrhous texture, afterward died of fungus hæmatodes in the same situation.—ED.

† The fungus hæmatodes of Hey, is the *medullary sarcoma* of Abernethy, the *matière cérébriforme*, or *encéphaloide* of Laennec, the *spongoid inflammation* of John Burns, and the *soft cancer* of several other writers. As it is not till an advanced stage of the disease that any fungus or ulceration occurs, medullary sarcoma is one of these first of these terms. Fungus hæmatodes is, at all events, totally inapplicable, until the morbid mass projects through the skin and bleeds; and even then it is not truly a fungus, but a soft medullary substance.—ED.

ed from the cancriform or crab-like ramifications of the dark distended veins of the cancerous tumour. The question is of some consequence, whether cancer be a constitutional or a local, whether an hereditary or merely an occasional disease. Much has been said, and well said, on both sides. Till of late years, the disease was generally regarded as a constitutional affection, and will, for the most part, therefore, be found in the division of cachexies, from Sauvages to Macbride, though Dr. Cullen has introduced it into his class *locales*; and since his time, many of the best writers of the present day, among whom are Dr. Baillie and Mr. Abernethy, concur in regarding it as local alone. If the disease be merely local, it is difficult, and perhaps insuperably difficult, to say why a blow on a conglomerate gland, as the breast for example, should sometimes produce a cancer, but more generally not; or what that power is that excites the cancerous action in one person, from which another, or perhaps a hundred others, remain free upon an application of the very same injury to the same organ. A blow on the knee often produces a white swelling, but ten thousand children receive blows on the knee without any such effect following. In this case we resolve the difference of result, without a controversy, into the presence or absence of a scrofulous constitution; and without this view of the subject we should find ourselves at a loss for an answer. And unless we apply the same reasoning to cancer, we shall ever, I fear, remain at an equal loss. The cases, moreover, in which cancerous tumours are found in other parts of the body, after one or more than one has been extirpated, lead us by an easy thread to the same conclusion, provided the tumour has been removed in an early stage of the disease, and before ulceration has taken place; for it is possible that the specific matter of a cancer, generated and matured locally, may be absorbed and deposited on the organs which are afterward affected.* But if the extirpation have taken place before the formation of the specific matter, it is not easy, except by a constitutional diathesis, to account for any subsequent appearances.†

* The impossibility of communicating cancer from one person to another by inoculation with the matter of cancerous ulcers, is a strong fact in opposition to this last hypothesis. The existence of a specific cancerous matter, or virus, is denied by M. Roux, as the editor conceives, upon very sufficient grounds.—ED.

† Dr. Carswell joins our author in considering cancer as a constitutional disease:—"It may," says he, "be regarded as a law, that the speciality of a morbid product, of the nature of those I am now treating of (carcinoma, &c.), is entirely independent of any local agency whatsoever. The trite, but important remark, that hundreds and thousands of individuals are daily affected, for example, with inflammation, without this local disease being followed by any other than its usual effects, places in the clearest light the necessity of a *previously existing modification of the economy, as the immediate and essential condition of the speciality of the heterologous formations, when they occur in conjunction with inflammation.*"—See Illustrations of the Elementary Forms of Disease, fasc. ii.—ED.

It is still stronger in proof of an hereditary predisposition, that various members of the same family have exhibited the same disease, either simultaneously or in succession; and that the descendants of those who have been afflicted with it, seem to have more frequently suffered from it than others. It is not necessary to advance individual instances in support of these positions, though it may be noticed, in passing, that Bonaparte died of a cancer in the stomach, his father of a scirrhous pylorus.—(*Account of the last illness, decease, &c. of Napoleon Bonaparte, by Archibald Arnot,* 1822.) The same remarks have been made upon a general survey of the disease in most ages; and the doctrine of an hereditary influence, in consequence, descended to us as a result of such remarks from the time of the Greeks and Romans.

Since the first and second editions of the present work, in which these remarks occur as now again presented to the reader, they have received no inconsiderable degree of confirmation by the publication of Sir Astley Cooper's Lectures on Surgery, in which the same line of pathology is pretty closely adopted. With respect to the constitutional character of the disease, he tells us, from numerous dissections, that "it seldom happens, when a tumour of this kind exists in the breast, that only one is found, for there are generally several smaller, in different parts of the glandular structure," and that not only the glands in the axilla, but those above the clavicle are changed in their internal appearance from the deposite of a scirrhous secretion resembling that in the breast, and that most of the viscera, in different cases, participate in the same morbid change, especially the lungs, the liver, the uterus, the ovaria; while in proof of its hereditary influence, he observes as follows:—"There are sometimes several persons in the same family who will be affected with this disease. A physician had three relations, sisters; the first of whom had a scirrhous tubercle of the breast, of which she died. A second had the disease, which was removed by Mr. Lucas senior; the disease returned, and she died. The third had applied to me, for a very painful swelling in the breast. They were unmarried. Therefore," continues he, "in a family in which one is affected, the first dawn of complaint should be carefully watched, and the general health be well attended to in others."—(*Tyrrel's edition,* vol. ii., pp. 183, 186, 189, 8vo., 1825.)

How far a predisposition to cancer, whether original or derived, may manifest itself by external signs, I am not able to determine. Such an outward character is by no means constant in the list of hereditary diseases. It is, perhaps, generally visible in those that affect the mind, but far less so in those that affect the body. In phthisis, the predominant diathesis has a striking exterior; in scrofula, the outward and visible sign is far less distinct, though such a sign seems to p evail generally: in gout, there is no specific exterior that we can depend upon. Dr. Parr, however, has conceived that cancer has its outward character as well as phthisis, and that it is indelibly marked in the complexion:

F 2

"for we have found," says he, "cancers more frequent, in the dark cadaverous complexions, than in the fairer kind. The complexion we mean is distinct from the darkness of the atrabilious or melancholic habits: a blue teint seems mixed with the brown, and is chiefly conspicuous under the eyes, or in the parts usually fair. This may, perhaps, be a refinement without foundation, but we think we have often observed it. There is certainly no constitutional symptom by which it can be predicted, if, in women, a scanty and a dark-coloured catamenial discharge be not a prognostic of the future disease. Cancer has certainly been traced in females of the same family; and those who have escaped suffer from irregular anomalous pains, and different, often unaccountable complaints."—(*Medical Dict. in verbo.*) The picture thus ingeniously drawn is worth bearing in mind, but I have never been able sufficiently to appropriate it; and, in the last two or three cases of cancerous breasts that have occurred to myself, the patients have been of fair complexion, and light hair; one of them, indeed, peculiarly so; the lady was about fifty, and had a large and very handsome family, all of whom were so fair as to make a near approach to the phthisical exterior, though none of them have ever exhibited its pathognomonics.

Cancer has also been imagined by many practitioners of high respectability to be contagious, of whom we may mention Bierchen, Sinnert, and Gooch; but there seems no sufficient ground for the continuance of such an opinion. Inoculation has been said to have produced the complaint: but this is contrary to the results of later investigations; for M. Alibert inoculated both himself and several of his pupils, without any other effect than that of local inflammation, and even this did not always ensue.—(*Maladies de la Peau,* &c.) The discharge from cancers has been swallowed by dogs without any mischief.

The parts most usually affected by cancer are the excretory glands, and especially those that separate the fluids to be employed in the animal economy, rather than those that secern the excrementitious parts of the blood. The lymphatic glands are seldom primarily affected, though they may become so secondarily, that is to say, in consequence of the effect of a neighbouring cancerous tumour or ulcer upon them; but whether this is on the principle of irritation or absorption, is not quite clear. "I never yet," says Mr. Pearson, "met with an unequivocal proof of a primary (cancerous) scirrhus in an absorbent gland."—(*Principles of Surgery,* &c., vol. i., p. 209' &c.) And hence we behold a striking difference between the nature of cancer and scrofula. But, though the secernent glands are most open to the attack of cancer, any part of the body may become its seat. We meet with it, however, chiefly in the breasts of females, the uterus, the testes, the glans penis, the tongue, stomach, cheeks, lips, and angles of the eyes. The diseased action commences in the minuter vessels, and the adjacent parts are affected in consequence.

Women are more subject to cancer than men,

and in these the mammæ and the uterus are the organs most predisposed to its influence. Celibacy, as well as the cessation of the menses, conduces to its production or appearance, and hence antiquated maids are mostly affected with it, and, next to these, mothers who have not suckled their children; for we may lay it down as an axiom, in the language of Dr. Parr, that a milk abscess never becomes a cancer. Then follow women who are past child-bearing, and, lastly, women who have borne children, and suckled them with their own milk, and males incidentally exposed to its occasional causes. To which we may add that, when cancer occurs in men, it is chiefly in the lips, and, when in children, in the eyes.[*]

Of the remote cause of cancer we know nothing. While scrofula has been supposed by some to be the result of an acid acrimony, cancer has by others been supposed to be produced by a peculiar alkali. Dr. Crawford, from a series of very curious experiments upon the matter of cancer, thought he had ascertained this to consist principally of hepatized ammonia, and found that this matter effervesced with sulphuric acid.—(*Phil. Trans.*, vol. lxxx., 1791.) Ploucquet, however, affirms that it sometimes effervesces with alkalis as well.—(*Init. Biblioth.*, tom. ii., p. 202.) The taste discovers nothing; for to the tongue it is insipid and mawkish rather than acid or alkaline. Yet Parr, laying hold of Crawford's experiments, has boldly ventured to assert that the remote cause, or rather the cause of the cancerous diathesis, consists in an excess of ammonia, with a redundant development of sulphur.

When it was popular in the Linnæan school to resolve almost all diseases into the irritation of worms, grubs, or insects existing parasitically in different organs of the body, cancer was by some theorists supposed to depend upon a like cause; and the hypothesis has been since adopted by several writers in our own country, as Mr. Justamond, who ascribed it to the larvæ of a particular species of insects, and Dr. Adams, who referred it to hydatids.—(*Observations on Morbid Poisons.*) Vermicles, or the larvæ of insects, have at times been found in the open ulcer of a cancer, as in the fetid discharge of many other malignant ulcers. These, as in other cases, have undoubtedly proceeded from eggs deposited in the sore as a nidus, though the worm or insect that has so deposited them has never been detected.[†] Such appears to be the

foundation of this hypothesis, which we have no authority for carrying further, and which is rarely advocated in the present day.

The occasional or exciting causes are numerous, but to account for their efficiency, it seems indispensable, as we have already observed, to suppose the existence of a cancerous predisposition or diathesis, since we see the same causes acting in innumerable instances daily without betraying any tendency to such a result. Where this is present, it may be produced by an external injury upon any of the parts most susceptible of cancer; by an indurated and chronic tumour incidentally inflamed or irritated; an accumulation of acrid filth in the rugæ of the skin, which is a frequent cause of cancer in the testes, and particularly among chimney-sweepers; the hard and pungent pressure of a wart or corn in an irritable habit, of which the medical records offer various examples; the general disturbance produced in the system by a severe attack of smallpox, or several other exanthems; a sudden suspension of a periodical hemorrhoidal flux, and a cessation of the menses; and, when in the stomach, by a previous life of ebriety or irregular living. With these, severe cold seems also to co-operate, as the disease is generally admitted to be both more frequent and more virulent in the high northern latitudes than in the southern regions of Europe.

When cancer takes place in the breast, it usually commences with a small indolent tumour that excites little attention. In process of time this tumour is attended with an itching, which is gradually exchanged for a pricking, a shooting, and at length a lancinating pain, a sense of burning, and a livid discoloration of the skin. And however difficult it may be to determine the precise point of time in which the scirrhus first becomes converted into a cancer, where these symptoms are united there can be no risk in calling the tumour by the latter name. Adhesive bands are now formed in the integuments, which become puckered, while the nipple is drawn inwards by suction, and, in some instances, completely disappears; the tumour rises higher towards the surface, and feels knotty to the finger, at the same time that the subcutaneous vessels are distended with blood, and show themselves in dark, cancriform varices. The march of the disease may be slow or rapid, for it varies considerably in its pace; but at

---

[*] The cases which used a few years ago to be set down as cancers of the eyes of children, are now well ascertained to be in reality examples of fungus hæmatodes.—ED.

[†] The great attention now paid to morbid anatomy has dispelled for ever these sports of the imagination. In cancer there is a deposite of what is termed heterologous matter, quite different from any of the normal tissues. The carcinomatous substance may exist in the molecular structure of organs or on free surfaces, and in the blood, and it always forms for the greater bulk of the disease. When the carcinomatous matter is deposited on free surfaces, the fibrous tissue is not often met

with as an anatomical element of the disease; but the serous tissue is frequently present, and may form either a capsule or interior cyst, filled with gelatinous, albuminous, or other fluids. However, in the molecular structure, the quantity of cellular and fibrous tissues which intersect a scirrhus in various directions may be very considerable. In dense organs, like the breast, uterus, ovaries, liver, walls of the stomach, &c., these tissues are often very abundant.—(See Dr. Carswell's Illustrations of the Elementary Forms of Disease, fasc. iii.) According to this author's investigation, the blood vessels seen in scirrhus are only branches belonging to the neighbouring tissues, and which have become enclosed within the morbid substance. —ED.

length the integuments give way in a few points to the ulcerative process, and a small quantity of caustic ichor, or of lymphatic fluid tinged with blood from eroded vessels, is thrown forth, sometimes with a short and deceitful relief (*Prysschriften Uitgegeven door het Genootsch. ter bevondering der Heelkunde*, Amsterdam, 1791): the ulcerative process in the meantime advancing and spreading more widely and deeply, till a considerable extent of surface becomes exposed, and a broad excavation is scooped out, with a discharge of a peculiar and most offensive fetor.* Here again the ulcer sometimes affords a delusive hope of recovery by its granulating; but the granulations are soft and spongy, and not unfrequently bleed, from the loose texture of the new vessels, or their erosion by the cancerous matter. It is rarely, moreover, that they extend over the entire surface of the sore; for, more generally, while one ' part is covered with them another part is sloughing, and each of the parts runs alternately into the action of the other.† And, not unfrequently, the lymphatic vessels become affected as high up as the axilla, and in their course betray a few smaller tumours. But whether this be a mere result of contiguous sympathy or of cancerous taint is uncertain. Cancer, as we have already observed, rarely, if ever, commences in lymphatic glands, but they, at length, partake of the disease in the course of its ravages; and hence all such suspected tumours are prudently removed when the knife has been resolved upon. Where the disease has spread widely or continued long, some of the muscles of respiration participate in the irritation, and the breathing is performed with difficulty.‡

When cancer attacks the uterus, it is known by tensive lancinating pains in this organ shooting through the region of the pelvis, indurations in the part sensible to the touch, a preceding and immoderate leucorrhœa or menstruation,

* C. Bell on the Diseases comprehended under the name of Carcinoma Mammæ.—See Medico-Chir. Trans., vol. xii.

† Both in cancer and fungus hæmatodes sloughing is a common occurrence, and arises from various causes, such as the pressure of the morbid substance on the veins, the irritation of it on the neighbouring tissues, or even the constriction of a portion of the disease by a narrow opening in a fascia, through which it protrudes. " Congestion, hemorrhage, softening, and sloughing," as Dr. Carswell observes, " take place in both cases of carcinoma. In scirrhus, however, they originate in the vascular system of the tissues included within the carcinomatous matter; but are not, on that account, less frequent and destructive than those which arise in the proper and collateral circulation in cephaloma (fungus hæmatodes). In general the softening is less complete, the hemorrhage not so considerable, and the sloughing more extensive in the former than the latter."—(See Dr. Carswell's Illustrations, fasc. iii., 4to., Lond., 1833.) Nerves, he says, have never been detected in either of these diseases, *as a new formation.* —ED.

‡ This probably depends on the absorbent glands under the sternum becoming diseased. Hence likewise the cough that usually takes place in the advanced stage of cancer of the breast.—ED.

sometimes both. The ulcerative process, as far as we are acquainted with it, is the same as already described; and as soon as it has worked to the surface of the organ, there is a sanious, or bloody, or mixed discharge, characterized by the peculiar stench of the disease. By degrees the labia swell and become œdematous, and if, as sometimes happens, the inguinal glands be obstructed, the œdema extends down the thigh, and the ulceration proceeds often to the bladder and rectum.—(*Clarke, Obs. on the Diseases of Females*, &c., 8vo., 1821.)

Cancer in the vagina, which, however, rarely takes place, can easily be felt; and in the rectum, the distinction is not difficult. The nature of the discharge, and the other symptoms just noticed, are sufficient to decide its existence. It is still more obvious in the penis.

None of these symptoms assist us in determining its presence in the stomach: and hence, how confidently soever it may be conjectured from the marks of an acute and burning pain, tenderness of the epigastrium upon pressure, nausea, and rejection of food, and even an offensive fetor in the breath, the disease can seldom be completely ascertained till after death. It is sometimes accompanied with vomiting, and sometimes not; and ordinarily the absence of vomiting is an unfavourable sign, as it has often been found to proceed from an induration of the coats of the stomach generally, which has rendered it incapable of contracting, or from a cancerous ulceration and enlargement of the pylorus (*Mém. sur le Vom., par M. Piedagnel*, &c. ; *Journ. de Phys. Exp., par M. Magendie*, 1821, Paris), which, upon the slightest pressure, readily admits the contents of the stomach into the duodenum. There is here, however, usually habitual nausea, though without vomiting.

The progress of cancer in the testicle is often slower than in many other parts. In chimney-sweepers we can trace an obvious cause, which is that of soot lodged in its rugæ, and irritating as well from its own acrimony, as from that of the perspiratory fluid with which it comes in contact and forms a union. A painful ragged sore, with hard rising edges, is first produced; or sometimes a little indurated wart; which, from inattention, increases in size, is repeatedly rubbed off by the exercise of climbing, enlarges and deepens its sphere of irritation, grows more malignant, and at length is converted into a real cancer, and affects the whole scrotum, or the body of the testis. In whatever part of this complicated organ, however the disease commences, it is progressively communicated to the rest; the scirrhosity increases in size and hardness, till the tumour often acquires an enormous and irregular magnitude, studded externally with numerous protuberances, and the shape of the testis, even before ulceration, is entirely lost. In the progress of the disease the spermatic cord becomes affected, and the taint or irritation is communicated more or less to the viscera and lymphatic glands of the abdomen.

From the cancerous effect of a highly irritable wart or crack on the scrotum of chimney-sweepers and smelters of metals, we may derive some idea of the formation of cancers on other superficial parts of the body from a similar beginning. These most frequently occur on the lips, nose, or eyelids ; and oftener from a crack than from a wart. The edges of the sore become hard, and one or more tumours issue from them, which increase in size, and gradually evince a cancerous character.

On the tongue the same disease sometimes shows itself, and more usually commences with a small wart or pimple near the tip, which hardens by degrees, grows highly irritable and malignant, and spreading its influence through the entire organ, swells it to a prodigious size, and renders it of a scirrhous induration.

These local tumours are seldom entitled to be called cancers on their origin. They are almost always produced, as Mr. Earle has justly observed, by local irritation, and exacerbated by a continuance of the same cause ; and hence they rarely give much trouble on extirpation, and perhaps never endanger the constitution. A chronic malignancy may, however, convert them into genuine carcinomata.—(*Medico-Chir. Trans.*, vol. xii., art. xxii.)

Cancer is said, in a few instances, to have terminated spontaneously. De Haen gives us one example of this (*Epist. De Cicutâ*, p. 43), and Parr affirms that he has seen six cases of the same in his own practice. But he adds, in proof of its being a constitutional affection, that in every case the cure was followed by some other disease, as an enteritis, fixed pains in the limbs, a sciatica, or an apoplexy ; in one of these cases the apoplectic attack occurred twice, and the last was fatal.*

In general, however, a cure is rarely affected but with the knife or caustic, the use of which it does not belong to the present course of study to explain. Yet the progress of the complaint may perhaps be arrested ; and we are often able, without cutting, to render it at least tolerable for a series of years. In an early stage of the disease relief may often be obtained by topical bleeding, as with leeches ; and topical refrigerant applications, as saturnine lotions, or sheet lead in very thin layers, as the linings of tea-packages, an application which has of late been brought forward as something new, but which was employed long ago, and may be found recommended in many of the older journals of established reputation.† The diet should be limited to the mildest nutriment, and wine be sedulously avoided. At this period, indeed,

whatever can prevent or lessen inflammation should be seriously studied and adhered to.

Ponteau relates the particulars of a cure produced by rigid abstemiousness alone, the patient taking nothing whatever but water for a period of two months.—(*Nuovo Metodo per curare sicuramente ogni Canchero coperto*, &c., Venezi, 1750 ; *Œuvres Posthumes*, tom. i.)

As, however, the disease advances, and assumes more of a chronic character, the activity of the smaller vessels may be gently urged, in order to relieve or prevent congestion. And, where the irritation is not great, we may by degrees apply gentle stimulants also externally, and let the saturnine lotion be superseded by the acetated solution of ammonia, tar-water as recommended by Quadiro, or the application of mercurial ointment, combined with a small portion of camphire, to the surrounding parts.

The internal medicines which have been chiefly trusted to for the cure of cancer, are the lurid and umbellate narcotics and the mineral tonics : the former apparently for the purpose of taking off irritation, and in some instances correcting the specific acrimony ; and the latter for supporting the living power, and thus enabling the system to obtain a triumph over the disease by its own instinctive or remedial energy.

Of the first class, the chief have been the belladonna and hemlock, and particularly the latter, which appears to have been most promising. When Dr. Stoerck of Vienna published his work upon the successful exhibition of hemlock in cases of confirmed cancer, many of which were vouched for by the Baron Van Swieten, every practitioner was eager for examples upon which to try the experiment for himself. Solanum had been in vogue, but was just sinking into disrepute from its numerous failures ; and corrosive sublimate was the medicine chiefly confided in at St. Thomas's Hospital. Dr. Akenside, who was at this time prescribing the corrosive sublimate in the hospital with what he thought a gratifying success, immediately exchanged it for the conium, or cicuta, as it was then called. He tried it upon a large scale in every stage and modification of the disease, and at first with the most sanguine expectations ; but his hopes gradually failed him as he advanced in the career of his experiments, and he was compelled to make very great drawbacks upon Dr. Stoerck's commendation of the medicine. He allows it, however, a certain portion of merit, and his account is drawn up with a degree of candour which entitles it to the fullest confidence, and appears to deal out the real truth. In recent states of the disease, where there was no ulceration, or none of any depth, he asserts that it often produced a favourable termination, and gives numerous examples to this effect. But in inveterate cases, where the cancerous ulcer had made considerable progress, its benefit was very questionable : it operated often for a very few days like a charm, diminished the pains, and improved the discharge ; but suddenly it failed to do the slightest good any longer, unless the

---

* Dict. in verb., vol. i., p. 329. The termination of carcinoma in mortification, from obliteration of veins, is stated by Professor Carswell as far from being a rare occurrence.—ED.

† Eph. Nat. Cur., dec. i., ann. iv., v., obs. 161. It is on the principle of diminishing the supply of blood for the nutrition and growth of cancerous tumours, that the frequent local abstraction of this fluid, the application of cold, the use of the ligature and compression, have been recommended as the most effectual means of arresting or retarding their progress.—Professor Carswell, op. cit., fasc. iii.—ED.

dose was very largely increased, upon which a like beneficial effect followed, but unfortunately of equally transient duration. The dose was in many instances again increased, and continued to be so, till at length the symptoms produced by the cicuta were as mischievous as those of the cancer itself, and Dr. Akenside was compelled to abandon it.—(*Transact. of the Coll. of Phys. of Lond.*, vol. i., art. vi., p. 64.)

We are hence in some degree prepared for the contradictory accounts of its effects. De Haen asserts that it affords neither cure nor relief of any kind (*Rat. Med.*, ii., 37); Bierchen, that it aggravates real cancer, though sometimes serviceable in scrofula; and Lange, that it is altogether inefficacious.—(*Diss. dubia Cicutæ vexata*, Helmst., 1764.) Fothergill is friendly to its use (*Works*, vol. ii., passim); and Bell (*On Ulcers*, part ii., sect. viii.) and Fearon (*On Cancers*, passim) recommend it both externally and internally, alone or in combination with opium.

For this discrepance of judgment, we have in some measure endeavoured to account. Yet the advocates of the medicine have doubtless, in some instances, suffered themselves to speak of it in exaggerated terms; and it is highly probable that in others, where it has seemed altogether inefficacious, the hemlock, whether in powder or extract, was administered in an imperfect state. Dr. Cullen gives a striking example of this last fact in a lady, who, being very particular in the use of this medicine, employed the powder as mostly to be depended upon, and weighed out her own doses, beginning with a small quantity at a time, and proceeding gradually till she took sixty grains at once. By this period her parcel of the powder was exhausted, and she had derived no beneficial effect. She supplied herself, however, with another parcel, and being warned that different samples were rarely of the same strength, she reduced her first dose of the new plan to a scruple: yet even this nearly killed her; for in ten or fifteen minutes she was affected with sickness, tremour, giddiness, delirium, and convulsions. Happily, the sickness proceeded to a vomiting, and the poison was rejected. But of the fresh supply she was never afterward able to take more than five or six grains at a dose, notwithstanding she had taken sixty grains of the preceding without any mischief.—(*Mat. Med.*, vol. ii., part ii., ch. vi., p. 264.)

Yet the quantities pretended to be given by some practitioners are far beyond this last amount. Thus, Dease informs us that he gave AN OUNCE AND A HALF of the powder every twenty-four hours (*Introduct. to the Theory and Pract. of Surg.*, i.), and performed a cure; and Rostard, that his ordinary allowance was six drachms of the extract for the same period, which is a still higher proportion.— (*Journ. de Méd.*, tom. xxxviii., p. 36.) Warner gave a drachm and a half, and thought it an enormous quantity, without mischief.—(*Treatise on the Eyes*, passim.)

Upon the whole, the balance of experiments

seems very much to confirm the candid report of Dr. Akenside. Schaeffer and many others contend, that even its beneficial influence is nothing more than a result of its narcotic power; but it does seem, in some instances, to act as a discutient, and to improve the quality of the secretion as well as to relieve the pains. Dr. Cullen advances further, and tells us that he has found it, in several cases, make a considerable approach towards healing the sore; "Though I must own," says he, "that I was never concerned in a cancerous case, in which the cure of the sore was completed."—(*Mat. Med.*, loco citat.)

Of the other narcotics, chiefly of the solanaceous order, that have been employed, it is hardly worth while to speak particularly. The same uncertainty has accompanied their use: and some of them, as aconite and dulcamara, have been rather supposed to effect whatever temporary benefit has flowed from their employment by the general disturbance they produce in the system, whereby a transient stop is put to every other anomalous action, than by their sedative power.

Of the metallic oxydes that have been brought into use, the only ones it is necessary to notice are those of mercury, iron, and arsenic. The first has been uniformly found mischievous when carried to the extent of salivation. Loss asserts, that by this means he cured a cancer of the nose and face (*Observ. Med.*, b. iv., Lond., 1672); but this was probably a spurious disease of zaruthan, as it has been called by some writers. It has more generally been employed as a gentle stimulant or alterant. Many practitioners have preferred the corrosive sublimate in small doses, but the submuriate is a far better preparation. And even this is given with more advantage in the form of Plummer's or the compound calomel pill, than alone; a form that conveniently unites a mild stimulant with a mild relaxant. To this, if the pain be acute, should be added a small quantity of opium; at the same time carefully guarding the bowels against constipation by any convenient aperient, if the pill itself should not prove sufficient.

Iron has been tried in almost every state of combination. The ferrum ammoniatum appears to have been the most successful, and is still the most popular. Under the name of flores martiales, it was introduced for this purpose before the public as far back as the middle of last century, by Francis Xavier de Mars, obtained, however, by a very uncouth and operose process. Dr. Denman was particularly attached to this metal, in whatever form administered; and broadly affirms that, after having employed almost all the medicines recommended for this disease in every different stage, he has never found any of them possess the pretensions of iron; and that the rest may be generally regarded as totally unavailing.—(*Observations on the Cure of Cancer*, p. 77.) Its greatly stimulant power rather recommends it to us on the present occasion, than proves an objection; for it is the kind of stimulus we stand in need of to excite a new local action. It is said to produce a very speedy mitigation of pain, an improved discharge, and a less fetid smell ; and, even in hopeless cases, to render the disease less malignant and distressing ; unfortunately, however, its effects, like those of conium, have rarely been found permanent ; and it has closed its career as a palliative, rather than as an antidote.

But of all the medicines of this class, arsenic has acquired the highest and most extensive reputation. This is a strictly oriental remedy, employed, as we shall have occasion more fully to observe when treating of elephantiasis, for every impurity of the blood. Who first ventured upon it in Europe for the disease before us, is not very satisfactorily known. It was common in the time of Hildanus, who ascribes its introduction into practice to the monk Theodoric, who flourished about the beginning of the eleventh century.—(Cent. vi., obs. 81.) It has formed the basis of almost all the secret remedies for cancer which have at any time been current, whether external or internal, from that of Fuschius, in the fourteenth century, who united it with soot and serpentary, to that of Richard Guy, who wrote upon the disease (*Essay on Scirrhous Tumours and Cancers*, 1759) in the middle of the last century, and whose boasted arcanum was found to be a composition of arsenic, sulphur, hogsfennel (*peucedanum officinale*), and crows-foot (*ranunculus sylvestris*.)—(*Richter*, *Chir. Bibl.*, band v., p. 132.)

Of the real effects of arsenic, as of several of the preceding medicines, we labour under great obscurity from the discrepant reports which have been communicated. Le Febure, with a host of practitioners antecedent to and contemporary with himself, employed it both externally and internally, and regarded it as a specific.—(*Remède eprouvé pour guérir radicalement le Cancer occulte, et manifesté ou ulcéré*, 8vo., Paris.) Smalz thinks it serviceable.—(*Seltene chirurgische und medicinische Vorfälle*, Leips., 1784, 8vo.) Schneider (*Chir. Geschichte*, Theil. v.) and Justamond declare it to be useless, though the latter employed it locally as an escharotic. Hildanus (*Account of the Methods pursued in the Treatment of Cancerous and Scirrhous Disorders*, Lond., 1780) and Delius (*Dissert. Observat. et Cognit. nonnulla Chirurg.*, fasc. vi.) assert it to be injurious ; and Schenck (*Observ.*, lib. ii., N. 304) and Meibom (*Blumenbach*, *Bibl.*, band viii., p. 724) give examples of fatal effects from its employment.

Fatal effects, indeed, it is easy to produce, provided a sufficient degree of caution be not employed in experimenting upon it. And, in truth, it is not till lately that any very convenient form has been devised for trying its virtues without a risk of mischief ; but the arsenical solution of the London College, for which we are indebted to Dr. Fowler, has given us a preparation of this kind. Yet, even with this advantage, we cannot boast of any certain success in the use of arsenic. It acts very differently on different constitutions, though, generally speaking, it proves beneficial, and in some cases may produce a radical cure. But more commonly, like the preparations of hemlock and iron, it unfortunately loses its effect as soon as the habit has become accustomed to its influence, and the cancerous action resumes its victorious career. And perhaps the only power that is capable of neutralizing cancer, or keeping it permanently in subjection, is the existence of a predominant diathesis of some other kind. How far the remark may have been made antecedently I know not, but from a pretty close attention to the subject within my own sphere of observation, I have been led to conclude that cancer does not often make its attack upon those who are constitutionally subject to gout, and seems to be restrained by its influence.

The list of external applications is still more numerous than that of internal. We have already glanced at the local treatment before ulceration has taken place. After this period sedative applications do not succeed, and moderate stimulants alone seem to afford any material degree of relief. In fact, the inflammation has now acquired much of the character of a malignant erythema, and requires warmer applications than phlegmonic sores.* Yet a cure is rarely to be effected, except by the caustic or the knife. When the poison was supposed to be of an acid character, a solution of the alkalis was employed to correct it. It was afterward conceived to be of an alkaline nature ; and various acids, and particularly the carbonic acid gas, were regarded as the best antagonists. Who first employed it for the present purpose is not known ; but it stands recommended as early as 1776, in an article of Magellan, inserted in Rosier's Journal ; and an easy and convenient mode of application has lately been contrived by Dr. Ewart of Bath. Dr. Crawford, however, for the same purpose, preferred a lotion of muriatic acid diluted with three or four times its weight of water. Carminati and Senebier applied the gastric juice of animals ; but poultices of carrots or charcoal have been in more general reputation. [A solution of the chlorides of lime or of soda, has also been of late years employed.]

All these have a considerable influence in correcting the oppressive fetor, and keeping the sore clean ; but whether they go beyond this has been doubted. Yet even this is of great importance, since such an effect must necessarily give some check to the spread of the ulceration, afford solace to the patient, and probably improve the nature of the discharge itself. And hence many writers have been sanguine enough to expect an entire cure from such processes ; and others have given accounts of such cures nearly accomplished, but which seem seldom, if ever, to have been rendered complete.

Fomentations of hemlock and various other narcotics have been also had recourse to, and sometimes tepid baths of the same, in which

* The editor has known the liquor opii sedativus preferred, in some instances, to every other dressing ; and, on other occasions, nothing was found to afford so much ease as the simple ung. cetacei.—ED.

the patient has been ordered to sit for twenty minutes at a time; and temporary benefit has sometimes followed the use of these means; but they have often been tried with as little avail as the suckling of toads, which was at one time a fashionable remedy, and esteemed of great importance, the animals being feigned to expire in agonies as the poison of the ulcer was drawn out, and its surface assumed a better aspect: Bouffey, who was a witness to their use, tells us, and probably with some truth, that they did more harm than good (*Journ. de Méd.*, tom. lxii.), and dealt out more poison than they took away. The era of this invention is unknown, but it was still in use about half a century ago in our own country, if we may judge from one of the private letters of Junius to Woodfall, who, alluding to the princess dowager of Wales, at that time afflicted with a cancer that destroyed her in January, 1772, asserts that " she suckles toads from morning till night."—(*G. Woodfall's edition*, vol. i., p. *241.)

One of the best detergents appears to be arsenic* finely levigated, and sufficiently reduced in strength by a union with calamine or some other ingredient. It is also one of the best caustics, in a simple or more concentrated state, and was freely employed as such by Mr. Justamond. Guy's powder, which we have already noticed, is used externally for the same purpose.†

[Mr. Carmichael some years ago strongly recommended the application of preparations of iron to ulcerated cancers, and gave a very interesting account of the good effects which he had seen arise from them. The plan has been repeatedly tried in this country, but its success here has not corresponded with that stated to have resulted from it in Ireland. When a medicine or application proves successful in the hands of one surgeon, and unsuccessful in those of another of equal skill, the inference is, that, if the medicine or application in each case be undoubtedly of similar qualities, but its effects different, the cases themselves cannot precisely correspond in their nature. No doubt, many alleged specifics for cancer have obtained their repute by the circumstances of their having

cured tumours and ulcers which only somewhat resembled, but were not really cancers.]

We have already observed that sheets of lead, among other preparations of this metal, were applied to the cancer about forty or fifty years ago, and bound over it with some degree of pressure. But a pressure of a much severer kind, together with the use of the same metallic sheeting, was employed a few years ago by Mr. Young, a fair and impartial trial of whose plan, however, by other surgeons, has completely proved that it is generally more hurtful than beneficial.

After all, when the cancerous character of the tumour is once decidedly established, little dependance is to be placed upon any plan but that of extirpation with caustic or the knife. The actual cautery, as employed by M. Maunoir, of which we shall have to speak more at large when discussing the genus ULCUS, may, perhaps, be most advantageously made use of in small cancers of the face; but the knife is the preferable instrument where the organ is large and extensively affected. Mr. Bell advises an early performance of the operation; Mr. Pearson, that we should wait till the extent of the disease has fully unfolded itself, so that no morbid part may be left behind.* Yet some parts may be doubtful even at last, and, wherever there is the least suspicion of this, they should unquestionably be removed along with the more decided portion of the morbid structure.

Even this remedy, however, can only apply to exterior organs, or to organs that can be brought down to the surface; for the uterus has been occasionally extirpated with success, but, far more frequently, without any benefit, perhaps from the operation having been postponed till too late.† In all other instances, the practice is melancholy from the first. The die is cast; and all we can hope to accomplish is to postpone the fatal result, to mitigate the sufferings of the day, and soften the harsh passage to the tomb.

GENUS VII
LUES.
VENEREAL DISEASE.

ULCERS ON THE GENITALS, INGUINAL BUBOES, OR BOTH, AFTER IMPURE COITION; SUCCEEDED BY ULCERS IN THE THROAT, COPPER-COLOURED SPOTS ON THE SKIN, BONE-PAINS, AND NODES.

THE term LUES is derived from the Greek λύω, " solvo, dissolvo"—"to macerate, dissolve, or corrupt;" and, agreeably to the common rule

---

* In consequence of many patients having fallen victims to the absorption of arsenic from the surface of cancerous and other anomalous sores, few modern practitioners now venture to apply powdered arsenic to carcinomatous ulcers.—ED.

† Baron Dupuytren uses arsenical applications, prepared so as to modify the diseased surface, without acting as a caustic. The formula of the powder which he applies is 4 parts of arsenical acid and 96 of the submuriate of mercury in every 100. Occasionally the proportion of arsenic is increased to 5 or 6 in 100. When the baron uses a liquid, or paste, he merely blends the above powder with distilled water, or gumarabic powdered and moistened. When, however, the lotion is employed, 6, 8, 10, or even 12 parts of arsenic may be the proportion of it to the calomel. It is chiefly for phagedenic or inveterate ulcerations about the nose, lips, and face, that Baron Dupuytren has recourse to this *heroic* remedy, as he calls it.—See Leçons Orales de Clinique Chirurgicale, tom. iv., p. 471, et seq., 8vo., Paris, 1834.—ED.

---

* The maxim of every surgeon of judgment in the present day, is to recommend the removal of every truly cancerous disease as soon as its nature is manifest. This proves the general inefficiency of all medicines and local applications, and the dangers resulting from delay.—ED.

† In cancers of the rectum Lisfranc has succeeded in extirpating the diseased structure with perfect relief to the patient. In a memoir read by

of expressing the power of the Greek υ by a Roman _y_, should be written LYES, as in the case of _Lyssa_ and _Paralysis_, both of which are derived from the same root ; but lues has been employed so long and so generally, that it would be little less than affectation to attempt a change, and in allucinatio, or hallucinatio, from the Greek ἀλύω, or ἀλυσις, we are supported by a similar example of deviation from the common rule.

It appears to have been known to the world from an early age, as I have remarked in the running comment to the volume of Nosology, that acrimonious and poisonous materials are at times secreted by the genitals, capable of exciting local, and, perhaps, constitutional affections, in those who expose themselves to such poisons by incontinent sexual intercourse. Celsus enumerates various diseases of the sexual organs, most of which are only referable to this source of impure contact ; but the hideous and alarming malady which was first noticed as proceeding from the same source towards the close of the fifteenth century, and which has since been called almost exclusively VENEREAL DISEASE, has suppressed, till of late, all attention to these minor evils, in the fearful contemplation of so new and monstrous a pestilence, to various modifications of which most of the anterior and slighter diseases of the same organs seem to have been loosely and generally referred, as though there were but one specific poison issuing from this fountain, and consequently but one specific malady. On which account, much confusion has arisen in the history and description of the disease ; and syphilis, its most striking species, though commonly admitted, as we shall see presently, to be comparatively of recent origin, is by Plenck (_Beobacht._, &c., ii.), Richter (_Chir. .Bibl._, band i., sect. ii., p. 163), Stoll (_Prælect._, p. 94), and other writers of considerable eminence, regarded as of far higher antiquity : asserted by Lefevre- de Villebrune (_Retz. Annales_, iv.) to have existed eight centuries before the expedition of Columbus to America, and by De Blegny (_L'Art de guérir les Mal. Vén._, &c.) to have been extant in the Mosaic age.

The keen and comprehensive mind of Mr. John Hunter first called the attention of practitioners to the idea of different poisons and different maladies ; and the subject has since been pursued by Mr. Abernethy with a force of argument, and illustrated by a range of examples, that seem to have put the question at rest. Mr. Abernethy has sufficiently established that, independently of the specific disease now generally recognised by the name of syphilis, there are numerous varieties of some other disease, perhaps other specific diseases, which originate from a distinct, possibly from several distinct, poisons secreted in the same region from pecu-

liarity of constitution or causes hitherto undiscovered, and which are accompanied with primary and secondary symptoms that often vary in their mode of origin, succession, and termination, from those of genuine syphilis, though, in many instances, they make a striking approach to it, and to which, therefore, Mr. Abernethy has given the name of pseudo-syphilitic diseases.*

The approach, indeed, is often so close as to render it difficult, and occasionally, perhaps, impossible, to decide between them ; and hence, whether these really constitute distinct species, issuing from distinct sorts of infection, or are mere varieties or modifications of one common species produced by one common morbid secretion, has not yet been sufficiently determined. In this ignorance upon the subject, it is better, for the present, to regard them in the latter, as being the more simple view ; and, with this preliminary explanation, the expediency of allotting the two following distinct species to the genus lues will, I think, be obvious to every one.

1. Lues Syphilis.   Pox.
2. —— Syphilodes.   Bastard-pox.

SPECIES I.
LUES SYPHILIS.
POX.

ULCERS ON THE GENITALS CIRCULAR, UNGRANULATING, THICKENED AT THE EDGE ; THOSE OF THE THROAT DEEP AND RAGGED ; SYMPTOMS UNIFORM IN THEIR PROGRESS ; SPEEDILY AND UNIFORMLY YIELDING TO A COURSE OF MERCURY WHERE IT AGREES WITH THE CONSTITUTION ; LESS CERTAINLY AND WITH MORE DIFFICULTY YIELDING WITHOUT IT.

THE vulgar term for the ulcers is _Chancres_, and the vulgar name for the disease is _Pox_, formerly _Greatpox_,† as contradistinguished from VARIOLA or SMALLPOX, on account of the larger size of its blotches. It was also very generally called French pox, as being supposed to be a gift to Europe from the French nation.

There is some uncertainty concerning the

---

him to the Royal Acad. of Medicine at Paris, he gives the details of a case in which three inches of this intestine were successfully removed.—See his memoir on Excision of the Rectum, trans. by Doane, in the U. S. Med. and Surg. Journ., vol. i., p. 294.—D.

* Had Dr. Good taken a correct view of the facts, disclosed in the paper on syphilis, inserted by the late Mr. Rose in the Medical and Chirurgical Transactions of London, he would have perceived that nothing could be more conducive to error, than the circumstances which Mr. Abernethy regarded as tests of the true venereal disease. One notion which he adopted was, that the venereal disease always became progressively worse, unless mercury were prescribed ; and, consequently, another part of his creed was, that if a sore or other complaint got well without the aid of the specific, fancied to be quite essential to the cure of every real form of the venereal disease, the fact was an adequate proof that the case could not have been of the latter nature. All these, and several other doctrines formerly entertained, have been annihilated by the plain and impartial details published by Mr. Rose. Most of Mr. Abernethy's syphiloid cases are now generally believed to have been truly _syphilitic_ ones.—ED.

† De Henry, La Méthode curative de la Maladie Vénérienne, vulgairement appellé la Grosse Vérole, &c., Paris, 8vo., 1552.

origin of the specific term SYPHILIS, which Swediaur ascribes to Fernelius, but which assuredly existed long before his day ; and was probably invented by Fracastorio about the close of the fifteenth century, from the Greek ὦ, and φιλέω, importing " mutual love ;" for such is the title by which he has designated his celebrated and very elegant poem upon this very inelegant subject.

There is an equal uncertainty as to the quarter in which the disease originated. It is usually ascribed to the American continent, and believed to have been imported into Europe by the crews of Columbus on his first or second return home in 1493 and 1496 ; a belief, however, which seems to be altogether without foundation, for, at the period even of the first return of this celebrated circumnavigator in March, 1493, it seems to have preceded his return by some weeks ; since, on his reaching Seville in the ensuing month of April, in order to join the Spanish army, it had already arisen, and was spread over Auvergne, Lombardy, and various other parts of Italy ; as, in the course of the summer months, it was observed in Saxony, Brandenburg, Brunswick, Mecklenburg, and especially Strasburg, as all the German writers concur in admitting ;[*] and even at Cracow, in Poland, according to Strykowsky's Chronicle of Lithuania ; while Fracastorio, who was an eyewitness of the entire progress of the disease, and, from his high medical reputation, and residence almost on the spot of its first appearance, more largely engaged in the cure of it than any physician of his day, asserts, that it was even ravaging a considerable part of Asia and Africa, as well as of Europe ; " Europam," says he, " ferè omnem, Asiæ verò, atque Aphricæ, partem non parvam occupavit."—(*De Contag. Morbis.*) The writer proceeds to notice the dispute that was then hotly engaged in, as well concerning the nature as the origin of the disease, and again expresses his disbelief in its having been imported from America by the crews of Columbus. On this account he feels himself at liberty to give it a very early origin in his poem upon the subject, and describes his fictitious hero Syphilus as having brought down the disease upon himself and the world at large as a curse for having insulted Apollo, while tending the flocks of King Alcithous.

" Protinus illuvies terris ignota profanis
　Exoritur: primus, regi qui, sanguine fuso,
　Instituit divina, sacrasque in montibus aras,
　SYPHILUS ; ostendit turpes per corpus achores,
　Insomnes primus noctes, convulsaque membra
　Sensit, et à primo traxit cognomina morbus :
　SYPHILIDEMQUE ab eo labem dixère coloni."

One of the earliest German writers who ascribed the disease to the return of Columbus, is Leonard Schmauss, a physician of Strasburg, whose works were published in 1518 ; but neither his history nor his arguments are in any degree satisfactory : while his countryman,

Matern Berlen, a clergyman of Ruffach, and an eyewitness of the disease on its first appearance, assigns it a very different origin ; and, in his history of the Italian expedition of Charles VIII., declares it to have been a punishment inflicted by the Almighty on this monarch and his subjects, in consequence of his having carried off the Dutchess Anne of Bretagne from the Emperor Maximilian, to whom she had been betrothed.

Among the Spanish writers, there are two chiefly who ascribe the origin of syphilis to an American source ; while others, by their silence upon the subject when detailing the particulars of the return of Columbus, give sufficient evidence that they disbelieved the report. Of the two who thus contributed to spread it, one of them, Gonçalvo Hernandez de Oviedo, affirms that it was conveyed into Italy by Cordova's fleet, which, however, did not arrive in Italy (Messina) till May 24, 1495, and, consequently, not till two years after the disease had existed there. The other is Sepulveda, who, in a history of America, written in a good Latin style, towards the middle of the sixteenth century, roundly asserts that " ex *Barbaricarum* mulierum consuetudine Hispani morbum contraxerunt." But as this writer does not, like his contemporary Fracastorio, enter into the particulars of the controversy, his assertion can go no farther than to the weight of his own individual opinion in a controverted case.

Among those who have been most full in their accounts of the voyages of Columbus and the discovery of America, we may certainly reckon Antonio de Herrera. He fixes the return of Columbus at the period above specified ; and is very particular in detailing the order sent to Lisbon to him, on the moment of his arrival, to follow the Spanish court to Barcelona, to which city it was then removed ; the highly honourable reception the great navigator received ; the preparations which were immediately made for his second voyage ; the speed with which these preparations were accomplished ; and the instructions given to him on the occasion. Yet not a hint is added that his crews were unhealthy, that the new recruits had any dread of the plague, to which, had he brought it home, they must have known they were about to be exposed, nor a single instruction to be provident of their health in this respect. He took leave of the royal pair with every mark of distinction, the whole court accompanying him to his house, as well at the time as when he quitted Barcelona. " *Despidóse*," says Herrera, " *de los Reyes, y aqual dia le acompanó toda la corte de palacio á su casa, ỹ tambien quando salió de Barcelona.*"—(*Hist. Gen. de las Ind. Occ.*, dec'ad. i., lib. li., ch. v.)

Linnæus stands alone in arranging syphilis as an exanthem, along with smallpox and measles. He thought himself justified, from the fever which occasionally accompanies the copper-coloured spots on the skin, in an advanced stage of its secondary symptoms ; or perhaps from the fever which, on the first appearance of the disease, unquestionably accompanied it, and uniformly preceded the eruptions. For it is an extraordinary fact, to which all the contemporaneous writers bear witness, that syphilis, when it first broke forth upon the world, and, indeed, as it is described in Fracastorio's poem, was not only called the plague, but was, in truth, a specific fever, attended with most violent putrid symptoms, together with carbuncles, buboes, and other glandular abscesses, which discharged a malignant sanies often fatal, and. even when recovered from, leaving the most melancholy marks of its ravages.

And hence, in many places, the infected were as much exiled from the community by a line of circumvallation drawn around them, as in the case of plague: In Scotland, indeed, they were strictly prohibited all medical assistance, and inhumanly left to the effects of their own licentiousness: for Mr. Arnot gives the copy of an order from the privy council of Edinburgh, which equally banished to the Island of Inchkeith those who were affected with the disease, and those who undertook to cure it.*

By degrees, however, the disorder appears to

* History of Edinburgh, by Hugo Arnot, Esq., 4to., 1789. With reference to the origin of syphilis, the editor is skeptical about the correctness of the doctrine which attempts to refer the first commencement of the complaint only to one source. Is it rational to believe that all the syphilitic mischief that has scourged the various cities, kingdoms, and generations of the world, has arisen from the amours of a single unfortunate individual in whom the virus was first produced? Are we to fancy that the disease never had but one primary source? and that it is to the mysterious concoction of the poison in one individual alone, that all quarters of the world are under obligations for the gift of the venereal disease? No doubt syphilis must have had a beginning, like every thing else; but probably it has had numerous beginnings. Various considerations would lead us to expect (what is, indeed, the fact), that in every country where the population is numerous, and promiscuous sexual intercourse exists, the venereal disease would be prevalent. Mr. Travers has consequently declared it to be his belief, that if all the syphilis in the world were to be now annihilated, a never-failing source of the disease would still remain, in the action of the matter of superficial or gonorrhœal ulcers of the penis on the human constitution.—(See his Pathology of the Ven. Disease.) In relation to this part of the subject, Mr. Wallace also considers it not in opposition to the general laws of nature, that the venereal disease may have arisen on different occasions spontaneously.—(See Treatise on the Ven. Disease and its Varieties, p. 8, 8vo., Lond., 1833.) At the same time he adds:—"No cases have occurred to me, nor have I heard or read of any, in which the evidence was quite satisfactory, that a deranged state of general health, or simple local irritation, or other accidental causes, either local or constitutional, ever produced by their influence on the system any effects which resembled in their series or order the constitutional symptoms of the venereal poison."—(P. 12.) The question, however, more immediately under our consideration is, not whether this poison exists at all, but whether the reality of its existence, whether it has had one or numerous origins? and whether it can originate under the circumstances adverted to by Mr. Travers?—ED.

have assumed a chronic form, and at length so far changed its nature, as to make its attack without fever, and to remain local except from absorption. It seems still, indeed, to be continuing its course of melioration, notwithstanding the assertion of Dr. Swediaur (*Beobachtungen*, &c., p. 172), that it has not assumed a more mitigated character at present than in former times; for very severe cases are now much rarer, not only in private practice, but even in public hospitals, than they were thirty or forty years ago.

It is possible that this change may have been produced by two causes; firstly, by the virus wearing out its own strength and becoming milder as it descends to different individuals and generations, and has to cope with the force of sound constitutions, and, perhaps, also, with a perpetual instinctive power or vis medicatrix naturæ, constantly labouring to subdue it : of which we shall hereafter have occasion to offer other examples than the present. And, secondly, it is also highly probable, that the frequent and indeed universal use of mercury for its extermination has succeeded, as a specific, in softening its violence, in the same manner as we know the virus of cowpox succeeds in giving a milder character to smallpox, even where it does not altogether answer as a prophylactic.

Syphilis shows itself under two distinct sets of symptoms, local and constitutional, the latter of which is commonly, but not always, a sequel of the former.

In which way soever it is produced, it is usually by means of impure coition; though we shall have occasion to show presently, that syphilitic matter coming in contact with any part of the surface of the body, where it is capable of burrowing and meeting with a little mucus, sweat, or, perhaps, any other natural secretion, is capable of assimilating it to its own nature, and hence of introducing the disease into the system by absorption, and consequently without any breach of surface. And hence, as other parts than the sexual organs may be a medium of communication, no local symptoms may in some instances ensue, and the constitutional signs be the first to manifest themselves.

The earliest ordinary mark, however, that infection has taken place, is the appearance of one or more minute pimples of a peculiar kind, which are called chancres; having a hard inflamed base, of a pale red hue, and irritable apex, which next opens with a small eyelet, becomes ulcerated, and discharges a small portion of limpid virus, that produces fresh chancres wherever it spreads. In the common mode of infection, the chancre shows itself on the prepuce, glans, and orifice of the urethra in men, and about the labia, nymphæ, clitoris, and lowermost part of the vagina in women. This mark sometimes appears as early as the third or fourth day after coition, more generally, however, a few days later; and in some instances, where the cutaneous absorbents possess little irritability, not till a lapse of several weeks. The chancre occasionally degenerates into a hard and irritable wart, with which the genitals are frequently studded, sometimes as low down as the anus.

Another local symptom is the formation of a bubo in one or both groins, evidently produced by an absorption of the virus first deposited, or, as is more commonly the case, multiplied in the ulcerated chancre, communicated to the lymphatics, and hence to the inguinal glands, which, in consequence, become inflamed and tumefied. The tumour, when first perceived, is small, but hard, fixed, and diffused, with a somewhat obtuse pain. It enlarges gradually, and becomes more acutely painful, so as to render walking troublesome ; and, if not opened by the lancet, generally bursts by the time it has reached the size of a pullet's egg, and discharges a copious quantity of pus from a single hollow. In a few instances the suppurative inflammation does not follow, and the tumour, as it augments, acquires considerable induration.

Sometimes, also, the inflammation extends by sympathy to the spermatic cord, which is inflamed and rigid through a great part of its course, while the testes themselves are tender and considerably swollen.

And occasionally, from sympathy also, or an entrance of a part of the received virus into the urethra, its mucous membrane becomes inflamed, and pours forth a considerable secretion of pus or purulent mucus, resembling that of blennorrhœa, or gonorrhœa, as it is commonly called, or the discharge from the eyes in purulent ophthalmia.

This was at one time mistaken for a genuine gonorrhœa, and the two diseases were very generally regarded as only different modifications of one and the same species. And some practitioners continue to be of the same opinion still, notwithstanding all the facts that have been adduced in proof of their being distinct maladies, produced by distinct kinds of contagion.* The local symptoms of syphilis, chancres, and buboes, are perpetually occurring without gonorrhœa, and gonorrhœa without chancres and buboes. Insomuch that there are not wanting practitioners who affirm that they never occur together, unless the two venoms are received simultaneously. And there is no doubt that this assertion is true in regard to a genuine gonorrhœa ; but, from the cause already stated, a large flow of pus or purulent matter, and a general irritation and enlargement of the body of the penis, in appearance strongly resembling the symptoms of a genuine gonorrhœa, sometimes coincide with the primary signs of a syphilis, of which a very marked case occurred to the author not long ago, which he showed to an eminent surgeon of the metropolis, who had antecedently been incredulous upon this point. And hence a like admission of Professor Frank, who, however, does not speak very decidedly

upon the subject ; and has strangely placed syphilis not only with gonorrhœa, but with leucorrhœa, mucous piles, hernia humoralis, and a variety of other diseases, under one and the same indistinct genus, to which he has given the name of medorrhœa.—(*De Cur. Hom. Morb. Epit.*, tom. v., p. 149, Manuh., 8vo., 1792.) But the clearest and most incontrovertible proof of distinction between the two complaints immediately before us is, that in no instance whatever has a simple gonorrhœa, unconnected with bubo or chancre, produced those secondary or constitutional symptoms to which the proper local signs of syphilis are sure to lead, if not corrected in their progress.*

These symptoms are, a progressive soreness and ulceration of the tonsils, uvula, palate, and tongue ; the voice being rendered hoarse, and the swallowing difficult. The ulcers about the fauces are of a distinctive character, being foul and rugged, with an excavated centre covered with a brown or whitish slough, and surrounded with a hard, red, elevated, and erythematous outline.

Sometimes the mucous membrane of the conjunctive tunic of the eyes next suffers in the same way, and displays an inflamed surface, with ulcerations on the eyelids and angles of the eyes.† The skin is in various parts covered over with copper-coloured spots, which at first desquamate in scurfs, afterward in scales, and still later in scabs ; each of which leaves a foul ulcer, that gradually grows deeper, and discharges an offensive fluid.

As the disease advances, irregular pains shoot through the limbs, and are felt so severely at night as to prevent sleep. By degrees they strike into the bones, which become diseased, and in many places swell into nodes, which at length grow carious : while the ulcerations about the fauces spread at the same time, or even before this, to the adjacent bones of the palate and nostrils, which are gradually eroded and carried away ; so that the speech is rendered nasal and imperfect, and the nostrils are flattened to the level of the cheeks.

Finally, the countenance grows sallow, the hair falls off, the appetite is lost, the strength decays, and a low hectic preys upon the system, and at length destroys it.

It is not easy to say how long the matter of syphilis, when once communicated, may remain limited to the local symptoms of chancres or

---

* Thus, in an enumeration of the morbid states or actions produced by the direct application of the venereal poison, we find included, by one of the latest writers on the subject, " an increased and morbid secretion from the diseased surface of the urethra, constituting the state commonly called gonorrhœa."—Wallace, on the Ven. Disease, p. 45, 8vo., Lond., 1833.—Ed.

* The earlier American physicians generally believed that gonorrhœa and lues syphilis arose from two distinct poisons, and necessarily demanded different modes of treatment ; that mercury was indispensable to cure the latter, while it was unnecessary, if not pernicious, in treating the former. This opinion, however, was somewhat questioned when the treatise of John Hunter was published in this country ; and his authority is so great, that some still maintain the identity of all venereal poisons.—D.

† Among the secondary symptoms Dr. Good should have mentioned iritis, which is a far more unequivocal effect of syphilis than the affections of the conjunctiva and eyelids, to which he has alluded.—Ed.

buboes, or continue inert in the system where no local symptoms have taken place ; or what period must intervene before a patient may be pronounced safe after having exposed himself to contamination. We have already seen that the primary or local signs generally manifest themselves within four or five days ; and, where the constitution has become infected without them, we have reason to expect the appearance of the secondary symptoms soon after three weeks, or from this time to six months : and if this latter interval have passed without the slightest manifestation of mischief, locally or generally, we have little reason to fear for the issue. It has been said, however, that the poison has lurked unperceived for several years ; yet it is rarely that such an assertion is made, except for the purpose of excusing some fresh infection. I should, indeed, have been disposed to think it had never been made otherwise, but that Dr. Hahnemann has referred to an instance or two to the contrary, in which he places full confidence (*Unterricht für Wundarzte über die Venerischen Krankheiten*, 8vo., Leips., 1789) ; and particularly that the late Mr. Hey of Leeds, whose authority is indisputable, has offered it as his opinion, formed from a variety of cases that had occurred to him during an extensive practice of nearly threescore years, that a man may communicate the disease after all the symptoms have been removed, and he is judged to be in perfect health ; and that a mother who has been once affected may convey it, notwithstanding an apparent cure, to two, three, or four children in succession, each of whom he supposes will have it in a milder form than the preceding one ; as though it were gradually ceasing in the constitution, though it still continues to show some degree of activity.*

* Facts illustrating the Effects of the Venereal Disease, by William Hey, Esq., F. R. S., 1816. The doctrines here adverted to, particularly that of the poison *lurking* unperceived in the constitution for many years, and that of a man in perfect health, or without any perceptible ailment about him, being able to communicate the disease to a woman, may be considered as now having few advocates. As the disease may be transmitted from the mother to the fœtus through the medium of the blood, a suspicion has frequently been entertained that it is likewise communicable through the medium of the natural secretions, the saliva, milk, semen, &c. With respect to the fœtus, we may infer that it receives the infection by means of the circulating blood, in the same manner as the mother herself receives her secondary symptoms ; but, with regard to the saliva, semen, and milk, it is difficult to pronounce how far these secretions will serve as means for the transmission of the disease, till the power of the secondary symptoms in general to do so is better made out. The editor believes with Mr. Travers, that none of the natural secretions of a contaminated individual can communicate the disease to other persons. The following statement in this gentleman's work (Pathology of the Ven. Disease) is interesting : a man who has syphilis in the secondary form, provided he be free from all affections of the genitals, will communicate no taint to his progeny any more than to his wife ; but a healthy wet-nurse, getting a sore nipple, in consequence of suckling a

It is obvious, however, that in syphilis, as in various other diseases produced by the absorption of a specific virus, different constitutions are differently affected, and that some are far more susceptible of the morbid action than others. In many instances it is received by simple contact alone, and through an unbroken skin. It is generally, perhaps, thus received in the ordinary course of connexion ; but still more evidently thus in other cases, and by other organs : for it has been very frequently caught by sucking the nipple of an infected wet-nurse ; by infected saliva communicated in kissing ; by drinking out of a cup that has previously been used by a syphilitic patient (*Reid, Diseases of the Army*, &c. ; *Grüner, die Ven. Anst. durch gemeinschaff. Trinkge., Weissenfels*, 1787) ; and it is said to have been produced by receiving infected breath, and lying in a bed which had been antecedently occupied by a person labouring under the disease (*Horstius*, opp. ii., p. 315) : in some of which cases, however, it seems necessary to suppose the existence of a cut or crack, or some other breach of-surface in the skin, and particularly about the lips, with which the syphilitic virus must have come into union. And it is hence easy to conceive how much more readily it may be communicated by the insertion of an exotic tooth (*Watson, Medical Transactions*, vol. iii., p. 325), by bleeding or scarification with an infected lancet (*Girtanner, die Venerischen Krankheiten*, &c., p. 165), or by the attendance of an infected midwife (*Act. Nat. Cur.*, vol. vii., obs. 75 ; vol. ix., obs. 94),* who has sometimes given the complaint both to the mother and the child.†

A very melancholy instance of infection is related by Dr. Barry of Cork, communicated by a woman who was in the habit of drawing the

pocky child, and having secondary symptoms, will communicate the disease to the fœtus of which she may become pregnant. This, we see, is agreeable to the usually received opinions, that the blood will contaminate the embryo though all genital sores may be absent, and though the party cohabiting with the woman is actually beyond the sphere of the influence of the disease in her. As far as the present state of our knowledge of the subject reaches, we may conclude that the disease is only communicable through the medium of a purulent fluid, and not an ordinary secretion, with the exception of the mode of its transmission to the fœtus, which receives the infection through the circulation, and may therefore be regarded as under the same circumstances with respect to the secondary effects of the disorder as the mother herself.—Ed.

* In the Westphaelischer Anzeiger, a case is stated where leeches, having been applied to a syphilitic patient, and afterward to an infant, the latter was affected with lues.—D.

† The faith to be put in several of these alleged modes of infection must be regulated by the well-established fact, that the venereal disease cannot be communicated unless the infectious matter be directly applied and lodged upon some part of the body of the person who catches the disease. The communication of the disorder through respiration, or by sleeping in a bed in which a venereal patient has previously lain, would not generally be credited by surgeons of the present time.—Ed.

breasts of puerperal patients; and who, upon examination, was found to have chancres on the lips and roof of her mouth, probably caught from some impure person in the course of her vocation. From the numerous engagements of this woman, the disease had spread very widely; and the rapidity of its progress was as striking as the manner of its communication. "The nipple," says Dr. Barry, "first became lightly inflamed, which soon produced an excoriation, with a discharge of a thin liquor; from whence red spreading pustules were dispersed round it and gradually spread over the breast, and, where the poison remained uncorrected, produced ulcers. The pudenda soon after became inflamed, with a violent itching, which terminated in chancres that were attended with only a small discharge; and in a short time after, pustules were spread over the whole body. It finished this course, with all these symptoms, in the space of three months. The disorder made a quick and rapid progress in those who first received it, they not being apt to suspect an infection of this nature in their circumstances. The husbands of several had chancres, which quickly communicated the poison, and produced ulcers in the mouth, and red spreading pustules on the body. But some of them escaped, who had timely notice of the nature of the disease, before the pudenda were affected. Some infants received it from their mothers, and to the greatest part of them it was fatal.'"*

---

* Edin. Med. Essays, vol. iii., art. xxi., p. 297. The real nature of the disease here spoken of is very ambiguous, and much doubt must be entertained respecting its syphilitic character; for, according to received opinions, it is not the ordinary course of the venereal disease to be communicated through the medium of any other secretion than the matter of a chancre, nor to attack the pudenda secondarily, after the infection has been originally communicated through some other quarter. According to Mr. Hunter, the matter of secondary venereal sores cannot impart the disease. However, it should be noticed, in opposition to the doctrine of the venereal disease being only communicable by the application of the matter of a chancre to the body of the person who catches the disease, that many cases are recorded of infants contracting the complaint, as was supposed, through the milk of infected nurses; and that other examples are related, in which most severe effects, resembling those of the worst forms of syphilis, have followed the transplantation of a tooth. In such instances, if the disease communicated were truly venereal, they were of course transmitted through the medium of the milk and the secretions of the mouth; but it is not a view in which the editor places any confidence. Various statements in the writings of Mr. Evans and the late Dr. Hennen, tend also to prove that the matter of true chancre in one person does not always communicate to another individual a sore of the same character; that the common secretions of the genitals, in unclean females, will cause in other persons who have connexion with them, sores of a very anomalous and infectious nature; and that several individuals who cohabit with a particular female that has, perhaps, merely a discharge, as ascertained by careful examination, may have, in one example, a true chancre; in a second, a superficial ulcer with elevated edges; in a third a clap, without any

Where a wet-nurse and the infant she suckles are both affected, and there is a doubt which has communicated it to the other, collateral circumstances will assist us much: but where the one, as is usually the case, has constitutional symptoms, and the other only local, the former must have had the disease the longest, and consequently have been the source of contamination.*

Such, however, is the insusceptibility of some idiosyncrasies, that the matter of syphilis, like that of smallpox, seems to have no effect upon them, and they are proof against its activity. I once knew a young physician, who, finding himself to be thus naturally protected, fearlessly, and for the sake of experiment, associated himself with females in the rankest state of the disease, and escaped in every instance. In like manner, Schenck (Obs., lib. vi., N. 21) gives us a case of an infant rendered syphilitic through a diseased father, while the mother remained unaffected; and Mauriceau and other writers give cases of infants which have been fortunate enough to avoid infection, though born of syphilitic mothers (Mau.iceau, ii., p. 100, 377; Eph. Nat. Cur., cent. iii., iv., obs. 18); while Pallas asserts that the Ostiacks have a general immunity from the disease, under whatever form it offers itself.—(Reisen, iii., p. 50.)

---

sore; and in a fourth, no ulceration, discharge, nor any complaint whatever. These facts certainly tend to prove that the nature of the complaint may be very considerably modified by some inexplicable peculiarity, either in the constitutions of different individuals, or in the state of the parts to which the infectious matter is applied.—Eᴅ.

* The hereditary transmission of lues will hardly be questioned, even by the most skeptical; and linical practice might controvert the opinion of Mr. Travers, that none of the natural secretions of a contaminated individual can communicate the disease to other persons. We have good authority for stating the following case, which occurred in the practice of the late Dr. Post, of New-York. A gentleman, who deemed himself cured of syphilis, married: his child exhibited the disease soon after birth, and imparted it to the wetnurse, whose character was beyond suspicion; the wet-nurse infected another female who drew her breasts, in consequence of which she was treated by mercurials, and was subjected to a surgical operation for an affection of her upper lip. The vision of the wet-nurse was impaired by the disease. In Dr. Hosack's Medical Essays, vol. ii., several cases are recorded of the communicability of syphilis to the fœtus in utero. In speaking of the remarkable fact that Dr. Denman never saw a decided instance of a child born with venereal disease, Dr. Francis remarks, "The diseased mother may affect the fœtus while in utero; the diseased infant may, by sucking, infect the nurse; the infected nurse may, in turn, communicate the complaint to the infant suckling at her breast. All this has occurred where the organs of generation, both male and female, were unaffected." "I have had under my care three cases of the venereal disease communicated to the fœtus in utero: two of these cases occurred where the genital system appeared in a perfectly sound state; in the other, there were ulcers of the labia and constitutional disease."—See Francis's Denman, 3d edit., New-York.—D.

And, after all, the symptoms that characterize the disease, as well in its first as its second stage, are at times so nearly approximated by those which are occasionally traced in the second species of this genus, syphiloid lues or spurious syphilis, that it is often extremely difficult to distinguish them, and we are obliged to enter minutely into the history of the case, in order to assist our decision.

It was regarded by Mr. Hunter as a pathognomonic character of syphilis, firstly, that it never ceases spontaneously ; secondly, that it is uniform and progressive in its symptoms ; and thirdly, that it is only to be cured by mercury. And such were the doctrines of a few of his warmest advocates, almost down to the present time.*

How far these characters may have applied to it on its first appearance in Europe, under the influence of European excitements, and when the general constitution of European nations was fresh to its virus ; or how far such characters may have descended to the middle of the last century, not long after which Mr. Hunter was so deeply engaged in drawing up those masterly views of this disease which he at length gave to the public in 1786, it may be difficult to determine. But to maintain any one of these doctrines without much modification, and especially as criteria of genuine syphilis in the present day, after the wide field of experiments which has been opened to us, both at home and abroad, would be the height of incredulity. For we have hundreds and perhaps thousands of proofs, that instead of "never ceasing spontaneously," it has occasionally disappeared without any other care than that of cleanliness and a reducent diet ; that instead of being uniform and progressive in its symptoms, it has occasionally retrograded, or disguised itself under a variety of peculiarities, according to the influence of habit, climate, or idiosyncrasy ; and that, instead of being only to be cured by mercury, various other modes of treatment have been quite as successful ; while, in numerous cases, mercury has added to the virulence of the disorder, and introduced many of those very symptoms which have usually been regarded as indicative of its secondary stage. Insomuch that it has been almost as seriously made a question in France, whether there is any such disease as syphilis,† as it has been in our own country, whether there ever was such a disease as plague : the former being as much resolved into local uncleanliness or constitutional irritation, as the latter has been into some modification of typhus with incidental influences.

This, however, is to run from one extreme of opinion to another ; and all we can fairly collect from such a collision of facts and opinions, is a confirmation of the conjecture I have already

ventured to throw out, that syphilis, like many other diseases, is capable of being greatly modified by contingent or habitual concomitants, or that it has actually changed its character, and is in a progressive course of melioration.

In truth, it is well known that Mr. Hunter himself found at times the secondary symptoms of syphilis intractable to a mercurial course, and had the candour to acknowledge as much. Dr. Adams, indeed, with all his warmth of attachment to the Hunterian code of doctrines, has given an impressive case of this very kind, in which, in spite of the mercury, the disease carried its assault from the first to the second order of parts, by which is meant the bones. But then this anomaly is accounted for by their ingeniously telling us, that if a constitutional disposition to the disease be formed, the mercury cannot cope with it till such disposition comes into action ; which seems, as Mr. Guthrie has justly observed, to mean nothing more, in plain language, than that ," the disease cannot be prevented in certain constitutions from running its own course, when it may at last be cured."

Of all the profession, the medical officers of the British army seem to have been first impressed with the expediency of re-examining and revising the established doctrines upon the subject before us, from having observed that mercury is little used in Southern Europe, especially in Spain and Portugal, and that syphilis is there suffered in a very considerable degree to take its natural course ; or at most to be treated locally as ordinary sores, and constitutionally with only herbaceous diluents or diaphoreties ; while the primary symptoms evidently vanish under this simple remedial course, and secondary symptoms are at times not more common than where mercury is had recourse to and solely depended upon. Mr. Rose, surgeon to the Coldstream regiment of guards, was determined to put the question to a test, and upon such a scale as might lead to something of a decisive result. He forbore, in consequence, about the year 1815, to employ mercury for the cure of any case of syphilitic affection, or suspected to be such, among the soldiers of his own regiment ; and soon sufficiently perceived, that though the cure did not advance so rapidly as under a judicious use of mercury, it nevertheless in every instance did advance ; that it was not more severely followed by secondary symptoms or a syphilitic dysthesy, than where mercury is trusted to as a specific ; and that, of course, it was without the risk of those mischiefs to the general health, which mercury is so well known to introduce where it disagrees with the constitution.*

Having persevered in this mode of treatment, in his own opinion very successfully, for a period of nearly two years, he communicated its

---

* The late Mr. Rose had the merit of establishing more accurate views of the nature of this Protean disorder, especially with regard to the points which are here specified.—ED.

† See the anonymous but ingenious pamphlet, " Sur la Non-existence de la Maladie Vénérienne," Paris, 8vo., 1811.

* Many facts tending to show that syphilis is curable without mercury, might be seen in the large work entitled the Aphrodisiacus of Lusitanus and others, edited by Boerhaave, and published more than a century ago. The voyages of Don Ulloa contain evidence of the kind influence of climate in this disease.—D.

result to the public (*Med. Chirurg. Trans.*, vol. viii., p. 349, 1817), with a long list of well-diversified cases and observations that cannot fail to make an impression on every one who reads them.

The experimental course laid down by Mr. Rose was soon adopted by others, and, on various occasions, carried into establishments which afforded ample space for a satisfactory examination. It was tried in other battalions of the guards, as well in France as at home; was introduced into the York Hospital at Chelsea, and various other hospital establishments, as at Dover, Chatham, and Edinburgh. "From these hospitals," says Mr. Guthrie, "I have seen the reports of nearly four hundred cases which have been treated with the same result, as far as regards the cure of primary ulcers; each ulcer appears to have run a certain course, which, as to extent, was much the same as in one of the same appearance where mercury was supposed to be necessary, and, at an indefinite period of time, to have taken on a healing action, and, in the greater number of instances, skinned over rapidly, leaving a mark or depression showing a loss of substance. With us, where the ulcer had the characteristic appearance of chancre, dry lint alone was generally applied to it. Where these signs were less prominent, a variety of applications were used. But there were a great number of sores, both raised and excavated, on which no application made the least favourable impression for many weeks. They did, however, yield at last to simple means, after remaining for a considerable time nearly in the same state, several of them having become sores of a large size previous to or in the first days of their admission. If they were ulcers without any marked appearance, and did not amend in the first fortnight or three weeks, they generally remained for five or seven weeks longer; and the only difference, in this respect, between them and the raised ulcer of the prepuce was, that this often remained for a longer period, and that ulcers possessing the true characters of chancre required in general a still longer period for their cure, that is, from six or eight, to ten, twenty, and, in one case, to twenty-six weeks, healing up and ulcerating again on a hardened base. Those that required the greatest length of time had nothing particular in their appearance that could lead us to distinguish them from others of the same kind that were healed in a shorter period. Neither were any of these ulcers followed by a greater number of buboes, nor did they suppurate more frequently than in the same number of cases treated by mercury. On the contrary, the ulcers were not so frequently, on the average, followed by them, neither did they so often suppurate. But this may also be attributed to the antiphlogistic means employed both generally and locally for their relief."—(*Medico Chirurg. Trans.*, vol. viii., p. 557.)—And to this it may be added, that M. Cullerier, the first surgeon in the Venereal Hospital at Paris, has been for years in the habit of demonstrating to his pupils the possibility of curing every kind of ulcer that

falls under his notice without mercury. He usually, indeed, has recourse to this medicine *afterward*, but for the mere purpose of guarding against secondary symptoms.

It is very candidly admitted, however, by Mr. Guthrie, that although these experiments give the strongest proof of the possibility of curing venereal ulcers without mercury, yet that a much longer period of time is required for the cure. "I have every reason," says he, "to be certain, from former experience, that almost all these protracted cases would have been cured in one half or even one third of the time, if a moderate course of mercury had been resorted to after common applications had been found to fail."

The result of this inquiry therefore should by no means induce us to relinquish the use of mercury as of specific influence in general practice; but it is of great importance as offering solid consolation to those who may be labouring under the disease with an idiosyncrasy or acritude of constitution that forbids the use of this specific, and converts it into a poison, instead of receiving it as a remedy.

It is admitted, also, that the cases of secondary symptoms occur more frequently in the cure of primary symptoms without mercury than where the last has been had recourse to. Upon the former plan of treatment, Mr. Guthrie calculates the secondary symptoms to occur about once in ten times; in the latter, once in about fifty-five times. But it is singular that, in the former case, the secondary symptoms are for the most part far milder than in the latter, the bones being rarely if ever affected. "Insomuch," says Mr. Guthrie, "that some of my friends, of great talents and experience, have been induced from this to suppose, that the greater severity of symptoms which are frequently met with have been caused by the exhibition of mercury in the first instance, which aggravated the constitutional disease." Mr. Guthrie, however, ascribes this more lenient show and course of the symptoms to the stricter antiphlogistic means resorted to in the simple than in the mercurial treatment, and endeavours to prove that mercury has no tendency to produce any such aggravation, except when injudiciously employed, or it does not harmonize with the idiosyncrasy, or actual state of the constitution.

It has been asserted, indeed, that in Portugal, where, as we have already observed, mercury is rarely had recourse to, both the primary and the secondary appearances are much more virulent than in England, or under a course of mercury: that the local ulcers are far more apt to slough and become gangrenous, and to run into that encircling phagedænic sore about the glans which has been vulgarly denominated *black lion*, and that a greater proportional number of British soldiers, and even officers, suffered irremediable injury from syphilis during the Peninsular war than are in the habit of suffering in this degree at home. These facts have been especially noticed by Dr. Fergusson in a valuable paper on the subject (*Med.-Chir. Trans.*, vol. iv.), and they are virtually admitted by Mr. Guthrie, who, however, ascribes the malignity, in every instance, to the accidental circumstances of change of climate and intemperance of habit, rather than to the absence of mercury. "I do not think," says he, "the disease which the troops contracted in Portugal was in the slightest degree more violent than the same kind of complaint at home, neither do I place the least reliance on what has been said by others about a distemper called the black lion of Portugal, which I do not believe exists. But I perfectly coincide with him (Dr. Fergusson) in opinion that the change from the climate of Great Britain to that of Portugal in the summer, with the different mode of life, does act most powerfully on our northern constitutions, and disposes strongly to inflammatory affections. It is this that rendered the same kind of wounds more dangerous to the British soldiers than to the natives, and it was to this disposition, increased by the greatest irregularity of conduct and often by intemperance, a vice the natives are not addicted to, that we were indebted for the mutilations which ensued from the venereal disease."

The following calculation of results seems to be a fair expression of the general facts, and, in the present state of the question, they are too important to be omitted. They comprise the conclusion of the same able writer's remarks upon the subject.

1. "Every kind of ulcer of the genitals, of whatever form or appearance, is curable without mercury. This I consider to be established as a fact, from the observations of more than five hundred cases which I am acquainted with, exclusive of those treated in the different regiments of guards, and which occurred in consequence of promiscuous intercourse.

2. "Secondary symptoms (and I exclude trifling pains, eruptions, or sore throats), that have disappeared in a few days, have seldom followed the cure of those ulcers without mercury, and they have, upon the whole, more frequently followed the raised ulcer of the prepuce, than the true characteristic chancre of syphilis affecting the glans penis.

3. "The secondary symptoms in the cases alluded to, amounting to one tenth of the whole, have hitherto been nearly confined to the first order of parts, that is, the bones have in two instances only been attacked, and they have equally been cured without mercury.

4. "As great a length of time has elapsed in many of these cases without the occurrence of secondary symptoms, as is considered satisfactory where mercury has been used, viz., from six to eighteen months.

5. "The primary sores were of every description, from the superficial ulcer of the prepuce and glans to the raised ulcer of the prepuce, the excavated ulcer of the glans, and the irritable and sloughing ulcer of these parts. In the inflammatory stage, attended by itching, scabbing, and ulceration, they were treated, for the most part, by antiphlogistic and mild remedies; in the latter stage, when the ulcers were indolent, whether raised or excavated, by gentle stimulants.

6. "The duration of these stages is very different, is often increased by caustic and irritating applications, and is much influenced by surgical discrimination in the local treatment.

7. "The last or indolent stage often continues for a great length of time, especially in the excavated chancre and raised ulcer of the prepuce. And it appears to me that in these particular cases, a gentle course of mercury, so as slightly to affect the gums, will materially shorten the duration of it, although in others it is occasionally of no service.

8. "Although the secondary symptoms do for the most part yield to simple remedies, such as venesection, sudorifics, the warm bath, sarsaparilla, &c., without much loss of time, that is, in the course of from one to four or six months, yet, as in the primary ulcers, a gentle course of mercury will frequently expedite, and in particular persons and states of constitution is necessary to effect a cure; and that a repetition of it will even in some cases be requisite, to render it permanent."*

There is yet one singular feature which remains to be noticed before we close the history of syphilis, and which, so far as I know, has never yet been fully brought before the public eye, although established by many of the best reports in the possession of the Army Medical Board'; and that is, the great difference which exists in the facility with which syphilis, and, I may add, the affections that make a near approach to it, as bastard syphilis and gonorrhœa, are propagated in the East, compared with their propagation in the West Indies. These reports have been submitted to me by the friendship of the director general; and the chief conclusion I have been able to draw from them —and it is a conclusion that Dr. Gordon, who was kind enough to go over these reports with me, has long since arrived at from the same documents—is, that every two regiments in the East Indies furnish, at least, as many cases of both genuine and doubtful syphilis, as are furnished by the whole army in the West Indies.

But the following tables will give the reader an opportunity of calculating for himself, and will show that the difference is sometimes much greater. The report from the whole of the West Indies for the year 1823 is as follows :—

Cases of syphilis unaccompanied with

secondary symptoms	16
Doubtful or bastard syphilis	15
Simple buboes	5
Annual number of cases for the whole of the West Indies in 1823	36

Now, the report from the 1st or royal regiment alone, for the same year, stationed at Trincomalee, gives 177 cases of syphilis, without any subdivision into genuine and doubtful.

In like manner, during a preceding year, while the 12th regiment of light dragoons furnished the following report—

---

* Medico-Chir. Trans., vol. viii., p. 576. Also, R. Carmichael's Essay on Venereal Diseases, and the Use and Abuses of Mercury in their Treatment, ed. 2, Lond., 1825.—ED.

Cases of syphilis　　-　-　- 44
　　Secondary symptoms -　　- 6
　　Doubtful ulcerated penis　- 5
　　Buboes　-　-　-　- 2
　　Cachexia syphiloidea -　ᷝ 7
　　Gonorrhœa　-　-　- 26
　　Hernia humoralis　-　- 15
　　　　　　　　　　　　　　　———
　　　　　　　　　　　　　　　105

the report for the same year from the whole of the West Indies, gives

Cases of syphilis　-　-　- 41
　　Buboes　-　-　- 29
　　Hernia humoralis　-　- 40
　　　　　　　　　　　　　　　———
　　　　　　　　　　　　　　　110

From the uncertainty which still prevails respecting the specific nature of several of the above affections in the minds of many practitioners, they are returned as of a common family ; and however unscientific such an arrangement may be in itself, it at least enables us to draw a more satisfactory general conclusion, as showing that none of the forms of disease which, in the widest latitude of the term, can be referred to a syphilitic origin, are here kept back.

I was, in effect, not a little surprised at finding how few reports respecting syphilis have been sent home from the West Indies, compared with those from the East, till Dr. Gordon convinced me, from the nature of those which have been received, of the difficulty of making out any such reports whatever in particular years ; and pointedly directed my attention to a remark in one of them, transmitted by Mr. Tegart, a highly intelligent inspector of hospitals at Barbadoes, as though offering an apology for the scantiness of his returns upon this subject. " One gentleman, Mr. Taylor, of much learning, and great experience in this island, who has resided here nearly thirty years, says that in that long period he has only seen two cases of primary disease. The fact is," continues Mr. Tegart, " that syphilis is almost unknown in this country :" alluding to the West Indies generally.

To what then are we to ascribe the wonderful contrast presented to us in these two colonies of the same empire ? Is syphilis regulated by some such law as that of plague, which, as we have already observed, seems incapable of existing in an atmospheric temperature above 80°, or much below 60° ; and hence has never been able to obtain a footing in Abyssinia or the south of Arabia, while it has rarely appeared earlier, as an epidemy, than June or July, in our own country ? or is it affected by any other meteorological influence ? The question is of no small moment : for if it be either the atmospherical temperature or temperament of the West Indies that produces so striking and beneficial an effect upon the specific poison of syphilis, it may be found that the best asylum we can provide, even for those who are actually labouring under the disease, and in its rankest form, is the same quarter : so that Barbadoes

and Jamaica may in process of time become as general a resort for syphilitic patients, as Madeira or the south of France for consumptive.

Till we are further acquainted, however, with the cause and nature of these discrepances than we are at present, we must continue to provide for syphilis the best means of cure we may be able to do at home. And in pursuing this object it is not to be wondered at, from the observations already offered, that plans of very different kinds, and medicines of very different classes, should not only be had recourse to in our own day, but should have been adventured upon at all times, even when the disease may be supposed to have raged with a far greater degree of malignity than at present.

From the number and repugnance even of those that have acquired any considerable degree of reputation, there is no small difficulty in reducing them to any thing like an intelligible classification. Yet, upon the whole, we may observe that the medicines which have been chiefly had recourse to, or have been found most serviceable in curing syphilis or arresting its progress, are narcotics, diluent diaphoretics, diuretics, drastic purgatives, and those which introduce a large portion of oxygen into the system.

Of the narcotics, recourse has been chiefly had to opium, conium, solanum, and belladonna, manifestly upon the principle of their being sedatives, and hence rendering the system inirritable to the syphilitic virus. This some of them accomplish in a very considerable and desirable degree ; and particularly opium, which has been mostly trusted to, and tried upon a wider scale than any of the rest. It moderates and alleviates every symptom ; and, from a cause not well ascertained, may be taken in very large doses with less inconvenience in syphilis than in almost any other disease. From its palliative effects, it has been supposed by many practitioners capable of producing a radical cure ; and numerous histories to this purpose have been published by those whose judgments have been unduly prejudiced in its favour. On these histories it is not necessary to enlarge : they have been long before the world, and have called forth other trials, which have not proved equally successful. Narcotics in general, and opium beyond the rest, add considerably to the efficacy of other means, and particularly of mercury ; but of themselves they are not competent to remove the complaint, and consequently are not to be depended upon.[*]

The list of warm and diluent diaphoretics

---

[*] As, from what has been said in the foregoing pages, every form of the venereal disease seems to admit of a spontaneous cure, without the specific influence of any medicine whatsoever, the question about opium should rather relate to its useful or injurious effects on the disease than to its power of curing it ; and if the disorder will get well of itself when no opium is given, and will not do so when this medicine is exhibited, the conclusion must absolutely be that opium is injurious, and prevents the cure. No doubt our author did not mean to maintain this doctrine.—Eᴅ.

that have been employed as remedies in syphilis are very extensive; but it may be sufficient to enumerate the following: mezereon, guaiacum, sarsaparilla, saponaria, bardana, smilax, and one or two species of asclepias, or swallowwort.

All these are supposed to be serviceable by exciting a determination to the skin, and throwing off the syphilitic poison, as various other poisons are thrown off, from the surface; and in very warm climates many of them are said to operate a radical cure, though the statements to this effect are rarely such as we can depend upon.*

They have all had their day, and the only one at present in much request is sarsaparilla, of the actual amount of whose virtues it is difficult to speak with precision. Like the *lobelia syphilitica*, or blue cardinal-flower, which is a purgative plant, it owes its earliest reputation to the American tribes; and when first imported into Europe by the Spaniards, about the year 1563, it had the character of being a specific for the venereal complaint. From being extolled, however, too highly,—for it never fulfilled this character in the old world,—it has since sunk, like many other useful medicines, into a very unmerited contempt, insomuch that Dr. Cullen allows but eight lines to its history and qualities, in the course of which he tells us that if he were to consult his own experience he would not give it a place in the Materia Medica, as he has never found it an effectual medicine in syphilis or any other disease.— (*Mat. Med.*, part ii., chap. v., p. 200.) The London College, however, have evinced a different opinion, for they have adopted it under various forms: and Professor Thomson, of Edinburgh, has been so highly satisfied with its antisyphilitic powers, that he has for some years relinquished the use of mercury altogether, in favour of a mode of practice which consists chiefly in the employment of sarsaparilla.— (*Edin. Med. and Surg. Journ.*, No. liii., p. 84.) Upon a very large scale, he has met with very great success; though, like Mr. Rose, he candidly acknowledges that the secondary symptoms of the disease have required a longer time to be overcome under the new treatment than they would under a mercurial.

There is also a much more powerful objection to its use; namely, that the secondary symptoms are in many cases apt to return soon after the new treatment has been relinquished, or other symptoms not essentially different. The fair pretensions of sarsaparilla appear to be those of a mild stimulant and diaphoretic. It is hence in many cases a useful auxiliary to mercury:

but I have chiefly found it succeed in chronic cases, where the constitution has been broken down, perhaps equally, beneath a long domination of the disease, and a protracted and apparently inefficient mercurial process. In connexion with a milk diet and country air, and with a total abandonment of mercury, I have here often found it of essential importance, and have seen an incipient hectic fall before a free use of it in a week. Its best form is the old one of the decoction of the woods, of which three or four pints should be taken daily.

In France the same plan has been long in general use, and has been found equally successful. On account of the dearness of sarsaparilla, when genuine, M. Etienne Sainte-Marie has been induced to try the *carex arenatia*, or German sarsaparilla of our old dispensatories, as Gleditch of Berlin had done before him; and though he does not, like Gleditch, regard it as more efficacious, he affirms, after employing it for ten years, that it is at least of equal value.—(*Méth. pour guérir les Mal. Vén. invét.*, &c., Paris, 1818.)

The syphilitic poison has also been often attempted to be thrown out of the body by exciting the excretories of some other organ than those of the skin, or in conjunction with them. Thus the flammula Jovis, or upright traveller's joy, the *clematis recta* of Linnæus, which acts powerfully both on the surface and on the kidneys, is said to have been employed with great advantage, and was at one time in high and extensive estimation. It was given in the form of an infusion of the leaves; and Dr. Stoerck, with his usual liberality, assigns it an extravagant praise, informing us that it effectually subdues all the secondary symptoms of inveterate headaches, bone-pains, nodes, ulcerations of the throat, and cutaneous eruptions.—(*Libell. quo demonstr. herb. vet. dict. flamm. Jovis posse tutò exhiberi*, Vienna, 1769.)

The *lobelia syphilitica* of the American Indians has a still fairer claim to notice. It is a drastic purgative, uniting something of the stimulant and narcotic powers of tobacco, to which it has some resemblance in its taste. In the simple life and inirritating diet of the American tribes, it is possible that it may have proved as successful as it is stated to have been; but it has completely failed in Europe.*

Of the antisyphilitics whose influence seems to depend on their being loaded with oxygen, the principal are the mineral acids and the metallic oxydes.

Of the first, the nitric has chiefly been made a subject of experiment in our own country, though the sulphuric has been employed abroad. —(*Crato.*, epist. v., p. 293.) Its general effects are, as we might expect them to be, tonic and sedative; whence the appetite is increased, a greater rigidity or firmness is given to the liv-

---

* Now, however, that the curableness of the venereal disease without any medicine, or with only such as are quite inert, and destitute of any specific power, is considered to be an established fact, the doubts here expressed concerning the subsidence and effectual dispersion of venereal complaints under a course of warm diaphoretic medicines, are quite inconsistent with the view which the author has taken of what was made out by Mr. Rose's investigations.—Ed.

* According to the best information, the lobelia is still used by the Indians. The ravages of this disease among them, however, have recently led them to employ mercury. Barton says (Veg. Mat. Med.), that the antisyphilitic powers of lobelia are no longer credited.—D.

ing fibre, and a greater density to the coagulable lymph: the action of the bowels, and even of the bladder, being diminished. Besides these, it has a particular effect on the mouth, approaching to that of ptyalism, for the gums are rendered slightly sore, the mouth and tongue become moist, and in India and other warm climates a real salivation is said to ensue. Under this change, the syphilitic symptoms assume a better appearance, and especially those that belong to the primary set; but we have no decided case in which a perfect cure has been accomplished in our own country,* though Dr. Scott affirms that in India this has been common. The acid he was in the habit of employing was a direct aqua regia, as already noticed in the treatment of jaundice (Cl. I., Ord. II., Gen. I., p. 205.;) and with the internal use of this he combined that of the acid bath, as there also particularly specified. His object was to effect a cure without incurring any of the evils so frequent upon a mercurial course; and to this object the proposed plan has, in his opinion, given complete success. It would have been happy for the world if this success had been permanent and universal; but the plan has since fallen in its reputation, not much less in India than in Europe.

The metallic oxydes have offered a large field for experiment; and almost all the metals have been had recourse to in rotation, as copper, iron, antimony, mercury, arsenic, and even gold.

The pretensions of arsenic are certainly considerable: it forms the ordinary medicine employed in syphilis by the cabirajahs or native Indian physicians, who depend upon it as a specific. They give it in the form of white arsenic, in combination with black pepper, as we shall notice more at large when treating of elephantiasis, for which also it is esteemed a powerful remedy. The only auxiliary is a cathartic of manna dissolved in a decoction of nymphæa Nelumbo.

Of the effects of any of the preparations of gold, we know but little. Many of them were in high repute formerly as a cure for various cachexies, and are said to have been used with success in syphilis.—(Agricola, Comment. in Pappium, Num., 1643.) They have since been tried in France,† and also in this country.‡

Antimony, and perhaps a few other metals, are useful auxiliaries: but, in fact, the only

metal, and I may add the only medicine, on which we can confidently rely for a general cure of syphilis in all its stages, in our own climate, is MERCURY.*

This has been tried from an early period in almost every variety of preparation; and, provided a sufficiency of it is introduced into the system, in every variety it has been found to succeed; so that, in the present day, the peculiar form is regarded of less importance than on its first use; though we may observe, that it seems to be most rapidly efficacious in those forms that introduce the largest proportion of oxygen into the system. And as it operates chiefly, like most other medicines, through the medium of the circulation, when it once becomes mixed with the current of the blood, it is equally efficient in the cure of a recent chancre and a chronic ulceration of the throat.

Mercury is a universal stimulant, and increases the action of all the secretories at one and the same time; for it operates simultaneously on the intestines, the skin, the salivary glands, and even the bladder; though it displays itself chiefly by its action on the salivary glands. It has also, when given in moderate doses, considerable pretensions to a tonic power, though this is overwhelmed by its stimulant effects when the dose is considerably increased. And it seems, therefore, to unite most of the virtues of the preceding remedies, excepting the sedative; and hence it is greatly improved by the addition of opium and camphire, which give it the quality it stands in need of.

Independently, however, of its combining in itself many of the virtues of the preceding remedies, mercury seems also to possess some specific virtue unknown to the rest; for we can associate all the general qualities by a combination of different medicines without producing the same result. Mercury, indeed, to these general qualities adds that of peculiarly stimulating the salivary glands, which the other remedies employed in syphilis do not at all, or never in an equal degree; but that its specific power as an antidote does not depend upon its being a sialagogue is clear, because, while it has sometimes excited salivation without effect, it has at other times produced a perfect cure without any salivation whatever; for, in some idiosyncrasies, the salivary glands are not affected by its irritation.

Dr. Cullen, however, who had a mortal aversion to considering any medicine in the character of a specific, denies that mercury is a specific in syphilis, as he does also that it is an antidote to the disease. It is in vain to point out to him its specific influence upon the salivary glands, or its specific action upon the mouth;

---

* As syphilis in most of its forms, if not all, has been fully proved to admit of a spontaneous cure, we should be obliged to suppose the nitric acid to be not only useless, but an impediment to the cure, if our author's statement were substantially true. This is not, however, suspected; nor can there be any foundation for the suspicion, while Mr. Rose's facts continue to dispel various prejudices concerning the incurable nature of the disease without the aid of mercury.—ED.

† See the Report of A. S. Duportal, M. D., and Th. Pelletier, Apoth. Annales de Chimie, tom. lxxviii., p. 38. Delpech, Chir. Clin., 4to., 1823.

‡ See a paper by Mr. R. D. Forster, on the Employment of the Chloride of Gold and Soda in Syphilis, published in Lancet for Feb., 1834.—ED.

---

* The preparations of gold and platina have been tried with perseverance by M. Cullerier, but without success. They are difficult to manage on account of their activity, and also of the facility with which they are decomposed. In this country, too, results have not warranted the reliance placed on them by Chrestien.—See Eberle's Am. Med. Review, vol. i.; also Dyckman's edition of the Edinburgh Dispensatory.—D.

he denies the whole, and contends that mercury might travel, and perhaps would travel for ever in some other direction, were it not for the friendly interposition of the ammoniacal salts of the blood, which he fancies to have a close affinity with mercury, as he supposes they have also with the salivary glands ; in consequence of which, they take the mercury by the hand, and introduce the one stranger to the other (*Mat. Med.*, part ii., chap. xvii., p. 443–450) ; thus solving the difficulty like divinity in the catastrophe of a drama. The result of the whole, in the opinion of Dr. Cullen, is, that mercury cures the venereal disease, not by producing any change in the state of the fluids, but entirely by giving a stimulus to the excretories at large, by whatever contrivance it reaches them, and thus increasing the excretions, and washing out the poison from the body.

That it does this is highly probable ; but this alone is not sufficient, for fresh poison is continually forming by the process of assimilation, or the conversion of some part of the fluids it comes in contact with into its own nature ; since, if it were not so, and the minute drop of virus that excited the disease at first remained without any increment, there can be no question that such a general scouring of the system would be unnecessary, and that the ordinary evacuations would be sufficient to throw it off. And hence we have not only to carry away the poison that is actually present in the vessels, but to prevent the formation of new.

Now it is in this power of prevention that the specific virtue of mercury seems to consist ; and this it is that renders it paramount to all other remedies in the cure of syphilis. It is not only an evacuant, but an antidote : for, as we have already seen, it quickens the action of other remedial means when united with them, and far more speedily effects a cure even by itself than any of them. By what means, however, it becomes an antidote, or exerts its specific power, we know not. The matter of a chancre, mixed up with a quantity of Plenck's gummy solution of mercury, has been applied to a sound person without occasioning either a chancre or any other syphilitic symptoms. And it has hence been supposed that mercury neutralizes the syphilitic virus, and produces a third and harmless substance ; as it has been further supposed, that it is by the disengagement of the oxygen which the various preparations of mercury introduce into the system, that this effect is accomplished. All this is ingenious, and may be true ; but the evidence does not come home to the conclusion. Even the experiment with chancrous matter and the mercurial solution has not been satisfactorily performed ; and if the result were as here stated, the matter, while it has no power of assimilating the solution into its own nature, as it has the fluids of the human body, may only have been rendered inert by simple dilution.

[Instead of these chymical hypotheses, the belief most commonly adopted by modern practitioners is, that mercury excites a new and peculiar action in the system, whereby the syphilitic action is destroyed. This, however, is only a theory ; and though it originated with Mr. Hunter, it should be regarded rather as an attempted than a well-proved explanation of the *modus operandi* of mercury.]

We have said that, provided a sufficient quantity of mercury be introduced into the system, the particular preparation is of no great importance. Van Swieten preferred the oxymuriate, and every one followed his example. The calcinated mercury came next into popularity, and triumphed over every other form. It was the leading article of most of the secret remedies that were sold for the complaint, and especially of Keyser's pills ; the receipt for which was purchased with great formality by the French government, with an express provision not to make it public till the inventor's death.[*] These pills, however, which consisted of nothing more than mercury calcined by needlessly operose elaboration and mixed up with manna, were found in many cases to irritate the bowels, even when united with aromatics and opiates ; and hence they gradually yielded on the continent to Plenck's solution, which still holds a considerable sway.

In our own country it is now most usual to employ the mercurial pill, or calomel, either alone or together with mercurial ointment. Yet, whatever plan is preferred, much caution is necessary in carrying it into effect ; for the older practitioners, who employed larger doses, frequently did as much mischief to the constitution by the antidote as it had received by the infection. If calomel be employed, about two grains a day will commonly be found sufficient, guarded when necessary by a grain of opium ; and if the ointment be preferred, half a drachm of the strong mercurial ointment may be rubbed in night and morning. If the disease be not severe or of long standing, it will not be necessary, with a little management, to produce salivation, which in most instances may be regarded only as a test that the system is thoroughly impregnated with the medicine ; but, in chronic cases, we ought not to be satisfied without it.

In the course of the present work—and the observation is applicable to other doctrines than those of medicine—we have often seen that extremes lead to extremes : and hence, while many practitioners have been reviving the attempt to cure syphilis entirely without mercury, others have revived that of attacking it with very large doses. The last has chiefly been confined to those who have been employed in warm climates, and been friendly to the same practice in dysentery and yellow fever. In syphilis, however, they seem to have been somewhat more successful than in the other diseases, doubtless from the more decidedly specific influence of mercury over the former. The dose, with these gentlemen, is the usual one of a scruple, which in our own climate is repeated daily for three or four days in succession ; but in warmer climates, four or even five times in

---

* Des Dragées, ou Pilules de M. Keyser, par Richard de Hautesierck. Recueil d'Observations de Médecine des Hôpitaux Militaires, &c., Paris, 1766.

twenty-four hours. In various cases the effects on the stomach and bowels are severe, and in all cases a considerable degree of nausea is excited, and the appetite is entirely suppressed. But, upon the whole, the bowels and general system are for the most part less affected than might be supposed ; ptyalism is often excited in two or three days, and a constitutional improvement speedily shows itself. So that, where the treatment does not disagree with the idiosyncrasy, the cure is rapid and perhaps radical ; the individual being usually set at liberty in a fortnight or three weeks.* But such a practice must not be attempted indiscriminately, and should indeed be used with great caution : for it has fallen to the author's lot to know of not a few instances, in which the constitution has been so completely broken down by the very onset of this energetic plan, as to require not two or three weeks, but many months, before the patient was re-enabled to take his station in society ; to say nothing of the virulence which has been added to all the symptoms of the case, whether primary or secondary, in dyscrasies or idiosyncrasies which are hostile to the use of mercury. There can be no doubt, indeed, that a long perseverance even in small doses, under like circumstances, will not unfrequently produce as lamentable an effect. But, in this case, we can hold our hand much more easily on the first appearance of mischief.

In all cases of the use of mercury, but particularly in cases of salivation, care should be taken to avoid cold, and flannel should be worn next the skin. It is also of importance that the diet should be light and simple, as the pulse is usually accelerated, and, by a stimulating regimen, would be so much quickened as to do serious mischief. Mr. Hunter lays no stress on this point, but it ought by no means to be neglected.

If a bubo have formed in the groin, the mercurial ointment is best rubbed in a little below it, as it would increase the inflammation if applied to the tumour itself. In about a week or ten days the mouth will become slightly sore, when the further use and proportion of the ointment or other preparation must be regarded by the violence or duration of the complaint.

An injudicious use of mercury, or indeed any use of it in highly irritable habits, will sometimes excite a very troublesome erythema, that spreads itself in trails or patches over the whole surface ; commonly, however, commencing about the genitals and lower limbs. It is accompanied with a painful tenderness and itching of the skin, and as the erythema meanders onward, the trails or patches first observed heal as new ones make their appearance. We have already glanced at this affection under the vesicular species of ᴇʀʏᴛʜᴇᴍᴀ. Mercury must in this case be desisted from, the bowels be loosened with some gentle aperient, and the irritability opposed by

* Dr. S. A. Cartwright of Mississippi has employed calomel in this manner in many cases of syphilis, where small doses of mercury had been used without success.—See his Essay on Syphilis in the Am. Med. Recorder, vol. viii.—D.

sedative and mild cardiacs, as camphire, guaiacum, and sarsaparilla ; and particularly by the mineral acids.*

SPECIES II.
LUES SYPHILODES.
BASTARD-POX.

ᴛʜᴇ ɢᴇɴᴇʀɪᴄ ᴜʟᴄᴇʀs ɪɴᴅᴇᴛᴇʀᴍɪɴᴀᴛᴇ ɪɴ ᴛʜᴇɪʀ ᴄʜᴀʀᴀᴄᴛᴇʀs ; sʏᴍᴘᴛᴏᴍs ɪʀʀᴇɢᴜʟᴀʀ ɪɴ ᴛʜᴇɪʀ ᴀᴘᴘᴇᴀʀᴀɴᴄᴇ ; ᴜsᴜᴀʟʟʏ ʏɪᴇʟᴅɪɴɢ sᴘᴏɴᴛᴀɴᴇᴏᴜsʟʏ ; ᴠᴀʀɪᴏᴜsʟʏ ᴀꜰꜰᴇᴄᴛᴇᴅ ʙʏ ᴀ ᴄᴏᴜʀsᴇ ᴏꜰ ᴍᴇʀᴄᴜʀʏ.

I ʜᴀᴠᴇ already observed, at the opening of the present genus, that the species before us is designed to include a multiplicity of affections, which, in many of their signs, have a close resemblance to syphilis, but differ from it in the progress of the symptoms, as well as in the means that are necessary for a cure.†

Such affections are of high antiquity, far higher, indeed, than those of syphilis, and some of them appear to be glanced at in the sacred records. A few of them may perhaps have arisen in much later times, and may be arising at present.—(*Pearson, Obs. on the Effects of var. art. of the Mat. Med. in the Cure of L. Ven.*, 2d ed., p. 53.) By Celsus the subject is touched upon scientifically : it has been taken up in modern times by Mr. Hunter with that spirit of inquiry which peculiarly distinguished him, and has since been pursued by Mr. Abernethy (*Surg. Obs. on Dis. resemb. Syphilis*, Lond., 1810), Mr. Carmichael, and various other surgeons and physiologists, with a kindred comprehension and genius : and the track which they have traced out in England is precisely parallel with the march which M. Etienne Sainte-Marie has of late years pursued in France, conceiving himself, according to his own account, to have been the original discoverer of these distinctions ; which is the more extraordinary, since this writer, as we have already had occasion to observe, believes in the exploded doctrine of the identity of syphilis, and what is commonly called gonorrhœa.—(*Méth. pour guérir les Mal. Vén.*, &c., Paris, 1818.) The subject, however, is still in its embryo. Mr. Hunter considered his own remarks rather as hints for others to prosecute than as a com-

----

* In the U. States, syphilis is generally treated by mercurials ; and although some practitioners believe that it can be cured without this class of medicines, but very few have adopted the non-mercurial practice. The preparations of mercury most used are calomel, blue-pill, and corrosive sublimate. The latter remedy, notwithstanding the violent opposition of Mr. John Pearson of the Lock Hospital, London, is too well known, and has proved too efficacious, to be invalidated even by him. An able view of the Medical History and Curative Action of Mercury, by Dr. J. W. Francis, will be found in the Am. Med. and Phil. Register, vols. iii. and iv.—D.

† Many of these cases would be arranged by Mr. Wallace as degenerations of syphilis.—See his Treatise on the Venereal Disease and its Varieties, p. 60, where he enters into the consideration of what he terms the "degenerations of primary syphilis."—Eᴅ.

plete account of it. And though Mr. Abernethy has accumulated facts and cases, and ably illustrated them with observations that sufficiently establish these hints, and give something of a body to the outline, we are still in want, as we have already seen, of distinctive characters, and cannot determine with any degree of accuracy, whether the wide group of complaints that fall within the present range of contemplation are mere varieties of a common species produced by a common poison, or distinct species dependant upon distinct poisons, as discriminable from each other as all of them are from proper syphilis.

Under the last species, we had occasion to notice Mr. Hunter's pathognomonic criteria of genuine syphilis : first, that it never ceases spontaneously ; secondly, that it is uniform and progressive in its symptoms ; and thirdly, that it is only to be cured by mercury.

Could this view of the disease be strictly supported, we should have a tolerably distinctive character by which to discriminate the preceding from the present species ; but sufficient proof has been offered, that not one of the three points holds good with a considerable degree of modification, whether in respect to the primary or secondary symptoms of these maladies.

Very ingenious attempts have since been made to distinguish these diseases, not by their general march and mode of cure, but by their immediate and prominent signs ; that of the true syphilitic chancre in the first stage, and those of the peculiar nature of the spots, the nodes, or the ulcers, in the second. But the close approach to syphilis, at times, of misaffections, whose history, when minutely investigated, has clearly proved them to have issued from other sources than syphilis, has in a great measure levelled all such landmarks, and nearly left us in extreme cases without a clew.

It is after all, therefore, rather from the general history of the different examples in all their bearings, than from the individual symptoms, that we can alone arrive at any sound or satisfactory means of referring them to a syphilitic or a different origin. If we can strictly rely upon the assertion, or know, as a fact, that there has been no impure connexion ; if we cannot perceive that there has been any primary ulcer ; if we find that the symptoms, whether primary or secondary, readily give way spontaneously, or by other remedies than mercury ; or if we have proof from the first that they are exasperated by this last medicine, whatever be the approximation of such symptoms to those of genuine syphilis, we may rest pretty well assured that the disease is syphiloid, rather than syphilitic lues. In the first case, indeed, unquestionably so, and nearly uuquestionably so in the second and third.

It is well known that constitutional derangement, in an irritable habit or idiosyncrasy, will often follow from other local causes of various kinds, and often from what is ordinarily of very slight import. It is hence that the general health in some persons suffers from such cutaneous eruptions as rose-rash, herpes, or itch. Gonorrhœa has perhaps at times, as we have already remarked, affected the constitution in like manner, and even thrown over the skin spots that have been mistaken for those of genuine syphilis. And there is hence reason for believing, that even an incidental and unspecific irritation of the prepuce or the glans may, in the same way, occasionally so far simulate the march of the same disease, as to exbibit a very close semblance to the raised ulcer, or the excavated chancre, or even the phagedænic slough ; or, passing by these first symptoms, that it may mimic as closely those of the second stage of the disease, And as it is now pretty generally admitted on all hands, that morbid and irritative secretions of various kinds, independently of those of syphilis or even gonorrhea, are thrown forth and accumulate in the sexual organs of contact, we can trace a variety of sources of both local and constitutional affection, which, issuing from the same seat, may assume something of a family character ; to say nothing of those more wonderful resemblances of the secondary symptoms of syphilis which have sometimes been found to occur without any previous local contagion, and in the most unspotted purity of single life.

A consideration, therefore, of such diseases, or varieties of diseases, as are thus found to approximate the general character of syphilis, though issuing from sources widely distinct, and possessing, in the midst of such approximation, a few discriminative marks, perhaps at all times, and under all circumstances, however they may hitherto have eluded the prying eye of the pathologist, is evidently called for, and it is the object of the present subdivision to imbody them, as far as the footsteps of observation will at present allow.

We have thus far, however, followed them into their extremes, in which alone their symptoms appear merged in those of syphilis ; for, in the greater number of cases, a distinction is not very difficult, either in the local or the constitutional attack.

In illustration of these remarks I might refer to the observations of those who have been attentive to the subject on a large scale, but I refer more particularly to the collection of cases which Mr. Abernethy has printed in the work already alluded to.

The disease ordinarily commences with local symptoms, though not always ; but the local symptoms have a less resemblance to those of genuine syphilis than the constitutional by which they are succeeded. A few foul and highly irritable sores are unexpectedly discovered on the genitals, commonly larger than chancres, and less thickened and indurated, about the size of a sixpence, and frequently sprouting with fungous granulations. Rarely, but very rarely, they have the guise of a true chancre ; so rarely, indeed, that of the twenty cases contained in Mr. Abernethy's book, the fifth is the only one that answers to this description. These are sometimes succeeded by buboes and sometimes not. And where buboes take the lead, they run their course more rapidly, and with more violent inflammation, than in the true disease, and spread to a greater number of circumjacent glands. These mostly, if not always, heal by the ordinary means without mercury, or constitutional symptoms of any kind. But, not unfrequently, in a few weeks or months, they are followed by a soreness and ulceration of the tonsils, copper-coloured spots over the body, and nodes or swellings of the periosteum in various bones ; and sometimes these symptoms change their order of succession, or appear single.

In a few instances the constitutional symptoms take the lead and the local follow, of which Mr. Abernethy's fourth case affords an example. The patient here perceived first of all a small ulcer on the breast near the nipple, after having suckled a nurse-child about four months. It was of the size and shape of an almond, and was ascribed to the child's having a sore nose and lips. A gland in the axilla soon swelled and subsided, but, in about two months, the patient had a severe febrile attack, accompanied with a sore throat ; from this she soon recovered, but had shortly afterward a copper-coloured eruption scattered over the body, and upon the disappearance of this, white blisters about the pudenda, which gave her pain in walking. About a week afterward her husband found a sore on the penis, covered by a black scab, of about the size of a sixpence, with a base neither hard nor thick, but with the surrounding skin much inflamed. Another formed in the course of the lymphatics towards the groin ; the inguinal glands enlarged, and one of them suppurated ; and an eruption of a papulous erythema, ushered by a few febrile symptoms, followed in about three weeks. The sores were twice touched with lunar caustic, and, as well as the bubo, were afterward washed with calomel in lime-water : they gradually healed. Both patients recovered, the wife with little assistance from mercury, having taken only a few compound calomel pills with small doses of nitric acid ; the husband without mercury altogether, except that a dose of calomel was once administered with other aperient drugs as a purge.*

---

* These cases resemble some others quoted by the author under the preceding species as syphilitic ; but against which inference the editor has mentioned a few considerations which occurred to him at the time of reading them. With regard also to the present examples, set down as syphiloid, the conclusion that they were not venereal cannot be maintained by the mere fact that they got well with little or no mercury, for, as already explained, all forms of the venereal disease are generally curable without mercury, though this often accomplishes the cure with greater expedition, and diminishes the frequency of secondary symptoms. When we read in Mr. Abernethy's Observations on Diseases resembling Syphilis, p. 44, that " the fictitious disease, in appearance, so exactly resembles syphilis, that no observation, however acute, seems to be capable of deciding on its nature ;" and when we find him admitting, at p. 54, that all his reasoning is founded " upon the presumption that diseases which spontaneously get well are not syphilitic," we are compelled, in the present more accurate state of our knowledge upon the latter point, to confess that Mr. Abernethy completely failed in making out

In all these cases we meet with a virus that seems to be more active and irritating than that of genuine syphilis, but which, while it pursues, though with much irregularity, the same general path, runs through its course much more quickly, and is more effectually coped with by the natural strength or remedial instinct of the constitution. And hence, all that we are here called upon to do in the way of treatment is to support the general vigour and second the instinctive effort. This is best to be accomplished by tonics and gentle stimulants, and, where necessary, by sedatives. The mineral acids are the best means of supplying the first intention ; camphire, the decoction of the woods, and the compound calomel pill, where small doses of mercury do not irritate, the second ; and opium the third, though to this last it will rarely be necessary to have recourse at all.

The distinction between these affections and genuine syphilis is frequently difficult, but of importance ; since, as a full use of mercury seldom seems to do good, and often does serious mischief in the former, such a plan has a chance of overwhelming the constitution with a second disorder instead of freeing it from a first.

To this family of maladies we are probably to refer the disease which, for a century or two, has been known in Scotland by the name of SIBBENS, or SIVENS, literally rubula, or raspberry eruption, and which seems to be a variety of lues, rendered hybrid by passing through a constitution already contaminated with genuine RUBULA or yaws.* The local symptoms have a much nearer resemblance to those of bastard-pox than of genuine syphilis, but in its constitutional progress, after the ordinary affection of the fauces, the disease has a tendency to throw forth over the surface an eruption of tubercles, which speedily degenerate into fungous ulcers resembling yaws, rather than an eruption of copper-coloured spots ; which tubercles sometimes show themselves also in the throat itself. The constitutional disease spends itself chiefly on the surface, and the bones are rarely affected. With these exceptions we may agree with Dr. Gilchrist (Account of a very infectious Distemper, &c.) and Mr. Hill, of Dumfries (Cases in Surgery), that it has not a symptom which does

---

any peculiarities in his cases to justify their being denominated pseudo-syphilitic. When we are told of a disease being exactly like syphilis in appearance, we ought first to be informed what is the precise appearance of syphilis itself ; for it presents itself in so many shapes, and has so many varieties, or degenerations, as Mr. Wallace terms them, that they form a very obscure and complex subject. Frequently no judgment of any value can be given about the nature of a sore, suspected to be venereal, merely from the look of it, without any reference to other particulars in the history of the case. On this point there are some interesting remarks in Mr. Wallace's Treatise on the Venereal Disease, p. 84, et seq.—ED.

* Some few cases of sibbens occurred in 1819-20 among the ditchers employed on the grand canal between lake Erie and the Hudson. The persons affected were last from Canada, and were natives of Scotland or Ireland.—D.

not accompany the lues venerea (meaning syphilis) through all Europe; that both are equally infectious; both only communicated by sexual intercourse or other familiar contact; and both beneficially treated by mercury, which, they affirm, is the only remedy to be depended on. Mr. Hill tells us that it was introduced into the vicinity of Dumfries about the year 1772, " by some pocky soldiers, who, to prevent their debauching in town, were disposed through upon the neighbouring villages." Even upon his own showing, however, a much looser and blander exhibition of mercury than is sufficient for the cure of a confirmed syphilis,* will effect this in sibbens; for he adds, that "by the employment of a mild preparation of this metal he has cured numbers without confining them to their houses, even in frosty or snowy weather." It is probable, therefore, that sibbens might be eradicated by other means as well; but these gentlemen, notwithstanding the peculiarity of many of its symptoms, regarded it as a genuine syphilis, and, in consequence, did not direct their attention to any other mode of treatment.†

GENUS VIII.

ELEPHANTIASIS.

ELEPHANT-SKIN.

SKIN THICK, LIVID, RUGOSE, TUBERCULATE; INSENSIBLE TO FEELING; EYES FIERCE AND STARING.; PERSPIRATION HIGHLY OFFENSIVE.

THE Greeks denominated this disease ELEPHAS, or ELEPHANTIASIS, because the skin of persons affected with it resembles that of the elephant in thickness, ruggedness, insensibility, and dark hue. Thus applied, therefore, the term imports *elephant-skin*, in the same manner as the same national school denominated dandruff pityriasis, or *bran-skin*, from the skin, under this disease, resembling branny scáles; and another sort of scaly malady, ichthyiasis, or *fish-skin*, from the resemblance óf the skin when thus affected to the scales of fishes. There are, however, two diseases of a very different kind, which occur in the translations of the Greek and Arabic writers under the name of elephas, elephantia, or elephantiasis; that immediately before us, and the thick leg of Barbadoes and other hot climates: and as the former of these has also, by many of the Arabian writers, been called lepra, or leprosy, and espe- cially black leprosy, though as distinct from genuine leprosy as it is from the thick leg; and as the common term lepra has been continued

in the translations of such writers, and copied from them by writers of our own times, an almost impenetrable confusion has been thrown around the whole of these diseases; and they have, even by modern writers, been strangely huddled together, and contemplated as mere modifications of one and the same malady, or as having some other connexion which does not in reality exist.

My attention was particularly called to this subject several years ago by an application from Dr. Bateman, who was then preparing his work on Cutaneous Diseases for the press, to assist him in unravelling it from the thorny maze in which it was at that time enveloped; and as the following letter from him, written in conse- quenco of my acceding to his request, shows the real difficulty of the case, and is highly creditable to the activity of his mind, the reader will be obliged to me for introducing it.

" In order to give you the least trouble pos- sible in the research which you were good enough to promise to make for me this morning, I wish to state, in a few words, the object of my inquiry. I believe the proper tubercular *elephan- tiasis* of the Greeks was called '*juzam* or *alju- zam* by the old Arabians (*dsjuddam* and *madsjud- dam* by the moderns, according to Niebuhr.)— (See *Avicen.*, quart. iii., or lib. iii., fen. iii., tract. iii., cap. i.)

" If so, do the other Arabian writers also designate the proper elephantiasis by the same appellation?—For instance, is it used by Haly Abbas?*

" Again, what is the Arabic term applied to the THICK LEG (which most of the translators call *elephantiasis*, but which the translator of Haly Abbas calls *elephas*, thus distinguishing it from *elephantia*)?—The *thick leg* is described by Haly Abbas (*Theoricè*, lib. viii., cap. xviii.), by Avicen (Lib. ii., fen. xxii., tract. i., cap. xvi. or xviii.), by Rhazes (*Ad Almanzor*, lib. ix., cap. xciii.), and by Avinzoar.—(Lib. ii., cap. xxvi.) The translators of the other works in these places used the word *elephantia*.

" Thus, the proper *elephantiasis* is called ele- *phantia* by (the translators of) Haly Abbas, and *lepra* by (the translators of) Avicen, Rhazes, and Avinzoar. And the *thick leg* is the *elephas* of the former, and the *elephantia* of the latter. My chief inquiry is, whether the difference is only among the translators, or whether there is likewise a want of uniformity in the nomencla- ture of the original writers.

" En passant, I may observe, that some far- ther confusion has arisen among the translators respecting another *leprous* disease, as it has been called, which the Arabians seem to have con- sidered as having some affinity with the proper elephantiasis (juzam), but yet is materially dif- ferent in its symptoms; and which they have denominated *baras* or *barras*, and *albaras*, and which appears to accord accurately with the *leuce* of the Greeks, and the *vitiligo* (species

---

* When it is recollected that the venereal dis. ease does not absolutely require mercury for its cure, but may be cured without it, the criterion here adverted to must be extremely fallacious. —ED.

† In the treatment of syphiloid affections, and in cases where mercury, through injurious man. agement or peculiarity of constitution, has proved detrimental, Plummer's pill will be found an effec- tual alterative. Carmichael's Essays on the Ve- nereal Disease contain satisfactory evidence of the valuable properties of antimonials in managing syphiloid disorders.—D.

† Theoricè, lib. viii., cap. xv., and Practicè, cap. iv. In which passages the translator has used the word Elephantia, and not Lepra, like the other translators.

3) of Celsus. If the Hebrews did not apply the term (translated) *leprosy* to several affections of the skin (such as the scaly lepra Græcorum, the psoriasis of Dr. Willan, and the *leuce*, which I suspect they did), this leuce or baras would seem to be the *unclean* leprosy described in Leviticus, chap. xiii.*

"If your knowledge of the oriental languages will enable you, together with your knowledge of these diseases, to disperse some of the thick mist in which the translators have enveloped them, I should be exceedingly glad to partake of a little of your light."

The substance of the author's reply to this letter, already given in a note to the volume of Nosology, but which ought not to be omitted on the present occasion, was as follows :—

The Greeks became first acquainted with the elephantiasis from their casual intercourse with Egypt. To this quarter Lucretius, adopting the common opinion, ascribes its origin :—

"Est ELEPHAS morbus, qui propter flumina Nili,
Gignitur Ægypto in mediâ, neque præterea usquam."†

High up the Nile, mid Egypt's central plains,
Springs the BLACK LEPROSY, and there alone.

Arabia, however, seems rather to have been the prolific source of this terrible scourge than Egypt ; if we may judge from what seems highly probable, namely, that this is the disease with which Job was afflicted in Idumea, a part of Arabia, as described in the sacred poem that bears his name under the appellation of צָרַעַת רָעַ, "the stroke of the scourge," and which affords, without question, the most ancient record in the world, composed in a mixed language of Arabic and Hebrew ; and if we add to this the still more powerful argument, that the Arabic name of the disease has extended itself all over the east, and is almost the only name by which it is known in Egypt, Persia, and India, in all which regions the disorder is about equally common. Yet the Arabic name is not *elephas* or *elephantiasis*, but juzam جُزَام literally "disjunction, amputation," vulgarly indeed, and more generally pronounced and written judam جُدَام, from جَدَ, a root which imports "erosion," "truncation," "excision ;" evidently referring to the destructive character of the disease, and the spontaneous separation of the smaller members, as the fingers and toes, when severe in its progress.

The Arabians, however, have a malady, but of a very different kind, to which THEY also give the name of *elephas*, or *elephant affection*, in their own language دَاءُ الفِيل dal fil,

which is literally *morbus elephas*, and which they sometimes contract to فِيل fil, or elephas, alone. It is the "swelled, tumid, or Barbadoes leg of modern writers, the *bucnemia tropica* of the present system." And, on this account, when learning, and especially medical learning, found an asylum during the dark ages at the splendid courts of Bagdat, Bassorah, and Cordova, and the best Greek writers were translated into Arabic, or the best Greek and Arabic into Latin, two different diseases were found to possess a like name ; for the Greeks, notwithstanding that they had elephantiasis to signify juzam, could only translate dal fil by elephantiasis also. And hence arose that confusion of the two maladies which has continued to the present moment, notwithstanding the wide distinction between them, the one being a tubercular affection of the whole body, while the other is a scaly affection of only particular parts, and commonly of not more than a particular limb.

The leprosy, properly so called, the *leuce* (λεύκη) of the Greeks, and the baras or beras بَرَص of the Arabians, was by many of the Arabian physicians, and very generally among the people, supposed, in various cases, to terminate in juzam or elephantiasis, as though this also was nothing more than a different stage or degree of the same disease. And hence another error and perplexity in medical study. Alsahavarius thus unites them, and they are jumbled together, or explained alike in nearly all the oriental dictionaries ; in which beras or leprosy, and juzam or elephant-skin, are, almost without an exception, regarded as convertible terms. This oriental confusion of two very different diseases was readily copied by the Latin translators, till at length both in the east and west, beras or lepriasis, though literally scale-skin, became a sort of family name for almost every disfigurement of the skin, whether tubercular or scaly, cutaneous or constitutional. And on this account, elephantiasis and leprosy, and several other diseases even in the nosology of Linnæus, are included under the term lepra ; all which the disciples of this school, extending a principle very widely adopted by them, ascribe to animalcules drunk in with the common beverage of water, especially the *gordius marinus*.

The author ought not to conceal Dr. Bateman's acknowledgment of this communication, and his assent to its explanation, contained in the following opening of a letter received a few days afterward :—

"I thank you sincerely for your ready and interesting communication, which satisfactorily explains the point respecting which I was the least able to obtain satisfaction from the translators ; viz., that the Arabians had applied the term *elephant (elephas,* according to the able translator of Haly Abbas), or fil, as you state, to the swelled leg. This is some apology for the appropriation of the Greek term elephantiasis (though it actually denoted a different disease) to the Arabian thick leg ; but the appropriation of *lepra*, which is never mentioned by

---

* This is the opinion of two learned old Germans, Leon. Fuchs, in his Paradoxa Medicinæ, lib. ii., cap. xvi. : and Gregor. Horst, in his Epist. to Hopner, inserted in his Observationes Medicinales, lib. viii., obs. xviii. And Sennert seems to be of the same opinion, Pract. Med. lib., v.; part i., cap. xl.

† De Rer. Nat., vi., 1112.

the Greeks but as a 'superficial, rough, and scaly affection,' to the tubercular Juzam, has unfortunately misled and confused us for a thousand years."

Dr. Bateman adds, that he apprehends the term elephantiasis had also a reference to the *magnitude* and DURATION of the disease, independently of the appearance of the skin. . And it is very probable, as the malady was likewise sometimes denominated *leontiasis*, that the formidable and frightful aspect of the patient labouring under it may have been hereby compared to the general exterior of both the elephant and the lion : for while Arctæus tells us, in describing it, that " it is disgusting to the sight, and in all respects terrible like the elephant," Avicenna affirms, " it renders the countenance terrible to look at, and somewhat of the form of the lion's visage."

The necessity of that stricter investigation into the nature of genuine elephantiasis, thus anxiously desired by Dr. Bateman, will be the more obvious when the reader learns, that in the classical work of Professor Frank it is arranged as a species of lepra ; as are also ichthyiasis, and various other cutaneous affections, that should take their station in distinct quarters.—(Op. cit., tom. iv., p. 211, 1792.)

Besides the elephantiasis of the Arabians, we have a disease of the same kind, or which seems to be of the same kind, common to some parts of Italy, and another common to some parts of Spain ; both which seem, indeed, to have issued from the Arabian stock. And hence elephantiasis, as a genus, offers us the three following species :—

1. Elephantiasis Arabica.   Arabian elephantiasis.
2. —————— Italica.   Italian elephantiasis.
3. —————— Asturiensis.   Asturian elephantiasis.

SPECIES I.

ELEPHANTIASIS ARABICA.

ARABIAN ELEPHANTIASIS. BLACK LEPROSY.

TUBERCLES CHIEFLY ON THE FACE AND JOINTS : FALL OF THE HAIR EXCEPT FROM THE SCALP : VOICE HOARSE AND NASAL : CONTAGIOUS AND HEREDITARY.

THIS species, which is the oldest of the three, is also the most inveterate : for we do not know that the Italian species is contagious, though, like the Arabian, it appears to be hereditary ; while the Spanish is, perhaps, neither contagious nor hereditary.

In some parts of the world, indeed, even the present species is said not to be contagious, though all the writers concur in its being hereditary in every quarter.* Thus Dr. Schilling,

* Dr. Kinnis mentions two patients whom he saw in the Isle of France, and who " stood in the relation of mother and daughter. The husband of the former had been dead eight or nine years : he had long been afflicted with palsy and dropsy, to which, only two years before he died, was su-

while he admits the latter effect, asserts that it is not contagious in Surinam, and Dr. T. Heberden asserts the same of this disease in Madeira. ."I not only," says he, ."am a daily witness of communication between lepers and other people without the least ill consequence, but know several instances where a leprous husband (afflicted with the Arabian leprosy or elephantiasis), married to a sound wife, has cohabited with her for a long series of years, and had several children by her, without her having contracted the least symptom of the disorder, although the children have inherited it ; and vice versâ between a leprous wife and sound husband."—(*Med. Trans.*, vol. i., p 35.)

That the disease, however, is contagious as well as hereditary in India and Arabia, we have the concurrent testimony of all the medical writers of both countries, native as well as foreign ; so that there can be no doubt upon the subject. And hence the Madeira and Surinam juzam should seem to be a variety of the oriental, influenced by peculiarity of climate or some other incidental cause.

This severe malady, wherever it shows itself, is sometimes slow in its growth, and continues many years without deranging the functions of the patient, yet great deformity is advancing upon his external make. The alæ of the nose become swelled and scabrous, and the nostrils are preternaturally dilated ; the lips are tumid ; the external ears, particularly the lobes, are enlarged and thickened, and beset with tubercles. The skin of the forehead and cheeks grows dense and hard, and forms large and prominent rugæ, especially over the eyes ; the hair generally, except on the head, falls off ; the voice becomes hoarse and obscure ; the external sensibility is obtunded or totally abolished, so that pinching or puncturing gives no pain. The tubercles at length begin to crack and ulcerate ; ulcerations appear in the throat and nostrils ; the breath is intolerably offensive ; the palate destroyed ; the nose falls off ; the fingers and toes, from the increased depth and virulence of the ulcerations, become gangrenous, and separate, and drop off one after another. [In the cases noticed in the Isle of France, the palms of the hand were seldom tuberculated, but had a dry, smooth, shrivelled appearance, as if the fat had been absorbed from under the skin. The backs of the hands, and more particularly

peradded elephantiasis. Her daughter was attacked about the time of her husband's death ; she herself about two years afterward ; and one of her sons had since fallen a victim to the disease. Her father was a Frenchman, her mother and maternal grandfather Creoles, and none of them was ever affected." Another patient is stated to have inherited the predisposition from the family of his maternal grandmother, who was never attacked herself, but lost two sisters and three nieces from the disease. None of his other relations, for three generations back, were ever known to have been affected. Dr. Kinnis saw his mother, with three other children, in the best health. She and her mother were Creoles, her grandparents Europeans.—See Edin. Medical Journal, No. lxxxi, p. 290.—ED.

of the fingers, were swollen, thickened, flabby, and beset with oblong tubercles, impeding the motion of the joints. One patient had lost four toes of the right foot, excepting a single phalanx, which three of them still possessed; and another had lost two phalanxes of the little finger. In one case the terminal bone of the great toe was exposed and dry; in another there was a circumscribed gangrenous spot on the fourth toe; and in most of the cases there were open indolent sores on the backs of the fingers, the bend of the ankle joints, the soles of the feet, or about the toes; sometimes superficial, and of a red colour; sometimes foul, discharging little, surrounded with hard, irregular edges, or overgrown with morbid cuticle.—(*Dr. Kinnis, Edin. Med. Journ.*, No. lxxxi., p. 288.)]

The mental powers suffer less than in the two other species; the dreams, however, are greatly disturbed, the manners, for the most part, morose and melancholy, and sometimes there is an inextinguishable desire of sexual intercourse.*

The disease is also known in the high northern latitudes of Norway and Iceland. In the last place it is peculiarly prevalent, produced, as Dr. Henderson justly observes, by the rancidity of the food usually fed on, wet woollen clothes, an insalubrious air, and want of cleanliness. It is called "Likthra," or "Putrefaction:" and an hospital is established for it in each of the four quarters of the island. It seems to be here both infectious and hereditary. "In its primary stage," says Dr. Henderson, "its symptoms are inconsiderable. A small reddish spot, scarcely larger than the point of a needle, breaks out at first about the forehead, nose, corner of the eyes, and lips; and in proportion as it increases, other pustules make their appearance on the breast, arms, armpits, which generally dry up in one place and break out in another without pain, till the disease has considerably advanced, when they cover almost the whole body, give the skin a scabrous appearance, stiffen it sometimes in shining scales, which fall off like dust, sometimes in malignant tumours and swellings. The patient in the meantime labours under lassitude of body, anæsthesia, and lowness of spirits." The miserable progress is nearly a transcript of the description just given. The patient is so worn out with fatigue and melancholy as to be often tempted to make away with himself. He sur-

renders one part of the body after another to the insatiable malady, "till at length," says Dr. Henderson, "death, the long wished-for deliverer, comes suddenly and puts an end to his misery."—(*Iceland, or the Journ. of a Residence in that Island*, vol. i., p. 295, 8vo., Edin., 1818.)

Mr. D. Johnson, of the Bengal establishment, ascribes the disease in India to nearly the same causes as Dr. Henderson in Iceland. It is found principally among the poorer castes, and "attacks chiefly such people as have their feet and hands frequently in cold water or earth, such as the peasants in the low marshy countries of Bengal and Orissa, Dobys (washerwomen) and Mollies (gardeners) in the upper provinces of India; and I conceive that cold and poorness of blood cause the circulation in the extreme capillary vessels to become too languid; the consequence is, a gradual decay or depolution of these parts." This writer admits that the disease appears in hereditary descent, but, as the different trades and occupations of the natives descend hereditarily also, he has some doubt whether the latter may not be the sole cause of its appearing in successive generations, instead of a family taint.—(*Misc. Obs. on certain Indigenous Customs, Diseases, &c. in India.*)

There seems to be a variety of this disease, in which a tumour of a larger size than the rest seats itself in the inguinal glands, sometimes in both groins, and is subject to a regular paroxysm of inflammation once in about every fourth month, preceded by shivering, and accompanied with a smart febrile excitement. These symptoms usually subside in three or four days, and leave the tumour as before. But, not unfrequently, that on the one side or on the other, rarely or never on both sides, advances to suppuration, and produces a troublesome sore. Dr. Adams met with cases of this kind in Madeira, and Dr. Kinnis has since observed the same in the Isle of France (*Obs. on Elephantiasis as it appears in the Isle of France*, Edin. Med. Journ., Oct., 1824, p. 289): thus giving the disease an approach towards BUCNEMIA TROPICA.

The cure is extremely difficult, but a course of warm diaphoretics succeeded by tonics, and especially the metallic tonics, seems to have constituted the most successful plan. Hence a free use of sarsaparilla, mezereon, or guaiacum, has been found beneficial, and mercurial alteratives still more so, though salivation appears to have

---

* According to Dr. Kinnis, who has given an interesting description of elephantiasis as it appears in the Isle of France, the wasting of the genitals, represented by Dr. Adam as attending the disorder in Madeira, did not take place in a single individual of the other island; "the testicles in males, and the breasts in females, being constantly of their natural size. With regard to the functions of these organs," says Dr. Kinnis, "neither the wonderful salacity ascribed to the miserable victims of this loathsome disease by some authors, nor the utter extinction of the venereal appetite so characterize them by others, existed in any case. One of the female patients, who had been affected with the disease only two years and a half, affirmed, that though she had ceased to menstruate from its commence-

ment, or to experience her former sexual propensities, she had yet suffered a miscarriage about twelve months before I saw her, and continued to cohabit with the person by whom she was kept. Another was the mother of two young children, one of whom I saw at the breast: she cohabited with a black," &c.—(Dr. Kinnis, in Edin. Med. Journ., No. lxxxi., p. 289.) In an example detailed by Mr. Lawrence, in the Med. Chir. Trans., the testes were unnaturally small and soft; and in four cases seen by Dr. Bateman, the venereal desire was lost. From the evidence collected on this point, we may conclude with Dr. Joy (Ency. clop. of Pract Med., art. ELEPHANTIASIS), that the affection of the mammary and seminal glands, like the femoral tumour, is at most only an occasional complication.—ED.

been uniformly mischievous· Even the lobelia has had its advocates, and, upon the ground of its proving salutary in syphilis, it has probably also been sometimes serviceable in elephantiasis. Dr. Schilling endeavours to increase the determination to the skin, by advising the use of the warm bath and gentle exercise, and embrocating the body with spirits of wine or rum, or exposing it to a vapour-bath of mastic, olibanum, benzoin, or lavender.

In India the cabirajahs, or native physicians, after bleeding and purging, immediately apply to the metallic tonics, and particularly to the white oxyde of arsenic, which they give, as in the case of syphilis, and indeed of various other impurities of the blood, in the form of pills ; mixing the arsenic, which, in Hindostanee, is sané hya, and in Arabic, shucc, with six times its weight of black pepper into a mass with a little water ; so that each pill may contain about two thirds of a grain of arsenic and four grains of pepper, which is to be taken twice a day : and this medicine is regarded almost as a specific antidote. It has no doubt proved often successful : and I have known various cases in our own country in which it has been found equally so in the form of the arsenical solution.·

In this quarter of the globe, however, Mr. Playfair has of late years revived the use of one of the species of asclepias or swallow-wort. In Europe, the a. *Vincetoxicum* was formerly in high favour as an alterant and alexipharmic, and was often denominated contrayerva Germanorum : but its virtues were not sufficient to support its character. The swallow-wort employed by Mr. Playfair is the a. *gigantea*, a native of the east, and appears, from an account lately published by Mr. Robinson (*Medico-Chirurg. Trans.*, vol. x.), to be possessed of more active and possibly more salutary qualities. It is the *muda*r or *midaur* of Hindostan, a shrub not yet systematically arranged, but found on all the uncultivated plains of India, producing a milky juice, which is the part employed medicinally, not only in this complaint, but in various herpetic affections, by being applied to the skin.— (*Misc. Obs.*, &c., *by Daniel Johnson, Esq.*)

The tonic found most useful by Dr. T. Heberden in Madeira was bark, which, however, has not proved of equal success in other places, or in the hands of other practitioners ; but he employed it in connexion with that course of external stimulants which has been found generally serviceable, and probably not a little contributed to its wonderful efficacy in the various cases he refers to, and particularly one of a confirmed and chronic attack. "I have," says he, "in this island experienced the use of the bark in four or five leprous patients with success. One had a confirmed elephantiasis ; the others were only incipient, having no other symptoms than florid or livid tubercles in the face and in the limbs. The confirmed elephantiasis was attended with livid and scirrhous tubercles, which had overspread the face and limbs ; the whole body was emaciated ; the eyebrows inflated ; the hair of the eyebrows fallen off entirely ; the bones of the nose depressed ; the alæ nasi tumefied, as

likewise the lobes of the ears ; with a suffusion in both eyes, which had almost deprived the patient of his sight. There was a want of sensation in the extremities, and a loss of motion in the fingers and toes."

For upwards of seven years, Dr. Heberden had used every medicine he could think of to relieve this patient, but in vain. Antimonials and mercurials of almost every kind, neutral salts, the warm diaphoretics, as sassafras and sarsaparilla, warm baths and medicated baths, were alike fruitless. On May 2d, 1758, he made his patient commence an electuary of powder of bark, with a third part bark of sassafras root, inspissated with sirup ; and of this the quantity of a large nutmeg was ordered to be taken *twice* a-day. The patient at the same time had his arms and legs bathed with an embrocation, consisting of an ounce of lixivium of tartar and two drachms of spirit of sal-ammoniac, inter-mixed with half a pint of proof spirit. By the latter end of May the tubercles were considerably softened ; by June 28th, they were dispersed ; a red scurfy efflorescence alone remaining behind, which in ten days lost its florid hue and peeled off, leaving the cuticle sound and clean. "The patient," says he, "gradually recovered the sensation in his legs and arms, and the use of his toes and fingers ; the hair has grown again on his eyebrows ; and the only remainder of the distemper which I can perceive is, that the nose continues somewhat flatter, from the depression of the bones. The suffusion is quite cured, and the patient is εὔσαρκος καὶ εὔχροος,* of a healthy skin and colour."

SPECIES II.

ELEPHANTIASIS ITALICA.
ITALIAN ELEPHANTIASIS.

TUBERCLES CHIEFLY ON THE BODY AND LIMBS, SOMETIMES DESQUAMATING : GREAT TENSION OF THE SKIN : VERTIGO : BURNING, LANCINATING PAIN IN THE HEAD : MELANCHOLY, AT FIRST REMITTING, AFTERWARD FIXED, TERMINATING IN ALIENATION OF MIND : HEREDITARY.

FOR a knowledge of this species we are almost exclusively indebted to the Italian physi-

---

* Med. Trans., ut suprà. Mr. Robinson represents the disease as presenting itself under two forms in Hindostan ; one characterized by the dropping off of the fingers and toes, the insensibility of the skin, and the extreme torpor of mind and body ; the other by tubercles, ulceration of the palate, and affections of the cartilages and bones of the face, together with the frequent occurrence of the oblong glandular tumour in the groin. The mudar, so useful in the first variety, is injurious in the second, which is benefited by arsenic.— (See Med. Chir. Trans., vol. x.) Iodine might be tried both externally and internally. Rayer recommends exciting a slight degree of inflammation in the diseased skin with ammoniacal liniments, tincture of cantharides, or ointment of the hydriodate of potass. If they produce too much irritation, they are to be used alternately with the warm bath.—ED.

clans, who have generally given it the name of pellagra or pelagra. The first writer upon the subject appears to have been Francis Frapolli, a physician of Milan, whose work, "In morbum vulgò Pelagram dictum," was published at Milan in 1771, and who expresses himself doubtful whether the disease, though not antecedently described, is not referred to occasionally by earlier writers, although he does not think that the pilarella, as the syphilis was called when it proved depilatory to the chin and eyebrows, was the disease in question, notwithstanding this seems to have been an extensive opinion at the time. The next tract of any note upon the subject was published at Venice in 1784, by G. M. d'Oleggio, under the title of "A Theoretical and Practical Treatise on the Diseases of Vernal Insolation, commonly called Pellagra."[*] But the best account we have received of this complaint is from the pen of Dr. Jansen, of Leyden, which appeared in 1788, and asserts that it is endemic in the Milanese territory.—(De Pellagra mòrbo in Mediolanensi Ducatu endemio.) It is, in truth, common to both the Milanese and Venetian territories, as well as to other districts widely differing in soil and temperature ; and can scarcely therefore be referred to either of these sources. There is little doubt of its being hereditary, but not contagious ; and it does not seem to have existed earlier than the middle of the last century.[†] It is commouly ascribed, as we have observed above, to the heat of the sun's rays (J. P. Frank, op. cit., tom. iv., p. 43) after the chill of winter, and is hence called mal del sole, which we have just seen-was the view taken of it by D'Oleggio ; while by Odoardo it is attributed to a scrofulous habit (D' una spezia particolare di Scorbuto, Venet., 1776), and by Videmari and others, who have too much limited themselves to the nature of the eruption, to an impetiginous impurity.—(De quâdam Impetiginis specie, 8vo., 1790.) But none of these explanations seem to rest on any very solid foundation ; and, upon the whole, we have more reason for regarding it as produced by the debilitating causes of hot, confined air, want of cleanliness, and bad diet, operating in many cases upon a diathesis hereditarily tainted. It is found chiefly among the Milanese and Venetian peasantry, whose hovels are full of wretchedness, and rarely makes its appearance till after the age of puberty. Alibert, in his "Diseases of the Skin," has denominated it, but with little accuracy, Ichthyosis Pellagra.—(Desc. des Mal. de la Peau, p. 175.)

The first symptoms of the disease are general languor, listlessness, gloom, feebleness, and stupor in the legs, and hence unsteady walking, vertigo, and confusion of ideas. Domeier, another writer upon the subject, extends the stupor of the legs to the entire frame, and asserts that anæsthesia is a characteristic symptom of

this species.—(Baldinger, Journ., vol. xxvi., p. 9.) But this assertion is not confirmed by the history of other pathologists, though the languor and inertness are often very great, as well as universal.

These symptoms usually take place in the spring ; and as the summer approaches, a sense of tension, burning, and itching is felt in every external organ except the head, followed by an eruption of rosy papulæ, scattered over the skin generally,[*] which terminate in tubercles of a shining red colour. After some days the tubercles desquamate, and the skin appears at first red, but soon recovers its natural colour. As the summer, however, advances, every symptom commonly subsides, and the strength is renewed with the winter ; but the symptoms return with increased violence with the return of the spring, and this for several years in succession. But if the symptoms do not thus subside, they soon become even on the first attack considerably exasperated, and form a second stage of the disease, in which the itching grows more pungent ; the heat more fiery ; the skin harder, cracked, and chapped ; the debility is greater ; the mental functions are disturbed generally ; the appetite is irregular ; the sleep broken with acute pain in the head and spine, soon followed by delirium. The cutaneous affection now diminishes, but the nervous symptoms are greatly augmented. The vertigo increases ; the patient is sad and loves solitude, and melancholy delirium alternates with furious mania. The tædium vitæ is insupportable, and self-murder is a frequent consequence. Strambi remarks, that those who labour under this disease have the greatest tendency to drown themselves, "as by a hallucination," says he, "opposite to that of hydrophobia."—(De Pellagra, Obs., ann. i., ii., iii., Mediol., 1785.) Coercion is at last necessary ; and a diarrhœa, dysentery, or dropsy, closes the dreadful scene, if the patient do not sink earlier from corporeal and mental exhaustion.[†] Dr. Holland tells us that at one time

---

* Tratto teoretico-pratico delle malattie dell' insolato di primavera volgarimente dette della Pellagra.

† Paralleli fra la Pellagra ed alcuna malattie, che più lo rassomigliano, del F. Fanzago. Padova, 1792.

---

* Dr. Holland says :—"The local symptoms very generally show themselves, in the first instance, early in the spring, at the period when the mid-day heat is rapidly increasing, and when the peasants are most actively engaged in their labours in the fields. The patient perceives on the back of his hands, on his feet, and sometimes, but more rarely, on other parts of the body exposed to the sun, certain red spots or blotches ; which gradually extend themselves, with a slight elevation of the cuticle, and a shining surface, not unlike that of lepra in its early stage."—See Med. Chir. Trans., vol. viii., p. 321.

† Besides exhibiting, at different periods in the same individual, many varieties in the appearances of the skin, as erysipelas, lepra, psoriasis, elephantiasis, and ichthyosis, it is liable to terminate in the production of several constitutional or general derangements of the system,—tetanus, chorea, epilepsy, convulsions, dropsy, melancholia, mania, marasmus, &c. "Hence," as Dr. James Johnson has observed, "we see written over the beds in the Milan Hospital the various diseases to which pellagra forms the adjective, as atrophia pellagrina, phthisis pellagrina, hydrops pellagrinus, paralysis pellagrina, mania pellagrina, &c."—

in the lunatic hospital at Milan, of five hundred patients more than one third were *Pellagrosi* (*Medico-Chir. Trans.*, vol. viii., part ii., p. 326); and he also informs us, that morbid dissections have thrown little light on the pathology of this disease; that the liver and spleen have at times evinced indurations and enlargements; and traces of disease have been occasionally seen in the intestines and mesenteric glands; but by no means constantly, and rather as effects than causes of the disorder.

The treatment needs not essentially differ from that of the preceding species. Pure air, habitual cleanliness, warm bathing, and a nutritious diet, with such tonics, whether vegetable or mineral, as best agree with the constitution, have proved most successful where the disease has not advanced beyond the reach of recovery. At Milan, the lichen Islandicus is one of the most popular remedies.

[Antimonials are also in repute, and attention is paid to the diarrhœa with which the disease is frequently accompanied. Bloodletting is rarely practised, except when mania or some local inflammation comes on. In some instances, according to Dr. Holland, the cutaneous affection forms the principal indication of the complaint for several successive years; being renewed every spring, and disappearing again in the autumn. In other cases, he says, where it has been found possible to remove the patient to a new situation and mode of life, the disease is still further arrested in its progress. "It rarely happens, however, that these means can be practically adopted; and the constitutional malady is generally so far established in the third or fourth year, that little hope remains of benefiting the patient, either by medicine or change in the mode of life."]

SPECIES III.
ELEPHANTIASIS ASTURIENSIS.
ASTURIAN ELEPHANTIASIS.

TUBERCLES CHIEFLY ON THE HANDS AND FEET; CRUSTACEOUS, DESQUAMATING: CONTINUAL TREMOUR OF THE HEAD AND UPPER PART OF THE TRUNK: BALDNESS OF THE SCALP, AS WELL AS OF OTHER PARTS: GLOOM AND TERROR OF MIND.

THIS species agrees in many of its symptoms with the Italic, and it is only worth while to notice the points in which they differ. Upon the whole, we may observe, that all the species coincide in being founded on an exhausted constitution, in the general character of the tubercles, and in their fatal termination by dropsy, atrophy, or some other asthenic disease. The Arabian species attacks the face, the roots of the hair, and the palate-bones, before the remaining parts on which it preys are diseased, and the affection of the skin increases with the increase of the other symptoms. In the Italian species, the affection of the skin diminishes as the nervous and mental commotion augments.

Change of Air, or the Pursuit of Health, p. 75.— EDITOR.

The pellagra also is distinguished by thick urine, double vision, and a peculiar mouldy smell of the sweat. In the Asturian species the crustaceous tubercles are peculiarly painful, highly fetid, more deeply furrowed with cracks, and more disgusting to the sight; attacking the head as well as other parts indiscriminately, and destroying the roots of the hair. The mind is less affected than in the last, and with melancholy and terror rather than with raving delirium.

This species constitutes the Asturian leprosy of Thiery, Vandermonde, and Sauvages; but genuine leprosy is rarely a constitutional complaint; and the present is its proper place. As the tubercles desquamate, the skin appears of a glossy leprous red, and the disease is hence called by the Spaniards Mal de la Rosa.

The causes are, extreme poverty and its attendants, filth, bad diet, and crowded unventilated rooms in the deep and swampy valleys of the country, almost impervious to the rays of the sun; and hence the medical treatment and general regimen recommended under the preceding species, will here afford the fairest promise of success.

GENUS IX.
CATACAUSIS.
CATACAUSIS.
GENERAL COMBUSTIBILITY OF THE BODY.

THE peculiar state of the constitution which lays a foundation for the present genus of morbid affections, is of a very singular and mysterious kind; and the only medical work that has referred to it in our own country, antecedently to the author's own system of Nosology, is Dr. Young's Medical Literature, in which it is noticed under the Greek name here applied to it, derived from καταϰαίω, "exuro." One species only has hitherto been discovered as belonging to it; which, from the peculiar habit under which it occurs, may be distinguished by the name of

1. Catacausis Ebriosa. Inebriate Catacausis.

SPECIES I.
CATACAUSIS EBRIOSA.
INEBRIATE CATACAUSIS.

THE LIVING BODY INFLAMMABLE IN CONSEQUENCE OF A LONG AND IMMODERATE USE OF SPIRITUOUS LIQUORS: THE COMBUSTION EASILY EXCITED, OR SPONTANEOUS.

IN this wonderful malady, the art of medicine can be rarely of any avail; since the mischief is, in almost all instances, only to be discovered after a cessation of life, and the destruction of some part of the body by an actual flame or fire, in many instances spontaneously issuing from its surface. There may be some difficulty in giving credit to so marvellous a diathesis; yet examples of its existence, and of its leading to a migratory and fatal combustion, are so numerous and so well authenticated, and press upon us from so many different countries and eras, that it would be absurd to withhold our assent. In almost every instance, the combustion seems to have taken place in females, advanced in life, and immoderately addicted to spirituous liquors.—(*Bartholin, Act. Hafn.*, i., obs. 118.) In some cases, the heat that has set them on fire appears to have originated in themselves; in others, to have been communicated by a stove, or a candle, or a stroke of lightning (*Fouquet, Journ. de Méd.*, tom. lxviii.); but in no case has the fire or flame hereby excited in the body been so powerful as essentially to injure the most combustible substances immediately adjoining it, as linen or woollen furniture. The body, in several instances, has been found actually burning, sometimes with an open flame flickering over it; and sometimes with a smothered heat or fire, without any open flame whatever: while the application of water has occasionally seemed rather to quicken than to check the igneous progress.

This is the more extraordinary, as the human body, in every other state we are acquainted with, whether of health or disease, is scarcely at all combustible of itself, and cannot be reduced to ashes without the assistance of a very large pile of fagots or other fuel, as universal experience in this very ancient mode of sepulture, and the history of martyrs who have been condemned to the flames, abundantly testify.

The event has usually taken place at night, when the sufferer has been alone; and has commonly been discovered by the fetid, penetrating scent of sooty films, which have spread to a considerable distance; the unhappy subject has in every instance been found dead, or more or less completely burnt up; the burnt parts being reduced to an oily, crumbly, sooty, and extremely offensive matter. "I confess," says M. Pierre-Aime-Lair (*Journ. de Physique,* an. viii.), "that these accounts at first appeared to me to be worthy of very little credit; but they are presented to the public as true, by men whose veracity is unquestionable. Bianchini, Maffei, Rollin, Le Cat, Vicq d'Azyr, and other men distinguished by their learning, have offered certain testimony of the facts. Besides, it is not more surprising to meet with such incineration, than a discharge of saccharine urine, or an appearance of the bones softened to a state of jelly."

Those who are desirous of pursuing this curious subject farther, and of entertaining themselves with the very extraordinary histories connected with it, as also of examining the various hypotheses by which they have been accounted for, may consult the Philosophical Transactions (see especially vols. xliii., xliv.), which contain numerous examples; as also a variety of foreign journals of established reputation, referred to and cited in the running commentary to the author's volume of Nosology.—(*Ploucquet, Littérat. Méd.; Dupont, de Corporis Hum. Incendiis Spontaneis.*) We have not space to enter into these separate cases, though many of them are highly interesting; but in a general course of medical study, the phenomenon ought not to be passed by: it forms one of

the most curious links in the long chain of morbid affections, and equally demands our attention as pathologists and physiologists.*

GENUS X.

PORPHYRA.

SCURVY.

LIVID SPOTS ON THE SKIN FROM EXTRAVASATED BLOOD: LANGUOR, AND LOSS OF MUSCULAR STRENGTH: PAINS IN THE LIMBS.

PORPHYRA is in Greek what purpura is in Latin, literally, "the purple or livid disease." The latter has been very generally made use of; but the former is here preferred on two accounts. First, that of technological simplicity,—the names of the genera under the present system being uniformly of Greek origin. And secondly, because the Latin purpura has been used in senses so numerous, so vague and unconnected, that at this moment it conveys no definite idea whatever. "The term purpura," observes Dr. Bateman, most correctly, "has been employed by different writers in so many acceptations, that some ambiguity would perhaps have been avoided by discarding it altogether; for some authors have used it as an appellation for measles, others for scarlet fever, for miliaria, strophulus, lichen, nettle-rash, and the petéchiæ of malignant fevers; while formerly it was applied to petechial spots only by Riverius, Diemerbroeck, Sauvages, Casson, and some others."—(*Synopsis of Diseases*, p. 102.)

The usual synonyme for purpura is *scorbutus*; but to this there are still stronger objections. For, as a term, it is neither Greek nor Latin, nor any language whatever; but an intolerable barbarism, derived, as is commonly supposed, from the German compound *schar-bocke*, literally "aggregate-pox," "cluster-pox;" but more likely from *scharf-pocke*, "violent," or "vehement-pox;" or *schorf-pocke*, "scurf," or "scurvy-pox," to which the inventor has endeavoured to give a sort of Latin termination. Independently of which, scorbutus, as employed at present, only indicates a particular species of scurvy; and could not, therefore, without imprecision, be used in a generic signification.

The sense here expressed by porphyra, runs, as nearly as possible, parallel with the range assigned by Dr. Willan to purpura. "With Riverius and some other authors," says he, "I propose to express by the term *purpura* an efflorescence consisting of some distinct pur-

---

* Cases of catacausis ebriosa are recorded in several American periodicals. A paper on the subject may be found in the Am. Med. Recorder, vol. v. The author of it, Dr. J. K. Mitchell of Philadelphia, maintains "that combustible gases are generated in the systems of drunkards by the decomposition of alcoholic potions; that these gases, and even the identical spirituous liquors, are distributed to every part of the system, and that these gases inflame spontaneously, just like gases out of the body, without the aid of fire"—See also the Elements of Med. Jurisprudence, by Prof. J. R. Beck and Trotter on Drunkenness.—D.

ple specks and patches, attended with general debility, but not always with fever." And again: " Cases of the purpura seem to have been studiously multiplied in periodical publications, and in medical or surgical miscellanies. I consider it under all the forms described as pertaining to the scurvy, though it is *not always* attended with sponginess of the gums, and a discharge of blood from them, according to the definition of scorbutus in nosology."—(*On Cutaneous Diseases*, Ord. III., p. 453.)

Porphyra, in its present signification, is intended to include every description of petechial eruption and spontaneous ecchymosis, not dependant on fever as their cause, in which case these affections are only symptomatic.

The genus, thus explained, will associate under its banners the three following species:—

1. Porphyra Simplex. . Petechial Scurvy.
2. ——— Hæmorrhagica. Land Scurvy.
3. ——— Nautica. Sea Scurvy.

SPECIES I.

PORPHYRA SIMPLEX.

PETECHIAL SCURVY.

SPOTS NUMEROUS, BUT SMALL AND FLEABITE-SHAPED : CHIEFLY IN THE BREAST, ARMS, AND LEGS : PALENESS OF VISAGE.

PULICOSE or petechial spots were at one time supposed to be, in every instance, the result of debilitating and putrid fevers. Riverius is perhaps the earliest author who distinguishes between simple petechiæ and petechial fevers. Vascular debility or relaxation is, however, the predisposing cause in both cases.—(*Plumb, Practical Treatise on the Diseases of the Skin*, p. 100, 8vo., 1824.) They necessarily, indeed, accompany each other, and, wherever they exist in any considerable degree, they lay a foundation for those minute extravasations which constitute the present species ; and which may take place either from occasional ruptures of the weakened coats of the minute subcutaneous bloodvessels, in consequence of their being incapable of resisting the impetus of the blood that flows through them ; or from the mouths of many of them, which should give forth only the finer and limpid particles of the blood, yielding and allowing an exit to the red globules.

Both these may follow atonic fevers ; but the usual remote causes, in the species before us, are severe labour with innutritious or spare diet, and especially with impure air ; an empoverished state of the system from a sudden and profuse loss of blood ; a sedentary and inactive life, or some chronic and exhausting disease, by which the general strength has been broken down. To these Riverius adds suppression of the catamenia, and a certain mild ebulliency of the blood in boyhood—levem quandam sanguinis ebullitionem—a phrase, apparently importing an excess of sanguineous temperament ; from both which, he tells us, he has frequently seen the disorder originate. And he is confirmed in the last by a case hinted at by Dr. Perceval in his manuscript comment on the author's Nosology,

in which he observes, under the present species, that " in a young lady of a full habit and florid complexion, if the skin of the face or neck were touched, even slightly, blood oozed from the pores."

The disease seems also to be produced at times by some unknown cause ; of which Cullen has given a striking instance in his Materia Medica. " The patient," says he, " was a woman who had lived very constantly upon vegetable aliment, and had not been exposed, so far as could be judged, to any febrile or putrid contagion ; and yet, without a feeling of any other disorder, was affected with numerous petechiæ over the whole surface of her body. After these had continued for some days, without any symptoms of fever, she was affected with swelled and bleeding gums, with fetid breath, and much thirst ; and, in the course of a week or two more, almost every symptom of a putrid fever came on, and in a few days proved fatal."

It is possible in this case, that the brain may have lost its energy, and the blood become empoverished by too low a diet, though the history is not given with sufficient fulness to speak with much decision upon this point. The fever was evidently produced by the irritability of weakness, and necessarily ran into a typhous type from the same cause.

The disease, as it commonly shows itself, appears under two forms, which may thus be described as varieties :—

α Pulicosa. Simple pulicose scurvy.	Exhibiting from the first a pulicose or fleabite appearance.
β Urticaria. Nettle-wheal scurvy.	The fleabite spots preceded by reddish, rounded, and nettle-sting wheals, but without the nettle-sting itching ; fugacious and migratory.

The FIRST VARIETY is not only produced by debility, but attended with languor and pains in the limbs, and chiefly affects women and children, in consequence of their greater laxity of fibre.

The SECOND VARIETY may possibly be accompanied with more constitutional affection ; for there is usually a loss of appetite, and an œdematous swelling of the hands and ankles, while the spots are brighter at night and darker in the day, evidently proving great irritability in the capillaries, and especially towards the period of the natural evening paroxysm of fever. This variety often continues for five or six weeks.

Better diet, freedom from hard labour, pure air, sea-bathing, the mineral acids, and other tonic medicines, afford a pretty certain process of cure.

SPECIES II.

PORPHYRA HÆMORRHAGICA.

LAND SCURVY.

SPOTS CIRCULAR, OF DIFFERENT SIZES ; OFTEN IN STRIPES OR PATCHES, IRREGULARLY SCATTERED OVER THE THIGHS, ARMS, AND TRUNK ;

OCCASIONAL HEMORRHAGE FROM THE MOUTH, NOSTRILS, OR VISCERA: GREAT DEBILITY AND DEPRESSION OF SPIRITS.

THIS species, the morbus maculosus Werlholfii of the German writers (*Gesch. eines glücklich geheilten Morbus Maculosus Werlholfii, von Dr. Marquett*, &c., Magdeburg), is sometimes marked by febrile paroxysms, with variable intervals, but usually occurring in the evening. It has no regular or stated termination. Dr. Willan has found it run on, in different cases, from fourteen days to a twelvemonth and upwards. It is met with at every period of life, but chiefly affects persons of a weak and delicate habit, often children, principally women.

The precursive symptoms are lassitude, faintness, and pains in the limbs, so that business, or even company, is found fatiguing. After this, there are often shiverings, nausea, and vomiting. The purple eruption, for the most part, appears first on the legs, and afterward, at irregular periods, on the thighs, arms, and trunk of the body; the hands and face generally remaining free. The spots, however, are frequent on the interior of the mouth, and particularly the tonsils, gums, and lips, where they are sometimes raised or papulated. It is here the first hemorrhage commonly issues, though, as the disease advances, blood flows also from the nostrils, lungs, stomach, intestines, and uterus; all which organs, together with the heart, are sometimes found studded with spots on their surface, on examination after death.—(*Edin. Med. and Surg. Journ.*, July, 1822.) The hemorrhage is often profuse, and cannot easily be restrained, and is accompanied with anasarcous swellings. It sometimes precedes the purple spots, but more commonly takes place a few days afterward. It is this rapid erosion or ulceration of the bloodvessels, and consequent discharge of blood, often accompanied with diarrhœa or dysentery, where the intestines associate in the complaint, by which land scurvy is chiefly distinguished from sea scurvy, and acquires the distinctive name of *hemorrhagic;* since, though these symptoms may also occur in the latter, they do so rarely, except in the last stage of the complaint.*

* There is no sponginess of the gums, as in common scurvy, nor are the limbs affected in the manner often exhibited in the latter disease. Rayer, in his Traité des Maladies de la Peau, tom ii., has described purpura under the name of hémacélinose (derived from αἷμα, blood, and κῆλις, a spot, and νόσος, disease), and arranged it with cutaneous and subcutaneous diseases. But, as Dr. Watson has justly observed, purpura cannot be regarded merely as a cutaneous disease; for the effusion of blood is not confined to the skin or subcutaneous textures, but may happen likewise on internal surfaces, and in the parenchymatous texture of the viscera.—(See Med. Gaz., vols. vii. and x.) Frequently, as Dr. Elliotson remarks, there is a bleeding from the mucous surfaces, bleeding from the mouth, from the stomach, and from the intestines. There is no inflammation nor tenderness of the particular parts. The white of the eye and inside of the mouth are often spotted. The disease occurs under the most op-

H 2

[In the dissection of a highly interesting case recorded by Dr. Fairbairn, the sides of the neck and upper parts of the chest were found swollen and livid, with a feeling of crepitus and considerable œdema over the trunk. In some places the cellular and muscular textures of the neck and chest were injected with blood, and emphysematous. The thorax contained about a pound of a fluid resembling blood, of a very dark colour and viscid consistence. The lungs, bronchial tubes, and trachea, contained a large quantity of bloody, serous fluid, and, beneath the internal coat of the latter, there was a slight effusion of dark venous blood. Between the folds of the anterior mediastinum and of the pericardium, a considerable quantity of very dark blood was effused in the cellular texture. Under the lining of the cavities of the heart, and under that of the aorta, there was a large bloody effusion. The floating abdominal viscera presented a dark leaden colour, and on the intestines were a few petechiæ. The inner coat of the stomach, towards the pylorus, was also thickly studded with them. The liver, spleen, and right kidney were softer than natural.—(See *Edin. Med. Chir. Trans.*, vol. ii., p. 161.)]

The most usual remote causes of the present, as of the preceding species, are poor diet, impure air, anxiety of mind, and a sedentary mode of life: and if women under these circumstances and affected with this complaint be wet-nurses, their infants participate in the disease from the milk not being sufficiently nutritious. It is also produced by habitual gluttony, and particularly by an habitual and immoderate use of spirits, which have the strongest tendency to render torpid the collatitious organs of digestion, and especially the liver, whence congestions and other obstructions, and whence, too, the larger and more dangerous hemorrhages that occur in this species.

[The causes of purpura, and its pathology, are not well ascertained. In the very remarkable example of the disease recorded by Dr. Fairbairn, the blood drawn presented a striking peculiarity in colour and consistence: it was florid like arterial blood, slow in coagulating; and the coagulum soft and tremulous, without separation of serum. What was drawn, however, at the third bleeding, coagulated more firmly, and showed a small portion of serum.*]

posite circumstances; occasionally with great debility, weakness of the pulse, exhaustion, and sometimes with an inflammatory state of the system, the blood being buffy and cupped, and the patient greatly relieved by venesection. In some other examples of the disease, such treatment would be death. In severe cases, the patient looks as if he were in a state of anæmia. On the other hand, Dr. Elliotson informs us that he has seen children with many hundreds of purpural spots upon them, running about perfectly well. Frequently no cause whatever can be assigned for the disease, and the pathology is a perfect mystery.—See Dr. Elliotson's Lect. at Lond. Univ., as published in Med. Gaz., vol. xi., p. 342.—ED.

* See Edin. Med. Chir. Trans., vol. ii., p. 163. Some of the best arguments in favour of the doctrine that purpura is dependant upon changes in

As these causes are widely different in their mode of action, though they concur in producing the same effects, the treatment must vary in like manner.

Where the source of the disease is poverty, with its miserable train of attendants, poor diet, impure air, hard labour, grief of mind, the mode of cure recommended for the preceding species will be found equally serviceable : but the tonic and stimulant plans may be carried to a higher range : the bark should be freely administered, wine be liberally allowed, and lemons, or citric acid in any other form, be used to an extent of three or four ounces of lemon-juice daily ; which, however, is the smallest quantity from which any essential benefit may be expected. Of all the antiscorbutics, this is by far the most effectual, and by some writers is regarded as a specific. [In Dr. Fairbairn's case, fifteen drops of diluted sulphuric acid were frequently given in cold water.] And, as the weak action of the vessels is extreme, the terebinthinate stimulants, as camphire and the rectified oil of turpentine, are often peculiarly advantageous. The last has been strongly and judiciously recommended by Dr. Whitlock Nichol ; and other practitioners have fully confirmed his views.*

The worst symptom is the tendency to hemorrhage, which is sometimes profuse, and restrained with great difficulty, and has been known to prove fatal. Occasionally, however, an accidental hemorrhage has had a contrary effect, and carried the complaint away ; and hence Dr. Parry of Bath, and Dr. E. Gairdner of Edinburgh (*Edin. Med.-Chir. Trans.,* vol. i., p. 671, &c.), have found venesection serviceable. In some of these cases we may reasonably suspect visceral congestion, and especially that of the liver, to lie at the foundation ; and dissections have proved this to be no uncommon cause of the disorder.—(*Plumbe on Diseases of the Skin,* p. 108, 8vo., 1824.) The symptoms of visceral obstruction, indeed, are often sufficiently clear ; and where these occur antecedently to the tonic plan, we must freely and repeatedly evacuate the bowels, and may advantageously have recourse to the lancet :† and the more so, as this form of the disease is sometimes accompanied with inflammatory action, and is chiefly what is referred to by Dr. Stoker under the name of dynamic purpura.—(*Path. Obs.,* &c., p. 110, Dublin, 1823, 8vo.)

the composition and properties of the blood, may be found in Dr. Watson's Lecture on Purpura.—See Med. Gaz., vol. x., p. 498.—ED.

* See Dr. Magee's case of purpura hæmorrhagica successfully treated with spirit of turpentine ; Edin. Med. and Surg. Journ., No. lxxxv., p. 307. He prescribes for an adult half an ounce, with an equal quantity of oleum ricini, and a little peppermint or cinnamon water. Rayer applies to the petechiæ and ecchymoses on the surface of the body, linen wetted in spirituous lotions, a solution of the chloride of soda, or vinegar and water.—See Traité des Mal. de la Peau, tom. ii.—ED.

† One of the most severe and successful cases that Dr. Elliotson ever saw treated, was under Dr. Roots, in St. Thomas's Hospital. There were petechiæ, vibices, and ecchymoses, in every part

[The case attended by Dr. Fairbairn, led him to consider it as having a striking resemblance to active hemorrhage ; and hence, he is an advocate for the depleting system.]

In some cases, the disorder appears to be relieved by metastasis. Willan has related a singular case, which it is difficult to account for otherwise. A lady, aged thirty-six, of the sanguine temperament, after experiencing for several days a painful inflation of the stomach, was seized, on the 17th of June, 1792, with violent vomiting, which continued almost incessantly through the 18th and 19th, and was accompanied with excruciating pains in the bowels. The fluid discharged was clear, strongly tinged with green bile, and amounted to three or four quarts a day. The vomiting abated about the 20th, and she had loose stools of a green colour, intermixed with black coagulated blood. This kind of discharge continued till the 25th, producing great languor and faintness, thirst and restlessness, with a cool skin and remarkably slow pulse. On the evening of the 25th her extremities became suddenly cold, the pulse scarcely discernible, a cold sweat trickled from every part of the body, her voice was indistinct, and her breathing laborious. From this alarming state she recovered in the course of the night ; and, on the following day, a rash appeared over the whole body in small and circular patches, confluent on the neck, shoulders, and nates, but in other places distinct. The eruption diminished in two or three days, and assumed a livid colour ; and the discharge of blood ceased from this time. She improved generally, but for two months suffered greatly from languor and debility : the extremities were for a long time anasarcous, and two of the spots became gangrenous. In the Trans. of the Medico-Chirurgical Society of Edinburgh, vol. i., p. 680, is a brief history of a case that proved fatal in less than forty-eight hours. The patient was a strumous child ; on dissection, the pericranium and dura mater were found covered with petechial spots. Blood was also effused on the brain ; and the serous membranes in the chest and abdomen were universally studded, like the dura mater, with dark livid spots.*

The account now given of the causes of this

of the body ; great congestion of the liver, so that the right hypochondrium was distended ; and blood was poured forth from different cavities. The patient was bled, and took oil of turpentine, and he got rapidly well. In another case, under Dr. Elliotson himself, treated in the same way, the patient became apoplectic, and a clot of blood was found on the brain. In proof that the disease may be inflammatory, it is alleged that the blood is sometimes buffy and cupped. In such cases, Dr. Elliotson finds that purging the patient with colchicum is a good practice. Where the pulse is strong, he approves of bleeding ; but would in each case adapt the mode of treatment to the particular circumstances of it ; and he admits the frequent necessity for bark, wine, and good nourishment.— See Med. Gaz., vol. xi., p. 343.—ED.

* Similar pathological appearances are recorded by Rayer, Traité des Mal. de la Peau, tom. ii., obs. 174, &c.—ED.

species, corresponds to such as we usually meet with in the present day. But if we look back into the history of, this disease as far as the seventeenth century, and especially to the state of this metropolis, we shall find hemorrhagic or land scurvy making a much nearer approach to sea scurvy than in our own time ; not only in its symptoms, but from the peculiar causes that seem to have given rise to it, and which are now, for the most part, removed. The population within the walls of the old city was at that period far greater than at present, since the streets have been very extensively widened, and many of them entirely pulled down ; and fashion, which does not always operate so usefully, has led all who are capable of following its steps into the more salubrious air of the neighbouring villages. Independently of this, the supply of fresh vegetable food for man, and of winter-fodder for cattle, was, at the period before us, so scanty as to render it necessary to salt a great quantity of the cattle that was killed in the summer season for winter use. To which we have to add a far greater degree of dampness and uncleanness, not only in the public streets, but also in private houses.

All these are also causes of sea scurvy ; and we find from the description of Willis and others, that they produced conjointly very similar effects ; and that the mortality hence ensuing was very great. The monthly deaths, according to the bills of mortality, occasioned by what is there called scurvy, were seldom less than fifty, and frequently as high as ninety. In the period of the plague, they are only set down at a hundred and five from this last cause for the year. It was not, indeed, till the beginning of the sixteenth century, that any great progress was made in the art of kitchen-gardening in our own country. At this last period, so low was the knowledge of this art, that Queen Catharine of Aragon could not procure a salad till a gardener was sent for from the Netherlands to raise it : nor were the most common articles of the kitchen-garden, such as cabbages, cultivated till this reign.—(Anderson's History of Commerce ; Sir G. Blane's article, Med.-Chir. Trans., vol. iv., p. 96.) And such was the prejudice at one time entertained against pitcoal, from its being supposed to load the atmosphere with unhealthy fumes, but which is now become one of our most powerful ventilators, and consequently one of our most active agents in promoting the general health of the city, that a law was formerly in existence which made it a capital offence to burn it within the city walls ; so that it was only allowed to be used in the forges of the environs. Sir Gilbert Blane informs us that the late Mr. Astle, keeper of the records in the Tower, told him that he had there discovered a document importing that, under the operation of this law, a person had been tried, convicted, and executed for this offence in the reign of Edward the First. We learn also from Davenant (page 351, ed. 1673), that heaps of the most noisome filth were suffered to accumulate in consequence of the imperfection of the public sewers ; and that particular places were marked

out and assigned for such accumulations, which were called lay-stalls ; and hence the name of Lay-stall-street, which exists in one or two parts of the metropolis even in the present day.

The same happy. causes, therefore, which have delivered us so generally from dysentery, remittent fevers, and even the plague itself, have freed us also from land scurvy. And it has operated over all the other large cities of England as well as over the metropolis ; and over the open country as well as over the towns. Even the remote districts of Somersetshire, not more than a century ago, formed a striking theatre for the exhibition of this tremendous scourge, as we learn from Dr. Musgrave's work (De Arth. Sympt.), published in the year 1703. "Agri Somersettenses, uliginosi magnâ parte et depressi, aërem crassum et humidum trahentes, incolæ, maculis subnigris, ulceribus malignis, crurum dolore, respiratione difficili, lassitudine spontaneâ, nervorum debilitate, hydrope, gangrænâ, et istiusmodi aliis SCORBUTI exquisiti signis CREBERRIME divexantur."

The picture is strongly and fearfully sketched, and precisely corresponds with the definition just offered. How then comes the country, as well as the town, to be so wonderfully and beneficially changed in our own day ? "The same spirit of improvement," says an admirable writer (Dr. Heberden, Med. Transact., vol. iv., art. vii.), from whom I have often had occasion to quote, and whose words I would always give rather than my own, "which has constructed our sewers, and widened our streets, and removed the nuisances with which they abounded, and dispersed the inhabitants over a larger surface, and taught them to love airy apartments, and frequent changes of linen, has spread itself likewise into the country ; where it has drained the marshes, cultivated the wastes, enclosed the commons, enlarged the farmhouses, and established cottages. Few, perhaps, even among physicians, are aware of the extensive influence of these measures. Few have adverted, with the attention it deserves, to the prodigious mortality occasioned formerly by annual returns of epidemical fevers, of bowel complaints, and other consequences of poor and sordid living, to which we are now entire strangers."

In consequence of this extraordinary improvement in the best branch of physical philosophy, the same attentive pathologist tells us, that "for ten years, during which time he was one of the physicians to St. George's Hospital, the cases of genuine scurvy that were brought into that establishment, and fell under his care, did not amount to more than four, not one of which was severe. In St. Bartholomew's Hospital, however, about the year 1795, owing to the very great severity of the preceding winter, various poor patients were received with all the characters of true porphyry ; which, in one man, were carried to such a height, that he died in a most offensive state the day after he was admitted."

We have lately, however, and to the astonishment of every one, witnessed a most severe and even fatal renewal of this disease, in the Penitentiary prison for convicts, established on the side of the Thames at Milbank : and this to such an extent, that at one time there were not fewer than about four hundred and fifty on the sick-list, out of a prison population of about eight hundred and fifty (*Report of a Select Comm. of the House of Commons*, 1823, p. 242), chiefly labouring under dysentery or diarrhœa, from the effects of the disease on the stomach and intestines, which, on post-obit examinations, were generally found to be pulicose or ulcerated in various parts; the complaint being at length apparently propagated by contagion.

The cause of this disease has hitherto been involved in much doubt. The prison was throughout ascertained to be cleanly, and, for the most part, well warmed, the cells lofty and unobjectionable, and the courts airy and paved with flagstone. The original soil was swampy, but it is generally believed at present to be free from damp, in consequence of the enormous expense of draining and other means of exsiccation that have been bestowed upon it: and the surrounding neighbourhood is undoubtedly healthy. It was at first mainly attributed to a reduced scale of diet, and particularly of animal food, which had been suddenly laid down for the prison; but a return to a richer scale produced no advantage; and was accompanied with an extension rather than a diminution of the diarrhœa or dysenteric form of the disease. So that at the end of six months, after every remedial plan which the physicians to the establishment could devise in succession, that of mercury being the chief, at first given in small and alternate doses, and afterward more freely, and for the express purpose of producing salivation, the whole prison population, as well male as female, was removed from the Penitentiary, and transferred to the hulks at Woolwich.

The real cause of this mischief has hitherto puzzled the ablest and most acute physiologists, and is supposed to bid defiance to all conjecture.—(*An Account of the Disease at the General Penitentiary, by P. M. Latham, M. D.*, &c., p. 217, 8vo. 1825.) Yet I think it is by no means impossible to follow it up, and drag it from its obscurity.

In a population so large as that we are now considering, it is not enough that the courts should be airy, and the air not manifestly loaded with moisture; but it is equally necessary that such air should be free from confinement; that it should be in a constant state of perflation, and refreshed and purified by renewal: for without this, large as the courts are, the air they contain must equally be drained of its vivifying power, and tainted with the azotic vapour that every individual is perpetually pouring forth from his skin and his lungs: and consequently must tend in a greater or less degree to a generation of the disease before us, or rather to all those morbid effects which the Milbank Penitentiary has so strikingly unfolded.

Now it appears to me almost impossible to take a survey of this prison, without coming to an admission that it is, with respect to ventilation, in the very condition just described. The inhabitants of the neighbourhood are healthy,

because, notwithstanding the lowness and original swampiness of the ground-soil, and its exposure to exhalations, the fanning breezes which are daily playing around them carry off the rising moisture, and supply them with a perpetual current of pure air. But the height of the terminal and intersecting walls of the prison, with only a few small openings for doors, and no opposite outlets, effectually prevent this within its limits. Air will here, indeed, find its way, as it will everywhere else, unless opposed by an hermetical seal; but as soon as it enters the courts of the Penitentiary, it is almost as much imprisoned as the convicts themselves: it is in a considerable degree bottled up; and the only change it can undergo is that of parting with its vivifying principle, and receiving a mischievous principle in return. Were it indeed entirely bottled up in the manner here spoken of, the result would be obvious instantaneously: but this is not the case, for a part of it must necessarily fly off in consequence of its higher temperature and greater specific levity, and its place be supplied with air from without. But the supply does not seem to be in proportion to the demand; the balance is not duly preserved, and the expired and tainted air is not sufficiently carried off. It is very possible, also, that some degree of humidity, though not manifest to the senses, is perpetually ascending from the low and once swampy soil beneath, which should be swept away by the winnow of a stirring breeze. Where a large population is immured in a boundary of any extent, if the supply of pure air be in the least degree below the supply of foul air, the health of such population must be encroached upon: and the less the difference, the more insidious the effeet, because the more invisible. It is, however, an effect that must go on: its influence must at length become obvious, and challenge attention; and the result, as already observed, must be, if I mistake not, a combination of symptoms more or less approaching to those which have of late been exhibited at the Penitentiary before us.

If the real cause be thus correctly traced out,[*] the remedy will not be difficult in the hands of an able pathologist, and a *skilful architect*.[†]

[*] The difficulty of acceding to the author's views arises from the fact that other prisons, quite as much crowded as the Penitentiary, less dry, and not so well ventilated, have not been visited by the disease in question.—Ed.

[†] This form of porphyra sometimes attends intemperance in ardent spirits, as well as the circumstances connected with indigence, bad food, vitiated air, &c. In many instances the epidemic termed spotted fever, which prevailed so extensively in the United States a few years since, exhibited in some individuals the characteristics of porphyra, and, as our author admits, cases of the complaint occasionally appear in jails, hospitals, &c. Mr. Eddy, in his account of the State Prison of New-York, has mentioned many instances of it, arising from errors in diet and confinement in impure air. Porphyra hæmorrhagica, though often marked by great debility, is sometimes relieved by venesection and purgatives, followed by tonics and stimulants.—D.

SPECIES III.
PORPHYRA NAUTICA.
SEA SCURVY.

SPOTS OF DIFFERENT HUES INTERMIXED WITH LIVID, PRINCIPALLY AT THE ROOTS OF THE HAIR; TEETH LOOSE; GUMS SPONGY AND BLEEDING; BREATH FETID; DEBILITY UNIVERSAL AND EXTREME.

This species is denominated SEA SCURVY, not from its being exclusively limited to mariners and extensive fleets, but from its being most common to persons thus occupied, and raging in such situations with the most fatal havoc. For the peculiar, as well as the general causes which produce it at sea, may also operate on shore, and have at times operated with merciless ravage in besieged garrisons, and among armies reduced to short provisions, or of unwholesome kinds, and worn down by fatigue, anxiety, and exposure to a damp atmosphere. Such seems to have been the condition of the Roman army under the command of Germanicus, as related by Pliny; whose account of the disease that preyed upon it, though vague and unsatisfactory, coincides with the general appearance of sea scurvy. We have similar descriptions in several of the expeditions that took part in the Holy Wars, and particularly that of St. Louis, as related by Joinville. We may hence conclude that sea scurvy is not a disease of recent times alone (*Richter, Pr. Disquisitio in Hippocraticas Scorbuti antiquitates*, &c.); though it does not appear to have attracted any very general attention till the melancholy result of the famous voyage of Vasco de Gama in 1497. The spirit of maritime discovery was at this time in full vigour and activity: the Portuguese, the Spaniards, the Dutch, and the English, vied with each other in their efforts to explore remote and unknown countries; the means of providing suitably for voyages of so great length were little understood; and hence the disease frequently made its appearance during the progress of the next half century, and raged with tremendous violence. It is well known, indeed, that so late as 1741, the fleet under Captain (afterward Lord) Anson, lost half its crew in the space of six months from the time it left England.

The diagnostics and progress of the disease are neatly and accurately concentrated by Dr. Parr. Its first appearance is evinced by a pale, bloated complexion, lassitude, and a disinclination to motion, with diminished energy in the muscular fibres: to which may be added, some degree of stiffness or induration, and an intumescence of the lower limbs. If the gums, even in this early stage, be examined, they will be found spongy and apt to bleed on being touched, while the teeth are loosened in their sockets. The skin is sometimes rough, but more generally smooth and shining, covered with bluish or livid spots, which do not rise above it; and these spots often coalesce in large blotches, particularly in the legs and thighs. About the same period, old ulcers often break out again, and the slightest mercurial preparation quickly produces

salivation. The ulcers discharge often a fetid sanies, or are covered with a coagulated crust, which is renewed whenever it is separated. The edges are livid, with irregular granulations, which sometimes run into a bloody fungus. During the whole of this period the appetite continues good, and though tensive pains arise, and are necessarily distressing, yet, on the whole, the patient feels little inconvenience.

The state of the bowels is very various. The stools are often frequent and offensive; but there is sometimes an obstinate costiveness. The urine is commonly high-coloured and fetid; the pulse feeble, but rarely quick. A weakness in the joints appears early, and increases with the disease; and a shrinking of the flexor muscles renders the limbs useless: producing scorbutic paralysis of Dr. Lind. The calves of the legs fall away, with sometimes an irregular hardness, and at length become œdematous, while the bones themselves, no longer supplied with a sufficiency of calcareous earth, give way at the callus of fractures; and those which have been formerly broken and re-united, become again separate at the line of re-union.[*]

The last stage is truly distressing. Blood is frequently discharged from the intestines, bladder, and other organs. The slightest motion brings on faintness, and often immediate death. Catchings of the breath and syncope, sometimes slightly experienced, indeed, at an earlier period, are now frequent and dangerous; yet the sense of weakness is so much less than its real amount, that the patient often attempts exertion, and dies in the very effort: though, more frequently, he survives the attempt for a short time, and especially when animated by any powerful and pleasant motive, as the hope of getting on shore, or even of engaging in fight with an enemy.

The most obvious of the remote causes of sea scurvy is salt provisions; and, perhaps, the most obvious of its proximate causes is a putrescent state of the blood: and hence these are the causes that have been commonly assigned, from the time of Sir John Pringle to the present day.

That an excess of salt, and particularly of salted meat, is a powerful cause in the production of scurvy, is unquestionable; yet not more perhaps from its tendency to dissolve the fluids, —for the blood retains a buffy crust even to the last,—than from its rendering the salted meat less nutritious. But it is by no means the only

---

* Aitken, Essays on several Important Subjects in Surgery, &c.; Lord Anson's Voyage, &c. Scorbutic ulcers have the following character:—Instead of pus, they excrete a thin, fetid, sanious fluid, mixed with blood. Their edges are generally of a livid colour, and swollen; a coagulum is soon formed on their surface, which can with great difficulty be wiped away, or separated from the subjacent parts. These are soft, spongy, and putrid. When, however, the removal of the coagulum is effected, another shortly afterward forms again, followed by a soft bloody fungus of considerable size, termed by sailors bullock's liver. According to Lind, it is as difficult to repress almost as fungus hæmatodes, and, when destroyed by the cautery or the knife, is reproduced again in a few hours.—ED.

cause. In the preceding varieties, we have already seen it produced on land as well as at sea, and in some cases where there was no employment of salt provisions. And even sea scurvy itself has occasionally been found to arise where the diet has by no means been saline; and in damp situations, whatever have been the diet, unless where peculiarly generous and stimulating; and we have one instance of its having occurred in a young woman who had subsisted almost wholly on tea.

In like manner, though the fluids of the body are loose and incoagulable, the muscular fibres are equally loose and incontractile; so that the latter, as justly observed by that excellent practical writer, Dr. James Lind (*Treatise on the Scurvy*, &c., p. 277), are as much affected as the former: and, if we attend to the course of the symptoms as they arise, we shall find that they are affected soonest; for the earliest signs of the disease are those of languor, debility, and dejection; though, upon the whole, the mental depression is less considerable than in land scurvy; and, as we have already observed, there is a sense of mental energy to the last, which is far more than commensurate with the actual strength of the body.

How far salt provisions alone might produce sea scurvy, is scarcely worth while to inquire; for there is no extensive history of the disease in which they have acted solitarily; having always been more or less united with a cold or damp atmosphere, great fatigue, or a want of proper and invigorating exercise, want of ventilation, neglect of cleanliness, and very generally short rations, or an unwholesome diet of other aliments besides salt meat.*

Now these are causes which must have a direct influence on the fibrous structure, and consequently on the whole organization of the body, before the fluids can become affected; and it is easy to trace the changes which occur in them subsequently to, and through the medium of this influence.

Under the circumstances we are now contemplating, the digestive organs suffer first; they become weakened in their power, and for the reasons already stated when treating of MARASMUS, the weakness will extend through the whole range of the digestive chain, and influence all the organs of assimilation; while the lungs, the brain, the heart, and the skin, unite in the general debility. Hence none of the secretions will be sufficiently elaborated, or, perhaps, in sufficient quantity; there will be a less supply of sensorial energy, and a less vigorous action of the vascular system: a smaller formation of gluten, and elimination of carbon from the lungs. And hence, as a necessary consequence, the looser texture and deeper hue of the blood.

On this account Girtanner (*In Blumenbach, Bibl.*, band iii., p. 527) and other pathologists, who refer sea scurvy exclusively to a looseness of the solidum vivum, have more to advance in

their behalf than those who refer it exclusively to a looseness of the fluids. But both are affected, and affected equally, though the former takes the lead. Sea scurvy is therefore a disease, whose proximate cause is a putrescent, though not a putrid state of the animal solids and fluids, produced by an assemblage of antecedents co-operating to a common effect.*

It is assuredly, however, not necessary that all the causes we have adverted to should operate at the same time. But it is of the utmost importance, both in preventing the appearance of the disease, and effecting its cure where it is present, to have the eye cautiously directed to every one of them, and to destroy its agency as far as we are able. And it is owing to the unremitting attention which is paid to these points in the navy of our own country, that sea scurvy has long been rarely heard of in English fleets or English merchant ships; and that the globe is perpetually sailed over, and the highest as well as the hottest latitudes coasted and cruised in, without the generation of this destructive plague. And thus it has been ever since the celebrated and extraordinary circumnavigation of Captain Cook in the Resolution; in which, by first laying down a code of regulations for the government of his crew, founded on the soundest judgment, and afterward persevering in them with an unremitting spirit, directed to all the subjects before us, he was enabled to fulfil his voyage of three years and eighteen days, with a company of a hundred and eighteen men, traversing all climates, from fifty-two degrees north to seventy-one south, with the loss of only one man by disease, and that man apparently labouring under a consumption before he left home.

The regulations and management adopted by Captain Cook, are contained in his paper communicated to the Royal Society.—(*Phil. Trans.*, vol. lxvi., year 1776, p. 402.) It is a production of the highest merit, and was justly honoured with the Copley medal for the year. In conjunction with Sir John Pringle's additional remarks upon it,† it has laid the chief foundation for the present mode of treating this disease, and particularly of providing against its attack. The principles it unfolds should be canvassed by the nautical student in the communications themselves, in conjunction with the later works of Sir Gilbert Blane (*Treatise on the Diseases of Seamen*) and Dr. Trotter.—(*Medicina Nautica.*)

With the auxiliaries of cleanliness, proper ventilation, a dry atmosphere, and fresh provisions, the medical treatment of sea scurvy is

---

* An insufficient supply, or total want of fresh succulent vegetables, might here have been noticed among the exciting causes of scurvy in long voyages.—ED.

* That scurvy is a disease of the whole system is now universally believed. In post-mortem examinations, p   g   find extravasations of dark-coloured , not merely in the sub-cutaneous cellular membrane, but in several of the viscera, and also between the fibres of the muscles. Some interesting specimens of the latter fact may be seen in the Museum of the London University. —ED.

† A Discourse upon some late Improvements of the Means for preserving the Health of Mariners, &c., 4to., London.

sufficiently simple, and the disease is found to yield easily. The means more immediately effectual are the native vegetable acids,.and above all that of lemons, upon which we shall speak more at large presently ; all sorts of fermented liquors ; the alkalescent plants, as garlic, scurvy-grass, water-cress, garden-cress, brook-lime, which, notwithstanding their alkalescence, contain a great quantity of acescent matter, and by their acrid property promote the excretions of urine and perspiration ; and the spruce-fir,* as well as other plants of the coniferous tribe that contribute to the same purpose.

The fruit of the *rubus Chamæmorus*, or cloudberry, found on boggy mountains in our own as well as in more northern countries, is also a cheap and valuable antiscorbutic. In Sweden, from the recommendation of Linnæus principally, the berries are eaten very largely as a confection ; the Laplanders, in whose gloomy region the plant grows in great abundance, preserve considerable quantities of the fruit in snow, and export them to Stockholm in casks.

The burdocks were formerly very much extolled in scorbutic and almost every other disease of the present order, and especially the *arctium Lappa*, clotbur, or great burdock, common to the wastes of our own country, which was supposed to possess all the powers of the China and sarsaparilla roots. The root, given in decoction, is certainly a diuretic and diaphoretic ; but, as an antiscorbutic, it is of far inferior merit to the plants already mentioned.†

The infusion of malt, as recommended by Dr. Macbride, does not seem to have answered all the expectations entertained concerning it. Dr. Trotter never saw it do good ; and Dr. John Clark affirms freely and candidly, that in various cases in which he tried it, with all the concomitants of pure air and good nutriment, it had no influence either in removing the disease or in checking its progress ; in consequence of which he preferred Dr. Silvester's antiscorbutic drink, which is made by boiling three ounces of cream of tartar, four ounces of juniper-berries, two drachms of ginger in powder, and five pounds

---

* The essence of spruce, or rather spruce beer, is admitted by Sir Gilbert Blane to possess antiscorbutic virtues, as well as beer or porter ; but the great remedy on which he insists is lemonjuice. The essence of spruce, a little diluted, produced surprising benefit in the West Indies. It acted as a purgative, and remained on the stomach when every thing else was rejected.—See Trotter's Med. Naut., vol. i., p. 349.—Ed.

† Sugar has sometimes proved useful in cases of scurvy. The following instance is recorded, and deserves notice :—

"A vessel came from the West Indies heavily laden with sugar. A calm that had not been foreseen, prolonged the passage till all their provisions were exhausted. The sugar was the only resource left to the crew, and, nourished by it, they at length arrived safely in port. Some sailors had died of scurvy during the voyage, and many were threatened with death from the same cruel malady. The scurvy ceased when its victims were from necessity reduced to the sugar diet, and the remedy was at the same time an agreeable aliment."—D.

of coarse sugar, in six gallons of water. After boiling half an hour, the whole is poured into a tub and allowed to ferment. It may be drank as soon as the fermentation commences, from one to three pints daily.—(*Obs. on Diseases in Long Voyages*, &c., 8vo.)

Captain Cook, however, thought very highly of malt sweetwort, and esteemed it one of the most powerful antiscorbutics. The Russians, for want of sweetwort or table-beer, employ a brisk acidulous liquor called quas, formed by fermenting small loaves made of ground malt and rye meal. Dr. Mounsey tells us, that this is the common drink of both the fleets and armies of the Russian empire. Oatmeal is also occasionally used for the same purpose, in the form of an acidulated gelatinous food denominated *soins ;* made by infusing the meal in water till a fermentation commences and the liquor grows sourish, which in a moderate temperature will take place in about eight-and-forty hours. The liquor is then poured off from the grounds, and boiled to the consistence of a jelly, which, sweetened with sugar and mixed with a little wine, yields an aliment not less palatable than medicinal.

Pure fresh water is also another material of great importance, not only in curing this disease, but in guarding against it : and of so much moment did Captain Cook esteem its purity, as well as its freshness, that he had the old stock poured away, though procured only a few days before, whenever he had an opportunity of obtaining a new supply. And at a time when it was universally conceived that the frozen water of the icebergs consisted of salt water, or was unwholesome, as formed of frozen snow, it was matter of most agreeable surprise to him to find that the melted ice of the sea, from whatever quarter derived, is not only sweet, but soft, and as wholesome as the purest spring or river water ; thus affording him a supply he had no expectation of finding.

The best means of preserving water pure, is by keeping it in casks charred for the purpose on their inner surface ; and the best means for restoring it to purity when it has become foul and offensive, is by mixing a little fresh powdered charcoal with every cask before it is tapped, and in drawing it off through a stone filtering-cistern, containing a bed of the same material.

As fermented liquors have been found serviceable, many of the gases have been tried in their simple form, and some of them have been thought serviceable ; but their carriage, or the means of obtaining them extemporaneously, is highly incommodious : and it was well observed by that excellent navigator La Pérouse, that seamen may be gorged with bottles of them without deriving a thousandth part of the benefit produced from a good slice of fresh meat, fruits, and herbs.

Of all the antiscorbutics, however, that have thus passed under our survey, the citric acid, or that of lemons, is the only one that can make an approach towards the character of a specific for sea scurvy ; and how well entitled this medicine is to the maintenance of such a claim, now that the mode of preserving it in a state of activity, first suggested by Dr. Lind, has been fully established, the following brief but triumphant narrative of Dr. Baird will sufficiently evince :—" The next time I saw this disease in a very spreading degree, so as to affect the whole fleet, at a period when the existence of the country depended upon that fleet keeping the sea, was in the year 1801, when my Lord St. Vincent took the command of the Channel fleet. A short time after we sailed, and in not more than a fortnight, the scurvy made its appearance, and spread very rapidly through the fleet. Fresh provisions were not then supplied to it as now, nor vegetables. Being aware that lemon-juice was then in store, and could be drawn for the fleet, I expressed to the commander-in-chief my great anxiety that a fresh supply should be had as fast as possible. The fleet was then blockading Brest : a cutter was despatched to communicate the state of the health of the fleet ; a supply of lemon-juice came out, and we gave it freely to those labouring under the disease, and daily, mixed with water and sugar, to the whole of the crews of the ships, and continued its use during the time we were at sea, which was nearly seventeen weeks ; during which time the fleet had not, as a fleet, a single fresh meal, nor any thing in the shape of an antiscorbutic, but lemon-juice. The disease under the use of this totally disappeared ; we returned with twenty-four sail of the line into Torbay, out of which number there must have been ten or twelve three-deckers ; and I think, estimating fairly, there could not, upon an average, have been less than seven hundred men in each. When we arrived, the surgeons of the fleet were desired to make a return of the number of patients fit for the hospital. They made a return of twenty-four. I was directed by the commander of the fleet to examine them, to see whether they were subjects for the hospital. I found eight of them were cases of hernia, or surgical cases, that could not be benefited by the hospital. I selected sixteen from them. Out of twenty-four sail of the line, there was not a single case of scurvy ; and, what was extraordinary, to such a state of health was that fleet brought by the use of lemon-juice, that the Glory had only four men on her sick-list ; so that out of fifteen or sixteen thousand men, there were only sixteen subjects for the hospital ; and some of the ships had not lost a man at that time."—(*Report of the Committee of the House of Commons upon the Penitentiary at Milbank*, 1823, p. 199.)*

As the vessel of a tainted crew approaches

land, nothing is more common, or apparently more reasonable, than for those that are most affected to be the most anxious to be put on shore at the moment. Yet, for reasons we have already urged, this should rarely be complied with ; for the real debility is so much greater than the apparent, or, in other words, the energy of the mind is so much greater than that of the body, that they often sink under the labour of the removal, and sometimes die before they reach the asylum provided for them. In cases of extreme weakness, the external air alone, and especially when sharp or in a current, is sufficient from its pressure and stimulus to puff out the little flame that flickers in the vital lamp ; a fact which, to adopt the words of Dr. Trotter, "has been long observed, and recently confirmed by five men dying in the boat belonging to the Prince of Wales ship-of-war, between the Downs and Deal hospital."

<hr>

GENUS XI.
EXANGIA.

ENLARGEMENT, BREACH, OR OTHER MORBID PERFORATION OF A LARGE BLOODVESSEL, WITHOUT EXTERNAL OPENING.

THE expediency of placing this genus in its present situation, among diseases dependant on a "morbid state of the blood or *bloodvessels*," would be obvious to every one, even though the maladies it embraces were in every instance local. This, however, is rarely the fact ; for the first two species included under it result commonly from a peculiar diathesis ; and the last is productive of severe, and often fatal constitutional disorder. These species are as follow :—

1. Exangia Aneurisma.		Aneurism.
2. —— Varix.		Varix.
3. —— Cyania.		Blue-skin.

<hr>

SPECIES I.
EXANGIA ANEURISMA.
ANEURISM.

PULSATING TUMOUR OF AN ARTERY.

THE disease of aneurism, which consists in a permanent dilatation or breach of the coats of an artery, may be produced by external violence, as a strain or puncture, or by arterial debility. The last is the more common cause, and it may be local or general : it may be limited to the part in which the aneurismal swelling occurs, or it may extend through the whole range of the arterial system, which is sometimes found to be universally though irregularly feeble, and consequently feebler in some parts than in others. It is this last condition of the arteries which constitutes what has been called the aneurismal diathesis ; and, under its influence, aneurismal tumours not unfrequently occur in different arteries of the same individual simultaneously or in succession. De Haen gives a singular example of this in a boy of seventeen.—(*Rat. Med.*, iv., 2, § 7.)

* This form of disease seldom prevails in the United States Navy; doubtless on account of the liberal supply of fresh vegetables, the use of citric acid, and the free employment of the chlorides of soda and lime. The temperance observed in dispensing stimuli to the seamen, is also attended with advantages; and the practice of commuting, when possible, for their daily allowance of ardent spirits, as recently recommended by the Secretary of the Navy, deserves imitation.—D.

- [Sir A. Cooper has seen seven aneurisms in one person: one in each ham; one in the bifurcation of the aorta; one at the origin of the arteria profunda; one in the middle of the thigh; and two between the popliteal and the femoral. —(*Lectures on Surgery*, vol. ii., p. 37, 8vo., 1825.) But Pelletan the enormous number of sixty-three, from the size of a filbert to that of a hen's egg.—(*Clinique Chir.*, tom. ii., p. 1.) It is an observation made by the former experienced surgeon, that when aneurisms occur opposite a joint, a partial disease of the artery often gives rise to them; but that, when they are seated in other parts of the body, there is usually a disease in the arteries, which produces a general disposition to their formation; in other words, there is an aneurismal diathesis. The ultimate success of operations, he says, will depend very much upon the disposition to the disease being partial or general.—(*Lect.*, vol. cit., p. 40.) With respect to the cause of aneurism, which our author ascribes to what he terms arterial debility, if we exclude those cases which arise from the wound or rupture of an artery, it is certain that the generality of instances are preceded either by a steatomatous thickening, with ulceration of the internal coats of the artery, or by calcareous deposition between the middle and internal coats, attended with loss of elasticity in the affected part of the vessel, and a disposition to crack or give way. The blood then comes in contact with the external elastic coat, which is raised into an aneurismal swelling. At length, more or less of this coat is removed by absorption, or bursts, and the blood then receives a covering from the arterial sheath. As the disease advances, it presses upon and causes the absorption of all the surrounding parts, and is more or less diffused and circumscribed, according as it may happen or not to be confined or bounded by an entire cyst, formed by the adhesive inflammation, the remains of the original sac, or any ligamentous expansion.—(*First Lines of Surgery*, p. 255, 5th edit.)]

Aneurism is ordinarily represented as appearing under only two forms: the true, or, as Mr. B. Bell more particularly denominates it, the encysted (*Syst. of Surg.*, vol. i., ch. iv., p. 196), and the false or diffused. To these it is necessary to add the varicose of Dr. Hunter, and the cardiogmus of the Greek writers; thus presenting us with the four following varieties:—

α	Cysticum.	Encysted aneurism.
β	Diffusum.	Diffuse aneurism.
γ	Varicosum.	Varicose aneurism.
δ	Cardiogmus.	Aneurism of the præcordia.

The TRUE or ENCYSTED variety, forming the aneurism by dilatation of M. Petit (*Mémoires de l'Acad. des Sciences*, 1736), is characterized by the tumour being circumscribed or having a defined outline; and is produced by a yielding or dilatation of the coats of an artery so as to form a sac, which constitutes the sphere of the arterial enlargement. Where it does not occur suddenly from external violence, it is commonly the result of a diseased state of the arterial coats, by which the artery becomes changed in its general character, and especially thinner in its texture. This morbid condition sometimes extends to a considerable range, and the artery is in consequence dilated through its whole circumference, and, where the aorta has suffered, has been found to occupy its entire curvature, and even to extend beyond it. At times, indeed, and not unfrequently, as we have already observed, it is a constitutional affection, and various arteries fall a prey to its influence simultaneously or in succession. And hence Sir Astley Cooper has wisely cautioned his pupils never to operate upon an aneurism till they are satisfied that no others exist.—(*Lectures*, &c., ut suprà, vol. ii., p. 29.) The period of life at which they most usually occur is between thirty and fifty years of age, when the muscular system is yet strong, but the strength of the arterial tissues is beginning to be impaired. And we can hence readily perceive why males should be more subject to the disease than females; as also why persons in very advanced life, like the young, should less frequently suffer from its attacks. One man of eighty, and one boy of eleven years of age, form the extremes on which Sir Astley Cooper tells us he has ever had to perform the operation;—in the first the aneurism was popliteal; in the second, tibial; and both appear to have done well.—(*Id.*, vol. ii., p. 46.)

The tumour, when first observed, is small, and excites little attention; for there is no pain, the skin is of its natural appearance, and the tumour vanishes when pressed upon by the finger. But during the pressure a pulsation is clearly distinguishable, corresponding with that of the subjacent artery. As the disease advances, the tumour increases; and when it has gained considerable magnitude, the skin becomes pale, and even œdematous; the pulsation still continues, though the tumour yields less regularly to the pressure of the finger than heretofore, being soft and fluctuating in some parts, but, from coagula lodged and hardened in the sac, firm and resisting in others. The seat of the aneurism at length becomes distressingly painful from the increased coagulation and swelling; the skin assumes a livid hue, and seems verging to a gangrenous state; the bloody serum oozes from it, and it often ulcerates; when the walls of the arterial sac, meeting with less support than hitherto, give way, the blood bursts forth with violence, and, if the artery be large, soon produces death by inanition.

In an early stage of the disease, it cannot easily be mistaken for any other; for the signs of a regular pulsation, absence of pain, and disappearance of the tumour on pressure, are sufficient to distinguish it. But when in the progress of the complaint the pulsation becomes almost imperceptible, and the tumour hard, it has been confounded with other encysted tumours, scrofulous swellings and abscesses. The last is the most common error, and by leading to an injudicious opening, has sometimes proved a fatal one.—(*Reinesius, Schola Ictorum Med.*, p. 321.)

Pressure, under favourable circumstances, has

sometimes produced changes leading to a cure of the disease. Dr. Albers of Bremen gives an instance of this even. in an aneurism of the femoral artery.—(*Trans. of Medico-Chirurg. Soc.*, vol. ix.) It has commonly been said that the compress should never amount to more than an easy support to the weakened and enlarged organ (*Desault, Journ. de Chirurg.*, tom. ii.) : and it is very probable that tight bandages, by impeding the circulation in the adjoining veins, as well as arteries, have often proved injurious. Dr. Perceval, however, in the manuscript comment with which he has enriched the author's volume of Nosology, has the following notice under the present head ; seeming to show that even a tight compress has at times been of the highest advantage ; and a like success is related by Acrel in an aneurism of the aorta.— (*Chirurgische Vorfälle*, band i., 44.) "In the rebellion of 1798, an officer received a wound from a bayonet which grazed the left carotid artery and produced a pulsatory tumour ; this was kept down by a spring-collar, and at length disappeared. Many years after, having lived rather freely, he died dropsical. Previous to his death he had a most violent palpitation of the heart, and discharged by stool immense quantities of blood. The heart was not found enlarged, but the cavity of the left carotid was almost entirely obliterated." -

In connexion with pressure, great benefit has also frequently resulted from keeping the amount of the circulating fluid in a diminished state by occasional venesections, purgatives, and a spare diet. Morgagni relates a case in which such a regimen alone effected a cure when commenced early.—(*De Sed. et Caus.*, ep. xvii., art. 30, 31.) Yet it is obvious that in some habits a cure, even of the same artery, is obtained much more easily than in others : and hence it seems sometimes to have taken place spontaneously ; of which an example is given by Mr. Crampton (*Med.-Chir. Trans.*, vol. vii., p. 341), and by Mr. Ford in a journal of an earlier date.[*]

[Although it is the common course of aneurisms, when they are left to themselves, to increase in size, and at length to burst and destroy the patients by hemorrhage, sometimes things happen otherwise, and, in consequence of certain changes taking place, a spontaneous cure is the result. There are four modes in which this desirable event may be produced. 1. Sometimes the whole aneurismal swelling suddenly inflames and sphacelates ; in this state, if the inflammation extend its effects to a sufficient depth, the sac in the vicinity of the artery, and a portion of the canal of this vessel itself, may become completely blocked up by coagulating lymph, so that no more blood can get into the tumour, the pulsation of which is

extinguished. The mortified parts, together with the mass of congealed and sometimes putrid blood in the sac, are cast off ; and, if the patient's constitution holds out, the ulcer left by the detachment of the sloughs heals up, and the cure is completed. When, however, the inflammation and sloughing are confined to the skin and superficial portion of the sac, the patient bleeds to death on the separation of the dead parts. 2. The second process by which the spontaneous cure of an aneurism may be produced, is the increase of the lamellated coagula in such a degree within the sac as completely to fill it, in which case the blood also coagulates in the adjoining portion of the artery, which becomes impervious for a certain extent above and below the communication which it had with the aneurismal cavity. Similar changes happen when the cure is accomplished by pressure. 3. Until lately, it was believed by Scarpa and other eminent pathologists that no aneurism could be cured, unless the sac and an adjoining part of the artery were thus obliterated ; but the facts collected by Mr. Hodgson leave no doubt that when an aneurism of the aorta undergoes a cure, the sac alone may be filled up with coagula, while the vessel itself remains pervious. 4. The last manner in which a spontaneous cure may be brought about, is by the pressure of the sac itself upon the artery.[*]]

Every palliative means should be had recourse to before an operation is resolved upon ; for, even under the most favourable circumstances, such a step is hazardous, and it is peculiarly so when the aneurism is connected with a diseased state of the arterial trunk, or the whole arterial system, of which it is seldom possible for us to form a correct judgment. To describe the nature of the operation would be to travel into the province of surgery. I may, however, observe that, in cases of necessity, it has often been performed with full success, and even a perfect use of the affected limb, in trunks of a very large calibre. Sir Astley Cooper has given an account of two cases in which the operation was effected on the carotid artery. The first proved unsuccessful from the long standing and size of the sac, which pressed with perpetual irritation on the larynx and pharynx, exciting frequent fits of coughing, and preventing deglutition. The second case terminated favourably, but the tumour was smaller and of more recent growth.[†]

In the SECOND VARIETY, OF DIFFUSE ANEURISM,

---

[*] London Medical Journal, vol. ix. Other instances have occurred to Dr. Baillie and to Sir Astley Cooper. "I have seen," observes the last writer, "spontaneous cures of aneurism produced without any circumstance which would readily explain the cause."—Lectures, &c., vol. ii., p. 48, 8vo., 1825

[*] See Sir A. Cooper's Lectures, &c., vol. ii., p. 47. The pressure of one aneurism on the artery leading to another aneurism, has sometimes cured the latter. Thus, Mr. Liston records one example, in which the pressure of an aneurism of the arteria innominata on the subclavian artery cured an aneurism in the axilla.—Ed.

[†] When the simultaneous existence of several aneurisms, the state of the health, or other particular circumstances, do not forbid the operation, the maxim of the best modern surgeons is to operate, if possible, before the aneurismal tumour has attained a large size, which always renders the cure more remote and uncertain.—Ed.

the aneurism by infusion of M. Petit (*Desault, Journ. de Chirurgie*, p. 321), the coats of the artery, instead of being dilated into a sac, are divided, and the blood flowing at large into the cellular or other surrounding parts, the tumour is extensive and undefined.

This is usually the result of external violence; the swelling often spreads to an unlimited range, and the progress towards a rupture of the integuments is more rapid than in the last. Here pressure is of no avail, and even mischievous, since it will more effectually obstruct the course of the blood in the surrounding veins than in the divided artery, and increase the chance of mortification. The cure should be conducted on the same principles by which the treatment of a wounded artery is regulated. Sometimes, however, a single ligature above the wound or rent in the vessel will suffice and does generally suffice in the false aneurism at the bend of the arm, not unfrequently occasioned by the unskilful use of the lancet.

The THIRD VARIETY, or VARICOSE ANEURISM, or ANEURISMAL VARIX, was first distinctly pointed out by Dr. Hunter, who characterized it by this name. It is produced by puncturing an artery through a vein that lies immediately above it and upon it, as in bloodletting at the arm, so that the arterial blood flows from the arterial puncture, not through the cellular substance, but into the superincumbent vein through the corresponding venous puncture. In this case the tumour is elongated, taking the course of the vein, which is hereby distended and rendered varicose. Sometimes, indeed, where the venous communications are frequent, all the adjoining veins participate in the distention, and are equally affected. The tumour, as in the first variety, disappears upon pressure, and as soon as the pressure is removed, the blood issues from the arterial puncture with a whizzing sound and a tremulous motion, rather than a distinct pulsation.*

This is the least dangerous of all the varieties of aneurism; and that in which pressure may be most successfully applied. It has sometimes produced a radical cure; but generally so far succeeded as to render the operation unnecessary, provided the patient passes a quiet and unfatiguing life; for it has been known to exist twelve, twenty, and even thirty years without any serious injury to the general health.†

* The varicose aneurism does not always correspond to this simple account of its nature; for, not unfrequently, between the vein and artery an aneurismal sac is produced, out of which the blood passes into the vein. This complication materially influences the principles of treatment, because the sac may enlarge to a considerable size, more particularly if its communication with the vein happen to be obliterated, while its communication with the artery remains free.—ED.

† The simple form of aneurismal varix, left to itself, usually attains the size of a pigeon's egg, and then continues stationary. In consequence of a good deal of the arterial blood, destined for the supply of the hand and forearm, passing directly into the vein, those parts are weakened, and sometimes colder than natural

The FOURTH VARIETY is distinctly a constitutional affection, and usually of considerable distress and oppression. It is characterized by an obtuse intumescence and constant disquiet of the præcordia, with a sense of internal weight and pulsation, increased on the smallest motion: according to Corvisart, the carotids throb, the pulse is strong, hard, and vibrating. It is the CARDIOGMUS* of Galen and Sauvages; the aneurisma præcordiorum of many authors, and the polypus cordis of others. The symptoms are usually found on dissection to proceed from an aneurismal enlargement of some part of the substance of the heart, or the larger vessels in its immediate neighbourhood; but whether, as Corvisart affirms, the enlargement be more common to the left than the right ventricle (*Sur les Maladies et les Lésions Organiques du Cœur*, &c.), is not satisfactorily determined.† It is sometimes accompanied with, and perhaps produced by, a polypous concretion; and sometimes without any such substance whatever: and, where the larger vessels are affected, they are here, more than in any other variety, thickened and rendered rigid by irregular deposites of calcareous or ossific matter. [Two remarkable examples of blood in the heart having become vascular, were published by M. Bouillaud in his and the pulse at the wrist enfeebled or imperceptible.—ED.

* Cardiogmus is used by some medical writers in two senses:—1. That of a partial enlargement of the heart, forming a sac in which coagulable lymph is deposited, and which is sometimes called an aneurism of the heart. 2. That of a general dilatation of the natural cavities of this organ.— (Bateman, Rees's Cyclopædia.) In the present work the term is more comprehensively employed, as under this head we find arranged dilatations of the cavities of the heart, aneurisms of the great vessels near it, and a thickening of the substance of the heart (hypertrophy), just as if they were only modifications of the same disease, and were marked by no material difference of symptoms. Now, although practitioners, even with the aid of the stethoscope and percussion, are not familiar enough with the pathognomonic symptoms of dilatations of the natural cavities of the heart and of hypertrophy to be able to give such a delineation of them as can be fully depended upon, yet it may be confidently asserted, that a dilated ventricle with an attenuation of its parietes, cannot present the same kind of pulse, and cause the same general effects on the circulation, respiration, and system at large, as a ventricle the muscular substance of which is enormously thickened. This must be perfectly obvious, notwithstanding the fact remarked by Andral (Anat. Pathol, tom. ii., p. 283), that the strength and hardness of the pulse do not depend altogether upon the greater or lesser thickness of the parietes of the left ventricle. The two diseases, in fact, are quite as different from one another as they are from aneurism of the arch of the aorta, with which they are classed.—ED.

† A thickening of the parietes of the heart, when partial, mostly affects the left ventricle (see Andral, Anat. Pathol., tom. ii., p. 284); but the walls of all the four cavities may be similarly changed. An attenuation of the parietes, with dilatation of the cavities, forming the passive aneurism of Corvisart, is more common on the right than on the left side of the heart.—Op. cit., p. 289.—ED.

valuable memoir on the obliteration of veins. In one, the right auricle was occupied by a coagulum, in which were an infinite number of red vessels. In the other, the right cavities of the heart contained masses of organized, albuminous, fibrinous matter, adherent to the parietes of the heart by means of filaments, and inseparable without breaking them. The patient died of symptoms resembling those of aneurism of the heart. Another case has been published by Dr. Rigacci.—(*Bulletin des Sciences Méd.*, Sept., 1828.)]*

Cardiogmus is sometimes a result of violent exertion; and is then mostly an affection of the young and the strong, of those who engage in manly exercises, or are subject to violent passions. But it is more frequently a result of debility, and chiefly to be met with in persons of advanced age. It is well observed, indeed, by M. Rostan, that a dilatation and thickening of the walls of the heart are not a consequence of great power or strength of constitution with energy of healthy action; but are generally caused by that state of the arteries which is an ordinary consequence of old age, in which they lose their natural elasticity, and become ossified, thick, inorganic tubes.—(*Nouveau Journ. de Médecine*, tom. i., p. 367.) This ossification affects the valves of the heart as well as the vessels in its neighbourhood, whence the heart is perpetually oppressed, and called upon for increased action; which increased action itself is another cause of increased thickening in the cardiac coats.†

* Laennec (De l'Auscultation Médiate, vol. ii., p 244) relates several cases of this kind; he terms them globular excrescences of the heart. Breschet thinks that their organization takes place in the same manner as those of the false membranes, and depends on the same cause.—See note to Doane's translation of Meckel's Anatomy, vol. ii., p. 217.

† Hypertrophy is not always the original cause of palpitations of the heart, but often the effect of them. They take place in three very different states of the animal economy, which Professor Andral advises to be carefully discriminated, as they call for different methods of treatment. The first is a state of plethora, that makes the heart beat with too much violence, giving rise to dizziness, vertigo, &c. Here low diet and copious bleeding are indicated. The second condition promoting the occurrence of palpitations, is that in which there is a deficiency of blood; and in a person thus circumstanced, the palpitations and dyspnœa cease as soon as he is fed well, and more blood has entered the system. In a third condition, the centres of the nervous system are primarily disordered, and then palpitations may be the only indication of the diseased modification of the nervous action; or sometimes merely a secondary effect, among many others, of which most organs may be the seat, as in hysteria. Here neither bleeding nor tonics will answer; but the patient must be submitted to such treatment as will bring about some change in the state of the nervous system. Thus, as Andral explains, there are many affections of the heart which morbid anatomy only shows us, as it were, the terminations of; and what is observed in the dead body is not always the original cause of the symptoms. It is not hypertrophy of the heart that has at first oc-

This, however, is the *passive* enlargement of M. Corvisart; who gives us also a thickening and enlargement which he calls *active*; in which the increased action of the heart, instead of being confined to itself, is extended to its parietes, to the vessels that issue from it, and, consequently, to the pulse generally. Laennec has acceded to this last form of disease (*De l'Auscultation Médiate*, &c., Paris, 1819), and it constitutes his *hypertrophia*.* In this case, the stethoscope, of which we have spoken under *marasmus phthisis*, may often be advantageously employed as a diagnostic.—(Suprà, p. 523.)

The disease not unfrequently proceeds from a distinct cyst, sometimes traced in the substance of the heart, as that of the right auricle, of which an example is given by Bartholin (*Act. Hafn.*, iv., obs. 47); or of the left ventricle, as stated by Dr. Douglas (*Phil. Trans.*, vol. xxix., p. 1414–1416); but more usually in the arch of the aorta.

And in some instances this cyst, or some other morbid structure, has been found to become so much enlarged as to encroach in a casioned the palpitations, but these have often been the cause of the hypertrophy. Moreover, although in the enlarged heart it seems as if a more active vitality existed, since there is an excess of nutrition, this local condition of the heart does not always prove the condition in which the constitution was at the period when merely an increase of pulsations existed, without any augmentation of nutrition. Here morbid anatomy might lead to error, if the inference were made, that because the heart is thickened and enlarged, debilitating treatment was indicated in the commencement of the disorder. The therapeutic means must often be determined by the states of the nervous and sanguiferous systems then existing.—See Andral, Anat. Pathol., tom. ii., p. 346.—ED.

* Hypertrophy of the left ventricle has several degrees. Thus, it may be quite restricted to the carneæ columnæ, or merely affect the pillars of the mitral valve. In some instances it is only the septum ventriculorum that is thickened; while in others, the whole of the parietes of the left ventricle may be in this condition. It is particularly in cases where the septum is in a state of hypertrophy, that the capacity of the right ventricle is singularly lessened, this cavity seeming, indeed, sometimes like a small appendage, of very narrow dimensions, attached to the left ventricle. The same effect, however, now and then proceeds from hypertrophy affecting only its fleshy pillars. The right ventricle seldom attains a considerable thickness, though Laennec has seen it five times thick, and MM. Bertin and Bouillaud fifteen. Hypertrophy of the auricles is rare, and when it happens, it is almost always accompanied by the same affection of the ventricles. In hypertrophy of the parietes of the heart, its substance may either retain its natural consistence, which is most common; or it may be indurated, which is very unusual; or softened, which is still less frequent. In hypertrophy of the parietes of the heart, its cavities may continue of their natural size; be dilated, constituting the active aneurism of Corvisart, the eccentric hypertrophy of MM. Bertin and Bouillaud; or, lastly, they may be diminished, so as to form the concentric hypertrophy of the two latter pathologists.—Andral, Anat. Pathol., tom. ii., p. 284.—ED.

very considerable degree upon the natural capacity of the heart. And hence, though the general substance of the organ, with its diseased increase of growth, has weighed upon dissection fifteen pounds, the cavity, in a few rare instances, has hardly equalled that of a walnut. Portal, who is disposed to admit of Corvisart's division of the disease into active and passive, seems chiefly to object to the term dilatation as applied to the heart in this state of engorgement.*

In many of these cases, we can trace the cause; for the aneurismal artery is at times as contracted in the vicinity of the sac, as if it had been tied by a ligature. The aorta has occasionally, in this manner, been rendered altogether impervious, the circulation being continued by an enlargement of the anastomosing vessels.—(*Cooper and Travers's Surgical Essays*, i., p. 125.)

On this account, Morgagni ascribes the disease before us to a narrowness of the larger arteries as its common cause; and hence explains why it is so frequently found among tailors and other sedentary workmen.—(*De Sed. et Caus.*, Ep. xxi., 49; xxvi., 31–33.)

The medical treatment can be rarely more than palliative. Fatigue and great exertion must be sedulously avoided, together with keen mental excitement. The diet should be light, the meals and hours of rest regular, and the exercise should be that of a carriage. The bowels must be attended to; and, where the palpitation or other distress is peculiarly troublesome, it may sometimes be relieved by camphire, ammonia, and tincture of hyoscyamus.

We may observe, before quitting the subject, that the largest aneurisms have been those of this quarter, and particularly of the aorta, as there is here the greatest force of action. Littre gives a description of one of the superior trunk, that ascended as high as the maxilla (*Mém. de l'Acad. Royale des Sciences à Paris*, Ann. 1707), and Teichmeyer of another that burst into the pericardium.—(*Dissert. de Stupendo Aneurysmate Brachii*, &c., Jen., 1734.) From their extent and pressure, they often erode the cartilaginous and even bony substance of the ribs; and La Faye relates a case in which a part of the sternum, as well as two cartilages of the ribs, was hereby destroyed.—(*Phil. Trans.*, N. 287.) In an enormous aneurism of the abdominal aorta, Morgagni mentions that the pos-

terior wall of the artery itself was destroyed, the neighbouring parts supplying the place of a wall (*De Sed. et Caus. Morb.*, Ep. xl., 26): and, in a like aneurism of the thoracic aorta, he found the bones in the vicinity broken and demolished by the force of its pressure.—(Ep. xvii., 25–27.)

SPECIES II.
EXANGIA VARIX.
VARIX.

SOFT, LIVID TUMOUR OF A VEIN.

THIS disease is to veins what the true or encysted aneurism is to arteries. The coats of the veins are preternaturally dilated, and more in some parts than in others, so that a vein thus enlarged to any considerable extent often appears to be a chain of venous cysts; and as contiguous veins often communicate, the enlargement is not unfrequently extended from one to another, till the whole forms a plexus of varices, and every part seems ready to burst. In some instances, they do actually burst.

This affection mostly occurs in the veins of the lower extremities, in consequence of their being the most dependant part. They often arise spontaneously in persons of lax fibres; but are far more frequently a consequence of undue fatigue, strains, cramps, or pressure. The most frequent cause is a pressure of the fœtus in pregnancy against the external iliac veins, in consequence of which the blood ascends with difficulty from all the inferior veins, which become distended and weakened by its accumulation.

From strains and other causes, however, varices have been occasionally traced in other large veins than those of the extremities. Thus Tozzetti discovered one after death in the *vena azygos* (*Prima Raccolta di Osservazioni Medici*, Firenze, 1752); and Michaelis describes another, that terminated fatally, in the jugular vein.* They are also met with in the spermatic veins; and, in this position, have very generally been described under the incorrect name of circoceie or varicose rupture. Morgagni asserts that the spermatic varix appears more frequently on the left than on the right side, from the insertion of the spermatic vein into the emulgent.—(*De Sed. et Caus. Morb.*, Ep. xliii., art. 34.) They are often possessed of considerable irritability in themselves, and almost always add in a high degree to the irritability of diseased

---

* Mémoires sur la Nature et le Traitement de plusieurs Maladies, tom. iv., 8vo., Paris, 1819. The cysts or partial dilatations of the heart here spoken of vary in size, from that of an almond to that of a hen's egg. Sometimes the parietes of the heart around them are thickened, sometimes remarkably attenuated. These pouches contain very solid layers of concrete fibrin, just as a common aneurismal sac does, to which they correspond in more than one point. M. Breschet, who has drawn up an interesting memoir on this form of disease, names it *false* consecutive aneurism of the heart; an appellation disapproved of by M. Andral, because dissection does not always exbibit a laceration of the lining of the heart.—Anat. Pathol., tom. ii., p. 290.—ED.

* See Richter's Chirurgische Bibliothek, in loco. The best modern pathologists make a distinction between simply enlarged and tortuous veins, and those which are varicose. The former are not attended with any disease of their coats, or with any changes disqualifying them for the due performance of the blood; whereas true varicose veins are accompanied with disease of their coats, and more or less obstruction of their canals. In Cruveilhier's Anat. Pathol., livr. xvi., may be seen an interesting representation of an enormous enlargement and tortuosity of all the subcutaneous veins on the forepart of the abdomen, causing a swelling, which he compares to a Medusa's head; the case was simple dilatation, not varix.—ED.

parts in the vicinity, so that if an ulcer take place contiguously, it will rarely admit of a cure till the varix be first removed.—(*Mém. de l'Acad. Royale des Sciences à Paris,* Ann. 1707.)

The best remedy, in all cases where it can be applied, is a moderate, steady, and continued pressure, which, where the varix occurs in the legs, is easily accomplished by an elastic stocking, or, which is preferable, a circular bandage of fine elastic flannel. Dauter's plan of using cold water is also a very simple, and, where the varix is fresh, not unfrequently a very efficacious remedy (*Von dem äuserlichen ortlichen Gebranche des Kalten Wassers,* &c., Leips., 1784, 4to.) ; but how far a solution of mineral acids or metallic salts may add to its virtue, as recommended by some practitioners, the author cannot affirm from his own practice.

[In cases which resisted compression, and were attended with a painful ulcer that would not heal, Sir Everard Home tied the trunk of the vena saphena, as it passes over the knee-joint. Many severe and fatal consequences, however, having resulted from this practice, Mr. Brodie conceived that it would be safer to cut the vein completely through, leaving the superincumbent skin undivided, a plan easily accomplished with a narrow, sharp-pointed, slightly-curved bistoury.*] The attempt to cure varices by the knife or ligature has succeeded where there is neither local nor constitutional irritability, but it has more frequently failed, and the inflammation hereby produced has occasionally proved fatal.† Yet, where the effect is less extensive, it is apt to be followed by a serious and far more diffuse enlargement of the vein, with varicose prominences, similar to that which sometimes occurs in drawing blood from the arm, of which, till of late years, no very intelligent explanation has been given, and which I shall, therefore, endeavour briefly to illustrate.

This singular and painful line of swelling was at first supposed to arise from the prick of a nerve, and it is perfectly clear that the tingling and shooting pains which succeed venesection are sometimes produced by a partial division of a nerve, from an interesting case of Mr. Sherwen, of Enfield, that only yielded to an entire division of the nerve by a transverse section above the orifice, after every other attempt had been tried in vain.‡ But the nerves of the arm liable to be wounded in bleeding are mostly small and unimportant ; while others are often pricked and wounded in many of the common operations of surgery, without any serious consequence whatever. The mischief has by other writers, as Heister, Garengeot, and Haller, been ascribed to wounding a tendon or its aponeurosis, but, unluckily for such physiologists, tendons in other places are often torn or wounded with very little inconvenience. Even the Achilles tendon, the largest in the body, is frequently broken without any of the severe symptoms that sometimes arise from bloodletting. Besides which, the accident from bleeding occurs as frequently when a person has been bled in a vein which has no tendon near it, as where there is reason to expect that a tendon may have been wounded. It happens as often that a swelled arm is the consequence of bleeding in the cephalic or cephalic-median vein as of bleeding in the basilic or basilic-median.

Mr. J. Hunter was the first physiologist who ascertained the real cause of the mischief before us, and traced it to a general principle, which he laid down as applicable to all internal cavities, namely, that when injured or rendered otherwise imperfect, they are often apt to inflame at the injured part, and to have the inflammation spread rapidly over their whole extent, as I have already had an opportunity of observing under peritonitis, puerperal fever, and on various other occasions. He was first led to this view of the cause in the case of veins from noticing what occasionally happens to horses. It is no uncommon thing for hostlers, out of an unnecessary or ill-judged care, to bleed these animals in the neck, even when in perfect health ; and, in several instances of this kind, Mr. Hunter had observed that the neck swelled and the horse died ; and, on examining the nature of the disease by dissection, he found that the cavity of the vein was inflamed, and that the inflammation had spread along its internal surface to the chest, sometimes even to the heart itself. And he afterward found a like effect produced in the veins of the human arm, where inflammation had succeeded to bleeding, and particularly in one case that occurred in St. George's Hospital, being that of a man who died suddenly on the eighth day after having been bled in the basilic vein of the right arm, and having suffered from inflammation as a consequence. On dissecting the arm, he found not only that the cavity of the vein had inflamed, but that the inflammation had extended from the puncture which had been made by the lancet in bloodletting, as high as the axilla, proceeding also to some distance below the puncture. About the middle of the arm the vein had suppurated, and, from the ulceration or absorption of parts which attends abscesses, the vein was divided into two, and each extremity, like the internal surface of the abscess, was irregular and jagged.

Mr. Hunter was disposed to think that the principal cause which produces the inflammation of a vein after bleeding is the want of a disposition to heal, arising either from its being exposed, or in consequence of the lips of the orifice in the skin not being properly brought together. And he hence strongly advises that the sides of an opened vein should at all times be made to approximate as accurately as possible, and that the orifice in the skin should be drawn to one side of that in the vein, so as to make the skin do the office of a valve to the venal opening.—(*Edin. Med. Com.,* vol. iii., p. 430.)

---

* See Med. Chir. Trans., vol. vii., p. 195. Mr. Mayo obliterates varicose veins by applying a caustic paste over them.—ED.

† Observations on Varix, &c., by Richard Carmichael, &c., Trans. King's and Queen's Coll., Dublin, vol. ii., p. 345, 1824.

‡ Edin. Med. Comment., vol. v., p. 430.—See also Stud. of Med., vol. i., Cl. III., Ord. II., Gen. VI., Spe. 5.

There seems, however, in this explanation, to be a something wanting, and I cannot avoid thinking, as in the case of puerperal fever, that there must be, at the same time, some peculiar local or constitutional irritability predisposing the injured part to run into an inflammatory action; a striking instance of which, already slightly alluded to, occurs in a case communicated by Dr. A. Duncan. The patient, himself of the medical profession, twenty-eight years of age, had opened a boil on his hand with a lancet which had been applied to an obscure sore on the back of another person about a month previously, but against which no proof of being either poisoned or unclean could be brought forward. The inflammation, instead of subsiding after opening the tumour, increased, and spread up the arm to the axilla; but the swelling was attended with little redness, and no acute pain, though with considerable fever and restlessness. The affected arm, three days afterward, exhibited one or two red streaks running up from the elbow to the shoulder, in the course of the cephalic vein; the breathing was much affected, quick and short, but without pain in the chest; there was a troublesome cough, and the expectoration, though small in quantity, was tinged with blood. The countenance was anxious, depressed, and of a leaden hue; the features sharpened; the eyes sunk and dull; tongue foul; pulse a hundred and ten strokes in a minute. These symptoms increased in violence, with transient fits of delirium and subsultus tendinum; the intumescence of the arm, however, remaining to the eye much the same, with little complaint of pain. The patient sunk gradually in just a week from the first appearance of local affection, and ten days after using the lancet.

On examining the body, much chronic disease was found in the chest; the cartilages of the ribs on one side were slightly ossified: there was a general adhesion of the lungs to the costal pleura, pericardium, and diaphragm, with a recent effusion of coagulable lymph; in some places a little coloured, and occasionally evincing a few fibrous shreds. The substance of the lungs appeared also generally unsound, and in some parts contained tubercles and calculi, one of the tubercles being as large as a nut, and filled with a yellow, purulent-looking fluid.

The general health had borne up under all these chronic sappings, undisturbed, to the time of the local affection of the hand, as also under a protracted fatigue, through the whole of the preceding winter, from a course of hard professional study, augmented, still more lately, by great mental anxiety and disappointment. All these seem to have produced a morbid excitement of habit, which, though not fatal of itself, gave a fatal tendency to the inflammation on the hand, or rather to the irritation of the cephalic vein, which was probably pricked on opening the bile, as will be sufficiently obvious from the appearances of the limb on dissection. Many livid spots were observed externally: the opened and unhealed ulcer was found to be accompanied with a swelling of the cellular substance, extending, more or less, up the whole arm: and,

VOL. II.—I

on making a long incision from this ulcer to the top of the shoulder, a small abscess was accidentally entered into at the bend of the arm, which proved to be the cephalic vein accidentally divided, and unfolded the immediate seat of mischief. The vein appeared full of purulent matter, and, in consequence, was carefully traced through its entire range. "The disease of the vein consisted in external redness, arising from the increased size of the vasa vasorum; thickening of all its coats, so that it remained, like an artery, round without collapsing; increased size, especially in the forearm; its containing no blood in any part of its course, and being generally filled with purulent matter, except in a few places where it seemed empty; and in the inner coat being everywhere red and thickened. The veins coming from the back of the forefinger, middle, and ring-finger, were all diseased, but that from the little finger was healthy."*

PHLEBITIS is far more easily produced than ARTERITIS, as veins are more irritable than arteries; but we hence learn that even the former is occasionally influenced by constitutional excitements

---

SPECIES III.
EXANGIA CYANIA.
BLUE-SKIN.

SKIN MORE OR LESS BLUE; LIPS PURPLE; GENERAL HEBETUDE AND INACTIVITY.

THIS species is designed to express that singular appearance and diseased state of the entire system, produced mostly by a connate communication of the two ventricles of the heart, and consequently, an imperfect discharge of the carbon of the blood at the lungs, which constitute the proper organ of its elimination. From the Greek κύανος, or "blue," Sir Alex-

* At the present day, our knowledge of the frequency and nature of phlebitis has been much increased. We are now aware that it may arise not merely from the puncture or mechanical irritation of a vein, but may arise as a consequence of any surgical operation or accidental injury, and of any suppurative disease. Cruveilhier seems to the editor to claim the merit of having given the most rational explanation of the cause of its severe and often fatal character. When a vein inflames and suppurates, or pus is introduced into it, this fluid circulates with the blood, and reaches the venous capillaries, in which it excites obstruction, inflammation, and abscesses. Cruveilhier found, that when he introduced any extraneous fluid or matter into veins which communicate with the vena portæ, abscess in the liver was excited; but if the veins so treated were of the system more directly connected with the vena cava, the abscess often formed in the lungs, joints, serous cavities, &c. If it be asked why the absorption of pus from common abscesses has no such effects, the answer which Cruveilhier would make is, that here the pus is so altered or modified by the action of the organs of absorption upon it, that the evil is thus prevented. Some of the best observations on phlebitis are contained in Cruveilhier's Anat. Pathol.—ED.

ander Crichton, in allusion to the colour of the skin by which it is peculiarly distinguished, has elegantly named it CYANIA, and the term has been adopted as a specific appellation on the present occasion.*

Antecedently to birth, the lungs are of small comparative importance to the functions of life and growth, and hence no more blood seems to circulate through them than is necessary for their development and health. The florid or decarbonated blood, instead of being received from the lungs by the pulmonary veins, is received from the placenta by the venæ cavæ, and passes for the most part at once into the general circulation, chiefly by means of the foramen ovale, by which the two ventricles communicate, and partly by means of the ductus arteriosus, by which the pulmonary artery at this time anastomoses with the aorta; that portion of blood only which escapes through this canal flowing forward into the collapsed substance of the lungs; amounting probably to not more than a third or a fourth part of the whole.

Immediately on birth, however, the plan of decarbonization is immediately changed. The fœtal duct and foramen are closed, and the whole mass of blood flows, black instead of florid, from the venæ cavæ into the heart, and is sent by the pulmonary artery to the lungs for ventilation, instead of to the placenta, in which organ, by the disengagement of the carbon with which it is loaded, and partly perhaps by the absorption of oxygen from the respired air (for the subject is still open to controversy), it acquires its perfeet elaboration and florid hue.

Hence if, in consequence of any aberration from the common law which regulates the functine heart and its attached vessels at the time of birth, either of these communications should remain open, the venous or black blood must wholly, or in a very considerable degree, be thrown back again into the general circulation, instead of passing to the lungs: and the minute arteries on the surface, which give to the complexion its tinge, being filled with the same, the general hue must be changed from a florid to a blue or purple, more or less deep, according as the pulmonary circulation is more or less impeded. This natural defect constitutes the disease before us. In the varicose aneurism, a small part of the florid or arterial blood flows through an accidental opening into the veins, but never in such a quantity as to disturb the economy of general health. In cyania a much larger, but variable proportion, of the black or venous blood, flows by a physical opening into the arteries; and usually with serious inconvenience to the general health, most commonly indeed with fatal effects.

* A variety of cyania, not noticed by the author, is found to result occasionally from the internal use of the nitrate of silver. This fact was known to Fourcroy.—(See Médecine éclairée par les Sciences Physiques, tom. i., p. 342.) The cases detailed by Drs. Albers and Roget are highly interesting and curious.—See Med. Chir. Trans., vol. vii., p. 284, et seq.—ED.

How far the ordinary disengagement of carbon from the blood may be dispensed with, or, in other words, to what extent these connate communications may remain, and the present disease take place, without endangering the life, we have no exact means of ascertaining. Dissections have shown us that the foramen ovale has continued partially open to old age, without much or even any interference with the common functions of health (*Geschichte einer Chirurg. Privatgesellschaft in Kopenhagen; Bertholin, Anal. Reform.*, lib. li., cap. 8): but we may confidently assert that, whenever so large a portion of venous blood is thrown into the arterial circulation as to give a blue or purple tinge to the lips or the skin generally, all the functions will be performed feebly, and there is great danger that the infant will never reach the age of puberty. There may be living power enough in the blood to support the growth of the frame during the retired and quiet tenour of infancy, in which there are no sudden exertions or calls for a more than ordinary expenditure of sensorial power; and hence it is no uncommon thing for a child to survive the first three or four years of life with a skin completely blue, and consequently with a full proof that the foramen ovale, or the ductus arteriosus, or both, are open to a very considerable extent, and that not more than perhaps a third or fourth part of the general current of the blood passes into the lungs and undergoes the process of ventilation. But as soon as a more active period of life commences, and the child is trusted to its feet, and engages, or should engage, in the pursuits or even amusements of boyhood, with all its physical and moral excitements, the living power is not adequate to the demands made upon it, and he sinks beneath their oppression, and generally expires in a fainting fit. There is commonly, moreover, through the short and pitiable term of his existence, the clearest proof of general torpitude and deficient energy; every exertion is a trouble, every stimulus produces fatigue; the muscles enlarge, but they want vigour and elasticity; and so far as I have seen, the faculties of the mind are equally blunted. The celebrated blue-boy, described by Dr. Sandifort, advanced farther towards an adult age than is by any means common. Here the aorta took its rise from both ventricles; the pulmonary artery was scarcely pervious to a small probe, and the difficulty of passing the probe from the heart to the lungs was greater than in the contrary direction. The patient was affected with an asthma from his second year, and terminated the miserable series of his sufferings in his thirteenth.—(*Observationes Anatomico-pathologicæ*, Lugd. Bat., 1777, 4to.) In the case of a young female, related by Morgagni, the term of life was protracted to the sixteenth year; but there appears to have been a somewhat freer communication with the lungs, notwithstanding that the foramen ovale was wide enough to admit the little finger. The patient, however, was sickly from her birth, and laboured under great general debility; her respiration was difficult, and her whole skin of a livid colour.—(*De Caus. et Sed.* ep. xvi.) Dr. Holmes has lately communicated a similar case, but where the passage was somewhat more free; the patient in consequence reached the age of twenty-one, and then died of dropsy.—(*Trans. of the Medico-Chir. Soc. of Edin.*, vol. i., art. vi., 8vo., 1824.)

Life, however, for a short time, has been maintained under still more complicated misformations of the heart and adjoining arteries. Mr. Standert gives the case of a blue-child, that lived ten days, in which the two ventricles communicated; there was no pulmonary artery, but its place was supplied by an artery that branched off to the lungs from the aorta in the situation of the ductus arteriosus, the blood from which was returned by four small pulmonary veins.—(*Phil. Trans.*, 1805, p. 228.) And, in Dr. Baillie's Morbid Anatomy, is a still more complicated case of a child that lived about two months, in which the two ventricles communicated, but seemed to change their respective offices; the aorta arising from the right ventricle, and the pulmonary artery from the left. The arterious duct was also open.—(Plate vi., p. 21.) Richerand, however, gives an example, and it is the only one I am acquainted with, of a man who, under this disease, reached the age of forty-one: his flesh was of a relaxed fibre, his colour uniformly blue; and he could only sleep in a sitting position.—(*Physiology*, &c.)*

In a few instances this disease has been suspected to arise subsequently to birth, from some injury or diseased condition of the heart. Corvisart has related a case of this kind, that terminated fatally, in a boy twelve and a half years old, and who had manifested no symptoms of the disease till five months before he saw him, which was on his admission into the Clinique Interne, April 21, 1797. His countenance was puffed, his lips violet, his restlessness extreme. He died on the 25th of the same month. On dissection, a foramen was found between the two ventricles, capable of admitting the little finger.†

---

* In the Archives Générales de Médecine, Sept., 1827, a still more curious case is mentioned. The subject lived till he was 35 years of age, was married, and was the father of five children. He had been affected with extreme agitations, palpitations, paroxysms of asthma, and even syncopæ. On dissection, it was found that the septum between the ventricles of the heart was deficient.—D.

† Cyania may occur, however, without any open communication between the right and left cavities of the heart; a fact particularly pointed out by Corvisart. On the other hand, such communication may exist without cyania being produced. Dr. Crampton has seen several cases of this description. In one the communications were so capacious, that the heart might have been regarded as consisting of only one auricle and one ventricle.—(Med. Trans. of Dublin College, vol. i., new series.) Breschet met with an instance in which the subclavian arose from the pulmonary artery, and yet there was no blue nor purple discoloration of the parts supplied by the ramifications of that vessel. Cyania of the face sometimes originates, as Corvisart explains, from the influence of organic disease in the right cavities of the heart upon the whole venous system. Under the same circumstances, the mucous tissues

In distressing affections of this kind the art of medicine is unavailable, and all we can advise is perfect tranquillity; a light diet, and attention to the state of the bowels. In one instance, and only one, I have seen the blueness of the skin gradually disappear a few months after birth, and the child grew stout; evidently proving that the morbid communication, whether in the foramen or the arterious duct, was closed by a natural process.*

GENUS XII.

GANGRÆNA.

GANGRENE.

THE DEATH OF A PORTION OF THE BODY, WHILE THE REST CONTINUES ALIVE, OFTEN IN A SOUND STATE.

GANGRÆNA, sphacelus, and necrosis, have been hitherto used in very indefinite senses, sometimes as synonymes, and sometimes as different stages of a common disease. And even in this last view they have rarely preserved their gradations with any thing like a uniform consent; the whole of them sometimes expressing the highest, and sometimes an inferior degree of the malady they equally import: For reasons stated in the volume of Nosology, the first of these terms is here employed in a generic sense, and the two latter as subdivisions or species included under it: sphacelus importing mortification, as it occurs in its ordinary form, with lividity, vesication, ulceration, and fetor; and necrosis, that insensibility and shivering of the flesh which occasionally occur in paralytic limbs. The genus will also extend to two other species: as the gangrene which commences in a bone, and is usually called a caries; and that peculiar form of the disease which begins insensibly in the extremities, and spreads without fever in an ascending direction, till the affected limbs drop off in succession.

All these will therefore be treated of in the following order.

1. Gangræna Sphacelus.   Mortification.
2. —————— Ustilaginea. Mildew mortification.

---

are liable to become injected, in old persons, with dark blood. Obstruction to the free passage of blood through the aorta, joined with hypertrophy of the heart, retardation of the pulmonary circulation, and plethora of the right ventricle and auriele, may likewise bring on cyania, or, as it is more frequently named, cyanosis.—ED.

* The details of fifty-six cases of cyanosis may be seen in Gintrac, Observations et Recherches sur la Cyanose, Paris, 1824; and Meckel, in Archiv. f. d. Physiol., vol. i., p. 221, has given a table of seventy-seven separate observations. Cases of the same have been recorded by American writers, as Jackson, Dorsey, and Thaxter, in the N. E. Journ. of Med. and Surg., vols. i., iii., and v.; by Perkins and Hoffman, in New-York Med. and Phys. Journal, vols. ii. and vi., and by Coates and Mauran, in Phil. Journ. of the Med. and Phys. Sc., vols. ix. and xiv.—See likewise Blue Disease, in a Dict. of Pract. Medicine, by James Copland, Boston, 1834.—D.

3. Gangræna Necrosis·   Dry Gangrene.
4. ———— Caries.   Caries.*

SPECIES I.
GANGRÆNA SPHACELUS.
MORTIFICATION.

THE DEAD PART SOFT, MOIST, CORRUPT, AND HIGHLY OFFENSIVE.

MORTIFICATION signifies the death of a portion of the soft parts, sometimes including also the bones, as when the whole limb mortifies. It is not, however, simply the death of parts occasioned in any kind of way, for when a piece of flesh is removed from the body by excision, its vital principle soon ceases; yet this is not mortification in the technical sense of the term. On the contrary, mortification is preceded by certain changes in the parts about to perish, which are generally converted into a brown or black, fetid, cold, insensible mass, with which the general nervous and vascular systems have no longer any organic connexion. The parts thus altered and deprived of vitality are called sloughs. In consequence of the discontinuance of the living principle, the laws of animal chymistry, previously held in subjection by its superior sway, acquire an ascendency; a play of chymical affinities takes place; and putrefaction, or a decomposition of the organized substance, and a restoration of its constituent parts to their elementary forms, necessarily ensue.

It is from this cause the affected part becomes soft, corrupt, and offensive, and is called *moist gangrene*; and not from an accumulation of animal juices, as stated by Professor Frank; "ob succorum stagnantium aut corruptorum abundantiam."—(Op. cit., tom. ii., p. 18.)

The total debility, insensibility, or torpitude, attending gangrene, may be produced by too much or too little action or excitement; for the vital flame may be supplied so rapidly as to destroy by its own violence, or there may be no supply whatever. And we are hence furnished with the two following varieties of the disease:

α Inductus.   Superinduced mortification.
β Atonicus.   Atonic mortification.

The ordinary causes of the first are fever, inflammation, local violence, or severe cold. Those of the second are old age, impure air, scanty or innutritious food; and for the same reason, as Sir Clifton Wintringham has observed, ossification in the arteries of the part affected; which is, indeed, chiefly a consequence of old age.— (*Comment. de Morbis quibusdam, &c.*, No. liv.)

Where mortification originates from a severe contusion or other injury, in a person of florid and vigorous health, and in the prime of life, we have an example of the FIRST VARIETY. There is in this case high inflammatory action, great heat, swelling, and pulsation; the vessels are supplied with a superabundance of living power (the excitability of the Brunonians), and are in consequence excited beyond their strength; they are hence worn out by the impetuosity of the toil, lose their tone, and the parts become torpid and insensible from the vehemence of their own exertion.*

The SECOND VARIETY may be illustrated by the mortification which so frequently takes place in the extremities of persons already exhausted by hard labour, intemperance, or advanced years, and whose extremities are bloated and anasarcous. In this case, instead of a superabundant supply of living power, there is little or no power whatever; for the whole circulation is languid, and the nervous energy now scarcely reaches the extremities, and particularly the lower limbs, the muscular fibres of which, however, are in themselves so inirritable, that a more than ordinary excitement is scarcely capable of rousing them; and hence they yield to the process of putrefaction from a cause the very reverse of what operates in the preceding case.†

Under the first form there is more pain and fever, as there is more sensibility and violence, than under the second; and, on this account, the destructive march is more rapid; but, with these exceptions, the symptoms, which are the ordinary ones of putrefaction, are the same. The colour of the skin changes to a dark red or livid hue; the cuticle is separated from the true skin by the interposition of an ichorous fluid, contained in vesicles, or bullæ, or diffused generally; it bursts by degrees; and the subjacent integuments are cold, black, flaccid, sloughy, and insensible; with a sanious or bloody discharge of a most offensive smell.—(*Frank, De Cur. Hóm. Morb.*, class ii., sect. 130.)

---

* The mere torpidity or insensibility of parts would not amount to sphacelus, or complete mortification, or even to any degree of it whatever; for, as the editor has elsewhere explained, the entire and unalterable cessation of every action and function in the part is absolutely essential to what is understood by sphacelus. Sensibility and power of motion may be annihilated, and yet the part affected continue to live, as is daily exemplified in cases of paralysis. In a palsied limb, the temperature of the parts and the force of the circulation are also lessened; yet the fluids pursue their usual course, nutrition and absorption are carried on, and the parts continue to retain, for an indefinite length of time, an inferior degree of vitality. Gangrene, however, in the sense in which it was used by Galen, and is still often used by the moderns, signifies the first stage of mortification, when there seems to be a partial but not total destruction of the parts, when the blood still circulates through some of the larger vessels, and the nerves retain a portion of their sensibility.—See First Lines of the Practice of Surgery, p. 37 and 39, 5th edit.

† "Mortification always spreads more extensively in cellular membrane than in the skin and muscles; a fact particularly worthy of recollection when amputation is to be performed."—Op. cit., p. 39.

---

* The sense of the term *necrosis*, as employed by the author, does not coincide with that commonly assigned to it by modern writers, and which is a mortification of a more or less extensive portion, or even of the whole of a bone; while *caries*, instead of being promiscuously used to denote either the mortification of bone, or the process in this structure analogous to ulceration of the soft parts, is now restricted by many judicious pathologists exclusively to the latter affection.—ED.

[One remarkable circumstance always attending sphacelus, but not noticed by the author, appears to merit attention, as it demonstrates the friendly effort made by nature for the preservation of the patient : when a limb sphacelates, the blood coagulates in the large arteries leading to the parts affected, and this for some distance from the line which marks the extent of their destruction. Now if this were not the case, the patient would inevitably bleed to death as soon as the process takes place by which the sloughs are thrown off; but, except in hospital gangrene and phagædenic sloughing, hemorrhage is rarely to be feared in mortification.]

If the sphacelus meet with no check from art or nature, it spreads rapidly in every direction, particularly under the first variety ; and more especially when aided by an impure or unventilated atmosphere, of which the hospital gangrene, as it is called, furnishes us with a fearful example. "I have seen," says Dr. Hennen, "the external ear and the palpebræ destroyed in this manner, as if in a series of concentric circles. Even upon surfaces barely contiguous, as the fingers and toes, it generally spreads in a similar way ; so that the sore which might have been on the middle finger or toe, and confined entirely to it in the morning dressing, by night engaged the adjoining sound ones, and in less than twelve hours more embraced the whole foot or hand. The gangrene still advancing, fresh sloughs[*] were rapidly formed, the increasing cup-like cavity was filled up and overtopped by them, and the erysipelatous livor and vesication of the surrounding skin gained ground, while chains of inflamed lymphatics could be traced from the sores to the adjoining glands ; thus exciting inflammation and suppuration, which often furnished a new nidus for gangrene. The face of the sufferer assumed a ghastly, anxious appearance ; his eyes became haggard, and deeply tinged with bile ; his tongue loaded with a brown or blackish fur ; his appetite entirely failed him ; and his pulse was considerably sunk in strength, and proportionally accelerated."

During this state Dr. Hennen adds, that the bravest soldiers betrayed "the greatest imaginable impatience of pain and depression of spirits. Men who had borne amputation without a groan, shrunk at the washing of their sores, and shuddered at the sight of a dead comrade ; or even, on hearing the report of his death, predicted their own dissolution, and sunk into sullen despair. The third and last stage was now fast approaching. The surface of the sore was covered with a bloody oozing ; and on lifting up the edge of the flabby slough, the probe was tinged with dark-coloured grumous blood, with which also its track became immediately filled : repeated and copious venous bleedings now came on, which rapidly sunk the patient ; the sloughs, whether falling off spontaneously or detached by art, were quickly succeeded by others, and discovered on their removal small thickly-studded specks of arterial blood. At length an artery sprung, which, in the attempt to secure it, most probably burst under the ligature : the tourniquet or pressure was now applied, but in vain ; for while it checked the bleeding it accelerated the death of the limb, which became frightfully swelled and horribly fetid. Incessant retchings soon came on, and with cauma, involuntary stools, and hiccough, closed the scene." —(Principles of Military Surgery, 2d edit., 8vo., Edin., 1810.)

In this severity of attack and debility of the system, the most compact parts of the solids fall a prey, as well as those that are more loose ; but when the atmosphere is purer or more bracing, and the strength firmer, the cellular texture first and chiefly suffers. And we are hence able to understand the meaning of Dr. Riberi, of Turin, who, in describing a similar gangrene in the hospital of San Giovanni in that city, during the years 1817–1820, tells us that it often alternated from a sphacelating to an erysipelatous inflammation, the latter appearing as the former began to cease; on the return of a cooler or drier air ; or, where both co-existed, the slighter erysipelatous affection being limited to the more robust patients, or those who were fortunate enough to lie in the best ventilated parts of the sick wards.—(Sulla Gangrena Contagiosa o Nosocomiale, Turino, 8vo., 1821.)

In this extreme form of gangrene a septic principle appears to be developed, capable of propagating the same disease by contagion ; for not only "upon surfaces barely contiguous" was it found to obtain an existence, but "the skin of other persons, although perfectly sound, which had been touched with a sponge employed in washing the gangrenous sores, ulcerated, and soon became itself a slough. This," adds Dr. Hennen, "was often observable among the orderlies and nurses ;" and the description of Riberi does not essentially differ.

The treatment belongs rather to the department of surgery than that of medicine. It is obvious, however, that, under the above two varieties, it must be greatly varied to meet the variety of cause and constitution. Where an inflammatory diathesis is present, evacuants of every kind must be had recourse to, as venesection, purging, and relaxants, while the local applications should consist of refrigerant epithems till the entonic action is completely reduced ; after which, bark and the mineral acids, with a nutritive, but not a stimulant diet, should be chiefly relied upon ; and if the fetor be considerable, powdered charcoal, or the yest or carrot poultice, should be applied topically. But where, on the contrary, the mortification is that of atony, the warmest tonics and stimulants are demanded, both locally and generally, from the first.

---

* In hospital gangrene the sloughs are not like those of common sphacelus ; but the disease is attended with a rapid and singular mode of decomposition in the mortified parts, of which hardly any vestiges appear. No ordinary sloughs are seen ; but, in lieu of them, the surface of the diseased part is covered with a whitish or ash-coloured viscid matter, which exhibits at particular points specks of blood.—See First Lines of the Practice of Surgery, p. 40, 5th edit. ; Delpech, Précis des Maladies Chirurg., tom. i., p. 75 ; R. Welbank, in Med. Chir. Transact., vol. ii. ; and Blackadder on Phagedæna Gangrænosa, Edin., 1818.

If the limb be frostbitten, and there be danger of mortification from this source, a plan of treatment will be requisite, different from both the above, the advantage of which is known to every one, though the principle upon which it acts has never been clearly explained.

The torpitude or insensibility of the part affected is in this case evidently produced by the exhausting power of the cold, which destroys or extinguishes the irritable and sensorial principle as rapidly as it is supplied. Putrefaction, however, or a decomposition of the organic structure, does not readily ensue, because the auxiliaries of this change, and which are absolutely necessary to its production, such as heat, air, and moisture, are not present; for, as the parts become frozen, they lose their moisture or fluidity, and as there is no breach of surface, there is no communication with the external air. When a limb in this state is suddenly brought before the fire, it becomes gangrenous almost instantly; for, by this means, putrefaction obtains possession of these auxiliaries, and, in its process, gains the start of the remedial or restorative power of nature. And hence it is well known, that the worst thing that can be done to a frozen limb is to bring it into such a situation. On the contrary, if we give time to this restorative power to exert itself, while we prevent the process of putrefaction from taking place, by keeping the limb very nearly in the same condition of freezing, or rather by raising it out of this condition by slow and imperceptible degrees, we shall have the best chance of recovering it to life; since we hereby afford an opportunity for the warm and circulating blood and the active principle of irritability to push forward once more into the vessels of the frozen structure, which, however weakened and insentient, have not yet become decomposed.

The advantage of plunging a frozen limb first into ice-water, and afterward into water raised just above the freezing point, and in this manner advancing it gradually to a common temperature, is of general notoriety; and it is this plan which forms the usual treatment. In what way the benefit is accomplished has been a frequent subject of inquiry; the remarks just offered may perhaps afford a satisfactory explanation of the subject.

[The treatment of hospital gangrene differs very materially from that of other cases of mortification; but, as the subject is strictly surgical, all that need be mentioned in the present place is, that the local applications by which it is most effectually checked, are the undiluted mineral acids, strong arsenical lotions, and, according to Delpech, the actual cautery.]

SPECIES II.

GANGRÆNA USTILAGINEA.

MILDEW MORTIFICATION.

GANGRENE DRY, DIFFUSE, DIVERGENT, COMMENCING IN THE EXTREMITIES, WITHOUT FEVER OR INTUMESCENCE, AND SPREADING TILL VARIOUS LIMBS DROP OFF IN SUCCESSION:

GREAT HEBETUDE OF MIND AND BODY; OFTEN WITH VIOLENT SPASMS.

THIS is the *necrosis ustilaginea* of Sauvages, the specific epithet being derived from the cause to which it has commonly been ascribed, and from which, in various cases, it seems to take its rise; I mean the use of grain vitiated or poisoned by the growth of parasitic plants in the interior of the culm or straw, chiefly the "ustilago," "blight or mildew;" whence the name of "*mildew mortification*" among ourselves, as that of ergot, or *spur*, among the French, from the resemblance which the mildewed or blighted corn bears to the spur of a cock, in Latin clavus, which is the name borne by this parasitic plant in the language of many botanists.

Grain, thus injured by some fungus or other, has been found, when employed as food, productive of two dreadful diseases, to both of which, indeed, the French have given the name of *ergot*, as occasioned by a common cause; as they have also that of *mal des ardens*, from the burning internal heat which is felt in either case. The one of these disorders is a typhus fever, with the general character of pestis, or what Sauvages calls *erysipelas pestilens*, which is synonymous with the third variety of PESTIS in the present work: the other is the migratory gangrene before us, which commences without fever in the hands and feet; with a sense of numbness and external coldness, a dusky or livid cuticle, great debility of mind and body, often violent spasmodic contractions (*Morgagni, De Caus. et Sed. Morb.*, Ep. lv., art. xxiv.; *Bresl. Sammlung.*, 1724, i., p. 643); and spreads rapidly over the system, till the fingers, arms, nose, legs, or thighs are affected, and some of them drop off spontaneously.

Mr. Pott has described a variety of dry or chronic mortification often met with in practice, but without appearing to satisfy himself with any particular cause. "Beginning," says he, "at the extremity of one or more of the small toes, in more or less time it passes on to the foot and ankle, and sometimes to a part of the leg, and, in spite of all the aid of physic and surgery, most commonly destroys the patient. It is very unlike to the mortification from inflammation, to that from external cold, from ligature or bandage, or to that which proceeds from any known and visible cause, and this as well in its attack as in its process. In some few instances it makes its appearance with little or no pain; but in by much the majority of these cases, the patients feel great uneasiness through the whole foot and joint of the ankle, particularly in the night, even before these parts show any mark of distemper, or before there is any other than a small discoloured spot on the end of one of the little toes.* Each sex is

------

* In a remarkable case of this species of mortification which the editor attended in the summer of 1828, with Mr. Hughes, of Newman's Row, Lincoln's Inn Fields, and which was also visited by Sir Astley Cooper, both feet and legs were attacked, and gradually destroyed, nearly up to the knees. The pulse varied from 100 to 130;

liable to it : but for one female in whom I have met with it, I think I may say that I have seen it in at least twenty males. I think, also, that I have much more often found it in the rich and voluptuous than in the labouring poor ; more often in great eaters than free drinkers. It frequently happens to persons advanced in life, but is by no means peculiar to old age. It is not in general preceded or accompanied by apparent distemperature either of the part or of the habit."

In its severer attacks, however, the constitution seems to be generally contaminated, the mind and body become equally debilitated, there is great irritability, and a tendency to convulsive action.

According to some statements, this singular disease is connected with a diseased state of the digestive organs, from excess of living, deleterious food, or some other cause in connexion with great nervous debility (*Home, Facts and Experiments,* p. 18 ; Ludwig, Adversar. i., i., 7, p. 188) ; and the tendency to gangrene proceeds rather from a deficiency of sensorial power than from any morbid condition of the circulating system,† whether atonic or entonic. And hence we find it best relieved by

---

and the stomach was so little disturbed that the patient used generally to eat a mutton chop for dinner until the last two or three days preceding his death, which took place about a month from the commencement of the disease. Until the final stage the patient had but little delirium. Two circumstances were particularly remarked: first, that the disease never extended itself without being preceded by violent pain in the part about to be destroyed, so that a judgment could always be formed beforehand, from the degree of suffering, whether the spreading of the disorder would be considerable or not ; secondly, that the process of mortification, and its appearance in one leg, were totally different from those exhibited in the other. In the left, the disorder began on the inside of one of the toes, and followed the course described by Pott ; in the right, a general diminution of the temperature of the foot and leg occurred, without any discoloration of the skin, or any vesications, or particular affection of the toes. The coldness was followed by total loss of sensibility in the parts, and cessation of the circulation and every other action in them ; the flesh was, in short, little more altered in appearance than that of the limb of a dead subject. It was a specimen of the *gangræna necrosis albida* of the present system.—Ed.

† An ossified state of the arteries leading to the mortified parts, and organic disease of the heart, have been detected in some examples of this species of chronic mortification ; but not so constantly as to appear to be an unequivocal cause of the disorder, especially as this is frequently not present where they exist. Yet, with old age and an impaired constitution, it is often suspected that they are capable of bringing on, or having some share in the production of this kind of mortification. Such were the ideas prevalent in this country about the causes of gangræna senilis ; but, of late, a new doctrine has been promulgated by the Baron Dupuytren, namely, that this variety of mortification is dependant upon arteritis, or inflammation of the small arteries leading to the parts affected.—(See Leçons Orales de Clinique Chirurgicale, tom. iv., p. 481, &c., 8vo., Paris, 1833.)

---

free doses of opium, in conjunction with a generous and even stimulant diet. Bark is of no avail, and the local use of spirituous fomentations and cataplasms, warm pungent oils and balsams, of as little. Mr. Pott tried them in every form, but without the smallest success ; and at length employed no other topical application than smooth, soft, unirritating poultices, and confined himself to the use of opium alone, of which he sometimes gave a grain every three hours. And under the influence of this medicine the progress of the gangrene has often become checked in a few days, and a line of separation distinctly marked ; soon after which the mortified parts have sloughed away, the diseased bone dropped spontaneously from the affected joint, healthy granulations succeeded, and in due time a cure has been effected.

SPECIES III.
GANGRÆNA NECROSIS.
DRY GANGRENE.
THE DEAD PART DRY, SHRIVELLED, HARD, AND DUSKY.

This singular species of gangrene seems to proceed from a marasmus or atrophy of the affected limb, in consequence of which, as in the atrophy of the body at large, the animal oil, flesh, and fluids also, are gradually absorbed, and the limb becomes emaciated and withered : " mummiæ instar pars affecta" (*De Cur. Hom. Morb. Epit.*, tom. ii., p. 18, 8vo., Mannh., 1792), says Professor Frank. During the progress of this change it necessarily grows feebler and more torpid, till at length it is no longer capable of receiving the nervous energy, and its different parts turn dead and rigid. In palsied limbs a termination of this kind is by no means uncommon.

In some instances of this affection the blood-vessels have collapsed, perhaps become obliterated, without a retention of any of the constituent principles of the circulating fluid, and consequently the withered limb has preserved something of the natural colour of the skin. In others, the red particles of the blood, changed, as in the veins, to a dark or livid hue, have, to a certain degree, remained in the vessels and given to the limb a purple or variegated die. And hence the species has laid a foundation for the two following varieties :—

α Albida.　　Retaining something of the White gangrene.　natural colour of the skin.
β Discolor.　　The natural colour changed Black gangrene.　to a livid, or a mixture of hues.

In consequence of such inflammation they are rendered impervious, and mortification is the result. The baron alleges that this view has been confirmed by *post-mortem* examinations, and, what is important to be taken into the account, be declares that, by having recourse to bleeding as well as opium, he stops the disorder, and saves not less than two thirds of his patients. When the notorious ill success with which this species of mortification is treated in Great Britain is recollected, we are bound to put Baron Dupuytren's statements to the test of experience.—Ed,

It has never hitherto been satisfactorily explained how it happens that, under this kind of mortification or death, the parts should not, as in the preceding species, fall a prey to putrefaction. Perhaps the following remarks may afford some clew to this singular exception. ·

We have already had occasion to observe, under the first species, that a frostbitten limb does not putrefy so long as it continues frozen, because the accessories or co-operative powers of putrefaction, without which this process cannot take place, are not present, such as warmth, moisture, and a free influx of air. Now none of these are present in the species before us ; for the limb is cold, completely emptied of its fluids, and impervious to atmospheric influence ; and, consequently, there are the same obstructions to putrefaction in dry gangrene as in a limb killed by the biting power of frost.

So in the burning sands of Egypt, a buried corpse is often found, if dug up a month or two after interment, with as few marks of putrefaction. I have said that warmth is a necessary auxiliary, but it must be warmth to a certain degree only ; for if it exceeds this, all the interior fluids will by the heat itself be raised towards the surface, and pass off rapidly in the form of vapour ; in consequence of which the animal substance whence they issue will be as destitute of moisture as if it were frozen, and hence as incapable of putrefying. Now this is the case with a body interred in the sultry sands of the Delta : all its fluids are so highly rarefied as to evaporate and be drunk up by the bibulous soil by which it is surrounded, before any organic decomposition takes place : and hence the buried corpse, instead of crumbling into dust, is converted into a kind of natural mummy, some parts of which exhibit proofs of that waxy fat to which the French chymists have given the name of adipocire ; but no part of which undergoes the decomposition of putrefaction. I do not mean that this is always the case, but that it has occurred in a variety of instances where the antiseptic incidents have been peculiarly favourable to such an effect.

And hence Dr. Frank tells us, that the dry gangrene sometimes changes to what is called humid, and, at others, converts the parts affected into a kind of mummy.—(*De Cur. Hom. Morb. Ep.*, class ii., § 130.)

Dr. Alix, of Altenburg, gives a singular example of the second variety of this species, in a man seventy-two years of age, which commenced, contrary to its usual course, with inflammatory symptoms. The back of the left hand was attacked with heat, swelling, and pain, accompanied with thirst, a smart fever, and delirium. At the time Dr. Alix saw him a blackness had spread over all the hand and part of the forearm, which were of a gangrenous hue, but without pain, and as hard as wood. The pulse was small and the spirits low. Amputation was advised, but not agreed to. About six months afterward he saw the patient again accidentally : the gangrene had spread up the elbow-joint, the limb was still without pain, the pulse was better, and there was no want of ap-

petite. As it was not supposed the man could live long, no further inquiries were made about him till a full year afterward, when he was found to be as firm and stout as ever, although he at this time laboured under a tertian inter-. mittent, and had lost one of his eyes. The gangrene had spread over the whole arm up to the shoulder-joint ; the limb still continued hard, and as black as smoked meat, but did not emit any cadaverous smell. In about a month from this time the arm dropped off spontaneously, without the least hemorrhage ; the exposed surface of the shoulder dried without any discharge whatever, and the old man, at the time of publishing the case, four years afterward, was in the enjoyment of a very good share of health.—(*Matthæi Francisci Alix, Med. et Chir. Doct.*, &c., *Observat. Chirurg.*, fasciculus i., 8vo., Altenburg, 1778.) In this instance the small proportion of living power, which continued after the inflammation had subsided, preserved the limb from putrefaction, aided by the hard and shrunk condition into which it had fallen from absorption, and a paralysis of the secernents.

Where there is no inflammation, topical stimulants, and especially of the oleaginous kind, as camphorated oils and warm balsams, with per- severing friction, are sometimes found useful in the commencement of this disease. Repeated blistering and setons have also proved serviceable, and the voltaic trough still more so, in conjunction with a nutritive and generous diet. But when the gangrene has established itself, medical skill can do nothing more than look on and lament its want of power.

SPECIES IV.
GANGRÆNA CARIES.
CARIES.

THE DEAD PART ORIGINATING IN A PORTION OF THE SUBJACENT BONE : PAIN DEEP-SEATED, SUPERJACENT INTEGUMENTS FLACCID AND DISCOLOURED.

BONES, notwithstanding their solidity, possess the same living power, and are subject to the same diseases, as are the soft parts. Like these, they are subject to a cessation or loss of this living principle, and the disease is in this case usually called a CARIES,* a Latin term, probably derived from the Hebrew כרה "*careh*," "to dig into, penetrate, or erode," "to scoop, or hollow out." It may originate in a bone itself, which constitutes a proper caries ; or it may be communicated from a superjacent ulceration, in which form it is more correctly denominated a carious ulcer.

The history and treatment of caries belong rather to the department of surgery than that of medicine, and are to be learned from writers on this branch of the profession who have expressly

---

* More frequently at the present day a *necrosis*, as already mentioned ; while the word caries is used by the best surgical writers to signify ulceration of bone.—See Dr. Cumin's Arrangement, &c., of Diseases of the Bones, in Edin. Med. Journal, No. lxxxii., p. 6.—ED.

treated of it, among whom may especially be mentioned Wiseman (*Surgery*, book ii., ch. 7), Petit (*Maladies des Os.*, tom. ii., ch. 16), and Monro ;* particularly the last, as his learned and ingenious essay on this subject ought to engage the attention of every one. The remarks, therefore, to which the author will limit himself, will be general and pathological, and as summary as possible.

Most of the causes that produce a gangrene in the soft parts, may produce a caries or gangrene in the bones : as external injuries, cold, and a deficiency of nutrition in consequence of old age or deleterious food. It is also not unfrequently produced by lues, porphyra, or scrofula. It is usually first ascertained, where there is no external ulcer, by an obtuse and deep-seated pain, which appears to issue from the bone ; an exostosis or protuberance of the bone or periosteum in the part affected, tenderness to the touch, a loose and flabby feel of the superincumbent integuments, and a discoloration of the skin. On being laid bare it evinces all the different modifications of sphacelus, which we have just noticed in the soft parts : for it is sometimes moist and wormeaten, forming the *caries vermoulé* of M. Petit, the cells being filled with a corrupt sanies or spongy caruncles, so that the whole assumes a quaggy appearance ; and sometimes dry and wasted ; and the dry variety, as in necrosis, is sometimes of a pale white, and sometimes of a black or livid hue. And hence M. Petit has subdivided the disease into four distinct species or varieties, founded on these remarks, but into which we have not space to follow him. The dry caries is generally the most superficial, and consequently exfoliates most easily ; the history and laws of which very curious process we have already pointed out under the genus APOSTEMA ; for the economy pursued by nature in the separation and removal of a dead soft part, is precisely the same as that pursued in the separation and removal of a dead portion of bone. The ancients attempted to expedite this by various means ; some of which were puerile, but others certainly calculated by their power to do either much good or a great deal of mischief ; particularly the destruction of the integuments by the potential cautery, and afterward an application of the actual cautery to the dead bone itself. Celsus gives a detailed account of this operation, which, when the caries was deep, was accompanied with numerous perforations into the bone, into each of which the hot iron was passed in succession.

[Instead of these formidable measures, which would destroy the bone if it were not already destroyed, and which are calculated to extend the destructive process in it farther than would otherwise be the case, modern practitioners are generally content either with simple unirritating applications, and awaiting the completion of ex-

foliation ; or, where this is too tedious and hopeless, they sometimes cut down the diseased portion of bone, and remove it by manual operation. Many surgeons are also in the habit of applying to dead and carious portions of bone the mineral acids, more or less diluted, with the view of expediting the exfoliation, and exerting a healthy action in the carious part ; but the practice should be adopted with caution, because such applications, if they do not fulfil the object proposed, will certainly increase the mischief. Mr. Nicol, of Inverness, has published some observations, recommending the external use of the nitrate of silver, and the internal exhibition of sarsaparilla, in the treatment of caries : his remarks deserve attention.—(See *Edin. Med. and Surg. Journ.*, No. xciv., art. 1.)]

When the restorative power of art or of nature has succeeded in forming a healthy line of separation, and detaching the dead part from the living, the former is usually thrown off in a cylindrical plate ; and before the exfoliation is accomplished, we are able to hear, as Severinus has justly remarked, a shrill sound whenever the carious plate is struck with a probe, as if it were hollow. Soon after this the edges of the exfoliating part rise a little, and a little pus, or even blood, is easily pressed out at the margin. Here also granulations begin at this time to appear, which spread over the sound bone underneath, and seem to assist the separation of the dead plate above ; so that it gradually becomes loose, and can soon afterward be taken away without violence.

The dead part of a bone is sometimes detached and thrown off to a very great extent, and especially in the cylindrical bones.—(*Bartholin, Act. Hafn.*, obs. 1 ; *Nicholai, Diss. Observ. quædam Medic.-Chir.*, Jen., 1786.) The whole body of the tibia has in this manner been occasionally detached by nature from its extremities, and its place supplied by a vicarious callus, which has run down the whole of the interior groove hereby produced, and acquired the hardness of bone. Several cases of this kind are given in the Edinburgh Medical Essays (vol. i., p. 192-194 ; vol. v., p. 370) ; in one of which the caries appeared in both legs : the total tibia of one limb, as the writer, Mr. W. Johnson of Dumfries, informs us, being separated and thrown off at once ; while that of the other was detached in small pieces, and thrown out gradually. In five months from the removal of the entire tibia, the patient, a boy of eleven years of age, was able to walk without crutches, continued well afterward, and was fit for any country work ; the legs being straight, with only a little thickness at the ankles. Justamond gives a similar case of the humerus, and Sherman of the thigh-bone. I have occasionally seen this natural process imitated successfully, both in the tibia and the bones of the forearm, and the diseased part taken out by a saw, by which process a very long period of pain and confinement has been saved to the patient.

If the caries commence in the internal laminæ, the superjacent sound part has sometimes been opened through its whole length by the trephine applied in a line of succession : the carious part

---

* Edin. Med. Essays, vol. v., p. 279. Besides these works, the valuable treatise of F. P. Weidmann, *De Ossium Necrosi*, fol. Francofurti ad Mœnum, 1793, deserves particularly to be consulted, as being more modern, and comprising the most approved doctrines.—ED.

has thus obtained an easy exit as soon as detached, and the entire bone has soon been renewed. The humerus was thus treated successfully in the case of a negro boy, as related by Mr. Walker.*

A caries of the spine, from the tumid, and, so to speak, *inflated* appearance of the superincumbent integuments, was formerly denominated *spina ventosa :* and the term has, with great inconsistency, been since applied by many writers to all bones whatever affected in the same manner, and particularly those of the tarsus and carpus; as it has by others been applied, with equal incorrectness, to a general softness or flexibility of the bones, as in *perostia flexilis*, or cyrtosis.

Of vertebral caries, Mr. Brodie has given cases which make it probable that here also the disease sometimes commences in the bones, and sometimes in the intervertebral cartilages; ·for in various instances the loss of substance was greater in the former, and in others in the latter.†

* Med. Trans., vol. iii., p. 27.   In a work devoted to medicine, a minute account of the process by which the dead bone, or sequestrum, as it is termed, becomes included in a new bony tube, may not be expected; but it is right to mention, that the mode hinted at ·by Dr. Good does certainly not generally take place; that is to say, the new shaft is not produced by a separation of the external lamina of the original bone. Numerous preparations in almost every museum prove, that at all events, in many instances, the sequestrum actually consists of the whole thickness of the original shaft, from which the periosteum has separated, assumed increased vascularity, and been converted into the organ for the new bony formation. After the osseous tube has been produced, a highly vascular substance begins to line its interior, lying between it and the outer surface of the sequestrum, and seemingly possessing a considerable absorbent power, which it exerts on the dead bone in contact with it. Under favourable circumstances, the greater part of the sequestrum will sometimes be gradually removed. The new osseous shell always has one or several apertures in it, termed *cloacæ*, through which any purulent matter and small particles of dead bone find their way to the outside of the new bony formation, whence· they pass through the fistulæ, and are discharged.—ED.

† Pathological and Surgical Obs. on the Diseases of the Joints, 2d ed. Caries, in the sense of ulceration of bone, is, as Dr. Cumin has correctly observed, of two kinds. In the *first*, a·process of destruction is going forward, without any attempt to repair the injury. In the *second*, the process of absorption of the osseous substance is accompanied by the formation of a new bony deposite, which is much more irregular in its arrangement, and imperfect in its organization, than the original bone. The first is· named by Dr. Cumin *caries expedens*; the second, *caries ossificans*. A simple absorption of bone, unaccompanied with the secretion of pus, he terms *osteo-anabrosis*. "Instances of this affection are presented by bones which have suffered from the pulsating action of aneurismal tumours; and remarkable examples of the disease have been occasionally met with in the bones of the cranium. Mr. Russell has detailed several cases, in which portions of bone were separated by this process of erosion. He has also seen the absorption proceed in such a manner as to leave an aperture in the cranium, without the separation of any bone, or any appearance of ulceration.—

GENUS XIII.
ULCUS.
U L C E R.

A PURULENT OR ICHOROUS SORE, PRODUCED BY THE SEPARATION OF A DEAD PART; BY THE BURSTING OF AN ABSCESS; BY A WOUND THAT HAS SUPPURATED; OR BY THE PROCESS OF ULCERATION.

THIS genus of diseases is, in every species, a subject of manual attention, and chiefly to be remedied or cured by external means. Its mode of treatment, therefore, must be learned under a course of surgical lectures; and it is only noticed in the present place, to show the exact station which it ought to bear in a general system of nosology founded on a physiological basis. Ulcus is, strictly speaking, a Greek term, with a mere change of one convertible vowel. for another, to give it more of a Latin form : the derivative noun being ἕλκος, probably, as conjectured by Eustathius, from ἕλκω, "traho," in the sense of "distraho," hereby producing what the Greeks called a λύσις συνεχείας, which is, literally, a "solution of continuity."

Ulcers have been treated of by different writers under a great variety of divisions and subdivisions; sometimes as being connected with the state of the constitution, or as being a mere local disease; sometimes as recent or chronic; and sometimes as mild or malignant: but, as local ulcers may become constitutional, the constitutional may assume various forms, the recent be rendered chronic, and the mild and the·malignant change places, none of these characters are calculated for clear or permanent distinction. And hence another principle has been appealed to in the volume of Nosology, derived from the variety of their external form, and they have been contemplated under the following species :—

1. Ulcus Incarnans.	Simple Healing Ulcer.
2. —— Vitiosum.	Depraved Ulcer.
3. —— Sinuosum.	Sinuous Ulcer.
4. —— Tuberculo-	Warty Excrescent Ulcer.
	sum.	
5. —— Cariosum.	Carious Ulcer.

SPECIES I.
ULCUS INCARNANS.
..SIMPLE HEALING ULCER.

THE DISCHARGE PURULENT, THE SURFACE HEALTHY AND GRANULATING.

WHEN an ulcer assumes this form, it is hardly

(Edin. Med. Chir. Trans., vol. i., p. 74.) A remarkable instance of the same disease is given by Mr. Wilmer from the practice of Mr. Harrold. —(Cases and Remarks, p. 40.) It is by the process of *osteo-anabrosis*, that nature produces the removal of the milk teeth; and a corresponding disease is sometimes met with in the adult, where the teeth become loose, and, when extracted, their fangs are found extensively absorbed, although by no means in a state of ulceration."—(Cumin, in Edin. Med. Journ., No. lxxxii., p. 8.) When a fungous tumour grows from the dura mater, the superincumbent part of the scull is generally absorbed without suppuration, and the swelling projects under the scalp.—ED.

to be called a disease; being nothing more than the ordinary process of the remedial power of nature to restore the substance that has been lost by external violence, or some internal morbid action, and to endow it with the same attributes of vascularity, feeling, and motion. It is to this form that all the other species of ulcer must be reduced, before a cure can be accomplished or hoped for. Even the surgeon has here little upon which to employ himself; for with cleanliness, a light and easy dressing, plain, unirritating diet, and regular hours, the processes of incarnation and cicatrization, which we have already explained under the genus APOSTEMA, will proceed spontaneously and without obstruction, and a cure be speedily completed.

SPECIES II.
ULCUS VITIOSUM.
DEPRAVED ULCER.
WITH A VITIATED SURFACE AND SECRETION.

THIS degenerate condition exhibits itself under various forms, and results from various causes. The modifications most worthy of notice are the following:—

a Callosum.	The edges indurated and retracted.
Callous ulcer.	
β Spongiosum.	With fungous or spongy excrescences, often from a medullary base.
Fungous ulcer.	
γ Cancrosum.	With a hard, livid, lancinating, irregular, and frequently bleeding tumour at its base.
Cancerous ulcer.	

The causes in each of these may be constitutional or local; and, in managing the ulcer, it is of great importance to determine this point; for the patient may otherwise be put very needlessly upon a long course of alterants, or may omit such a course when absolutely necessary. If there be a cancerous, a scrofulous, a scorbutic, a venereal, or any other constitutional disorder, it will be imperative upon us to pursue the respective modes of treatment already laid down for these several complaints, since otherwise no topical applications can be of the least avail. There may be also a considerable degree of constitutional debility and relaxation, to which the depraved state of the ulcer is owing; and, in truth, this is the most common of all the constitutional causes, and one which demands quite as much attention as any of the rest. In treating of abscess, we endeavoured to show that one of the uses of pus is to promote the formation of healthy granulations; and in treating of inflammation, we observed that a certain degree of vigorous and entonic, as well as inflammatory action, is necessary for the secretion of that fluid. And hence, if the system be without this condition, the ulcer cannot heal; and, instead of genuine pus and healthy granulations, we shall find a watery, ichorous fluid poured forth, of no advantage whatever, and often of an acrimonious quality, that irritates and thickens, and sometimes erodes and extends the edges of the ulcer; or a thin imperfect pus, accompanied with flabby and fungous granulations, that sprout up, indeed, rapidly and luxuriantly, but want firmness of texture, show a weak and morbid sensibility, and bleed and die away almost as soon as they are formed.

Where this is the case, the ulcer, whatever modification it assumes, can only be brought into a healing train by increasing the health and vigour of the constitution. This, however, it is often difficult to accomplish; for, in very numerous instances of obstinate ulcers, we find the constitution has been exhausted and worn out by hard labour, hard drinking, or protracted exposure to a tropical sun, and is labouring under a long train of dyspeptic, hepatic, or podagral symptoms. It is not necessary to repeat the plan it will be incumbent upon us to pursue under these circumstances, as we have already detailed it under the constitutional affections themselves. And if, by persevering in such general treatment, we can give to the constitution a sufficient degree of vigour, the only difficulty we shall have to encounter is the vitiated state, and perhaps habit, to which the ulcer has been reduced in consequence of the constitutional affection.

We hence come to the local treatment of ulcers, which forms a direct branch of surgical, and even manual attention. And I shall hence only further observe, that the principles which seem to have been productive of the best success, are those of changing the nature of the vitiated action, by a local application of irritants;[*] and increasing the tone of the vessels by warm suppuratives and astringents, and the pressure of elastic bandages, which should be made of calico or the finest flannel. Mr. Baynton preferred the former on every occasion, as less cumbrous and more cleanly, and as being "a better conductor of that morbid heat which so constantly affects inflamed parts." In many cases, however, and particularly in cold, œdematous limbs, it is rather desirable to accumulate than to carry off heat; and here the use of flannel will be preferable to that of calico: it possesses, moreover, more elasticity, and, when thin and fine, is neither more cumbrous nor more uncleanly.

Formerly, the actual cautery was frequently used in this country, as it is now abroad, as the most effectual as well as the shortest means of extirpating cancerous scirrhosities about the lips and other parts of the surface. And it is sometimes considered peculiarly calculated for radically destroying many of those irregular and spongy excrescences, which have a tendency to bleed freely from the slightest cause.

Fungus hæmatodes, classed in the present system with ulcers, has been regarded by some writers, and especially by M. Roux, as a soft and fungous cancer; but it seems to be without any of the pathognomonic signs by which cancers are distinguished. It is not known to be hereditary, nor to become scirrhous in any

* Extensive experiments with kreosote have proved this agent to be very valuable for this purpose.—D.

stage,* nor does it chiefly affect a glandular situation.

[Although fungus hæmatodes was in former days generally confounded with cancer, it is a disease of a very peculiar nature. Instead of being hard and unyielding, like a scirrhous tumour, it is generally soft and elastic. Instead of being intersected by the same kind of ligamentous fibres or bands which exist in a scirrhus, fungus hæmatodes consists of a soft pulpy matter, which mixes readily with water, and is hardened by acids or by being boiled in water. When the skin gives way, instead of the morbid growth being destroyed by ulceration, as in cancer, a quick-growing fungus arises from it, and the tumour increases with augmented rapidity. Fungus hæmatodes, instead of having a firm texture like the fungus of a cancerous ulcer, is a dark-red or purple mass, of an irregular shape and of a soft texture, easily torn, and bleeding profusely when slightly injured. A cancer, in its primary form, seems to be confined to certain organs and textures; and, while in some of these fungus hæmatodes, in its primary state, has not been seen, it has been detected in other parts where no truly cancerous disease has ever been noticed. While cancer is also rather a disease of advanced life, many of the patients attacked by fungus hæmatodes are young.— (See *Wardrop on Fungus Hæmatodes*, chap. xii., and *First Lines of the Practice of Surgery*, p. 215, 5th edit.) No remedy, external or internal, seems to have the power of checking this formidable disease. Abroad, the actual cautery has indeed been alleged sometimes to have answered; but in this country, all escharotics, and even concentrated sulphuric acid, have been found incapable of destroying the fungus as fast as it is regenerated. The only chance of cure depends upon the early removal of the whole of the disease by amputation or excision; but even this is frequently impracticable, in consequence of the particular seat of the disease; and often unavailing, on account of so many parts being affected, that the disease may be said to pervade the system.†]

In the treatment of depraved ulcers, some practitioners depend almost entirely for the cure on a restoration of the constitutional health; and contend that, with the accomplishment of this, the remedial power of nature is adequate to all the rest, with local cleanliness, rest, and the use of warm or cold water, according to the nature of the case. Such especially is the practice of

Professor Kern in the Imperial Hospital at Vienna, who makes a boast of proscribing ointments, plasters, lotions, charpie, caustics, and even bandages themselves, except in a few cases, trusting entirely to the use of water and a simple covering of linen, and this too even in gangrenous, scrofulous, and venereal ulcers.—(*Ann. der Chirurg. Klinik*, 2 vols., 8vo., Wien., 1809.) This practice is too simple to become very popular, but his success is undisputed.

SPECIES III.
ULCUS SINUOSUM.
SINUOUS ULCER.

COMMUNICATING WITH THE NEIGHBOURING PARTS BY ONE OR MORE CHANNELS.

WE have already seen that inflammations of every kind propagate themselves by continuous sympathy, and hence one cause of the spread of those that are ulcerated. But ulcerative inflammations do not spread equally; for those parts are most subject to their action, and consequently give way soonest, where the living principle is weakest, or the structure is most loose and cavernous. And hence a more frequent origin of hollows and sinuses in the cellular substance, particularly in the more dependant parts, as about the rectum and the urethra.

When these sinuosities are first formed or scooped out, their walls are soft, irritable, and of the common cellular web; but when they have remained for a considerable period of time, they become callous and insensible, forming the two following varieties, noticed in the volume of Nosology:—

α Recens.	The channel fresh and yield-	
Recent sinus.	ing.	
β Fistulosum.	The channel chronic and in-	
Fistulous sinus.	durated.	

The form assumed by a sinus is determined by the course of the probe; its capacity, by the quantity of water or any other fluid it will contain, when injected by a syringe.

Three modes of cure have been attempted: that of incarnation, or filling up the hollow by sound granulations issuing from the bottom; that of coalition, or a union of the walls of the sinus; and that of destroying it, by an opening down its entire length. The first is sometimes accomplished by warm lotions, where the sinus is shallow. The second is more usually had recourse to where it is deeper; and attempted first by irritant and even erosive injections, so as to excite a new inflammation down the whole course of the canal; and afterward by pressure, applied at first to its lowest part, and advanced gradually to its mouth; or, which is better, by a seton passed from the orifice of the ulcer to the utmost depth of the sinus, leaving here an opening sufficiently large for the escape of whatever matter might otherwise collect and become stagnant. The third mode of cure is effected by the knife; and where unaccompanied with danger or inconvenience from the vicinity of large bloodvessels, is by far the speediest and most decisive of the whole.

---

* These observations are partly incorrect. Sir Astley Cooper mentioned a case to the editor a little while ago, where a lady, after having had a scirrhous breast removed, died of a fungus hæmatodes. Professor Carswell, as already noticed in the section on Carcinus, regards fungus hæmatodes as a species of carcinoma; and he speaks of the two diseases as occasionally met with together, not only in the same individual, but in the same organ.—See his *Illustrations of the Elementary Forms of Disease*, 4to., Lond., 1833.—ED.

† The material deposited in scirrhus is not disposed to become organized, and vessels are rarely perceptible in it; but the brain-like substance of fungus hæmatodes abounds with them.—ED.

SPECIES IV.

ULCUS TUBERCULOSUM.

WARTY EXCRESCENT ULCER.

WITH TUBERCULOUS EXCRESCENCES, AND RAGGED AND SPREADING EXULCERATIONS.

THIS is the NOLI ME TANGERE (*Dartre Rongeànte* of M. Alibert) of many writers, and the LUPUS of others ; evidently referring to its unmanageable character, and the ravenous or wolf-like ferocity with which it preys on the neighbouring organs, spreading in ragged and fungous lobes, or with cracking and callous edges, and destroying the skin through an extensive range, and sometimes even the muscles, to a considerable depth.

A valuable practical paper upon this disease (*Phil. Trans.*, vol. xlix., year 1755) was addressed to the Royal Society by M. Daviel, surgeon to Louis XV. of France ; who describes it as a cancer, to which, indeed, from its tendency to ramify, and the virulence of its discharge, it has some resemblance ; and whence Sauvages denominates it *cancer lupus.* [The disease generally commences on the alæ of the nose, with small tubercles, which gradually change into ulcerations. These throw out a discharge, which dries and produces scabs, under which the sores are sometimes much concealed, and burrow more deeply into the part. In general, a portion of the disease will be healing, while another is extending itself ; and afterward, the parts previously healed break out again. In this manner all the skin of the nose suffers, and sometimes other parts of the face : in bad cases, even the cartilages are destroyed, and little of the nose is ultimately left but its bridge. According to Dr. Bateman, the disease sometimes appears on the cheek, in the form of a sort of ringworm, destroying the substance, and leaving a deep and deformed cicatrix ; and he had seen a similar circular patch of the disease dilating itself at length to the extent of a hand-breadth or more over the pectoral muscle.—(*Bateman's Cutaneous Diseases,* p. 296, 3d ed., 1814.)]

When the case is recent, and there is no morbid irritability in the habit, the diseased action has yielded to a skilful application of counter-stimulants, as a dilute solution of the nitrate of silver or aromatic vinegar ; after which the tar ointment has been found most serviceable.

[In particular examples, the most successful local applications have been solutions of arsenic or sulphate of copper, and the unguentum hydrargyri nitratis. Frequently, however, nothing will avail without internal alterative medicines, such as the compound decoction of sarsaparilla, nitrous acid, the muriate of barytes ; and, above all, the liquor arsenicalis. In obstinate cases, the practice of dissecting away all the diseased parts has sometimes been adopted.]

SPECIES V.

ULCUS CARIOSUM.

CARIOUS ULCER.

THE ULCER EXTENDING INTO THE SUBSTANCE OF THE SUBJACENT BONE

WHEN a portion of a bone is killed by an ulcerative process commencing in itself, it forms, as we have already observed, a CARIES properly so called. When it is destroyed by the spread of a sore commencing in the integuments or muscles above it, the disease is called a CARIOUS ULCER ; and when the ulceration extends to the medulla of the bone, it is often denominated an arthrocace.

Upon this subject, however, it is not necessary to enlarge in the present place, as we have already discussed the general nature and the ordinary forms of ulceration under the SECOND SPECIES of the genus before us; and the mode by which the death and separation of one portion of bone from another are effected, under the FOURTH SPECIES of the preceding genus.

CLASS IV.

NEUROTICA.

DISEASES OF THE NERVOUS FUNCTION.

ORDER I.

PHRENICA.

AFFECTING THE INTELLECT.

II.

ÆSTHETICA.

AFFECTING THE SENSATION.

" III.

CINETICA.

AFFECTING THE MUSCLES.

" IV.

SYSTATICA.

AFFECTING SEVERAL OR ALL THE SENSORIAL POWERS SIMULTANEOUSLY.

CLASS IV.

PHYSIOLOGICAL PROEM.

THE numerous and complicated train of diseases we are now entering upon, appertains to the highest function of visible beings : the possession of which emphatically distinguishes animals from plants, and the perfection of which as emphatically distinguishes man from all other animals : these are diseases of the NERVOUS FUNCTION ; which, in the sphere of its activity, embraces the powers of intellect, sensation, and muscular motion. Each of these powers evinces diseases of its own, and will consequently lay a foundation for a distinct order under the class before us. While, as there are also other diseases that affect several of them simultaneously, we become furnished with a fourth order, which will complete the series.

All these diversities of vital energy are now well known to be dependant on the organ of the brain,* as the instrument of the intellectual powers, and the source of the sensific and motory. Though, from the close connexion and synchronous action of various other organs with the brain, and especially the thoracic and abdominal viscera, such diversities were often referred to several of the latter in earlier ages,

and before anatomy had traced them satisfactorily to the brain as the fountain-head. And of so high an antiquity is this erroneous hypothesis, that it has not only spread itself through every climate on the globe, but still keeps a hold on the colloquial language of every people ; and hence the heart, the liver, the spleen, the reins, and the bowels, generally, are among all nations regarded either literally or figuratively as so many seats of mental faculties or moral feeling. We trace this common and popular creed among the Hebrews and Arabians, the Egyptians and Persians, the Greeks and Romans ; among every savage as well as every civilized tribe ; nor is there a dialect of the present day that is free from it : and we have hence an incontrovertible proof that it existed as a doctrine of general belief at a time when mankind, few in number, formed a common family, and were regulated by common notions.

The study of anatomy, however, has corrected the loose and confused ideas of mankind upon this subject ; and while it distinctly shows us that many of the organs popularly referred to as the seat of sensation do and must, from the pe-

---

* Perhaps, instead of the expression, " organ of the brain," it would be more correct to say, "nervous system ;" for it is not every animal that has a brain, and certain functions of the nerves, even in the human subject, seem to be independent of this organ. " A nervous system appears essentially composed of two parts : of a central organ, consisting of two cords ; one corresponding with either half of the body, upon which nodular mass- es are generally placed ; and, secondly, of other cords, called nerves, derived from the central organ to the sentient surfaces, or contractile parts of the animal. In the star-fish, a radiated animal, the central organ consists of a ring of white nervous matter, which surrounds the orifice of the stomach, and gives off opposite to the centre of each ray nerves for its supply."—See Mayo's Outlines of Physiology, p. 252, 2d edit., 1828.—ED.

culiarity of their nervous connexion with the brain, necessarily participate in the feelings and faculties thus generally ascribed to them, it also demonstrates that the primary source of these attributes, the quarter in which they originate, or which chiefly influences them, is the brain itself.

We are speaking, however, of man and the higher classes of animals alone : for, as the scale in animal life descends, the organ of a brain is perpetually diminishing in its bulk, till at length it totally disappears, and its place is supplied by other fabrications, as we shall have occasion to observe in the sequel of this introduction : which will lead us to take a brief notice of the following subjects :—

I. The General Nature of the Brain, its Ramifications and Substitutes.
II. The Principle of Sensation and Motion.
III. The Intellectual Principle.

I. In man, and those animals whose encephalon approaches the nearest to his in form, the brain is of an oval figure, surrounded by various membranes of different firmness and density, and consists of three principal divisions : the cerebrum, or brain, properly so called, the cerebel, or little brain, and the oblongated marrow. The first forms the largest and uppermost part : the second lies below and behind ; the third lies level with the second, and in front of it ; it appears to issue equally out of the two other parts, and in turn to give birth to the spinal marrow ; which may hence be regarded as a continuation of the brain, communicating with its different parts by the aid of numerous commissures, the *querbänder* of the German writers, and extended through the whole chain of the back-bone. They are similarly accompanied with a cineritious or ash-coloured substance, which forms the exterior of the three first divisions, but the interior of the spinal marrow, and appears to derive its hue from the great number of minute vessels that appertain to it.

It is still, however, a contested opinion, as it was among the Greek physiologists, whether the brain or the spinal marrow be the parent organ. Vesalius, Fallopius, Winslow, Haller, and Portal, concur with Galen in regarding the spinal marrow as an appendix of the brain. Malpighi, Reil, Tiedemann, and Gall, contend, on the contrary, as Plato and Praxagoras contended formerly, that the brain is an efflorescence of the spinal marrow, which takes the lead in the process of organization : while M. de Serres has still more lately thrown out a third hypothesis, and derived not only each of these organs from a different source, but even the cerebellum as well : the spinal marrow issuing from the intercostal arteries, the cerebellum from the vertebral, and the proper brain from the carotids. Time alone, and more minute examination, must settle these discrepances.*

According to Mr. Bauer's very delicate microscopic experiments, when the substance of

the brain is made a subject of examination immediately after death, "abundance of fibres," to adopt the words of Sir Everard Home in relating these experiments, "are met with in every part of it ; indeed, it appears that the whole mass is a tissue of fibres, which seem to consist entirely of an accumulation of globules, whose union is of so delicate a nature, that the slightest touch, even the mere immersion in water, deranges and reduces them to that mass of globules of which the brain appears to be composed, when examined with less accuracy, or under less favourable circumstances." Mr. Bauer found that the globules of the brain, as well as those of pus, are exactly of the same size as those of the blood when deprived of their colouring matter.—(See *Sir Everard Home's Croonian Lecture, Phil. Trans. for* 1818.) And hence the doctrine of Prochaska (Op. Min., tom. i., p. 342) and the Wenzels (*De Structurâ Cerebri*) respecting the globular form of the ultimate particles of the brain, seems sufficiently confirmed.*

[When we cut into the interior of the brain, we find it to be composed of two substances, which differ in their colour and consistence, and are named the *cortical* or *cineritious*, and the *medullary*. The cortical, as its name imports, is on the outside, and is of a reddish-brown colour ; and is softer than the medullary, and considerably more vascular. The medullary matter is, both from its aspect and relative position, generally considered as constituting the nervous substance in its most perfect state : and Gall and Spurzheim conjecture, that the use of the cineritious is to form or secrete the medullary part.—(*Recherches sur le Système Nerveux*, § 2.) The particular facts, says Dr. Bostock, from which they derive their hypothesis, are, that the nerves appear to be enlarged when they pass through a mass of cineritious matter, and that masses of this substance are deposited on all the parts of the spinal cord, where it sends out nerves. In opposition to the above opinion, however, Professor Tiedemann states, that in the fœtus the medulla is formed before the cortex ; and he limits the use of the latter to the conveyance of the arterial blood, necessary to support the energy of the perfect nervous matter.†]

Sir Everard Home, from the above-mentioned microscopic disclosures, endeavours to show that muscular fibres are minute chains, formed by an attachment of one globule of blood to an-

---

* Paragraph found among the author's MSS. subsequently to the publication of the third edition.

---

* According to Prochaska, the nervous pulp consists of flocculi, which are composed of globules, about eight times less than the red particles of the blood (Op. Min., p. 342) ; and this account, in its essential parts, has been confirmed by the more recent and elaborate investigations of the Wenzels.—(De Structurâ Cerebri, p. 24, et seq.) Bauer, whose researches confirm the existence of globules, found them larger and in greater proportion in the medullary than in the cortical substance.—See Phil. Trans. for 1818 and 1821 ; also, Bostock's Physiology, vol. i., p. 234.—Ed.

† See Anatomie du Cerveau, traduite par Jourdan, p. 128 ; Bostock's Physiology, vol. i., p. 223 ; Magendie, Physiologie, tom. i., p. 162, &c.

other; and that vascularity in coagula or extravasated blood, or in granulations produced by pus, is effected by the escape of minute bubbles of carbonic acid gas from the living fluid ; which hereby opens a path to a certain extent into the tenacious blood or pus that is extravasated or secreted.

From the lower part of the brain, or, according to the latest researches, rather from the medulla oblongata, and also from the spinal cord, arises a certain number of long, whitish, pulpy strings, or bundles of fibres, capable of being divided and subdivided into minuter bundles of filaments or still smaller fibres, as far as the power of glasses can carry the eye. These strings are denominated nerves; they are enclosed in sheaths of membrane ; and, by their various ramifications, convey different kinds or modifications of living power to different parts of the body, keep up a perpetual communication with its remotest organs, and give motivity to the muscles. [The nerves are most copiously distributed to the organs of sense and voluntary motion ; the viscera are much more sparingly supplied with them ; the glands have still fewer nerves ; and some of the membranous parts are sometimes conjectured to be destitute of them. Generally speaking, the nerves which supply the organs of sense proceed immediately from the base of the brain, or rather from the medulla oblongata ; while most of the muscles (but not all) receive their nerves from the spinal cord. As Dr. Bostock has observed, there is more irregularity with respect to the course of the nerves which go to the viscera ; they generally derive their immediate origin from some of the ganglia and plexuses forming part of the great sympathetic nerve, and they are connected with each other in a great variety of ways. The nervous system, viewed as a whole, however, and comprising the brain, spinal cord, and all their ramifications, is in general so symmetrical, that if the body were longitudinally divided into two equal halves, the arrangement of the brain and nerves in each half would, with the exception of a few deviations from this rule, caused by the situations of particular viscera, precisely correspond.—(*Bostock's Physiology*, vol. i., p. 228.)

In various examples, the fibrils of which adjacent nerves are composed are reciprocally thrown across from one to the other, forming what is termed a *plexus*. As Mr. Mayo has explained, the nerves which proceed from the further side of a plexus may be more numerous or fewer than those which enter it ; but the essential result is, that nervous fibrils from different sources are brought together to form new trunks.* A ganglion is a small nodule, usually

flattened, of an oval or circular shape, and of a reddish-gray colour, which is found either on the trunk of a single nerve, or where two or more branches coalesce. Sir Charles Bell's opinion respecting the ganglions will be presently noticed. Scarpa supposes that a ganglion is but a bed of gelatinous membrane, in which the smallest fibrils of the nerves are arranged in new combinations. Others believe that nervous filaments originate in the gray matter of ganglions. —(*Mayo's Physiology*, p. 324, 2d edit.)]*

As the brain consists of three general divisions, it might at first sight be supposed that each of these is allotted to some distinct purpose ; as, for example, that of forming the seat of intellect or thinking ; the seat of the local senses of sight, sound, taste, and smell, and the seat of general feeling or motivity. The investigations and experiments of Sir Charles Bell and M. Magendie, to which we shall presently advert, pave the way to some important doctrines in respect to a few of these points, but leave us quite in the dark with respect to various others ; and particularly as to the source of intellect : while it is difficult to reconcile even the doctrines which have been thus fairly deduced with the motific, and even with the sentient powers that must exist in numerous cases of an extensive disorganization of the brain, and in acephalous animals. The first and second nerves, and the portio mollis of the seventh, sufficiently attest their exclusive uses as nerves of the special senses ; while the distribution of the greater part of the third, of the fourth, and of the sixth nerves to voluntary muscles, which receive fil-

plexus is intricate in proportion to the number of muscles to be supplied, and the variety of combinations into which the muscles enter, while the filaments of nerves, which go to the skin, regularly diverge to their destination. The nerves on the face and those on the side of the neck form plexuses ; but the grand plexuses are near the origins of the nerves of the upper and lower extremities. By the interchange of filaments, the combination among the muscles is formed.—See Med. Gaz. for Feb., 1834, p. 777 ; also, Exposition of the Natural System of the Nerves of the Human Body, 8vo., 1824.—ED.

* " The most probable conjecture as to the use of the ganglia seems to be that they are points of nervous communication, in some respects similar to the arterial communications, as they serve to diffuse more equally the nervous influence ; or to lymphatic glands, which collect parts and change their mode of distribution."—See A Comparative View of the Sensorial and Nervous Systems in Men and Animals, by John C. Warren, M. D., Prof. of Anat. and Surg. in Harvard University, Boston, 1822.—D.

† It is a remark made by Sir Charles Bell, that the principles and facts unfolded in his views of the nervous system, lead us to understand the " use of all the intricate nerves of the body, with the exception of the sixth. The sixth nerve stands connected with another system of nerves altogether ; I mean the system hitherto called the sympathetic, or sometimes the ganglionic system of nerves; and of this system we know so little, that it cannot be matter of surprise if we reason ignorantly of the connexion of the sixth with it." —Natural System of the Nerves of the Human Body, p. 64.—ED.

---

* In explaining the cause of the complexity of the nerves, Sir Charles Bell remarks, that some degree of irregularity in their distribution must arise from their being compound ; but, says he, the principal cause is the necessity of arranging and combining a great many muscles in their different offices. Wherever we trace nerves of motion, we find, that before entering the muscles they interchange branches, and form an intricate mass of nerves, or what is termed a *plexus*. This

aments from no other source, proves clearly that these nerves are voluntary nerves, as well as conducive to muscular sensation. "Perhaps," says Mr. Mayo, "it is not unfair to argue analogically from the preceding instances, that the same surface of the brain or spinal cord furnishes to each voluntary muscle of the body its voluntary and sentient nerves, *if the two are not identical.*"—(*Anat. and Physiol. Commentaries*, No. ii., p. 1., 8vo., Lond., 1822.) There is in like manner reason for believing that the fifth nerve, which at its origin consists of two portions, is not only a nerve of voluntary motion, but furnishes branches to the special senses, and even communicates general sensation to the muscular fibres ; and that its gustatory twig is a nerve of both touch and taste at the same time.*

The remarks of Sir Charles Bell upon this subject are well entitled to attention. "The trigeminus, or fifth nerve," says he, "bestows upon all the surfaces of the head and face, external and internal, that sensibility which is enjoyed by the rest of the body through the spinal marrow" (*Phil. Trans.*, 1823, pp. 289, 290); and, in proof of this, he describes various experiments which show that, on dividing its branch to the cheek and lips, or on its destruction by disease, insensibility instantly takes place in these organs. Yet some of its branches prove motific as well as sensific, and draw the muscles of the eye into a state of mutual action to expel offensive particles that have found admission to its surface : while, of the nine nerves that proceed from the brain, constituting the whole number that thus originate, six of them are distributed in a greater or less proportion to the single organ of vision, and co-operate in giving perfection to its powers ; as the third, fourth, part of the fifth, sixth, and seventh.

Several of these phenomena may indeed be resolved, though not the whole, into that close interunion which some parts of the brain maintain with other parts by means of ganglions, commissures, and decussations of nerves ; whence injuries on one side are often accompanied with loss of motion or feeling in the organs of the other side. So the curious and ingenious experiments instituted by Dr. Philip (*Phil. Trans.*, 1815, pp. 5–90), and to which we shall have occasion to return presently, sufficiently prove, that stimuli of a certain kind, as spirit of wine, applied to the posterior part of the naked brain

of an animal, produce the same effect on the heart, and equally increase its action, as if applied to the anterior part. To affect the heart, however, it seems necessary that the stimulus should spread over a pretty large extent of the brain ; so as to take in, by the range of its excitement, some of the ganglions of the brain, whose office, as Dr. Philip conceives, is "to combine the influence of the various parts of the nervous system from which they receive nerves, and to send off nerves endowed with the combined influence of those parts."* He hence accounts for some organs of the frame being affected by every part of the nervous system, and others by only certain small parts of it ; and the wide influence possessed by the great sympathetic nerve, which is less a single nerve than a string of ganglions. We are also hereby shown why the intestines, like the heart, sympathize with every portion of the nervous system.

From all this, however, it is clear, that there, is much yet to be learned concerning the actual arrangement of the brain, or of its partition into three divisions, and of the respective shares which the different parts take in producing a common effect : and consequently it seems to be altogether a wild and idle attempt to subdivide these perceptible regions of the brain into still smaller and merely imaginary sections, and to allot to each of them a determinate function and faculty.

That a sensorial communication, however, is maintained between some part or other of the brain and every part of the body, and that this communication is conducted by the nerves, is unquestionable from the following facts :—If we divide, or tie, or merely compress a nerve of any kind, the muscle with which it communicates becomes almost instantly paralytic ; but upon untying or removing the compression, the muscle recovers its appropriate feeling and irritability. If the compression be made on any particular part of the brain, that part of the body becomes motionless which derives nerves from the part compressed. And if the cerebrum, cerebellum, or medulla oblongata be irritated, excruciating pain or convulsions, or both, take place over the whole body ; though

---

* The fact of the same nerve seeming to answer both for motion and sensation, is accounted for by the important discoveries of Sir Charles Bell and M. Magendie. Mr. Mayo's experiments and arguments tend to prove that "the *ganglionless* portion of the fifth, and the hard portion of the seventh nerve, are voluntary nerves to parts, which receive sentient nerves from the larger or *ganglionic* portion of the fifth." By the expression *sentient* nerves, Mr. Mayo means those, the division of which is followed by instantaneous loss of sensation in a part ; by *voluntary* nerves, he means those upon the division of which the will ceases to influence the muscles they supply.—Outlines, &c., p. 331, &c.—ED.

---

* Phil. Trans., 1815, p. 436. An opinion formerly prevailed, that ganglia were intended to cut off sensation ; but Sir Charles Bell noticed that every one of the nerves, which he took to be instruments of sensation, had ganglia on their roots. " Some very decided experiment," he says, " was necessary to overturn this dogma. I selected two nerves of the encephalon ; the fifth, which had a ganglion, and the seventh, which had no ganglion. On cutting across the nerve of the fifth pair on the face of an ass, it was found that the sensibility of the parts to which it was distributed was entirely destroyed. On cutting across the nerve of the seventh pair on the side of the face of an ass, the sensibility was not in the slightest degree diminished. By pursuing the inquiry, it was found that a ganglionic nerve is the sole organ of sensation in the head and face ; and thus my opinion was confirmed, that the ganglionic roots of the spinal nerves were the fasces or funiculi for sensation."—C. Bell's Nat. Syst. of the Nerves, p. 34.—ED.

chiefly when the irritation is applied to the last of these three parts.* For, according to the laws of the nervous action, as collected from a variety of experiments by Dr. Philip (*Phil. Trans.*, 1815, p. 444), and stated in a subsequent paper to that just referred to, " neither mechanical nor chymical stimuli (irritating the brain by a knife, or pouring spirits of wine upon it) applied to the nervous system excites the muscles of voluntary motion, unless they are applied near to the origin of the nerves and spinal marrow." It is from the medulla oblongata that all the nerves of respiration take their rise; and hence, any sudden injury or accident that interrupts its course, by putting a close to the respiration, induces death instantly.—(*On the Nerves*, &c., *by Sir Charles Bell.*, *Phil. Trans.*, 1822, p. 284.)

The nerves issue in pairs, one of each pair being alloted to either side of the body. The whole number of pairs is forty, of which nine rise immediately from the great divisions of the brain under which we have just contemplated it, and are *chiefly*, though not wholly, appropriated to the four local senses; and thirty-one from the spinal marrow.

We have thus far represented the spinal marrow as issuing from the brain, in conformity with the general doctrine that has hitherto been held upon the subject. It has of late years, however, been contended by various physiologists (*Tiedemann*, *Anatomie du Cerveau*, *trad. par A. J. Jourdan*, &c., Paris, 1823 ; *Serres*, *Anat. Comparée du Cerveau*, &c.), and particularly by Drs. Gall and Spurzheim, that the spinal marrow itself is the origin or trunk of the nervous system, and that, instead of issuing from the brain, it gives birth to it. The argument is derived from the existence of a spinal marrow alone in acephalous monsters, and a nervous cord without a brain, answering the purpose of a spinal marrow, in most invertebral animals. Whence it is inferred that the nervous column is the radical part of the system, and that the brain is an increment from it in the more perfect classes.†

The question is not of much importance, though there is something ingenious in thus tracing animal life from its simpler forms. Yet the opinion seems to be in direct opposition to a well-ascertained fact we shall have to advert to presently, namely, that the magnitude of the brain and the extent of its intellectual powers hold an inverse proportion to the size of the spinal marrow, and consequently, upon this hypothesis, to their apparent means of supply. Nor

is it the mode of induction usually adopted by physiologists on like occasions ; since they generally describe the arteries as issuing from the heart, instead of giving rise to it, notwithstanding that the heart, like the brain, has been found totally wanting in some monsters, and the circulation carried on by an artery and a vein alone, of which Mr. Hewson gives a very singular instance (*On the Lymph. Syst.*, part ii., p. 15); and that most of the worm genera are equally without a heart, though they are in possession of circulatory vessels. We only see in these arrangements, that neither a brain nor a heart is essentially necessary to animal life : and that the great Author of nature is the lord, and not the slave of his own laws; and is capable of effecting the same general principle by a ruder, as well as by a more elaborate design.

There is one part, however, of the system of nervous power, in the more perfect classes of animals, that is particularly worthy of our attention, as furnishing a rule peculiar to itself, and being without a parallel in any other part ; and that is, the origin, structure, and extensive influence of the great sympathetic or intercostal nerve, which forms a kind of system in itself, an epicycle within the two cycles of cerebral and vertebral influence. It is connected both with the brain and spinal marrow, and may be said to arise from either. Admitting the brain to be its source, it is an offset from the sixth pair of nerves on either side, and in its course receives a small tributary twig from the fifth, and branches from all the vertebral, from whose union and decussation it is studded with numerous ganglions or medullary enlargements, of which there are not less than three in the neck alone, teinted by an addition of cineritious substance, a larger number in its line through the chest, and others as it descends still more deeply, independently of various confluences of smaller branches that unite and form extensive networks. Having reached the hollow of the os coccygis, it meets its twin from the opposite side, which has pursued a similar course, and been augmented by similar contributions.

Thus equally enriched with the nervous stores of the brain and the spinal marrow, it sends off radiations, as it takes the course of the aorta, to all the organs of the thoracic, abdominal, and hypogastric regions, to the lungs, the heart, the stomach and intestines, the bladder, uterus, and testes ; and thus becomes an emporium of nervous commerce, and an instrument of general sympathy : and, what is of infinite importance in so complicated a frame as that of man, furnishes to the vital organs streams of nervous supply from so many anastomosing currents, that if one, or more than one, should fail or be cut off, the function may still be continued. To this it is owing, in a very considerable degree, that the organs of the upper and lower belly exhibit that nice fellowship of feeling which often surprises us, and that most of them are apt to sympathize in the actual state of the brain.

There is no animal whose brain is an exact counterpart to that of man : and it has hence been conceived, that by attending to the dis-

---

* Some of the observations of Flourens and Hertwig on this subject will be presently noticed. —Ed.

† Anatomie et Physiologie du Système Nerveux, &c., par. F. J. Gall et G. Spurzheim, 4to., Paris, 1810. The later investigations of Tiedemann and Serres into the development of the nervous system of the human fœtus, represent the spinal cord, the medulla oblongata, the cerebellum, and the cerebrum, as formed in the succession here specified.—Béclard, Additions à Bichat. —Ed.

tinctions between a human brain and that of other animals, we might be able to unfold a still more mysterious part of the animal economy than that of sensation or motion, and account for the superior intellect with which man is endowed.

But the varieties are so numerous, and the parts which are deficient in one animal are found connected with such new combinations, modifications, and deficiencies in others, that it is impossible for us to avail ourselves of any such diversities.

[The principle of improvement in the nervous system, throughout the ascending scale of animals, is the progressive accumulation of nervous matter in larger masses upon that part of the central organ which is nearest the head or mouth. In proportion as this alteration from the simplest type of organization is effected, the animal becomes more and more individualized, portions separated from it are found to be less capable of independent existence, and the destruction of one organ is observed to produce more derangement of the rest.—(See *Mayo's Outlines of Human Physiology*, p. 257, 2d ed.)]

Aristotle endeavoured to establish a distinction, by laying it down as a maxim that man has the largest brain of all animals in proportion to the size of his body; a maxim which has been almost universally received, from his own time to the present period. But it has of late years, and upon a more extensive cultivation of comparative anatomy, been found to fail in various instances: for, while the brain of several species of the ape kind bears as large a proportion to the body as that of man, the brain of several kinds of birds bears a proportion still larger. Söemmerring has carried the comparison through a great diversity of genera and species:* but the following brief table will be sufficient for the present purpose. The weight of the brain to that of the body forms

In man from . . .	1-22 to 1-33 part.	
Several simiæ . .	.	1-22
Dog . . .	.	1-101
Elephant . . .	.	1-500
Sparrow . .	.	1-25
Canary-bird . .	.	1-14
Goose . .	.	1-360
Turtle (smallest) .	.	1-5688

Söemmerring has hence endeavoured to correct the rule of Aristotle by a modification under which it appears to hold universally; and, thus corrected, it runs as follows; "Man has the largest brain of all animals in proportion to the general mass of nerves that issue from it." Thus, the brain of a horse gives only half the weight of that of a man, but the nerves it sends forth are ten times as bulky. The largest brain

* Diss. de Basi Encephali., Götting., 1778, 4to. G. R. Treviranus has given the results of a series of observations on the relative weight and breadth of the brain to that of several of its parts in different mammiferous animals; also a table of the proportion of the several parts of the brain to the greatest breadth of the spinal cord. The particulars may be found in the Edin. Med. and Surgical Journ. for January, 1829.—Ed.

which Söemmerring ever dissected in the horse kind weighed only 1 lb. 4 oz., while the smallest he has met with in an adult man was 2 lb. 5¼ oz.

But the remark applies farther than to man: for this acute physiologist has been able to trace a direct proportion between the degree of intelligence in every class of animals and the bulk of the brain, where the latter bears an inverse proportion to the nerves that arise from it. And we may hence observe, in passing, as, indeed, we have already hinted, that the nerves seem rather to be a product of the brain, than the brain of the nerves: for it is much more easy to conceive how a fountain may become exhausted in proportion to the magnitude of its streams, than how a reservoir can be augmented in proportion to the minuteness of its channels.*

Upon a general survey I may observe, that the nervous structure of all vertebral animals, comprising the first four classes of the Linnæan classification, mammals, birds, amphibials, and fishes, is characterized by the two following properties:—Firstly, the central organ of the nervous system consists of a brain, with a long cord or spinal marrow descending from it; and, secondly, that both are securely enclosed in a bony case or covering.

In man, as I have already observed, the brain is (with a few exceptions) larger than in any other animal in proportion to the size of the body; and, without any exception whatever, in proportion to the size of its dependent column.

In other animals, even of the vertebral classes, or those immediately before us, we meet with every variety of proportion, from the ape, which in this respect approaches nearest to that of man to tortoises, and fishes, in which the brain does not much exceed the diameter of the spinal marrow itself.

It is not, therefore, to be wondered at, that animals of a still lower description, and without a vertebral column, should exhibit proofs of a nervous cord or spinal marrow, without a brain of any kind at the top; and that this cord should even be destitute of its common bony defence. And such is actually the conformation of the nervous system in insects, and, for the most part, in worms; neither of which are possessed either of a cranium or a spine; and in none of which we are able to trace more than a slight enlargement of the superior part

* The doctrine that the nerves arise from or are a production from the brain, has of late years been considerably weakened, if not quite refuted, by various facts, among which it is only necessary to mention here the existence of nerves in acephalous monsters. One of the most interesting cases of this kind formed the subject of a memoir, published not long ago by M. Spessa, surgeon of Treviso. A female infant was born totally destitute of brain, cerebellum, and medulla oblongata. It was not at all under the ordinary full size of a child at birth, being a foot in length; and, notwithstanding its acephalous condition, it exhibited, directly after birth, manifest signs of life, for it breathed, cried, and moved its limbs. The heart and arteries pulsated in the usual manner. The infant suddenly ceased to live at the end of eleven hours.—See Lond. Med. Gaz., vol. xi., p. 559.—Ed.

of the nervous cord, or spinal marrow, as it is called, in animals possessing a spine ; often consisting of one, and sometimes of two ganglions, designed, apparently, to correspond with the organ of a brain ; the descending column chiefly taking the course of the œsophagus, and surrounding it. The nervous cord however, in these animals, is proportionally larger than in those of a superior rank ; and though sometimes simple, as in molluscous worms, in other cases, as in insects, is possessed at various distances of minuter ganglions, or little knots, from which fresh ramifications of nerves shoot forth like branches from the trunk of a tree, and which have sometimes been regarded as so many distinct cerebels, or little brains : having a close resemblance to the subordinate system of the intercostal nerve in man, as we have already traced it in its various ramifications and connexions.*

In worms of apparently the simplest make, as zoophites and infusory animals, no distinct structure can be discerned, and particularly nothing like a nervous system. The hydra, or nearly transparent polypus, found so frequently in the stagnant waters of our own country, with a body of an inch long, and arms or tentacles in proportion, seems, when examined by the largest magnifying glasses, to consist of a congeries of granular globules or molecules, not unlike boiled sago, surrounded by a gelatinous substance ; in some tribes solitary, in others catenated. And hence, whatever degree of sensation or voluntary motion exists in such animals, can only be conceived as issuing from these molecules acting the part of nervous ganglions, detached or connected. And on this account M. Virey has elegantly divided all animals into three classes, according to the nature of their nervous configuration ; as, first, animals with two nervous systems, a cerebral and sympathetic, including

mammals and birds, amphibials and fishes. Secondly, animals with a sympathetic nervous system alone, surrounding the œsophagus, as mollusca and shellfishes, insects and proper worms. And, thirdly, animals with nervous molecules, as echini, polypes, and infusory animalcules, corals, madrepores, and sponges ; all which, in M. Virey's classification, are included under the term zoophites.*

The only sense which seems common to animals, and which pervades almost the whole surface of their bodies, is that of general touch or feeling ; whence M. Cuvier supposes that the material of touch is the sensorial power in its simplest and uncompounded state, and that the other senses are only modifications of this material, though peculiarly elaborated by peculiar organs, which are also capable of receiving more delicate impressions.† Touch, however, has its

---

* See Sir E. Home's Croonian Lecture on the Internal Structure of the Human Brain, when examined in the microscope, as compared with that of fishes, insects, and worms.—(Phil. Trans., 1824, p. 1.) On this part of the subject, Sir Charles Bell has presented some different, but very ingenious views. In animals which do not breathe by a uniform and general motion of their bodies, he observes, there is no spinal marrow, strictly speaking, but only a long compound and ganglionic nerve, extending through the body for the purpose of sensation and motion. In such creatures, the cord does not actuate the animal machine with alternate dilatation and contraction. There may be a motion of some part which admits and expels air from a cavity, or agitates the water, and which motion is subservient to oxygenation of the blood ; and there may be a nerve supplied to that apparatus, with sensibility and power suited to the function thus to be performed, and resembling our par vagum in office ; but there is no regular and corresponding distribution of a respiratory system of nerves to both sides of the body, and no arrangement of bones and muscles for a general and regular motion of the frame, like that which takes place in vertebral animals, and which is necessary to their mode of existence.—Sir Charles Bell's Exposition of the Natural System of the Nerves of the Human Body, p. 23, London, 8vo, 1824.—ED.

* When the nerves, the spina marrow, and medulla oblongata (as Mr. Mayo observes) are proved to be sufficient for the continuance of sensation, volition, and the commonest instincts, we naturally suppose that the cerebral masses which seem to grow in the scale of animals with their approximation to reason, are the seat of the higher affections of the mind. When, indeed, we read over an enumeration of the different affections of consciousness, and compare the phenomena of the mind with the anatomy of the brain, we see not the most remote correspondence between the structure of the organ and the mutual dependance of the mental phenomena. When, again, we compare the brain in man with the brain in the higher animals, we are surprised to find exactly the same complexity of structure, the same series and order of internal parts, the same general exterior structure in both. The brain, however, in the higher animals (contrasted with their other organs in general, and their spinal cord and medulla oblongata in particular) is relatively smaller than in man, and its external structure much less complicated. The brain of the monkey, for example, has the internal parts of the same general form with those of the human brain ; but the surface of the hemispheres, instead of the numerous intricate furrows and sinuosities, by means of which the quantity of cineritious matter upon the cerebrum and cerebellum in man is so prodigiously increased, exhibits but a few straight depressions, and has proportionately a vastly less extent of the cortical superficies, and of the immediate medullary substratum. " It is here, then, that we are tempted to place the seat of reason ; and, as it appears that the human brain excels that of the monkey by the number and intricacy of its folds and convolutions, so should we analogically be led to suppose, that the difference in mental endowments between one man and another may be connected with a greater amplitude of the surface of the brain in those who are most highly gifted." —Outlines of Physiology, p. 298, 2d edit.

† Anatom. Comparat., i., 25. In the writings of Sir Charles Bell will be found many interesting observations upon the doctrine of *common sensibility.* " The sensibility of the skin," says he, " is one thing ; the sensibility of the surface of the eye is another ; the sensibility of a third part (as the throat) differs again from these ; the sensibility of internal parts differs from the sensibility of external parts ; and each degree and kind of sensibility is benevolently bestowed for a definite purpose. When you compare the external and

peculiar local organ, as well as the other senses, for particular purposes, and purposes in which unusual delicacy and precision are required : in man, this peculiar power of touch is well known to be seated in the nervous papillæ of the tongue, lips, and extremities of the fingers. Its situation in other animals I shall advert to presently.

The differences in the external senses of the different orders and kinds of animals consist in their number and degree of energy.

All the classes of vertebral animals possess the same number of senses as man. Sight is wanting in zoophites, in various kinds of molluscous and articulated worms, and in the larvæ of several species of insects. Hearing does not exist, or at least has not been traced to exist, in many molluscous worms and several insects in a perfect state. Taste and smell, like the general and simple sense of touch, seem seldom to be wanting in any animal.

The local sense of TOUCH, however, or that which is of a more elaborate character, and capable of being exercised in a higher degree, appears to be confined to the three classes of mammals, birds, and insects : and, even in the last two, it is by no means common to all of them, and less so among insects than among birds.

In apes and macaucoes, constituting the quadrumana of Blumenbach, it resides partly in the tongue and tips of the fingers, as in man, but equally, and in some species even in a superior degree, in their toes. In the racoon (*ursus lotor*) it exists chiefly in the under surface of the front toes. In the horse and cattle orders, it is supposed by most naturalists to exist conjointly in the tongue and snout, and in the pig and mole, to be confined to the snout alone : this, however, is uncertain ; as it is also, though there seems to be more reason for such

the internal parts, you find that it is not a common sensibility which they partake of. What would be your condition, were the parts within and around the knee-joint, or the ankle-joint, as sensitive as the surface of the body ? You would be creeping home as if you had inflammation in the joints. You could not walk, if the parts that were bruised in the motions of the body possessed sensibility like the integuments. On the other hand, what would be the consequence if there were no sensibility there ? You would have no guidance in the measure of your exertions ; you would have nothing to tell you how much power in using the limbs was compatible with the texture of your body ; you would be subject to injury, not from without, but from within, to rupture and to laceration. Thus, you will ever find, that the sensibility which is to guard the body is suited to the particular part." Sir Charles Bell afterward adverts to another illustration of his doctrine, afforded by that delicate organ the eye ; the sensibility of whose surface has a relation to the protecting apparatus, so that the fine structure and transparency of the globe may be preserved ; while the sensation of the retina is adapted to the varieties of light and colour only. In the operation of couching, the pain from the passage of the needle through the retina is not so great as that which proceeds from a particle of sand under the eyelid. —See Clinical Lecture in Med. Gaz. for Feb., 1834, p. 760.—Ed.

a belief, that in the elephant it is seated in the proboscis. Some physiologists have supposed the bristly hairs of the tiger, lion, and cat, to be an organ of the same kind, but there seems little ground for such an opinion. In the opossum (and particularly the Cayenne opossum) it exists very visibly in the tail ; and M. Cuvier suspects that it has a similar existence in all the prehensile-tailed mammals.

Blumenbach supposes the same sense to have a place in the same organ in the platypus, or ornithorhyncus, as he calls it, that most extraordinary duck-billed quadruped which has lately been discovered in Australasia, and, by its intermixture of organs, confounds the different classes of animals, and sets all natural arrangement at defiance.

The local organ of touch or feeling in ducks and geese, and some other genera of birds, appears to be situated in the integument which covers the extremity of the mandibles, and especially the upper mandible, with which apparatus they are well known to feel for their food in the midst of mud, in which they can neither see nor perhaps smell it.

We do not know that amphibials, fishes, or worms, possess any thing like a local sense of touch : it has been suspected in some of these, and especially in the arms of the cuttlefish, and in the tentacles of worms that possess this organ ; but at present it is suspicion, and nothing more.

In the insect tribes, we have much reason for believing such a sense to reside in the antennæ or in the tentacles ; whence the former of these are denominated by the German naturalists, *fühl-horner*, or feeling-horns. This belief has not been fully established, but it is highly plausible from the general possession of the one or the other of these organs by the insect tribes, the general purpose to which they apply them, and the necessity which there seems for some such organ from the crustaceous or horny texture of their external coat.

The senses of TASTE and SMELL in animals bear a very near affinity to the local sense of touch ; and it is difficult to determine whether the upper mandible of the duck tribe, with which they distinguish food in the mud, may not be an organ of taste or smell as well as of touch : and there are some naturalists that in like manner regard the cirrous filaments or antennules attached to the mouths of insects as organs of taste and touch equally. Taste, in the more perfect animals, resides jointly in the papillæ of the tongue and the palate ; but I have already had occasion to observe that it may exist, and in full perfection, in the palate alone, since it has been found so in persons who have completely lost the tongue from external force or disease.*

* The brilliant discoveries of Sir Charles Bell, with respect to the Nervous System, prove very clearly that the fifth pair is not only the nerve of sensibility to the head and to the tongue,—not only the *gustatory nerve*,—but has branches which go to the muscles, and those muscles are connected with the act of mastication.—Ed.

In animals that possess the organ of nostrils, this is always the seat of smell; and in many quadrupeds, most birds, and perhaps most fishes, it is a sense far more acute than in man, and that which is chiefly confided in. For the most part it resides in the nerves distributed over the mucous membrane that lines the interior of the bones of the nostrils. Generally speaking, it will be found that the acuteness of smell bears a proportion in all animals to the extent of surface which this membrane displays, and hence, in the dog and cattle tribes, as well as in several others, it possesses a variety of folds or convolutions, and in birds, is continued to the utmost points of the nostrils, which, in different kinds, open in very different parts of the mandible.

The frontal sinuses, which are lined with this delicate membrane, are larger in the elephant than in any other quadruped, and in this animal the sense is also continued through the flexible organ of its proboscis. In the pig the smelling organ is also very extensive; and in most of the mammals possessing proper horns, it ascends as high as the processes of the frontal bone from which the horns issue.

It is not known that the cetaceous tribes possess any organ of smell: their blowing-holes are generally regarded as such, but the point has been by no means fully established. We are in the same uncertainty in respect to amphibials and worms: the sense is suspected to exist in all the former, and in several of the latter, especially in the cuttlefish; but no distinct organ has hitherto been traced out satisfactorily.*

In fishes there is no doubt: the olfactory nerves are very obviously distributed on an olfactory membrane, and, in several instances, the snouts are double, and consequently the nostrils quadruple, a pair for each snout. This powerful inlet of pleasure to fishes often proves fatal to them from its very perfection; for several kinds are so strongly allured by the odour of marjoram, asafœtida, and other aromas, that, by smearing the hand over with these substances, and immersing it in the water, they will often flock towards the fingers, and in their intoxication of delight may easily be laid hold of: and hence the angler frequently overspreads his baits with the same substance, and thus arms himself with a double decoy.

* According to the researches of Sir Charles Bell, the act of smelling is not simply the exposure of the odoriferous particles floating in the atmosphere to the olfactory nerve; but they must rush with a certain violence over it. "There is," says he, "a sort of double or internal nostril; and a change is produced in the figure of the passage when you breathe simply, and when you smell. This configuration of the tube is that which, in the act of taking snuff, gives force to the stream of air upwards. If a man were putting his nose to his snuff-box, and simply breathing, all the snuff would go into the throat; but when he snuffs with the nostril it goes upwards, and stimulates the higher part of the Schneiderian membrane. This is effected by the action of the muscles of the nostril, which depends upon the portio dura. Hence, when the influence of this nerve is lost, there is an imperfection in the act of smelling."—Sir Charles Bell, in Med. Gaz. for Feb, 1834, p. 701.—Ed.

There can be no doubt of the existence of the same sense in insects, for they possess a very obvious power of distinguishing the odorous properties of bodies, even at a considerable distance beyond the range of their vision; but the organ in which this sense resides has not been satisfactorily pointed out. Reimar supposes it to exist in their stigmata, and Knoch in their anterior pair of feelers.

The general organ of HEARING is the ear, but not always so; for in most of those who hear by the Eustachian tube only, it is the mouth: in the whale tribes, it is the nostrils or blow-hole. It is so, however, in all the more perfect animals, which usually for this purpose possess two distinct entrances to the organ; a larger and external surrounded by a lobe, and a smaller and internal opening into the mouth. It is this last which is denominated the Eustachian tube. The shape of the lobe is seldom found even in mammals similar to that in man, excepting among the monkey and the porcupine tribes. In many kinds there is neither external lobe nor external passage. Thus in the frog, and most amphibious animals, the only entrance is the internal or that from the mouth; and, in the cetaceous tribes, the only effective entrance is probably of the same kind; for, though these may be said to possess an external aperture, it is almost imperceptibly minute. It is a curious fact, that among the serpents, the blind worm or common harmless snake is the only species that appears to possess an aperture of either sort; the rest have a rudiment of the organ within, but we are not acquainted with its being pervious to sound.

Fishes are well known to possess a hearing organ, and the skate and shark have the rudiment of an external ear; but, like other fishes, they seem chiefly to receive sound by the internal tubule alone.

That insects in general hear is unquestionable; but it is highly questionable by what organ they obtain the sense of hearing. The antennæ, and perhaps merely because we do not know their exact use, have been supposed by many naturalists to furnish the means; it appears fatal, however, to this opinion to observe, that spiders hear, though they have no true antennæ; and that other insects which possess them naturally, seem to hear as correctly after they are cut off.

The sense of VISION exhibits perhaps more variety in the different classes of animals than any of the external senses. In man, and the greater number of quadrupeds, it is guarded by an upper and lower eyelid, both of which in man, but neither of which in most quadrupeds, are terminated by the additional defence and ornament of cilia or eyelashes. In the elephant, opossum, seal, cat kind, and various other mammals, all birds and all fishes, we find a third eyelid, or nictating membrane as it is usually called, arising from the internal angle of the eye, and capable of covering the pupil with a thin transparent veil, either wholly or in part, and thus defending the eyes from danger in their search after food. In the dog this membrane is narrow ; in oxen and horses it will extend over half the eyeball ; in birds it will easily cover the whole ; and it is by means of this veil, according to Cuvier, that the eagle is capable of looking directly against the noonday sun. In fishes it is almost always upon the stretch, as in their uncertain element they are exposed to more dangers than any other animal. Serpents have neither this nor any other eyelid, nor any kind of external defence whatever but the common integument of the skin.

The largest eyes, in proportion to the size of the animal, belong to the bird tribes, and nearly the smallest to the whale ; the smallest altogether to the shrew and mole, in the latter of which the eye is not larger than a pin's head.

The iris, with but few exceptions, partakes of the colour of the hair, and is hence perpetually varying in different species of the same genus. The pupil exhibits a very considerable, though not an equal variety in its shape. In man it is circular ; in the lion, tiger, and indeed all the cat kind, it is oblong ; transverse in the horse and in ruminating animals ; and heart-shaped in the dolphin.

In man, and the monkey tribes, the eyes are placed directly under the forehead ; in other mammals, birds, and reptiles, more or less laterally ; in some fishes, as the genus pleuronectes, including the turbot and flounder tribes, both eyes are placed on the same side of the head ; in the snail they are situated on its horns, if the black points on the extremities of the horns of this worm be real eyes, of which, however, there is some doubt ; in spiders the eyes are distributed over different parts of the body, and in different arrangements, usually eight in number, and never less than six. The eyes of the sepia have lately been detected by M. Cuvier ; their construction is very beautiful, and nearly as complicated as that of vertebrated animals.—(*Animal Kingdom, trans. by H. M'Murtrie, M. D.*, New-York, 1833.) Polypes and several other zoophites appear sensible of the presence of light, and yet have no eyes ; as the nostrils are not in every animal necessary to the sense of smell, the tongue to that of taste, or the ears to that of sound. A distinct organ is not always requisite for a distinct sense. In man himself we have already seen this in regard to the sense of touch, which exists both locally and generally : the distinct organ of touch is the tips of the tongue and of the fingers, but the feeling is also diffused, though in a subordinate and less precise degree, over every part of the body. It is possible, therefore, in animals that appear endowed with particular senses without particular organs for their residence, that these senses are diffused, like that of touch, over the surface generally ; though there can be no doubt that, for want of such appropriate organs, they must be less acute and precise than in animals that possess them.

Whether there be any other than the five senses common to man and the higher classes of animals, may be reasonably doubted ; but we occasionally meet with peculiarities of sensation that can hardly be resolved into any of them.

Thus the bat appears to be sensible of the presence of external objects and obstructions that are neither seen, smelt, heard, touched, or tasted ; for it will cautiously avoid them when all the senses are purposely closed up. And hence many naturalists have ascribed a sixth sense to this animal. It is equally difficult, by any of the known senses of fishes or of birds, to account for the accuracy with which their migratory tribes are capable of steering their annual course through the depths of the ocean or the trackless regions of the atmosphere, so as to arrive at a given season on a given coast, or in a given climate, with the precision of the expertest mariner. While, with respect to mankind themselves, we sometimes meet with persons who are so peculiarly affected by the presence of a particular object that is neither seen, smelt, tasted, heard, or touched, as not only to be conscious of its presence, but to be in great distress till it is removed. The presence of a cat not unfrequently produces such an effect ; and the author has himself been a witness of the most decisive proofs of this in several instances. It is possible that the peculiar sense may, in such cases, result from a preternatural modification in some of the branches of the olfactory nerve, which may render them capable of being stimulated in a new and peculiar manner ; but the individuals thus affected are no more conscious of an excitement in this organ of sense than in any other ; and, from the anomaly and rare occurrence of the sensation itself, find no terms by which to express it.

In Germany it has of late been attempted to be shown that every man is possessed of a sixth sense, though of a very different kind from those just referred to ; for it is a sense not only common to every one, but to the system at large ; and consists in that peculiar kind of internal but corporeal feeling respecting the general state of one's health, that induces us to exult in being as light as a feather, as elastic as a spring, or to sink under a sense of lassitude, fatigue, and weariness, which cannot be accounted for, and is unconnected with muscular labour or disease. To this sensation M. Hubner has given the name of cænesthesis, and several of his compatriots that of *selbstgefühl*, and *gemeingefühl*, "*self-feeling* or *general-feeling ;*" and its organ is supposed to exist in the extremities of all the nerves of the body, except those that supply the five external senses.* I scarcely know why these last should have been excepted ; for the sensation itself is nothing more than a result of that general sympathy which appears to take place between different organs and parts of the body, expressive of a pleasurable or disquieting feeling, according as the frame at large is in a state of general and uninterrupted health, or affected by some cause of disquiet.

II. As the nerves thus generally communi-

* Comment. de Cænesthesi ; Dissert. Aug. Med. Auct. Chr. Fred. Hubner, 1794. This is totally different from what has been termed *common sensibility*, the objections to which expression, as brought forward by Sir Charles Bell, have been alluded to in a previous note.—ED,

cate with each other, and with the brain where this organ exists, it has been a question in all ages by what means they maintain this communication, and what is the nature of the communicated influence? or, in other words, what is the fabric of the nerves, and the quality of the nervous power?*

Upon these points, two very different opinions have been entertained from an early period of the world, which, under different modifications, have descended to our own times: for by many physiologists, both ancient and modern, the nerves have been regarded as solid capillaments, or tense and elastic strings, operating by tremours or oscillations, like the chords of a musical instrument; and by others, as minute and hollow cylinders conveying a peculiar fluid. The word NERVE, which among the ancients was applied to tense cords of every kind, and especially to bow-strings and musical strings, affords a clear proof how generally the former of these hypotheses prevailed among the Greeks. It was not, however, the hypothesis either of Hippocrates or Galen: for by them, while the nerves were regarded as the instruments of sensation and motion, the medium by which they acted was supposed to be a fine ethereal fluid, elaborated in the organ of the brain; to which they gave the name of animal spirit, to distinguish it from the proper fluid of the arteries, which was denominated vital spirit. "Not," says Galen, "that this animal spirit is of the substance of the soul, but its prime agent while inhabiting the brain."—(*De Hippocratis et Platonis Decretis*, lib. vii., A, tom. i., p. 967, ed. Basil, 1542.) But, with respect to the manner in which the animal spirit operates upon the nerves, they spoke with great modesty; for though they thought they had been able to trace a tubular form in some of the nerves, and particularly those of vision, they had not been able to succeed in others. "And hence," says Galen, "it is impossible for us to pronounce absolutely, and without proof, whether a certain power may not be transmitted from the brain through the nerves to the different members; or whether the material of the animal spirit may not itself reach the sentient and moving parts; or, in some way or other, so enter into the nerves as to induce in them a change, which is afterward extended to the organs of motion."—(Id., sect. C, p. 969.)

In a state not much less unsettled remains the subject at the present moment. Dr. Hartley, in the beginning of the seventeenth century, revived the hypothesis, that the nerves are bundles of solid capillaments conveying motion, sensation, and even perception, by a vibratory power, and supported his opinion with great in-

genuity and learning (*Observations on Man, his Frame, &c., his Duty and his Expectations*, 2 vols., 8vo., 1749); but the opposite hypothesis, that they are minute tubes filled with the animal spirit of the Greek physiologists, had acquired so extensive a hold ever since the discovery of the circulation of the blood, which presupposes the existence of tubular vessels too subtile to be traced by the senses, that it never obtained more than a partial and temporary assent; and hence, from the times of Sydenham and Boerhaave almost down to our own day, the last has been the popular doctrine.

In effect, no fibres of the animal frame can be less adapted to a communication of motion by a series of vibrations than those of the nerves, since none exhibit a smaller degree of elasticity; and though we have little reason to confide in their tubular structure, or to believe that any kind of fluid is transmitted in this way, the close affinity which the nervous power is now known to hold with several of the gases that chymistry has of late years unfolded to us, and the wonderful influence which some of them possess over the moving fibres of the animal frame, seem to leave no question that the nervous power itself is a fluid,* though not, perhaps, of their precise nature, yet resembling the most active of them in its subtilty, levity, and rapidity of movement. Nor is there, upon this supposition, any difficulty in conceiving its transmission by solid fibres or capillaments of a particular kind, the *neurilemma* of Bichat, while we behold the ethereal fluids now referred to transmitted in the same way by substances still more solid and unporous.

But there is another question, closely connected with the present subject, which has also greatly interested physiologists both in ancient and modern times, and is not yet settled in a manner altogether satisfactory.

It has appeared that the nerves are instruments both of sensation and motion. Are these two effects produced by the same nervous fibres, or by different? or by the same fluids, or by different? That there must be two distinct kinds of fibres or of fluids is clear, because, as we shall have more particularly to observe when we come to treat of paralysis, the muscles of a limb are sometimes deprived of both sensation and motivity at the same period, sometimes of sensation alone while motivity continues, and sometimes of motivity alone while sensation continues. And hence Hippocrates and Galen, the last of whom has treated of the subject with great minuteness in many of his writings, while they speak of only one kind of animal spirit, speak of two kinds of nerves, those of sense and of motion; equally issuing from the brain, and mostly accompanying each other, and forming parts of the same organs.†

This distinction is supported by the concurrent observations and experiments of physiolo

---

* "The question," says Dr. Bostock, "may be thus stated in direct terms:—When an impression made upon an organ of sense is transmitted by a nerve to the brain, or when the exercise of volition is communicated to the nerve, so as to produce the corresponding effect upon the muscle, what change does the nerve experience, or in what way is it acted upon so as to admit of this transmission?" —Elem. Syst. of Physiology, vol. i., p. 250.—ED.

* The editor's opinion of this hypothesis will appear in the sequel.

† The curious fact of most of the nerves of motion (though not all) originating from the spinal marrow, has been already stated.—ED.

gists, and especially by the curious investigations of many of those of our own day, among whom should be particularly noticed the names of Flourens, Rolando, Charles Bell, Magendie, and Shaw. M. Rolando attempted to show, by a long train of interesting but very painful experiments, carried on through animals of almost every kind, that the cerebrum is the ordinary source of sensation, and the cerebellum of motion: for, according to his observations, in every instance in which the former is much broken down, or in any other way injured, drowsiness, stupor, or apoplexy is sure to follow; the animal being still capable of exercising locomotive power, but without any guidance or knowledge of what it is about, or where it is moving to. But the moment the cerebellum is wounded, the locomotive power is instantly lost.— (*Saggio sopra la vera Strutt. del Cervello*, &c., *e sopra le Fonz. della Sist. Nervosa*, Sassari, 1809.) These investigations were valuable, as leading on to others more accurately conducted, and followed up by more correct conclusions. That these distinct portions of the brain are endowed with separate powers, as observed by Rolando, has been sufficiently ascertained by other pathologists; and especially by M. Flourens (*Arch. Gén. de Méd.*, i., ii.; also, *Recherches Exp. sur le Syst. Nerveux*, Paris, 1824), who does not seem at the time to have been acquainted with Rolando's experiments, and consequently gives us the weight of an unconnected testimony. But it seems to M. Magendie (*Exp. sur les Fonctions*, &c., *Journ. de Physiologie*, tom. ii., iii., passim, 1822, 1823) to be now better established, that the converse of M. Rolando's constitutes the law and order of nature: sensation appearing to be dependant upon the cerebellum instead of upon the cerebrum; while motivity takes its rise from the cerebrum instead of from the cerebellum.

[If, however, the researches and experiments of Magendie oppose those of the foregoing physiologists, let it be remembered that the results of his investigations disagree with many observations made on this subject by physiologists of high reputation. According to Sir Charles Bell, the nerves of the greatest number of the voluntary muscles are derived from the medulla spinalis, and the best modern anatomists trace the origins of most of the other nerves to the medulla oblongata. If, therefore, the origins of the nerves could be taken as a criterion, Magendie's views would not be at all tenable. But it is not by this test that the question can be settled, because the inquiry here refers, not to what nerves are concerned in sensation and voluntary motion, but to what part of the brain or cerebellum the power of regulating the voluntary action of the muscles is to be ascribed. It is a question, therefore, that can only be settled by experiment.

In order to determine the exact uses of particular parts of the brain and its appendages, numerous experiments have been performed, which consisted in observing very carefully the effects resulting from the injury of definite portions of those organs. The first researches of

this description were those of Molinelli (*Comment. Bononiens*, p. 130), and they have been followed up by the more important experiments of Boerhaave, Haller, Zinn, Zimmermann, Fodera (*Magendie, Journ. de Physiologie*, vol. i., 1823), Legallois (*Exp. sur le Principe de la Vie*), Krauss (*Diss. de Cerebri læsi ad motum Volunt. relatione*, Vratisl., 1824), Hertwig (*Hecker's Litterarische Annalen*, &c., May, 1826), and those of the physiologists already enumerated. Of all the experiments made on this subject, those of Flourens are perhaps the most valuable. From them, which, indeed, confirm earlier observations, it results that each strongly developed part of the brain is intended for the performance of particular functions, the hemispheres of the cerebrum being the organ of the mental faculties (understanding, memory, and will), and the centre of all the perceptions;[*] while the cerebellum is the organ in which the different muscular motions are regulated and directed to one common object. In the corpora quadrigemina is seated the original active principle of the iris, the retina, and optic nerves. Irritation of the corpora quadrigemina, medulla oblongata, and medulla spinalis, shows that these are the only parts of the nervous system connected with muscular contractions. Another inference is, that the power of sensation is a single one, and resides in a single organ.

According to Hertwig's still more recent investigations, although the substance of the hemispheres is the centre of all the perceptions, it is insensible of external irritations. Irritations and even injuries of the hemispheres, he found, produce no involuntary motions of the muscles, merely weakness and paralysis of them; and always on the side of the body opposite to that on which the injury was inflicted. Hertwig's experiments also confirm the doctrine that the operation of the hemispheres is in a crossed direction, that the *consensus communis* is not dependant on them alone; since it remains after they have been destroyed; and that the respiration and circulation are also independent of them.

With respect to the cerebellum, Dr. Hertwig found that its substance was not sensible to immediate external irritations, by which also no motions of the muscles were excited; but that the undisturbed operation of this organ is necessary to the production and co-operation of the muscles for a particular purpose, as flying, walking, &c. His experiments likewise tend to prove that the action of the cerebellum on the voluntary muscles takes place in a cross direc-

---

[*] The following criticism is entitled to consideration:—"One of the most important points which M. Flourens attempts to establish is, that the lobes of the cerebrum are the exclusive seat of sensation and volition; yet it seems quite evident, from the result of the experiments, that, after the removal of these lobes, sensation, although rendered feeble or obtuse, was by no means extinguished; while the functions which depend upon volition, such as the various kinds of locomotion, were still executed by the animal, although it was difficult to excite them into action."—See Bostock's Physiology, vol. iii., p. 374.

tion; and that the uses of the senses and all the other functions depend very little on the action of the cerebellum.

According to Dr. Hertwig, a superficial irritation or wound of the pons varolii produces in animals some pain and temporary convulsions; but deep, penetrating injuries cause, independently of the other effects, a permanent irregularity in the voluntary motions of the body, arising from a disturbance in the balance of the powers between the two sides of the body, or between its anterior and posterior parts. The pons exerts considerable influence over the voluntary locomotive organs for the preservation of the balance between them. Another conclusion to which Dr. Hertwig's experiments led him is, that the pons varolii has little influence over the senses and consciousness. With regard to the medulla oblongata, Dr. Hertwig's experiments corroborate the opinion that it has great influence over respiration, and also partly over the circulation. Hence its complete division destroys life by interrupting respiration. The same experimenter infers, that, as injuries of this organ do not disturb the senses, the intellectual functions can have no dependance upon it.]*

Sir Charles Bell has successfully followed up the distinct and established powers of the two departments of the brain (*Idea of the Anatomy of the Brain*, 1809) into the spinal marrow, which he has sufficiently proved to consist of a double cord;* an anterior connected with the crura of the cerebrum and productive of locomotion, and a posterior connected with the crura of the cerebellum, productive of sensation.† And he has further shown, that these two distinct powers are communicated to every part of the body by nervous fibres, according as they issue from the one or the other of these respective channels: that, for the most part, every nervous fascicle distributed over the body and limbs has a double origin, and issues equally from both the anterior and posterior trunk of the spinal marrow, and is, consequently, alike sensific and modific; while those which proceed from one alone are limited in their power to the peculiar property of their source,‡ of which the

---

* According to the learned Professor Jackson, of Philadelphia, "the cerebrum is the seat of the organs of the intellectual, and affective or moral faculties. The cerebellum is the organ for co-ordinating or combining the muscular contractions required to produce locomotive motions and equilibration or station. The ash or gray substance, the most vascular portion of the nervous structure, is that which is active in the production of the nervous phenomena. It originates the power or agent, the cause of the sensations and voluntary movements, that excites the muscular contractions requisite to the performance of respiration, the expressions, &c., and which would appear to be generated by this substance in the medulla oblongata; and finally, in the cerebrum it constitutes the organs exercising the intellectual and moral faculties, &c. The white medullary or fibrous substance is subservient to the offices of the ash or gray substance, conveying to it impressions excited on the external and internal surfaces of relation by the nervous cords composed of this substance, and reconducting from the ash substance the nervous force, agency, influence, or whatever name may be given to this unknown principle or agent, into the different organs and tissues, and probably fluids of the organism. The white medullary or fibrous substance of the cerebrum and cerebellum is encephalic nerves, executing the same office as the same substance has been shown to perform in nerves and the spinal marrow; and it transmits the actions excited in the medulla oblongata, by sensible impressions proceeding from the senses, to the gray substance composing the intellectual and affective organs in the cerebrum constituted for that purpose; and reconveys the actions of these organs into the medulla oblongata, whence they are directed into the organism, causing locomotions, the expressions, and even disturbances, when violent, of the organic and functional actions of the viscera."—See the Principles of Medicine, founded on the Structure and Functions of the Animal Organism, by Samuel Jackson, M. D., &c., Philadelphia, 1832.—D.

* The following is Sir Charles Bell's description: "Different columns of nervous matter combine to form the spinal marrow. Each lateral portion of the spinal marrow consists of three tracks or columns; one for voluntary motion, one for sensation, and one for the act of respiration. So that the spinal marrow comprehends in all six rods, intimately bound together, but *distinct in office*; and the capital of this compound column is the medulla oblongata. No doubt," he adds, "these grander columns contain within them subdivisions; for if we lift up the medulla spinalis from the cerebellum, and look at its back part, we shall see more numerous cords, the offices of which will one day be discovered."—See Exposition of the Natural System of the Nerves, p. 20, 8vo., London, 1824.

† "The anterior column of each lateral division of the spinal marrow is for motion, the posterior column is for sensation, and the middle one is for respiration. The two former extend up into the brain, and are dispersed or lost in it, for their functions stand related to the sensorium; but the latter stops short in the medulla oblongata, being in function independent of reason, and capable of its office independent of the brain, or when separated from it.

"It is the introduction of the middle column of the three, viz., that for respiration, which constitutes the spinal marrow, as distinct from the long central nerve of the animals without vertebræ, and which is attended with the necessity for that form of the trunk which admits of the respiratory motions."—Op. cit., p. 22.

‡ The following observations were published by Mr. Mayo:—"When a spinal nerve is divided in its course through the body, the parts supplied by it beyond the division are paralyzed: they lose sense and motion. If the two origins of the spinal nerves are exposed in a young animal, and separately divided, different effects are produced. The section of the anterior root deprives of voluntary motion the part supplied by the nerve; the section of the posterior root deprives the corresponding part of the body of sensation, voluntary motion being left." These experiments were made by M. Magendie, and published by him in his Journal of Physiology. But many years earlier, Mr. Bell had made experiments upon the spinal nerves, some account of which had been printed and circulated among his friends, as well as delivered in his lectures. The following is an extract from this account:—"On laying bare the

portio dura of the seventh nerve affords a striking example : being, when uncombined, simply a nerve of motion, without the attribute of sensation, but exercising motion over all the organs of the face that are connected with the function of respiration, whether in the cheeks, lips, or nostrils ; and hence operating equally in the acts of speaking, singing, sucking, drinking, spitting, coughing, and sneezing. And he has confirmed these discoveries by the striking fact, that the nerves of the head, which issue, like the spinal medulla, from both departments of the brain, possess the same double power, and are, in like manner, nerves of sensation and motion ; of which the fifth pair offers a notable example, bestowing at the same time sensibility on the head

and face, and performing various muscular motions common to all animals, so as to be analogous to a double spinal nerve, or rather to the spine itself, and enriched, like the spine, with ganglions in particular parts. Many of these experiments have since been repeated, and the results to which they have thus led, though in some respects opposed by other experiments of M. Fodera (*Rech. Exp.*, &c., *Journ. de Physiologie*, Juillet, 1823), have generally been confirmed by M. Magendie, Mr. Shaw, Mr. Broughton, and various other anatomists ; and we hence see the reason of those frequent decussations and other interunions of nerve with nerve, by which those possessing a single origin, and consequently a single property, hereby exchange

roots of the spinal nerves," observes Mr. Bell. "I found that I could cut across the posterior fasciculus of nerves, which took its origin from the posterior portion of the spinal marrow, without convulsing the muscles of the back ; but that, on touching the anterior fasciculus with the point of the knife, the muscles of the back were immediately convulsed." Mr. Bell was carried by these experiments, says Mr. Mayo, very near to the truth, but he failed at that time to ascertain it : he inferred from his experiments, indeed, that the anterior and posterior roots of the spinal nerves have different functions ; but in the nature of these functions he was mistaken. Upon the anterior root he supposed both sensation and motion to depend ; the posterior he considered an unconscious nerve, which might control the growth and sympathies of parts. When Mr. Bell published a further account of the functions of these nerves, M. Magendie had already given to the world the true theory of their uses.—(See Mayo's Outlines of Physiology, p. 325, 2d edit., 1828.) However this may be, the editor believes that if it had not been for the original train of experiments instituted by Sir Charles Bell, we should yet have remained ignorant of the distinction between nerves of sense and nerves of motion. Nor does Sir Charles Bell admit some part of the foregoing statements. As for Magendie, his claim is also put in a different light by certain important explanations recently published. In the tract printed long before 1811, Sir Charles Bell declares that he distinctly inculcated the great principle, "*that a nerve, whatever its nature may be, cannot perform two functions at once ;* it cannot convey sensation inwards to the sensorium, at the same time that it carries outwards a mandate of the will to the muscles, whether it be through the means of a fluid, or an ether, or a vibration, or what you will, that it performs its functions. Two vibrations cannot run counter through the same fibre, and at the same instant. Two undulations cannot go in different directions through the same tube at the same moment ; and therefore," says Sir Charles Bell, " I conceived that the nerves must be different in their kind. This led me to experiment upon the nerves of the spine ; for, I said, where shall I be able to find a nerve with the roots separated ? where shall I be able to distinguish the properties of a compound nerve ? By experimenting upon the separate roots of the spinal nerve. So then, taking a fine instrument, the point of a needle, and drawing it along one set of roots, and then along another, I found that as I touched one set, the anterior roots, it was like touching the key of a pianoforte—all the chords, as it were, the muscles, were in vibration ; and when I touched the other, there was pain and struggling. That would not do ; the

animal being alive to sensation, there was confusion ; and therefore I struck the animal on the head, and then I made my experiments clearly ; by which it was shown that *the roots of these nerves were of different qualities : one obviously bestowing motion ;* and, by inference, the other bestowing *sensibility.*" Having come to the conclusion that *the roots of the spinal nerves were double, that each might have a double function,* he inquired of himself, How is the head supplied ? Is there any nerve in the head that has a resemblance to the nerves of the spine, one root of each of which nerves has a ganglion, and the other not ? Then, he said, what nerve of the head has a ganglion ? The fifth has a double root, with a ganglion on one of these roots, like a spinal nerve. Now the function of the posterior root of the spinal nerve, or that which did not excite motion when irritated, he thought might be illustrated by considering the fifth pair as nerves of the same class. Experiments were made upon the three branches of the fifth pair in the face ; and what was incomplete in the experiments upon the spinal nerves was made perfectly clear by them. It was established, that *branches proceeding from a ganglion, in all respects the same in structure as the ganglions of the spinal nerves, were the only nerves which bestowed sensibility on the head.* "It has been said," observes Sir Charles Bell, "that I gave out that *sensation and motion belonged to the anterior roots.* How could that be ? The principle upon which I proceeded, the idea which I entertained for many years, that which forced me on to all my experiments, was, *that one filament could perform only one function ;* and for me to say that the anterior roots performed two functions, was just giving the whole matter up. It has been my misfortune to put all these things down in a large, heavy, dear book : were it generally read, which I learn from my bookseller that it is not, I should have no occasion at any time to vindicate the originality or correctness of my observations. When M. Magendie took up this subject he had in his hands my original paper, in which the classification of the nerves, and the principles on which that classification is founded, 'that nerves arising from distinct roots are endowed with distinct functions,' are all stated. He had copies of these plans which are now hung up beside me. The experiments upon the fifth nerve, which are detailed in that paper, and which were suggested to me by my previous experiments upon the roots of the spinal nerves, were repeated before him in Paris by Mr. John Shaw, who had on various occasions made the experiments on the spinal nerves before my pupils in Great Windmill-street, previously to visiting Paris."—See Medical Gazette for February, 1834.—Ed.

filaments, and become enriched with a new power, the respective filaments being enveloped in the same sheath.

[In elucidating the uses of the fifth pair of nerves and the portio mollis of the seventh, Mr. Mayo merits considerable honour. From a series of experiments detailed by him (*Anat. and Physiol. Commentaries*, 1822), the conclusion is made, that *the portio dura of the seventh nerve is a simple voluntary nerve*, and that *the facial branches of the fifth are exclusively sentient nerves*. In pursuing this subject, Mr. Mayo was led to observe that there are muscles which receive no branches from any nerve but the fifth : these muscles are the masseter, the temporal, the two pterygoids, and the circumflexus palati. These muscles, he further remarked, are supplied with branches from the third division of the fifth, that is to say, from the particular division of the fifth with which the *smaller fasciculus or root of the nerve is associated.* After some careful dissection, in the greater part of which he found that he had been anticipated by Palletta, he made out that *the smaller fasciculus of the fifth is entirely consumed upon the supply of the above-mentioned muscles,* to which it is to be borne in mind that twigs from the ganglionic portion are likewise distributed. " But," says Mr. Mayo, " I had already ascertained by experiment, that almost all the branches of the larger or ganglionic portions of the fifth were nerves of sensation. I proved this point in the ass, the dog, and the rabbit, respecting the second and third divisions of the fifth ; in the pigeon, respecting the first division. It was therefore thoroughly improbable that the twigs sent from the same part of the nerve to the muscles of the lower jaw should have a different quality, and be nerves of motion. For this function it was reasonable to look to the other nervous fibrils which the masseter, and temporal, and pterygoid muscles receive ; in other words, *to the branches of the smaller fasciculus or root, or ganglionless portion of the fifth.* All this was made out before the publication of M. Magendie's discovery of the parallel functions of the double roots of the spinal nerves."— (*Mayo's Physiology,* p. 331, et seq., 2d edit.)

At the same time that praise is due to others for what they have done on this intricate subject, the world and posterity will never forget the matchless claims of Sir Charles Bell to the glory of having first pointed the path that led to all the success with which the nervous system has been examined in latter times. It is not fair that his merit should be lost sight of, and even his originality questioned, because other physiologists have contributed to establish and perfect the system which he first suggested. Sir Charles Bell has most ably explained, that the great error which misled anatomists in their conceptions concerning the nerves, consisted in following, though with some license, the old hypothesis, that the nerves receive their influence from the brain, and confer it on remote parts of the body, and that they are endowed with the same powers. For (says he) whether we look upon the intricacy of the parts

on dissection, or attempt to unravel the mystery of sensation and voluntary and involuntary motion performed by a single nerve, there is a complete discrepance between the fact and the hypothesis. In the view which Sir Charles Bell takes of the nerves of the human body, there are, besides the nerves of vision, smell, and hearing, four systems combined into a whole. Nerves, entirely different in function, extend through the frame : those of sensation ; those of voluntary motion ; those of respiratory motion ; and lastly, nerves which, from their being deficient in the qualities that distinguish the three others, seem to unite the body into a whole, in the performance of the functions of nutrition, growth, and decay, and whatever is directly necessary to animal existence. These nerves, Sir Charles Bell remarks, are sometimes bound together ; but they do not in any case interfere with or partake of each other's influence. A nerve is seen to consist of distinct filaments, but there is nothing to distinguish them or indicate their offices. One filament may be for the purpose of sensation, another for muscular motion, a third for combining the muscles in the act of respiration ; but the subserviency of any particular filament to its proper office can only be made out by tracing it and observing its relations, and especially its origin in the brain and spinal marrow.

The key to Sir Charles Bell's system is in the simple proposition, that *each filament has its peculiar endowment, independently of the other filaments bound up along with it ;* and *that it continues to have the same endowment throughout its whole length.* Thus, if its office be to convey sensation, that power shall belong to it in all its course, wherever it can be traced ; and at whatever point, whether in the foot, leg, thigh, spine, or brain, it may be bruised, pricked, or otherwise injured, sensation, and not motion, will result ; and the perception arising from the impression will be referred to that part of the skin where the remote extremity of the filament is distributed.

There is much, however, in this recondite subject, that still requires elucidation ; and particularly in regard to that continuation of sense and motion in many cases which we shall hereafter have to notice, in which the brain, through a very considerable extent, both in its white and cineritious substance, has been found in a mollescent or pulpy state ; often, indeed, entirely disorganized, and as soft as soap : while, in other instances, the spinal marrow, through an extent of six or seven inches in length, has been found equally dissolved, and its chain completely destroyed ;* one set of limbs being rendered

---

* This point requires further investigation. When the spinal cord is divided in experiments upon warm-blooded animals, or is compressed or lacerated, the lower part of the body is totally paralyzed. This result, as Mr. Mayo observes, is so uniform, that we are bound to suppose an error in the narrative of two well-attested cases, on record, of sensation and voluntary motion continuing after the division of the spinal marrow. Some violence is scarcely avoidable in opening the spinal canal;

rigid and motionless, with an augmented sensibility, at the same time that the sensation and mobility of the rest have been scarcely interfered with. And hence a separate and specific power has, from an early age, been ascribed to the nervous fibres themselves, while the brain has been contemplated as their radix. This, in truth, was the peculiar hypothesis of Glisson, and nearly so of Haller, with respect to the motory power; and Girtanner, who trod in the same footsteps, with a clear and comprehensive mind, considerably enlarged upon it, and gave to the moving energy the name of vis insita, as, by way of distinction, he applied that of vis nervea to the energy or power of feeling.* And as he believed that other organs besides muscles, and indeed plants† as well as animals, are possessed of fibres endowed with the same power, and that a brain is by no means essential for their production, he in like manner changed the name of muscular to that of irritable fibre; and contended that a principle of irritability is common to fluids as well as to solids, and co-extensive with organized nature.—(*Mém. sur l'Irritabilité, Journ. de Phys.*, 1790.)

By what means these fibres unite into solid masses or hollow coats, and what are their respective powers when thus complicated, shall be glanced at hereafter;‡ at present we must confine ourselves to their actuating principle, whatever that may consist in.

Oxygen was at this time the popular aura of the philosophers, as caloric had been a short time before. Lavoisier had just proved its close connexion with several of the vital functions, and hence the chymical divinity of Girtanner was oxygen. He paid unbounded homage to its influence; attempted to show that irritabili-

ty, and even life itself, are dependant upon it; and that in the animal system it is distributed to every part by means of the circulating blood.

But the still more striking properties of the galvanic fluid began now to be discovered, and to captivate the general attention; and the time drew nigh in which oxygen was doomed to fall as prostrate before the shrine of galvanic aura, as caloric had fallen before that of oxygen. And it is curious to remark how nearly this discovery was not only made but completed in all its bearings, and by the very same means, about fifty years before the attention of Galvani was directed to the subject; for we are told in the Philosophical Transactions for 1732 (vol. xxxvii., p. 324), that the queen's physician, Dr. Alexander Stuart, being engaged in a course of experiments upon the frog, observed, upon thrusting the blunt end of a probe into the spinal marrow after decapitation, that the muscles of the animal's body were thrown into convulsive contractions; and that the same happened to the muscles of the head when the probe was thrust into the brain. And by additional experiments he advanced so far as to infer that what the nerves contribute in muscular motion cannot be produced by oscillations or elasticity, but must be owing to a fluid contained in them: but which fluid he was unfortunate enough to conceive was a pure and perfectly defecated elementary water; using the word water, however, in a general sense, as merely opposed to sal volatile or fermented spirits, which he thought the term animal spirits was calculated to import.

Whatever be the nature of the active and ethereal fluid which was thus supposed to exist by Stuart, and has since been attempted to be established by Galvani, it is presumed to have a powerful influence upon many branches or divisions of the nervous system, though not upon all.* Its effects upon the muscles of an animal for some hours after death are too well

---

and if the spinal cord be already partially divided, the operation of exposing it may easily complete the rupture. How slight a continuity of nervous fibre is sufficient to sustain the communication between parts of the medulla spinalis, must be known to those who have attempted to destroy animals by pithing: a very slender layer of nervous substance will enable the animal to continue breathing, which, however, ceases instantly on its division.—See Mayo's Outlines of Physiology, p. 285, 2d edit.—Ed.

* The doctrines involving the respective properties of the vis insita and vis nervea formerly attracted much attention, and the views of Whytte and Haller were treated with some severity. The manner in which Mr. Abernethy has discussed many topics connected with the intricate questions of human physiology and comparative anatomy, will always recommend his writings, and more particularly his lectures delivered before the Royal College of Surgeons in 1817, as worthy of an attentive perusal.—D.

† The seeming analogy between the life of animals and that of plants has led vegetable physiologists to a comparative investigation of the subject. Besides light, heat, and oxygen, the common stimuli of plants, electricity has been mentioned as an official agent by which plants are excited to increased development. De Candolle remarks that the discharge of electricity is one of the most powerful stimulants to the vital action of plants.—D.

‡ See the introductory remarks to Order III. of the present Class, Neurotica, Cinetica.

* Although our author, as we shall presently find, makes the judicious distinction between the hypothesis of galvanism and electricity being identical with the imaginary nervous fluid, and the doctrine of their being only stimulants, by which the secretion of this fluid may be excited, and the action of the nerves continued, he does not seem to entertain the slightest doubt of the actual existence of a nervous fluid, and of its being a secretion, as if these circumstances had been satisfactorily proved and demonstrated. The editor often regrets that Dr. Good should have assumed these hypotheses as positively established facts, and that he did not rest satisfied with the less objectionable expressions, nervous power, nervous energy, or nervous influence, instead of the phrases, more frequently introduced into the second edition than the present, of "secretion of sensorial power, of the nervous fluid," &c. &c., involving him in the most visionary speculations. The hypothesis of a nervous fluid, the product of secretion, is not essentially different from the notion of the existence of animal spirits. The principal ground of the latter, as Dr. Bostock remarks, "seems to have been the idea that the brain is a secretory organ; an idea which was suggested by the great quantity of blood sent to it, and by some supposed resemblance in its structure to other secreting glands.—(Descartes, Tractus de Homine, § 14.)

known to be particularized; and Dr. Philip seems to have shown, by various trains of experiments (*Phil. Trans.*, 1814, pp. 5–90), that it is equally capable of maintaining respiration, and the operation of several of the animal secretions, especially those that induce digestion, for as long a period. But in drawing from such facts the corollary, that the "IDENTITY of galvanic electricity and nervous influence is established by these experiments," he seems, like those who have anticipated him in the same doctrine,* to proceed farther than he is warranted: for we have no right to say more than that galvanic electricity is a stimulus exciting the nervous influence into a state of continued secretion or continued action, which may possibly

---

Yet, as nothing cognizable by the senses is produced by it, it was concluded that it must secrete something of a subtile or ethereal nature, peculiarly suited to the performance of the functions which belong to the brain, and which are so unlike those of other material substances. It must be recollected that about two centuries ago, every thing that could not be otherwise explained was referred to the agency of some kind of refined spirit; an idea which appears to have been originally derived from the alchymists; and after being incorporated with the metaphysics of the age, gave rise to a long train of mysticism. Almost every philosopher of that period adopted more or less of these notions. . Newton's ether is well known to have proved an abundant source of speculation to multitudes of those who called themselves his followers, and who seem unfortunately to have copied almost the only error which this great man committed. Upon this slender foundation was built the hypothesis of the nervous fluid, or the animal spirits, as they have been termed; yet their existence was assumed as an ascertained fact, and even their different affections and diseases were spoken of with as much confidence as if the authors had been treating upon something which was the immediate object of their senses, and with which they were perfectly familiar. The doctrine of the animal spirits has likewise become a subject of popular belief, and has given rise to a variety of expressions that are every day employed in our common language. There does not, however, appear to be the least shadow of proof of their existence, either from experiment or observation; there is no analogy in their favour; the structure and physical properties of the nerves do not seem adapted to the office that has been assigned them; and, in short, the whole is an hypothesis entirely unfounded and quite gratuitous."—See Bostock's Physiology, vol. i., p. 253.
* The researches of Valli led him also to conclude that electricity and the nervous fluid were identical.—(Journ. de Phys., tom. xli.) And, as is remarked by Dr. Bostock, Mr. Abernethy goes still further; for he regards some subtile fluid, analogous to electricity, not merely as the prime agent in sensation, but even as constituting the essence of life itself. " Singular as it may appear, we find this highly respectable and intelligent writer sliding into materialism at the very time when he is directing the force of his genius against this doctrine.—(See Lect. on H$_{unter}$ s Physiology, pp. 26, 30, 35, 80, &c.) It is scarcely necessary to observe, that, metaphysically speaking, the subtile or ethereal agents that are called in to aid in our explanation of the vital phenomena, are as truly *material* as the densest stone or metal."—See Bostock's Physiology, vol. i., p. 256.

be done by various other stimuli as well as by that of galvanism. M. Rolando, however, has proceeded farther than this; for while he regards the nervous fluid and that of galvanism as identic, he contemplates the cerebellum and its appendages as a galvanic machine, in which the cerebellum itself constitutes the formative pile, the medulla oblongata the conductor in which the fluid is accumulated, and the spine and nerves the channels through which it is conveyed to the muscles for the purpose of exciting *voluntary motion*. But this puts us into possession of only one half of the powers of the brain,—the *motific*. For the *sensific* powers, M. Rolando has revived the old doctrine of vibrations already noticed, and conceives that all sensations are commenced at the extremities of the nerves, and are conveyed from the circumference to the centre of the system by vibrating cords.—(*Coster, Archives Gén. de Méd.*, Mars, 1823.)*

Upon the whole, the nervous system seems to present itself, in the different classes of ani-

---

* Messrs. Dumas and Prevost have made some curious observations on the part taken by the nerves in muscular contraction. Their experiments, as stated by Prof. Dunglison (Human Physiology, by Robley Dunglison, vol. i., p. 313, Philadelphia, 1832), are as follow :—" By a microscope magnifying ten or twelve diameters, they first of all examined the manner in which the nerves are arranged in a muscle; and found, as has been already observed, that their ramifications always entered the muscle in a direction perpendicular to its fibres. They satisfied themselves that none of the nerves really terminate in the muscle; but that the final ramifications embrace the fibres like a noose, and return to the trunk that furnishes them, or to one in its vicinity: the nerve setting out from the anterior column of the spinal marrow and returning to the posterior. On farther examining the muscles at the time of their contraction, the parallel fibres composing them were found by the microscope to bend in a zigzag manner, and to exhibit a number of regular undulations: such flexions forming angles, which varied according to the degree of contraction, but were never less than fifty degrees. The flexions, too, always occurred at the same parts of the fibre, and to them the shortening of the muscle was owing, as MM. Dumas and Prevost proved by calculating the angles. The angular points were always found to correspond to the parts where the small nervous filaments enter, or are fixed into, the muscle. They therefore believed that the filaments, by their approximation, induce contraction of the muscular fibre: and this approximation they have aseribed to a galvanic current running through them, which, as the fibres are parallel and very near each other, ought to cause them to attract each other, according to Anpere's law, that two currents attract each other when they move in the same direction. The living muscles are consequently regarded by them as galvanometers of an extremely sensible kind, on account of the very minute distance and tenuity of the nervous filaments.

" They moreover affirm, that by an anatomical arrangement, the nerve is fixed in the muscle in the very position required for the proper performance of its function; and they esteem the fatty matter which envelops the nervous fibres, and which was discovered by Vauquelin, as a means of insulation, preventing the electric fluid from passing from one of the fibres to the other."—D.

mals, under various scales of elaboration; but, in every scale, to be a secernent organ through its entire range; operating by means of two or more different sets of fibres, which may be secretories or conductors of as many different fluids, or modifications of the same fluid.*

In the higher and more complicated classes of animals it consists of a cylindrical cord or spinal marrow, a central or ganglionic compages, and a brain, all communicating and acting in harmony.—(*De Nervi Symp. hum. fabricâ, usû, et morbis,* &c., *Auctore, J. Lobstein,* Paris, 1823.) In some of the inferior classes we find the cylindrical cord alone, and in others the ganglionic compages; while, in the lowest of all, we trace a variety of distinct and granular molecules, which seem to act the part of nervous ganglions, though we cannot discover their connexion.

The brain has so much of the general structure and character of a gland, as to be admitted by many to be an organ of this kind.† This is a point conceded even by Dr. Cullen, notwithstanding that, by supposing the energy of the brain to be a mere quality rather than a specific essence, and to be incapable of undergoing any change of recruit or exhaustion, he finds no adequate use for its glandular conformation. As we are justified, however, by all the force of analogy in regarding it as a gland, though unquestionably a gland of a peculiar kind, and as we are equally justified, on the same ground of analogy, in regarding the nervous power or energy by which it maintains a communication with every part of the system as a fluid of a peculiar kind, we are almost driven to the necessity of contemplating it as the source from which this fluid issues, and by which it is supplied as it becomes exhausted: and more especially when we reflect upon the enormous proportion of blood which is sent from the heart to the head, as the

* One objection to this hypothesis depends upon the fact, that, if it were admitted, we should not then have any clearer notions of the mode in which the brain and other parts of the nervous system perform their functions, than if no such hypothesis had ever been started. As Mr. Lawrence has observed, " who understands muscular contraction better by being told that an Archeus or subtile matter sets the fibres at work?"—Eᴅ.

† This doctrine, though adopted by some physiologists, is not espoused by others. When the comparison of the brain to a gland is made, we may inquire whether it be intended to assume that the nervous fluid is secreted by the brain, and thence transmitted through the nerves? or whether the brain only secretes its own nervous fluid, and the nerves theirs? Lastly, we may ask, who has ever seen this wonderful fluid? and how many kinds of it are fancied to exist? for the several parts of the brain have different functions; and some nerves are for sensation, and others for motion. In short, it is better to confess that we know nothing of the way in which the brain and other parts of the nervous system execute their functions; and, instead of talking about the secretion of the nervous and sensorial fluid, it may be wiser to rest satisfied with the less objectionable phrases of nervous action, nervous energy, nervous influence, sensorial power, &c.—Eᴅ.

most extensive laboratory of the entire frame, and which, according to Haller (*Elem. Physic.,* x., v., 20), amounts to one fifth, or, on the lower estimate of Monro (*On the Nervous System,* p. 3), to one tenth* of the entire current poured forth from the left ventricle of the heart, while it is well known that the weight of the human brain is not more than one fortieth part of the entire body.

It is probable that the nervous fluid, on its first secretion and in its simplest state, is as homogeneous as that of the blood; but that, like the blood, it becomes changed by particular actions, either of the particular parts of the brain, or of particular nerves themselves, into fluids possessing different powers, and capable of producing very different effects. And as modern experiments have induced us to believe, with Galen, that the nerves are a continuation of the matter of the brain (*Hippocr. et Plat. Decret.,* lib. iii., tom. i., p. 921), it is not improbable that many or all of them are endowed with something of its secernent power, and are capable of assisting in the secretion of the same fluid in its simplest state, or in some of its simpler modifications. And we may hence see the reason of that complicated mechanism which distinguishes the higher classes of animals, and how it is possible for a nervous system to exist, though with inferior powers, under a less composite fabrication.

This, however, is not mere conjecture; for in acephalous and anencephalous monsters we are compelled to admit it as a fact; and in different ramifications of the nerves we can trace such different effects actually produced: and as it has sufficiently appeared that the operative power is a quick and subtile fluid, we are directly led to conclude that such difference of effects must depend on a diversity of fluids, or on various modifications of a common fluid in different trunks or ramifications; the last of which explanations is by far the simplest and easiest.† And hence, in certain parts of the system, the nervous influence becomes capable of producing the effect of sensation; in others, of motion. And hence, again, the sensific influence is rendered capable of exciting in one set of organs a sense of sight; in others, of hearing, smell, or taste; while that of touch is diffused over the surface generally.

This last, by its extensive diffusion, is by Mr. Hunter called *common sensation;* and his view of the subject is in perfect consonance with the present. "It is more than probable," says he, " that what may be called organs of sense (local

* Boerhaave's estimate of the proportional quantity of the blood sent to the head is greater even than that named by Haller.—D.

† These hypotheses are at once refuted by the consideration that the different attributes of different nerves or nervous filaments are ascertained by the best modern physiologists, and particularly by the important experiments of Sir Charles Bell and those of M. Magendie, to depend upon the nature of their origin or roots, and the particular manner in which they are connected with certain portions of the brain, spinal cord, &c. Their connexion or not with ganglions, is another circumstance seeming to have much influence.—Eᴅ.

organs) have particular nerves, whose mode of action is different from that of nerves producing common sensation, and also different from one another; and that the nerves on which the peculiar functions of each of the organs of sense depend, are not supplied from different parts of the brain. The organ of sight has its peculiar nerve: so has that of hearing; and probably that of smelling likewise: and, on the same principle, we may suppose the organ of taste to have a peculiar nerve, although these organs of sense may likewise have nerves from different parts of the brain; yet, it is most probable, such nerves are only for the common sensations of the part, and other purposes answered by nerves."—(On the Animal Economy, p. 261.)

We see farther, that, for the purpose of elaborating the exquisitely fine and active fluid that, differently modified, excites the local organs of sense, and excites* them in perfection, it is necessary that the nervous system should exist in its highest scale of fabrication, and be crowned with the apparatus of a brain, though this is not the only use to which the brain is subservient: and hence it was long ago pointed out by Galen, that it is from the brain alone the nerves appropriated to the local senses take their rise (De Instrumentis Odoratûs, edit. Basil, tom. i., p. 381); for though we have instances of the existence of a few of these senses where the nervous system is found in a much less finished form, they are never complete in number, nor apparently in acuteness.

The sense of touch, on the contrary, which, as we have already observed, is regarded by Cuvier as produced by the sensific fluid in its simplest and least compounded state, or, as Galen has it, " is the dullest and rudest of all the sentient powers," flows, for the most part, as the latter has also remarked, from the spinal marrow alone, since it is from this column that the nerves of touch almost exclusively arise. And hence we have little difficulty in conceiving how a sense of this kind may exist in mollusca, shellfishes, and the larvæ of insects, which have no other nervous system than a medullary column, with a slight increment at the upper extremity, or no increment whatever; and have no other sense, or none but in a very imperfect degree.

The nervous power producing motion, and which has properly been denominated irritative, appears to be of a still lower description than that of touch. It is hence common to the great

mass of muscular fibres, and is probably capable of being secreted by these fibres generally; so that every fibre supplies itself where it receives no supply from any other source. Yet the proper source or reservoir of this modification of nervous fluid seems to be a ganglionic system; that which, in the higher classes of animals, we have already noticed as formed by the curious structure and ramifications of the intercostal nerve, and that which appears to be a copy of it in worms and zoophites, which have no other nervous organization whatever. From the copiousness with which this central system furnishes a recruit to the involuntary organs, with which it is peculiarly connected in mammals, we may see why these organs are able to persevere in one uninterrupted train of action, without exhaustion or weariness, from the beginning to the end of life; and why several of them, as the heart, the lungs, and the stomach, should be able to exhibit proofs of irritative power for a considerable period of time after the death of the system, and especially when roused by particular stimulants. Fishes in general have few pretensions to this structure, and hence they die sooner than most other animals, and exhibit little muscular irritability afterward. Yet it is remarkable, that in those genera which make the nearest approach to a ganglionic system, as the cod and carp, we have examples of a like power. The fishmongers of the metropolis have taken advantage of this endowment in the cod-kind, and introduced the fashion of crimping or corrugating the flesh by the stimulus of transverse incisions; and in some curious experiments on the carp, lately instituted by Mr. Clift, he found its heart leaping, when out of water, four hours after a separation from the body.—(Phil. Trans., 1815, p. 90.) If the apparently isolated molecules found in the make of the polype and various worms are ganglions of nervous irritation, extending their vital influence through certain ranges or peripheries, we are also hence enabled to account for the peculiar tenacity with which the principle of life adheres to them, and that wonderful power of reproduction which belongs to detached segments.

The curious and striking experiments which have lately been made upon animals by Dr. Philip and M. le Gallois, confirm the general view now offered so far as they bear upon it. These have consisted in an examination into the different effects produced on the heart and lungs by suddenly destroying or cutting off the communication of the whole brain; by slowly destroying it; by destroying it in the posterior part alone, and in the anterior part alone; and by destroying, in like manner, the spinal marrow at the neck, or where it unites with the brain; in its middle or dorsal, and in its lumbar region. The animals operated upon were chiefly rabbits.

According to the experiments of M. le Gallois (Exp. sur la Principe de la Vie, &c.), after the destruction of the brain, the action of the heart still continues for a considerable period of time unimpaired; while, on the destruction of

---

* Here it is to be observed that the author speaks of the "fine and active fluid" as merely exciting the organs of sense, and not as the means by which the impressions received by those organs are communicated to the sensorium. But if we ask whether vision is excited by this imaginary fluid, or by the rays of light impinging upon the retina, the invalidity of the hypothesis, even in this shape, is immediately self-evident. On other occasions the nervous fluid is used in a different meaning, being nothing less than synonymous with nervous or sensorial power itself. In all this a great want of precision attends the hypothesis, which, to increase the confusion, extends itself also to the explanation of muscular action.—ED.

the spinal marrow at its upper or cervical extremity, this action becomes instantly so debilitated as to be no longer capable of supporting the circulation. Whence he infers that it is from the cord of the spinal marrow, and not from the brain, that the heart derives the principle of its life and motions.

The experiments of Dr. Philip (*Phil. Trans.*, 1815, pp. 15 and 444) are at variance with the above of M. le Gallois, and his conclusions are therefore somewhat different. They seem to show that both the brain and spinal marrow may be destroyed, and yet the heart continue to act forcibly and steadily, provided the lungs be excited by the artificial breath of a pair of bellows.

The brain and spinal marrow were destroyed by a hot wire, the animal being first stupified by a blow on the occiput. Frogs and a few other animals were here employed, as well as rabbits. It is not exactly stated how long, under this process, the heart continued to beat. Yet, contrary to what Dr. Philip seems to have expected, but in perfect concurrence with the hints I have just thrown out, he found that certain stimuli applied to the brain, whether in the anterior or posterior part of the head, increased very sensibly the action of the heart, the animal being still prepared as just stated. The same effect ensued when the same stimuli were applied to the cervical and even the dorsal part of the spinal marrow, but not when applied to the lumbar.

Dr. Philip hence concludes that there are three kinds of vital power :—muscular, possessed by the lowest kinds of animals that are destitute of both the others ; nervous, or that which is here denominated the medium of touch or simple feeling, chiefly derived from or dependant upon the spinal marrow, and possessed by animals somewhat more advanced in the scale of life ; and sensorial, constituting what we have just regarded as the medium of the local senses, and appertaining to the higher classes. He adds, that each of these may exist alone, and consequently independently of the rest ; but admits that where the nervous principle co-exists with the muscular it exerts an influence over it, so that the latter may even be overborne or destroyed by such influence ; and that when the sensorial co-exists with both, it exercises over both an equal degree of control.

III. But the nervous organ in its most elaborate and perfect state, as in man, is not only the seat of sensation and motion, but of intelligence ; it is the instrument of communication between the mind and the body, as well as between the body and the objects by which the body is surrounded. And as a failure or irregular performance of its functions in various ways lays a foundation for an extensive division of corporeal diseases, so a like failure or irregularity of performance in other ways lays a foundation for as numerous a train of mental maladies.

Of the nature of the mind or soul itself, we know little beyond what REVELATION has informed us : we have no chymical test that can reach its essence ; no glasses that can trace its mode

Vol. II.—L

of union with the brain ; no analogies that can illustrate the rapidity of its movements. And hence the darkness that in this respect hung over the speculations of the Indian gymnosophists and the philosophers of G$_{reece}$ continues without abatement, and has equally resisted the labours of modern metaphysicians and physiologists. That the mind is an intelligent principle, we know from nature ; and that it is a principle endowed with immortality, and capable of existing after death in a state separate from the body, to which, however, it is hereafter to be reunited at a period when that which is now mortal shall put on immortality, and death itself be swallowed up of victory—we learn from the God of nature. And, with such information, we may well rest satisfied ; and, with suitable modesty, direct our investigations to those lower branches of this mysterious subject that lie within the grasp of our reason.

I cannot, however, drop the subject altogether, without observing that the discussion concerning the particular entity of the mind seems to have been conducted with an undue degree of heat and confidence on all sides, considering our present ignorance of whatever substance has been appealed to as constituting its specific frame.

Is the essence of the mind, soul, or spirit, material or immaterial ? The question, at first sight, appears to be of the utmost importance and gravity ; and to involve nothing less than a belief or disbelief, not, indeed, in its divine origin, but in its divine similitude and immortality. Yet I may venture to affirm that there is no question which has been productive of so little satisfaction, or has laid a foundation for wider and wilder errors, within the whole range of metaphysics : and for this plain and obvious reason, that we have no distinct ideas of the terms, and no settled premises to build upon. Corruptibility and incorruptibility, intelligent and unintelligent, organized and inorganic, are terms that convey distinct meanings to the mind, and impart modes of being that are within the scope of our comprehension. But materiality and immateriality are equally beyond our reach. Of the essence of matter we know nothing, and altogether as little of many of its more active qualities ; insomuch that, amid all the discoveries of the day, it still remains a controvertible position, whether light, heat, magnetism, and electricity are material substances, material properties, or things superadded to matter, and of a higher nature.

If they be matter, gravity and ponderability are not essential properties of matter, though commonly so regarded. And if they be things superadded to matter they are necessarily immaterial, and we cannot open our eyes without beholding innumerable proofs of material and immaterial bodies co-existent and acting in harmonious union through the entire frame of nature. But if we know nothing of the essence, and but little of the qualities of matter, of that common substrate which is diffused around us in every direction, and constitutes the whole of the visible world, what can we know of that which is immaterial? of the full meaning of a term that, in its strictest sense, comprehends all the rest of the immense fabric of actual and possible being, and includes in its vast circumference every essence and mode of essence of every other being, as well below as above the order of matter, and even that of the Deity himself?

Shall we take the quality of extension as the line of separation between what is material and what is immaterial? This, indeed, is the general and favourite distinction brought forward in the present day: but it is a distinction founded on mere conjecture, and which will by no means stand the test of inquiry. Is space extended? every one admits it to be so. But is space material? is it body of any kind? Descartes, indeed, contended that it is body, and a material body; for he denied a vacuum, and asserted space to be a part of matter itself: but it is probable that there is not a single espouser of this opinion in the present day. If, then, extension belong equally to matter and to space, it cannot be contemplated as the peculiar and exclusive property of the former ; and if we allow it to immaterial space, there is no reason why we should not allow it to immaterial spirit. If extension appertain not to the mind or thinking principle, the latter can have NO PLACE of existence : it can exist NOWHERE ; for WHERE or PLACE is an idea that cannot be separated from the idea of extension. And hence the metaphysical immaterialists of modern times freely admit that the mind has NO PLACE of existence ; that it does exist NOWHERE ; while, at the same time, they are compelled to allow that the immaterial Creator, or universal Spirit, exists EVERYWHERE, substantially as well as virtually.

Nor let it be supposed that the difficulty is removed by adding to matter the quality of solidity in conjunction with that of extension, and hence distinguishing it as possessed of SOLID EXTENT ; for the quality of solidity is less characteristic of it than any we have thus far taken notice of, and is perpetually fleeing from us as we pursue it. That matter is infinitely divisible we dare not say, because we should hereby reduce it to mathematical points, and because, also, there would in such case be no certain or permanent basis to build upon, and to ensure a punctuality of material cause and effect; and hence Sir Isaac Newton was obliged to suppose that it is possessed of ultimate atoms which are solid and unchangeable. But of these the senses can trace nothing, and our admission is nothing more than conjectural.

Let not the author, however, be misunderstood upon this abstruse and difficult subject. That the mind has a DISTINCT NATURE and is a DISTINCT REALITY from the body, that it is gifted with immortality, endowed with reasoning faculties, and capacified for a state of separate existence after the death of the corporeal frame to which it is attached, are, in his opinion, propositions most clearly deducible from revelation, and, in one or two points, adumbrated by a few shadowy glimpses of nature. And that it may be a substance strictly IMMATERIAL and ESSEN-TIALLY DIFFERENT from matter is both possible and probable, and will hereafter, perhaps, when faith is turned into vision, and conjecture into fact, be found to be the true and genuine doctrine upon the subject. But till this glorious era arrive ; or till, antecedently to it, it be proved, which it does not hitherto seem to have been, that matter, itself of divine origin, gifted even at present, under certain modifications, with instinct and sensation, and destined to become immortal hereafter, is physically incapable, under some still more refined, exalted, and spiritualized modification, of exhibiting the attributes of the soul ; of being, under such a constitution, endowed with immortality from the first, and capacified for existing separately from the external and grosser frame of the body ; and that it is beyond the power of its own Creator to render it intelligent, or to give it even brutal perception, the argument must be loose and inconclusive : it may plunge us, as it has plunged thousands already, into errors, but can never conduct us to demonstration. It may lead us, on the one hand, to the proud Braminical and Platonic belief, that the essence of the soul is the very essence of the Deity, and consequently a part of the Deity himself; or, on the other, to the gloomy regions of modern materialism, and to the cheerless doctrine that it dies and dissolves in one common grave with the body.

It is no fair objection, however, against the immaterialist, that, by contemplating the mind as a distinct essence from that of the body, man is hereby rendered a compound being, possessing at one and the same time two distinct lives mysteriously united in an individual frame, and running in parallel lines till the hour of death. For while the known and obvious laws and faculties of the mind and body are so widely different as they are acknowledged to be on all hands, some such composite union has been and must be allowed under every hypothesis whatever. And least of all have the skeptical physiologists of the present day any right to triumph upon such an objection ; who, drawing no light from nature, and rejecting that of sacred writ, contemplate the mind as formed of the same gross modification of matter as the body, and doomed to fall with it into one common and eternal dissolution. For even these acute materialists, with all the aid of physiological, anatomical, and chymical research, instead of simplifying the human fabric, have made it more clumsily complex, and represented it sometimes, indeed, as a duad, but of late more generally as a triad, of unities, a combination of a corruptible life within a corruptible life two or three deep, each possessing its own separate faculties or manifestations, but covered with a common outside.

This remark more especially applies to the philosophers of the French school, and particularly to the system of Dumas (*Princ. de Phys. iol.*, 4 tomes, 8vo.; Paris, 1800–3) as modified by Bichat ; under which more finished form man is declared to consist of a pair of lives, each distinct and co-existent, under the names of an organic and an animal life ; with two distinct assortments of sensibilities, an unconscious and a conscious. Each of these lives is limited to a separate set of organs, runs its race in parallel steps with the other, commencing coetaneously and perishing at the same moment. This work appeared at the close of the past century, was read and admired by most physiologists, credited by many, and became the popular production of the day. Within ten or twelve years, however, it ran its course, and was as generally either rejected or forgotten even in France ; and M. Richerand first, and M. Magendie since, have thought themselves called upon to modify Bichat, in order to render him more palatable, as Bichat had already modified Dumas. Under the last series of re-modelling, which is that of M. Magendie, we have certainly an improvement, though the machinery is quite as complex. Instead of two distinct lives, M. Magendie presents us with two distinct sets or systems of action or relation, each of which has its separate and peculiar functions ; a system of nutritive action or relation, and a system of vital. To which is added, by way of appendix, another system, comprising the functions of generation.—(*Physiologie*, 2 tomes, 8vo., Paris, 1816, 1817.) Here, however, the brain is not only the seat, but the organized substance of the mental powers ; so that we are expressly told a man must be as he is made in his brain, and that education, and even logic itself, is of no use to him. "There are," says M. Magendie, "justly celebrated persons who have thought differently, but they have hereby fallen into grave errors." A Deity, however, is allowed to exist, because, adds the writer, it is comfortable to think that he exists, and on this account the physiologist cannot doubt of his being. "L'intelligence de l'homme," says he, "se compose de phénomènes tellement différens de tout ce que présente d'ailleurs la nature, qu'on les rapporte à un être particulier qu'on regarde comme une émanation de la Divinité. Il est trop *consolant de croire à cet être*, pour que le physiologiste mette en doute son existence ; mais la séverité de langage ou de logique que comporte maintenant la physiologie, exige que l'on traite de l'intelligence humaine comme si elle était le résultat de l'action d'un organe. En *s'écartant* de cette marche, des hommes justement célèbres sont tombés dans des *graves erreurs ;* en la suivant, on a, d'ailleurs, le grand avantage de conserver la même méthode d'étude, et de rendre très-faciles des choses qui sont envisagées généralement comme presque au-dessus de l'esprit humain."—"Il existe une science dont le but est d'apprendre à raisonner justement, c'est *la logique ;* mais le jugement erroné ou l'esprit faux (for judgment, genius, and imagination, and therefore false reasoning, all depend on organization) tiennent à l'organization. Il est impossible de se changer à cet égard ; nous restons tels que *la nature* nons a faits."—(*Précis Élémentaire*, &c., ut suprà, passim.)

Dr. Spurzheim has generally been considered, from the concurrent tenour of his doctrines, as belonging to the class of materialists ; but this is to mistake his own positive assertion upon the subject, or to conclude in opposition to it. He speaks, indeed, upon this topic with a singular hesitation and reserve, more so perhaps than upon any other point whatever ; but as far as he chooses to express himself on so abstruse a subject, he regards the soul as a distinct being from the body, and at least intimates that it *may be* nearer akin to the Deity. Man is with him also possessed of two lives, an AUTOMATIC and an ANIMAL : the first produced by organization alone, and destitute of consciousness ; the second possessed of consciousness dependant on the soul, and merely manifesting itself by organization. "We do not," says he, "attempt to explain how the body and soul are joined together and exercise a mutual influence. We do not examine what the soul can do without the body. Souls, so far as we know, may be united to bodies at the moment of conception or afterward ; they may be different in all individuals, or of the same kind in every one ; they may be emanations from God, or something essentially different."—(*Physiognomical System*, &c., p. 253, 8vo., London, 1815.) The mind of this celebrated craniologist seems to be wonderfully skeptical and bewildered upon the subject, and studiously avoids the important question of the capacity of the soul for an independent and future existence ; but, with the above declarations, he cannot well be arranged in the class of materialists.

The hypothesis adopted by Mr. Lawrence (*Introduction to Comp. Anat. and Phys.*, &c., 8vo., 1816), and which is nearly the same as that of Bichat* and Cuvier,[†] is altogether of a different kind ; and, though undoubtedly much simpler than any of the preceding, does not seem to be built on a more stable foundation. According to his view of the subject, organized differs from inorganized matter merely by the addition of certain PROPERTIES which are called vital, as sensibility and irritability. Masses of matter endowed with these new PROPERTIES become organs and systems of organs, constitute an animal frame, and execute distinct sets of PURPOSES or FUNCTIONS, for functions and purposes carried into execution are here synonymous. "Life is the assemblage of ALL the functions (or purposes), and the general result of their exercise."—(Ibid., p. 120.)

Life, therefore, upon this hypothesis, instead of being a twofold or threefold reality, running in a combined stream, or in parallel lines, has no reality whatever. It has no ESSE or independent existence. It is a mere assemblage of PURPOSES, and accidental or temporary PROPERTIES : a series of phenomena (Ibid., p. 122), as Mr. Lawrence has himself correctly expressed it ;— a name without a thing. "We know not," says he, "the nature of the link that unites these phenomena, though we are sensible that a con-

---

* "La vie est l'ensemble des fonctions qui résiste à la mort."—Recherches Physiologiques sur la Vie et la Mort, art. 1.

 † "Dans chaque être, la vie est un ensemble qui résulte de l'action et de la réaction mutuelle de toutes ses parties."—Le Règne Animal, tom. i. ; Introd., p. 16.

nexion must exist ; and this conviction is sufficient to induce us to give it a NAME, which the VULGAR regard as the sign of a particular principle : though in fact that name can only indicate the ASSEMBLAGE OF THE PHENOMENA which has occasioned its formation."—(Ibid.)

The human frame is, hence, a barrel-organ, possessing a systematic arrangement of parts, played upon by peculiar powers, and executing particular pieces or purposes ; and life is the music, produced by the general assemblage or result of the harmonious action. So long as either the vital or the mechanical instrument is duly wound up by a regular supply of food or of the winch, so long the music will continue : but both are worn out by their own action ; and when the machine will no longer work, the life has the same close as the music ; and in the language of Cornelius Gallus, as quoted and appropriated by Leo X.,

" — redit in nihilum, quod fuit ante nihil."

There is, however, nothing new, either in this hypothesis or in the present explanation of it. It was first started, in the days of Aristotle, by Aristoxenus, a pupil of his, who was admirably skilled in music, and by profession a physician. It was propounded to the world under the name of the system of HARMONY, either from the author's fondness for music, or from his comparing the human frame to a musical instrument, and his regarding life as the result of all its parts acting in accordance, and producing a general and harmonious effect.

How far Mr. Lawrence's revised edition of this hypothesis may prove satisfactory to other classes of materialists I cannot tell : but if he should succeed he will be more fortunate than Aristoxenus, who pleased neither the other materialists nor the immaterialists of his day: From the latter, indeed, he could expect no countenance : but even the Epicureans, though they held that the mind was corruptible, as formed of matter, which they had no reason to believe was then or ever would be otherwise than corruptible under any modification whatever, held, at the same time, that it had a substantive existence, distinct from that of the grosser frame of the body, and possessed of other and far higher properties ; being formed of the finest, lightest, smoothest, and most moveable material elements, and hence exquisitely etherealized and volatile :

" — est animi natura reperta . Mobilis egregie, perquam constare necesse est Corporibus parvis, et lævibus, atque rotundis."*

The atomic philosophers, therefore, joined with the Platonists and Stoics in opposing the system of harmony, and that chiefly upon the two following grounds, which will apply with as much force to its present as to its primary form. First, admitting that an assemblage and exercise of ALL the functions of the machine are necessary to maintain the phenomena of life, we are left as much in the dark as ever concerning the nature of the principle by which this harmonious instrument becomes gradually developed, and is

---

* Lucret., De Rer. Nat., iii., 204.

kept in perpetual play. And next, that the life or wellbeing of the animal frame does not depend upon an assemblage and exercise of ALL its functions or purposes ; since the mind may be diseased while the body remains unaffected, or the body may lose some of its own organs, while the mind, or even the general health of the body itself, may continue perfect.—(Ibid., iii., 105–266 ; Lactant. in Vit. Epicur. Polignac. Anti-Lucret., lib. v., 923.)

In the darkness, therefore, which continues to hang over the mysterious subject before us, I feel incompetent to enter into the question concerning the actual essence of the mind, and am perfectly content to take its general nature, powers, and destiny, from the only volume which is capable of giving us any decided information upon the subject ; to follow it up as far as that volume may guide us ; and to stop where it withdraws its assistance.

Closely connected with the present question is another of nearly as much perplexity, and the consideration of which has not been attended with much more success, but which must not be passed by on the present occasion without being glanced at.

Whatever be the nature or substance of the mind, the brain is the organ in which it holds its seat, and whence it maintains an intercourse with the surrounding world. Now it must be obvious to every one who has attended to the operation of his senses, that there never is nor can be any direct communication between the mind, thus stationed in the brain, and the external objects the mind perceives ; which are usually, indeed, at some distance even from the sense that gives notice of them. Thus, in looking at a tree, it is the eye alone that beholds the tree, while the mind only perceives a notice of its presence, by some means or other, from the visual organ. So, in touching this table, it is my hand alone that comes in contact with it, and communicates to my mind a knowledge of its hardness and other qualities. What then is the medium by which such communication is maintained ? which enables the mind to have a perception of the form, size, colour, smell, and even distance of objects, correspondent with that of the senses which are seated on the surface of the body ? and which, at the same time that it conveys this information, produces such an additional effect, that the mind is able, at its own option, to call up an exact notion or idea of those qualities at a distant period, or when the objects themselves are no longer present ? Is there, or is there not, any resemblance between the external or sensible object, and the internal or mental idea or notion ? If there be a resemblance, in what does that resemblance consist ? and how is it produced and supported ? Does the external object throw off representative likenesses of itself in films, or under any other modification, so fine as to be able, like the electric or magnetic aura, to pass without injury from the object to the sentient organ, and from the sentient organ to the sensory, or mental presence-chamber ? or has the mind itself a faculty of producing, like a mirror, accurate countersigns, intellectual pictures or images correspondent with the sensible images communicated from the external object to the sentient organ? If, on the contrary, there be no resemblance, are the mental perceptions mere notions, or intellectual symbols excited in the mind by the action of the external sense; which, while they bear no similitude to the qualities of the object discerned, answer the purpose of those qualities, as letters answer the purpose of sounds? or are we sure that there is any external world whatever; any thing beyond the intellectual principle that perceives and the sensations and notions that are perceived; or even any thing beyond those sensations and notions, those impressions and ideas themselves?

Several of these questions may perhaps appear in no small degree whimsical and brainsick, and more worthy of St. Luke's than of a work of physiological study; but all of them, and at least as many more, of a temperament as wild as the wildest, have been asked and insisted upon, and supported again and again in different ages and countries, from the zenith of Grecian science down to our own day, by philosophers of the clearest intellects in other respects, and who had no idea of labouring under any such mental infirmity, nor ever dreamed of the necessity of being blistered and taking physic.

The nature of the questions themselves, therefore, when put by the characters referred to, sufficiently manifests the obscurity of the subject to which they relate: and to enter into the discussions to which they have given rise, would lead us to an irrecoverable distance from the path before us. Those who are desirous of following them up, and of witnessing an exposure of their absurdity, cannot do better than apply themselves to the metaphysical writings of Dr. Reid, Dr. Beattie, Dr. Campbell, and Professor Stewart; who if, on the overthrow of so many 'Babel-buildings, they have not been able to raise an edifice much more substantial in their stead, have only failed from the insuperable difficulty of the attempt.

No man was more sensible of this difficulty than Mr. Locke, nor has taken more pains both to avoid what is unintelligible and unprofitable, and to elucidate what may be turned to a good account and brought home to an ordinary comprehension. It was his imperishable Essay on Human Understanding that gave the first check to the wild and visionary conceits in which the most celebrated luminaries of the age were at that time engaged; recalled mankind from the chasing of shadows to the study of realities, from a pursuit of useless and inexplicable subtleties to that of important and cognoscible subjects: or rather to the only mode in which the great inquiry before him could be followed up with any reasonable hope of success or advantage.

To this elaborate and wonderful work, which has conferred an ever-during fame, not only on its matchless author, but on the nation to which he belonged, and even the age in which he lived, the physiologist cannot pay too close an attention. It is, indeed, of the highest importance to every science, as teaching us the elements of all science, and the only mode by which science can be rendered really useful, and carried forward to ultimate perfection; but it is of immediate importance to every branch of physical knowledge, and particularly to that which is employed in unfolding the structure of the mind, and its connexion with the visible fabric that encloses it. It may, perhaps, be somewhat too long; it may occasionally embrace subjects which are not necessarily connected with it: its terms may not always be precise, nor its opinions in every instance correct; but it discovers intrinsic and most convincing evidence, that the man who wrote it must have had a head peculiarly clear, and a heart peculiarly sound: it is strictly original in its matter, highly important in its subject, luminous and forcible in its argument, perspicuous in its style, and comprehensive in its scope. It steers equally clear of all former systems: we have nothing of the mystical archetypes of Plato, the incorporeal phantasms of Aristotle, or the material species of Epicurus; we are equally without the intelligible world of the Greek schools, and the innate ideas of Descartes. Passing by all which, from actual experience and observation, it delineates the features and describes the operations of the human mind with a degree of precision and minuteness which has never been exhibited either before or since; and stands, and probably ever will stand, like a rock, before the puny waves of opposition by which it has since been assailed from various quarters. The author may speak of it with warmth, but he speaks from a digested knowledge of its merits: for he has studied it thoroughly and repeatedly; and there is, perhaps, no book to which he is so much indebted for whatever small degree of discrimination or habit of reasoning he may possibly be allowed to lay claim to.

Upon one point he is perfectly clear; namely, that the chief objections at any time urged against this celebrated production have proceeded from an utter mistake of its meaning, of which he could give numerous instances, if such a digression were allowable, from the writings of many who have the credit of having studied it profoundly. The remark applies to several of the most popular psychologists of both North and South Britain, but especially to those of the continent, and more particularly still to M. Condorcet, from whom the French in general have received an erroneous idea of several of its leading doctrines. It is to this book the medical student ought to turn himself for a knowledge of the laws that regulate the development and growth of the mind, as he should do to the labours of Haller or Hunter for a knowledge of those that regulate the development and growth of the body; and I shall hence draw largely upon it through the remainder of this introduction.

The whole, then, of the metaphysical rubbish of the ancient schools being cleared away by the purging and purifying energy of the Essay on Human Understanding, mankind have since been enabled to contemplate the body and mind as equally, at birth, a *tabula rasa*, or unwritten sheet of paper; as consisting equally of a blank or vacuity of impressions; but as equally capable of acquiring impressions by the operation of external objects, and equally and most skilfully endowed with distinct powers or faculties for this purpose : those of the body being the external senses of sight, hearing, smell, taste, and touch ; and those of the mind, the internal senses of perception, reason, judgment, imagination, and memory.

It is possible that a few slight impressions may be produced a short time antecedently to birth ; and it is certain that various instinctive tendencies, which, however, have no connexion with the mind, are more perfect, because more needful, at the period of birth than ever afterward ; and we have also frequent proofs of an hereditary or accidental predisposition towards particular subjects. But the fundamental doctrine before us is by no means affected by such collateral circumstances.

External objects first impress or operate upon the outward senses ; and these senses, by means hitherto unexplained, and perhaps altogether inexplicable, immediately impress or operate upon the mind, or excite in it perceptions or ideas of the presence and qualities of such objects ; the word idea being here employed, not in any of the significations of the schools, but in its broad popular meaning, as importing " whatever a man observes, and is conscious to himself he has in his mind" (*Locke, on Human Understanding*, b. i., ch. i., § 3), whatever was formerly intended by the terms archetype, phantasm, species, thought, notion, or conception, or whatever else it may be which we can be employed about in thinking.—(Id., b. i., ch. i., § 8.) And to these effects Mr. Locke gave the name of *ideas of* SENSATION, in allusion to the source from which they are derived.

But the mind, as we have already observed, has various powers or faculties as well as the body, and they are quite as active and lively in their respective functions ; in consequence of which the ideas of external objects are not only perceived, but retained, thought of, compared, compounded, abstracted, doubted, believed, desired : and hence another fountain, and of a very capacious flow, from which we also derive ideas ; viz., a reflex act or perception of the mind's own operations, whence the ideas derived from this fountain are denominated *ideas of* REFLECTION.

The ideas, then, derived from these two sources, and which have sometimes been called OBJECTIVE and SUBJECTIVE, constitute all our experience, and, consequently, all our knowledge. Whatever stock of information a man may be possessed of, however richly he may be stored with taste, learning, or science, if he turn his attention inward, and diligently examine his own thoughts, he will find that he has not a single idea in his mind but what has been derived from one or the other of these two channels. But let not this important observation be forgotten by any one ; that the ideas the mind possesses will be fewer or more numerous, simpler or more diversified, clear or confused, according to the number of the objects presented to it, and the extent of its reflection and examination.

Thus a clock or a landscape may be for ever before our eyes ; but unless we direct our attention to them, and study their different parts, although we cannot be deceived in their being a clock or a landscape, we can have but a very inadequate idea of their character and composition.

The ideas presented to the mind, from which soever of these two sources derived, are of two kinds—SIMPLE and COMPLEX.

SIMPLE IDEAS consist of such as are limited to a single notion or perception ; as those of unity, darkness, light, sound, simple pain or uneasiness. And in the reception of these the mind is passive ; for it can neither make them to itself, nor can it, in any instance, have any idea which does not wholly consist of them ; or, in other words, it cannot contemplate any one of them otherwise than in its totality.

COMPLEX IDEAS are formed out of various simple ideas, associated together or contemplated derivatively. And to this class belong the ideas of an army, a battle, a triangle, gratitude, veneration, gold, silver, an orange, an apple ; in the formation of all which it must be obvious that the mind is active, for it is the activity of the mind alone that produces the complexity out of such ideas as are simple. And that the ideas I have now referred to are complex, must be plain to every one ; for every one must be sensible, that the mind cannot form to itself the idea of an orange without uniting into one aggregate the simple ideas of roundness, yellowness, juiciness, and sweetness ; and so of the rest.

Complex ideas are formed out of simple ideas by many operations of the mind ; the principal of which, however, are some combination of them, some abstraction, or some comparison. Let us take a view of each of these.

And first of complex ideas of COMBINATION. Unity, as I have already observed, is a simple idea ; and it is one of the most common simple ideas that can be presented to the mind ; for every object without, and every notion within, tend equally to excite it : and being a simple idea, the mind, as I have also remarked, is passive on its presentation : it can neither form such an idea to itself, nor contemplate it otherwise than in its totality ; but it can combine the ideas of as many units as it pleases, and hence produce the complex idea of a hundred, a thousand, or a hundred thousand. So beauty is a complex idea ; for the mind, in forming it, combines a variety of separate ideas into one common aggregate. Thus Dryden, in delineating the beautiful Victoria in his Love Triumphant,

" Her eyes, her lips, her cheeks, her shape, her features,
Seem to be drawn by Love's own hand ; by Love Himself in love."

In like manner the mind can produce complex ideas by an opposite process ; and that is by ABSTRACTION or separation. Thus chalk, snow, and milk, though agreeing, perhaps, in no other respect, coincide in the same colour ; and the mind, contemplating this agreement, may abstract or separate the colour from the other properties of these three objects, and form the idea which is indicated by the term *whiteness*; and having thus acquired a new idea by the process of abstraction, it may afterward apply it as a character to a variety of other objects; and hence particular ideas become general or universal.

Other complex ideas are produced by COMPARISON. Thus, if the mind take one idea, as that of a foot, as a determinate measure, and place it by the side of another idea, as the idea of a table, the result will be a formation of the complex idea of length, breadth, and thickness. Or, if we vary the primary idea, we may obtain, as a result, the secondary ideas of coarseness and fineness.

And hence complex ideas must be almost infinitely more numerous than simple ideas, which are their elements or materials; as words must be always far more numerous than letters. I have instanced only a few of their principal kinds, and have applied them only to a few of the great variety of subjects to which they are referable, and by which they are elucidated in the great work on Human Understanding.

It must, however, from this imperfect sketch, appear obvious, that many of our ideas have a NATURAL CORRESPONDENCE, congruity, and connexion with each other; and as many, perhaps, on the contrary, a NATURAL REPUGNANCE, incongruity, and disconnexion. Thus, if I were to speak of a cold fire, I should put together ideas that are naturally disconnected and incongruous; and should consequently make an absurd proposition, or, to adopt common language, talk nonsense. I should be guilty of the same blunder if I were to talk of a square billiard-ball, or a soft reposing rock; but a warm fire, on the contrary, a white or even a black billiard-ball, and a hard rugged rock, are congruous ideas, and consequently consistent with good sense. Now it is the direct office of that discursive faculty of the mind which we call reason, to trace out these natural coincidences or disjunctions, and to connect or separate them by proper relations: for it is a just perception of the natural connexion and congruity, or of the natural repugnance and incongruity of our ideas, that shows a sound mind, and constitutes real knowledge. The wise man is he who has industriously laid in and carefully assorted an extensive stock of ideas; as the stupid or ignorant man is he who, from natural hebetude, or having had but few opportunities, has collected and arranged but a small number. The man who discovers the natural relations of his ideas quickly, is a man of sagacity; and in popular language is said, and correctly so, to possess a quick, sharp intellect: the man, on the contrary, who discovers these relations slowly, we call dull or heavy. If he rapidly discover and put together relations that lie remote, and perhaps touch only in a few points, but those points striking and pleasant, he is a man of wit, genius, or brilliant fancy, of agreeable allusion and metaphor: if he intermix ideas of fancy with ideas of reality, those of reflection with those of sensation, and mistake the one for the

other, however numerous his ideas may be, and whatever their order of succession, he is a madman; he reasons from false principles, and, as we say in popular language, and with perfect correctness, is out of his judgment.

Finally, our ideas are very apt to ASSOCIATE or run together in trains; and, upon this peculiar and happy disposition of the mind, we lay our chief dependance in sowing the seeds of education. It often happens, however, that some of our ideas have been associated erroneously, and even in a state of early life, before education has commenced; and hence, from the difficulty of separating them, most of the sympathies and antipathies, the whims and prejudices, that occasionally haunt us to the latest period of old age.

Such, then, is the manner in which the mind, at first a sheet of white paper, without characters of any kind, becomes furnished with that vast store of ideas, the materials of wisdom and knowledge, which the busy and boundless fancy of man paints upon it with an almost endless variety. The whole is derived from experience, THE EXPERIENCE OF SENSATION OR OF REFLECTION; from the observations of the mind employed either about external sensible objects, or the internal operations of itself, perceived and reflected upon by its own faculties.

These FACULTIES are to the mind what organs are to the body; they are its ministers in the production, combination, and resolution of different trains of ideas, and in supplying it with the results of its own activity. We sometimes, however, are apt to speak of them as distinct and separate existences from the mind, or as possessing a sort of independent entity, and as controlling one another by their individual authorities, and occasionally, indeed, as controlling the mind itself: for we accustom ourselves to describe the will as being overpowered by the judgment; or the judgment as being overpowered by the imagination; or the mind itself as being carried headlong by the violence of its own passions. By all which, however, we only mean, or should only mean, that the mind does not, on such occasions, exert its own faculties in a fitting or sober manner, or that from some diseased affection it is incapable of doing so. For the faculties of the mind are so many powers; and, as powers, are mere attributes of the being or substance to which they belong, and not the being or substance itself. These, therefore, being all different powers in the mind or in the man to do several actions, he exerts them as he thinks fit; but the power to do one action is not operated upon by the power to do another action: for the power of thinking operates not on the power of choosing, nor the power of choosing on the power of thinking; any more than the power of dancing operates on the power of singing, or the power of singing on the power of dancing (*Locke*, p. 129), as any one who reflects on these things will easily perceive.

The body has its feelings, and the mind has its feelings also; and it is the feelings of the latter which we call PASSIONS, a mere Latin term for the feelings or sufferings of colloquial language. The feelings of the body are numerous and diversified, as those of simple ache or ease, hunger, thirst, heat, cold, and a multitude of others. Those of the mind are still more numerous and more diversified, for they comprise the multifarious train of grief, joy, love, hatred, avarice, ambition, conceit, and perhaps hundreds more : all which, whether of body or mind, Mr. Locke has endeavoured to resolve into different modifications of pleasure or pain, according as they are productive of good or evil.

But the analogy we are thus conducting between the mind and the body holds much farther ; for as the latter is subject to DISEASES OF VARIOUS KINDS, so also is the former. The body may be enfeebled in all its powers, in only a few of them, or in only a single one. So also may the mind :—" The powers of perception and imagination," observes M. Pinel, " are frequently disturbed without any excitement of the passions. The functions of the understanding, on the other hand, are often perfectly sound, while the man is driven by his passions to acts of turbulence and outrage." And these infirmities, whether of body or mind, may be constitutional and permanent, periodical or recurrent, or merely incidental and temporary. The body may be of a sanguineous temperament, of a plethoric temperament, of a nervous or irritable temperament ; and the mind may, in like manner, possess an overweening confidence and courage, be characteristically dull and inactive, or be ever goaded on by restlessness and eager desire : it may be quick in apprehension and taste, but weak in memory ; strong in judgment,

but slow in imagination ; or feeble in judgment, but rapid in imagination : its feelings or passions may be sluggish, or all alive ; or some passion may be peculiarly energetic, while the rest remain at the temperate point.

When the corporeal deviations from the standard of high health are but slight, they are scarcely entitled to the name of diseases ; but when severe or extreme, they become subjects of serious attention. It is the same with the different states of the mind, with which I have just contrasted them. While several, or even all the mental faculties are slightly weak or sluggish, or inaccordant with the action of the rest, they are scarcely subjects of medical treatment—for otherwise half the world would be daily consigned to a strait waistcoat : but when the same changes become striking and strongly marked, they are real DISEASES OF THE INTELLECT ; and, in the ensuing order, the genera will be found taken from the peculiar faculties of the mind that chance to be thus affected.

The mind and the body bear also, in many cases, a reciprocal influence on each other ; which is sometimes general, and sometimes limited to particular faculties or functions. It is hence that fever or cephalitis produces delirium, and vapours or low spirits dyspepsy.

The mind, therefore, like the body, becomes an interesting field of study to the pathologist, and opens to his view an additional and melancholy train of diseases. It is these which will constitute the subject of the first order of the class we have now entered upon, and which are entitled to a deep and collected attention.

CLASS IV.

NEUROTICA.

ORDER I.

PHRENICA.

DISEASES AFFECTING THE INTELLECT.

ERROR, PERVERSION, OR DEBILITY OF ONE OR MORE OF THE MENTAL FACULTIES.

THE word PHRENICA is Greek, from the Greek noun φρὴν, " the mind" or " intellect." The diseases comprised in the order are so closely associated with each other, that, however the ordinal names may differ in different systems of nosology, they are for the most part grouped in some form or other under a correspondent division. And hence the present order will be found to run nearly parallel with the Deliria of Sauvages, the Mentales of Linnéus, the Paranoiæ of Vogel, the Vesaniæ of Cullen, and still more with those of Crichton, and the Aliénation mentale of Pinel : although the generic divisions are widely different from all of them, and are attempted to be rendered something clearer and more exact. The order comprehends the six following :—

Each of these will be found to include various distinct species of disorder, proceeding from a morbid condition of one or more of the mental faculties or feelings, or an irrespondence of them to others ; sometimes originating in a diseased state of the body, and sometimes producing such a state as has already been explained in the preceding proem.*

* The different forms of madness, or insanity, are classified by Dr. Prichard under the following divisions :—1. *Moral insanity*, or madness consisting in a morbid perversion of the natural feelings, affections, inclination, temper, habits, and moral dispositions, without any notable lesion of the intellect, or knowing and reasoning faculties, and particularly without any maniacal hallucination. 2. *Intellectual insanity*, or madness attended with hallucination ; in which the insane person is im-

GENUS I.

ECPHRONIA.

INSANITY. CRAZINESS.

DISEASED PERCEPTION, WITH LITTLE DERANGE-
MENT OF THE JUDGMENT, OCCASIONALLY SHIFT-
ING INTO DISEASED JUDGMENT WITH LITTLE
DERANGEMENT OF THE PERCEPTION ; DIS-
TURBING THE MIND GENERALLY ; DIMINISHED
SENSIBILITY ; IRREGULAR REMISSIONS.

THE generic term ECPHRONIA, in the Greek writers ἐκφρώνη or ἐκφροσύνη, is derived from ἔκφρων, " extra mentem"—literally " out of one's mind," as ἔμφρων is "mentis compos," or "in one's mind." It is here used, as among the Greeks, generically alone, in the ordinary sense of insanity ; and is designed to include the two following species :—

1. Ecphronia Melancholia.　　Melancholy.
2. ————— Mania.　　　　Madness.*

Each of these species has been regarded by many nosologists as forming a genus of itself, for which there seems to be no just reason. Dr. Cullen has thus arranged them in his Synopsis ; but has given them a different arrangement and a very subordinate place in his Practice of Physic, so that, in the two works, he is in this respect altogether at variance with himself. In both, his order is entitled vesaniæ, which, in the first, includes fatuity, mania, melancholy, and sleep-disturbance (oneirodynia), as distinct genera ; but, in the last, takes for its genera de-

pressed with the belief of some unreal event, as of a thing which has actually taken place, or in which he has taken up some notion repugnant to his own experience and to common sense, as if it were true and indisputable, and acts under the influence of this erroneous conviction. 3. Another well-marked variety, *incoherent madness*, as it was called by Dr. Arnold, in which the whole mind seems to be equally deranged. The most striking phenomena of this case are the rapidity and disorder with which the ideas follow each other, almost without any discoverable connexion or association, in a state of complete incoherence and confusion. It is impossible to fix the attention of the patient long enough to obtain a reply to the most simple question. His understanding is wholly lost in the constant hurry of ideas which crowd themselves upon him, and which appear to exceed the power of distinct utterance, while his habits betray a corresponding degree of restless activity and extravagance.—See Cyclop. of Pract. Med., art. INSANITY.

In the truth of the following observation we must all concur :—" The interests of the public greatly require that medical men, to whom alone the insane can ever properly be intrusted, should have opportunities of studying the forms of insanity, and of preparing themselves for its treatment, in the same manner in which they prepare themselves for the treatment of other disorders. They have at present no such opportunity. During the term allotted to medical study, the student never sees a case of insanity, except by some rare accident. While every hospital is open, every lunatic asylum is closed to him : he can study all diseases but those affecting the understanding—of all diseases the most calamitous."—(See Dr. Conolly's Inquiry concerning the Indications of Insanity, 8vo., Lond., 1830, Introd.) No doubt, it was the consideration of the necessity of making some attempt to remedy this defect in medical education now spoken of, that induced the governors of Guy's Hospital to attach a lunatic establishment to it. Dr. Conolly admits, however, that insane patients are not always in a state to be visited by pupils, and that a very strict discipline would be necessary to prevent disorder or impropriety ; but he argues that such arrangements might be made as would at once guard those patients from disturbance whom it might injure, and present a sufficient number of instructive examples to the student.—ED.*

* The various forms of insanity have been treated with much learning by Dr. Rush in his work on the diseases of the mind ; be there considers derangement of the intellect under several heads : as *hypochondriasis*, or *tristi-mania* ; *ameno-mania*, or partial intellectual derangement, accompanied with pleasure, or not accompanied with distress : *mania* ; *manicula* ; which, according to Dr. Rush, is a second grade of general mad-

ness, and differs from mania, as chronic rheumatism varies from that which is acute, that is, in being accompanied with a more moderate degree of the same symptoms : *manalgia* ; the symptoms of which are taciturnity, downcast looks, a total neglect of dress and person, and insensibility to heat and cold. Dr. Rush treats also of derangement of the memory, fatuity, incubus, somnambulism, illusions, revery, the derangement of the passions, the morbid state of the sexual appetite, and of the disorders of the moral faculties.

Dr. T. Y. Simons (Observations on Mental Alienation, &c., Charleston, 1828) considers insanity under various grades, as, 1st, *Mania*, a total hallucination on all subjects, or a total perversion of the intellectual faculties, accompanied with furor. 2. *Melancholia*, a total or partial hallucination, accompanied with extreme dejection, fear, and false apprehensions. 3. *Monomania*, a false reasoning or conception on one subject, which, when it completely overcomes the other operations of the mind, produces either melancholia or mania, according to the cause and the temperament of the individual. 4. *Hypochondriasm*, a continued apprehension of the physical health, regardless of worldly affairs, connected with dyspeptic symptoms.—D.

* The word *mad* is stated by Dr. Armstrong to be derived from the Gothic word *mod*, which signifies rage ; and the word *mania*, which the Greeks apply to madness, has the same signification. Melancholy etymologically signifies black bile. Hence, in the ancient writers, the term mania is applied to that form of madness in which there is excessive excitement of the system, with violent emotions of the mind ; and the term melancholia, to that form in which the body and mind are depressed. Hence, also, the terms high madness and low madness. Insanity, from *insanus, unsound*, and derangement, from the French *dérangement*, signifying disorder, are common names for madness. The word lunatic was originally applied only to patients who had lucid intervals, and who were supposed to be under the influence of the moon. Idiocy signifies the condition of those who are imbecile from their birth, or become so in consequence of injury or disease of the brain. Delirium, derived from the Latin words *de lirâ*, out of the track, is now generally restricted to the wanderings attendant upon fever.—See Armstrong's Lectures on the Morbid Anatomy, Nature, and Treatment of Acute and Chronic Diseases, edited by Joseph Rix, p. 703, 8vo., Lond. 1834.—ED.

lirium, fatuity, and oneirodynia. He contemplates delirium, moreover, as of two kinds ; one combined with fever, and one without : the latter, he tells us, is what we name insanity ; and under this latter kind alone, the apyretic delirium or insanity, running synonymously with the present genus ecphronia, he proceeds to treat of melancholy and mania as species or subdivisions of it : throwing back the other kind of delirium to the class of fevers, as unconnected with the subject before him. So that, properly speaking, Dr. Cullen's order of vesaniæ should run parallel with the present order phrenica ; the genera of which should be delirium and fatuitas ; while mania and melancholy should be the species of delirium or the first genus.

Crichton, Parr, Young, Pinel, and most of the German writers, contemplate these diseases under the same sort of specific subdivision. Parr, indeed, in his article MANIA, asserts that both constitute nothing more than VARIETIES of one common species : yet, with an inconsistency which, among much that is excellent, is too frequently met with in his Dictionary, he changes his opinion in the article NOSOLOGY, makes vesania the genus, and arranges melancholia, mania, and even oneirodynia, as separate species under it.

The distinguishing characters, as the two species are contemplated by the generality of nosologists, are clear. In melancholy the alienation is restrained to a few objects or trains of ideas alone ; in madness it is general ; in reference to which distinction M. Esquirol has exchanged the term MELANCHOLY for that of MONOMANIA. And it hence follows, that gloom, gayety, and mischievousness may equally exist under both species ; according as these propensities are limited to a single purpose, or are unconfined and extend to every thing. Occasionally, however, among ancient writers, we find melancholy insanity limited to insanity accompanied with gloom or despondency, without any attention to the universality or partiality of the disease : for an undue secretion of melancholia, which is only a Greek term for black bile or choler, was supposed to be a common cause of mental dejection, and where it became habitual, to produce a low or gloomy temperament ; to which the term melancholic has continued to be applied to the present day. And hence the vulgar sense of the term, which is in unison with this view, is at variance with the technical and pathological. Yet the pathologists themselves have not been uniformly true to their own import : for even Dr. Cullen, who has followed the technical signification in his Synopsis, by defining melancholy as "insania *partialis* sine dyspepsia," sometimes adopts the colloquial meaning in his Practice of Physic, and hereby betrays a confusion which rarely belongs to him ; while Sir Alexander Crichton has given himself over completely to the popular, or, as he would perhaps call it, the ancient interpretation of the terms ; distinguishing mania, not by the generalization of the delirium, but by its raving fury or elevated gayety ; and melancholy, not by a limitation of the delirium to single objects or trains of ideas, but by its concomitant dejection and despondency.

There seems to be an equal incorrectness, though of a different kind, in M. Pinel, whose book is, nevertheless, of great merit. Delirium or wandering is made a pathognomonic symptom in his definition of the genus ; in other words, a want of correspondence between the judgment and the perception : and consequently this symptom should be found in every species which he has arranged under it. M. Pinel, however, has given us one species which has no such symptoms, and which is purposely intended to include cases of what he calls mania without any such discrepance ; on which account he has denominated it *mania sans délire*. All such cases, however, are reducible to modifications of rage or ungovernable passion, and ought by no means to be confounded with mania ; the judgment being, in these instances, not at variance with the perception, but overpowered by the predominant fury or passion that has been excited. They all belong properly to our next genus ; under which they will be considered.

Much difficulty has also been felt in defining ecphronia or insanity, so as to draw the line between real disease and habitual waywardness or oddity ;* and hence, while some definitions are so narrow as to set at liberty half the patients at Bethlem or the Bicêtre, others are so loose and capacious as to give a strait waistcoat to half the world.

M. Dufour undertook, with great learning and ingenuity, to prove that, as all our knowledge of an external world is derived from the action of the external senses, while mental sanity depends upon the soundness of these senses, mental insanity is alone to be referred to a diseased condition of one or more of them. And, in proof of this, he gives the case of a person who lost his senses because he could not be persuaded that the objects he saw in consequence of an incipient cataract arose entirely from that complaint. "When he found that he could not remove the dark web which appeared to him to be constantly floating before his eyes, he fell into such frequent fits of violent passion that he became quite insane. But as soon as the disease was completed he became more tractable, and submitted to the operation like a reasonable man."

---

* The following are distinctions insisted upon by Dr. Conolly, between eccentricity and insanity :—" The man who is merely eccentric can, if he exert himself, act rationally, and leave off his eccentricity ; the lunatic cannot. The eccentric man also commonly justifies his eccentricity more speciously and more calmly ; or perhaps laughs at it himself ; the madman seldom justifies his peculiarities with much skill, is provoked by contradiction, and is very seldom capable of joining in a laugh which is raised against himself."—(Inquiry concerning the Indications of Insanity, p. 139.) Dr. Conolly acknowledges, however, that there are cases on its boundary-line, between eccentricity and madness, which seem to bid defiance to all definition ; but generally resolvable into the effects of habit in confirming trifling actions, at first performed on some insufficient ground of reasoning.—ED.

But this only shows us that

"Ira furor brevis est,"

or else that the insanity was caused, not by the cataract, but by the frequent fits of violent passion. Thousands of persons have had cataracts in every form, and other external senses than the eye diseased in every form, and have been born defective in several of these senses, without the least mark of insanity ; while other persons, apparently in the most perfect possession of all the five senses, have been stark mad. Hence, the doctrine of M. Dufour boasts of few advocates in the present day.

In insanity or delirium without fever, it is far more obvious that there is a morbid condition of the judgment, or of the perception, or of both. Mr. Locke, and after him M. Condillac, refers it to the former alone, and characterizes madness, in the general sense of the term, by *false judgment ;* by a disposition to associate ideas incorrectly, and to mistake them for truths ; and hence, says Mr. Locke, "madmen err as men do that argue right from wrong principles."— (B. ii., ch. xi., § 13.) Dr. Battie, on the contrary, refers madness to the latter faculty alone, and characterizes it by *false perception ;* but the perceptions in madness seem, for any thing we know to the contrary, to be frequently as correct as in health, the judgment or reasoning being alone diseased or defective.*

It is difficult to say which of these two explanations of madness is most imperfect. It is sufficient to observe, that neither of them, taken alone, describes a condition of the faculties strictly morbid, and consequently neither of them defines madness. For we are daily meeting with thousands of mankind who are under the influ-

* Of those lunatics whose intellectual faculties are manifestly disordered (says Dr. Prichard), there is always a considerable proportion in whose minds it is impossible to trace any particular hallucination, or erroneous perception, or recollection. The rapid succession of thoughts, the hurried and confused manner in which ideas crowd themselves into their mind in a state of incoherence, or without order or connexion, is in very many instances among the most striking phenomena of madness. There are likewise cases of a different description, in which the intellectual faculties appear to have sustained but little injury, while the feelings and affections, the moral and active principles of the mind, are strangely perverted and depraved ; the power of self-government is lost or greatly impaired ; and the individual is found to be incapable, not of talking or reasoning upon any subject proposed to him, for this he will often do with great shrewdness and volubility, but of conducting himself with decency and propriety in the business of life. His wishes and inclinations, his likings and dislikings, have all undergone a morbid change ; and this change appears to be the originating cause, or to lie at the foundation of any disturbance, which the understanding itself may have sustained, and even in some instances to form throughout the chief character or constituent features of the disease.—(See Cyclop. of Pract. Med., art. INSANITY.) Whether these morbid changes, however, in the inclinations and wishes, likings and dislikings, are strictly the originating cause, may very well be disputed.—ED.

ence of false judgments, who unite incongruous or discrepant ideas, and draw from false associations right conclusions, yet whom we never think of regarding as out of their senses. While, on the contrary, if false perceptions be sufficient to constitute madness, every man is insane who mistakes at a distance a square for a round tower, the bending azure sky that terminates an extensive landscape for the sea, or the distant rumbling of a heavy wagon over the streets for a peal of thunder : and we should none of us be safe from such a charge for a single day of our lives.

Dr. Cullen seems to have embraced Mr. Locke's view of the subject ; for his definition of insanity (vesaniæ) in the latter editions of his Synopsis is, "injured functions of the mind in judging (*mentis judicantis*) without pyrexy or coma." Dr. Crichton, on the contrary, seems rather to adhere to Dr. Battie's view, though he enlarges and improves upon it ; and hence his definition is, "general derangement of the mental faculties, in which *diseased* perceptions are mistaken for realities ; with incoherent language and unruly conduct."

Diseased is certainly a better term than *false,* which is that of Dr. Battie ; but "unruly conduct" does not essentially belong to madness, even under this excellent writer's own explanation ; for of the three species which he comprehends under this disease as a genus, viz., *mania furibunda, mania mitis,* and *melancholia,* the last, as he afterward illustrates it (*Of Mental Derangement,* book iii., ch. iii., vol. ii.), evinces these symptoms only occasionally, he expressly tells us of the second, that the diseased are "all happy, gay, and cheerful ; that good-humour characterizes this insanity, and hence the patients are in general very tractable."—(Id., book i., ch. v., pp. 181, 182, vol. i.)

But the chief objection to Sir A. Crichton's definition of insanity, is his limiting it, in respect to the mental faculties, to the power of perception, while the judgment remains totally unaffected. "In regard to lunatics," says he, in another place, "and men who are of a sound mind, the faculty of judging *is the same in both ;* but they have different perceptions, and their judgments therefore must be different."

Now, if the faculties of perception, attention, and memory be liable to derangement, as the same writer admits, and there be "a *general* derangement of mental faculties in insanity," there seems no sufficient ground for exempting the faculty of judgment. And a little attention to the history of an insane patient will, I think, sufficiently support the opinion of Mr. Locke and Dr. Cullen upon this point, and show that this, if not the faculty chiefly diseased, labours under at least as much disease as that of perception.

We have already observed, in the proem to the present class, that all the powers of the mind are as liable to be affected with diseases, and diseases of various kinds, as those of the body ; and that either the body or the mind may be enfeebled at the same time in the whole of its powers, a few of its powers, or in a single power. A sound mind supposes an existence of all the mind's feelings and intellectual powers in a state of vigour and under the subordination of the judgment, which is designed by nature to be the governing or controlling principle. And, thus constituted, the mind is said to be in a state of order or arrangement. It often happens that this order or arrangement is slightly broken in upon by natural constitution or some corporeal affection ; but, so long as the irregularity does not essentially interfere with the mental health, it is no more attended to than slight irregularities or disquietudes of the body. Yet, whenever it becomes serious and complicated, it amounts to a disease ; and the mind is said, and most correctly so, to be deranged or disordered.

This derangement may proceed from a morbid state of any of the intellectual or any of the impassioned faculties of the mind ; for the perception may not correctly convey the ideas we receive by the external senses, or the judgment may lose its power of discriminating them, or the memory may not retain them, or the imagination or the passions may be in a state of unruly excitement—all which will lay a foundation for different kinds or genera of diseases, and, in fact, form the foundation of those appertaining to the present order.

Now, an attentive examination into the habits of an insane person will show, first, that the judgment and the perception are BOTH injured during the existence of insanity ; and next, that though, from a violent or complicated state of the disease, the morbid condition often extends to some other, or even to all the other mental faculties, yet it does not necessarily or essentially extend to them ; for a madman may be furious or passionate, yet every madman is not so ; his memory may fail, or his attention be incapable of fixing itself, or his imagination be wild and extravagant, but these do not always occur. The faculties, however, of the judgment and the perception are affected in every case, though they are not always equally affected at one and the same time ; for the morbid power seems, for the most part, unaccountably to shift in succession from the one to the other, so as alternately to leave the judgment and the perception free, or nearly free, from all estrangement whatever ; the disease being, however, always accompanied with irregular remissions, and often with such a diminution of sensibility that the patient is uninfluenced by the effects of cold and hunger, and very generally insusceptible of febrile miasm.

Thus, a madman will often mistake one person who is introduced to him for another, and, under the influence of this mistake, will reason correctly concerning him ; and although he may have been for years his next neighbour, will ask him when he came from China or the East Indies, by what ship he returned home, and whether his voyage has been successful—in all of which the error may be that of the perception alone. But if, as is frequently the case, the patient address his visiter by his proper name, he gives a ground-for believing that he perceives him aright, and that the error is that of the judg-

ment, which thus unites incongruous ideas, applying a visionary history to a real and identified person. At another time, he may from the first perfectly recognise the individual so presented to him, and, to prove his recollection and the correctness of his perception, may rapidly run over a long list of his relations, and a long string of anecdotes respecting his former life ; after which he may suddenly start, and, looking at the visiter's walking-stick, tell him that that drawn sword will never save him from destruction, nor all the men that slept with him in the same bed the night before—that his rival is now pushing forward with all speed on a black horse with a large army behind him, and that to-morrow he will fight and lose his crown.*

In such a case, and it is by no means an extreme one, the perception and the judgment travel soundly and in harmony at the outset of the interview, but they soon separate and abandon each other as far as the east and west. It is not always easy to say whether the first paroxysm of insanity that thus suddenly displays itself is limited to the one faculty or the other, or is common to both. For, if the perception suddenly wander, the judgment has a new train of ideas presented to it, and must necessarily take a new direction. Yet it is difficult to conceive how the judgment can be thus abruptly led astray, if it continue sound ; and hence it is more probable that the judgment itself is at

* The definition of madness adopted by Dr. Conolly is, "a loss or impairment of one or more of the mental faculties, accompanied by the loss of comparison."—(Inquiry concerning the Indications of Insanity, p. 114.) The cases of Nicholai and Dr. Bostock prove that persons may be conscious of the appearance of phantoms and other illusions, and know them to be false. If the foregoing gentlemen, as Dr. Conolly remarks, had for one moment lost the power of comparing, they must have believed the illusions to be real ; and "from the moment of such belief they must have been mad, and the same so long as the belief remained." Dr. Conolly introduces the following observations in his illustration of his theory :—"In a fever, the patient's bed will seem in flames ; or voices will whisper in his ear ; or the smell of a banquet assail him ; or his sense of touch seem opposed by moving bulky bodies ; or the sense of sight will be harassed by the rapid succession of imaginary faces, already spoken of, appearing and disappearing in endless trains and variety. If we talk with patients thus affected, some will tell us, in a very quiet way, that they are thus tormented. Others will seem confused, and make a visible effort of sight and hearing before they tell us how they are troubled ; and others will tell us what they see and what they hear, with an expressed belief, on their part, of the reality of what we know to be delusions. Of these three classes of patients," says Dr. Conolly, "the last are in a state of delirium ; the second are approaching to it ; the first are in a state of sound mind."

In another part of his interesting publication (P. 123), Dr. Conolly admits that it is not always easy to determine, in the case of the insane man, whether his sensation or his attention be impaired ; but the effect remarked, which may arise from either impairment, is the want of power of comparing one object with another, and this, in such cases, produces the insanity.—Ed.

fault, and admits a train of ideas which, however congruous to themselves, are incongruous to those furnished by the faculty of perception ; or both may equally wander and accompany each other in the visionary scene, as they at first associated in the real. It is obvious, however, if I mistake not, that both faculties are affected in the derangement of insanity, jointly or in irregular succession.*

How far a morbid state of the mental faculties may in any case depend upon the mind itself, as distinct from the sensorium or instrument by which it is connected with the body, it is impossible for us to know till we become acquainted with the nature of this connexion, and perhaps also with the essence of the mind, which, in our present state of information, seems to be a hopeless subject of inquiry. But we may possibly obtain some insight into the manner in which correct ideas of perception are changed in their nature and rendered incorrect or incongruous by a diseased judgment, by attending to a process of variation that is frequently occurring in perfect sanity and acuteness of mind. " The ideas we receive by sensation," says Mr. Locke, in adverting to this process, " are often in grown people *altered by the judgment* without our taking notice of it." And he explains this position by observing that, when a ball of any uniform colour, as of gold, alabaster, or jet, is placed before the eye, the idea thereby imprinted in the mind is that only of a flat circle variously shadowed, with different degrees of light and brightness coming to the organ of

sight. " But, having by use been accustomed to perceive what kind of appearance convex bodies are wont to make in us, what alterations are made in the reflections of light by the difference of the sensible figures of bodies, the judgment presently, by an habitual custom, alters their appearances into their causes ; so that from that which truly is variety of shadow or colour, collecting the figure, it makes it pass for a mark or figure, and *frames to itself the perception* of a convex figure and a uniform colour."—(*Human Underst.*, book ii., ch. ix., § 8.). And the same change occurs still more conspicuously in looking at an engraving or a picture, in which the only idea presented by the eye to the perception is that of a plane variously shaded or coloured, but which the judgment immediately changes and multiplies into other ideas of life and motion, and running streams, and fathomless woods, and cloud-capt mountains. And if in a sane state we find the judgment capable of thus varying the ideas of perception presented to it, we can have no great difficulty, I think, in conceiving by what means such a variation may be produced, and may ramify into incongruities of great extravagance in a judgment deranged by disease.

Nor is there much difficulty in conceiving how the paroxysm should be subject to remissions or even intermissions more or less regular, or the derangement be limited, as we frequently find it, and especially in melancholy, to particular subjects or trains of ideas. For, first, all diseases have a tendency to remissions or in-

---

* According to Dr. Conolly's views and arguments, which are replete with truth, each of the faculties of the mind may be impaired, and impaired without insanity ; at the same time, when the impairment of them, or any one of them, is such as to bring on inability to perform the act of comparison, or is accompanied by the loss of this faculty, insanity is the direct and inevitable result. The decisions are then no longer correct, the judgment no longer sound, and the actions no longer rational. —(See Inquiry concerning the Indications of Insanity, p. 170.) And, in a subsequent part of the work, when speaking of cases in which the sensations are morbid, Dr. Conolly observes, that, in numerous instances, the hallucination of the sense arises from an imagination previously over-excited ; that over-excitement is disease, but not madness ; it produces a hallucination, but, *if the hallucination is known to be a hallucination*, still there is no madness; *if it is mistaken for reality*, then the man is mad.—(P. 307.) Dr. Conolly gives from Shakspeare a fine illustration of the struggle between sanity and insanity. When the dagger first appears to Macbeth, although apparently sensible that it is a delusion, he attempts to seize it ; and failing to do so, says,—

" I have thee not, and yet I see thee still.
Art thou not, fatal vision, sensible
To feeling, as to sight ? or art thou but
A dagger of the mind, a false creation,
Proceeding from the heat-oppressed brain ?"

" The exercise of one sense to correct the suspicious evidence of another, the comparison, and the questioning which follows, are very striking. As Macbeth proceeds, it will be observed that he is struggling to exercise the comparison, which will prevent his belief in the delusion ; and that

when he becomes fully able to do it, he triumphs over the delusive appearance. The struggle is begun in the lines already quoted ; it is continued in the following :—

" ' I see thee yet, in form as palpable
As this which now I draw.
Thou marshall'st me the way that I was going ;
And such an instrument I was to use.
Mine eyes are made the tools o' the other senses,
Or else worth all the rest.'

" Here we observe that the delusion is powerful, but that Macbeth compares it with the reality of his own dagger ; he is evidently connecting the appearance with the cause of it ; with his actual intentions, and mentally accounting for it by associating it with his hidden thoughts ; yet he reasons with himself concerning the possibility of the evidence of his eyes being finer and truer than any other evidence, or the greater probability that by his state of commotion, and his disturbed feelings, his eyes are made 'the tools o' the other senses.' In this state of agitation the vision assumes some variety, while it maintains its distinctness ; but the words which follow show us that the mental process, the reasonings, the comparisons which Macbeth has made, effect a triumph over the delusion :—

" ' I see thee still ;
And on thy blade and dudgeon gouts of blood,
Which was not so before.—*There's no such thing.*
It is the bloody business, which informs
Thus to mine eyes.' "

These passages, and the comment on them by Dr. Conolly, certainly present a beautiful illustration of some of the doctrines concerning insanity contained in his valuable publication.—ED.

termissions; but those connected with the brain or nerves more than any others, as is evident in hemicrania, epilepsy, hysteria, and palpitation of the heart. And, next, there is no man in a state of the most perfect sanity whose judgment is equally strong and exact upon all subjects, and few whose judgments are not manifestly influenced and led astray by partialities or peculiar incidents of a thousand kinds : insomuch that we dare not, on various occasions, intrust to a man of the strictest honesty and the clearest head a particular subject for his decision, whom we should fly to as our counsellor upon every other occurrence. And it is not, therefore, very extraordinary, that in a morbid state of mind, and particularly of that faculty which constitutes the judgment, there should be an aberration in some directions or upon some subjects which does not exist upon others.

The corporeal indications differ as much as those of the mind, and generally as being governed by the latter. We have hence sometimes, as an opening symptom, an extraordinary flow of high spirits ; at others extreme terror. The countenance is pale and ghastly, and strongly expressive of inward emotion ; the speech hurried and tremulous ; and the extremities bedewed with a cold sweat. In other instances the eye glares malignantly ; the face is flushed, and evinces a dreadful ferocity ; the objects of terror become objects of vengeance ; and the patient is furious. In some there is an unusual degree of suspicion, and an anticipation of evil, and a belief in imaginary plots or conspiracies. In others, great irascibility and malignity, and a desire to commit some act of desperation, vengeance, and cruelty. All this is often combined with headache, giddiness, throbbing of the temples, or impaired vision. There is little or no sleep, for the mind is in a state of too much excitement ; though at times the patient lies listless, and refuses to be roused.—(*Annual Report of the Glasgow Asylum for Lunatics,* 1821.)

Concerning therefore the remote or even the proximate cause of the disease, we have yet much to learn. From the view we have taken in the proem of the close connexion between the mind and the brain, it seems reasonable to conceive that the remote cause is ordinarily dependant upon some misconstruction or misaffection of the cerebral organs ; and hence every part of them has been scrutinized for proofs of so plausible an hypothesis, but hitherto to no purpose whatever. The form of the cranium, its thickness, and other qualities ; the meninges, the substance of the brain, the ventricles, the pineal gland, the commissures, the cerebellum, have all been analyzed in turn, by the most dexterous and prying anatomists of England, France, Germany, and Italy, but with no satisfactory result. The shape or thickness of the scull has been started, indeed, as a cause, by many anatomists of high and established reputation ; but the conjecture has been completely disproved by others, who have found the very structures supposed to be most certain of producing madness, exist in numerous instances with perfect soundness of intellect. A particular shape of the scull seems, indeed, to be often connected with idiotism from birth or soon after birth, but with no other species of mental derangement whatever.

Morgagni engaged in an extensive course of dissections upon this subject, and pursued it with peculiar ardour ; and his results are given in his eighth epistle, from the second to the eighteenth article. In some cases the brain was harder, in some softer, than in a healthy state ; occasionally the dura mater was thicker, and was studded with soft, whitish bodies on the sides of the longitudinal sinus. This sinus itself sometimes evinced polypous concretions ; and the pineal gland, or several of the glands in the plexus choroides, were in a diseased state. Dr. Greding (*Vermischte Medicinische und Chirurgische Schriften,* Altenb., 1781), with a like spirit of investigation, arrived at a like diversity of facts. Meckel found the brain denser and harder than usual (*Hist. de l'Acad. Royale des Sciences,* &c., Ann. 1760, Berol., 4to., 1761); Dr. Smith (*Med. Observ. and Inquir.,* vol. vi.) descried a bony concretion, and Plenciz and several others represent the brain as bony or calculous in various parts ; while Jones, in the Medical Commentaries, found it softer than usual, with a thickening of the membranes and a turgescence of the ventricles. From all which, nothing precise or pathognomonic can be collected, since all such morbid appearances have been traced under other diseases as well as under insanity.

M. Pinel is firmly decided upon this point ; and after a very extensive course of investigations, he asserts, with respect to the cranium, that there are no facts yet clearly established which prove the faculties of the mind (except in the case of idiotism) to be in any degree influenced by its size, figure, or density : while with respect to the contents of the cranium, " I can affirm," says he, " that I have never met with any other appearances within the cavity of the scull, than are observable on opening the bodies of persons who have died of apoplexy, epilepsy, nervous fevers, and convulsions :" and his successors M. Esquirol and M. Georget concur in the same remarks. The last, after having examined three hundred lunatics on their decease, to settle the point before us, thus concludes : " Toutes les altérations que nous avons observées sur les aliénées de la Salpétrière sont consecutives au développement de la folie, excepté celles des cerveaux d'idiotes, qui sont primitives et liées à l'état intellectuel."

The observations of Haslam are nearly to the same effect : for they concur in showing that, except in so considerable a misformation of the scull or its contents as to induce idiotism from an early period of life, as in the case of cretinism, nothing decisive can be obtained in reference to insanity from any variations of appearance that have hitherto been detected.*

---

* From the dissections recorded by Dr. Haslam, his own inference is, that madness is always com-

The dissections of Greding extended to not fewer than two hundred and sixteen maniacal patients, the whole of whom, however, died of disorders unconnected with their mental ailments: three of the heads were exceedingly large, two exceedingly small; some of the scullbones extremely thick, others peculiarly thin; in some, the frontal bones were small and contracted; in others, the temporal bones compressed and narrow.

In a table containing an aggregate of the patients received into the lunatic asylum at Bicêtre during a considerable part of the French revolution, from 1784 to 1792, by far the greatest number admitted were between the ages of thirty and forty: next, those between forty and fifty; next to these, patients between twenty and thirty; then those from sixty to seventy;

nected with disease of the brain or its membranes. Indeed, he expresses a decided opinion that insanity is not a *disease of ideas*, and is among the first who in modern times have regarded it as connected with disease of the brain or its membranes. —(See Obs. on Madness and Melancholy, &c., p. 238, &c.) A similar opinion had been previously delivered by Dr. Marshall.—(See Morbid Anatomy of the Brain in Mania, &c.) According to Greding, the pia mater and arachnoid membrane were hardly ever sound. The same fact was noticed by Dr. Haslam in thirty-seven out of thirty-eight dissections; also by J. Werzel, of Mentz (Obs. sur le Cervelet, &c., trad. par M. Breton, Paris, 1811); and Chiarugi, of Florence (Della Pazzia, &c., in Firenze, 1794). M. Bayle considers *chronic meningitis*, a form of meningeal inflammation essentially and primarily chronic, as the most frequent pathological cause of mental derangement.—(Traité des Maladies du Cerveau, &c., Paris, 1826.) The frequency of disease of the brain in insane persons is confirmed by the researches of M. Calmeil.— (De la Paralysie considéré chez les Aliénés, &c., Paris, 1826.) Dr. Conolly also agrees in "ascribing mental disorders to corporeal disease; not to any specific corporeal disease, but to any disease capable of disturbing the functions, or impairing the structure of the nerves:" yet he adds, "we do not find in insanity, as in consumption, such invariable disorganization or impairment as would account for the long continuance of the malady, or for the small proportion of cures."—(An Inquiry concerning the Indications of Insanity, p. 14.) When insanity proceeds from adversity, domestic calamity, and other external influences on the mind, and especially when the alteration of the mind is suddenly produced by such causes, the connexion of the mental change with any organic or visible disease must be, at least in the first instance, beyond all suspicion, unless disturbance of the innervation and circulation, and other functional disorders, not necessarily accompanied by change of structure, be comprehended under the denomination of corporeal diseases. As Dr. Uwins observes,—"Who shall pronounce upon the precise nature of that change in the sentient organization, when unexpected intelligence instantaneously destroys a keen appetite? when madness occurs as the immediate result of some heartrending disappointment? when the whole man is thoroughly and in a moment revolutionized by a change of scene and circumstance? or when faith in a physician at once breaks down the strongholds of hitherto confirmed disease?"—On Disorders of the Brain and Nervous System, p. 11, 8vo., Lond., 1833.—Ed.

and lastly, those from fifteen to twenty; below which we have no account of any admission whatever. Hence different stadia of life seem to exercise some control, and the period most exposed to the disease is that in which the influence of the passions may be conceived to be naturally strongest and most operative. "Among the lunatics confined at Bicêtre," says M. Pinel, "during the third year of the republic, and whose cases I particularly examined, I observed that the exciting causes of their maladies, in a great majority of instances, were extremely vivid affections of the mind; as ungovernable or disappointed ambition, religious fanaticism,* profound chagrin, and unfortunate love. Out of one hundred and thirteen madmen, with whose histories I took pains to make myself acquainted, thirty-four were reduced to this state by domestic misfortunes; twenty-four by obstacles to matrimonial unions which they had ardently desired to form; thirty by political events connected with the revolution; and twenty-five by religious fanaticism." Those were chiefly affected who belonged to professions in which the imagination is unceasingly or ardently engaged, and not controlled in its excitement by the exercise of the tamer functions of the understanding, which are more susceptible of satiety and fatigue. Hence the Bicêtre registers were chiefly filled from the professions of priests, artists, painters, sculptors, poets, and musicians: while they contained no instances of persons whose line of life demands a predominant exercise of the judging faculty: not one naturalist, physician, chymist, nor geometrician.

But there are other organs that also betray very prominent signs of diseased action in insanity as well as the brain, as those of the epigastrium and the adjoining regions; and hence other physiologists have sought for a remote or even a proximate cause of the malady in these, rather than in the encephalon. This was the case among several, though not the majority, of the Greek physicians, as we have seen already; and it is to this quarter that M. Pinel refers the proximate cause in almost every instance in our own day. It is here he supposes the disease to commence, and contends that the affection of the brain and of the mental faculties is subsequent to the abdominal symptoms, and altogether dependant upon them; and, in proof of this, he adverts to various dissections which have shown a considerable derangement, not only in the function, but even in the structure of one or more of the abdominal organs, and particularly a displacement of the transverse colon.

But this is to give a weight to the morbid appearances occasionally manifested in these organs, above what is allowed to like misformations in the cranium. Yet there can be no doubt that, in most cases of insanity, the brain

* According to Dr. Burrows, there are five times as many females insane from this cause as males.— See Commentaries on the Causes, Forms, Symptoms, and Treatment, moral and medical, of Insanity, 8vo., 1828.—Ed.

and epigastrium suffer jointly; and that the disease may, and often does, commence in some
structural or functionary affection of the abdominal organs, is perfectly clear from the frequency of this complaint during pregnancy and
in childbed: its being connected with a peculiar state of the genital organs, as we shall presently have occasion to show, and its following
upon a sudden suppression of the menstrual or
hemorrhoidal discharge.

Nor is it difficult to account for this association of influence from the extensive distribution
of the par vagum, and more particularly of the
intercostal nerve over the abdominal viscera:
on which account a like sympathy is by no
means uncommon in various other disorders.
Thus, while a concussion or compression of the
brain produces nausea, sickness, and constipation, worms are frequently found to excite convulsions or epilepsy.

The fair result of the whole inquiry appears
to be, that insanity, in every instance, to adopt
the language of Sir A. Crichton, "arises from a
diseased state of the brain or nerves, or both"
(*Of Mental Derangement*, vol. i., p. 138); but
that in many instances this diseased state is a
primary affection, and in others a secondary,
dependant upon a morbid condition of the epigastric or some other abdominal organ: for, in
whatever this morbid condition may consist, and
whatever symptoms it may evince, it is not till
the sensorium has by degrees associated in the
chain of unhealthy action, that the signs of insanity are unequivocal. And, in like manner,
dyspeptic and other abdominal symptoms are
not unfrequently brought on by a previously diseased state of the mind: and it is hence peculiarly difficult, and perhaps in some cases altogether impossible to determine, where we are
not acquainted with the incipient symptoms,
whether melancholy or hypochondrias has originated in the state of the abdominal viscera or
of the cranium; or, in other words, whether the
one or the other be a primary or a secondary
affection.

---

* The ensuing passage conveys Dr. Conolly's
mode of viewing one part of this mysterious subjcet, which has defied, and, as Dr. Good states,
will continue to defy, all attempts at a satisfactory
explanation:—"The manifestation of the mind
must depend upon, and be modified by, the development of the brain in each individual. The
same intellectual light may be given to all; but,
in some, obscured by a gross organization; and in
others, more happily organized, shining forth more
brightly. Itself out of the reach of physical injury,
it works by physical instruments; and the exactness of its operations depends on the growth, maturity, integrity, and vigour of its instruments,
which are the brain and nervous system. If the
nervous agents of sensation are unfaithful, the
mind receives false intelligence, or transmits its
orders by imbecile messengers; if the seat of
thought, the centre of intellectual and moral government, is faultily arranged, the operations of
the understanding are impeded and incomplete."—
(See An Inquiry concerning the Indications of
Insanity, p. 62.) The editor cannot discover the
agreement between the tenour of these observations, and the doctrine to which the author of the

When, however, we are made acquainted
with the history of the incipient symptoms, we
have a tolerable clew to guide us; and for the
most part may safely decide, that the region
primarily affected is that which first evinces
morbid symptoms; and hence, while we shall
have little scruple in assigning the origin of
most cases of hypochondriacism to a morbid condition of one or more of the digestive organs,
we need have as little in assigning the greater
number of cases of mania to a primary misaffection of the brain or the nerves.

In what that misaffection consists is a question that has never been settled to the present
hour; and from our total unacquaintance with
the nature of the connexion between the brain
and the mind, it never will be in any very satisfactory manner.* The morbid changes, indeed,
which we have already seen are frequently to
be traced in the structure of the brain, show
very sufficiently that a considerable degree of
diseased action has been taking place there; but
as these changes are often found in other disorders of the head as well as in mania, and more
especially as we cannot tell whether they have
preceded or been produced by such action, they
give us little information as to the nature of the
diseased action itself.

Dr. Cullen has offered a series of ingenious
arguments to prove that mania consists in some
inequality in the excitement of the brain (*Prac.
Phys.*, vol. iv., Aph. 1562), or of the nervous
power (Id. 1544), and, in most cases, in an increased excitement. Dr. Cullen's idea of the
nervous power, as we have already had occasion to observe, is very far from being explicit:
for he defines it "a subtile very moveable fluid,
included or *inherent* in a manner *we do not
clearly understand*, in every part of the medullary substance of the brain and nerves." While,
in other parts of his writings, he represents it
as never either recruited or exhausted, and thus
conceives it to possess qualities beyond the
ordinary endowments of living matter. Yet
his general principle appears to be well founded, and Sir Alexander Crichton has availed him-

---

foregoing excellent work inclines, that mental disorders may be ascribed to any corporeal disease
capable of disturbing the functions, or impairing
the structure of the brain. The incongruity which
is here manifest, depends upon the term *mind* being made to signify also the *soul*. But the intellectual organization and functions certainly constitute a very different subject from that of the
theological doctrines of our immortal nature.
Hence, also, the following passage cannot be correct:—"Nay, so dependant is the immaterial soul
upon the material organs, both for what it receives
and what it transmits, that a slight disorder in the
circulation of the blood through different portions
of nervous substance, can disturb all sensation, all
emotion, all relation with the external and living
world; can obstruct attention and comparison;
can injure and confound the accumulations of the
memory, or modify the suggestions of imagination." The statement is not accurate in relation
to the soul; but unobjectionable, perhaps, if applied to the mind. Our souls, it is to be hoped,
will exist, when our brain, nerves, circulation,
&c., are no more.—ED.

self of it in giving a fuller explanation of this highly probable hypothesis : and, after appealing to the doctrine which has already been advanced and supported in the preceding pages of the present work, that the nervous power is a peculiar fluid secreted in the medullary substance of the brain or the nerves, he endeavours to show that the cause of insanities is a specific morbid action of the vessels which secrete the nervous fluid in the brain (*Of Mental Derangement*, vol. i., p. 174) ; and which may hereby be altered not only in quantity but in quality.*

From the quickness of the external senses, the irascibility, heat of the skin, flushed countenance, and uncommon energy which maniacs evince, we have reason to believe this morbid action to be, for the most part, a preternaturally increased action; and we are hence able to account for the various exacerbations and remissions which it evinces, sometimes periodically, and sometimes irregularly. Yet as the health of the faculties of the mind must depend upon a healthy energy of the vessels, too scanty a secretion of nervous fluid must be as effectual a cause of mental derangement as too copious a flow ; and hence torpor of the vessels of the brain may prove as certain a cause of a wandering mind as entony, and, consequently, typhus fever may become a source of delirium as well as inflammatory. And as the various secretions can only be elaborated from the blood, and are often affected by its condition, we may see also how madness may be a result of acrid narcotics and other poisons introduced into the blood by absorption, or a transfusion of blood from animals of a different nature, of which Dionis has given some very striking examples.

That there is a tendency not only to an increased secretion of sensorial power in the head in most cases of insanity, but to an accumulation of it from all parts of the body, and especially from the surface, is clear from the patient's

diminished sensibility to external impressions, and his being able to endure the severest winter's cold, and a fasting of many days, without inconvenience or indeed consciousness. But that there is, in some cases, a diminished secretion of this fluid, producing a general debility of the living fibre, is also clear from the great tendency manifested by some maniacs, whose brain gives no proof of increased excitement, to a gangrene in their extremities, and, where they are uncleanly, about the buttocks. The insensibility from this cause is sometimes so considerable as to affect not only the diffuse organ of feeling, but some of the local senses as well. And hence some patients lose their hearing, and others are capable of staring at the meridian sun without pain, or any change in the diameter of the iris.—(*Blumenb.*, bibl. i., p. 736.) Sometimes, however, the increased secretion of sensorial power is so considerable as not only to affect the head, but to augment the corporeal sensibility generally. And hence Hoffmann makes accumulated sensation an ordinary symptom of this disease (*Opp.*, Suppl. ii., 2), mistaking the exception for the general rule : and Riedlin gives us an instance of a maniac, who, instead of calling for and being able to endure large quantities of snuff, sneezed and was convulsed on smelling the mildest aromatics.*

It is a melancholy reflection, that insanity is often the result of an hereditary predisposition. This, indeed, has been denied by a few writers, but their opinion has unhappily been confuted by the concurrent voice of those who have thought differently, and the irresistible evidence of daily facts. Mysterious as the subject is, we have perpetual proofs that a peculiarity of mental character is just as propagable as a peculiarity of corporeal ; and hence wit, madness, and idiotism, are as distinctly an heirloom of some families, as scrofula, consumption, and cancer of others.† In most of the latter we have already observed that something of a constitutional make or physiognomy is often discernible ; and the

---

* Id., vol. i., p. 169. With respect to the hypothesis here laid down, the editor has already delivered his opinion in the Physiological Proem. That the brain is an organ receiving a very great supply of blood; that its vessels are large and numerous ; that an increased determination of blood to the brain, or, on the contrary, a diminution of the quantity conveyed to it, must have an effect upon the cerebral functions; that the vessels secrete from this blood the medullary and cortical substances, the fluid in the ventricles, and every kind of matter composing the various tissues of the brain ; and that the perfect or imperfect state of the intellectual and nervous powers is intimately dependant upon the condition of the circulation within the head, are facts of which no doubt can be entertained. But when the venturesome physiologist proceeds farther, and first assumes the existence of a nervous fluid as synonymous with sensorial or nervous power, represents it as a secretion, and mental derangement as arising from its altered quality or quantity; he is getting out of his depth, and only contenting himself with an hypothesis, which, if it were admitted, would, after all, not render the subject at all more intelligible. Instead of the "secretion of the nervous fluid," it might be better, therefore, to read, " the production of nervous or sensorial power."—Ed.

* Lin. Med., 1696, p. 29. Such occurrences are only accidental accompaniments of insanity, by no means essential to it, or even indicative of its existence. Were the contrary view adopted, the modern Romans, who are greatly annoyed by a perfumed handkerchief, might be set down as lunatics, as well as others whose sense of smell is so inconveniently acute, that they almost " die of a rose in aromatic pain."—Ed.

† In six sevenths of the cases which have come under the observation of Dr. Burrows, hereditary predisposition was traced. He does not consider that the several forms of insanity tend to transmit each its own kind from one generation to another ; but, on the contrary, that they mutually transmit one another, so that mania, melancholia, and hypochondriasis, may be all remarked in different individuals of the same family. He admits, however, one exception to this rule in the instance of suicidal insanity. Probably, hypochondriasis may be another exception. Dr. Burrows does not consider hereditary insanity more difficult to cure than other forms of it, which statement disagrees with what is commonly believed.—See Commentaries, &c., and Edin. Med. Journ., No. xcviii., p. 123.

same is contended for by many authorities in the disease before us. Yet, if we examine the marks accurately, we shall find that they merge, for the most part, into the common symptoms of a sanguineous or melancholic temperament : either of which constitutions exercises such a control over the disease as to give it a peculiar modification, whatever be the nature of the exciting cause, which is, in truth, of little importance to the constitutional turn the malady may take, though well worth attending to in the moral treatment. " The violence of the maniacal paroxysm," observes M. Pinel, " appears to be independent of the nature of the exciting cause ; or, at least, to be far more influenced by the constitution of the individual, and the peculiar degree of his physical and moral sensibility. Men of a robust constitution, of mature years, with black hair, and susceptible of strong and violent passions, appear to retain the same character when visited by this most distressing of human misfortunes. Their ordinary energy is augmented to outrageous fury. Violence, on the other hand, is seldom characteristic of the paroxysms of individuals of more moderate passions, with brown or auburn hair. Nothing is more common than to see men with light-coloured hair sink into soothing and pleasurable reveries ; while it seldom or never happens that they become furious or unmanageable. Their pleasing dreams, however, are at length overtaken by and lost amid the gloom of an incurable fatuity. Those of the greatest mental excitement, of the warmest passions, the most active imagination, the most acute sensibility, are chiefly predisposed to insanity. A melancholy reflection !—but such as is calculated to call forth our best and tenderest sympathies."

It has long been a current opinion, that insanity is a disease more common to our country than to any other : and this opinion has of late been rendered more seriously alarming by the following assertion of Dr. Powell, secretary to the commissioners for licensing lunatic establishments, and which is given as the result of his official tables of returns from 1775 to 1809 inclusive, divided into lustra or periods of five years each. "Insanity appears to have been *considerably* upon the increase : for if we compare the sums of two distant lustra, the one beginning with 1775, and the other with 1809, the proportion of patients returned as having been received into lunatic-houses during the latter period, is to that of the former nearly as 129 to 100."—"The facts also," says he, "which present themselves to the observation of the traveller, whatever direction he may take through this country, and all the local information which we receive upon the subject, supply us, as I am led to think, with sufficient proof, that the increase must actually have been *very considerable*, though we cannot ascertain what has been its exact proportion."*

The first part of this opinion, or that which

* Med. Trans., vol. iv., p. 131, art. Observations on the Comparative Prevalence of Insanity at different Periods.

regards insanity as a disease PECULIARLY PREVALENT in England, does not seem to rest on any established basis ; for, calculating with Dr. Powell, that the number of lunatic paupers, and those received into public hospitals, which, under the act of parliament, are not cognizable by the commissioners, together with those neglected to be returned, compared with the returns entered into the commissioners' books, bear the proportion of three to two, which is probably far above the mark, still the aggregate number of insane persons for the year 1800, contrasted with the general census for the same year, will only hold a ratio of about 1 to 7300 ; while if we take with Dr. Burrows the proportion of suicides committed in foreign capitals as a test of the extent to which insanity is prevalent in the same towns, which is nevertheless a loose mode of reckoning, though it is not easy to obtain a better, we have reason to conclude that insanity is comparatively far less frequent among ourselves than in most parts of the continent : the suicides of Paris, Berlin, and Copenhagen, as drawn from tables collected by Dr. Burrows for this purpose, being, in proportion to the relative population of London, as 5 to 2 for the first, 5 to 3 for the second, and 3 to 1 for the third.—(*Inquiry into certain Errors relative to Insanity,* &c., p. 93, 8vo., 1820.)

Nor does the idea that insanity is an INCREASING DISEASE in our own country appear to rest on a stabler foundation. Taking Dr. Powell's result as drawn from full and incontrovertible data, and comparing the supposed march of the disease with the acknowledged march of the population, although the former may possibly be said to have overstepped the latter by a few paces, the difference will hardly justify the assertion, that "insanity is considerably upon the increase." And if we take into view the intensity of interest with which this subject has, for the last twenty years, been contemplated by the public, the operation of those feelings of humanity which have dragged the wretched victims of disease from the miserable abodes of prisons and neglected workhouses, and placed them under the professional care of the superintendents of licensed establishments, and, above all, the augmented number of such establishments in consequence hereof, and the great respectability of many who have the management of them, thus giving the commissioners returns which, by the power of the act of 26 Geo. III., they could not otherwise have been in possession of, we may, I think, fairly conclude, that this apparent overstep, be it what it may, in the march of insanity beyond that of the population of the country, is a real retrogression.

At this conclusion we might, I think, fairly arrive, even if the data selected by Dr. Powell were full and incontrovertible ; but he himself has candidly admitted that, instead of being full and incontrovertible, they " are subject to numerous inaccuracies, and that any deductions which may be made from them must be imperfect." It is still more consolatory to learn, that the direct deductions from the parochial and district establishments are not only in accordance with Dr. Powell's, but such as seem to show that a retrogression, instead of an advance, has actually taken place. Dr. Burrows has industriously collected many of these, and, as far as they go, they lead to such an inference almost without exception.—(*Inquiry*, &c., ut suprà, p. 66, et alibi.) Yet it is probable that even this inference does not give us the precise fact, and that it is as chargeable with an error on the favourable side, as the opposite account is on the unfavourable ; since the increase of licensed houses, whose returns seem to have swelled the list of the commissioners beyond its proper aggregate, has been considerably supported by a transfer from the establishments which have thus fallen off. And hence, allowing the error on the one side to compensate that on the other, we are brought to the conclusion which, after all, appears more natural, that the career of insanity is only varied in its uniformity by temporary contingencies, but that it is by no means a prevalent disease in our own country.*

---

* Dr. Burrows thinks that climate does not appear to be an exciting cause of insanity ; but it cannot be denied, he adds, that the seasons are so ; and that, when the thermometer is highest in temperate regions, the number of insane is greatly augmented. Thus, in Paris, on taking the average of nine years, the number of insane increased in May, arrived at its maximum in July, and gradually decreased till January, when it was at its minimum. Dr. Burrows also remarks, that the species of insanity termed suicidal always prevails most in the hottest season. From registers published in the cities of Westminster, Paris, and Hamburgh, suicides are most frequent in June and July ; in short, whenever the thermometer ranges near 84° F. Hence, he concludes, that it is not climate, but a high temperature, which exposes the intellectual functions to derangement.

It would seem, at first view, from many circumstances, that females are more liable to insanity than males. Dr. Rush remarks, that women, in consequence of the greater predisposition imparted to their bodies by menstruation, pregnancy, and parturition, and to their minds by being much alone in their families, are more predisposed to madness than men. Yet, according to the statistics given by Dr. Burrows (if we except large cities, as Paris, Lyons, Milan, &c., where immorality and habits prejudicial to the female prevail), the majority of the insane are men. In the Royal Asylum at Charenton in France, from January 1, 1815, to January 1, 1823, 1453 lunatics were admitted ; of these there were 847 males, 606 females. Of 2507 insane admitted to the Parisian hospitals, 1095 were men, and 1412 were women. At Lyons, the proportion was, men 60, women 150. In England, the number of lunatics confined in private houses from 1812 to 1824, was 7804 : of these, 4461 were males, and 3343 females. But, according to an analysis published of the Pauper Lunatic Asylum in the county of Middlesex, including the metropolis, in 1827, the proportion was stated to be, men 307, women 546. In Scotland, in 1818, the proportion was, men 2311, women 2339. In the Dublin House of Industry in 1824 and 1827, nearly the same number of both sexes were admitted. The same was true of Zurich in 1823. In Germany, the men exceed. In Vienna, in 1812, the number of men insane was 177, of women 94. In Berlin, in 1816, the number of insane males was 242, of females 177.—

M 2

ECPHRONIA MELANCHOLIA.

MELANCHOLY.

THE DISCREPANCE BETWEEN THE PERCEPTION AND THE JUDGMENT LIMITED TO A SINGLE OBJECT, OR A FEW CONNECTED OBJECTS, OR TRAINS OF IDEAS : THE WILL WAYWARD AND DOMINEERING.

WE have already stated, that whatever be the exciting cause of mental alienation, the symptoms are in every instance greatly modified by the prevailing idiosyncrasy ; and hence, though a love of solitude, gloom, fear, suspicion, and taciturnity, are the ordinary signs of the present species, these signs often yield to symptoms widely different, and sometimes even of an opposite character ; and we hence become possessed of the four following varieties :—

a Attonita.		Mute, gloomy, retiring melancholy.
Gloomy melancholy.		
β Errabunda.		Roving, restless melancholy, evincing a constant desire to change the abode.
Restless melancholy.		
γ Malevolens.		Morose or mischievous melancholy, occasionally terminating in suicide, or the injury of others.
Mischievous melancholy.		

(Burrows's Comment on Insanity, p. 241, London, 1828.) We must regret the imperfect statements of the number of insane in the United States. Dr. A. Brigham of Hartford, taking the ascertained number of insane in Connecticut as the basis of his calculation, estimates the whole number in the United States to be 50,000 ; which is certainly very large, and probably exceeds the true amount. —(See Remarks on the Influence of Mental Cultivation on Health, by Amariah Brigham, Hartford, 1832.) According, however, to the reports of the Bloomingdale Asylum, New-York, the number of insane in that institution, including those remaining at the end of December, 1830, and those admitted and discharged during part of 1831, was 98 ; in 1832 and 1833, 216 ; of whom 145 were males, and 73 females ; in 1834, 103 ; of whom 67 were males, and 36 females.

Dr. Burrows asserts that indulgence in ardent spirits is the cause why insanity prevails most among males, and in the U. States we have unfortunately too many instances of this truth. Dr. Rush remarks, that on inquiring in regard to the insane confined in the Pennsylvania Hospital, he found that one third of the whole number had become deranged from intemperance. The most frequent cause of insanity, says the report of Dr. Woodward, the able superintendent of the Lunatic Asylum at Worcester, Mass., is intemperance ; and we have reason to think the same is true as respects the inmates of the Lunatic Asylum at Bellevue and at Bloomingdale.

If these facts be well founded, and there is reason to think they are, philanthropists have cause to be gratified with the salutary results which must follow from the extension of the temperance system in the United States ; an abstinence from alcoholic drinks would diminish the number of the insane at least one half : hence, with the present exertions of the friends of temperance, insanity must be comparatively on the decrease in this country.—D.

δ Complacens. - Self-complacent and affable Self-complacent melancholy; occasionally melancholy. rejoicing in a visionary superiority of rank, station, or endowment.

The same variety of symptoms, as chiefly modified by the prevailing temperament, are noticed by Fracastorio. "The phlegmatic," says he, "are heavy; the sanguine lively, cheerful, merry, but not witty; the choleric are in rapid and perpetual motion, impatient of dwelling upon any subject. An acuteness of wit belongs to most of the varieties, but not to all."—(De Intellectione, lib. ii.) And hence Diocles, in opposing Galen for holding, after Hippocrates, that gloom and terror are pathognomonic signs of melancholy, observes, "Upon serious consideration I find some patients that have nothing of these qualities, and others that exhibit every diversity of feeling; for some are sad without being fearful, others fearful without being sad; some neither, and some both."

Besides these modifications there is another of a very peculiar kind, noticed by Dr. Spurzheim, in order to show that the faculties of the mind are double, and that each hemisphere of the brain contains a distinct set. As I have never met with an instance of this variety, I must describe it in his own words. "Tiedemann," says he, "relates the example of one Moser, who was insane on one side, and who observed his insanity with the other. Gall attended a minister who, having a similar disease for three years, heard constantly on his left side reproaches and injuries, and turned his head to that side in order to look at the persons. With his right side he commonly judged of the madness of his left side, but sometimes, in a fit of fever, he could not rectify his peculiar state. Long after being cured, if he happened to be angry, or if he had drunk more than he was accustomed to do, he observed in his left side a tendency to his former alienation."— (Physiognomical System, &c., p. 144, 8vo., 1815.)

It may appear strange to those who have not studied the subject with much attention, that persons who are possessed of a diseased, or even defective judgment, should at any time be of quick and lively apprehension, and thus be witty without being wise. But the faculty of wit is dependant not so much on the judgment as on the imagination, and particularly on the memory; on the possession of a large stock of ideas stored up for ready use, and brought forth with rapidity. "And hence," says Mr. Locke, "some reason may perhaps be given of that common observation, that men who have a great deal of wit, and prompt memories, have not always the clearest judgment or deepest reason. For wit lying most in the assemblage of ideas, and putting those together with quickness and variety, wherein can be found any resemblance or congruity, thereby make up pleasant pictures and agreeable visions in the fancy; judgment, on the contrary, lies quite on the other side; in separating carefully, one from another, ideas wherein can be found the least difference, thereby to avoid being misled by similitude, and by affinity to take one thing for another."—(On Human Understanding, book ii., chap. xi., sect. 2.) And hence we may easily account for that gayety and those ebullitions of a vivid fancy, which so often assume the character of wit in persons whose minds are deranged, and especially in the sober faculty of the judgment.

Mirth and wit, however, though sometimes found in the present species of insanity, are by no means its common characters: but, on the contrary, as we have already observed, a love of solitude, gloom, and taciturnity, and an indulgence in the distressing emotions of the mind. And hence, whenever hypochondriacism merges into actual insanity, it almost always takes this form; as melancholy, from a sort of natural connexion between the two, often assumes many of the symptoms that essentially appertain to the hypochondriac disease; the morbid state of the brain influencing the abdominal organs in the latter case, as the morbid state of the abdominal organs influences the brain in the former.

The disease shows itself sometimes suddenly, but more generally by slow and imperceptible degrees. Among the earliest symptoms may be mentioned headaches, frequent attacks of giddiness, sudden confusion of ideas, a great disposition to anger, violent agitations when irritated, and an uncommon sensibility of nerves, whereby the patient is apt to be carried to as great excesses from causes of joy as from those of grief. There is a desire of doing well, but the will is wayward and unsteady, and produces an inability of firmly pursuing any laudable exertion, or even purpose, on account of some painful internal sensation, or the perverseness of the judgment, led astray by false or erroneous ideas which command a firm conviction in the mind.—(Crichton, of Mental Derangement, passim.) And if the disease occur in a person possessing that temperament which has been conceived to predispose to it, and was by the Greeks denominated melancholic, the external signs become peculiarly marked and prominent: "the patient," says Hippocrates, in his book on insanity, "is emaciated, withered, and hollow-eyed, and is at the same time troubled with flatulence and acid eructations, with vertigo and singing in the ears, gets little sleep, and when he closes his eyes is distracted with fearful and interrupted dreams."

The FIRST VARIETY most commonly commences with this character, and creeps on so gradually that it is for some time mistaken for a mere attack of hypochondriacism or lowness of spirits (Falret, de l'Hypochondrie et du Suicide, passim, 8vo., Paris, 1822), till the mental alienation is at length decided by the wildness of the patient's eyes, the hurry of his step whenever he walks, his extraordinary gestures, and the frequent incongruity of his observations and remarks. The first stage of the disease is thus admirably expressed by Hamlet:—"I have of late, but wherefore I know not, lost all my mirth, foregone all custom of exercise; and, indeed, it goes so heavily with my disposition, that this goodly frame, the earth, seems to me a steril promontory ; this most excellent canopy, the air, look you, this brave o'erhanging firmament, this majestical roof, fretted with golden fire, why it appears no other thing to me than a foul and pestilent congregation of vapours."

But while the external world is thus in general falsely recognised by the perception, or falsely discriminated by the judgment, the mind is so completely possessed by some particular trains of imaginary ideas, that the attention is perpetually turned to them, and the judgment mistakes them for substances; and, so far as it is sensible of surrounding objects or scenery, is perpetually blending the vision with the reality. It is not that the patient's ideas are incongruous with themselves, but with the world around him ; for the remarks of the melancholy man, when his attention is once correctly fixed, are for the most part peculiarly shrewd and pointed. But in the gloom that hangs over him under the variety we are now contemplating, he can rarely be brought into conversation, seeks for solitude, sits moping in one continued posture from morning till night ; or, if he walk at all, seeks for orchards, back lanes, and the gloomiest places he can find. "One of the chief reasons," says Hippocrates, in his epistle to Philipœmenes, "that induced the citizens of Abdera to suspect Democritus of craziness, was, that he forsook the city and lived in groves and hollow trees, upon a green bank by a brookside, or by a confluence of waters, all day and all night."*

Sauvages, under the variety of *melancholia attonita*, gives an extreme case of the present modification, though not from personal knowledge. "The patient," says he, "never moves from place to place, nor changes his posture ; if he be seated, he never stands up ; if standing, he never sits ; if lying, he never rises. He never moves his feet unless they are pushed aside by a by-stander ; but he does not shun

the presence of man ; if asked a question he does not answer, and yet appears to understand what is said. He does not yield to admonition, nor pay any attention to objects of sight or touch ; he seems immersed in profound thought, and totally occupied by foreign matters. Yet at times he is more awake ; if food be put to his mouth, he eats ; if liquor be presented, he drinks." M. de Sauvages then adds, that this rare modification of the disease occurred once to Dr. James, physician to the Elector of Saxony, in a man about thirty years old, who was terrified with the thought that the Deity had condemned him. It continued for four months, during the autumn and winter, but the patient was at length restored to his right understanding.—(*Nosol. Med.*, class viii., ord. 3.)

Grief, and particularly for the loss of friends, discontent, severe disappointment, the dread of some real or imaginary evil, a violent and long-continued exertion of any of the passions, and deep uninterrupted study, have frequently proved accidental causes or accessories of this variety of melancholy, where the peculiarity of the constitution has formed a predisposition, and have sometimes produced it even where no such predisposition can be traced. M. Magendie met with a singular exemplification of this from a cause few would expect, though not difficult of solution. The patient, an intelligent and agreeable man, though of a highly nervous temperament, had the misfortune, at the age of thirty-six, to meet with various crosses in business, and to have his wife become deranged in her confinement with her first child. All his energies were devoted to the recovery of his wife, whom he accompanied in travelling, which was recommended to her ; he nursed her with tender assiduity, and was a witness to all her sufferings of body and mind. In time she recovered ; but he himself, instead of giving way to joy, fell into a state of the most distressing melancholy—believed himself ruined, pursued by the officers of police, and about to take his trial for some heinous offence. Upon every other subject his mind was sound. We have already observed that the sudden cessation of any habitual drain, or other corporeal irritation, has occasionally proved a cause of melancholy ; and we here find that there is at times as much danger in a sudden cessation of mental as of corporeal irritation ; the excited mind being as little capable of bearing the change in the one instance as in the other. And hence, whenever such an effect occurs in an irritable frame, the individual should be instantly roused to some new pursuit, that may swallow up, though more agreeably, the whole of the surplus of sensorial power that has habitually been produced. In the state above described M. Magendie's patient continued many months, when, from some unknown cause, the disease upon the mind was thrown upon the motific fibres, and he was attacked with a chorea ; the intellect recovering its powers as the muscles of locomotion were more and more thrown into the most ridiculous but involuntary gesticulations. He was restored from this, and to perfect health, by the use of

---

* A gentleman residing in a part of the country with which Dr. Conolly is well acquainted, easy in his circumstances, and not unhappy in his family, conceived an aversion to interchanging a word with anybody whatever. He would avoid people whom he saw approaching, or leave the room when they entered it. He generally had his hands clasped before him, and used to deal much in short exclamations, such as "Lord have mercy upon us!" "What a wicked world this is !" and so forth. Yet this man, when circumstances compelled him into conversation, wanted none of the powers, and had lost none of the information requisite for performing his part in it with credit. His aversion to meeting or speaking to people was a mere aggravation of what nervous persons are very subject to : but there appeared also to be in him an inaptitude of the nervous system to be so acted upon by ordinary impressions as to attend to them ; but when the impression was increased, his faculties, and especially his attention, were roused into healthy action, and consequently he was not insane, according to the principles laid down by Dr. Conolly.—See Inquiry concerning the Indications of Insanity, p. 124.—Ed.

tonics, and especially the sulphate of quinine.—
(*Magendie, Journal de Physiologie,* Avr., 1822.)

Other excitements by which the present species is produced, are immoderate exercise, insolation, or long exposure to the direct rays of the
sun, sudden transitions from heat to cold, powerful stimuli applied to the stomach.

In the case related by Sauvages, the disease
appears to have proceeded from a heated imagination exercised upon false views of religion :
and perhaps there is no cause more common or
more operative, especially in timid minds ; and
more particularly still where the conscience is
alarmed by a review of a long catalogue of real
delinquencies, and a dread of eternal reprobation.

Few persons have given a more striking example of this than the Abbé de Rancé when first
touched with remorse for the enormity of his
past life, and before the disturbed state of his
mind had settled into that turn for religious seclusion and mortification which produced the
appalling austerities of La Trappe. "To this
state of frantic despair," says Dom Lancelot in
his letter to La Mère Angélique of Port Royal,
"succeeded a black melancholy. He sent away
all his friends, and shut himself up in his mansion at Veret, where he would not see a crea-
ture. His whole soul, nay, even his bodily wants,
seemed wholly absorbed in a deep and settled
gloom. Shut up in a single room, he even forgot to eat and drink : and when the servant re-
minded him that it was bedtime, he started as
from a deep revery, and seemed unconscious
that it was not still morning. When he was
better, he would often wander in the woods for
the entire day, wholly regardless of the weather.
A faithful servant, who sometimes followed him
by stealth, often watched him standing for hours
together in one place, the snow and the rain
beating on his head ; while he, unconscious of
them, was wholly absorbed in painful recollections. Then, at the fall of a leaf, or the noise
of the deer, he would awake as from a slumber,
and wringing his hands, hasten to bury himself
in a thicker part of the wood ; or else throw
himself prostrate, with his face in the snow, and
groan bitterly."

The same causes operate in the production
of ROVING or RESTLESS MELANCHOLY, forming
the second variety, and exhibiting a modification
which often depends obviously upon a difference
of idiosyncrasy, though the cause is not always
to be explained, and under the operation of which
the patient has a constant desire to change his
pursuit or his residence. And hence, while Albert Durer is entitled to the approbation he has
so long received for his admirable picture of
melancholy, under the guise of a pensive female
leaning on her arm with fixed looks and neglected dress, Shakspeare has equally copied from
nature in his description of the beautiful and interesting Ophelia, who, instead of shutting herself up from the world, and seeking silence and
solitude, is represented as peculiarly busy and
talkative, and unwittingly divulging the fond secret of her distraction to every one she meets,
as well in verse as in prose. Sadness is the
prevailing colour of the mind; but it is often,

as Jaques expresses it, "a most humorous sadness," so blended with sallies of pleasantry and
wit, that is impossible to listen to them without
smiling, notwithstanding the gravity of the occasion. "Humorous they are," says Burton
(and, unhappily for himself, no one knew how to
describe the disease better), "beyond all measure ; sometimes profusely laughing, extraordinarily merry, and then again weeping without a
cause ; groaning, sighing, pensive, and almost
distracted. Multa absurda fingunt et à ratione
aliena (*Frambes.* Consult., lib. i., 17) ; they feign
many absurdities, void of all reason : one sup-
poseth himself to be a dog, cock, bear, horse,
glass, butter. He is a giant, a dwarf, as strong
as a hundred men, a lord, duke, prince. Many
of them are immoveable and fixed in their conceits ; others vary upon every object heard or
seen. If they see a stage-play, they run upon
that for a week after ; if they hear music or see
dancing, they have naught but bagpipes in their
brain ; if they see a combat, they are all for
arms ; if abused, the abuse troubles them long
after. Restless in their thoughts and actions,
continually meditating,—

———'velut ægri somnia, vanæ
Finguntur species ;'———

more like dreamers than men awake, they feign
a company of entire fantastical conceits : they
have most frivolous thoughts, impossible to be
effected ; and sometimes think verily that they
hear and see present before their eyes such phantasms or goblins they fear, suspect, or conceive ;
they still talk with and follow them. 'They
wake,' says Avicenna, 'as others dream.'
Though they do talk with you, and seem to be
very intent and busy, they are only thinking of
a toy ; and still that toy runs in their mind, whatever it be ; that fear, that suspicion, that abuse,
that jealousy, that agony, that vexation, that
cross, that castle in the air, that crochet, that
whimsey, that fiction, that pleasant waking dream.
If it be offensive, especially, they cannot forget
it ; they may not rest or sleep for it ; but still
tormenting themselves, Sisiphi saxum volvunt
sibi suis."

How melancholy a reflection, that the writer
of this spirited description should have drawn
many of its features from himself ; and that the
work from which it is copied, engaged in for the
purpose of diverting his thoughts, and replete
with genius, learning, and the finest humour,
should only have exasperated the disease, and
urged the pitiable patient, as there is too much
reason to fear, to an untimely end ! "He composed his book," says Mr. Granger, "with a
view of relieving his own melancholy ; but it increased it to such a degree that nothing could
make him laugh but going to the bridge-foot, and
hearing the ribaldry of the bargemen, which
rarely failed to throw him into a violent fit of
laughter. Before he was overcome with this
horrid disorder, he, in the intervals of his vapours, was esteemed one of the most facetious
companions in the university."

The THIRD VARIETY, in which the alienation
assumes a morose or mischievous character, is

perhaps the most common form under which the disease makes its appearance. Sometimes the patient is extremely passionate, and will quarrel furiously with every one alike, in whatever tone or manner he is addressed, and expresses himself with great violence of language, occasionally with gross unqualified abuse, but occasionally also in a style of repartee that never was evinced in a sane state. More generally, however, he selects his objects of resentment; which are, for the most part, unaccountably taken from his nearest relations and kindest friends. Against these he harbours the blackest suspicion and jealousy, believing that they are haunting him to take away his money or his life, or to put him to torture. He loads them with every term of the deadliest hatred, or scowls at them with contempt, and denounces them as fools and idiots. Under the distressing influence of this horrid form of the disease, the mother abominates her infant family, and the wife her husband; the most chaste become lascivious; and lips which have hitherto uttered nothing but the precepts and the language of piety, become grossly profane, and are the vehicles of oaths and impudence. The unhappy individuals are, at the same time, not only sensible of what they say or do, but occasionally, sensible of its being wrong, will express their sorrow for it immediately afterward, and say they will not do so again. But the waywardness of the will, and its want of control by the judgment, urge them forward in spite of their desire, and they relapse into the same state almost as soon as they have expressed their regret. Mr. Locke has, with great ability, pointed out the proper distinction between these two faculties of the DESIRE and the WILL, and has exemplified it by the chastisement with which an indulgent father frequently finds himself called upon to visit an offending child, and which he wills to perform; though his desire is in the utmost degree reluctant. The disease before us is pregnant with examples of the same kind, and strikingly shows the correctness with which this great master of his subject analyzed the human mind.

We have already observed that the peculiar turn or modification of the malady depends in general far less upon the immediate and exciting cause, than upon the constitutional temperament, or some operative principle which we cannot always develop. And in proof of this it may be hinted that I have drawn the principal lineaments of the description just laid down from the case of a lady of about sixty years of age, respecting whom I was lately consulted, and whose exciting cause has been, manifestly, suppressed grief for the death of an only son, and separation from a daughter who was the remaining solace of her advancing years, in consequence of her having married a gentleman whose station is in a remote part of the globe. Possessed by nature of a high and commanding spirit, and of a peculiar degree of energy and activity, she effectually succeeded, by a violent internal struggle, in subduing the pangs that at first suffocated her; and has for several years talked of her daughter, and her daughter's children,

for the latter has since become a mother, without emotion. But with the loss of fine feeling for her daughter, she has lost, at the same time, all fine feeling upon other subjects; and her judgment has sunk amid the general wreck. The love of her nearest relations has turned to contempt or hatred; the ardour and animation of her mind, which restrain her from taciturnity and retirement, have rendered her forward and invective; rational expostulation has yielded to sudden and unmeaning fits of violence and blows, and the voice of piety to exclamations that would formerly have shocked her beyond endurance. She, too, is often sensible of her doing wrong, and, in letters of great sobriety and excellence, often complains of her own conduct, and the burden she is become to her friends; but the intervals of sanity are only of a few hours' duration, and with all her calmness, she is sure to relapse.—(Compare with the Report of the Glasgow Asylum for Lunatics, 1821.) For many months she was intrusted in her own house to the control of a professional female attendant, who, with great dexterity, at length succeeded in obtaining a due degree of authority over her without personal restraint; and, under the regimen of perfect quiet and seclusion from the world, she seemed to be in a fair way of recovery; but the mischievous fondness of her nearest relations has since removed this faithful watchwoman, and her senses have again been bartered for her liberty.

The symptoms most afflictive to the relations of the patient in this variety of insanity are the tendency to behold them with indifference or even violent aversion, and to utter exclamations and employ language of the most offensive kind to a serious and a delicate ear; and it is the symptom apparently most unaccountable to those who have not studied the disease with much attention. I have already remarked that, in insanity, the corporeal sensibility is greatly diminished, but it is not more so than the moral sensibility; and as the moral sensibility disappears, all moral restraint disappears also: and for the reason that the insane man has little feeling of cold or hunger, he has also little feeling of decency or religion. In the present variety, the worst passions are in a state of excitement, and the language most freely employed is the language of the passion that predominates; and there being no longer any moral restraint, it is employed in its utmost vehemence and coarseness. And as the fond affections have given way to the irascible, it should seem to follow, of course, that the greater the love or friendship formerly, the greater the hatred at present.

There is one consolation, however, though a small one, that we may reap from this distressing contemplation, and to which the friends of the sufferer should not be indifferent. It is that, with this blunted sensibility of mind, the patient has no pain from a consciousness of his degraded condition. And it is singular to observe, what may also contribute to alleviate the distress of the sympathizing heart, how completely his unconsciousness prevails even after a patient's restoration to health, so that few look back upon what they have undergone with the horror that would be expected; while many, even in the apprehension of a relapse, contemplate it, and turn their eye to the abode of misery where they were lately inmates, without dread.

The FOURTH VARIETY, or SELF-COMPLACENT melancholy, is perhaps less frequent than any of the rest; but it occurs occasionally, and is often accompanied with a high-coloured and ruddy complexion, and other marks of a sanguineous habit: "Such persons," says Burton, "are much inclined to laughter, are witty and merry, conceited in discourse, pleasant, if they be not far gone, and much given to music, dancing, and to be in women's company." Aristotle gives the case of an inhabitant of Abydos, who, labouring under this variety of the disease, would sit for a whole day as if he had been upon a stage, listening to visionary actors; sometimes acting himself, and occasionally clapping his hands and laughing as overjoyed with the performance.—(*Lib. de Reb. mir.*) Such persons have not unfrequently thought themselves called upon to undertake some desperate adventure, and are exquisitely elated with the new and lofty character they are about to embrace.

These stimulant feelings are not unfrequently connected with erroneous ideas of religion, and excite in the mind of the patient a belief that he is supernaturally endowed with the power of working miracles, or undergoing the severest mortifications without injury. The German Psychological Magazine is full of examples of this kind; and, among others, relates the case of a gens-d'armes of Berlin, whose name was Gragert, of a harmless and quiet disposition, but rather of a superstitious turn of mind. From poverty, family misfortunes, and severe military discipline, he brought on a series of sleepless nights, and a mental disquietude that, according to his own report, nothing could dissipate but a perusal of pious books. In reading the Bible, he was struck with the book of Daniel, and so much pleased with it, that it became his favourite study; and from this time the idea of miracles so strongly possessed his imagination, that he began to believe he could perform some miracles himself. He was, persuaded more especially that, if he were to plant an apple-tree with a view of its becoming a cherry-tree, such was his power that it would bear cherries. He was discharged from the king's service and sent to the workhouse, where he conducted himself calmly, orderly, and industriously for two years, never doing any thing that betrayed insanity; at which time Dr. Pike examined him, that he might be discharged and sent to his family. He answered every question correctly, except when the subject concerned miracles: in regard to which he retained his old notions; adding, however, at the same time, that if he found, upon trial, after he was at home, that the event did not correspond with his expectation, he would readily relinquish the thought, and believe he had been mistaken; and confessed that he had already removed one error in his mind in this way; for there was an old woman whom he had at

one time considered as a witch, but whom he afterward discovered, upon trial, to be no such thing.

Upon the medical treatment of diseases of this kind, we shall not have to say much; but as the plan chiefly advisable for the present species is equally advisable for the ensuing, it will be most expedient to reserve the discussion of it till the latter has been described in its order.

SPECIES II.
ECPHRONIA MANIA.
MADNESS.

THE DISCREPANCE BETWEEN THE PERCEPTION AND THE JUDGMENT GENERAL; GREAT EXCITEMENT OF THE MENTAL, SOMETIMES OF THE CORPOREAL POWERS.

THIS species appears under almost infinite varieties of character, of which, however, it may be sufficient to mark the following, modified for the most part by the predisposing causes that we have already noticed, as modifying the preceding species:—

α Ferox.	Furious and violent madness.
β Exultans.	Gay and elevated madness.
γ Despondens.	Gloomy, despondent madness.
δ Demens.	Chaotic madness.

The exciting causes, like the predisposing, are chiefly those already enumerated under ecphronia melancholia: as sudden and violent mental emotion; bad passions indulged habitually; false views of religion, especially the dread of reprobation and eternal punishment; sudden reverse of fortune, whether from bad to good, or from good to bad; preying anxiety, or lurking discontent; deep protracted study, unrelieved from week to week by an interchange of exercise or society, and breaking in upon the hours of sleep; unkindly childbed; a suppression of various periodical evacuations; and sometimes even a virtuous restraint of sexual orgasm in a vigorous constitution, without taking purgative or other means to reduce the irritative entony.

Of these one of the most frequent causes is that of childbed, and recovery from childbed, though it is not always easy to develop the immediate mode by which this change in the constitution acts upon the brain; for it has occurred not only where there has been some organic affection from puerperal fever, a sudden cessation of the lochia, or a sudden relinquishment of nursing, but where the recovery has been unattended with a single unfavourable symptom, and the mother has ardently persevered in the office of a nurse. It shows us, however, very sufficiently, how strong is the chain of sympathy between the brain and many remote organs of the body, and especially those subservient to the function of generation.

M. Esquirol, not long ago, communicated a paper to the Société de Médecine upon this important subject, enriched with the results of the Hospital de la Salpêtrière, for the years 1811, 12, 13, and 14. During these four years eleven hundred and nineteen women were admitted, labouring under mental derangement: of whom ninety-two (nearly an eleventh part of the whole) had become deranged after, delivery, during or immediately-subsequent to the period of suckling. In the higher ranks of society, the proportion of puerperal maniacs he calculates to be not less than a seventh of· the whole. Of the above 92 cases, 16 occurred from the first to the fourth day after delivery; 21 from the fifth to the fifteenth; 17 from the sixteenth to the sixtieth day; 19 from the sixtieth to the twelfth month of suckling: and in 19 cases it appeared after voluntary or forced weaning.*

· Of the above 92 cases, 8 were-idiotic, 35 melancholic, and 49 maniacal. The respective ages were as follows : 22 from 20 to 25 years; 41 from 25 to 30 years; and 12 above 30. Fifty-six out of the ninety-two were entirely cured, and thirty-eight of these within the first six months. Fright was the most frequent cause. —(Quart. Journ. of· For. Medicine, No. i., p. 98.)†

I have said that a virtuously restrained orgasm, in a full habit, and where no steps have been taken to reduce the entonic vigour, has occasionally induced mania. There is a curious instance of the powerful effect of such a state related by Kemnesius in his history of the Council of Trent, which, though it did not terminate in madness, proved quite as fatal. In the year 1419, Rossa, nephew to the King of Portugal, and archbishop elect of Lisbon, was taken seriously ill at Florence. His physicians told him that his disease proceeded from an excessive irritation of the genital·organs, and that he would certainly die unless he committed fornication or married. With a courage worthy of a happier issue, he resolved on death, and met it without breaking his vow of celibacy.—(Kemnes. Concil. Trident.; part iii.; De Cœlibatû Sacerdotum.)

The following instance, however, will prove that mania itself is sometimes the consequence of the same firmness of mind. A clergyman of exemplary character, and one of the most distinguished preachers I have the pleasure of being acquainted with, was, many years ago, very unexpectedly attacked with a paroxysm of mania, the cause of which it seemed impossible to unfold. He recovered in about six months, and returned to a regular and punctilious discharge of clerical duty. He is a man of exquisite taste, warm imagination, exalted and highly cultivated

* In the New-York Med. Journal, vol. i., p. 280, Dr. McDonald, physician to the Bloomingdale Asylum for the insane, has published some observations on puerperal mania, and concludes, " That young women are much more obnoxious to this malady than those more advanced, and that the susceptibility of females to it diminishes in about the same ratio that their years increase ; that wo. men are more liable to this disease at the first than at subsequent parturitions ; that an hereditary predisposition to insanity exists in less than one sixth of the cases; that moral causes are co-operative only ; that puerperal insanity is one of the most curable forms of mental disorder."—D.

† There is a greater predisposition to madness, says Dr. Rush, between twenty-five and fifty, than at any of the previous or subsequent years of human life.—D.

mind. With these qualifications, in less than a year after his recovery, he married his maid-servant, and the world imagined he was gone or going out of his senses a second time. A confidential statement of his situation soon proved to myself that nothing could be more prudent or praiseworthy than the step he has thus taken, and which had excited so much astonishment among his friends. He was fully convinced, he said, though he had never communicated it to any one, that the cause of his unfortunate malady was a genital irritation, exciting to a constant desire of matrimony, which he was not in a situation to comply with, and which compelled him to exercise from day to day a severe restraint upon his feelings. On being fully restored to health, he found the same morbid propensity beginning to return. I felt, said he, it would again drive me mad if I did not relieve it, and my principles forbade me to think for a moment of relieving it immorally. To what respectable family could I now offer myself, having so lately been discharged from private confinement ? The servant who lived with me was a very excellent young woman; her disposition was amiable, her mind well capable of cultivation, and her form and manners by no means unpleasing ; and hence, after mature deliberation, I determined upon marrying her, if she herself would venture upon so perilous a risk. He married her accordingly ;—has ever since, for upwards of twenty years, enjoyed an almost uninterrupted share of health, and has been more than ordinarily happy in his family. Other examples of a like kind are to be found in Paullini (Cent; iii , obs. 14), Martini (Osservazioni, ch. ii., 10), and Vogel (Beobachtungen, p. 9): but it is unnecessary to copy them. And hence, castration . has been often advised and submitted to, and occasionally with success.

It is from a like sympathy of action between the brain· and other parts of the ·body that we meet with instances of the one or the other species of disease before us, produced occasionally, and perhaps in habits of great sensibility, by suppressed irritations of much smaller moment ; as cutaneous diseases,* a suppressed hemorrhoidal flux (Santacruz, De Melancholia, p. 29 ; Lentilius, Miscell., i., p. 36), or an ulcer of long standing suddenly dried up.—(Forestus, lib. x., obs. 24.)

Furious· mania, constituting the first variety, sometimes makes it attack very abruptly, and commences with the patient's being sensible of some indescribable movement in his head, which excites him to loud and sudden shrieks, at the same time that he runs up and down the room, and mutters something to himself that is altogether unintelligible : though the symptoms, even in this abrupt and violent attack, admit of much diversity.

More commonly, however, the disease is the work of time ; and its growth is thus admirably described by Dr. Monro in his reply to Dr. Battie :—" High spirits, as they are generally term-

* Act. Nat. Cur., vol. viii., obs. 28. Descottes, Journ. de Méd., tom. lxvi. Petit, Œuvres posthumes, tom. iii.

ed, are the first symptoms of this kind of disorder. These excite a man to take a larger quantity of wine than usual, and the person thus afflicted, from being abstemious, reserved, and modest, shall become quite the contrary, drink freely, talk boldly, obscenely, swear, sit up till midnight; sleep little, rise suddenly from bed, go out a hunting, return again immediately, set all his servants to work, and employ five times the number that is necessary. In short, every thing he says or does betrays the most violent agitation of mind, which it is not in his own power to correct. And yet, in the midst of all this hurry, he will not misplace one word, or give the least reason for anyone to think he imagines things to exist that really do not, or that they appear to him different from what they do to other people. They who but seldom see him admire his vivacity, are pleased with his sallies of wit and the sagacity of his remarks; nay, his own family are with difficulty persuaded to take proper care of him, till it becomes absolutely necessary from the apparent ruin of his health and fortune."

This picture is drawn from a rank of life something above that of mediocrity, but its general features of ebullient spirits, and hurry and bustle, and "much ado about nothing," will apply to every rank. Such a person, says Sir A. Crichton, in allusion to the present description, cannot be said as yet to be delirious, but that event soon follows, and he has then the symptoms common to the disease, symptoms which only differ from a difference in the train of thoughts which are represented in his mind. He begins to rave, and talk wildly and incoherently; swears as if in the most violent rage, and then immediately afterward bursts into fits of laughter; talks obscenely; directs offensive and contemptuous language against his relations and those around him; spits at them; destroys every thing that comes in his way; emits loud and discordant screams; and continues this conduct till he is quite exhausted. The state of rest which follows is generally short and sleepless; the patient is obstinate; he will not speak a word, and clinches his teeth if any thing be offered him to swallow; or else cunningly pretends to drink a little, but immediately squirts it out on the person who offers it. Instantly he again breaks out into all the wild and extravagant language and actions he committed before. If kept in strict coercion, he has often so much command over himself as to behave mildly and modestly; and were it not for the general expression of his countenance, and the peculiar glistening appearance and rapid movement of his eyes, he might impose on many of the by-standers, and make them imagine that the phrensy was over. The length of the paroxysm and of the interval varies greatly in different individuals.* But, generally speaking, the more violent the fit the sooner it ceases, from exhaustion; and hence sometimes it ceases in a day or two, and sometimes runs on to a month or

even more; returning at the distance of a few weeks, or at certain periods of the year.

In the SECOND VARIETY, or ELEVATED MADNESS, the passions, and especially the irascible ones, are less busy, and the imagination is chiefly predominant, and at work without ceasing. It is here we most frequently trace something of the ruling pursuit of their former lives, so that the covetous man is still conversant about purchasing lands and tenements, and amuses himself with perpetually augmenting his possessions; while the devotional character is for ever engaged in a routine of prayers, fastings, and ceremonies, visions and revelations, and fancies himself to be inspired and lifted into heaven.* The phantoms are all of a pleasurable kind, and mostly such as afford the deluded sufferer a vast opinion of his own rank or talents. Donatus gives a case of a lady at Mantua, who conceited she was married to a king, and would kneel down and affect to converse with him as if he were present with her attendants; and if she found by chance a piece of glass in the street, she would hug it as a jewel sent her from her royal lord and husband.—(De Hist. Med. Mirab., lib. ii., cap. i.) He relates another case, from Seneca, of Senecio, a madman of considerable wealth, who thought himself and every thing about him great; that he had a great wife, and great horses, and could not endure little things of any kind; so that he would be served with great pots to drink out of; great hosen, and great shoes bigger than his feet : "Like her," says Burton, "in Trallian, that supposed she could shake all the world with her finger, and was afraid to clinch her hand lest she should crush the world to pieces like an apple."— (Anat. of Melancholy, part i., sect. 3.)

Yet even here the train of thoughts or ideas which occupy the mind of the maniac, in many instances throw no light whatever on the nature or origin of the complaint; and we can still less avail ourselves of them than in various cases of melancholy.

This is particularly observable in the THIRD VARIETY, or DESPONDENT MADNESS; for though this modification of the disease may occasionally be produced by suspicion, terror, or a guilty conscience, it is far more frequently the result of a melancholic idiosyncrasy, or a debilitated state of the constitution at the time of the attack, in consequence of which the sensorial fluid is secreted* perhaps even less freely, instead of more so, than in a condition of health; so that the patient sinks by degrees into a state of insensibility; unless he should be roused with false courage, and find means to put an end to his existence before this period arrives.

In DEMENTIA, or CHAOTIC MADNESS, this state of sensorial exhaustion and consequent insensibility are still more obvious, though there is, perhaps, less constitutional tendency to the de-

---

* In some instances, the person labouring under this variety of elevated madness has imagined himself to be the Messiah.—D.

† As this expression is quite an improbable hypothesis, it would be better to exchange it for "sensorial power is generated."—ED.

* The paroxysm is accurately and powerfully described by Spenser, Fairie Queen, b. ii., cant. iv., xv.

pressing passions: The judgment here is more diseased and weakened than in any other form, and none of the kindred faculties assuming a paramount power, there is a general anarchy and confusion in the ideas that flit over the sensory, without connexion or association of any kind. And hence Pinel has admirably characterized it as consisting in a " rapid succession or uninterrupted alternation of insulated ideas and evanescent and unconnected emotions ; continually repeated acts of extravagance ; complete forgetfulness of every previous state ; diminished sensibility to external impressions : abolition of the faculty of judgment ; perpetual activity without object or design, or any internal sense of its taking place."—(*De l'Aliénation Mentale,* ch. iii., iii., § 176.)

These maniacs are often ungovernable except by means of coercion ; but they are more easily restrained than those who are in a state of phrensy. They are intractable, and neither listen to entreaty or to menaces. Fear of corporeal punishment, however, makes them obey. They willingly avoid the light, burying themselves under the bedclothes, or under the straw of their cells. They are totally regardless of decency and cleanliness, and, from some strange motive, are often found smearing themselves over with their excrement. For the most part, they have little appetite, and refuse the food offered them ; yet a sense of hunger seems sometimes to return with great keenness, when they will greedily devour their feces. Of the nature of the ideas that take place in the sensory, and are expressed by an unintelligible mutterin, we know nothing further than that, from the screams and howlings with which their jargon is accompanied, there can be no doubt that they are often excited by painful sensations of body or mind.

It is happy for those who suffer under this as well as under the preceding form, that they rarely sustain a long conflict ; the exhaustion of sensorial power by repeated paroxysms soon leading to a total torpitude, and consequently a death of the sensorial organ ;* though there are instances in which a paroxysm of more violence than usual has produced a favourable change, and suddenly restored the patient to his senses.

In gloomy madness, in which there is often a chronic affection of some of the abdominal organs co-operating with a diseased condition of the brain, we find least to justify hope ; the patients generally become weakened by fresh paroxysms, and often sink into a state of idiotism.

The first variety, on the contrary, if the constitution have not been seriously broken down by intemperance, or the patient be not suddenly

carried off by the violence of the attack on its commencement, will often work its own cure by its own ardour ; and will gradually soften into a more sober state from simple mental fatigue. While in the milder and more pleasurable modification of the second variety, in which the production of sensorial power is upon the whole perhaps less than in a condition of sanity (since, though the stimulus of the disease may tend to increase it a little, the total privation which the patient enjoys of all the vexations, and anxieties, and wearing vicissitudes of real life, reduce it to a moderated and even tenour it could not otherwise possess), nothing is more common than for maniacs to continue to a very advanced age. I am at this moment interested in the case of a clergyman who has reached his ninety-sixth year, and has been in a state of quiet insanity for more than half a century.

For the most part, those are most easily as well as most rapidly cured, whose insanity, of whatever kind it be, has been produced by accidental causes, as intoxication, sudden transition from cold to heat, retention of habitual discharges, or a revulsion by a transfer of morbid action from other organs. And hence the comparative facility with which a cure is effected in insanity after childbirth. While, on the contrary, those are least likely to obtain a permanent recovery who possess an hereditary taint ; the disease may indeed leave them for a time, but, the predisposition remaining, they commonly fall victims to fresh attacks after intervals of a year or two, or even of a few months.

"Mania and melancholy," says Dr. Greding, writing while he was physician to the workhouse at Waldheim, "have continued half a year with some, and remained forty years and upward with others, among whom one patient only in this workhouse attained the age of eighty-five."—(*Vermischte Schriften,* ut suprà, &c.)

The chance of recovery is considerably greater upon the first than upon any subsequent attack, and especially if the disease have not exceeded three months' duration when the patient is first put under medical treatment. If it have at this time lasted a twelvemonth, the prospect of success is diminished by half ; if two years, not above a fourth part as many recover ; and if more than two years, the expectation is small, though, where the second year is not much exceeded, a cure is by no means to be despaired of.*

The treatment of ecphronia has generally been discussed under the two heads of ᴍᴇᴅɪᴄᴀʟ and ᴍᴏʀᴀʟ. Both have undergone a very great improvement within the last twenty or thirty years : the first by being considerably simplified ; the second, by being more thoroughly studied and raised to a higher degree of importance.†

---

* " Death of the sensorial organ" seems by no means an eligible expression, as it may be understood to signify that the brain, in the case here described, dies first, and the rest of the system perishes afterward, in consequence of the death of the sensorial organ. In the examples referred to, the violence of the paroxysms may be said to derange the functions of the whole nervous system, disturb all the operations of the animal economy, and thus bring on debility, various forms of disease, and speedy dissolution.—Eᴅ.

* The instructive volume of Dr. Rush, " On the Diseases of the Mind," mentions many cases of most of the prevalent forms of mania. Knapp's Life of the late Thomas Eddy contains the interesting particulars of the case of Count Renauld St. Jean d'Angély, from the pen of Mr. Colden. This distinguished French orator died of mania.—D.

† When a medical practitioner is consulted re-

Nothing can be more injudicious than the ordinary routine of MEDICAL TREATMENT, which, till within a few years, was equally employed in almost all the larger lunatic establishments in our own country and on the continent, especially at Bethlem, the Hospice d'Humanité, and the Hôtel Dieu ; and which consisted in a course of venesections, emetics, and purgatives, administered in every case indiscriminately, and often, indeed, without even the personal inspection of the consulting physician or other superintending medical officer ; and if, to these means of cure, we add the occasional use of bathing in various forms and various temperatures, we shall very nearly have exhausted the merely medical process that till of late was ordinarily had recourse to.

Upon the cruel and disgusting scenes which, from the late parliamentary inquiry and the report of the committee which followed, are well known to have occurred not long ago in the largest and most celebrated receptacle of lunatics in this metropolis, it is now unnecessary to dwell. But from the official communication of M. Esquirol to the French government concerning the residences for lunatics throughout France, it is perfectly clear that we have not transgressed in a greater degree than our neighbours. Filth, straw, and dirty rags, were all

specting a person suspected to be insane, his whole duty, as Dr. Conolly explains, resolves itself into two parts :—1. To determine whether the individual in question be of sound mind. 2. To give an opinion respecting the treatment required, and especially concerning the necessity of restraint, and *the degree and nature of such restraint.*

The aid of medicine is required in most cases of disturbed mind ; personal restraint may be required in many ; but the degrees of it which are required in different cases vary, as the cases themselves vary, from the slightest to the most complete ; and complete restraint is very rarely required. Whether the person ought to be confined at all will rest, as Dr. Conolly very properly insists, upon the consideration, whether the degree or character of the mental disturbance is such as to make the patient dangerous to himself or others, either as regards person or property.—(See Dr. Conolly's Inquiry concerning the Indications of Insanity, pp. 365, 386, &c.) This talented writer adverts to the frequency of cases in which patients become more and more susceptible of all impressions, and more and more irritable, in consequence of habitual indulgence in diet which disagrees with them. Certain articles of food, or of drink, which produce a temporary disturbance of the whole system, are taken so frequently, that the body and mind are never left quite free from their effects. During the early stage of such cases, restraint may be productive of a complete cure ; and even when insanity has become declared, but has not long existed, it will recede and disappear, if the habits which are destroying the mind are resolutely broken. The cure depends partly upon physical, and partly upon moral treatment ; and Dr. Conolly gives it as his opinion, that both may often be better administered out of an asylum than in it. Long-continued superintendence and occasioual restraint are necessary ; but seclusion, confinement among lunatics, deprivation of property, long separation from friends, are quite uncalled for and improper.—Op. cit., p. 393.—ED.

these miserable beings possessed in many depôts to mitigate the coldness of the air, and the dampness of their paved, crammed, and suffocating cells. And in some instances they had neither straw nor rags, and were perfectly naked, except from a layer of dirt. " J'ai vu," says M. Esquirol, with just indignation, " un malheureux imbécile, tout nu et sans paille, couché sur le pavé. Exprimant mon étonnement d'un pareil abandon, le concierge me répondit que l'administration ne lui passait, pour chaque individu, qu'une botte de paille tous les quinze jours. Je fis remarquer à ce barbare que le chien qui veillait à la porte des aliénés étoit logé plus sainement, et qu'il avoit de la paille fraîche et en abondance. Cette remarque me valut un sourire de pitié. Et j'étois dans une des grandes villes de France."—(*Des Etablissemens des Aliénés en France, et des Moyens d'ameliorer le Sort de ces Infortunés,* Paris, 1819.) It is satisfactory, however, to know, that a more judicious and discriminative practice has in all these asylums been introduced since the above period, and that it has been followed by an abundant success.*

Admitting the proximate cause of insanity to be in most cases an increased action of the vessels secreting the nervous fluid [or supplying with blood the organs by which the sensorial power is produced], venesection and cathartics, and a general reducent regimen, seem indicated as an ordinary means of relief ; and are unquestionably called for when the pulse is full and strong, and the temperament is sanguineous : and the success which has so frequently accompanied this practice, stamps it with the highest sanction it can receive. But there is great reason to believe, from even where the demand for bloodletting is unequivocal, it has been carried to a mischievous extent, and ruined its own benefit. Thus Plater made a point of repeating it once a week, and sometimes had recourse to it for seventy weeks in succession.—(*Observ.,* lib. i., p. 86.)

Much caution, however, is necessary even in the first trial ; for as a sound intellect depends apparently upon a certain degree of excitement in the sensorial vessels, and a certain quantity of the fluid secreted [or intellectual power generated], derangement may take place also,

---

* In Dr. Conolly's Inquiry into the Indications of Insanity, many judicious reflections will be found on the disadvantages of the common system of lunatic asylums. Every humane mind will also incline to his opinion, that it is not every form of mental derangement that justifies confinement in such establishments. A man may fancy his legs to be butter, and take all due care of them; without injury to himself, his family, his property, or the property and persons of others, and no one can have a right to interfere with him.—(Op. cit., p. 305.) He may, on seeing his doctor, address him as if he were Jesus Christ ; or he may fancy that a princess is in love with him, and do many extravagant things in consequence of the delusion ; yet his conduct will not justify restraint, unless his mental disorder lead him to neglect his affairs and his family, or to inflict injury either on others or on himself.—Op. cit., p. 384.—ED.

as we have already observed, from diminished instead of from increased action, and diminished instead of increased secretion or production. And such we have reason to believe is the cause of delirium whenever it occurs in profuse hemorrhage and in typhus fevers : in all such instances, a reducent plan must necessarily tend to augment instead of to carry off the disease. And hence, the patient's general habit and temperament, the nature of the exciting cause, the probability of visceral congestion, the violence or mildness of the maniacal symptoms, the progress they have made, and the length of time he has laboured under them, are all to be taken into consideration before we can determine upon the expediency of bleeding even at first. And if, when we have decided upon its propriety, no benefit be produced from a second or a third repetition, we have no encouragement to proceed further, and should withhold the lancet altogether.

To a series of purgative medicines there is less objection, provided they are not rendered too violent. The abdominal viscera, it has already appeared, form in many instances an important link in the morbid chain of action, and are sometimes the primary cause of the disease : and it is hence of great moment that they should be effectually cleared of any matter that may irritate or clog them up. But beyond this, by keeping up such an increased action in the abdominal region as the organs may bear without debility, we may diminish or change the morbid action in the head by remote sympathy, or entirely withdraw it by a revulsion. A spontaneous diarrhœa has been known in various cases to carry off the disease as by a charm : and the use of this class of medicines is the more necessary, as the bowels of maniacal patients are apt to be extremely costive. If the black hellebore of the ancients, which appears to have been a different plant from that of the modern dispensatories, were ever entitled to half the antimaniacal virtues ascribed to it, it was most probably upon the obvious ground of its being a purgative attenuant and deobstruent.

Dr. Dubuisson has lately revived the use of the modern black hellebore in various species of mental alienation, as chronic mania, melancholy, and hypochondriacism : in all which he speaks of its effects, after an extensive trial, as highly successful. He has given it also in every form, as that of powder, decoction, watery extract, and tincture ; but prefers the extract as least irritating.—(*Des Vesanies, ou Maladies Mentales*, Paris, 1816.) His opinion, however, is not supported by the result of general practice, and appears to be by far too sweeping and indiscriminate. Spleissius, nevertheless, affirms that in his hands, when given freely, it proved sedative and produced sleep.—(*Annotat. in Zapat. Mirabil.*, p. 136.)

Upon no other description of medicines can we place any rational dependance. Emetics, narcotics, and other sedatives and antispasmodics, have been tried for ages in every form and in every proportion ; sometimes alone, and sometimes in conjunction with blisters and the warm or cold bath. There are instances in which they have all appeared to produce some benefit ; but the far greater number, in which they have failed, prevents us from placing any reliance upon them.

Of the narcotics, the chief that have been had recourse to are opium, aconite, belladonna, and the stramonium. Far more mischief than good seems to have followed from the use of all of them, with the exception of the first, which would probably be found a remedy of high value if we could duly discriminate the proper states or modifications of the disease for its use. Dr. Cullen's experience of it in mania he admits to be small, but he has correctly estimated its general effects in telling us that, in some cases, he found it useful in moderating the violence of the disease, but that in others he found it manifestly hurtful. A monographist upon this malady could not, perhaps, be engaged more usefully, than in turning his attention to the peculiarities which produce this difference. On the continent, it has also been given sometimes alone ; but, more usually, in conjunction with nitre or camphire, or both ; but in all these forms, also, with variable success. —(*Fribourg, Coll. Soc. Med. Hafn.*, ii., p. 176.)

Upon what ground St. John's wort was ever advanced to the rank of a powerful sedative I know not ; but in this class it at one time took the lead, and held it for ages. Its antispasmodic powers were regarded of so high a character as equally to put to flight hysterics, hypochondriacism, and madness of every kind, and especially that which was formerly described under the name of dæmonomania (*Abrah. Mayer, Archiv. der Practischen Arzneykunde*), whence, indeed, its technical name of *hypericum*, or fuga dæmonum, under which it was also celebrated. It occupied a place in a late edition of the Pharmacopœia of the London College, and was at one time noticed as an antispasmodic even by Dr. Cullen, who rejected it, however, most deservedly, in his maturer courses of lectures. Its only sensible qualities are those of a slight resinous bitter, not worth the trouble of extracting.

Camphire is a sedative far better entitled to attention, and appears to have been tried with more extensive success than any other medicine of the same tribe. It has been given alone, and in union with other sedatives, chiefly with opium, nitre, and the mineral acids, none of which, however, seem to have improved its powers. Berger, Fischer, and Herz, speak favourably of its effects abroad ; and, in our own country, it has had equal commendations from physicians of distinguished talents. Dr. Mead thought highly of it ; Sir Clifton Wintringham tells us that he found it, given to the amount of half a drachm in the evening, diminish the phrensy, procure sleep, and produce perspiration. Unfortunately, however, here, as in the case of opium, we have so many proofs of its utter inefficacy, as to render us at present incapable of placing any dependance upon it in any quantity or with any auxiliary. Dr. Cullen had a patient who began with five grains for the night's dose, and advanced it gradually to thirty, without any benefit, though without any increase of the pulse. At this time it was carried by accident to forty grains, which produced syncope, and nearly proved fatal. The patient, however, recovered from the accidental symptoms, but unhappily no impression was made on the constitutional disease.—(*Mat. Med.*, vol. ii., p.294.)

The warm and cold bath have also had their votaries, but no certain benefit appears to have been derived from either. The last may be useful as a tonic in a . state of convalescence, but has rarely produced real benefit during the progress of the disease. Weber, however, thought it useful, and published several cases to this effect.—(*Obs. Med.*, fascic. i., p. 26; see also, *Act. Med. Berol.*, dec. i., vol. vii., p̄. 61.)

From an idea that the disease consists in an undue determination to the head, or an undue excitement of the vessels supplying the organs of sensorial power, Wendt (*Nachricht, Von dem Klinischen Institut. zu Erlangen*, 1783, 8vo.) surrounded the head with cataplasms of pounded ice in the form of a nightcap ; and Daniel, with a still more ingenious spirit of adventure, applied cataplasms of the same kind to the head, while the body, with a view of encouraging a revulsion more effectually, was plunged into a warm bath. The process will be found described in his Beyträge zur Medicinischen Gelehrsamkeit, published in quarto at Halle in 1749. And I mention the fact as an act of justice to the author, since the same process has of late years been revived in France and in our own country as a new discovery. Daniel thought it highly beneficial ; and by its recent revivers it was at one time held up as a specific ; but whatever success may, in a few rare instances, have attended it, the practice has not been able to work itself into public favour ; and a sober attention to its effects does not seem to justify its further continuance. M. Pinel was at one time favourable to an employment of jets of cold water directed upon the head, while the body was immersed in tepid water ; but his successor, M. Esquirol, is decidedly of opinion that it is injurious ; and in many cases has induced disorganization of the cerebrum, and rendered the madness incurable.*

After all, we have chiefly to depend on MORAL TREATMENT. Firmness on the part of the attendant, with conciliatory manners, has done wonders ; but a sense of authority must be maintained, though occasional severity should be necessary for this purpose : yet it will rarely be needful to exceed the coercion of the strait waistcoat. It is needless to add, that the diet should be of the simplest kind, that every thing which can tend to produce excitement should

be prohibited, and that, in public institutions, the patients should be divided into proper classes. Amusements of every kind that may engage the attention and encourage exercise in the open air, without rousing the passions or producing fatigue, should be promoted by every contrivance that can be thought of. And if the turn or previous occupation of the patient point to any particular pursuit, and especially to handicraft trades, and those that employ the mind without exhausting it, as that of sawing, gardening, bookbinding, or watchmaking, he should be enabled to pursue it according to his own desire. The desire itself is a favourable symptom, and has often led to the most beneficial results.

Judicious conversation and cheering advice are also of great importance ; and regular daily attendance on religious services in the bosom of a private family, or with a few patients of a like standard in a public institution, may be allowed, where the disease has assumed a convalescent shape, and the service is performed soberly and dispassionately.—(*Report of the Glasgow Asylum for Lunatics*, 1820.) This will at first, perhaps, be only of use as promoting a habit of moral order and quietism ; but every good man will indulge the hope, that it may afterward introduce into the mind the higher blessing of spiritual peace and consolation. Yet the attempt must not be begun too soon, and in no case till the patient has acquired not only a spirit of subordination, but of tranquillity. Before this period, nothing can be so absurd as to attempt devotional instruction of any kind ; for the subject of religion can only be addressed to the reason, or to the passions : the former of which does not exist in a state to be influenced ; and the latter of which, if they could be influenced at all, would only add to the excitement and increase the disease. The clear duty of the priest and of the physician is in this case one and the same : it is to bring the mind home to the world around it ; to draw it down and fix it upon things of time and sense, instead of rousing it to things invisible and eternal ; to enable it to behold God in the materialities of his works, instead of urging it to a contemplation of him in the spiritualities of his word. To instigate to an abstract and elevated communion with his Creator a madman, who is incapable of holding an intercourse upon ordinary topics with his fellow-creature, is to cure a frozen limb by pouring boiling water upon it, or to teach the Optics of Newton in a nursery.

In many cases, the cure mainly depends upon withdrawing the patient's mind as much as possible from every former scene and every former companion ; in setting before him a new world, and giving an entire change to the current of

---

* The treatment of mental disorder must be determined in a great measure by the cause of the affection. That cause will probably be found to be " one of those producing temporary inequalities of mind, but the operation of which has, in the case of the insane person, more deeply affected the understanding. Some stimulus may have been withdrawn, or some emotion may have acted too much as a stimulus. Disease, or age, may have produced disturbance or debility. If

the undue exercise or the too great neglect of any one faculty, as of the attention, the memory, or the imagination, has brought on the malady, the object must be to excite or to sooth, to rouse or to restrain such faculty ; or if the irregularity seems dependant on some bodily inaptness or disorder, to this, of course, attention must be immediately given."—See Dr. Conolly's *Inquiry concerning the Indications of Insanity*, p. 388.—ED.

his recollections and ideas. There are particular cases, however, and perhaps particular periods of the disease, if we could accurately hit upon them, in which the sudden admission of a well-known friend or relation, and a sudden recall of the mind to its former images and habits, tend to produce a most salutary excitement, and disperse the maniacal cloud like a dream. Dr. Gooch has given an interesting illustration of this remark in the case of a lady, twenty-eight years of age, of a good constitution but susceptible mind, who fell into a state of melancholy, in the ordinary sense of the term, a few months after a second childbirth, and at length became furious. "She was now," says he, "put under the care of an experienced attendant, separated entirely from her husband, children, and friends; placed in a neat cottage surrounded by agreeable country (it was the finest season of the year), and visited regularly by her physician. For several weeks she manifested no improvement; sometimes she was occupied with one notion, sometimes with another; but they were always of the most gloomy description. At length it became her firm belief that she was to be executed for her crimes in the most public and disgraceful way; every noise she heard was that of the workmen erecting the scaffold; every carriage, the officers of justice assembling at the execution. But what affected her most deeply was, that her infamy had occasioned the disgrace and death of her children and husband, and that his spirit haunted her. As soon as the evening closed, she would station herself at a window at the back of the cottage, and fix her eyes on a white post that could be seen through the dusk; this was the ghost of her husband; day and night he was whistling in her ears. Several weeks passed in this way. The daily reports varied, but announced nothing happy. At length her husband became impatient, and begged to have an interview with her, thinking that the best way to convince her he was not dead was to show himself. This was objected to. He was told the general fact, that patients are more likely to recover when completely separated from their friends; and that if she saw him, she would say it was not himself but his ghost. But the husband was obstinate, and an interview was consented to. When he arrived at the cottage he was told that she had had a tolerable night, was rather more tranquil, but that there was no abatement of her gloomy notions. 'As soon as I entered the drawing-room, where she usually spent the day' (I copy his own statement, which I have now before me, and which he wrote down at the time of the occurrence), 'she ran into a corner, hid her face in a handkerchief, then turned round, looked me in the face, one moment appearing delighted at the thought that I was alive, but immediately afterward assuming a hideous expression of countenance, and screaming out that I was dead, and come to haunt her. This was exactly what Dr. —— had anticipated, and for some minutes I thought all was lost. Finding that persuasions and argument only irritated and confirmed her in her belief, I desisted, and

tried to draw off her attention to other subjects. It was some time since she had either seen me or her children: I put her arm under mine, took her into the garden, and began to relate what had occurred to me and them since we parted. This excited her attention; she soon became interested; and I entered with the utmost minuteness and circumstantiality into the affairs of the nursery, her home, and her friends. I now felt that I was gaining ground, and when I thought I had complete possession of her mind, I ventured to ask her, in a joking manner, whether I was not very communicative for a ghost. She laughed. I immediately drew her from the subject, and again engaged her attention with her children and friends. The plan succeeded beyond my hope: I dined, spent the evening with her, and left her at night perfectly herself again.' He went the next morning in a state of intense anxiety to know whether his success had been permanent; but her appearance at the window with a cheerful countenance soon relieved his apprehensions. While he was there, Dr —— came in. He went up stairs without knowing the effect of the interview, and came down, saying, 'It looks like magic!' With the view of confirming her recovery, she was ordered to the seaside to bathe. As soon as the day of her departure was fixed she began to droop again, the evening before it she was very low, and on the morning of her setting off was as bad as ever. This state continued for several weeks, in spite of sea-air and bathing; and ceased as suddenly as it had done before, apparently in consequence of interviews with friends, calculated to remove the apprehensions by which her mind was haunted. She has since then continued perfectly well, and has had another child, without the slightest threatening of her former malady."—(*Med. Trans.*, vol. vi.)*

---

* On the medical treatment of mania we would remark, that whether the results of American practice be more or less favourable than those abroad, yet that neither in our public nor private institutions have those afflicted with insanity ever experienced such harsh and injurious treatment as the late parliamentary reports have brought to light. The moral treatment of the insane was adopted at the Bloomingdale Asylum about twenty years since, and was warmly advocated by the late Thos. Eddy (See his Hints and Life, by S. L. Knapp, New-York, 1834); and if philanthropists have relied more upon it than on medical treatment, we have cause to be gratified with the benefits they have conferred on the cause of humanity. Perhaps a more active mode of medical practice is generally pursued by American physicians in the acute forms of insanity than is recommended in the text; and this would seem to be justified by the results. The following remarks, however, deserve attention. Dr. Francis observes,

"There is another circumstance I can hardly allow to be passed over on this occasion without a remark, and which, I think, has been a concurring cause of the too hasty and too general adoption of moral management, as of itself alone the essential means of cure of maniacal subjects. The delirium of inebriety, and the more advanced forms of diseased action denominated *delirium tremens*, have inadvertently been confounded with *idiopathic mania*; and inasmuch as the right use of

This was a bold venture, and the physician must be of a temper more than ordinarily sanguine who would predict a like success upon every similar attempt. Yet we have already had occasion to observe, that puerperal insanity is more easily recovered from than most other forms of the disease.*

---

reason is for the most part, in those cases, restored by mere abstraction from noxious potation, which is effectually secured by confinement, moral management, without other aid, has been allowed an undue weight in the curative process of genuine mania. I am aware that permanent cerebral disorganization may arise from intemperance in drink, as dissection has repeatedly shown ; but the neglect of a distinct pathognomonic difference between the ravings of inebriety or delirium tremens, and mental derangement, strictly so considered, has led to gross miscalculations in our prognosis. As alcoholic insanity is engendered in every country where drunkenness prevails, it is perhaps more frequently seen in our *mixed* population than in that of Europe. Hence we have sometimes been led to pronounce hastily and erroneously that our success in the management of lunacy is greater than that of other nations. We, however, must be supplied with more extensive and more accurate tabular views of the comparative results of practice in different institutions abroad and at home, before we can come to a satisfactory conclusion on this contested head. It is cheering to the feelings of the philanthropist to know, that by remedial measures, much more is accomplished at the present day than was at a former time imagined practicable."—D.

* In the foregoing talented observations, Dr. Good has omitted to notice a subject which has been most eloquently treated of by Dr. Conolly, namely, the many circumstances which, in places for the reception of lunatics, retard or prevent the patient's return to the full enjoyment of reason. In particular, Dr. Conolly adverts to the neglect of making a proper classification of the inmates of such establishments. "There is," says he, "sometimes a mere separation of the rich from the poor ; or of the noisy from the quiet ; or of the paralytic and idiots, or, at the best, of convalescents from the rest. Even this case is not common. Not only so long as it is neglected, but so long as one lunatic associates with another lunatic, supposing the cases to be curable, so long must the chances of restoration to sanity be very materially diminished. Convalescents should not even associate with convalescents, except under the strict watching of persons of sound mind : they can hardly assist, and they may retard, recovery of one another."—(Inquiry concerning the Indications of Insanity, p. 28.) Dr. Conolly also points out a class of patients for whom a lunatic asylum is a most improper place, viz., those who become affected with various degrees of weakness of intellect. In such persons there is little or no extravagance, still less is there any thing in their condition to render their liberty dangerous. As this infirmity of mind is diversified by intervals of amendment, it is clear that confining such individuals with lunatics is the most likely thing both to afflict them and to shut out every hope of restoration to mental strength. The maxim which Dr. Conolly everywhere inculcates is, that restraint, with reference both to the person and to the management of affairs, can never be justified, except by probable danger to the person of the patient or to others, or to his property or the property of others.—(P. 430.)

GENUS II.
EMPATHEMA.
UNGOVERNABLE PASSION.

THE JUDGMENT PERVERTED OR OVERPOWERED BY THE FORCE OF SOME PREDOMINANT PASSION ; THE FEATURES OF THE COUNTENANCE CHANGED FROM THEIR COMMON CHARACTER.

THE term EMPATHEMA is derived from the Greek πάθημα, "passio," "affection," whence ἐμπαθὴς, "cui insunt affectus seu perturbationes ; affectû percitus vel commotus."

We have already had occasion to observe, that the various faculties of the mind are just as liable to be separately diseased as those of the body : for, as the faculty of digestion may be impaired, while that of respiration or secretion remains in perfect health ; so may the perception or the judgment be injured, while the memory or the imagination continues in its former activity. It is the same with the pathetic faculties. These, I have stated, are to the mental part of the human frame, what feelings, properly so called, are to the corporeal : and hence both may be excited pleasurably or painfully ; they may be in morbid excess or in morbid diminution ; and their influence may equally vary, according to the peculiarity of the passion or the sense affected. Each will therefore furnish a distinct division of diseases : the first constitutes the genus before us ; the second will be found in the ensuing order.

The present genus, however, has never hitherto been properly arranged or digested. Pinel is constantly describing the species that belong to it in his general remarks and illustrative cases, but allots no place to it in his nosological arrangement, with the exception of the third species ; which, as I have already observed, he has irregularly ranked as a subdivision of mania, under the name of manie sans délire ; although he admits that the judgment and perception, and, indeed, all the reasoning faculties

---

" If an insane man believes that he has communication with angels, or is an emperor, or a general, his happiness may be very harmless ; he may require no restraint. But, in the angelic revelations made to him, he may be ordered to kill his children ; or, in his capacity of emperor or general, he may put his supposed subjects or soldiers to death. The disposition to do this may arise suddenly, and nothing but watching and superintendence can lead to a discovery of it. Yet, to restrain this poor man at all times from walking about the fields, or partaking of any of the common enjoyments of society of which he is capable, because such a thing may happen, is not to be justified. Unless he is known to be mischievous, it is unnecessary and cruel. A man must not be made a prisoner for life because he chooses to wear a coat the wrong side outwards, or a pointed hat. It may be more necessary to protect him from others, than others from him ; and therefore an asylum to him may be what its name imports, —a sanctuary and a refuge ; but unless he is disposed to injure others or himself, he must not be subjected to severe restraint. If he has property, and can take care of it, no one ought to touch that property on account of his peculiar dress."—Op. cit., p. 430.—ED.

of the mind, are in most cases undisturbed. In like manner, Sauvages has incorrectly merged the whole family into a single species under the genus mania, to the utter confusion of both.

It is not a little singular that Dr. Crichton, who has written so excellently on the diseases of the passions, and has illustrated his observations with such a variety of examples, should, both in his "Inquiry into the Nature of Mental Derangement," and in his "Synóptical Table," either have assigned no place to these diseases, or have transferred them, like Sauvages, to insanity, under his nomenclature, *delirium ;* although, as I have just remarked, the perception and the judgment (a diseased condition of which is usually appealed to as constituting pathognomonic symptoms of insanity) are, for the most part, strikingly clear in empathema, and often peculiarly acute. This last faculty, indeed, is frequently *perverted* by the prevailing emotion or passion of the hour ; as where a man, under the influence of despair, reasons himself into the lawfulness and expediency of suicide ; but the argument, though deflected, runs still in a right line ; or, in other words, consists of correct reasoning built on a perception of false ideas as its premises, of which we have had various examples in the philosophical suicides of Germany. In the greater number of cases, however, the judgment, instead of being perverted, is merely overpowered by the impassioned emotion ; there is neither false judgment nor false perception.

Ungovernable passion, or empathema, nevertheless, though not strictly insanity, is as much a mental derangement as insanity itself.

"Ira FUROR brevis est,"

is as clear a truth as is to be found in the whole learning of the Roman empire ; and hence the elegant and fanciful mind of the Greeks added the term mania to that expressive of any passion or emotion whatever, when in a state of violence or misrule, as doximania, erotomania, chrysomania ; and, in this sense, mania is often used in the colloquial language of our own day. For poetry or vernacular speech, mania, thus employed, is intelligible enough ; but it is not sufficiently correct for medical or physiological purposes, under which predominant passion must necessarily be distinguished from delirium.

The genus EMPATHEMA has three species : the first characterized by the rousing power of the prevailing passion ; the second, by its depressing power ; the third, by symptoms different from both, and which will be explained in its order.

1. Empathema Entonicum. — Impassioned Excitement.
2. ————— Atonicum. — Impassioned depression.
3. ————— Inane. — Hairbrained passion.

SPECIES I.

EMPATHEMA ENTONICUM.

IMPASSIONED EXCITEMENT.

THE PREDOMINANT PASSION ACCOMPANIED WITH

INCREASED EXCITEMENT, ARDOUR, AND ACTIVITY ; EYE QUICK AND DARING ; COUNTENANCE FLUSHED AND TUMID.

THE varieties are innumerable : the chief are as follow :—

α Lætitiæ.	Ungovernable joy.
β Philautiæ.	Self-love. Self-conceit.
γ Superbiæ.	Pride.
δ Gloriæ famis.	Ambition.
ε Iracundiæ.	Anger.
ζ Zelotypiæ.	Jealousy.

All these, and, indeed, all other passions whatever, are as much direct and indirect stimulants to the mind, as provocative foods or drinks are to the body. Employed occasionally, and in moderation, both may be of use to us, and are given to us by nature for this purpose : but when urged to excess, they throw the system off its healthy balance, rouse it by excitement, or depress it by exhaustion ; and weaken the sensorial vessels by the wear and tear they produce.

As those we are now contemplating are attended with increased action, they have some few symptoms in common, how widely soever they may differ in others ; of which the chief are, an augmented temperature and an accelerated pulse. If carried to such a degree that the judgment loses its power, or, in other words, the man has no longer any command over himself, they betray themselves by their effect on particular features and particular organs, according as the emotion is of a painful or a pleasurable character, or as the pain or the pleasure predominates in those cases which partake of both.

There are some organs, however, that seem to be equally affected under a vehement excitement of whatever may be the prevailing passion, as the brain, the heart, and the lungs ; for headache and apoplexy, palpitation and anhelation, are alike common to sudden fits of extreme joy, terror, and rage. The thoracic effects are, indeed, the most striking ; and hence it is that the præcordia has been more generally supposed in all ages and countries to be the seat of mental emotion than the encephalon ; and the state of the heart as light and jumping for joy, oppressed and breaking with grief, or black and bilious with hatred, has been more commonly appealed to than that of the animal spirits ; though the latter is the cause, and the former the mere effect.

It may be thought, perhaps, that the vulgar character of the heart, as indicative of hatred or revenge, is merely figurative, and has no foundation in nature. But this is not the case : for anger, when long indulged, is well known to affect the functions of the liver, and has often laid a foundation for jaundice, and consequently for a deeper colour as well as other properties of the blood that circulates through the heart ; a fact so well known, that the seat of anger has, in the poetical language of most countries, been transferred to this organ, and bilious or choleric and irascible are convertible terms in the popular language of our own day.

We have endeavoured to account for the difference of effect produced by the sensorial fluid in the different organs of local sensation, by supposing some degree of change to take place in the nature of this fluid by the action of the respective sentient nerves at their origin or extremity.* It is possible that other changes may take place in the sensorium, from the influence of peculiar mental impressions, and that certain classes or ramifications of nerves may be more affected by particular impressions than others. And we may hence account, not only for the sympathy of the liver with the sensorium when urged by anger, but for that of other organs, under other impassioned excitements ; and this not merely whether pleasurable or painful, but according to the peculiarity of the pleasure or the pain which forms the source of incitation. Thus, while anger stimulates the liver, fear has a tendency to produce a diarrhœa and incontinence of urine ; grief disorders the stomach, and affects the lachrymal glands ; sudden fright divests the muscles of locomotion, and produces palsy ; while mirth throws them into involuntary action, and compels a man to leap, laugh, and sing.

This, however, is to digress ; for our present business is to contemplate the mental, rather than the corporeal, effects of the passions, when urged to excess, or intemperately protracted.

The instances of derangement produced by a sudden FIT OR IMMODERATE FLOW OF JOY are numerous, and not difficult to account for. As this impassioned emotion, when indulged with a rampant domination over the judgment, is a direct stimulus of a very powerful kind, acting not only on the nerves but on every part of the body, it cannot take place without producing great sensorial exhaustion, and consequently cannot be persevered in without remissions of languor and lassitude, like the effects of intoxication from strong wine or spirits. The misfortune is, that when the elevating faculties of the mind, and especially the imagination, are once let loose by the operation of this passion, and both run wild together, the mental excitement will sometimes continue after the strength of the body is completely prostrated. And when this strength is sufficiently recruited for the external senses to convey once more to the perception true and lively impressions of the objects that surround them, the perception, which has been also morbidly affected by the violence of impassioned paroxysms, will not receive or convey them in a true state, and a permanent derangement is the consequence. Cardan (*De Sapientiâ*, lib. ii.) gives the case of an artisan of Milan, who, having had the good luck to find an

instrument that formerly belonged to Archimedes, ran mad with a fit of transport into which he was hereby thrown : and Plutarch, in his life of Artaxerxes, has a like story of a soldier, who, having had the high honour of wounding Cyrus in battle, became so overjoyed that he lost his wits from the moment. Boerhaave (*De Morb. Nerv.*, lib. ix., cap. 12) and Van Swieten (*Comment.*, tom. iii., p. 144) relate cases of epilepsy that followed from the same cause.

Occasionally, the exhaustion of sensorial power hereby produced is so sudden and total, that the whole nervous system seems instantaneously to become discharged of its contents, like a Leyden vial loaded with electricity when touched with a brass rod, and death takes place at the moment. There are various instances on record, in which a like fate has followed upon the injudicious production of a pardon to a culprit just on the point of his being turned off at the gallows. Valerius Maximus relates two anecdotes of matrons, who in like manner died of joy on seeing their sons return safe from the battle at the lake Thrasis ; the one died while embracing her son ; the other had been misinformed, and was at that moment lamenting his death. The power of surprise was added, therefore, in this case, to that of joy, and she fell even before her arms could clasp him.—(Lib. ix., cap. 12.) Marcellus Donatus, Pechlin, and other collectors of medical curiosities, are full of incidents of this kind : and a case not very unlike occurred a few years since to the present author, in the person of an intimate friend and most exemplary clergyman. This gentleman, who had consented to be nominated one of the executors in the will of an elderly person of considerable property with whom he was acquainted, received, a few years afterward, and at a time when his own income was but limited, the unexpected news that the testator was dead, and had left him sole executor, together with the whole of his property, amounting to three thousand pounds a year in landed estates. He arrived in London in great agitation ; and on entering his own door dropped down in a fit of apoplexy, from which he never entirely recovered ; for though he regained his mental, and most of his corporeal faculties, his mind was shaken and rendered timid, and a hemiplegia had so weakened his right side that he was incapable of walking farther than a few steps.

Could this passion be employed as a medicine, and administered with a due regard to time and measure, from its powerful influence on the whole system, there can be no doubt that it might be made productive of the most beneficial effects. And there is hence no reason for hesitation in admitting many of the wonderful cures which are reported to have been occasionally operated by its sudden incursion. Corineus gives the case of a tertian ague thus removed ; Lory that of a stricture of the pylorus with incessant vomiting (*De Melancholiâ*, tom. i., p. 37); and Trellian, what we should less have expected, a radical cure of melancholy.—(Lib. xli., p. 17.)

In the SECOND VARIETY we have noticed the

---

* This and other hypotheses, founded on the presumed existence of a sensorial fluid, may satisfy readers disposed to be content or pleased with conjecture ; but until the reality of such fluid be proved, they can only be regarded as sports of the imagination. It is fortunate, however, that the occasional reference made to them in the text does not impair the generally valuable character of the author's matter.—Ed.

predominance of SELF-CONCEIT. The ordinary feeling here is still of a pleasurable kind, but never amounts to the paroxysms of the preceding ; its effects, therefore, on the soundness of the mind are more gradual, but in many instances quite as marked. It is a vain and preposterous estimation of one's personal powers or endowments, accompanied with so immoderate a love of one's own self on this very account, as to make the possessor blind to every instance of superiority in another person, and hence to save him in a considerable degree from the pain he would otherwise endure ; for the self-conceited man is not easily mortified or humiliated, and hence not easily cured of the malady. "A wise man," says Mr. Mason in his Treatise on Self-Knowledge, "has his foible as well as a fool : but the difference between them is, that the foibles of the one are known to himself, and concealed from the world ; the foibles of the other are known to the world, and concealed from himself. The wise man sees those frailties in himself which others cannot : but the fool is blind to those blemishes in his character which are conspicuous to every one else."— (Part i., chap. vii.) It was under the influence of this disease that Menecrates, as we learn from Ælian, became so mad as seriously to believe himself the son of Jupiter, and to request of Philip of Macedon that he might be treated as a god. But it is not always that the man thus deranged falls into such good hands as those of the Macedonian monarch ; for Philip, humorously determining to make the madman's disease work its own cure, gave orders immediately that his request should be complied with, and invited him to a grand entertainment, at which was a separate table for the new divinity, served with the most costly perfumes and incense, but with nothing else. Menecrates was at first highly delighted, and received the worship that was paid to him with the greatest complacency ; but growing hungry by degrees over the empty viands that were offered him, while every other guest was indulged with substantial dainties, he at length keenly felt himself to be a man, and stole away from the court in his right senses.—(Lib. xii., cap. 51.)

The passion of PRIDE has a close affinity to that of self-conceit : but is less confined to self-endowments, and is a relative as the former is a personal vanity. The proud man may indeed have the same preposterous estimation for some supposed gift of person, but the grasp of the passion does not terminate here ; for he carries the same estimation to every thing that in the remotest degree appertains to him, and is hence as vain of his birth, or family connexions, his wealth, his estates, his country, his office, his honour, or his religion ; and he is hence open to more numerous mortifications, and is in fact more frequently mortified, than the mere egotist. Examples of a deranged mind from ungovernable pride are to be found in every rank of life ; but as those in the loftiest have the cup of intoxication most frequently offered to them, and drink deepest of its contents, it is here, among kings, and courtiers, and prime ministers, and

commanders, that we are to look for the most striking instances of this malady. Many a crown won by good fortune, and which might have been preserved by moderation, has been lost by the delirium of pride and vain-glory ; of which the history of Demetrius of Macedonia furnishes us with one of the most memorable examples : who, in his disgraceful fall, was obliged to abandon, among the other idols of his heart, the unfinished robe which was to have hung over his shoulders, containing a magnificent embroidery of the sun, the moon, and all the stars of heaven, designed to have represented him as the sovereign lord of the whole.

There is, however, another kind of madmen, to adopt the words of Burton (*Anat. of Melanch.*, part i., sect. ii., vol. i., p. 189), opposite to these, " that are insensibly mad, and know nothing of it ; such as affect to contemn all praise and glory, and think themselves most free when they are most mad : a company of cynics, such as monks, hermits, and anchorites, that contemn the world, contemn themselves, contemn all titles, honours, offices, and yet, in that contempt, are more proud than any man living. They are proud in humility, proud in that they are not proud. They go in sheep's russet, many great men that might maintain themselves in cloth of gold, and seem to be dejected ; humble by the outward carriage, when as inwardly they are swollen full of pride, arrogance, and self-conceit. And therefore Seneca adviseth his friend Lucilius, in his attire and gesture, his outward actions especially, to avoid all such things as are most notable in themselves ; as a ragged attire, hirsute head, horrid beard, contempt of money, coarse lodging, and whatever leads to fame that opposite way."—(*Epist.* v.)

When the passion of pride is united with that of ardent desire after something beyond us and above us, it constitutes the next feeling of AMBITION : and hence this also is an inflating emotion, a tympany of the mind, and may be called *prospective* vanity, as pride is *relative* vanity, and self-conceit *personal*. It is the more dangerous to the understanding, in consequence of the double force with which it overpowers the judgment ; and hence the slave of inordinate ambition is far more restless, and in a far higher degree of excitement, than the slave of either of the other two kinds of vanity ; and as, being dependant upon a greater number of contingencies, he is most of all open to reverses and downfalls.

Examples are not necessary, and would be a waste of time. Whenever the stimulant ideas or thoughts that are connected with any one of this train of passions pass over the mind, the blood, as is justly observed by Sir A. Crichton, rushes with impetuosity to the head, the sentient principle is formed in preternatural quantity, and the excitement is at last so often renewed, and increases to such a degree, as to occasion an impetuous and permanent delirium. But when the expectations and high desires which pride or vanity naturally suggests are blasted ; when these passions are assailed by poverty, neglect, contempt, and hatred, and are unequal to the contest, they now and then terminate in despondency, or settled melancholy.—(*Of Mental Derangement,* book iii:, ch. ii.)

But if such be a frequent effect of the stirring passions of a pleasurable kind, it is not difficult to conceive that those accompanied with pain, as the passion of ANGER, and all its compounds, suspicion, revenge, and especially jealousy, must make a much wider inroad upon the domain of a well-ordered mind, and introduce confusion and derangement. Nor is the effect confined to the head ; for a stimulus thus violent affects the entire system, and as we have already observed, has a peculiar sympathetic influence on the liver ; producing in many instances a diseased secretion of bile, and altering it in a very short period, not only in its quantity but in its quality. At the same time, every vessel is exhausted of its irritability, and the whole strength is so prostrated as occasionally to lead on to obstinate faintings, convulsions, and death. The expressions and gestures are always violent and offensive, and are similar to those of maniacal rage ; the eyes are red and inflamed, the countenance is flushed, swollen, and distorted, and the person is ungovernable. Such was the case, in 1392, with Charles VI. of France ; who, being violently incensed against the Duke of Bretagne, and burning with a spirit of malice and revenge, could neither eat, drink, nor sleep for many days together, and at length became furiously mad as he was riding on horseback, drawing his sword, and striking promiscuously every one who approached him. The disease fixed upon his intellect, and accompanied him to his death.

In JEALOUSY, as in ambition, there is a combination of irritating passions, and the combination is still more complicated ; for it is a compound of suspicion, hatred, eager desire of revenge, occasionally intermixed with love. To hot climates it appears to be endemic ; and there is not, perhaps, an eastern dynasty that does not offer numerous examples of its sanguinary phrensy and diabolical career.

It is not often, however, that any of the varieties of this species terminate in permanent insanity, although the case of Charles VI. of France forms an exception to the general rule. As moral treatment appears to be of more benefit in the preceding genus than medical, it is almost the only treatment that can be recommended in ungovernable passion ; though the violence of the excitement should unquestionably be reduced by venesection and purgatives. After this, time and perfect quiet must be chiefly depended upon : yet judicious conversation, and more especially a judicious choice of subjects, may accomplish much. A deaf ear is generally turned to the precepts of the moralist ; but if attention can be obtained for them, Epictetus and Mason's Self-Knowledge, Pascal's Thoughts, and Lord Bacon's Essays, will furnish valuable remedies ; and so also, and of a much more powerful opcration, will the still better penned ethics of a book, which, in every Christian country, should be uppermost in the mind without any suggestion. Moral castigation, however, if not too

sudden or severe, is that which generally works most effectually ; and few madmen of this kind have been able to meet a serious reverse of fortune, or condition of life, without being the better for it, if not destroyed by its first shock. Self-conceit, which is a mere product of self-ignorance, is best removed by an acquaintance with the world, and especially with men of real talents and genius, in which sphere the man who labours under it will soonest learn his own emptiness, and the means of remedying this defect. And hence the advantage of a public education over a private one ; in which talents are brought into a fair competition with talents, and every one learns to appreciate his powers, not by the standard of his own vanity, but by the stamp of merit that has passed the mint.

SPECIES II.

EMPATHEMA ATONICUM.

IMPASSIONED DEPRESSION.

THE PREDOMINANT PASSION ACCOMPANIED WITH DIMINISHED EXCITEMENT, ANXIETY, AND LOVE OF SOLITUDE : EYE FIXED AND PENSIVE ; COUNTENANCE PALE AND FURROWED.

THE mental emotions productive of these effects, are at least as numerous as those which harass the frame by increased excitement. The following may serve as examples :—

a Desiderii.	Ungovernable Love.
β Auri famis.	———— Avarice.
γ Anxietudinis.	———— Anxiety.
δ Mœroris.	———— Heartache.
ε Desperationis.	———— Despondency.

As increased sensorial excitement produces various symptoms in common, whatever be the nature of the governing passion at the time, there are also various symptoms common to decreased sensorial excitement under each of these depressing passions : as a greater or less degree of torpor in every irritable part, especially in the circulating and absorbent systems ; whence paleness of the countenance, coldness of the extremities, a contraction and shrinking of the skin and general surface of the body, a retardation and smallness of the pulse, want of appetite, deficiency of muscular force, and a sense of languor which overspreads the whole frame.

The ardent desire which is distinguished by the name of LONGING, is directed towards objects of various kinds that are absent, and equally relate to places and persons. It is a painful and exhausting emotion, as compounded of hope, love, and fear, and peculiarly agitates the præcordia ; and hence the striking and beautiful apothegm of the wise man,—" Hope deferred maketh the heart sick." It is felt by children at a distance from home, and who are eager to return to the embraces of their parents ; by foreigners who have a strong and inextinguishable love for their country, and are anxious to return to the scenes and the companions of former times ; and by the youthful pair who have vowed an eternal attachment, and are sure that they cannot live without each other, but whose union is opposed by bars that are felt to be insurmountable. And hence the present variety includes the three modifications of HOME-SICKNESS, COUNTRY-SICKNESS, and LOVE-SICK-NESS. The first is for the most part transitory; the second, the *heimweh* of the Germans, has sometimes, and especially among the Swiss, when their manners were simpler, and their domestic virtues and feelings much stronger, than they seem to have been of late years, produced not only a permanent melancholy but hectic fever. Yet it is to the third that our attention is chiefly called on the present occasion, from the greater frequency of its occurrence, and the more severe and tragic effects to which it has led, where obstacles have arisen in its progress.

We have, on the present occasion, nothing whatever to do with the gross passion of concupiscence, which is as different from that of pure and genuine love as light from darkness. The man of lust has indeed his love, but it is a love that centres in himself, and seeks alone his own gratification; while the passion we are now speaking of puts self completely out of the field, and would voluntarily submit to every pain, and sacrifice even life itself, in promoting the happiness of the beloved object. Yet, constituted as we are by nature for the wisest and best of purposes, a pure corporeal orgasm still interweaves itself with the sentimental desire, though subordinate to it in virtuous minds, and the flame is fed from a double source. "Nuptial love," says Lord Bacon, "maketh mankind; friendly love perfecteth it; but wanton love corrupteth and embaseth it."—*(Essays*, No. x.)

What it is that first lights up this flame is of no importance to the present subject. A peculiar cast of form or of features, acknowledged by all to be moulded according to the finest laws of symmetry, and productive of a high degree of external grace or beauty; or a figure, or a manner, that to the eye of the enamoured beholder gives token of a mind adorned with all he can wish for; or an actual knowledge, from long acquaintance, of the existence of such internal cultivation and excellence, may be equally causes of the same common effect. And hence this is of little or no account; for the passion being once excited, the judgment runs a risk of being overpowered by its warmth and violence; and the moment it is overpowered, the new train of ideas that are let loose upon the mind are of a romantic character; and as soon as any obstacle starts up as a barrier in the vista of hope, instead of being damped or repressed, they grow wilder and more vivid, till at length the sensorial system is worn out by the vehemence of its labour; and though the excitement is really less than at first, because there is less vascular vigour for its support, it is still greater than ever, compared with the weakened state of the sentient organ.

Yet love-sickness itself, whatever mischief it may work in the corporeal frame by sleepless nights, a feverish pulse, and loss of appetite,[*] and however, from the exalted state of the ima-

gination and the increased sensibility of the body, it may transpose the reality of life into a kind of visionary existence, and so far produce mental derangement, rarely leads to direct insanity, so long as there is the remotest hope of the attainment of its object. But if hope be suddenly cut off by an inexorable refusal, the intervention of a more fortunate rival, the concealment of the object of adoration, or any other cause whatever, the mind is sometimes incapable of resisting the shock thus produced by the concurrent yet opposite powers of desire and despair; and in a moment in which the judgment is completely overwhelmed, the love-sick maniac calls to his aid the demoniacal passion of revenge, and, almost at hazard, determines upon a plan of murder directed against his rival, his mistress, or himself. The story of Mr. Hackman and Miss Rae will at once, perhaps, occur to the recollection of most of the author's reader's in proof of this assertion. He himself had some acquaintance with the former; and is convinced, from what he knew of him, that nothing but a paroxysm of insanity could have urged him to so horrible an act.

The operation of the passion of AVARICE, when it has once obtained an ascendency over the mind, is altogether of a different nature from that of the preceding variety, though it often produces a wider and more chronic alienation. It has not a stirring property of any kind belonging to it, but benumbs and chills every energy of the body as well as of the soul, like the stream of Lethe: even the imagination is rendered cold and stagnant, and the only passions with which it forms a confederacy, are the miserable train of gloomy fear, suspicion, and anxiety. The body grows thin in the midst of wealth, the limbs totter though surrounded by cordials, and the man voluntarily starves himself in the granary of plenty, not from a want of appetite, but from a dread of giving way to it. The individual who is in such a state of mind must be estranged upon this point, how much soever he may be at home upon others. Yet these are cases that are daily occurring, and have been in all ages: though perhaps one of the most curious is that related by Valerius Maximus of a miser who took advantage of a famine to sell a mouse for two hundred pence, and then famished himself with the money in his pocket.—(Lib. vii., cap. vi.) And hence the madness of the covetous man has been a subject of sarcasm and ridicule by moralists and dramatic writers, in every period, of which we have sufficient examples in the writings of Aristophanes, Lucian, and Molière.

There is another mental feeling of a very afflictive, and too often, like the last, of a chronic kind, which is frequently found to usurp a dominion over the judgment, and to imbitter life with false and visionary ideas, and that is, a habit of ANXIETY, or PREYING CARE; which not only drives the individual who possesses it mad, but runs the risk of doing the same to all who are about him, and are harassed with his complaints and discontents. This is sometimes the effect of a long succession of misfortunes or vexatious troubles; but seems in some persons

---

[*] Schurig. Gynealog., p. 94. Horstius, An Pulsus aliquis amatorius concedendus? Bilizer, De Naturâ Amoris, Gloss. 1611, 4to.

to depend on a very high degree of nervous sensibility, united with a choleric or melancholic temperament.* Their age, wealth, or situation in life is of no importance ; and though their digestive powers are good, and they are not hypochondriacs, they are always apprehensive and full of alarm, and flee from every appearance of joy as they would from an apparition, or even sooner. In the language of Burton, who knew too well how to describe them, " the old are full of aches in their bones, croups, and convulsions ; dull of hearing, weak-sighted, hoary, wrinkled, harsh, so much so that they cannot know their own selves in a glass ; a burden to themselves and others. If they be sound, they fear diseases ; if sick, weary of their lives. One complains of want, a second of servitude, another of a secret or incurable disease, of some deformity of body, of some loss, danger, death of friends, shipwreck, persecution, imprisonment, disgrace, repulse, contumely, calumny, abuse, injury, contempt, ingratitude, unkindness, scoffs, scouts, unfortunate marriage, single life, too many children, no children, false servants, unhappy children, barrenness, banishment, oppression, frustrated hopes, ill success ;

" ' Cætera de genere hoc, adeo sunt multa, loquacem,
Delassare valent Fabium.'

" ' In the meantime,' continues the younger Democritus, ! thus much I may say of them, that generally they crucify the soul of man, attenuate our bodies, dry them, wither them, rivel them up like old apples, and make them as so many anatomies.' "—(*Anat. of Melancholy*, part i., sect. ii., subs. x.)

Nothing can be more different than this constitutional pining, and the pains produced by HEARTACHE, or the reality of severe grief. The former is talkative and querulous ; the latter is dumb, and flies from company. The sensorial exhaustion is so considerable, that the mind, with its attention upon the full stretch, has scarcely strength enough to collect the train of ideas on which alone it resolves to dwell ; and hence all conversation is irksome, the presence of a friend disquieting, and the deepest solitude is anxiously sought for. And not unfrequently the discharge of nervous power is so considerable and sudden as to produce a general torpor of the brain ; which, if it do not happily terminate in quiet sleep, is the inlet of apoplexy. Even in the former case, the inirritability of the nervous fibres continues to such an excess, that the sufferer has no natural evacuation for perhaps several days, feels no hunger, cannot be persuaded to take food, is incapable of sighing, and sheds no tears. And hence the appearance of tears and sighing are good omens, and are correctly regarded as such ; since they show that the

generatl orpitude is giving way in the organs that most associate with this painful emotion of the mind, to a slight return to irritability. As soon as the flow of the sensorial principle is a little increased, the præcordia struggles with great anxiety, and the heart is overloaded and feels ready to break or burst,' whence the name of HEARTACHE, so appropriately applied to this variety of suffering. Sometimes, also, hysteric flatulence oppresses the respiration, and convulsions, and not unfrequently death itself, ensue. Of this last effect Erndtl has given numerous instances.—(*Relatio de Morbis anno* 1720 *Warsaviæ curatis*, Dresd., 1730.) But if recovery should take place, it is usually long before the judgment re-assumes its proper sway in the mind, and the temporary derangement altogether ceases. At times, indeed, this never returns, and the pitiable sufferer only lives through the shock to endure the severer evil of confirmed insanity ; of which Shakspeare has given us an admirable copy in the character of King Lear, finely imagined to be a result of filial ingratitude.

DESPAIR makes a near approach to heartache in the overwhelming agony it produces, and its pressing desire of gloom and solitude ; but, generally speaking, the feeling is more selfish, and the mind more hurried and daring. Despair, as it commonly shows itself, is utter hopelessness from mortified pride, blasted expectations, or a sense of personal ruin : heartache is either hopelessness from a sense of some social bereavement, or relative ruin. The gamester, who cares for no one but himself, may rage with all the horror of despair ; but the heartache belongs chiefly to the man of a warmer and more generous bosom, stung to the quick by a wound he least expected, or borne down, not by the loss of fortune, but of a dear friend or relative, in whom he had concentrated all his hopes. The well-known picture of Beverley is drawn by the hand of a master, and he is represented as maddened by the thought of the deep distress into which his last hazard has plunged his wife and family ; but if his selfish love of gaming had not triumphed over his relative love for those he had thus ruined, he would not have been involved in any such reverse. While Beverley was in despair, it was his wife who was broken-hearted.

The sources of this most agonizing emotion are innumerable ; and from the total shipwreck of all hope on which it is founded, there is no passion of the mind that drives a man so readily to an act of suicide. To live is horror : the infuriated sufferer feels himself an outcast from God and man ; and though his judgment may still be correct upon other subjects, it is completely overpowered upon that of his actual distress ; and all he thinks of and aims at is to withdraw with as much speed as possible from the present state of torture, totally regardless of the future, or falsely satisfying himself by a perversion of his judgment that there is no crime in his doing so.

One of the severest causes of despondency is a conscience labouring under a deep sense of guilt for some

" —— undivulged crime
Unwhipt of justice ;"

---

* One position maintained by one of the latest writers on mental derangement is, that mere nervousness and insanity are absolutely identical ; or, in other terms, that nervous derangements differ "in measure more than in kind."—Dr. Uwins on the Disorders of the Brain and Nervous System, pp. 5, 24, &c., 8vo., Lond., 1833.—ED.

and so severe has the anguish been in many cases, that the tormented wretch, thus haunted by himself, and hating the light of heaven, has been compelled, as the less evil of the two, to surrender himself to the laws of his country, and court the disgrace of a public execution. Yet the same miserable feeling has sometimes followed from an ideal cause, especially in a mind of natural timidity, or constitutionally predisposed to a gloomy view of nature : for such, by a mere exercise of their own meditations, but far oftener by the coarse but impassioned oratory of itinerant preachers, are induced to believe that the Almighty has shut them out for ever from the pale of mercy, and that the bottomless pit is yawning to receive them ; and under the influence of such an impression, they too frequently work themselves up into a state of permanent insanity, or hurry themselves by their own hands into the horrors of a fate from which they feel assured that no repentance nor power of religion can save them.

In the midst of great public calamities, the passion of ungovernable despondency is apt to become epidemic, and particularly, as M. Falret has well observed, where the constitution of the atmosphere, from being moist and hot, and consequently relaxing and debilitating, favours its spread. In 1806 the feeling of desperation was so common at Paris, that sixty suicides occurred during the months of June and July ; at Copenhagen, in the course of the same entire year, three hundred ; and in 1793 about thirteen hundred at Versailles alone.—(*Falret, de l'Hypochondrie et du Suicide*, 8vo., Paris, 1822.) The sensation, however, whether general or individual, is most acute where there is little corporeal exertion, and consequently where there is time to cultivate and brood over it. Hence suicide is frequent in the distress of sieges, in the first alarm of civil commotions, or when they have subsided into a state of calmness, and the mischiefs they have induced are well pondered ; but it seldom takes place in the activity of a campaign, whatever may be the fatigue, the privations, or the sufferings endured. On the fall of the Roman empire, and throughout the revolution of France, self-destruction was so common at home as at last to excite but little attention ; it does not appear, however, to have stained the retreat of the Ten Thousand under Xenophon, and, according to M. Falret, was rare in the French army during its flight from Moscow.*

In all these varieties of empathema, the art of the physician can do but little ; and, in many of them, nothing whatever. Yet, where the heart suffers acutely, and the mind is deeply dejected, sedatives and antispasmodic cordials may occasionally be found useful ; and, as the

abdominal viscera are greatly liable to be affected, the appetite to fail, the liver to be congested, and the bowels rendered costive, these organs must be watched, and such relief be afforded as they may stand in need of. Where aperients are required, the warm and bitter resins will generally answer the purpose best, alone or combined with rhubarb. Where love is the cause of disease, and the fair patient is young and delicate, suppressed menstruation or even chlorosis is by no means unfrequent, followed by hysteria and other nervous affections that produce considerable trouble.

In all cases of mental dejection, however, a kind and judicious friend is by far the best physician. Medicines may do a little, change of scene and country, of custom and manners, a little also ; but the soothing of tenderness and indulgence, and the voice of that friendship which knows how to discriminate opportunities, and seasonably to alternate admonition with consolation, will accomplish more in the way of cure than all the rest put together. The despondency produced by the real sense of a guilty conscience, or the visionary belief of eternal reprobation, may derive important and most salutary advantage from religious instruction, when conducted with a judicious attention to the exigency of the case. But much circumspection and adroitness are requisite upon this point ; for, so rooted is the feeling to be extirpated, that no ordinary means will suffice for its eradication ; while, if it be forcibly snapped off, it will shoot out the wider, and grow ranker than ever.

The excitement of an opposite passion or train of feelings has sometimes been accompanied with success ; for there are instances in which the slave of imaginary pain and misery has for ever forgotten his sense of visionary grievances under the stroke of poignant and real affliction ; and the miser, when reduced by a sudden reverse of fortune to actual beggary, and thus completely disencumbered of the load that has hitherto so much oppressed him, has returned to his sober senses, and learned a juster estimate of worldly possessions.

The same attempt has often been recommended in disappointments under the passion of love ; and, according to the concurrent report of the poets of ancient and modern times, many of whom profess to be well versed in this kind of discipline, it has very generally been attended with success. Where the emotion has more of a corporeal than a sentimental origin, this may easily be conceived ; and it is possible that it may also sometimes have occurred under a purer feeling ; though, for the honour of the human heart, I do not think this is much to be trusted to. Where the choice between two young persons of fair character is really imprudent, yet the affections are so riveted as to bid defiance to all forcible attempts to unfetter them, a promise of consent on the part of the reluctant parent at the distance of a given period of time, as a year and a half, or two years, with an undertaking on the part of the lovers neither to see nor correspond with each other in the meantime, an engagement easily fallen into, has

---

* Spurzheim remarks (Obs. on Insanity, p, 186, London, 1817), that "there are countries and districts where suicide is endemical. In Germany, about Hamburg, Pottsdam, Halle, Jena, it is much more common than in Austria ; and at certain periods it is more frequent than at others ; sometimes it is epidemic, so that in a short time there are a great number of instances, and then much fewer during a long interval."—D.

answered in many instances to which I have been privy. The ardour has gradually cooled on the one side or the other; the judgment has been more impressed with the nature of the imprudence; or a more attractive form has interposed, and irretrievably settled the question. While, on the contrary, if the fidelity should hold on both sides to the end, and the passion be heightened instead of depressed, as in this case there is most reason to suppose it would be, hard, indeed, must be the heart that would extend the restriction further, and that would not wish joy to so deserving a couple.

SPECIES III.
EMPATHEMA INANE.
HAIRBRAINED PASSION.

WAYWARD AND UNMEANING PASSION, URGING TO INDISCRIMINATE ACTS OF VIOLENCE: AIR HURRIED AND TUMULTUOUS; COUNTENANCE FLUSHED; EYES GLARING AND PROMINENT.

THIS is the *manie sans délire* of M. Pinel, a case of frequent occurrence, but incorrectly named in this manner; since, in the opinion of all other nosologists, and, perhaps, all other pathological writers, the character of delirium (that is, of diseased judgment, diseased perception, or both) is essential to mania.

M. Pinel ascribes this species principally, and with great force of reason, to a neglected or ill-directed education upon a mind naturally perverse or unruly, and gives the following striking example:—An only son of a weak and indulgent mother was encouraged in the gratification of every caprice and passion, of which an untutored and violent temper was susceptible. The impetuosity of his disposition increased with his years. At school he was always embroiled in disputes and quarrels; and if a dog or a horse offended him, he instantly put it to death. This wayward youth, however, when unmoved by passions, possessed a perfectly sound judgment. When he came of age he proved himself fully competent to the management of his family estate, as well as to the discharge of his relative duties; and even distinguished himself by acts of beneficence and compassion. But his deep-rooted propensity to quarrel still haunted him; and wounds, lawsuits, and pecuniary compensations were the general consequence. At last an act of notoriety put an end to his career of violence. Enraged at a woman who had used offensive language to him, he tumbled her into a well. A public prosecution followed, and, on the testimony of a great many witnesses, who deposed as to his furious deportment, he was condemned to perpetual confinement at the lunatic asylum of Bicêtre.

On the commencement of the French revolution, when the mob broke open the doors of the prisons and the lunatic hospitals to liberate all whom they thought unjustly confined and under restraint, a patient labouring under the present species in the Bicêtre asylum pleaded his own cause so rationally and pathetically, and so artfully accused the governor of the asylum of cruelty, that the armed rabble commanded him to be instantly liberated, and scarce suffered the governor to escape with impunity. The patient, thus restored to freedom, was led about in triumph amid reiterated shouts of "Vive la République!" The sight of so many armed men, their loud and confused noise and tumultuous conduct, soon roused the visionary hero to a fresh paroxysm of fury. He seized, with a vigorous grasp, the sabre of his next neighbour, brandished it about with great violence, and wounded his liberators indiscriminately. Fortunately, he was soon mastered, when the savage mob thought proper to lead him back to his cell, and with shame and reluctance acknowledged their own ignorance and misconduct. The mode of treatment may be collected from the preceding pages.

GENUS III.
ALUSIA.
ILLUSION. HALLUCINATION.

THE JUDGMENT PERVERTED OR OVERPOWERED BY THE FORCE OF THE IMAGINATION; THE SPIRITS PERMANENTLY ELEVATED OR DEPRESSED; THE FEELINGS OF THE MIND DEPICTED IN THE COUNTENANCE.

ALUSIA is here derived from the Greek ἄλυσις, "aberratio," from ἀλύω, "errabundâ mente afficior,"—"inquietus aberro:" whence the Latin term allucinatio or hallucinatio. According to the rule which renders the Greek υ by the Latin y, the name of this genus ought rather perhaps to be *alysis*; but as the Latins have themselves retained the υ in all*u*cinatio, it is here suffered to continue in alusia, making a similar exception to that already observed in *lues*. The Greek term is preferred to the Latin, as the name of the genus, for the sake of uniformity. Sauvages, and after him Sagar, have employed hallucinatio as the name of an order; Darwin and Crichton as that of a genus, and, consequently, running parallel with the genus before us. Wherever the genus exists, hypochondrias or hypochondriasis is usually placed under it. It is so by Sauvages, Sagar, and Crichton: and it occupies the same place in Linnæus, who has merely adopted the term imaginarii instead of hallucinationes.

Alusia embraces the two following species:—

1. Alusia Elatio. Sentimentalism.
   Mental extravagance.

2 ——— Hypochondrias. Hypochondriacism.
   Low spirits.

SPECIES I.
ALUSIA ELATIO.
SENTIMENTALISM. MENTAL EXTRAVAGANCE.

ROMANTIC IDEAS OF REAL LIFE; ARDENT AND EXALTED FANCY; PLEASURABLE FEELINGS; FREQUENT PULSE; GREAT ACTIVITY; EYE KEEN AND LIGHTED UP; COUNTENANCE CONFIDENT AND ANIMATED.

THE merit or demerit of this species, named

from the rhetoricians ᴇʟᴀᴛɪᴏ, and with them importing "elevated, exalted, magnificent style or imagery," must, I fear, mainly rest with the author himself. It is, however, strictly derived from nature, and is intended to fill up what has hitherto been left as a vacant niche by the nosologists. Alusia or hallucination, like ecphronia or insanity, comprises a list of affections that are characterized by two opposite states of nervous action, entonic and atonic, or, in the language of Dr. Cullen, excitement and collapse : elatio is intended to include the former of these, as hypochondrias, the ensuing species, is the latter. They stand in the same relation to each other as elevated and dejected madness or melancholy. Both are united with a peculiar modification of the digestive function, but possessing opposite bearings ; being in the former strikingly active and energetic, and in the latter strikingly sluggish and languid. Hence, under the first species, the patient is able to endure enormous fastings, and to support life upon the scantiest and least nutritive diet, either of which would be destructive under the second.

This species embraces the following varieties :—

α Heroica.	Chivalry.	Romantic gallantry.
β Facetosa.	Crack-brained wit.	
γ Ecstatica.	False inspiration.	
δ Fanatica.	Fanaticism.	

The age of the first of these varieties, that of ᴄʜɪᴠᴀʟʀʏ ᴏʀ ʀᴏᴍᴀɴᴛɪᴄ ɢᴀʟʟᴀɴᴛʀʏ, has nearly, if not altogether, departed. It may be regarded as a generous and high-spirited flight of the imagination, that gives a visionary colouring to the external world, and combines, without a due degree of discrimination, ideas of fact with those of fancy. Like many of the varieties of empathema or ungovernable passion, it may lead to or be combined with ecphronia or insanity.

I have sometimes had to attend patients who, having spent the greater part of their days and nights over the most captivating novels of the present day, had acquired so much of this falsity of perception as to startle their friends around them, and to give evident proof that they were of a mind occasionally deranged, though, when the attention could once be seriously engaged, capable of being brought down to the soberness of external objects and real life. These have commonly been ladies unmarried or without a family, about the middle or a little beyond the middle of life, of a nervous temperament, fine-taste and fancy, but whose education had been directed to subjects of superficial or external ornament rather than of intrinsic excellence. Their manner has been peculiarly courteous, their conversation sprightly and figurative, and their hand ready to aid the distressed. But it has been obvious that in all they were saying or doing they had some ideal character in their minds, whose supposed air, and language, and manners they were copying ; and the distressed were always most sure of relief, and of a relief often beyond the necessity of the case, whose story was combined

with some perilous adventure or sentimental catastrophe.

In former times, however, when the wild and daring spirit of romance formed the subject of popular study, and

"The spinsters, and the knitters in the sun,
And the free maids that wove their threads with
Were wont to chant it,"　　　.　　[bones,

this bewildering triumph of the imagination over the judgment was far more common, and carried to a much higher pitch. The high-toned and marvellous stories of La Morte d'Arthur, Guy of Warwick; Amadis of Gaul, The Seven Champions of Christendom, and the Mirror of Knighthood ; the splendid and agitating alternations of magicians, enchanted castles, dragons, and giants, redoubtable combatants, imprisoned damsels, melting minstrelsey, tilts and tournaments, and all the magnificent imagery of the same kind that so peculiarly distinguished the reign of Elizabeth, became a very frequent source of permanent hallucination. The historian of Don Quixote adhered strictly to the tenour of his times in representing the library of this most renowned knight as filled with romances of this description, and himself as being permanently crazed by an uninterrupted perusal of them. And that the same morbid effect was not confined to Spain, and was, indeed, common to our own country, we know from the severe but just invectives of Ascham against this class of writings, and his complaints against the disordered turn they had given to the public mind ; and still more from the necessity Shakspeare felt himself under in making all his maniacal characters, whether really or but pretendedly so, deeply versed in the prose or poetical romances of the day, and throwing forth fragments of exquisite force or beauty in the midst of their wildest and most disordered ravings : Lear, Edgar, and the heart-broken Ophelia are in this respect alike gifted, and show to what sources their reading had been directed. Without an attention to these casual glances it is impossible to understand the meaning of the sentiment, and its force or feeling is lost upon us, as in the following burst of Ophelia; which consists of a string of quotations, or allusions to picturesque customs :—

"You must sing *Down-a-down an you call him
- adown-a.* O, how the wheel becomes it ! It is the
false steward that stole his master's daughter."

We have not space for the explanation, but it may be found in the commentators, or in the interesting and elaborate history of " Shakspeare's Times," by my early and valued friend, Dr. Drake.

The ꜱᴇᴄᴏɴᴅ ᴠᴀʀɪᴇᴛʏ of the present species, that of ᴄʀᴀᴄᴋ-ʙʀᴀɪɴᴇᴅ ᴡɪᴛ, is derived rather from the peculiar temperament of the individual than from any particular habit or train of reading ; for, in general, few persons have given themselves less time to read, study, or even think, than those who are possessed by it. It is characterized by high spirits, a sportive and rampant imagination, and a flow of facetious ebullient wit incapable of restraining itself. It is hence often poured forth on most improper occasions, and hesitates not to sacrifice a friend at the shrine of a jest.

There are some persons who possess by nature so perpetual a tide of excitement, that their high spirits seem seldom or never to ebb ; and so irresistible a propensity to this kind of verbal merriment, that no change of circumstances can deprive them of it. Sir Thomas More, who perhaps overflowed with this disposition in a very high degree, is well known to have been facetious on his own scaffold.

It is not always, however, nor, as we have just observed, even for the most part, that the man of ready wit is, like Sir Thomas More, a man of ready judgment or sound learning. The apprehension necessary to constitute the one, is widely different from that necessary to constitute the other, as we had occasion to remark under a former genus : and hence vivacious sallies, taunts, and repartees, not only may co-exist with a deranged condition of mind, but are frequently a result of it. And on this account the court jester of former times, whose office succeeded to that of minstrel, was commonly denominated the king's fool, as uttering, from the unbridled liberty of speech that was allowed him, humorous flashes of rebuke which no man in his sober senses would have ventured upon ; and which seemed, to adopt the language of Jaques, who was himself not unjustly accused of wearing the same livery, to show that-

———— " in his brain,
Which is as dry as the remainder biscuit
After a voyage, he hath strange places cramm'd
With observation, the which he vents
In mangled forms."

The THIRD VARIETY, or ECSTATIC ILLUSION, is also a pleasurable hallucination ; and consists in a sense of false inspiration, or a visionary boast of some preternatural endowment, in the course of which the judgment is so far perverted as to mistake the energetic notions of the imagination for realities ; so that the victim of the delusion believes in apparitions, affects an intercourse with the world of spirits, or lays claim to a power of working miracles.

This morbid afflatus has often been aped by cunning impostors, to serve their own interests with the multitude : and there is no great difficulty in conceiving that it is in many cases a real and serious hallucination, when we reflect on the ease with which such impostors themselves are capable of deluding the populace and working them up into false ecstasies, and especially of inveigling them into a hearty belief of their own miraculous powers. When the passions of men are once set afloat, and the subject presented to them is full of the marvellous and the terrible, they are too apt to confound the false with the real, and are prepared to proceed to whatever extremities the magician may choose to lead them. We are told by Lucian that when Archelaus, a celebrated Greek actor, performed the part of Andromeda in the tragedy of Euripides, several of the spectators were seized with a delirium ; some at the time of performance, others a day or two afterward ; during which they did

nothing but declaim in a theatrical manner, and piteously lament the fate of the persecuted princess. Burton, therefore, has some reason for remarking, that what the impostors before us, or the brain-sick enthusiasts whom they imitate, once broach and set on foot, " be it never so absurd, false, and prodigious, the common people will follow and believe. It will run like murrain in cattle, scab in sheep. Nulla scabies superstitione scabior : as he that is bitten by a mad dog bites others, and all in the end become mad. Either out of affectation of novelty, simplicity, blind zeal, hope, and fear, the giddy-headed multitude will embrace it, and without farther examination approve it."—(Anat. of Melancholy, part iii., sect. iv., l. 3.)

The genuine enthusiast is always possessed of a warm imagination; and generally of a nervous temperament and delicate frame ; and a long series of elevated abstraction on religious subjects, combined with protracted fasting, has ordinarily been the harbinger of the fancied afflatus. Such was the discipline by which the lovely, and blooming, and sincerely devout Saint Teresa was prepared for ecstasies and visions, and led to impose upon herself and all that beheld her ; and seriously to believe, in the fervour of her mind, that her body was lifted from the earth : and that she heard the voice of God, saw our Lord with St. Peter and St. Paul standing on her left hand ; by the first of whom the cross which was at the end of her beads was miraculously transformed into four large gems, incomparably more precious than diamonds ; with many other marvellous revelations, which we cannot find room to detail. Though it should be noticed, that devils appeared to her as well as blessed spirits, whom she always kept at a distance by sprinkling holy water ; and that she was an eyewitness to the joyful escape from the flame of purgatory of the purified souls of Father Peter of Alcantara, Father Ivagnez, and a Carmelite friar.—(Butler's Lives of the Saints, in loco.)

It is not necessary to produce other examples, though many might be brought from our own times. A cure is extremely difficult to be obtained ; and I am afraid that even Mr. Locke's admirable chapter on Enthusiasm would be read to no purpose. In one instance, the enthusiast seems to have been brought home to himself by a pleasant and ingenious stratagem of his superintendent at Venice. This visonary had conceited himself to be Elias, and, like the prophet, had determined upon fasting forty days. The keeper, fearful that he would never hold out, and that he should lose his patient, dressed up a man in the attire of an angel, who was introduced to him in no ordinary manner, and informed him that he was commissioned from Heaven to bring him food. The supposititious Elias took it, was afterward allowed to find out the trick, and thus, at the same time, found out his own imposition upon himself.

From the influence which we have seen such enthusiasts, or even pretended enthusiasts, capable of producing upon the mind of the multitude, when roused by the solemnity and awful ness of the revelations that are supposed to be disclosed to them, we can easily see how FANAT-ICISM, constituting the FOURTH VARIETY of the present species, may obtain an ascendency, and even rage with all the ramifying power of an epidemic : consisting of religious flights of the imagination, predominant over the natural feelings as well as the judgment, excited by the calls or doctrines of those who affect to be preternaturally gifted, or who possess an equal influence over the mind by the high sanction of priesthood, profound learning, or any other respected authority : and often urging to a voluntary and inappropriate submission to severe privations, mortifications, and tortures ; or to the torture and massacre of those who profess different creeds.

Examples, as in the last variety, may be found in every age and religion, but chiefly in times of gross ignorance and barbarism ; where the general mind has been too little informed to distinguish between truth and sophistry, and the passions have been undisciplined to restraint. It is hence of no importance what religion or superstition is to be inculcated ; for those that are true and those that are false have been equally laid hold of by enthusiasts and impostors to produce the same end, and effect the same triumph by means and machinery that could only be furnished from the infernal regions. Hence the blood and raving of the prophets of Baal ; the Curetes or Phrygian priests, and the delirious votaries of the Indian Juggernaut ; the cruel and senseless penances and punishments sustained in many of the convents and nunneries of Lamism, and still more so in those of many Catholic countries. Hence the terrible sufferings of the Waldenses, the furies of St. Bartholomew's day, the fires of Smithfield, and the dark and doleful cells, the whips, and wires, and pincers, and pulleys, and all the infernal paraphernalia of the Inquisition. Hence, in ancient times, the matrons of Canaan and of Carthage were instigated to throw their own children into the flames, and sacrifice them to the gloomy deity whose anger it was held necessary to appease ; and hence, in more modern days, Philip II. of Spain was goaded to impeach a son, of whom he was little worthy, before the Chamber of Inquisitors, to bespeak their condemnation of him, and to take effectual care that he should be poisoned as soon as his sentence had been pronounced.

The cure of these diseases belongs rather to colleges of general instruction than of medicine. Individual cases of enthusiasm and fanaticism have existed, and will probably continue to exist, in all ages ; but when the general mind is well informed, and the social feelings and virtues are duly estimated and widely cultivated, the wildfire will burn in vain, and meet with little or no fuel to support its rage.

SPECIES II.

ALUSIA HYPOCHONDRIAS.

HYPOCHONDRIACISM. LOW SPIRITS.

ɢʟᴏᴏᴍʏ ɪᴅᴇᴀs ᴏғ ʀᴇᴀʟ ʟɪғᴇ ; ᴅᴇᴊᴇᴄᴛᴇᴅ sᴘɪʀɪᴛs ; ᴀɴxɪᴇᴛʏ ; ᴅʏsᴘᴇᴘsʏ ; ʟᴀɴɢᴜɪᴅ ᴘᴜʟsᴇ ; ɪɴᴅɪsᴘᴏsɪᴛɪᴏɴ ᴛᴏ ᴀᴄᴛɪᴠɪᴛʏ ; ᴇʏᴇ ᴏʙʟɪQᴜᴇ ᴀɴᴅ sᴄᴏᴡʟɪɴɢ ; ᴄᴏᴜɴᴛᴇɴᴀɴᴄᴇ sᴀᴅ ᴀɴᴅ sᴜʟʟᴇɴ.

THE term HYPOCHONDRIAS is taken from the anatomical compound hypochondria, to which region the disease was formerly supposed to be altogether confined. Hypochondrias is here used instead of hypochondriasis, the common name, because, as already observed on various occasions, *iasis* as a termination is limited, nearly with this single exception, to denote in the medical vocabulary a peculiar family of cutaneous diseases, as pityriasis, psoriasis, ichthyiasis, and many others. The author has felt the less difficulty in proposing this change, as hypochondriasis is of comparatively modern invention, and is not to be met with in the Greek or Latin writers, by whom the complaint is usually alluded to or described as a species of melancholy, or rather as a disease of the melancholic temperament.

It constitutes the third sort or species of this malady described by Galen, and which he regards as connected with a peculiar state of the stomach ; though, from its mental symptoms, he does not incline to contemplate it, as Diocles, a contemporary physician of reputation, had done in his Book on Gastric Affections, as a simple disease of this organ. The controversy has been in different times continued to our own day ; and it does not seem to be even yet universally settled whether hypochondrias should be regarded as a mental or a dyspeptic malady. M. Esquirol and M. de Villermay (*Traité des Maladies Nerveuses*, &c.) contemplate it in the latter light ; M. Georget (*Sur la Folie—Physiologie du Cerveau*) and M. Falret, though a pupil of M. Esquirol, refer it in every instance to the brain as its primary seat.—(*De l'Hypochondrie et du Suicide*, &c., 8vo., Paris, 1822.) In Pinel the disease seems to be included under *aliénation mentale*, and its different varieties to be distributed, though without particular remark, amid the five species into which he has divided that genus.

The present species bears so near a resemblance to several of the varieties of genuine melancholy as to be often distinguishable from them with great difficulty ; and the more so as it is no uncommon thing for hypochondrias to terminate in melancholy, or for melancholy to be combined with hypochondrias.—(*Falret, de l'Hypochondrie*, &c., ut suprà, passim.) Both may be the result of a predisposing constitution, or may be primarily induced by accidental causes where no such constitution exists : and the predisposition and the accidental causes of the one may become those of the other : for the temperament known by the common name of melancholic, and characterized by a lean and dry corporeal texture, small and rigid muscles, a sallow skin, brownish-yellow complexion, little relieved by redness of any kind, deep-black and coarse hair, eyes sunk in hollow sockets, large prominent veins, especially in the hands and arms, with a tendency to solitude and private musing, is a common precursor of both. And, in like manner, a sedentary life of any kind, and especially severe study protracted to a late hour in the night, and rarely relieved by social intercourse, exercise, or nugatory amusements; a debauched and dissolute habit, or excesses in eating and drinking, may become causes of either of these maladies, from accessory circumstances that cannot be traced out even where the predisponent temperament does not seem to exist. But it is very justly observed by Sir A. Crichton, that, even in those "whose health is much deranged, true melancholy seldom arises, except mental causes of grief and distress join themselves to the corporeal ones: and this constitutes one of the characters which distinguish *melancholia vera* from hypochondriasis. The former may be said to be always excited by mental causes, and consists in various phenomena of grief, despondency, and despair; whereas the latter most commonly arises from corporeal causes, and its mental phenomena consist of erroneous ideas entertained about the patient's own make or body."—(*Of Mental Derangement*, vol. iii., p. 235.)

The corporeal causes are usually a diseased condition of one or more of the digestive organs, and especially, as we shall presently have to observe, a displacement of some part of the colon. It is also not unfrequently a result of the sudden cessation of some periodical or other habitual discharge, as that, of an issue, or of a hemorrhoidal flux, a chronic ulcer, or some external eruption.

The melancholy man seldom lives long, and his disorder often commences in the meridian of life. He frequently terminates his days by violence, or, at the utmost, never attains old age. The hypochondriac seldom becomes affected till after the meridian of life, and very generally continues to the stage of longevity.

The common corporeal symptoms are, a troublesome flatulence in the stomach or bowels, acrid eructations, costiveness, a copious discharge of pale urine, spasmodic pains in the head and other parts of the body, giddiness, dimness of sight, palpitations, general sleeplessness, and an utter inability of fixing the attention upon any subject of importance, or engaging in any thing that demands vigour or courage. The mental feelings and peculiar trains of ideas that haunt the imagination and overwhelm the judgment exhibit an infinite diversity, and lay a foundation for the three following varieties:—

    a Antalgica.   Vapours.
    β Pertæsa.   Weariness of life.
    γ Misanthropica. Misanthropy. Spleen.

In the FIRST VARIETY, which is commonly distinguished by the name of VAPOURS, or LOW SPIRITS, the patient is tormented with a visionary or exaggerated sense of pains or some concealed disease; a whimsical dislike of particular persons, places, or things; or groundless apprehensions of personal danger or poverty.

Greding gives an account of a medical practitioner who applied to him for assistance, under an impression that his stomach was filled with frogs, which had been successively spawning ever since he had bathed, when a boy, in a pool

in which he had perceived a few tadpoles. He had spent his life in trying to expel this imaginary evil, and had travelled to numerous places to consult the first physicians of the day upon his obstinate malady. It was in vain to attempt convincing him that the gurglings or borborygmi he heard were from extricated and erratic wind. "He argued himself," says M. Greding, "into a great passion in my presence, and asked me if I did not hear the frogs croak."

I have under my care a hypochondriac of about fifty years of age, who affords a sufficient proof that Molière drew his Malade Imaginaire from nature, and hardly added an exaggerating touch. His profession is that of the law; his life has been uniformly regular, but far too sedentary and studious. Without having any one clearly-marked corporeal affection, he is constantly dreading every disease in the bills of mortality, and complaining, one after another, of every organ in his body, to each of which he points in succession as its seat: especially the head, the heart, and the testes. He now suspects he is going to have a cataract, and now frightens himself with an apprehension of an involuntary seminal emission. It is rarely that I have left him half an hour but I have a note to inform me of some symptom he had forgotten to mention, and I have often five or six of these in the course of the day. The last was to state that, shortly after my visit, he had a discharge of three drops of blood from the nose—a change which he thought of great importance, and requiring immediate attention. His imaginary symptoms, however, soon disappear, provided they are listened to with gravity and pretended to be prescribed for; but not otherwise. Yet, in disappearing, they merely yield to others that can only be surmounted in like manner. His head is too much confused to allow him to engage in any serious study, even if it were prudent to recommend it to him: but on all common subjects he is perfectly clear, and will converse with shrewdness and a considerable extent of knowledge. His bowels are sluggish; his appetite not good, though he eats sufficiently; his sleep is unquiet, but he has enough of it without opiates; his pulse is variable, sometimes hurrying on abruptly, and without any obvious cause, to a hundred strokes in a minute, but often very little quicker than in a state of health. His tongue varies equally, and is irregularly clean, milky, and brownish, and then suddenly clean again. He is irritable in his temper, though he labours to be calm; and is so rooted to his chamber that it is difficult to drag him from it. He has now been ill about ten weeks; but it is during the winter, and the season is too severe and inclement for him to venture abroad. I look forward to his restoration in the spring from exercise, change of air, and a course of tonic medicines. I have not found him complain of *dysphagia globosa*, or that sense of suffocation from the feeling of a constricting ball in the throat which is so common to hysteric patients, and which, from its being often also traced in the present disease, has been called by Pechlin *suffocatio hypochondriaca* (Lib. i., obs.

31); but his spirits are in a state of almost perpetual depression.

A superficial and injudicious perusal of medical books addressed to those who are not of the profession has been a frequent source. of this affection. M. Villermay distinctly states as one 'of its causes among his own countrymen 'a "lecture habituelle de Buchan." Rousseau admitted that this was a powerful cause of hypochondrias in 'respect to himself. "Having read," says he, " a little on physiology, I set about studying anatomy; and passing in review the number and varied actions of the parts which compose my frame, I expected twenty times a day to feel them going wrong. Far from being astonished at finding myself dying,'my astonishment was that I could live at all. I did not read the description of any disease which I did not imagine myself to be affected with; and I am sure that, if I had not been ill, I must have become so from this fatal study. Finding in every complaint the symptoms of my own, I believed I had got them all, and thereby added another still more intolerable—the fancy of curing myself."

The whims that are sometimes seriously entertained under this variety of the disease are so truly ludicrous, that "to be grave exceeds all power of face." One thinks himself a giant, another a dwarf; one is as ,heavy as lead, another as light as a feather. Marcellus Donatus makes mention of a baker of Ferrara who thought himself a lump of butter, and durst not sit in the sun nor come near the fire for fear of being melted. They are all extremely timid, and their fears are exercised upon trifles, or are altogether groundless. Some suspect their nearest and dearest friends of designing to poison them : others dare not be alone in the dark lest they should be attacked with ghosts or hobgoblins. They dare not go over a bridge, or near a pool, rock, or steep hill, lest they should be tempted to hang, drown, or precipitate themselves : and, if they come to a place where a robbery or a murder has been committed, they instantly fear they are suspected. Trincavellius had a patient that for three years together could not be persuaded but that he had killed a man, and at length sunk into a confirmed melancholy, and made away with himself for fear of the gallows.—(*Consil.*, xiii., lib. i.)

It is a melancholy reflection that the wisest and best of mankind are as open to this affliction as the weakest, and, perhaps, more so. Pascal himself was at one time so hallucinated with hypochondriacism as to believe that he was always on the verge of an abyss into which he was in danger of falling. And, under the influence of this terror, he would never sit down till a chair was placed on that side of him on which he thought he saw it, and thus proved the floor to be substantial.

It is frequently induced by too free a use of spirituous liquors, the stomach and other digestive organs being hereby debilitated and almost paralyzed; and, where this is the case, the disease is apt to terminate in that exhausted state of the nervous system generally, and delirious condition of the brain, which by some writers has been called delirium *tremens ;* in which the mind and body exhibit equal feebleness, combined with a high degree of irritability, and the patient often falls a sacrifice in a few days ; previous to which he is worn out with convulsive struggles, succeeded by a cold and general perspiration ; the pulse increases in rapidity and becomes thready, and the twitching of the tendons subsides into à tremour that spreads over the whole body ; the countenance is pale and anxious, the patient mutters with incessant rapidity, and the DELIRIUM is constant, though easily interrupted by questions addressed to him. In one case, says Mr. Blake, who has given a good description of the complaint, the mind was so diseased that the patient, after being desired to put out his tongue, continued for nearly half an hour to push it out and draw it in alternately in quick succession, whenever I looked towards him.—(*Edin. Med. and Surg. Journ.*, Oct., 1823, p. 501.) If, before this extremity takes place, a sound and refreshing sleep creep gradually over the frame, the irritability subsides, a healthful quiescence succeeds to general commotion, and the mind and the body become by degrees reinvigorated.

Under the SECOND VARIETY we meet with a totally distinct set of morbid feelings and ideas ; for the patient is here oppressed with a general listlessness and disgust ; an irksomeness and weariness of life, often without any specific reason whatever. This is the melancholia *Anglica* of Sauvages, who describes it as common to our own countrymen ; under the attack of which, says he, "languid, sorrowful, tired of remedies of every kind, they settle their affairs, make their wills, take leave of their friends by letters, and then put an end to their lives by hanging, poison, or some other means :. exhibiting a wish to die, not from insanity or severe grief, but tranquilly, from a mere tædium vitæ, or irksomeness of existence." This may occasionally be the case ; but by far the greater number of suicides in our own country proceed, not from hypochondriacism, but a despondency produced by real losses ; and belong, therefore, as I have already observed, to the genus empathema. Yet this miserable upshot occurs in a few instances from the feeling, or rather the want of feeling, here assigned ;' the perpetrators of the horrid deed being generally those who, having been actively engaged in the heyday and meridian of

---

* Delirium tremens is unfortunately very frequent in the United States. American practitioners have paid great attention to it, and have written many valuable treatises upon its nature and treatment. Our limits will not permit even an abstract of them. We would, however, refer the reader to a learned article by Dr. Coates, in the N. A. Med. and Surg. Journal, vol. v. ; to Dr. Brown's Essay in the Am. Med. Recorder, vol. v. ; to the communications of Dr. Drake and Dr. Klapp, in the first and second volumes of the same journal, and to a treatise on the same subject by Dr. John Ware, of Boston. Baron Dupuytren also has described the same disease in the first volume of his Clinical Lectures on Surgery, under the term nervous delirium.—D.

life, have retired upon their fortunes with a view of enjoying them in quiet, but who unhappily find themselves fitted for any thing rather than for quiet; who have no taste for reading, reflection, or domestic tranquillity, and are too proud to return to the bustle of the world and the excitement of nicely-balanced speculations. There is here a want of the habitual stimulus to a production of sensorial power; in consequence of which the individual sinks' into a state of low spirits, and becomes unhappy. A like issue frequently follows upon a life devoted to all the pursuits of sensual gratification, in the course of which the individual has exhausted his stock of enjoyments, and worn out his powers of body and mind before he has reached little more than the midway of his existence. Every thing now palls upon his senses, and he has neither taste nor energy to engage in more rational pursuits. " A ride out in the morning, and a warm parlour and a pack of cards in the afternoon, are all that life affords," said a patient of Dr. Darwins to him, a man of polished manners about fifty years of age. He got tired of these in a few months, and having no other resource, shot himself.—(*Zoonom.*, vol. iv., p. 90, edit. 8vo.)

Burton has well described the state of mind of many that are tormented with this most wretched malady (*Anatomy of Melanch.*, part i., sect. iii., i., 2), but still more so those affected with the THIRD VARIETY, which is strikingly accompanied with peevishness, general malevolence, and an abhorrence of mankind. " They are soon tired with all things : they will now tarry, now be gone ; now in bed, they will rise; now up, then go to bed ; now pleased, and then again displeased ; now they like, by-and-by dislike all, weary of all : sequitur nunc vivendi nunc moriendi cupido, saith Aurelianus (lib. i., cap. vi.) ; discontented, disquieted ; upon every light occasion or no occasion object ; often tempted to make away with themselves ; they cannot die, they will not live ; they complain, weep, lament, and think they lead a most miserable life : never was any man so bad. Every poor man they see is most fortunate in respect of them; every beggar that comes to the door is happier than they are ; jealousy and suspicion are common symptoms in the misanthropic variety. They are testy, pettish, peevish, distrustful, apt to mistake, and ready to snarl upon every occasion and without any cause with their dearest friends. If they speak in jest, the hypochondriac takes it in good earnest : if the smallest ceremony be accidentally omitted, he is wounded to the quick. Every tale, discourse, whisper, or gesture he applies to himself : or, if the conversation be openly addressed to him, he is ready to misconstrue every word, and cannot endure that any man should look steadfastly at him, laugh, point the finger, cough, or sneeze. Every question or movement works upon him, and is misinterpreted, and makes him alternately turn pale and red, and even sweat with distrust, fear, or anger."

As in this species the body is more affected than in any other division of mental alienation, more may often be accomplished by MEDICINE ; though we must by no means be inattentive to moral discipline. The skin is very frequently cold and without a free secretion, and hence general friction, with rubefacients and the warmer diaphoretics, have often been found serviceable. The digestive organs are almost always torpid, and several of them, especially the stomach and liver, secrete their respective fluids not only in too small a quantity, but of an unhealthy quality, so as to be too viscid, too dilute, or morbidly stimulant. Some kind of acrimony, indeed, is almost always found in the stomach, and particularly that of acidity. And hence aperients, carminatives, and particularly the tonic plan which has already been recommended under LIMOSIS *Dyspepsia*, are manifestly called for, and will often be found serviceable.

Post-obit examinations have also frequently pointed out another local cause, which otherwise we should little expect : and that is, a displacement of the transverse colon.* M. Pinel, as we have already observed, regards this as a very common cause of insanity in all its forms : but there can be no question that it is a powerful and ready cause of the present species of mental alienation. M. Esquirol, who has found it as frequently as M. Pinel, tells us that this displacement sometimes consists in an oblique, and sometimes in a perpendicular direction of the intestine, so that its sinister extremity lies behind the pubes ; while it has sometimes descended into the form of an inverted aorta even below the pubes and into the pelvis. No disease of the organization has been found in any instance, and hence the change of place must proceed from relaxation and debility alone where the misposition is not connate; on which account it may in some instances be an effect, as it is certainly a cause in others. It is under these circumstances that we chiefly meet with that pain in the epigastrium to which we have already adverted, and which gives the feeling of a tight cord surrounding the body in the line of distress ; and when such a symptom, therefore, occurs, we have reason to suspect the cause of the disease to be produced by some derangement of the colon in respect to position. Under the operation of such a cause, the art of medicine can do but little ; temporary ease, however, may be obtained by the pressure of a belt broad enough to support the whole of the lower belly ; and it is possible that the intestine may gradually right itself under a course of the warmer tonics, as columbo, canella alba, and cassum-muniar, or lose its morbid irritability by habit. But these are rare terminations; for more generally the

* The facts in support of this doctrine have not been so numerous in this country as in France ; and its correctness has even been doubted. In Paris, however, the opportunities of dissecting the bodies of insane persons have been for many years much greater than in London ; and when we find such authorities as MM. Pinel and Esquirol attesting, by recorded dissections, the truth of the cause here assigned for the present species of mental alienation, the fact, in relation to the natives of France, must at all events be admitted. —ED.

displacement increases, and the disease itself gains ground and becomes more incurable.

Congestions from weakness of vascular action in one or more of the abdominal viscera are a frequent result of the present complaint, and not unfrequently a primary cause ; and hence we may see why the bleeding piles should be serviceable in so many instances as to obtain from Alberti the name of *medicina hypochondriacorum* (*Dissert. de Hæmorrhoidibus*, Halle, 1716), and why leeches repeatedly applied to the anus, as recommended by Schoenheyder, should often have a like beneficial effect.—(*Act: Soc. Med. Hafn.*, ii., p. 313.) This is of the greatest importance where the disease has been preceded by a periodical flow of blood from the hemorrhoidal veins, and should point out to us the necessity of renewing any other discharge or external irritation to which the system may have been accustomed.

Opium is a very doubtful medicine, though strongly recommended by Deidier and other respectable writers, and readily had recourse to by hypochondriacs themselves to relieve their distressful sensations. Dr. Cullen asserts peremptorily that he has always found a frequent ruse of opiates pernicious in hypochondriacs (*Mat. Med.*, vol. ii., p. 245, edit. 4to.) ; and, in many instances in which I have myself been tempted to employ it, I have been compelled to withhold its further use from its doing more mischief than good. It has often in such cases been exchanged for other sedatives, but rarely with any decided advantage.

Exercise of all kinds should be encouraged in every modification of the disease, but especially exercise on horseback, though it is seldom, in the first and third varieties, we can succeed in getting a patient to try it. The diet should be governed by the principles already laid down for treating indigestion.

In the MORAL MANAGEMENT, assiduous kindness and consoling conversation produce a deeper effect than they seem to do. Loquacity is always hurtful ; but a talent for cheerful discourse, intermixed with interesting and amusing anecdotes, frequently draws away the patient's attention from himself, and becomes a most useful palliative. In the autalgic variety, in which he is perpetually haunted with a feeling of some dreadful disease which exists nowhere but in his own fancy, the hallucination, when we possess his confidence, should be removed by a candid statement of the fact, and, if necessary, friendly expostulation : but the moment we find the prepossession is too strong to be removed by argument, it is better to humour the conceit, and to pretend to prescribe for it. It is sometimes necessary, indeed, for the hypochondriac is often possessed of great cunning, to drop all pretensions whatever, and to put him in good earnest upon a course of medicines for a disease we know he is as free from as ourselves. Thus a firm belief that he has an inveterate itch is a common delusion with a patient of this kind, and it will be often found impossible to persuade him that he is cured till his whole body has been repeatedly rubbed over with sulphur or

hellebore ointment. I had lately under my care a special pleader of considerable eminence, who in the course of this affection would have it that he had the pox. I at first argued the point with him day after day, but to no purpose ; he felt certain that he should never be well till he was not only salivated, but had used tonic injections for a gleet which he said accompanied it, though he had no discharge whatever. It was in vain to deceive him by supposititious medicines ; for he was a man of considerable learning, and well acquainted with medical preparations ; and I hence allowed him his heart's desire : he rubbed in mercurial ointment every night, and for an injection used a solution of zinc. In a week he persuaded himself he was well, and begged permission to desist from a farther use of the remedies ; a permission which was readily granted him.

In the second variety, or tædium vitæ, where the time seems to hang intolerably heavy on the patient's hands from his having, in a mistaken search after happiness, relinquished a life of constant excitement and activity for the fancied delights of rural retirement and quiet, the best and most radical cure would be a return to the situation that has been so unfortunately abandoned ; but if this cannot be accomplished, the patient must be put into a train of pursuits of some other kind. If he be fond of the sports of the country, he should weary himself in the daytime with hunting or shooting, or even horse-racing, rather than be hypochondriacal from idleness ; and spend his evenings in the bustle of dinner-parties or cards. And if he be capacitated for higher and more useful occupations, let him plunge headlong into the public concerns of the parish and its neighbourhood, become a member of its select vestries, a trustee of the highways, or a magistrate of the district. The habit of excitement must for some time be maintained, though it be afterward let down by degrees : and the intermediate steps are of no great importance, so far as they answer their purpose. We are not at present arguing the case upon a principle of ethics or of religion, but merely upon a principle of moral medicine. Yet I have often known persons of the above description broken in by degrees to a love of domestic quiet for which they were by no means fitted when they first entered upon it ; and who, with a love of domestic quiet, have settled also, as a more sober stage of life has advanced, and reflection has gained ground upon them, into a love of strict moral order, and the higher duties of a conscientious Christian, to which one time they seemed as little disposed.*

* The following remarks by Dr. Conolly are exceedingly just :—" So many hypochondriacal persons are known to be at large who entertain strange opinions concerning their own form and nature, that it seems hardly necessary to caution the practitioner against treating such patients as madmen are commonly treated. That the mind of these individuals is impaired, is unquestionable ; but the character of the impairment is not dangerous. Yet when there is much anxiety to get rid of a troublesome member of a family, very great stress is laid on these fancies, to which,

GENUS IV.
APHELXIA.
REVERY.

INACTIVITY OF THE ATTENTION TO THE IMPRES-
SIONS OF SURROUNDING OBJECTS DURING
WAKEFULNESS.

APHELXIA is derived from ἀφίλκω, "abstraho,
retraho, avoco, abduco ;" and is in use among
the Greek writers.

The subject is almost, if not altogether, new
to nosology, and has seldom been dipped into by
physiologists. Dr. Darwin occasionally touches
upon it in various parts of his "Zoonomia," and
Dr. Crichton in his "Inquiry into the Nature
of Mental Derangement;" and it is well described and illustrated by La Bruyère in his
"Characters :" but it yet remains to be analyzed, and reduced to a nosological method, and
examined in a pathological view. A few leading ideas on this subject have already been
thrown out by the author, in his comment upon
the present definition in the volume of Nosology ; and of these he will avail himself in treating of it more at large.

In order to our becoming acquainted with the
existence of surrounding objects, or of an external world, as it is called by psychologists, three
things are necessary : sound external senses ;
a secretion of the nervous fluid (or, as it might
be perhaps more correctly expressed, a due
maintenance of the nervous and sensorial energy), apparently under different modifications,
whereby they are made capable of being roused
or excited by the different objects addressed to
them ; and an exercise of the faculty of attention to the impressions which are thus produced.
The will has, or ought to have, a power of calling this, as well as every other faculty of the
mind, into a state of exertion, or of allowing it
to be indolent ; and it is chiefly upon this want
of power, or the same power intensely exerted,
that the phenomenon of revery depends; thus
giving rise to the three following species of mental aberration :—

1. Aphelxia Socors.   Absence of Mind.
2. ———— Intenta.   Abstraction of Mind.
3. ———— Otiosa.   Brown-study.

In the first of these the attention is truant,
and does not yield readily to the dictates of the
will : in the second it is riveted, at the instiga-
tion of the will itself, to some particular theme
unconnected with surrounding objects : and in
the third it has the consent of the will to relax
itself, and give play to whatever trains of ideas
are uppermost or most vivacious in the sensory.

SPECIES I.
APHELXIA SOCORS.
ABSENCE OF MIND.

TRUANT ATTENTION ; WANDERING FANCY ; VA-
CANT OR VACILLATING COUNTENANCE.

THIS is an absence, or vacuity of mind, too

common at schools and at church ; over tasks
and sermons ; and there are few readers who
have not frequently been sensible of it in some
degree or other.

In reading books in which we are totally un-
interested, composed in a tedious and repulsive
style, we are almost continually immersed in
this species of revery. The will does not exert its power : the attention is suffered to wander to something of stronger attraction ; or the
imagination is left to the play of its own nugatory ideas ; and though we continue to read,
we have not the smallest knowledge of the argument before us ; and if the subject to which
the train of our thoughts is really directed be
of a strikingly ludicrous character, we may possibly burst into a laugh in the middle of a discourse of great gravity and seriousness, to the
astonishment of those around us.

This is a common case, and may lead to great
embarrassment. We have nevertheless thus far
supposed that the will does not exert its power,
and sufficiently rein in the attention to the subject addressed to it. It not unfrequently happens, however, that the will, for want of a proper
habit, has lost its power, either wholly or in a
very great degree, and cannot, with its utmost
energy, exercise a due control over the attention ; and it also happens in other cases, from a
peculiarity of temperament or morbid state of
body, that the faculty of the attention itself is
so feeble, that it is incapable of being steadily
directed for more than a few minutes to any object of importance whatever, with all the effort
of the will to give it such direction.

The mind, under either of these conditions,
is in a deplorable state for all the higher purposes of reflection and knowledge for which by
its nature it is intended ; since it is upon the
faculty of attention that every other faculty is
dependant for its vigour and expansion : without
it the perception exercises itself in vain ; the
memory can lay up no store of ideas ; the judgment draw forth no comparisons ; the imagination must become blighted and barren ; and
where there is no attention whatever, the case
must necessarily verge upon fatuity.

In early life, the attention, like every other
faculty of the mind, is weak and wandering, is
often caught with difficulty, and rarely fixed upon
any thing. Like every other faculty, however,
it is capable of being strengthened and concentrated ; and may be made to dwell upon almost
any object proposed. But this is a work of time,
and forms one of the most important parts of
education ; and, in the course of this discipline,
it should not be forgotten that the faculty of attention, when it first shows itself, is more readily
arrested by some subjects than by others, and
that it is hence of great moment to ascertain
those subjects, and to select them in the first
instance. The habit is what is chiefly wanted ;
and the quicker this is acquired, the more time
we gain for transferring the same habit to other
and perhaps more valuable purposes afterward.

This is a point seldom sufficiently considered
in the course of education ; and, for want of
such consideration, far more than half the time

_taken by themselves, the practitioner must not
attach great importance."—See Inquiry concerning the Indications of Insanity, p. 405.—ED._

of many boys becomes an entire blank, and is lost ; and not a few suffered to remain block-heads in the particular department to which their hours of study are directed, who might discover a considerable capacity and genius if the de-partment were changed for one more adapted to their own taste, or, in other words, more attract-ive to their attention.

There is a very singular instance of habitual absence of mind related by Sir A. Crichton in a young patient under the care of Dr. Pitcairn and himself, which, though some other circum-stances appeared to have combined with it, is ascribed considerably to the error of education we are now speaking of, that of not duly study-ing the peculiar bent of a mind in many respects singularly constituted, and drawing forth and strengthening the faculty of attention, which was in an especial degree weak and truant, by an employment of such objects and pursuits as were most alluring. This patient was a young gentle-man of large fortune, who, till the age of twenty-one (and he does not seem to have been much more at the time of describing his case), had en-joyed a tolerable share of health, though of a deli-cate frame. In his disposition he was gentle and calm, but somewhat unsociable. His absence of mind was extreme, and he would sometimes willingly sit for a whole day without moving. Yet he had nothing of melancholy belonging to him ; and it was easy to discover by his coun-tenance that a multiplicity of thoughts were con-stantly succeeding each other in his imagination, many of which were gay and cheerful ; for he would heartily laugh at times, not with an un-meaning countenance, but evidently from mental merriment. He was occasionally so strangely inattentive, that, when pushed by some want which he wished to express, if he had begun a sentence, he would suddenly stop short after getting half way through it, as though he had forgotten what else he had to say. Yet, when his attention was roused and he was induced to speak, he always expressed himself in good lan-guage and with much propriety ; and if a ques-tion were proposed to him which required the exercise of judgment, and he could be made to attend to it, he judged correctly. It was with difficulty he could be made to take any exercise ; but was at length prevailed upon to drive his curricle, in which Sir Alexander at times accom-panied him. He at first could not be prevailed upon to go beyond half a mile ; but in succeed-ing attempts he consented to go farther. He drove steadily, and when about to pass a carriage, took pains to avoid it : but when at last he be-came familiarized with this exercise, he would often relapse into thought, and allow the reins to hang loose in his hands. His ideas seemed to be for ever varying. When any thing came across his mind which excited anger, the horses suffered for it ; but the spirit they exhibited at such an unusual and unkind treatment made him soon desist, and re-excited his attention to his own safety. As soon as they were quieted, he would relapse into thought : if his ideas were melancholy, the horses were allowed to walk slow ; if they were gay and cheerful, they were

Vol. II.—O

generally encouraged to go fast.—(Of Mental Derangement, vol. i., p. 281.)

Perhaps, in this case, something might have been owing, as supposed by Sir A. Crichton, to an error in the mode of education ; but the chief defect seems to have been in the attentive fac-ulty itself, and its labouring under a natural im-becility, which no mode of education could en-tirely have removed. We have had frequent occasions to observe that the powers of the mind vary in different individuals as much as those of the body : and we have already offered exam-ples of weak or diseased judgment, weak or diseased perception, and weak or vehement im-agination. In the case before us, the mental dis-ease seems to have been chiefly confined to the faculty of attention ; and we shall presently have to notice a similar imbecility of the memory, and even of all the mental faculties conjointly.[*]

SPECIES II.
APHELXIA INTENTA.
ABSTRACTION OF MIND.

THE ATTENTION WOUND UP AND RIVETED TO A PARTICULAR SUBJECT ; WITH SYMPATHETIC EMOTION OF THE MUSCLES AND FEATURES CONNECTED WITH ITS GENERAL DRIFT.

In this species the faculty of attention, in-stead of being feeble or contumacious to the will, is peculiarly strong, and vehemently ex-cited, and acts in perfect co-operation with the will itself. And in many instances the senso-rial energy maintained is so great, and demands so large a supply of sensorial power, as appa-rently to exhaust the entire stock, except, in-deed, the reserve which is in almost all cases instinctively kept back for the use of the vital or involuntary organs. And hence all the ex-ternal senses remain in a state of torpor, as though drawn upon for their respective contri-butions of sensorial power in support of the pre-dominant meditation : so that the eyes do not see, nor the ears hear, nor does the flesh feel ; and the muser may be spoken to, or conversa-tion may take place around him, or he may even be struck upon the shoulders, without any knowl-edge of what is occurring.

Abstraction of mind may be produced by va-rious causes, but the following are the chief, and form two distinct varieties :—

α Aphelxia a pathe-　From some overwhelm-
　　mate.　　　　　　　ing passion.
β Aphelxia a studio.　From intense study.

Of THE FIRST VARIETY we have already of-fered abundant examples in the two preceding

* The absent man cannot spread his attention over many things at once : it is concentrated on one subject, or one train of thought ; and the most trivial thoughts are sufficient for its exclusive oc-cupation. He therefore commits a thousand ex-travagances ; puts on his friend's hat ; loses his way in his native town ; goes to bed in the mid-dle of the day, because he finds himself in his bed-room ; or forgets his own name when he knocks at a person's door.—See Conolly on Insanity, p. 121.—ED.

genera : and especially in the cases of ungovernable joy or rapture, grief and despondency ; under the influence of which the affected person is often as much lost to the world around him, as if he were in a profound sleep and dreaming ; and only hears, sees, and feels the vivid train of ideas that possess themselves of his mind, and rule it as a captured citadel. To these alone the attention is directed ; here it exhausts all its power, and the will concurs in the exhaustion ; insomuch that the patient is said in some cases to have stared at the meridian sun without pain (*Blumenb.*, bibl. i., p. 736) ; and in others to have been undisturbed by the discharge of a cannon.—(*Darwin, Zoonomia*, iii., i., ii., 2.)

We meet with like proofs of this variety of revery in many cases of intense study, and especially upon abstract subjects, as those of pure mathematics, in which all the reasoning and more serious faculties of the mind, as the perception, the memory, and the judgment, as well as the attention, are jointly called into action, and kept equally upon the stretch. Of the power of this variety of revery in rendering an individual torpid and almost dead to all around him, we have a decided instance in Archimedes at the time of his arrest. When the Roman army had at length taken Syracuse by stratagem, which the tactics of this consummate engineer prevented them from taking by force, he was shut up in his closet, and so intent on a geometrical demonstration, that he was equally insensible to the shouts of the victors and the outcries of the vanquished. He was calmly drawing the lines of a diagram when a soldier abruptly entered his room, and clapped a sword to his throat. "Hold, friend," said Archimedes, "one moment, and my demonstration will be finished." The soldier, surprised at his unconcern at a time of such extreme peril, resolved to carry him before Marcellus ; but as the philosopher put under his arm a small box full of spheres, dials, and other instruments, the soldier, conceiving the box to be filled with gold, could not resist the temptation, but killed him on the spot.*

SPECIES III
APHELXIA OTIOSA.
BROWN-STUDY.

LEISURELY LISTLESSNESS ; VOLUNTARY SURRENDER OF THE ATTENTION AND THE JUDGMENT TO THE SPORTIVE VAGARIES OF THE IMAGINATION ; QUIESCENT MUSCLES ; IDLE GRAVITY OF COUNTENANCE.

THE attention is equally summoned into action and dismissed at the command of the will. It is summoned in the last species : it is dismissed when a man voluntarily surrenders himself to ease and listlessness of mind ; during which period, moreover, in consequence of this indulgence in general indolence, the external senses unite in the mental quiescence, and a smaller portion of nervous energy is probably generated, for the very reason that a smaller portion is demanded ; and hence the active senses without are as vacant and unstrung as the active senses within, and as blunted to their respective stimuli. The first playful ideas that float over the fancy in this case take the lead, and the mind relaxes itself with their easy and sportive flow. It is the *studium inane* of Darwin (*Zoonom.*, iii., i., ii., 2 ; and again, iv., ii., iv., 2), who seems, however, to have in some degree misapplied the name, or to have confounded the aberration with that of ecphronia or alusia. Cowper has admirably described it in the following verses :—

"Laugh, ye who boast your more mercurial
          powers,
That never feel a stupor, know no pause
Nor need one : I am conscious, and confess,
Fearless, a soul that does not always think.
Me oft has fancy, ludicrous and wild,
Soothed with a waking dream of houses, towers,
Trees, churches, and strange visages, express'd
In the red cinders, while with poring eye
I gazed, myself creating what I saw.
Nor less amused have I quiescent watch'd
The sooty films that play upon the bars
Pendulous, and foreboding in the view
Of superstition, prophesying still,   [proach.
Though still deceived, some stranger's near ap-
'Tis thus the understanding takes repose
In indolent vacuity of thought,
And sleeps and is refresh'd. Meanwhile the face
Conceals the mood lethargic with a mask
Of deep deliberation, as the man
Were task'd to his full strength, absorb'd and
          lost."

In the indolent mind such indulgence is a disease ; and, if not studiously watched and opposed, will easily become a habit. In the studious and active mind it is a wholesome relaxation ; the sensory, in the correct language of the poet, "sleeps and is refreshed," grows fertile beneath the salutary fallow, and prepares itself for new harvests.

This is more particularly the case where, in conjunction with an attention "screwed up to the sticking-place," and long continued there, a spirit of ardent emulation is at the same time stirring, and distracted between the hope and fear of gaining or losing a distinguished honour or reward. I have seen this repeatedly in young men who have been striving night and day, and week after week, for the first prizes of our English universities ; some of whom have indeed succeeded, but with a hectic exhaustion that has been recovered from with great difficulty ; while others, in the full prospect of success, have been compelled to relinquish the pursuit, and to degrade.

---

* If the attention be much engrossed by one object, it is necessarily withdrawn from others ; and although readily transferred in general from one set of objects and ideas to another set of objects and ideas, it is sometimes so tenacious of one set as to refuse, as it were, to turn to a succession. We read that when Sir Joshua Reynolds, after being many hours occupied in painting, walked out into the street, the lamp-posts seemed to him to be trees, and the men and women moving shrubs.— See Dr. Conolly's Inquiry concerning the Indica tions of Insanity, p. 119.—ED.

· Yet even without this conflict of feeling, where the attention alone has been too long directed to one or to a variety of recondite subjects without relaxation, the mind suffers considerably, and its powers become shaken and confused ; of which we have an interesting example in the case of Mr. Spalding, a scholar of considerable eminence in Germany, as drawn by himself, and communicated to the editors of the Psychological Magazine.—(*Crichton's Inquiry into Mental Derangement*, i., 237.) His attention, he tells us, had been long kept upon the stretch, and had been still more distracted by being continually shifted from one subject to another, when, being called upon to write a receipt for money paid him on account of the poor, as soon as he had written the two first words, he found himself incapable of proceeding farther. He strove all he could, and strained his attention to the utmost, but to no purpose ; he knew the characters he continued to make were not those he wished to write, but could not discover where the fault lay. He then desisted, and partly by broken words and syllables, and partly by gestures, made the person who waited for the receipt understand that he should leave him. For about half an hour a tumultuary disorder reigned in his senses, so that he was incapable of remarking any thing very particular, except that one series of ideas of a trifling nature, and confusedly intermixed, forced themselves involuntarily on his mind. At the same time his external senses continued perfect, and he saw and knew every thing around him. His speech, however, failed in the same manner as his power of writing, and he perceived that he spoke other words than those he intended. In less than an hour he recovered himself from this confusion, and felt nothing but a slight headache. On examining the receipt on which the aberration first betrayed itself, he found that, instead of the words "fifty dollars, being one half-year's rate," he had written "fifty dollars, through the salvation of Bra—" the last word being left unfinished, and without his having the least recollection of what it was intended to be. /

GENUS V.

PARONIRIA.

SLEEP DISTURBANCE.

THE VOLUNTARY ORGANS CONNECTED WITH THE PASSING TRAIN OF IDEAS OVERPOWERED BY THE FORCE OF THE IMAGINATION DURING DREAMING, AND INVOLUNTARILY EXCITED TO THEIR NATURAL OR ACCUSTOMED ACTIONS ; WHILE THE OTHER ORGANS REMAIN ASLEEP.

PARONIRIA, from παρὰ and ὄνειρον, signifies "depraved, disturbed, or morbid dreaming." So in Dioscorides (vol. ii., p. 127), δυσόνειρος signifies "tumultuosis et malis somniis molestans." In treating of the genus EPHIALTES, or nightmare (Vol. i., Cl. I., Ord. II., Gen. V.), I endeavoured to explain its course and nature ; and hereby pointed out the essential distinction which exists between that disease and the present, and the impropriety of uniting the species which belong to both of them under one head, as Dr. Cullen has done in his genus oneirodynia ; since, with the exception of their occurring in the night, and during sleep, and therefore involuntarily, they have little or no connexion or resemblance, in cause, symptoms, or even mode of cure.

The three following species are so clearly and decidedly of one and the same family, as to prevent all dispute in their present position. They are here. however, associated for the first time in a genus distinct from ephialtes.

1. Paroniria Ambulans.   Sleep-walking
2. ————— Loquens.   Sleep-talking.
3. ————— Salax.   Night-pollution.

· The nature of these singular affections, and the means by which they are produced, have never yet been explained ; and rarely, so far as I know, has any explanation been attempted. To understand them fully, it would be necessary for us to enter into a minute development of the physiology of sleep and dreaming, which the limits of the present work will not allow. On some future occasion, the author may perhaps follow it up into such a detail ; but a few general remarks must suffice for the occasion before us.

In sleep, accompanied with dreaming, the faculties of the mind bear a pretty close parallel with those of the body, as to the effect produced upon them. Some of them, as the will, the perception, the judgment, are in a state of general torpidity, like the voluntary organs of the body ; while the memory and the imagination, like the vital or involuntary organs of the body, are in as high activity as ever. Hence, the sensory is as much crowded with ideas as at any time ; but, destitute of a controlling power, they rush forward with a very considerable degree of irregularity, and would do so with the most unshapeable confusion, but that the habit of association still retains some degree of influence, and produces some degree of consonance and proportion in the midst of the wildest and most extravagant vagaries. And hence that infinite variety which takes place in the character of our dreams ; and the greater regularity of some, and the greater irregularity of others. Hence a combination of thoughts or ideas, sometimes only in a small degree incongruous, and at other times most frantic and heterogeneous ; occasionally, indeed, so fearful and extravagant as to stimulate the external senses themselves into a sudden renewal of their functions, and consequently to break off abruptly the sleep into which they were thrown.

Now, as the stimulant force of our ideas in dreaming is often sufficient to rouse the external senses generally, and to awake us all of a sudden, it may be of such a kind, and just of such a strength, as to excite into their accustomed action the muscles of those organs or members only which are more immediately connected with the train of our dreams or incoherent thoughts, while every other organ may still remain torpid. And hence the muscles chiefly excited being those of speech, some persons talk, or the muscles chiefly excited being those of locomotion, other persons walk in their sleep, without being conscious, on their waking, of any such occurrence.* And by the same means we may easily account for the third species of the genus, or that which consists in dormant and involuntary salacity.

SPECIES I.
PARONIRIA AMBULANS.
SOMNAMBULISM. SLEEP-WALKING.
THE MUSCLES OF LOCOMOTION EXCITED INTO THEIR ACCUSTOMED ACTION BY THE FORCE OF THE IMAGINATION DURING DREAMING.

In profound sleep, all the faculties of the mind, as well as all the voluntary organs of the body, are in a state of inactivity or torpitude, and the only organs that preserve their active tenour are the involuntary ones ; so that, in this state, there is neither thought nor idea of any kind. In dreaming, some of the mental faculties only sleep or are torpid, while the others, like the involuntary organs of the body, continue wakeful or active : the somnolent faculties, we have already observed, are the will, the perception, and the judgment ; the wakeful are the memory and the imagination.

It would not be difficult, if we had time, to show why the involuntary organs do not require rest, or, in other words, become torpid like the voluntary ; nor why the will and the judgment sooner associate in the general sleep of the external senses than the imagination ; but this would carry us too far into the subject of animal physiology. There are two physiological remarks, however, which it is necessary to make, in explanation of the morbid affection immediately before us. The first is, that sleep is a natural torpitude or inertness, induced upon the organs of the body (with the exception of the involuntary) and the faculties of the mind by fatigue and exhaustion. And the next is, that, in the production of sleep, it is not necessary that all these powers of body and mind should have been equally exposed to exhaustion : for such is the effect of association and habit, that as soon as one faculty or organ feels fatigue or becomes exhausted, the rest participate in the same condition, and the sleep or torpitude becomes common to the whole. It is hence the body is made drowsy by mental study, and the mind by corporeal labour ; that muscular exercise wearies all the senses, and the exertion of the senses wearies the muscles : though there can be no doubt that the general tendency to sleep is also partly superinduced by the indirect exhaustion sustained by the organs or faculties that have been less employed, in consequence of the share of sensorial energy which, as from a common stock, they have themselves contributed towards the support of the more active and hence more debilitated powers.

---

* Hennings, von den Träumern und Nachtwandlem, Weimar, 1784. Horst, De Naturâ, Differentiis, et Causis corum qui dormientes ambulant, &c., Leips., 1593, 8vo.

Now it sometimes happens, either from disease or peculiarity of constitution, that all the external organs of sense do not associate in the general action that has taken place, or yield alike to the general torpor to which it gives rise ; and that the auditory, the optical, or some other sense, continues awake or in vigour while all the rest are become inert ; as it does also, that such particular sense, like the muscles of particular members, as observed a page or two above, is awakened or restimulated into action in the midst of the soundest sleep, by the peculiar force and bent of the dream, while the rest still sleep on and are unaffected.

If the external organ of sense thus stimulated be that of sight, the dreamer may perceive objects around him, and be able to distinguish them : and if the tenour of the dreaming ideas should as powerfully operate upon the muscles of locomotion, these also may be thrown into their accustomed state of action, and he may rise from his bed, and make his way to whatever place the drift of his dream may direct him, with perfect ease and free from danger. He will see more or less distinctly in proportion as the organ of sight is more or less awake : yet, from the increased exhaustion, and, of course, increased torpor of the other organs, in consequence of an increased demand of sensorial power from the common stock, to supply the action of the sense and muscles immediately engaged, every other sense will probably be thrown into a deeper sleep or torpor than if the whole had been quiescent. Hence, the ears may not be roused even by a sound that might otherwise awaken the sleeper. He may be insensible, not only to a slight touch, but a severe shaking of the limbs ; and may even cough violently without being recalled from his dream. Having accomplished the object of his visionary pursuit he may safely return, even over the most dangerous precipices, for he sees them distinctly, to his bed ; and the organ of sight being now quite exhausted, or there being no longer any occasion for its use, it may once more associate in the general inactivity, and the dream take a new turn, and consist of a new combination of images.*

---

* A remarkable instance of somnambulism occurred in 1833–4, at Springfield, Mass., in the person of Jane C. Rider, and was observed by Dr. L. W. Belden, of that town, from whose statement (An Account of Jane C. Rider, the Springfield Somnambulist, Springfield, 1834) we quote the following particulars:—The mother of Miss R. died suddenly of disease of the brain. The young lady, when these attacks commenced, was in her seventeenth year, and of a full habit. A small spot on the left side of her head has, from her earliest recollection, always been tender or painful on pressure, and much more so whenever she suffers from headache, with which she is occasionally affected. During the paroxysms of somnambulism, this spot is frequently the seat of intense agony. Her eyes are extremely sensible to the light.

The first paroxysm of somnambulism appeared in June, 1833 ; from this she was relieved by an emetic ; in a month, however, she was again affected, and the paroxysms recurred at different

Somnambulism occurs in many persons without any manifest predisponent cause, though it is generally connected with a considerable irritability of habit. A morbid state of the stomach, where this habit exists, has very frequently proved an exciting cause ; of which Dr. Yeates has given us an example in the case of a young gentleman of ten years of age.—(*Med. Trans.*, vol. v., art. xxviii., p. 444.) He was of a delicate frame, often troubled with sickness ; sometimes ejected his food undigested, after having lain two days in his stomach : his bowels were costive, and the stools were dark, offensive, and ill formed. The sympathetic symptoms were frequent headaches, with occasional stupor, general coldness of the skin, and limpid urine. After being in bed for about two hours, he was wont to start up suddenly, as if in a fright, dart rapidly into the middle of the chamber, or of the room adjoining, and walk about with much agitation. In this state he would run over quickly, but incorrectly, the transactions of the day ; and he once attempted to spell a word which in the. daytime he had spelled wrong, in doing which he jumbled a number of letters together. When spoken to he would make a rational re-

ply ; and, in one of his sleeping perambulations, he called for an epitome of the History of England, which he was in the habit of reading. The nurse brought him a book, but not the one he called for : on perceiving the difference he immediately threw it from him with great violence, and with expressions of anger and disappointment. On these occasions his eyes were wide open, though he did not seem conscious of seeing, nor of his situation at the time. It was, says Dr. Yeates, a perfect state of dream throughout, though partaking of the acts of the waking state, for he would avoid objects walking about the room. His face was quite pallid at the time.

In this case, much of the nervous hurry and agitation seems to have depended upon the debilitated and irritable state of the patient's frame. But where the affection proceeds from idiosyncrasy, or where there is no disturbance of the general health, the dreamer often proceeds far more coolly and collectedly ; and the eyes, instead of being wide open, as though staring, are often not more than half unclosed, in some cases even less than this ; which has given occasion to marvellous stories of somnambulists walking over dangerous places, or avoiding dan-

---

intervals until February, 1834. From the 6th to the 13th of December she had from one to three paroxysms daily. "At first they occurred only in the night ; and generally soon after she went to bed. As the disease advanced, they commenced earlier ; she then fell asleep, or rather passed into the state of somnambulism in the evening, sitting in her chair. At a still later period, the attacks took place at any hour during the day or evening. After she began to be affected in the daytime, the fit seldom commenced when she was in bed. The duration of the fits varied from a few minutes to forty-eight hours.

"The state of somnambulism was usually preceded by a full, heavy, unpleasant feeling in the head ; sometimes by headache, ringing in the ears, cold extremities, and drowsiness. To a spectator she seemed as if going to sleep ; the respirations became long and deep ; her attitude and the motions of her head resembled those of a person in a profound slumber. During the fit, the breathing, though sometimes natural, was often hurried, and attended with a peculiar moan. The pulse was at times accelerated, but generally it did not vary much from the natural standard. Occasionally the whole system was thrown into violent agitation, and she appeared like a person in hysterics. The eyes were generally closed, but at times they were open, and the pupil was then considerably dilated. These different states of the eye seemed to occasion no difference in the power of seeing—she saw apparently as well when they were closed as she did when they were open. All attempts to rouse her during a paroxysm were unsuccessful. She heard, felt, and saw ; but the impressions she received through the senses had no tendency to waken her.

"At the termination of a paroxysm she sunk into a profound sleep. The frown disappeared from her brow ; the respirations again became long and deep ; she soon began to gape and rub her eyes ; and in fifteen or twenty minutes from the first appearance of these symptoms she opened her eyes, and recollection was at once restored.

"Her manner differed exceedingly in different

paroxysms ; sometimes she engaged in her usual occupations, and then her motions were remarkably quick and impetuous—she moved with astonishing quickness, and accomplished whatever she attempted with unusual celerity. She attended to her domestic occupations, and was sometimes employed in sewing, reading, writing, &c. In the intervals of reading or talking, and even when thus engaged, her nods, her expression of countenance, and her apparent insensibility to surrounding objects, forced on the mind the conviction that she was asleep. Occasionally she was cheerful, but generally she was petulant and irritable. How far she was sensible to the presence of surrounding objects, it is very difficult to determine. Indeed, facts seem to prove that she was not in every paroxysm alike in this respect. In the early stage of her complaint she appeared to take little notice of persons unless they were connected with her train of thought ; but at a later period she seemed to comprehend more of what transpired in her presence. She recollected during a paroxysm circumstances which occurred in a former attack, though there was no remembrance of them in the interval. She occasionally imitated the manners, language, and sentiments of those around her with great fidelity ; though in her natural state she had no imitative powers, and could even sing accurately and agreeably, although when in health she can do neither."

The most remarkable feature, however, of this curious case, was the extraordinary power of vision attending the earlier paroxysms. Although her eyes were carefully covered by a white handkerchief folded so as to make eight or ten thicknesses, and the spaces below the bandage filled with strips of black velvet, yet she read, played backgammon, gave answers as to the colours of different objects presented to her, &c., with the utmost precision. She took a pencil, and while rocking in a chair wrote her own name, each word separately, and dotted the *i*.

In this case the disease evidently depended on a derangement of the digestive organs, and was cured by appropriate remedies.—D.

gerous objects, with their eyes completely shut all the time.*

The remedial treatment which it may be necessary to pursue we shall defer till we have briefly noticed the succeeding species, as the same treatment will apply to the whole.

SPECIES II.
PARONIRIA LOQUENS.
SLEEP-TALKING.

THE MUSCLES OF SPEECH EXCITED INTO THEIR ACCUSTOMED ACTION BY THE FORCE OF THE IMAGINATION DURING DREAMING.

IT is not necessary to dwell upon this species, as we have already explained the general principles of the inordinate action in the preceding pages. As the train of ideas which form the dream, when peculiarly lively and immediately connected with the organs of locomotion, may stimulate those organs into their accustomed activity, and thus give the dreamer a power of walking without consciousness; in like manner, if a similar train of dreaming ideas be immediately connected with the organs of speech, these may also be equally influenced, and the dreamer be able to talk without being conscious of it, or having any recollection of such exertion when he awakes. And as, for reasons already specified, the organ of sight is sometimes in the same way roused from a state of sleep or torpitude to a state of wakefulness, while all the other external senses continue somnolent, or from idiosyncrasy, or some local or accidental cause, do not join in the general repose, but continue vigilant during its dominion, the organ of hearing may be roused in the same manner, or exhibit the same anomaly; and in this case the dreamer, who, under the influence of the last species of affection, is able to see as well as to walk, is able, under the present, to hear as well as to speak.† Examples, in-

---

* It seems to Dr. Uwins, that the phenomena characterizing that remarkable condition of the brain and nerves which leads to sleep-walking, might be adduced in favour of the principle that one series of organs may be active while another is dormant. It is well known, says he, that the perceptions are so exceedingly acute in sleep-walkers as to enable them to pass over narrow bridges, &c., the contemplation of which they have shuddered at when awake. " Is not this superior adroitness referrible to the suspended agency of other parts of the brain, rather than to a positive augmentation of power in the parts in exercise? And is not this the pivot or main-spring upon which aberration turns and depends? Wake a sleep-walker, and he is immediately alive to his danger; prove to a maniac the untenable nature of his assumptions, and he is directly conscious of, or awake to, all his insane wanderings."—Dr. Uwins on those Disorders of the Brain and Nervous System usually called mental, p. 31, 8vo., London, 1833.—ED.

† Dreaming seems to Dr. Uwins to differ from the condition of actual madness, inasmuch as there are in it no correctives against aberration from the senses: "when these are called into exercise, all the lofty conceits and wild combinations

---

deed, are given, in which a by-stander, obtaining some clew into the train of thoughts of which the dream is composed, has been able not only to keep up an irregular conversation, but, by dexterous management, and the artful assumption of a character which he finds introduced into the dream, to draw from the dreamer the profoundest secrets of his bosom, the dreaming ideas generally consisting of those on which the dreamer is most employed when awake, or which lie nearest his heart. I have never met with a case of this kind in my own practice, but it is given as a fact by various physiologists from the time of the Greeks and Romans to our own day.*

SPECIES III.
PARONIRIA SALAX.
NIGHT POLLUTION.

THE SEXUAL ORGANS EXCITED INTO VENEREAL ACTION BY THE FORCE OF THE IMAGINATION DURING DREAMING.

BY Sauvages this affection is absurdly placed among the species of gonorrhœa, which, with great looseness of generic character, is defined " passio, cujus præcipuum symptoma est fluidi *puriformis* vel *seminiformis* effluxus stillatitius ex urethrâ." This definition is, indeed, wide enough to embrace the affection before us; but the absurdity consists in intermixing a natural discharge, produced by the ordinary orgasm, with morbid discharges, in which, in most cases, there is no orgasm whatever. Dr. Cullen, however, has continued to assign the same place and the same name to the present species, and this with still greater inconsistency: since he has struck out of his definition of gonorrhœa the epithet *seminiformis*, and confined it to a " fluxus humoris ex urethrâ *præter naturam*." So that he has been obliged to break his own bounds, to introduce this natural flux into the place he has allotted it. And hence, in laying down the treatment of gonorrhœa in his Practice of Physic, he takes no notice of his gonorrhœa *dormientium*, as though feeling that it was altogether a different subject.

We have already observed, that whatever part of the animal frame is immediately connected with the tenour of the somnolent vision, it is often roused, under particular circumstances, from the general sleep or torpitude in which it had participated, and becomes wakeful, while every other part perseveres in the common repose. During sleep, moreover, our ideas are often more lively and operative than during

---

of the dreamer are in a moment over; while they continue in the mad, despite of the sensual information; nay, the workings of the brain seem occasionally to change these sensual guards against aberration into actual ministers of misconception."—On Dis. of the Brain, &c., p. 31.—ED.

* The lectures on moral philosophy of Dr. Samuel S. Smith, the late president of Princeton College, contain many valuable remarks on the causes of the morbid phenomena adverted to by Dr. Good when treating of paroniria.—See likewise the ingenious work of MacNish on sleep.—D.

wakefulness, and this on two accounts; first, because from the uninterrupted activity of the involuntary organs, there is a more ready secretion of sensorial as well as of most other fluids in a state of perfect tranquillity; and next, because the ideas that predominate at the time are not broken in upon or weakened by exterior impressions and disturbances. It is on this account, when the faculty of the judgment is stimulated into activity instead of the ear or eye, or the motory powers, a man has sometimes been able to solve difficulties in dreaming which proved too hard for him when vigilant. And to this effect Dr. Spurzheim: "Somnambulists," says he, "even do things of which they are not capable in a state of watching; and some dreaming persons reason sometimes better than they do when awake."—(*Physiognomical System*, p. 175, 8vo., Lond., 1815.) A singular and amusing instance of this occurred not many years ago to a very excellent and justly celebrated friend of the author's, the Reverend William Jones, of Nayland, Suffolk, who, among other branches of science, had deeply cultivated that of music, to which, indeed, he was passionately attached. He was a man of irritable temperament, ardent mind, and most active and brilliant imagination; and was hence prepared by nature for energetic and vivid ideas in his dreams. On one occasion during his sleep he composed a very beautiful little ode of about six stanzas, and set the same to very agreeable music; the impression of which was so firmly fixed in his memory, that, on rising in the morning, he sat down and copied from his recollection both the music and the poetry.

It is hence not difficult to conceive, that members so irritable as the sexual organs, when once the imagination leads energetically to the subject of concupiscence, should occasionally participate in the vision and prove their sympathy by the result.

In some morbid states of the body, and especially when accompanied with local irritation, produced by inflammation, fibrous entony, the debility of old age, or a habit of vicious indulgence, a seminal flux has sometimes taken place without any connexion with the dream, and sometimes without either erection or turgescence; but this does not constitute the affection immediately before us; in which the stimulant power lies in the sensory, and is propagated from that organ to those of generation.

The Roman poet, who so admirably unlocked the NATURE OF THINGS to his contemporaries by following the footsteps of nature herself into most of her deepest recesses, directed his attention to this subject, among other physiological facts, and has elegantly explained it in the above manner; adducing at the same time another instance of the influence which the ideas of dreaming sometimes exercise over the organs connected with them, derived from the evacuation of the bladder, which frequently takes place in children, whose dream is directed to this natural want, and who image to themselves the ordinary vessel employed for such purpose as at hand for their use (*De. Rer. Nat.*, iv., 1020):—

"Pueri sæpe, lacum propter, seu dolia curta,
Somno devinctei, credunt se extollere vestem;
Totius humorem saccatum corporis fundunt;
Quom Babylonica, magnifico splendore, rigantur.
Tum, quibus ætatis freta primitus insinuantur,
Semen ubi ipsa dies membris matura creavit,
Conveniunt simulacra foris e corpore quoque,
Nuncia præclari voltûs, pulchrique coloris,
Qui ciet inritans loca turgida semine multo,
Ut, quasi transactis sæpe omnibus rebus, profundant,
Fluminis ingenteis fluctus, vestemque cruentent."

In the medical treatment of all these species of paroniria we must never lose sight of this principle, that although in many instances their predisponent cause is a peculiar idiosyncrasy or habit, their exciting cause is in all cases general or local irritation; and that this irritation is of two very opposite kinds, which it also becomes us very particularly to attend to, namely, that of entony, or excess of power, and that of atony, or deficiency.

It is to the former that Lucretius alludes, and which is by far the most common exciting cause; and where this exists, our first indication is to reduce the superabundant vigour by venesection, purgatives, laborious exercise, and a limitation to a plain and spare diet. While, on the contrary, where the exciting cause is debility, our attention should be directed to a tonic course of medicines, and particularly to those tonics which prove sedative at the same time that they strengthen the system. Several of the mineral acids are entitled to this character, and especially the sulphuric; and a still greater number of the vegetable bitters, and particularly the extracts of hop and lettuce. Dr. Cullen, indeed, as we have already observed, supposes a sedative power to exist in all the bitters, though not equally in all. How far the prussic acid might be usefully employed for this purpose, I cannot say from personal practice.

Our next object of attention should be to prevent all undue accumulation of the sensorial principle during sleep; and this may be accomplished in two very distinct and opposite ways. The first is the use of a hard mattress, with so small a covering of clothing that the sleep may be somewhat less sound than ordinary, and consequently more easily broken off. For the force of our dreaming ideas will always be in proportion to a certain degree of soundness in our sleep; I say a certain degree; because if the fatigue, or exhaustion, or torpitude be extreme, the sleep will become profound or lethargic, all the faculties of the mind will participate in it, and, as already observed, there will be no ideas or dreaming whatever.

And hence the second mode of preventing an accumulation of sensorial and especially of irritable power will be the employment of narcotics till the morbid habit is destroyed; for these, when carried to a sufficient extent, diminish vascular action, and consequently take off sense and motion so completely as to extinguish the vital principle altogether; and hence not only to suppress all power of dreaming, but even life itself.

I had lately under my care, for the last species, a very modest and regular young man, who was a student of Christ's College, Cambridge; and was alarmed at the idea of having his constitution undermined by its continuance. He was rapidly growing, of slender make, and of a relaxed habit. Nitre, which has been so often recommended as a sedative, in this case did no service; but, under the use of a pill composed of one grain of opium and five of camphire, taken nightly, and draughts of myrrh and infusion of columbo acidulated with sulphuric acid, he lost the tendency in a fortnight, after having been subject to the discharge for many weeks. His bowels were kept at the same time constantly stimulated by the pill of aloes and myrrh, and the cold bath formed a part of his regimen. Pagini and De Cazelles (*Journ. de Médecine*, tom. lxxiv.) have recommended electricity; but the author has never tried its effects, having uniformly succeeded without it.*

Where either of these species, but particularly the two former, are connected with a morbid state of the stomach, the disease must be attacked in this quarter; as it was with great judgment and a favourable issue in the case quoted from Dr. Yeates.

GENUS VI
MORIA.
FATUITY.

DEFECT OR HEBETUDE OF THE UNDERSTANDING.

MORIA is a Greek term, from μῶρος, "stultus, fatuus." It is here limited to its proper signification. Vogel employs it, though with a different termination (morosis instead of mória), in the same or very nearly the same sense; but he is almost the only medical writer that does so. By Neuter and Sauvages, mória is used to denote *melancholia complacens* (self-complacent melancholy), while by others it is employed synonymously with ancea or idiotism. To complete the confusion, morosis (*amentia morosis*) is the name given by Sauvages to mental imbecility (*mória imbecillis*), though, as already observed, he had just before used mória in the sense of melancholy. It is precisely in the signification now offered, that the term is employed by Erasmus in his celebrated treatise entitled "*Moriæ Encomium*," or "The Praise of Folly," which he dedicated to Sir Thomas More.

Mora, moror, morosus, morositas, are derived from this common source; and uniformly import "waywardness, tardiness, dulness, impediment;" though the lexicographers, not having hit upon the right path, have wandered in different directions without being able to satisfy themselves. In Sauvages and Sagar *morositates* are

* In the entonic state of paroniria salax, we are often obliged to employ the usual antiphlogistic remedies. When it depends on an opposite condition, which is more frequently the case, we rely on bark, iron, chalybeate waters, country air, and agreeable society. Blisters to the perineum are often serviceable, and so too with cold hip-baths. Opium, tobacco, and other narcotics are thought by some to possess an anti-aphrodisiac power.—D.

in fact "*corporeæ moriæ*," defects or hebetudes of the bodily faculties.

The preceding genera are founded upon a morbid perversion or misrule, a diminished or excessive excitement, of one or more of the powers of the mind, operating upon the mind itself or upon the body. The present is founded upon a natural or permanent dulness or hebetude of one or more of the same powers, producing a deficiency in the understanding, which, however, may be regarded as the general frame or constitution of the mind, in the same manner as the body is the general frame or constitution of the organs which form its separate parts. Mória, thus explained, will be found, as a genus, to embrace the two following species:—

1. Mória Imbecillis.   Imbecility.
2. —— Demens.   Irrationality.

SPECIES I.
MORIA IMBECILLIS.
MENTAL IMBECILITY.

THE DEFECT OR HEBETUDE PARTIAL, OR CONFINED TO PARTICULAR FACULTIES OF THE UNDERSTANDING.

WE have already observed that all the faculties of the mind are as subject to a diseased disturbance as the organs of the body; and hence all of them are liable to be affected by the present species. The whole of the varieties, therefore, under which mental imbecility is capable of being contemplated, might form an extensive list: but it will be sufficient to confine ourselves to the four following:—

α Stupiditas.   Dulness and indocility of the apprehension; torpitude and poverty of the imagination.
Stupidity.

β Amnesia.   Feebleness or failure of memory.
Forgetfulness.

γ Credulitas.   Weakness and undue pliancy of the judgment, with a facility of being duped.
Credulity.

δ Inconstantia.   Instability and irresolution of the will.
Fickleness.

In STUPIDITY, there is generally a dulness in several of the faculties besides the apprehension and the imagination; and sometimes, perhaps, in all of them: but then it originates in these, and the rest are for the most part only secondarily dull, as not being furnished with a sufficient number of ideas, or in sufficient rapidity for their use. Thus the judgment of a heavy or stupid man is often as sound in itself as that of a man of capacious comprehension; and more so, perhaps, for a reason we have already observed under *alusia facetosa*, or crack-brained wit, than that of a man of facetious quickness of parts: but the heavy man requires time and patience to collect his ideas, and compare them with each other; for they are neither furnished to him in a free current from his memory or his imagination, nor does he readily apprehend or lay hold of them as they are offered from external objects to his perception, which, in effect, is little more than a synonyme for the apprehension—the apprehension being the perception in a state of exercise or exertion. There is hence a material difference in physiology, though perhaps little in practice, between ignorance and stupidity. The former is want of knowledge from want of its ordinary means; and by the use of such means may perhaps soon be gotten the better of: the latter is dulness in the use of such knowledge as by ordinary means has been acquired, and exists in the sensory, though in a state of stagnation or dormancy. Mr. Locke has made the same distinction, though he has justly enough observed, that for all practical purposes, the man of stupidity had almost as well be without his knowledge as with it. "He," says this admirable writer, "who, through this default in his memory, has not the ideas that are really preserved there ready at hand when need and occasion call for them, were almost as good be without them quite, since they serve him to little purpose. The dull man, who loses the opportunity while he is seeking in his mind for those ideas that should serve his turn, is not much more happy in his knowledge than one that is perfectly ignorant. It is the business of the memory to furnish those ideas which it has present occasion for; and in the having them ready at hand on all occasions, consists that which we call invention, fancy, and quickness of parts."—(*Essay concerning Hum. Underst.*, b. ii., ch. x., sec. 8.)*

Stupidity or dulness of apprehension may be idiopathic; but it may also proceed from want of education, or education irregularly conducted; for all the faculties of the mind, like the muscles of the body, become invigorated and are rendered more alert by a well-disciplined exercise. And hence stupidity is a natural result of idleness; as it is more particularly of idleness in conjunction with an undue use of wine and fermented liquors, which have a proverbial power of besotting the understanding. It is also produced temporarily or habitually by various corporeal diseases; as hemicrania, chronic inflammation or dropsy of the head, gout in the head, and sometimes repelled cutaneous eruptions or habitual discharges.

Stupidity, like wit, is propagable; and hence we frequently see it run from one generation to another; and not unfrequently it forms a distinctive mark in the mental character of districts or nations: in many cases, indeed, where they border closely on each other. The Dutch have at least as much solid sense as their neighbours, the French; but they are certainly less quick, or, in other words, they have a duller fancy and apprehension. Bœotia, in respect to chorography, was merely separated from Attica by Mount Cithæron; but in respect to genius, the two countries were as far apart as the poles. So, in the Pacific Ocean, the natives of Otaheite

learn every thing with facility; the natives of New South Wales have no aptitude, and learn nothing. The residence of a few missionaries among them for a short term of years has nearly civilized the former: the actual possession of the country for a far longer period by a British public and a British government, with a perpetual intercourse and the kindest encouragement, has made little or no impression upon the latter.

A FAILURE OF MEMORY, however, which forms the SECOND SPECIES of mental imbecility before us, is a far more severe evil than dulness of perception with poverty of imagination; for as all the sources of information to which we have been privy cannot be always immediately before us to excite the perception, we must necessarily draw upon our recollection for those which are not so, and whose ideas or impressions we stand in need of. And hence the memory is the great storehouse of intelligence; and in one sense at least the Platonic doctrine is universally true, that "all knowledge is reminiscence." There are some minds in whom this faculty has been peculiarly retentive, as that of Newton, who made it answer the purpose of intuition; and of Pascal, who is said never to have forgotten, till his health failed him, any thing he had ever done, read, or thought of.*

Retention of memory, however, is a different property from that of quickness. They may and often do co-exist, but they are also found separate; for there are many persons who can well catch hold of an entire song, an entire sermon, or a series of speeches in parliament, and can recite them almost, if not altogether, verbatim immediately afterward, but who lose all recollection of them in a day or two; while there are others who are obliged to pause over the subject submitted to them, or to have it repeated for several times before they can get it by heart, yet who, when they have once fixed it in the memory, retain it as long as they live. Mr. W. Woodfall, the celebrated reporter of the parliamentary debates, was an instance of the former of these talents in regard to his powers of apprehension; the well-known Jedediah Buxton of the latter; though it should be remarked, that Mr. Woodfall retained with as much ease as he first fixed speeches in his memory.

Failure of memory takes place in a variety of ways.† It is sometimes general, and extends to every subject; but it is frequently far more

---

* As stupidity sometimes depends on mechanical causes, so, too, after the operation of the same causes in stupid persons, the mind sometimes manifests more energy. The celebrated Père Mabillon was considered as stupid till a tile fell upon his head: he then began to display great abilities.—D.

* Actors, who are compelled by their professional pursuits to cultivate the memory, often present remarkable examples of the powers of apprehension and retention of this mental faculty. Hodgkinson, a celebrated comedian, was able, by three or four readings, to recite the contents of a newspaper without error. The distinguished Dr. S. L. Mitchill could repeat, in earlier life, an entire sermon which he had heard a few hours previously.—D.

† The curious case related by Major Elliot of West Point, N. Y., merits attention:—

"The patient was a young lady of cultivated mind, and the affection began with an attack of somnolency, which was protracted several hours beyond the usual time. When she came out of it, she was found to have lost every kind of acquired

manifest on some subjects than on others. Salmuth mentions a case in which the affected person had forgotten to pronounce words, but could
nevertheless write them.—(Cent. ii., obs. 41.)
Mr. J. Hunter was suddenly attacked with a
singular affection of this kind in December, 1789,
when on a visit to the house of a friend in town.
"He did not know in what part of the house he
was, nor even the name of the street when told
it, nor where his own house was : he had not a
conception of any thing existing beyond the
room he was in, and yet was perfectly conscious
of the loss of memory. He was sensible of impressions of all kinds from the senses, and therefore looked out of the window, although rather
dark, to see if he could be made sensible of the
situation of the house. The loss of memory
gradually went off, and in less than half an
hour his memory was perfectly recovered."—
(Sir Everard Home's Life, prefixed to his Treatise on the Blood, Inflammation, &c., 4to., 1794.)
This might possibly be connected with a gouty
habit, to which Mr. Hunter was subject, though
not at this time labouring under a paroxysm.
The late bishop of Landaff, Dr. Watson, gives
a singular case of partial amnesia in his father,
the result of an apoplectic attack. "I have
heard him ask twenty times a day," says Dr.
Watson, " ' What is the name of the lad that is
at college ?' (my elder brother) ; and yet he
was able to repeat, without a blunder, hundreds
of lines out of classic authors."—(Anecdotes of
the Life of Richard Watson, D. D., Bishop of
Landaff.) And hence there is no reason for
discrediting the story of a German statesman, a
Mr. Von B., related in the seventh volume of
the Psychological Magazine, who, having called
at a gentleman's house, the servants of which
did not know him, was under the necessity of
giving in his name ; but unfortunately at that
moment he had forgotten it, and excited no small
degree of laughter by turning round to a friend
who accompanied him, and saying, with great
earnestness, " Pray tell me who I am, for I cannot recollect."*

From severe suffering of the head in many
fevers, a great inroad is frequently made upon
the memory, and it is long before the convalescent can rightly put together all the ideas of
his past life. Such was one of the effects of
the plague at Athens, as we learn from Thucy-
dides : τοὺς δὲ καὶ λήθη ἐλάμβανε παραυτίκα ἀναστάν-
τας τῶν πάντων ὁμοίως καὶ ἠγνόησαν σφᾶς τε αὐτοὺς, καὶ
τοὺς ἐπιτηδείους : " and many, on recovery, still
experienced such an extraordinary oblivion of
all things, that they knew neither themselves nor
their friends." A few years ago a man with a
brain-fever was taken into St. Thomas's Hospital, who, as he grew better, spoke to his attendants, but in a language they did not understand.
A Welsh milk-woman, going by accident into
the ward, heard him, answered him, and conversed with him. It was then found that the
patient was by birth a Welshman ; but had left
his native land in his youth, forgotten his native
dialect, and used English for the last thirty
years. Yet, in consequence of this fever, he
had forgotten the English tongue, and suddenly
recovered the Welsh.*

Boerhaave, however, gives a still more extraordinary instance of oblivion in the case of a
Spanish tragic author, who had composed many
excellent pieces, but so completely lost his memory in consequence of an acute fever, that he
forgot not only the languages he had formerly
learned, but even the alphabet ; and was hence
under the necessity of beginning to read again.
His own poems and compositions were shown
to him, but he could not be persuaded that they
were his production. Afterward, however, he
began once more to compose verses, which had
so striking a resemblance to his former writings,
that he at length became convinced of his being
the author of them.†

---

knowledge. She immediately began to apply herself to the first elements of education, and was
making considerable progress, when, after several
months, she was seized with a second fit of somnolency. She was now at once restored to all the
knowledge which she possessed before the first
attack, and without the least recollection of any
thing that had taken place during the interval.
After another interval she had a third attack of
somnolency, which left her in the same state as
after the first. In this manner she suffered these
alternate conditions for four years, with the very
remarkable circumstance that during one state she
retained all her original knowledge, but during the
other that only which she had acquired since the
first attack. During the healthy interval, for instance, she was remarkable for the beauty of her
penmanship ; but during the paroxysm wrote a
poor, awkward hand. Persons introduced to her
during the paroxysm, she recognised only in a
subsequent paroxysm, and not in the interval ; and
persons whom she had seen for the first time during the healthy interval, she did not recognise during the attack."—D.
    * The late Hon. Thomas Law of Washington

city, the brother of Lord Ellenborough, was a remarkable instance of this peculiarity. He frequently was unable to give his name when calling
at the postoffice for letters : yet on other occasions, as in respect to past events and on business
of importance, his powers of memory were strong
and acute.—D.
    * In a case occurring under the notice of Dr.
John Ware of Boston, where the patient had suffered excessively from sea-sickness, the memory
of recent events was entirely lost. The gentleman could recollect distinctly what had occurred
several years before, but retained no trace whatever of what had happened a few months previous
to his illness.—See Am. Journal of Med., Sc. &c.,
vol. v., p. 379.—D.
    † Prælect. Acad. in Instit. Med. ex edit. Haller,
tom. iv., p. 463. See also Crichton of Ment. Derangement, i., 370. Dr. Uwins considers the very
condition of madness as implying some sort of forgetfulness, or forgetfulness of something, which,
were memory to recall, the hallucination would be
over. " Both in actual dreams and in the day-
dreams of madness, we bring together into one
point of time the most extravagant alibis, and join
in conversation with those who have paid nature's
great debt many years before. The portions of the
brain implicated, if they tell us nothing but the
truth, but at the same time do not tell us the whole
truth, lead to all these misconceptions as to time,
and place, and circumstance. How they do this,
and how they leave that undone, constitutes the

The memory may also be prematurely impaired (for in age it is a natural defect)[*] by various other causes. Idleness or inattention will do it, as in the case of stupidity, as will also an over-exertion of the faculty, injuries of the head, rheumatic or gouty pains in it, dyspeptic maladies, various narcotic poisons, prostrating hemorrhages or want of food, and libidinous indulgence.—(*Dissert. de Memoriæ Læsione ex nimis Vener. Usu*, Alt., 1695.)

Dependant upon this last cause, Sir Alexander Crichton has given a single example of what may be called perverse oblivion in an old attorney, nearly seventy years of age, who, though married to a lady much younger than himself, kept a mistress, whom he visited every night. He was suddenly seized with great prostration of strength, giddiness, and forgetfulness; but the last was of a peculiar kind, and consisted in the mistaking the name of one thing for that of another; so that, if he wanted bread, he would ask for his boots; and though enraged at the latter being brought to him, he would still call out for his boots or shoes. In like manner, if he wanted a tumbler to drink out of, it was a thousand to one but he would call for the ordinary chamber utensil; or, if this were wanted, he would call for a tumbler or a dish. This gentleman, however, was cured of the complaint by large doses of valerian and other cardiacs.

In CREDULITY, constituting the THIRD VARIETY of the imbecility before us, the faculty of the judgment is the chief seat of disorder. It is unquestionably more generally to be found among ignorant people, than those whose minds are well stored with the elements of knowledge; but as we also frequently perceive among the former a most obstinate and wilful incredulity, and among the latter extraordinary proofs of the present failing, it cannot be regarded as altogether an effect of a general want of ideas: it is in reality a hebetude or indolence of the judgment or power of ratiocination, which induces a man to take things upon trust, and allow others to think for him, not for want of ideas, but for want of comparing one idea with another, those of probability with those of improbability, and fairly striking the balance; in consequence of which, under the influence of this mental osci-

taney, he readily yields himself, body and soul, to the opinions of others, and follows such opinions blindfold: as those who shut their eyes must be led by those who see, or else fall into the ditch.

This is voluntary credulity; yet many have been so long accustomed to it that it has all the effect of a chronic disease, and is as difficult of cure as the most obstinate. There are some men, however, whose judgment is more morbidly dull by nature than from inactivity or a neglected education; or may possibly have been rendered so by intemperance; who are deficient in natural skill to use the evidence they possess of probabilities: and being incapable of carrying on a train of consequences in their heads, and of weighing exactly the preponderance of contrary proofs and testimonies, are easily misled, and rendered the dupes of every plausible sophist, and the playthings of every impostor. "There are some men," says Mr. Locke, "of one, some but of two syllogisms, and no more; and others that can but advance one step further. These cannot always discern that side on which the strongest proofs lie; cannot constantly follow that which in itself is the more probable opinion."—(*Human Understand.*, book iv., ch. xix., § 5.)

There is another imbecility we have noticed, as strangely interfering with the integrity of the understanding: and that is FICKLENESS, or an instability and irresolution of the will. The faculty of the will requires not only to be directed aright in infant life, but to be fortified and strengthened by a course of exercise and discipline as much as any faculty whatever. This we may say as physiologists; but as moralists we may speak a bolder language, and maintain that it demands the spur and trammels of education even more than all the other faculties put together, since it is designed by nature to be the governing power, and to exercise an absolute sway over the rest, even over the desire itself, by which, however, it is moved in all ordinary cases.

A child whose inclinations have never been reined in is perpetually letting the will and the desire run together, and changing both every moment; and if this disposition be suffered to grow into a habit, it will produce the fickleness of which we are now speaking, and form a character on which there can be no reliance; whose determination of to-morrow cannot be known from that of to-day: because the will itself, void of all firmness or resolution, is the sport of every transient incident, every interposing uneasiness or pleasure; and which hence becomes its own torment still more than the torment of those around it; since, being ever instigated by the feelings of the moment, and sacrificing the future to the present, it often purchases a fleeting gratification, and of subordinate value, at an expense of permanent and substantial happiness.

Upon the REMEDIAL PROCESS for the mental infirmities which appertain to this species, little is to be said in a work of medical instruction. So far as they relate to corporeal causes, and we have pointed out various causes of this kind

---

great and still unsolved problem in mental philosophy."—Uwins on Mental Disorders, p. 44.—ED.

[*] The impairment produced by age is not so much insanity as imbecility or fatuity: the memory fails, but it only fails with the other mental powers. "Musicians have told me," says Dr. Conolly, "that as they became old, they found they could not play the music learned in later years without having the music before them; but could still go through long compositions learned in early life without the book, and without the mistake of a note. The susceptibility to sensations and emotions is diminished; the attention is less excited by them; they make a weak and fading impression on the memory. Those things which yet excite more attention are better remembered, even in old age. Old men, Cicero remarks (De Senect.), do not commonly forget where they have deposited their money."—See Inquiries concerning the Indications of Insanity, p. 282.—ED.

applicable to several of them, those causes should be minutely inquired into, and, as far as possible, removed or palliated ; and whatever will tend to invigorate the entire frame, as the metallic tonics, regularity of diet, sleep, exercise, and above all, cold bathing, must supply the rest. To the arms of mental and moral instruction, however, the sickly understanding must be chiefly intrusted ; and where these are properly applied, the mind may often be rendered sufficiently sound for all the ordinary purposes of life, and even for some of its elegances ; though it may never be distinguished for terseness, brilliancy, or comprehension. The leading aim should be to lay hold of the strongest faculty, and to make the direct cultivation of this an indirect cultivation of the rest.

———

SPECIES II.
MORIA DEMENS.
WITLESSNESS. IRRATIONALITY.
DEFECT OR HEBETUDE OF ALL THE FACULTIES OF THE UNDERSTANDING.

OF this species we have three varieties that seem to require a distinct notice :—

a Stultitia. Silliness. Folly.	Shallow knowledge, vacant countenance, light frivolous fancy; for the most part with good-nature ; sometimes with obstinacy.
β Lerema. Dotage. Superannuation.	Impotence of body as well as of mind, from premature old age ; childish desires and pursuits ; drawling speech or garrulous babble, composed of ideas for the most part associated by previous habit.
γ Anœa. Idiotism.	General obliteration of the mental powers and affections; paucity or destitution of ideas ; obtuse sensibility ; vacant countenance ; imperfect or broken articulation ; with occasionally transient and unmeaning gusts of passion.

The difference between the understanding of some men and that of others is extreme ; yet it is not every minute variation from the standard of soundness that constitutes a disease, whether in mind or body : but as soon as in either case such variation becomes a marked or serious evil, it is entitled to this name ; and, in the subject before us, falls within the range of the FIRST of the preceding varieties.

This, which is what we ordinarily denominate SILLINESS, is generally a natural infirmity, and in some families appears to be hereditary. A well-directed education, however, may do much, as there is commonly some faculty that will bear cultivating better than the rest, and which points to the particular line to which the study of the individual should be especially addressed, and in which he may appear respectable. He may have imitative powers, and make a good painter or engraver, though he may not have creative powers, and make a good orator or poet. He may be fond of arithmetic, and fitted for trade and accounts, though he may not possess a taste for scientific subtleties, or be well calculated for any one of the professions.

DOTAGE, when a mere result of old age, is hardly to be regarded as a disease, and is rarely accompanied by any effervescence of the passions. But it often appears prematurely,* and is especially accelerated by excessive indulgence in corporeal pleasures ; sometimes by violent mental emotion, as anger, or by long-continued grief. Under the two former of these causes, there is often combined with it an incessant garrulity, a very high degree of passionate but unmeaning effervescence and puerile mobility M. Pinel gives a striking example of this in a person whom he had frequently an opportunity of seeing. " His motions," says he, " his ideas, his broken sentences, his confused and momentary glimpses of mental feeling, appeared to present a perfect image of chaos. He came up to me, looked at me, and overwhelmed me with a torrent of words without order or connexion. In a moment he turned to another person, whom, in rotation, he deafened with his unmeaning babble, or threatened with an evanescent look of anger ; but as incapable of determined and continued excitement of the feelings as of a just connexion of ideas, his emotions were the effect of a momentary effervescence, which was immediately succeeded by a calm. If he went into a room, he quickly displaced or overturned the furniture, without manifesting any direct intention. Scarcely could one look off before he would be at a considerable distance, exercising his versatile fondness for bustle in some other way. He was quiet only when food was presented to him. Even at night he rested but for a few moments." A strong desire of food, however, is by no means common under this species : it is perhaps most frequently met with in the dotage of old age ; but in premature lerema, we often find the appetite entirely banished, and a resistance to food of all kinds when offered.

IDIOTISM, the THIRD VARIETY, is often the result, as we have already observed, of an original misformation of the cranium, sometimes in respect to thickness, more frequently in respect to shape ; by both which the internal cavity, and

———

* Much difference is observed in different individuals, with respect to the period of life at which the mental faculties acquire their ultimate degree of power, and at which they begin to decline. Some men attain that prudence at twenty, which others, with equal advantages of precept and example, do not acquire in less than ten years after that age. If the youthful temperament remain beyond the age of thirty-five, Dr. Conolly believes that the mind never acquires much intellectual tone. In some instances, the mind, after displaying considerable powers, has seemed to become exhausted soon after forty ; while in others of a more agreeable nature, minds of ordinary power have risen into greatness, or superior minds have preserved it, long after that period.— See Dr. Conolly's Inquiry into the Indications of Insanity, pp. 271–276.—ED.

consequently the capacity of the brain, are unduly diminished.

The internal causes are habitual inebriety, excessive and enervating pleasures, violent agitation of the passions, whether pleasurable or painful, as overwhelming joy, startling terror, deep and protracted grief, or furious anger; tumours within the cavity of the cranium; apoplectic attacks; injury of the brain from external violence; injudicious management in ecphronia; and especially an excessive use of the lancet.

Idiotism, however, is more frequently congenital than accidental; and it is melancholy to think that it is also sometimes hereditary. Of those who are idiots from birth, many, moreover, are sooner or later afflicted with palsy or epilepsy, or both; a clear proof of the existence of some organic affection of the brain or nerves, the former being sometimes partial, and confined to the face only, or extending down one of the sides. Idiots rarely attain old age; they seldom exceed the term of thirty years; and when paralysis or epilepsy is concomitant, they usually die at a much earlier period.

In idiotism the ideas of sensation and of reflection appear to be equally inaccurate. There is a vague, unsteady, wandering eye, seldom fixed for any length of time upon one determinate object; a stupid expression of countenance, in which no sign of intelligence is portrayed; a gaping mouth, from which the saliva flows continually; a perpetual rolling and tossing of the head; no memory, no language, no reason. The idiot has all the animal instincts, and some of the passions. Of the last, joy, fear, and anger, are those with which he is most frequently affected, but these are of a very limited kind. His joy is unmeaning mirth; his fear a transient qualm; his anger a momentary fit of violence. The toys of children, and the gratification of hunger and thirst, are his only pleasures; bodily pain, or fear of bodily pain, his only distresses. It is said that idiots have sometimes shown a strong sexual appetite; but this is not common, for they rarely seem to attend to any distinction of sex.—(*Crichton of Ment. Derangement*, i., p. 314.)

The treatment, where medical assistance can be of any use, must chiefly depend upon the nature of the case. Blistering and internal stimulants to increase the action of the nervous system, and augment the habitual torpitude of the abdominal viscera, which are usually affected in this malady, offer the fairest chance of advantage. Accidental commotion of the brain, an occasional cause, has occasionally also proved serviceable, as has likewise a fracture of the cranium. Hence, too, fevers have relieved the disease; and active paroxysms of mania have proved a complete cure; and I once knew a cure effected in a lad who fell from the first floor of a house into the street, the torpitude or obstruction, or whatever was the cause, being hereby removed.*

ORDER II.

ÆSTHETICA.

DISEASES AFFECTING THE SENSATION.

DULNESS, DEPRAVATION, OR ABOLITION OF ONE OR MORE OF THE ORGANS OF CORPOREAL SENSE.

ÆSTHETICA is derived from αἰσθάνομαι, "sentio, et propriè, sensû corporis." The term applies, however, to all the external senses, and, in the language of Galen, peculiarly expresses ἡ αἰσθητικὴ δύναμις, "the power or faculty of sensation." It must also be admitted that it is occasionally applied to mental sensation, as in Isocrates to Demonicus, οὕτω τὴν ἐκείνων γνώμην αἰσθῇση, "thus will you *feel* their mind or inclination."

The term has hence been used in different significations by different medical writers. It has seldom, indeed, been applied to the mind, but has strangely varied between expressing sensation generally, and the sense of touch alone. In Dr. Young's excellent volume on Medical Literature it runs for the most part parallel with its meaning in the present work, and imports diseased action of all the corporeal senses; but with this appropriation of the term, there seems to be an incorrectness in applying it, as the same author does immediately afterward, to defective memory, which he names *dysæsthesia interna*, and ranks in the same list or genus with defect of the external senses. Sauvages, and after him Sagar and Cullen, have applied *dysæsthesiæ* to a morbid state of the corporeal senses generally; whence *ánæsthesia* should, in their hands, have expressed atony or total inactivity of these senses generally. But while *dysæsthesiæ* extends to all the senses, *anæsthesiæ* is by the same writers limited to the single sense of touch, with no small perplexity to the young student.

In the Physiological Proem to the present class, we have taken so full a survey of the connexion which exists between the brain and the corporeal senses, by means of the nerves, that it is not necessary to say more upon the subject at present; and I shall only therefore further observe, in these preliminary remarks, that where one of the senses is deficient, and especially where naturally deficient, the rest have very frequently been found in a more than ordinary degree of vigour and acuteness; as though the sensorial power were primarily derived from a common source, and the proportion belonging to the organ whose outlet is invalid, were distributed among the other organs.†

---

* On this interesting subject Dr. Spurzheim's Observations on the Deranged Manifestations of the Mind, or Insanity, may be consulted with great profit. Dr. T. R. Beck also, in his able treatise on Medical Jurisprudence, has learnedly discussed the subject of mental affections.—*D.*

† Trinckhusius, De Cæcis, sapientiâ ac eruditione, claris mirisque cæcorum quorundam ac-

The genera, under the order before us, are taken in a regular series from the corporeal senses themselves in a state of morbid action, and are in number six; of which the first five are derived from the five external senses, and the last from a diseased state of particular branches of the nerves distributed over the frame generally, for the common and pleasurable feeling of health in the different organs through which they are dispersed.

I.	Paropsis.	Morbid Sight.
II.	Paracusis.	—— Hearing.
III.	Parosmis.	—— Smell.
IV.	Paragusis.	—— Taste.
V.	Parapsis.	—— Touch.
VI.	Neuralgia.	Nerve-ache.

GENUS I.
PAROPSIS.
MORBID SIGHT.

SENSE OF SIGHT VITIATED OR LOST.

PAROPSIS is literally "diseased or depraved vision," from παρά, male, and ὄψις, visus; as paracusis, "diseased or depraved hearing," from παρά, and ἀκουή.

The ophthalmic monographists, by making every variety of affection a distinct disease, have most unmercifully enlarged the list under this genus.—(*Campiani Raggionamenti sopra tutti i Mali degli Occhi descritti*, &c., Genoa, 1759.) To say nothing of Campiani, Taylor has in this manner mustered them at two hundred and forty-three (*Catalogue of two hundred and forty-three Diseases of the Eyes*, Edin., fol., 1749), while Plenck has contrived to multiply them to nearly six hundred.—(*Doctrina de Morbis Oculorum*, 8vo., Vienna, 1783, 2d edit.) Upon a comprehensive view of the subject, it will, I think, be found, that this formidable number may be reduced to the twelve species following :—

1.	Paropsis Lucifuga.	Night sight.
2.	—— Noctifuga.	Day sight.
3.	—— Longinqua.	Long sight.
4.	—— Propinqua.	Short sight.
5.	—— Lateralis.	Skew sight.
6.	—— Illusoria.	False sight.
7.	—— Caligo.	Opaque Cornea.
8.	—— Glaucosis.	Humoral Opacity.
9.	—— Cataracta.	Cataract.
10.	—— Synizesis.	Closed Pupil.
11.	—— Amaurosis.	Drop Serene.
12.	—— Strabismus.	Squinting.

tionibus, Geræ, 1672. Meckren. Observ. Med. Chir., cap. xx. Whether the principle adverted to in the text be true or not, the editor will not undertake to say; but it is more certain that another principle is generally concerned, resolvable into habit or practice. Thus, a blind man, whose eyes cannot apprize him of danger, or convey to him any kind of information, is habitually all attention with his ears; just as the organ of touch, in a deaf and dumb person, is, from necessity, continually exerted, and brought by habit to acquire a nice power of feeling and discrimination, far superior to what is enjoyed by the generality of mankind.—ED.

Most of these fall rather within the province of the ophthalmic surgeon than that of the physician; but as their general nature ought to be known to every practitioner, we shall proceed to give a glance at each of them in their order. The maladies of the eye dependant on inflammation, and constituting ophthalmia, have been already treated of in Class III., Order II., HÆMATICA PHLOGOTICA.

SPECIES I.
PAROPSIS LUCIFUGA.
NIGHT SIGHT.

VISION PAINFULLY ACUTE IN A STRONG LIGHT; BUT CLEAR AND PLEASANT IN A DEEP SHADE OR THE DUSK OF THE EVENING.

THE specific term *lucifuga* is so distinct as at once to point out the general nature of the affection, while constituting a very prominent symptom. The author, however, has found a necessity for introducing this new name, not more from its own clearness than from the confusion which has taken place among earlier writers in distinguishing the disease by two directly opposite terms, nyctalopia and hemeralopia, according as these terms have been used in a literal or a technical and implied sense. The Greeks called it by the former name, literally *night sight*, in consequence of the person labouring under it being only able to see at night or in a deep shade; while *nyctalopia* has been used by most modern writers in the opposite sense of night-sight*ache*, agreeably to the technical and implied meaning of *opia* when applied pathologically; in which case it always imports diseased vision, as though a contraction of the term paropia or paropsis; whence nyctalopia has necessarily been made to import *day sight* instead of *night sight*, or that imperfection of vision in which the eye can only see in the day, or whenever there is a strong light. And hence hemeralopia, the opposite to nyctalopia, has been used with the same confusion and contradiction of signification; by the Greeks importing *day sight*, being taken naturally or literally; by the moderns *day-sightache*, and consequently *night sight*, being taken technically or by implication; and hence Sauvages, "Græcis hemeralopia; neotericis nyctalopia." It is the *luscitas* of Beer (*Lehre von der Augenkrankheiten, als Leitfaden zu seinen offentlichen Vorlesungen entwurfen*; Twey bände, 8vo., Wien, 1817); the *day blindness* of various other writers.

The disease is dependant upon a peculiar irritability of the retina, produced by two very different causes; a sudden exposure to a stronger light than the eye has been wont to sustain, and a deficiency of the black pigment which lines the choroid tunic. If the iris be weak and torpid, it is enlarged; if strong and contractile, diminished.

From the first cause, this disease is common to those who live almost constantly in dark caverns or chambers, as mines, dungeons, or dark prisons, or who have recently had a cataract depressed or extracted, the growth of which has still more effectually excluded the light from the retina. And in all these cases we find it accompanied with a perpetual nictitation, from the sympathy which prevails between the retina and the orbicular muscles of the palpebræ.

Ramazzini asserts that this complaint is common to the peasants of Italy who are employed in agriculture ; but in whom he is able to trace no other peculiarity than a considerable enlargement of the pupil.—(*De Morbis Artificum*, &c.) It is not difficult, perhaps, to assign a reason for such an affection among these people, though Ramazzini is silent upon the subject. The sky of Italy is peculiarly bright, its atmosphere particularly clear, and its temperature relaxingly warm. The peasants of Italy, therefore, are exposed to the joint operation of almost every cause that can produce habitual debility in the iris, and irritability in the retina. And we find these causes acting with renewed power at the time when the disease chiefly makes its attack, which we are told is on the return of spring, or rather at the vernal equinox, when a double flood of day breaks on them. And such is the dimness it produces, that the peasants lose their way in the fields in the glare of noon ; but on the approach of night they are again able to see distinctly. It is hence necessary for them to keep for some weeks in the shade, or in comparative darkness, till the eyes recover their proper tone ; and the weakness, and consequently the disease, subsides. And hence Ramazzini tells us that in the course of the succeeding month, or in other words, after they have taken due care of themselves, the peasants recover their sight. The glare of the sun in tropical regions, and especially where reflected from bright chalk-hills, has often produced the same effect.

A deficiency of the black pigment is occasionally found in persons of a fair complexion and light hair ; and as the retina is hereby deprived of the natural shade that softens the light in its descent upon this very sensible membrane, its morbid irritability is not to be wondered at. Albinoes, who are without the common pigment that lies between the cuticle and cutis in other persons, are always deficient in this also : and hence they are painfully able to open their eyes in a strong sunshine ; they contract their brows, and keep the eyelids nearly closed during the day ; but no sooner does twilight come, than they are able to see quite distinctly. In old persons the same deficiency of black pigment is sometimes traced, but without painful vision ; for at this time of life the optic nerve is become more obtuse. In horses, this want of pigment constitutes what is called a *wall-eye*.

[There are many states of the organ in which vision is very imperfect, even to blindness, in the strong light of the day ; and much better sight is enjoyed in twilight and the dusk ; but Mr. Lawrence has never seen such a state as an amaurotic affection, or what is here called *night sight*, dependant on disease of the retina or optic nerve. In central leucoma of the cornea, in incipient opacity of the lens, in partial central opacity of the capsule, in contractions of the pupil from prolapsus iridis, or adhesion of the pupillary margin, connected with either of the former circumstances, the patient will see best in a weak light; and find vision very imperfect in a strong glare. The enlargement of the pupil in the former, and its contraction in the latter state, sufficiently account for this difference. On the same ground, sight is much improved in some of these circumstances by the use of belladonna. In strumous ophthalmia, the intolerance of light often amounts to blindness during the day ; the symptoms remitting in the evening, at which period the eyes are opened, and the patient sees well. Unnatural sensibility to light is the form which sympathetic affection of the retina sometimes assumes.—(See *a Treatise on the Diseases of the Eye, by Wm. Lawrence*, p. 570, 8vo., Lond., 1833.)

Acuteness of night vision is natural to various animals that prowl in the dark ; as cats, lynxes, lions, and perhaps all the feline genus ; which save their eyes from the pain produced by broad daylight, by a closer contraction of their pupils than mankind are able to effect ; expanding them gradually as the night shuts in, till, by the extent of the expansion, they are able to see much better than mankind in the dark. Owls, bats, cockroaches, moths, sphinxes, and many other insects, have a similar power.

Where the disease proceeds from an accidental irritability of the retina, sedative applications, as the tincture of belladonna and internal sedatives, as hyoscyamus and conium, have often proved serviceable, and the more so when combined with the bark. In old age, or an early deficiency of the black pigment that covers the choroid tunic, medicine has very little chance of success ; and all we can hope for is to afford occasional relief by palliatives, if the irritation be violent, or accompanied with inflammatory symptoms.

SPECIES II.
PAROPSIS NOCTIFUGA.
DAY SIGHT.

VISION DULL AND CONFUSED IN THE DARK ; BUT CLEAR AND POWERFUL IN BROAD DAYLIGHT.

This species, the nyctalopia of neoteric authors, or night blindness, is said to be endemic in Poland, the West Indies, Brazils, and the intertropical regions generally.—(*Hautesierck, Recucil d'Obs. de Médecine*, i., ii.) Its cause is precisely the reverse of that of the preceding species, and proceeds from too great instead of too small an habitual exposure to light, whence the retina becomes torpid, and requires a strong stimulus to raise it. At noontide, therefore, it is sensible to the impressions of objects ; but does not clearly discern them in the shade, or towards the close of day. [Hence the present complaint is rarely met with, except in climates or situations where the light is very powerful. Between the tropics, as Mr. Lawrence observes, the full glare of a vertical sun in an unclouded sky, and the strong reflection of the solar rays from the sea, or from a sandy soil, produces an excitement of the retina to which we are wholly unaccustomed in our latitudes; although, in some parts of Europe, analogous influences exist in a sufficient degree to cause the affection. Europeans in the West Indies, and particularly soldiers and sailors, who are much exposed to the sun, often have the complaint. In all the cases which Mr. Lawrence has seen, the disease commenced in the East or West Indies, and was brought to England.

In the commencement, the person can see by moonlight, or when the room is lighted by a candle; but as the disorder proceeds, he can see nothing after sunset; and in the morning, vision returns. There is no, change of appearance in the eye, and, of course, if the patient can see perfectly during the day, the organ can have undergone no important change. At first, a slight increase of irritability is remarked; but as the disorder increases, the pupil becomes rather dilated, and the case is alleged to terminate sometimes in amaurosis. The feeble light of night and twilight does not impress the retina, after it has been so strongly excited in the day, sufficiently for perfect vision.—(See *Lawrence's Treatise on the Diseases of the Eye*, p. 569.)]

Day sight is said to be endemic in some parts of France (*Mém. de la Soc. Royale de Méd.*, 1786); and particularly in the neighbourhood of Roche Guyon, on the banks of the Seine. And so general is its spread there, that in one village we are told it affects one in twenty of the inhabitants, and in another one in ten, every year. It makes its attack in the spring, and continues for three months; sometimes, though in a slighter degree, returning in the autumn; and there are individuals who have had annual returns of the complaint for twenty years in succession. It passes off, after having run its course, or rather, perhaps, after having been treated with due medical attention, without any inconvenience, excepting a weakness in a few eyes that renders them impatient of wind and strong light. The soil is here a dazzling chalk, and the keenness of the first reflected light, after the dreariness of the winter, is probably one cause of so general an evil. [According to M. de Hautesierck, the disorder at one time prevailed extensively among some French troops stationed in Belleisle, under a combination of local peculiarities calculated to act powerfully on the retina, and at a season of the year favourable to their influence.—(*Recueil d'Obs. de Méd. des Hopitaux Militaires*.)] Perhaps however, there is no part of the world in which this disease is found more commonly, or more decidedly, than in Russia: but then it is rarely found except in the Russian summer, when the eye is exposed, almost without intermission, to the constant action of light, as the sun dips but little below the horizon, and there is scarcely any interval of darkness. The malady, again, mostly makes its appearance at this time among the peasants, who protract their hard labour in the fields from a very early to a very late hour; and at the same time exhaust and weaken themselves by their daily fatigue. The sight is soon restored by rest, a proper shade, and bathing the eyes with an infusion of any bitter and astringent vegetable. Dr. Guthrie, in the Memoirs of the Medical Society of London, from which this account has been taken, gives also an example of the disease having appeared suddenly, a few springs before, in a detachment of Russian soldiers; who, being ordered to attack a Swedish post, at the moment of its incursion, had nearly destroyed one another by mistake. These men had been harassed by long marches, and been exposed night and day to the piercing glare of an uninterrupted scene of snowy mountains; both which causes had concurred in producing this effect.

Sir Gilbert Blane has found it occasionally occur in scorbutic patients; but no such diseases appeared in the Russian soldiery. Hens are well known to labour under this defect naturally; and, hence they cannot see to pick up small grains in the dusk of the evening, and so employ this time in going to roost: on which account the disease is sometimes called *hen-blindness*.

[All practitioners who have had opportunities of witnessing this disorder, concur in delivering a favourable prognosis. When it is recollected that Mr. Bampfield (see *Med. Chir. Trans.*, vol. v.), a naval surgeon, saw in the East Indies about three hundred cases, and that they were all easily cured without any permanent injury of sight, no doubt can be entertained of the generally favourable result of proper treatment, in which the avoidance of the cause of the affection is one of the most important things to be observed.]

Tonics and gentle stimulants have been much recommended. The bark may be freely employed internally, and blisters externally, with the vapour of camphire, ether, or carbonated ammonia; and a few drops of the tincture of opium, the citrine ointment, or a minute portion of prussiate of iron, also in the form of an ointment, occasionally applied to the ball of the eye. In most of the endemic cases it seems to be an intermittent, as the preceding species appears to be occasionally; and in such circumstances, a free use of the bark used to be the plan chiefly depended upon. [Of late years, however, in consequence of the great and decided success with which Mr. Bampfield cured every case by means of blisters on the temples, and aperient medicines, this practice is now generally preferred. With it, Mr. Lawrence has occasionally associated cupping from the temples or nape of the neck.]

When the sight is once stimulated by the full light of the day, it occasionally becomes peculiarly acute and vivid. Plenck asserts, that he has known some men labouring under this disease evince so high an excitement of vision as to be able to distinguish the stars at noon.

Dr. Heberden has communicated a singular case of this species, which it will be best to give in his own words.—(*Med. Transactions*, vol. i.) "A man about thirty years old had in the spring a tertian fever, for which he took too small a quantity of bark, so that the returns of it were weakened without being entirely removed. He therefore went into the cold bath; and after bathing twice, he felt no more of his fever. Three days after this last fit, being then employed on board of a ship in the river, he observed, at sunsetting, that all objects began to look blue, which blueness gradually thickened into a cloud; and not long after he became so blind as hardly to perceive the light of a candle. The next morning, about sunrising, his sight was restored as perfectly as ever. When the next night came on, he lost his sight again in the same manner; and this continued for twelve days and nights. He then came ashore, where the disorder of his eyes gradually abated, and in three days was entirely gone. A month after he went on board another ship, and after three days' stay in it the night blindness returned as before, and lasted all the time of his remaining in the ship, which was nine nights. He then left the ship, and his blindness did not return while he was upon land. Some little time afterward he went into another ship, in which he continued for ten days, during which time the blindness returned only two nights, and never afterward."

I have observed that *nyctalopia noctifuga* is often an intermittent affection. In the present case it was distinctly of this nature, and evinced a decided quotidian type. We are not acquainted with the exciting cause of this intermittent; but we know that when once a circuit of action has been established in a weakened and irritable habit, it adheres to the system with almost invincible tenacity, and is recalled with the utmost facility upon a repetition of such a cause. And hence the uniform return of the affection on shipboard, where it commenced, till a cure was obtained.*

SPECIES III.
PAROPSIS LONGINQUA.
LONG SIGHT.
VISION ONLY ACCURATE WHEN THE OBJECT IS FAR OFF.

This is the *dysopia proximorum* of Cullen, the *vue longue* of the French.

In both the preceding species the morbid affection seems chiefly to appertain to the retina; in the present species it belongs chiefly to the iris, which is habitually dilated, and not easily stimulated to a contractile action. "For it is well known," observes Dr. Wells, "to those who are conversant with the facts relating to human vision, that the eye in its relaxed state is fitted for distant objects, and that the seeing of near objects accurately is dependant upon muscular exertion."

* Dr. Davenport remarks, that "this disease is frequently, perhaps commonly, sympathetic of disordered stomach or derangement of the biliary organs." Three instances have been observed by him where p. noctifuga was *congenital*. In two of these the occurrence of *oblique* vision was noticed during the usual nocturnal paroxysm.—See the Boston Med. and Surg. Journal, vol. xi., p. 415.—D.

The species offers three varieties, as follow :—

α Vulgaris. Common long sight.	Iris relaxed, but moveable; cornea mostly too flat.
β Paretica. Unalterable long sight.	Iris incontractile, pupil unchangeable, from partial paralysis.
γ Senectutis. Long sight of age.	Cornea less convex; relaxation and hebetude common to all the powers of the eye.

The FIRST VARIETY is common to every period of life, in which the iris is affected with an habitual relaxation. [The truth of the foregoing statement, that long sight is dependant on the state of the iris, is not very manifest. No doubt, the pupil is often large; but it may be questioned whether this may not be only an effect of the infirmity; for nothing is more certainly established than that this defect of vision, as well as the opposite one, called short sight, is principally occasioned by a peculiarity in the refractive powers of the eye. In long-sighted persons the rays of light are not collected in the proper place, the focus in which they would meet being behind the retina. Like short sight, it is, as Mr. Lawrence has observed in his Lectures, " merely consequent upon some circumstances in the transparent media of the eye, which, in all other respects, is perfectly natural. Now the eye being in a great part of its functions a mechanical instrument, must be subjected to mechanical laws; and we find that a given configuration of the transparent media, a certain relation of them to each other, and their position at a determinate distance from the retina, are necessary to the formation of a distinct picture upon that nervous expansion. There is a certain distance from the eye which is called the point of distinct vision, at which we can see objects in all their details with perfect clearness. Every eye, considered as an optical instrument, has its point of distinct vision. The latter, therefore, varies in different persons, and is generally different in the two eyes of the same individual. Objects are not so distinctly seen when moved nearer to or further from the eye than this point. In ordinary well-constructed eyes, the distance ranges from fifteen to twenty inches." Too flat a configuration of the cornea or crystalline lens, too little distance between the retina and the lens, or too weak a refraction of the rays of light, from insufficient density of the humours and transparent media, total loss of the crystalline lens by operations for cataract, may be so many causes of long sight. It has been remarked by Mr. Wardrop, that when people advance in life, the cornea gradually loses its convexity, perhaps from the humours of the eye being diminished. The change, however, is not absolutely restricted to old persons; for the same writer speaks of a girl eight years of age, the cornea of whose eyes was observed to be remarkably flat, and her vision very imperfect from her infancy. In subjects much enfeebled by considerable evacuations, by numerous bleedings, or by disease, the quantity of the aqueous humour diminishes, the convexity of the cornea is lessened, and they can only see objects at a distance.—(See *Wardrop's Essays on the Morb. Anat of the Human Eye*, p. 115 ; *Portal, Anatomie Médicale*.) The ingenious experiments of Sir Everard Home and the late Mr. Ramsden, recorded in the Philosophical Transactions, prove, however, that the sphericity of the cornea is altered according to the distance at which objects are viewed. Hence, an impairment of this power of accommodation in the eye may sometimes be concerned in the present infirmity, as well as in the opposite one of near sight. In the present, the faculty which the eye has of adapting itself to near objects is presumed to be defective.]*

The SECOND VARIETY constitutes the disease called IMMUTABILITY OF SIGHT by Dr. Young (*Phil. Transact.*, year 1793) ; and is admirably described by Dr. Wells in the Philosophical Transactions, in an interesting case of a young person, about thirty-five years of age, whose retina was as sensible to the stimulus of light as ever ; yet who, from a paresis or permanent dilatation of the pupil, saw near objects with considerable confusion, but remote objects with perfect accuracy. The power of moving the upper eyelid was also lost. It was an extreme case of the disease before us, complicated with partial paralysis of the adjoining muscles, and may be imitated by applying the tincture of belladonna. It was easily remedied by the use of spectacles with convex glasses, by means of which the patient was able to read without difficulty in a printed book, whose letters he was scarcely able to distinguish from each other before the spectacles were applied.

The THIRD VARIETY, or that produced by old age, constitutes the presbytia and presbyopia of medical writers, from πρέσβυς, *senex*, and takes place in various degrees. The rays of light unite into a focus too late ; that is to say, they strike the retina before they have conjoined into a focus ; and the focus which they are calculated to form would be situated behind the retina. [The eyes undergo certain changes in age, which have the effect of diminishing their refractive power. Persons after fifty, and sometimes before that age, generally find that they cannot distinguish near objects so well as they have been accustomed to do. The rays of light are more divergent the nearer the object is to the eye : and the further it may be, the more do they approach to the parallel direction ; consequently, a greater refractive power is necessary in the former than in the latter case. Far-sighted persons can see distant inscriptions, or distinguish the hour by a distant church clock, when they cannot read a common print held in their own hands, or see the figures and hands of a watch. The custom of old persons to hold a

book or letter a long way from their eyes, and to draw back their heads, in order to be able to read it, when they have not their spectacles at hand, is familiarly known.]

In the present, as in the other varieties of this affection of the eyes, the best remedy for supplying the deficient convexity of the cornea, as well as the deficient irritability of the iris, is convex spectacles ; adapting their power to the precise demand of the eye, and increasing it as the demand grows more urgent.

They should be of that power which will enable the patient to see without straining the organ, and should only be worn for reading, writing, or the examination of near objects.

SPECIES IV.

PAROPSIS PROPINQUA.

SHORT SIGHT.

VISION ONLY ACCURATE WHEN THE OBJECT IS NEAR.

THIS (the myopia of many writers) is in most respects an opposite disease to the preceding ; for it not only produces an opposite effect, but proceeds, in the main, from an opposite cause. In the former, the iris is for the most part relaxed and weakly ; here it is sound, often too much contracted : in the former, the cornea is in almost all cases too much flattened ; in the present, it is too convex or polarized. The best palliative, therefore, is spectacles of an opposite character to those recommended under the preceding species ; and with these we must satisfy ourselves till age brings us a natural relief, by taking off the eutony and depressing the cornea. Unfortunately, however, this is a relief that does not always continue for many years, since the excess of tone becomes too much lowered as the age advances, and the sight grows imperfect from this cause.

Mice are said to have this kind of vision naturally, and hence one of the technical names for it is myopia or myopiasis, literally " mouse-sight."

[The explanation of the infirmity is, that rays of light are collected too soon, and brought into a focus before they reach the retina. Although a sound eye never discerns remote objects so clearly as near ones, inasmuch as the rays of light entering the eye from a distant thing are always fewer in proportion to its distance from the organ, yet a short-sighted eye sees objects at even a very small distance very indistinctly. The degrees of short sight are various : some individuals cannot discern things which are beyond two inches from their eyes. In the worst form, the person squints in examining an object with care ; for he is compelled to put it so close to the eyes that the visual axis of the two eyes cannot be made simultaneously to bring it within their scope. This defect of vision depends upon the refractive powers being too strong, the eyeball being too long, or the impairment of that faculty by which the eye accommodates itself to distant as well as to near objects. The premature formation of a focus within the eye some-

---

* See Farther Observations on Vision, by Dr. Hosack, published in the Trans. of the Royal Society for 1794 : in this paper the author attributes to the action of the external muscles of the eye its power of accommodation to objects of different focal distances. On this principle Mr. Ramsden formed his artificial eye.—D.

times depends on the great convexity of the cornea; a state which is always promoted by the humours being very abundant in the eye. Hence the reason why a short sight is most frequent in young persons; why it sometimes decreases with age; and why any accidental causes increasing or diminishing the quantity of humours in a sound eye may render it sometimes rather shortsighted, and sometimes oppositely disposed. It is a common opinion, that persons who are short-sighted from too great a convexity of the cornea always have objects depicted upon their retinæ in a larger and plainer way than is the case in the eyes of other individuals. This circumstance, which does not appear to be well founded, is ascribed to the strong refractive powers of the eye. According to Mr. Lawrence, there is no ground for the notion that a near sight is strong sight. Another thing generally promulgated by writers, and already mentioned here, does not coincide with this gentleman's observations. "The eye, in progress of age," he says (op cit., p. 580), "becomes presbyopic, and it might be supposed that this natural change in the organ would remedy the excess of refractive power in the near-sighted, and enable them to dispense with their concave glasses: but this is not the case; the near-sighted continue so in old age." As this account disagrees with that given by Richter (*Anfängsgr. der Wundarzn.*, b. iii., p. 487), and other men of great experience in disorders of the eye, it is noticed here as one meriting further investigation. Besides great convexity of the cornea, other causes of short sight are generally enumerated; as too great convexity of the lens; preternatural density of the transparent parts of the organ; too great a space between the cornea or lens, and the retina; or a loss of the power by which the eye accommodates itself to the varying distances of objects. On this subject there is an interesting passage in Mr. Lawrence's Treatise, in p. 578. "It may be a question," he says, "whether this state of the eye depends upon the habits of the individual. I am inclined to think that the habitual mode of employing the organ has some influence. In persons of a literary and studious character, who use their eyes much in reading or writing, and in others who are constantly occupied on minute objects near the eye, we observe that the sight is frequently myopic. I remember once attending a book-sale, at which I was struck by the number of persons wearing spectacles: having counted them, I found there were twenty-three gentlemen in the room, and that twelve of the number had spectacles on. Mr. Ware endeavoured to ascertain the proportional number of the near-sighted in the different ranks of society, and he consulted the surgeons of the different regiments of Guards in and about London, at that time comprehending about 10,000 men; and he was informed that near-sightedness was almost unknown among them; not six individuals had been discharged, nor six recruits rejected, on this account, in twenty years. He pursued the investigation at the Military Asylum at Chelsea, containing 1300 children,

among whom only three were near-sighted. He then made some comparative inquiries of the heads of colleges at Oxford and Cambridge, and found near-sightedness very prevalent in all those institutions. In one particular instance, where the society consisted of 127 members, thirty-two either wore spectacles or used hand-glasses.— (*Ware's Tracts on the Eye*, p. 201, &c.) From these facts, together with the well-known far-sightedness of sailors and country people, we may infer that the habitual mode of-employing the eyes has a decided influence in rendering them either myopic or presbyopic. Near-sightedness is not observed early in life; you never see persons trying to use glasses until towards the age of fourteen, or from that to eighteen." Mr. Lawrence admits, however, that the defect may exist previously without being noticed, as very young persons do not attend minutely to the state of their sight, er compare accurately their own vision with that of others.

The only assistance which a near-sighted person can obtain is from concave glasses, which should be such as will enable him to see distant objects distinctly, without producing any sense of painful exertion in the eye. As there is great reason to believe, with Mr. Lawrence, that the optical powers of the eye accommodate themselves to the circumstances under which vision is habitually exercised, near-sighted persons should not wear spectacles constantly, but only at periods when such aid is particularly required.—(See *Lawrence*, op. cit., pp. 579–580.)]

SPECIES V.

PAROPSIS LATERALIS.

SKEW SIGHT. SIGHT ASKEW.

VISION ONLY ACCURATE WHEN THE OBJECT IS PLACED OBLIQUELY.

In this species the patient can only see in an oblique direction, in consequence of some partial obfuscation of the cornea (usually, perhaps, from scratches or slight scars), or of the humours through which the light is transmitted, or from a partial paralysis of the retina. This must not be confounded with strabismus, or squinting, as it sometimes has been, but which proceeds from a different cause, and is accompanied with different phenomena. In skew sight, or lateral vision, the axis of the eye affected usually coincides with that of the sound eye, though it runs somewhat obliquely, to avoid the obstruction in the tunic. In strabismus the two axes do not coincide, and the judgment is formed from the strongest eye alone. If, however, in lateral vision, the obstruction be such as to make the optical axis of the affected eye at variance with that of the sound eye, squinting must be a necessary consequence of the disease.

SPECIES VI.

PAROPSIS ILLUSORIA.

FALSE SIGHT.

IMAGINARY OBJECTS FLOATING BEFORE THE

SIGHT; OR REAL OBJECTS APPEARING WITH IMAGINARY QUALITIES.

THIS species, thus defined, clearly includes two varieties, as follow :—

α Phantasmatum. Appearances of objects
Ocular spectres. before the sight that have no real existence.

β Mutationis. Real objects apparently
Ocular transmuta- changed in their natu-
tions. ral qualities.

Both these varieties offer a very numerous family of distinct illusory perceptions, which require to be noticed in their order.

Of the OCULAR SPECTRES, constituting the FIRST VARIETY, one of the most frequent forms is that of DARK SPOTS. These are the *muscæ volitantes* of many authors; and are "sometimes," says Dr. Young, "if not always, occasioned by an opacity of some of the vessels of the vitreous humour near the retina. They are seen in a full light, and cannot, therefore, as Sauvages has justly remarked, be caused by any thing in the anterior part of the eye; and they may often be observed to change their form with the motions of the eye; which they could not do if they did not depend on some floating substance. Their apparent change of position, when we attempt to follow them with the eye, is a necessary consequence of the motion of the eye itself which contains them."—(*Delius, Diss. Phantas. ante oculos volitantia,* Erlang, 1751.)

If, however, these phantasmata depended upon vascular opacity of any kind, it is difficult to account for their mobility. And hence Demours is perhaps nearer the mark, in ascribing them to small portions of Morgagni's humour that have acquired an increase of density, weight, and refractile power, without losing their transparency.—(*Traité des Maladies des Yeux,* p. 409.) And in this view of their formation Mr. Guthrie coincides.[*]

Another form these ocular spectres exhibit is that of NET-WORK; hence called *suffusio reticularis* by Sauvages, and *visus reticularis* by Plenck. This is sometimes permanent, sometimes transitory; and is probably, as conjectured by Sauvages, produced by a morbid affection of the arteriolæ of the retina.

A third form is that of SPARKS: and hence called by Sauvages *suffusio scintillans.* It proceeds generally from a blow, or excess of light.

---

[*] Lectures on the Operative Surgery of the Eye, p. 211, 1823, 8vo. Mr. Lawrence is of opinion, that the immediate cause of muscæ volitantes has not yet been satisfactorily explained. The notions of partial pressure on the nervous structure, by distention of vessels in the retina or the choroid, or by inequality in the surface of the latter membrane, he regards as purely conjectural. The explanation derived from minute particles supposed to be floating in the aqueous humour, seems to him to have no better foundation.—(See Lawrence's Treatise on the Diseases of the Eye, b. 567.) We know that muscæ volitantes are an early symptom in amaurosis; and probably in all cases they depend upon functional derangement of the retina, temporary or permanent. Such disorder may be combined with organic disease.—ED.

The eye is also troubled with an imaginary sense of DAZZLING, constituting the marmoryge of the Greek writers. Its usual cause is supposed to be a plethora of the minute vessels of the eye.

Sometimes, from the same cause, the ocular spectres assume an IRIDESCENT APPEARANCE; or exhibit, in splendid succession, all the colours of the rainbow. This Sauvages calls *suffusio coloris.* It is occasionally a regularly intermittent affection, or returns at stated periods, and particularly in the evenings; and occasionally the morbid appearance is confined to a single colour. Dr. Heberden has given a curious example of an affection of this kind in a lady of advanced age, who took lodgings on the eastern coast of Kent, in a house that looked immediately upon the sea, and was of course very much exposed to the glare of the morning sun. The curtains of the bed in which she slept, and of the windows, were of white linen, which added to the intensity of the light. When she had been there about ten days, she observed one evening, at the time of sunset, that first the fringes of the clouds appeared red, and soon after the same colour was diffused over all the objects around her, and especially if the objects were white, as a sheet of paper, a pack of cards, or a lady's gown. This lasted the whole night; but in the morning her sight was again perfect. The same alternation of morbid and sound sight continued the whole time the lady was on the coast, which was three weeks, and for nearly as long after she left it; at which time it ceased suddenly and entirely of its own accord. Excess of light upon a delicate and irritable habit appears to have been the cause of this singular affection. The retina was too strongly excited to throw off the impression easily; and that of the red rays of the descending sun constituting the last impression communicated, remained after the sun itself had disappeared. The circle of action may be easily accounted for by a uniform return of the same cause.

The SECOND VARIETY of FALSE SIGHT, or that in which real objects appear changed in their natural qualities, is by Plenck denominated, in consequence of such change, metamorphopsia.

Sometimes the change exhibits ERROR OF FORM; and the objects appear too large, too small, cut in half, or distorted.

Sometimes ERROR OF MOTION: in consequence of which they seem to be dancing, nodding, or in rapid succession.

Sometimes ERROR OF NUMBER: and then they appear double, triple, or otherwise increased or multiplied; constituting the diplopia of Sauvages and many other writers.

Sometimes ERROR OF COLOUR; in which case one hue is mistaken for another, as red for green, or green for yellow, or every hue appears alike. Examples of this imperfection are not unfrequent. Mr. Scott has given a singular instance of it (*Phil. Trans.,* vol. lxviii., 1778, p. 611), and Dr. Priestley another.—(Id., lxvii., 1777, p. 260.) The last is especially worthy of notice, as in some degree a family defect; and was communicated to Dr. Priestley by Mr. Huddart, of North America. Of five brothers and two sisters, all adults, three of the former were affected with it in a greater or less degree ; while the remaining two and the two sisters possessed perfect vision. One of the brothers could form no idea whatever of colours, though he judged very accurately of the form and other qualities of objects ; and hence he thought stockings were sufficiently distinguished by the name of stockings, and could not conceive the necessity of calling some red and others blue. He could perceive cherries on cherry-trees, but only distinguished them, even when red-ripe, from the surrounding leaves, by their size and shape. One of the brothers appears to have had a faint sense of a few colours, but still a very imperfect notion ; and upon the whole, they seem to have possessed no other distinguishing power than that of light and shade, into which they resolved all the colours presented to them ; so that dove and straw-coloured were regarded as white, and green, crimson, and purple, as black or dark. On looking at a rainbow, one of them could distinguish it as consisting of stripes, but nothing more.

Dr. Nicholl, of Ludlow, has published two papers* on the imperfection of vision producing a delusive appearance of colours. His cases were hereditary, and not symptomatic of amaurosis. In one, the imperfection seems to have been confined to one or two colours alone. The patient could easily distinguish the green of the grass, or the leaves of the trees.; but like those in Mr. Huddart's statement, he confounded with the green the red fruit or flowers which, happened to be intermixed with it. The false sight in this case was also connected with *paropsis longinqua ;* for the patient saw objects at a greater distance than other people, and more distinctly in the dark. The irides were here also gray, with a yellow tinge round the pupil.†

The causes of these varieties are not always assignable : many of them, however, are the same as have been pointed out under the variety

---

* Transact. of the Medico-Chir. Soc., vols. vii. and ix. For additional facts on this subject, consult Glasgow Med. Journ., vol. ii., art. 2.

† The following observations on the cause of this curious infirmity, are delivered by Mr. Lawrence :—" This peculiarity, which is an original defect, and not a pathological condition, is seated, according to the opinion of Drs. Gall and Spurzheim, in the sensorium. They conceive that the function of the eye is limited to the receiving certain impressions, but that the judging of these impressions, the power of understanding the relations which colours bear to each other, is the function of the sensorium ; and they assign this faculty to a particular part of the brain. It is certain that an eye may be excellent for the general purposes of vision, and capable of distinguishing the minutest objects, and yet the individual may not be able to judge of colours. The latter power, with the accurate perception of the harmony of colours, and their various relations to each other, is a higher endowment : indeed, only a few persons possess it eminently."—(See Treatise on Diseases of the Eye, p. 574.) The incapacity of distinguishing colours, viewed as an original defect, and one seated in the organization of the brain, must be incurable.—ED.

of ocular spectres. Diplopia, or errors of number, have often been occasioned by long exposure to severe cold ; sometimes by local spasm, sometimes by hydrocephalus.—(*Justi, Baldinger, N. Mag.*, bande xi., p. 446.) Baumer gives a case produced by a wrong position of the pupil.—(*Act. Hafn.*, i., bert. xxvii.) Raghellini another caused by a double pupil.—(*Lettera al S. Coechi sopra l' offesa della vista in una Donna*, Veneta, 1748, 1479.) In Letin is a singularly complicated example of objects seen triply.—(Lib. ii., obs. 20.)

The chief diagnostic of many of these illusions is their mobility (*Guthrie, Lectures*, &c., ut suprà, p. 212), which distinguishes them very decidedly from the fixed spots perceived in the eye, and which depend on an opacity of the lens. They are well known frequently to precede amaurosis. Sometimes, however, when they have reached a certain point, they cease to become more troublesome, or rather, from habit, to be troublesome at all, and are little attended to : for if amaurosis do not soon follow, there is no reason for expecting it ; a consolation of no small moment, as no certain remedy has hitherto been discovered.

In other cases, and especially where the misaffection is not structural, but dependant upon an entonic or an atonic condition of the optic nerve, muscular fibres, or bloodvessels, benefit has been derived in the first instance from local bleeding, blisters, and sedatives ; the sedatives being employed both generally and topically :* and in the last instance from stimulant collyriums and general tonics.

Many of these varieties of false sight, and especially ocular spectres, are also found as symptoms in several species of dinus, syspasia, syncope, plethora, cephalitis, dyspepsy, and various fevers : some few of the filaments, of the great sympathetic passing off, at its origin within the cavernous sinus, to the orbit, and uniting with the lenticular ganglion.—(*Cloquet, Traité d'Anat. Descriptive ; Bloch, Besch. des fünfter Nervenpaares*, &c., Leip., 1817.)

SPECIES VII.
PAROPSIS CALIGO.
OPAQUE CORNEA.

DIMNESS OR ABOLITION OF SIGHT, FROM OPACITY OF THE CORNEA OR SPOTS UPON ITS SURFACE.

THE Latin term CALIGO sufficiently explains the nature of the disease, by importing " dimness, darkness, cloudiness, obscurity." In old English, this opacity, as well as the pterygium, was denominated a " web of the eye," from its giving the idea of a film spreading across the sight ; whence Shakspeare in King Lear, "This is the foul fiend Flibbertigibbet : he gives the

---

* Several forms of paropsis illusoria, or false vision, depend on a disturbed state of the digestive organs or on plethora. Hence, too, some one of them is more apt to occur when the tone of the system has become impaired by previous illness, by a long course of inebriation, or by excess in eating and drinking, and also by great efforts of mind.—D.

ᴡᴇʙ and the ᴘɪɴ: squints the eye, and makes the hare-lip." The ᴘɪɴ is a variety of the synizesis, "closed or contracted pupil."

[Surgeons usually divide common opacities of the cornea into four varieties or kinds:—

a Nebula corneæ.	Superficial opacity.
β Albugo.	Deep-seated dense opacity.
γ Leucoma.	A white cicatrix.
δ Arcus senilis.	Circular loss of transparency, extending in old age from the margin of the cornea.

The first or simple opacity, or *nebula corneæ*, as it is often termed, is a diffused cloudiness of the whole or a part of that membrane, without any distinct or circumscribed boundary. Hence it is always greatest in its centre, and gradually diminishes towards its circumference. The iris and pupil are discernible through the dimness, and the patient yet has a degree of vision. It rarely extends to the deep lamellæ of the cornea, but is generally restricted to a cloudiness or milky thickness, arising from the albuminous secretion effused under the corneal conjunctiva, or in the texture of this delicate membrane itself.

When this superficial cloudiness of the cornea is accompanied with active inflammation of the eye, the treatment must be regulated by the principles applicable to ophthalmia in general. The disease is mostly attended with groups of turgid, knotty vessels in the conjunctiva. If this be the case, another indication presents itself besides that of diminishing inflammation; namely, to reduce the enlarged vessels; and if that be impracticable, to cut off all communication between the trunks of the most prominent of them in the conjunctiva, and the branches immediately distributed to the nebulous portion of the cornea. For the first purpose, Scarpa recommends the unguent. hydrarg. nitrat. and astringent collyria; for the second, the excision of a fasciculus of the enlarged vessels.* These measures may often be proper; but in Scarpa's practice the cause of the affection is not much considered; and if the treatment were regulated with reference to it, some of the plans which he proposes would not be needed. As a nebulous state of the cornea generally arises from inflammation or irritation, and is kept up by it, whatever removes the cause will also disperse the cloudiness of that membrane. Thus, the nebula is often dependant on the irritation of hard fungous granulations on the inside of the eyelid, a sequel of purulent ophthalmia: now, if these granulations are removed, the nebula soon disappears without any other proceeding. The first indication, when inflammation is present, is to put a stop to it. If we do this, and wait a little, we shall find that the opacity will diminish of itself. Afterward, coun-

* This practice is not approved by Mr. Lawrence: he has little confidence in its efficacy, and objects to it also on the ground that the vessels of the cornea are derived from the sclerotica, and not from the conjunctiva. Scarpa means, however, the vessels visibly extending to the opaque part of the cornea to be partially removed by excision, without any reference to their origin.—Eᴅ.

ter-irritation by issue, or seton in the temple, with attention to diet, and the state of the stomach and bowels, will be proper. Then the absorption of the opaque matter may be promoted by collyria containing the nitrate of silver in the proportion of two grains of it to one ounce of distilled water at first, the strength being gradually increased. It may be dropped into the eye, or applied to the opaque part with a camel-hair pencil.—(See *Lawrence on Diseases of the Eye*, p. 371.)

Albugo and *leucoma* are deeper opacities of the cornea, arising from previous severe ophthalmia, or an ulcer or wound of the cornea. The term *leucoma* is particularly applied to the pearl-coloured opacity, produced by the cicatrix of a wound or ulcer. In these deep opacities, the texture of the cornea is often so disorganized that they cannot be removed; for they do not consist merely of an effusion of a thin milky secretion, but of a dense lymph, which insinuates itself between all the lamellæ of the cornea, and becomes inseparably connected with them. When an albugo is recent, however, its dispersion may be attempted by applying the ung. hydrarg. nitrat. to it, and bathing the eye with a collyrium made of rose-water, and two grains of the nitrate of silver to each ounce of it. The leucoma occasioned by a cicatrix is evidently incurable.

The *arcus senilis*, or that opacity formed in persons of advanced years round the whole or part of the margin of the cornea, and sometimes extending considerably towards the pupil, so as to lessen the sphere of vision, is the effect of old age, and absolutely incurable. It comes on without any pain or uneasiness, and at length renders the texture of the cornea, in the part which it occupies, entirely impervious to light. This opaque circle, Mr. Lawrence observes (op. cit., p. 369), is not situated at the very margin of the cornea, but there is generally a transparent rim which intervenes between it and the sclerotic coat. In some cases, the opacity is very narrow; and in other cases, it becomes much broader; but he has never seen it interfere with vision, a sufficiency of the centre of the cornea for this purpose being left transparent. He describes it as a natural change in the part, from causes independent of disease. It shows itself, he says, much earlier in some cases than others; being occasionally seen between the ages of thirty and forty, but generally later. He compares it to the opaque knots which take place in the internal coat of the larger arteries of old persons.]

In newly-born infants spots on the cornea are occasionally met with, which soon vanish spontaneously (*Farr, Med. Commen.*, ii., 30): probably, the rays of light acting as a salutary stimulus upon the occasion.

SPECIES VIII.
PAROPSIS GLAUCOSIS.
HUMORAL OPACITY.

ᴅɪᴍɴᴇss ᴏʀ ᴀʙᴏʟɪᴛɪᴏɴ ᴏғ sɪɢʜᴛ ғʀᴏᴍ ᴏᴘᴀᴄɪᴛʏ
ᴏғ ᴛʜᴇ ᴠɪᴛʀᴇᴏᴜs ʜᴜᴍᴏᴜʀ.

Gʟᴀᴜᴄᴏsɪs is a Greek term, from γλαυκὸς, "bluish or greenish teinted," from the common colour of the obscurity. It was also called by the Greeks glaucóma, and by the Romans glaucédo. Glaucosis is here preferred to glaucóma, because the final oma imports usually, and, for the sake of simplicity and consistency, ought always to import, external protuberance; as in staphyloma, sarcoma, and various others noticed in detail in the volume of Nosology.

[It is remarked by Mr. Lawrence that the term glaucóma was formerly given to cataract, but is no longer so applied. We use it now to denote a certain change of the vitreous humour consequent on inflammation of that part of the eye, attended with an alteration in the colour of the pupil. The first symptom of glaucosis, as our author prefers to call it, is a pain in the head, usually situated over the brow. In conjunction with this pain, the patient begins to complain of dimness or of weakness of the sight; and, if the eye be now examined, the pupil presents a greenish, muddy-green, or yellowish-green colour, instead of its natural deep-black. In a strong light, the appearance resembles a yellowish metallic reflection from the bottom of the eye. At the same time, the pupil is generally rather dilated, and the motions of the iris sluggish. The state of vision is different in different instances: in some, an alteration of the pupil is distinctly produced, and yet the eyesight may be tolerably perfect; while in other cases vision is entirely lost, with apparently no more discoloration of the back part of the eye, or change of the pupil, than in the former instance. Glaucosis has of late years generally been regarded as an inflammation of the vitreous humour, the texture and colour of which are changed. As the retina lies close upon this humour, there is no difficulty in accounting for their both being inflamed; and whether they both suffer from the commencement or not, if the inflammation of the vitreous humour be not checked it will involve the retina, and produce such changes in its structure as to render the eye permanently amaurotic. The eyesight becomes gradually worse and worse; the discoloration behind the pupil grows more and more considerable; and the iris becomes more and more sluggish, until it is at last motionless, and vision is entirely lost. The lens also is sometimes attacked, and with it the iris propelled forward, so that, as Mr. Lawrence remarks, it is no uncommon thing for cataract to occur subsequently in an eye originally attacked by glaucosis.

Glaucosis, the precise causes of which are not known, occurs chiefly after the middle period of life, and in persons not of the most healthy character. It appears to Mr. Lawrence to be merely a chronic form of what is sometimes termed arthritic inflammation of the deep part of the eye; but he particularly mentions that it does not occur more frequently in gouty and rheumatic persons than in others; so that the expression arthritic cannot be very eligible.

In glaucosis, the colour of the pupil is green, or yellowish-green; and if the eye be viewed laterally, no discoloration can be seen; but in cataract, the pupil looks gray, or of a grayish

white, and it remains so, whether it be regarded laterally or not. The loss of vision in glaucosis is not in direct proportion to the change of colour of the pupil; for, with an inconsiderable change of this kind, vision may be entirely destroyed or very seriously impaired. But in cataract there is a direct proportion between the state of the opacity or change of colour, and the injury to sight. In cataract, vision is best in a weak light; but in glaucosis, sight is most perfect in a strong light.—(Lawrence, op. cit., p. 393.)

It is not yet decided among pathologists, whether the opacity in this disease be seated in the delicate membranous septa of the tunica hyaloidea, or in the fluid contained in the cells of the vitreous humour; or whether both are altered. Beer, in dissecting a glaucomatous eye, found the vitreous humour immediately surrounding the foramen of Soemmerring much more deeply coloured than the rest of it. Were this fact corroborated by further observations, we might perhaps infer that this is generally the original seat of the disease, and that the morbid changes extend from this point.[*]

Beer delivers a most discouraging prognosis, asserting that nothing will prevent glaucosis from terminating in amaurosis. All practical writers seem to agree that we possess no means of removing the opacity of the vitreous humour; but Mr. Lawrence is of opinion that the disease may be checked, and any degree of sight now enjoyed preserved, by having recourse to suitable treatment. There is, he says, a decided congestion about the brain and orbit, and the removal of that congestion is attended with considerable benefit. Hence, he recommends antiphlogistic remedies; cupping; active purgatives; alterative doses of mercury; a regulated diet; and repose of the eye. By such means, he has known cases kept for two or three years stationary.]

SPECIES IX.

PAROPSIS CATARACTA.

CATARACT.

DIMNESS OR ABOLITION OF SIGHT, FROM OPACITY OF THE CRYSTALLINE LENS.

THE cataract, as it is now called, was by old English writers named PEARL EYE, or PEARL IN THE EYE, and is so denominated by Holland,

---

[*] G. Frick, on Diseases of the Eye, p. 220, 2d ed. by Welbank, 1826. Mr. Mackenzie observed the following changes in eyes affected with glaucoma:—1. The choroid coat, and especially the portion of it in contact with the retina, was of a light brown colour, without any appearance of pigmentum nigrum. 2. The vitreous humour was in a fluid state, perfectly pellucid, colourless, or slightly yellow. There was no trace of hyaloid membrane. 3. The lens was of a yellow or amber colour towards its centre, its consistence firm, and its transparency perfect, or nearly so. 4. In the retina, no trace of limbus luteus, nor of the foramen centrale.—See Glasgow Med. Journ., vol. iii., p. 259; and Mackenzie's Treatise on Diseases of the Eye.—ED.

the faithful translator of Pliny. Cataracta, as a Greek term, is usually derived from καταῤῥάσσω, " to disturb, destroy, or abolish." Καταῤῥάκτης or καταράκτης, however, was employed by the Greek writers themselves to signify a gate, door, or loophole, and the bar which fastens it, and becomes the impediment to its being opened.' And it is probably from this last sense that the term cataract was first applied to the disease in question, as forming a bar to the eyes, which were called the loopholes or windows of the mind by various philosophers, as we learn from Lucretius, who thus closes his opposition to their view :—

" Dicere porro oculos nullam rem cernere posse, Sed per eos animum ut *foribus* spectare reclusis Difficile est."*

To deem the eyes, then, of themselves survey Naught in existence, while the interior mind Looks at all nature through them, as alone Through *windows*, is to trifle—

Whence, perhaps, Shakspeare, in the speech of Richmond :—

" To thee I do commend my wakeful soul, Ere I *let fall the windows* of mine eyes."

The Greeks themselves, however, called this disease indifferently hypochyma, apochysis, and hypochysis. The earlier Latins, suffusio : while cataracta seems first to have been made use of by the Arabian writers, and was probably introduced into the medical nomenclature by Avicenna. Yet the more common name among the Arabians was *gutta obscura*, as that for amaurosis was *gutta serena;* the pupil, in this last species, being serene or transparent.

The Arabians, who had adopted generally the humoral pathology of Galen, conceived both these diseases to be the result of a morbid rheum or defluxion falling on a particular part of the visual orb ; in the one case producing blindness with obscurity, whence the name of an obscure *rheum* or *gutta;* and in the other without obscurity, whence the contrary name of a transparent or serene *rheum* or *gutta*. But as various other diseases, and particularly of the joints, were also supposed to flow from a like cause, and were far more common, the terms *gutta* and *rheuma* were afterward emphatically applied and at length altogether limited to these last complaints, whence the terms *gout* and *rheumatism*, which have descended to the present day, as the author has already had occasion to observe under ARTHROSIA PODAGRA. For *gutta* the Arabian writers sometimes employed *aqua;* and hence cataract and amaurosis are described by many of them under the names of *aqua obscura* and *aqua serena;* and the former, by way of emphasis, sometimes under the name of *aqua* or *arqua* alone.

The opacity producing a cataract may exist in the lens alone, the capsule alone, or in both ; thus laying a foundation for the three following varieties :—

a Lenticularis. The opacity existing in the
`Lenticular cat- lens itself, and confined to
aract. it.

β Capsularis. The opacity confined to the
Capsular or capsule, or membrane of
membranous the lens.
cataract.
γ Complicata. The opacity common to the
Complicated lens and its capsule.
cataract.

We are told moreover by Richter (*Von der Ausziehung des Grauen Staars*, Gott., 1773, 8vo.), of a cataract of the humour of Morgagni, or the interstitial fluid which lies between the capsule and the lens : whence this has also been copied by Plenck, Beer, and Sir William Adams, into the list of modifications ; but rather as a possible than an actual case ; for none of these practitioners give a single example of such a variety ever having occurred to them with certainty, though Beer suspected it in one case. —(*Lehre von den Augenkrankheiten*, band ii., sect. 56.)

[Mr. Lawrence doubts the separate existence of this as a distinct species of cataract. How, he asks, could we determine that this fluid was opaque, and the lens transparent ? Can it be supposed that it could undergo this change, and the capsule and lens remain transparent ? He thinks, therefore, that in a practical consideration of the subject, this kind of cataract might be safely omitted.]

Cataract is sometimes accompanied with a sac, enclosing a small body of pus or ichor, and is probably the result of the inflammation that produced it. In this case it forms the cataracta capsulo-lenticularis cum bursa ichorem continente of Schmidt.—(*Ueber Nachstaar und Iritis*, &c., Wien, 1801.) Beer affirms that this sac is commonly seated between the lens and posterior part of the capsule, and very rarely between the former and the anterior part.— (*Lehre von den Augenkrankheiten*, band ii., p. 301, 1813.)

Professor Beer seems to have refined a little too much in his divisions and subdivisions of cataract ; for he not only assigns a distinct place to the Morgagnian and this pustular cystic, but to a cystic form without pus, to a siliquose, and a trabecular ; while he further partitions the capsular into two separate forms, according as it is before or behind the lens itself, thus giving us a catalogue of nine distinct forms of what he calls the *true* cataract, while he allots four other subdivisions to what he denominates the *spurious* cataract : meaning hereby some other obstacle to vision, the seat of which is without the crystalline capsule, between its anterior hemisphere and the iris.

[The most striking circumstances observable in cataract are an opaque body placed behind, or even filling up the pupil, and the impaired state of vision which is the result of that change. In both these respects it agrees in its incipient stage with glaucoma and some forms of amaurosis ; but as the treatment is essentially different in these several affections, it is very necessary to discriminate them accurately. In incipient cataract we can do little or nothing ; we must wait until the opacity has become complete before we perform an operation : but

* De Rer. Nat., iii., 260.

in the early state of amaurosis we must take means to arrest the affection; for if we should leave the case to itself, under the supposition of its being a cataract, loss of sight would be inevitable and irremediable. The diagnosis of cataract from other affections, Mr. Lawrence, therefore, very properly represents as an important subject; and in doubtful cases we shall be much assisted by the influence which the belladonna has in dilating the pupil, and affording as clear a view as possible of what lies behind that opening.—(Op. cit., p. 397.)

The situation of the opacity is the best ground of distinction between glaucosis and cataract: in the latter it is very near the pupil; but in glaucosis, and also amaurosis, the discoloration of the pupil is much more deeply seated; it looks as if it were at the back of the eye; and hence, when the eye is viewed laterally in glaucosis, no opacity is perceived. The discoloration cannot be seen unless the surgeon look directly into the pupil; it is also equally diffused, and sometimes the opacity has a concave appearance.

The following observations, by the same surgeon, are highly valuable to the practitioner. In cataract, the opacity begins generally in the centre of the pupil; consequently it is more dense in the centre, and less so towards the sides. Hence, some light passes through the circumference of the pupil, enabling the patient to see objects laterally, when he cannot see them directly in front of the eye. Dilatation of the pupil, by exposing the margin of the lens, which is sometimes transparent when the centre is opaque, and at all events is much thinner, and therefore less densely opaque, improves vision considerably, especially in incipient lenticular cataract. Such patients see best in the dusk or twilight, or when the pupil has been artificially dilated by the belladonna. They see best when their back is turned towards the window. These circumstances particularly distinguish cases of cataract from those of glaucoma and amaurosis; for, in the latter affections, the sensibility of the retina being impaired, the individual generally sees better in strong lights, and his sight is not improved by belladonna.

In the commencement of cataract, objects seem as if surrounded by a mist or fog; the patient fancies that there is something interposed between his eye and the object at which he is looking; while the haziness or cloudiness increases gradually in proportion to the degree of opacity. A cataract patient sees a lighted candle as if it were involved in a cloud, which becomes thicker as the opacity proceeds, and ultimately shrouds the flame so completely that its position only is discernible. To an amaurotic patient the flame of a candle would appear as if scattered into rays, like a star, or surrounded by a halo, or confused with prismatic colours. In cataract, the sight is impaired in proportion to the degree of opacity; but there is no such direct ratio in glaucosis and amaurosis; for, with only a slight greenish discoloration of the pupil, there may be a considerably impaired state of vision, such as the opacity would not

account for; indeed, sight may be entirely destroyed when there is only a trivial change in the colour of the pupil.

With respect to the iris and figure of the pupil, Mr. Lawrence observes, they are not generally affected by cataract, or at any rate, not in the early period of its formation. The iris continues to move as usual, and the pupil retains its circular shape. In some cases, indeed, where the bulk of the lens is increased, this body presses against the iris and impedes its motions; but this happens chiefly in soft cataracts, and not in the early stage of them. In cases of cataract, the margin of the pupil represents a black circle, formed by the uvea, in consequence of the white or grayish-white ground which the opaque lens constitutes behind that opening.—(Lawrence, op. cit., p. 399; also, Beer, Lehre, &c., b. ii., p. 281.)]

Cataracts are of different colours and of different degrees of consistency, from circumstances influencing the morbid action with which we are but little acquainted; and as little with the occasional causes of such action, though old age seems to be a common predisposing cause. They are therefore black,[*] white, leaden-hued, ferruginous, amber; as they are also fluid or milky, soft, firm, hard, horny, and even bony. They are not unfrequently the result of an hereditary taint, adhering to generation after generation, and appearing either congenitally, or by a very general predisposition afterward.

All ages are subject to cataracts; children are even born with them; and they may occur at any age, from infancy to the remotest period of life. Perhaps elderly persons are most subject to the cataract, especially from fifty, sixty, or upwards.[†] Cataracts are never hard in young persons; you will never meet with a hard lens below the age of puberty. They are not always hard in old persons; you may have soft cataracts in such, and hard ones during the middle period of life.—(Lawrence, op. cit., p. 410.)

Mr. Pott inculcated what experience has amply confirmed, that when the opaque crystalline is perfectly dissolved, so as to form a soft cataract, it is somewhat enlarged; and that when such dissolution does not take place, and a hard cataract is produced, the crystalline is in some degree lessened. The hard cataract has also

---

* The occurrence of black cataract is still a matter of dispute. Dupuytren, with his vast experience, has never seen a case of it.—See his Clinical Lectures on Surgery, translated by Doane, New-York, 1833, p. 39.

† The following table is compiled from the observations of Drs. Maunoir and Fabini.

Of 612 cases of cataract,

14	were between	1 and 10 years of age.				
16	"	"	11	"	20	" "
23	"	"	21	"	30	" "
21	"	"	31	"	40	" "
62	"	"	41	"	50	" "
127	"	"	51	"	60	" "
213	"	"	61	"	70	" "
136	above	70				

See the Rep. Ann. de Clinique Med. Chirurgicale, Deuxième Année, Paris, 1834.—D.

been distinguished by the name of *ripe*, as the soft by that of *unripe*. " But if we would think and speak of this matter," observes Mr. Pott, " as it really is, we should say that a dissolution or softening of the crystalline lens is by much the most common effect; and that seven times out of nine, when it becomes opaque and tends to form a cataract, it is more or less softened: the softening sometimes extending through the whole range of the lens, and sometimes through only a part of it; while, however, the part that remains undissolved is rarely, if ever, so firm as the centre of the sound crystalline." Mr. Pott proposes it as a question, whether cataracts which have been found perfectly soft have not in general grown opaque by slow degrees; and whether those which have been discovered to be firm have not become opaque hastily, and been preceded by or accompanied with severe and deepseated pain in the head, particularly in the back part of it?—(*Chirurgical Observations relative to the Cataract*, &c., 8vo., 1775, London.)

There is no ophthalmologist, however, who has paid so much attention to this subject as Professor Beer; and though his divisions are perhaps a little too minute, yet the microscopical accuracy with which he has followed up all the modifications of the cataract, is entitled to our most serious attention. He agrees with Mr. Pott that a hard cataract is always comparatively small, though he adds, that every small cataract is not necessarily hard. He is peculiarly minute in examining all the qualities which the disease may exhibit, of position, colour, shadow, shape, range; together with the mobility and degree of prominence of the iris; and till all these characters have been accurately weighed, he hesitates to determine as to the variety of the cataract; or, in effect, whether it be a cataract at all. The shadow cast by the iris constitutes his leading clew. If the lens in an opaque state maintain the size it possessed when transparent, there is a manifest shadow thrown back upon the surface of the cataract by the iris. If the cataract be less than the natural lens, this shadow is broader than usual. If the opaque lens be swollen, no shadow is present; as the capsule is pushed forward into contact with the iris, and the posterior chamber is abolished. And by carefully comparing all the signs that lie before him, he is able to indicate with certainty, in every instance, the seat, the size, and the consistence of the cataract.

[The most frequent species of lenticular cataract is that called hard or firm. In this state the lens the opacity has a grayish appearance, with more or less of the yellowish brown or amber teint towards the centre. In the firm and darker coloured portion it resembles wax in consistence, slightly softened by heat; the circumference is lighter coloured and softer, being about the consistence of soft jelly. The more of the amber colour is seen, and the deeper the teint, the harder is the cataract; the grayer its appearance, the softer is the consistence. The common firm cataract here described, presenting the amber teint in the middle, shaded off into a gray, is the ordinary form of the complaint in elderly persons. The lens in such a case is generally smaller than natural; and the capsule being unaffected, the opaque body appears at a small distance behind the pupil. There is a marked interval between that aperture and the cataract; the iris has its full play; and the patient retains the power of distinguishing objects during the formation of the cataract, by the passage of light through the less opaque circumference of the lens.—(See *Lawrence*, op. cit., p. 400; *Richter's Anfangsgr.*, &c., b. ii.) Mr. Pott's opinion, that the colour of a cataract affords no clew to its consistence, we find, from what has been here stated, to be at variance with modern experience.

In the *soft* cataract, the lens is not soft in the circumference only, but its whole texture is changed, having various degrees of consistence, as that of cheese, jelly, or milk. Soft cataracts are larger than the hard; so that they press against the iris and render its front surface convex. Their surface is distinguished by a bluish kind of white.

The opacity extends uniformly to the circumference of the lens; it intercepts the light more completely than the hard cataract does; and the patient at last retains merely the power of distinguishing light from darkness.

Capsular cataracts are those in which the front or back of the capsule of the lens is alone affected, and those in which the whole capsule is opaque. An opacity of the capsule does not begin in the centre, but in all parts of the membrane indifferently: it is not uniform, but in spots or streaks, with less opaque or transparent intervals. These opaque portions have a glistening chalky white, or bluish white, or pearly appearance. In the anterior capsular cataract, the opacity always projects as far forward as the edge of the pupil. The capsule cannot become extensively opaque without the lens being also affected; and when the anterior portion of the membrane is opaque, the lens is in the same condition. We may have, Mr. Lawrence observes, a single streak of opacity in the capsule after iritis; but that will not constitute a cataract: the capsule may be more extensively yet partially covered by a new adventitious membrane, the rest remaining clear; but there is no such case as a capsule, generally opaque, containing a transparent lens.—(*On Diseases of the Eye*, p. 404.)

When the posterior part of the capsule becomes opaque, while its front portion and the lens continue transparent, the opacity is situated at a marked distance behind the pupil: its situation corresponds to the known position of the capsule. It presents a concave surface, with partial streaks, the intervals of which are transparent. The posterior capsular cataract has not that glistening white colour which distinguishes the anterior, because it is seen through the lens, and acquires a yellowish and rather dull appearance. This change in the capsule is followed by opacity of the lens, which, however, may not occur for a considerable time. Mr. Lawrence adverts to two patients who were attending the Ophthalmic Infirmary, in whom posterior capsular cataracts could be very distinctly seen. One of them could read the large print of a Bible ; and when the pupil was dilated with belladonna, the spaces between the opaque radii, through which the light gained admission to the eye, were very manifest. As the lens becomes more opaque, vision decreases.*

What our author denominates *complicated cataract*, or the case in which both the lens and capsule are opaque, is very frequent. It is the *capsulo-lenticular cataract* of the Germans. Generally speaking, the lens in these cases is soft and the cataract large, often pushing forwards the iris, and impeding its motions. The streaks of the anterior portion of the capsule on a level with the edge of the pupil, the different teint of the opaque lens seen through the less opaque parts of the capsule, and the considerable degree in which sight is interrupted, owing to the bulk of the lens, are characteristic of this example of cataract. The varieties of appearance presented in the capsule-lenticular cataracts, have afforded the German oculists abundance of opportunity for minute distinctions. Thus they describe the *cataracta marmoracea*, where the opaque capsule exhibits a marbled appearance ; *c. fenestrata*, with bars, fancied to resemble those of a window ; *c. punctata*, with spots, &c. Also the *cataracta aridā siliquosa*, or *dry-shelled cataract*, in which the capsule has a thickened and corrugated appearance, and contains only the nucleus of the lens. This variety is often met with in children, and frequently mistaken for a congenital affection. In young infants, Beer says, it is manifestly produced by a slow and neglected inflammation of the lens and its capsule, excited by the stimulus of too strong a light. In adults, the case is generally the result of external violence. Schmidt supposed that in infants the siliquose cataract might be caused by convulsions, attended with violent action of the muscles of the eye ; but the correctness of this opinion is now beginning to be disbelieved.

In a cataract complicated with glaucoma, or glaucosis, as our author chooses to name it, the vitreous humour is first affected, and the lens subsequently. If, says Mr. Lawrence, the iris is altered in colour ; if the pupil is fixed in the dilated state ; if the sight was lost with considerable headache, and before the cataract had formed, the eye may be inferred to be glaucomatous.

The complication of cataract with amaurosis is denoted by the inability to discern light from darkness. The insensibility of the retina may not be totally destroyed, and thus the power of discerning the difference between light and darkness may exist with a cataract attended by imperfect amaurosis. Here, as Mr. Lawrence explains, the practitioner must attend to the symptoms under which the loss of sight has occurred, as well as to the present state of the eye. Simple cataract comes on without pain ; while, in amaurosis, there is often considerable pain in the head; or neighbourhood of the eye. In cataract unattended with enlargement of the lens or adhesion, the iris has generally its natural power of motion. A motionless or sluggish iris, and a fixedly dilated pupil, are therefore strong evidence of an amaurotic affection, when they are not accounted for by the particularities of the cataract itself.]

Like PAROPSIS *glaucosis*, or opacity of the vitreous humour, a cataract has sometimes, though very rarely, ceased spontaneously, or without any manifest cause.* Helwig gives an instance in which the cessation was not only spontaneous but sudden.—(*Observ. Physico-Med.*, 23, Aug. Vind., 1680, 4to.) It has also, at times, been carried off by a fever.†

There is hence specious ground for conceiving that some medicine might be discovered, capable, by some general or specific action, of producing a like change, and proving a remedy for the disease ; and the more so, as we find ganglions and other accidental deformities frequently removed from the extreme parts of the system by external or internal applications. But no such remedy has hitherto been discovered, or at least none that can be in any degree relied upon, excepting in those cases of supposed but miscalled cataracts which have consisted in a deposition of lymph from an inflammation of the iris and ciliary processes : for recourse has been had to mercurial preparations, both external and internal, as almost every other metallic salt, aconite, the pasque-flower, or pulsatilla, to protracted vomiting, electricity, and puncturing the tunics of the eyes, but without any certain advantage.—(*Beytr. zur Chir. änd Augenheilkunst; Von Franz Reisinger*, &c., Göttingen, 1814.) This is the more to be lamented, because, whatever surgical operation may be determined upon as most advisable, there is no guarding, on all occasions, against the mischievous effects which may result ; I do not mean from the complication or severity of the operation ; for this, under every modification, is simpler and less formidable than the uninitiated can readily imagine ; but from the tendency which is sometimes met with, from idiosyncrasy, habit, or other irritable principle, to run rapidly into a state of destructive inflammation ; and in a single night, or even a few hours, in spite of the wisest precautions that can be adopted, to endanger a total and permanent loss of vision. I speak from personal knowledge, and have in

---

* This kind of cataract seems particularly frequent in children; of fifty-four cases observed by Saunders, only twenty-three occurred in adults.—D.

* Haggendorn, Observ. Med., cent. i., obs. 50, Franc., 1698, 8vo. Ludolf, Miscel. Berol., tom. iv., 258. Walker on the Theory and Cure of a Cataract.

† Velschius, Episagm. 20. The cases which occasionally disappear spontaneously, are generally such as have been induced by injuries of the eye, followed by manifest inflammation. The attempt to disperse other cataracts is now deemed a hopeless experiment. "It may be asserted without any qualification, that no external application nor internal medicines with which we are at present acquainted, can alter the condition of the opaque lens and capsule."—Lawrence, op. cit., p. 411.—ED.

one or two instances seen such an effect follow, after the operation had been performed with the utmost dexterity, and with every promise of success ; and where a total blindness has taken place in both eyes, the operation having been performed on both ; neither of them being quite opaque antecedently, and one of them in nothing more than an incipient state of the disease, and the patient capable of writing and reading with it.* And hence it is far better, in the author's opinion, to have a trial made on one eye only at a time, and that the worst, where both are affected and one is still useful, than to subject both to the same risk ; for the sympathy between them is so considerable, that if an inflammatory process from any constitutional or accidental cause should show itself in either, the other would be sure to associate in the morbid action. [This advice is supported by that of Scarpa and Lawrence. The latter offers the following arguments for the decision. If you restore sight in one, it is sufficient for all useful purposes, and the patient will generally be satisfied. The other may be operated on afterward, or be retained as a reserve in case the restored sight should fail, or be lost by disease or accident. When both are operated on together, they are not both necessarily involved in any unfavourable subsequent occurrence ; yet they are likely to suffer together from common causes, and under such circumstances the patient loses all chance of regaining sight. On the other hand, if things go on unfavourably, it is a great consolation both to the patient and surgeon to know that one eye only is risked. These arguments seem perfectly convincing.

There are some cases, as Mr. Lawrence says, in which it is better for the patient to be content with very imperfect vision, than to submit to an operation which may end in total blindness. The restorative powers, he observes, are feeble in very old persons ; in them, and in cases where the propriety of operating may be doubtful for other reasons, it is best to employ the palliative aid of belladonna, as long as it will procure any degree of useful vision. He

advises no operation, in such cases, until the patient is quite blind ; until the sight is in that state in which the failure of the operation can make it no worse. In general, he thinks we should not operate till all useful vision is gone. At all events, says he, this rule is absolute in doubtful cases. He mentions one exception ; namely, where the cataract is mature in one eye and immature in the other the former may be operated upon, so as to give the patient the use of that eye while the cataract is forming in the other. Much difference of opinion prevails on the question, whether the operation should be done when only one eye is affected and the other is sound ; but on this topic we shall not enter, as it is generally discussed in surgical works ; and shall merely mention that this is a point of practice on which a candid statement of cases is much desired.]

The usual modes of operating for the cure of a cataract are three : that of couching or depression, that of extraction, and that of what is called absorption. The first was well known to the practitioners of Greece and Rome ; and is ably described by Celsus, who advises, in cases where the lens cannot be kept down, to cut it into pieces with the sharp-edged needle, by which means it will be the more readily absorbed. And from this last remark we have some reason for believing that even the third of the above methods, that of absorption, was also known at the same time ; as it is probable, indeed, that the second, or the operation by extraction, was likewise ; since we find Pliny recommending the process of simple removal or depression in preference to that of extraction or drawing it forth : "squammam in oculis emovendam potius quàm extrahendam" (*Nat. Hist.*, lib. xxix., cap. i.), which Holland has thus honestly, though paraphrastically translated : " a cataract or pearl in the eye is to be couched rather, and driven down by the needle, than quite to be plucked forth."

In the east, however, both these plans appear to have been pursued through a much longer period. Both are noticed by the Arabian writers in general, and especially by Avicenna and

---

* The prognosis, which should be regulated by circumstances, is here too discouraging. In order to counteract this impression, the judicious remarks of Mr. Lawrence upon this part of the subject are introduced. " The prognosis," he says, " is completely favourable when the affection is confined to the lens or capsule ; when the sensibility of the retina is undiminished ; when the motions of the iris are unimpaired ; when the constitution of the patient is sound, and the health is good at the time of operating ; and when the patient is of a spare rather than a full habit. Under these circumstances, the prognosis is completely favourable ; that is, supposing the operator to understand the subject well, to select the kind of operation most suited to the particular species of cataract, and to possess sufficient manual dexterity for performing it in the most advantageous way. The prognosis will be particularly favourable in congenital cataracts ; in those of young persons (in whom, however, it seldom arises, except in consequence of injuries), and in the firm lenticular cataract of elderly persons. It is bad when

the cataract is complicated with glaucoma or amaurosis ; with a fluid state of the vitreous humour ; with a varicose condition of the bloodvessels ; with dropsy of the eye ; or with a very contracted or closed pupil. Indeed, some of these circumstances would form decided objections to the operation. It is also bad when the cataract has been preceded or accompanied by severe pains in the head or in the eye ; by muscæ volitantes, sparks or flashes of fire before the eye ; as all these circumstances indicate affection of the nervous structure. The prognosis is doubtful when cataract is the result of internal inflammation of the eye, or of that vascular disturbance which comes under the head of congestion. Adhesions of the pupil are unfavourable, since the laceration and removal of them may excite inflammation in the iris and internal tunics ; particularly in gouty individuals, in whom such adhesions are most frequent, and who are most likely to suffer from inflammation after the operation. The prognosis is doubtful in cases of cataract affecting one eye, when the other is amaurotic or glaucomatous."—Ed.

Rhazes; and both seem to have been practised from time immemorial in India, and, according to the account of the cabirajahs, with wonderful success. Dr. Scott was informed by one of the travelling operators, who, however, spoke without a register, that in the operation of depression, this success was in the proportion of a hundred who were benefited to five who obtained no advantage whatever.

[*Extraction* consists in making an incision through the cornea, dividing the crystalline capsule, and letting the lens escape through the pupil, and the opening made in the cornea.

There is a particular modification of couching, or depression, that was first suggested and practised by Willburg, and named *reclination :* in this the lens is not pushed downwards in a straight direction, but is turned on its axis, so as to be placed horizontally in the vitreous humour, behind the lower part of the iris, or, as is sometimes advised, at the bottom of the vitreous humour, between the inferior and external straight muscles.—(*Frick, on Dis. of the Eye,* 2d edit., by Welbank, p. 200.) In this operation the posterior surface of the lens is turned downwards; the anterior upwards; the superior margin is backwards, the inferior forwards.]

One form of extraction was introduced as an improvement by Sir William Adams : after detaching the cataract, he first passed it through the opening of the pupil into the anterior chamber by means of his needle, and then extracted it by an opening on the outer side of the cornea, instead of by one in its inferior part. The method is now very properly abandoned.

The simplest and least irritating of these operations, however, is that by absorption, as it is now commonly called : it was named precipitation by Maitre-Jan (*Traité des Maladies de l'Œil.,* edit. sec., Troyes, 1711), on his first noticing the disappearance of portions of the opaque lens; but which in effect is neither absorption nor precipitation, but SOLUTION, or dissolution, as Mr. Pott correctly described it. But it should be known to the operator, that while the solvent power of the aqueous humour is wonderfully active, that of the vitreous is weak and inconsiderable : and hence the solvent or absorbent plan practised by Scarpa, consists in dividing the cataract, after its separation, into small fragments, and passing them with the needle by which they are thus divided through the pupil into the anterior chamber, which constitutes the seat of the aqueous humour, apparently in perfect coincidence with the method first practised by Gleize, and since recommended by Richter.—(*Chirurgische Bibliothek,* band x.) The fragments thus deposited are usually dissolved in a few weeks ; and where the cataract is fluid, they have often been dissolved and absorbed in a few seconds, and sometimes even before the needle has been withdrawn.

[In the proceeding by *absorption,* or *solution,* as it is sometimes termed, the needle may be introduced either through the cornea and pupil, or behind the iris, as it is in the operation of depression, the pupil having been first dilated with belladonna. These two methods are dis-

tinguished by the appellations of the anterior and posterior operations. The anterior operation, invented by Buchorn (*Buchorn de Keratonyxide,* Halæ, 1806), or rather by Conradi, has been named *keratonyxis,** a term derived from the Greek, and signifying puncture of the cornea. This practice was introduced into this country by Mr. Saunders, who does not seem to have been aware that it had ever been done abroad. No person who understands the subject would advise either of these operations to be exclusively employed. Each method has its advantages, and is eligible under certain circumstances : our object then should be, not to select one operation, with the view of practising it in all cases ; but to consider the circumstances which make one preferable to the other, and to select in each instance that which is best suited to the particular form of the complaint.—(See *Lawrence, on Dis. of the Eye,* p. 417.)

The principles which should determine the preference in individual cases, and the details, of the several operations, must be sought in works on surgery.],

---

SPECIES X.
PAROPSIS SYNIZESIS.
CLOSED PUPIL.

DIMNESS OR ABOLITION OF SIGHT FROM CONTRACTION OR OBLITERATION OF THE PUPIL.

THE term SYNIZESIS is derived from συνίζω, " consido, coëo, coalesco ;" and was used among the Greek grammarians, before it obtained its introduction into the medical vocabulary, to signify the coalescence of two or more syllables into one. [The pupil may be simply contracted or closed ; or these changes may be combined with opacity of the lens or capsule, with an adventitious membrane in the pupil, with adhesion of the iris either to the capsule (synechia posterior) or the cornea (synechia anterior), with protrusion of the iris, displacement of the pupil, or opacity of the cornea. All these conditions of the eye are the consequence of severe inflammation, either external or internal. As Mr. Lawrence correctly observes, it must also be recollected, that this serious inflammation may not have confined itself to the production of the foregoing evils, but extended its effects to the nervous structure of the eye, or to other parts of the organ. Hence, says he, it is necessary to ascertain correctly whether the loss of vision is produced by the changes of the pupil only, before a decision is made about an attempt to form an artificial pupil.] This species exhibits two varieties :—

α Simplex. Simple closure of the pupil.
Simple closed
pupil.

---

* M. Dupuytren has made a number of experiments to ascertain the value of this operation. Of twenty-one individuals operated upon by him in this mode, seventeen recovered their sight. For many valuable remarks on the nature and treatment of cataract, see his Clinical Lectures on Surgery, trans. by Doane, New-York, 1833.

β Complicata.   Closure of the pupil com-
Complicated clo- plicated with cataract,
  sed pupil.   opaque cornea, or other
                  changes specified above.

The pupil sometimes becomes closed or obliterated from a gradual contraction, and at length
coalition, of the muscular fibres of the iris, unattended with any other change or impairment of
the eye. In all these cases, it is a SIMPLE OB-
LITERATION OF THE PUPIL. It is COMPLICATED
when the obliteration is combined with an opacity of the cornea, with a cataract, with adhesions of the iris to the cornea or capsule of. the
lens, &c. When the disease is an effect of inflammation, it forms the ATRESIA IRIDIS of Dr.
Schmidt of Vienna, who further subdivides it
into *complete, incomplete,* and *partial,* according
as the vision is totally destroyed, impaired, or
confined to a part of the pupil.—(*Ueber Nachstaar und Iritis nach Staaroperationen,* 4to.,
Wien, 1801.)

The natural shape of the human pupil is circular, this being the natural form of the fine
fringe of the iris by which it is surrounded. But
in a few instances the fringe or rays of the iris
have evinced a different figure, and the pupil, in
consequence, has been found oblong or heart-
shaped.—(*Eph. Nat. Cur. Dec.,* iii., ann. vii.,
viii., obs. 21.) The first has occurred most frequently, and according to Albinus, has sometimes preceded loss of vision.—(*Anat. Acad.,*
lib. vi., cap. 3.) Bloch gives an instance in
which the disease was congenital and hereditary.—(*Medicinische Bemerkungen,* p. 1.)

If the iris contract irregularly, sometimes only
a few of its fibres spread across the pupil, while
others are retracted : and hence we have examples of double or more than double pupils,
though of smaller dimensions than the natural
circle. Solinus gives an instance of two pupils
hereby produced (Vide *Marcel. Donat.,* lib. vi.,
cap. 2, p. 619), and Janin not less than five.
—(*Mémoires.* &c.)

Medicines in this disease are of little avail.
In the first variety, an external application of
the tincture of belladonna, or a solution of stramonium, which is said to answer the same purpose,* has occasionally effected a cure by destroying the contractile action ; and so have dilute solutions of brandy, camphire, or sulphate of
zinc, by their tonic or stimulant power. When
the disease does not yield to this mode of treatment, or consists of the complicated variety, it
belongs manifestly to the art of surgery, and its
removal must be sought for in books on that subject : among the best of which may be mentioned, Mackenzie's Treatise on Diseases of the
Eye, Lawrence's work on the same subject,
Mr. Guthrie's Lectures on the Eye, and Beer's
Essay on Staphyloma and Artificial Pupil, published in 1804,† and his Doctrine of the Diseases

of the Eye, published in 1817.—(*Lehre von den
Augenkrankheiten,* &c., ut suprà.) According
to the nature of the coalition, Beer employs
three varieties of operation ; incision, excision,
and separation ; which he distinguishes by the
names of COROTOMIA, CORECTOMIA, and CORO-
DIALYSIS. The first is the simplest, and that
most usually had recourse to. In the second,
an incision being made with a cataract-knife,
close to the edge of the cornea, and not larger
than the third part of its circumference, the iris,
if it protrude, is laid hold of with the hook ; or,
if no protrusion take place, the hook, introduced
through the incision, is made to lay hold of the
pupillary edge of the iris, which drags it through
the wound when a sufficient portion of it is removed with a pair of scissors. In the third
method, which is that originally proposed by
Dr. Reisinger, the operation is performed with
a double hook or hook forceps.*

SPECIES XI.

PAROPSIS AMAUROSIS.

DROP SERENE.

DIMNESS OR ABOLITION OF SIGHT, RESULTING
FROM AN AFFECTION OF THE NERVOUS STRUC-
TURE OF THE EYE, WHETHER SEATED IN
THE RETINA, OPTIC NERVE, OR BRAIN ; AND
WHETHER DIRECTLY THE RESULT OF ORGANIC
CHANGES IN THOSE PARTS THEMSELVES, OR
INDIRECTLY THE EFFECT OF THEIR SYMPATHY
WITH DISORDER OF OTHER ORGANS.

THIS is the GUTTA SERENA of the Arabic
writers, whence the term "Drop Serene," of
our own tongue ; terms we have already explained under PAROPSIS CATARACTA. Milton is
well known to allude to this affection in his
beautiful address to light, as he does also to the
cataract, by him called *suffusion,* as the Latins
call it *suffusio;* but it is singular that, in the
course of this allusion, he seems doubtful as to
which of the two diseases he ought to ascribe
his own blindness :—

  "Thee I revisit safe,
And feel thy sovereign vital lamp ; but thou
Revisit'st not these eyes, that roll in vain
To find thy piercing ray, and find no dawn.
So thick a DROP SERENE has quench'd their orbs,
Or dim SUFFUSION veil'd."*

The term AMAUROSIS is derived from the
Greek ἀμαυρὸς, "obscurus, caliginosus, opacus."
The most common cause is a paralysis of the
retina, usually in conjunction with a paralysis
and dilatation of the iris. Occasionally, however, this is rigidly contracted. From the different degree in which the disease presents itself, and from its assuming at times an in-

---

* Annual Report of the Liverpool Institution for
Diseases of the Eye. By Alexander Hannay, M.
D., 1822.
† Ansicht der Staphylomatoien Metamorphosen
des Auges, und der Künstlichen Pupillenbildung.
Also, particularly, G. J. Guthrie on the Operations
for the Formation of an Artificial Pupil, 8vo., Lon-

don, 1819 ; and Lawrence's Treatise on Diseases
of the Eye, p. 452 et seq., 8vo., Lond., 1833.
* See also D. Weller's Treatise Ueber künst-
liche Pupillen, und eine besondere Methode, diese
fertigen ; published in Langenbeck's Neue Bibliothek, b. ii., st. 4. See also Dr. Schlagintweit
Ueber den gegenwärtigen Zustand der künstlichen
Pupillenbildung, &c., München, 1818.
† Par. Lost, iii., 21.

termittent type, it has three principal varieties :—

a Perfecta.　　　`Attended with total blindness.
Complete amaurosis.

β Imperfecta.　　　With vision impaired, but
Incomplete amaurosis.　　not altogether destroyed.

γ Intermittens.　　With periodical cessations
Intermittent amaurosis,　　and returns.

Plenck makes a distinct disease of an unalterable pupil, *with* or *without* injury of the vision, under the name of MYDRIASIS. When accompanied with injured vision, it is evidently a variety of amaurosis ; and it is questionable whether an unalterable pupil is ever to be traced without defective vision.

It is probably to the cases attended with contraction of the pupil, that Shakspeare chiefly alludes by the term *pin* or *pin-eye*, the pupil being sometimes contracted to nearly the diameter of a pin's head ; though the synizesis is equally entitled to the name. I have quoted one example already under P. Caligo, which he calls web-eye ; another is contained in the following couplet :—

> ——' Wish all eyes
> Blind with the PIN and WEB."

[In the former editions of this work, the author made the state of the pupil the ground of two of his varieties of amaurosis. When the pupil was dilated, the amaurosis was termed *atonic* ; when contracted, *spasmodic*. Thus the iris was more adverted to than the real seat of the disease, and incidental changes were mistaken for essential ones, and considered to be absolutely dependant upon atony and spasm. These errors the editor is happy to have the opportunity of expunging ; and in their place he has substituted the two varieties of *perfect* and *imperfect amaurosis*, as cases admitted by every modern writer on diseases of the eye, and the distinct consideration of which is highly useful in practice. The *intermittent* amaurosis, the third variety adopted by the author, remains ; though the principal examples of it are comprised in the subjects of day blindness and night blindness. Other better founded and more practical distinctions than those formerly given by our author, are the *organic*, and the *sympathetic* or *functional* ; the former depending upon a diseased state of the retina or optic nerve ; the latter consisting of a suspension of the functions of the nervous structure of the organ of vision, in consequence of the influence of the disease or disorder of some other part of the body on the eye. This last case is also sometimes denominated *symptomatic* amaurosis, being the mere effect of another disease, which is the primary one. In this point of view, the loss of vision or paralysis of the retina from various organic changes affecting the whole eyeball, as hydrophthalmia, fungus hæmatodes, &c., may be considered as a symptomatic amaurosis. Besides the important division of this disease into the *perfect* and *imperfect*, *organic* and *functional* varieties, some others, not noticed by our author, cannot be

overlooked by the practitioner, because they make very considerable differences in the prognosis. The further distinctions here alluded to are those of *recent* and *inveterate*, and of *complicated* amaurosis.

Amaurosis is generally characterized by a very dilated state of the pupil, which is frequently not affected by any degree of light that is made to fall upon the retina. Sometimes the pupil is extraordinarily contracted. Hence, as already stated, the varieties formerly selected by the author of this work were badly chosen ; because they were founded, not upon any intelligible differences in the condition of the retina, but upon incidental states of the iris. His second or *spasmodic* variety, indeed, as far as the definition went, might have signified rather synizesis, or impediment to vision from great and permanent contraction of the pupil. In amaurosis the pupil seldom retains its circular form, but becomes more or less irregular or angular. Neither does it commonly exhibit the clear appearance of a sound eye, but a grayish or dark green hue, resembling what is observable in the eye of a horse. In certain examples, a whitish or greenish-yellow spot is perceptible apparently in the fundus of the eye, and a little to one side of the visual axis, with a splendid disk, like the tapetum of sheep, or the coloured choroid of fishes. Another change in the pupil, noticed by Beer and all the most correct writers on amaurosis, is an alteration in its position : it is mostly drawn towards the internal and superior portion of the eye. The iris is in general very sluggish, or absolutely motionless ; but in a few cases it preserves its usual power of motion (*Caldani ad Haller, vide Richter, Nov. Comm. Soc. Goett.*, tom. iv., p. 79 ; *Hey, Med. Obs. and Inq.*, vol. v.), and sometimes acts with greater rapidity than in a healthy eye. Amaurosis is ordinarily preceded by certain defects in the sight, and illusive appearances before the eye. One of the most important is what is termed by writers the *visus interruptus*. Thus, in reading, it seems to the patient as if syllables, words, or whole lines were deficient ; and he is obliged to move the eye or head ere he can discern what seems wanting. If he look upon any other object he will seldom see the whole of it, unless he make a similar motion of his eye or head. On other occasions, he will see the whole of the object when it is held in a particular direction, but he loses it again as soon as this is altered.

A common precursor of amaurosis is an appearance as if motes or small bodies were incessantly moving about in front of the eye. This is the *visus muscarum*, or *muscæ volitantes* of surgical writers. When it is a dark-coloured speck that the patient fancies to interrupt his sight, it receives the technical name of *scotoma* ; for appearances of this kind may be either single or very numerous, and of diversified shapes. They are most troublesome when the patient looks at very bright or light-coloured surfaces. In incipient amaurosis every object frequently appears to the patient as if it were surrounded by a zone of variegated colours ; but sometimes things have a different look, seeming as if they were enveloped in a mist, gauze, or network. In many cases, single objects appear to be double: this defect of vision is termed *visus duplicatus*, and proceeds from impairment of the faculty by which the axis of vision in each eye is made to adapt itself to the object looked at.

Amaurosis may present itself as an uncombined local affection of the optic nerve or retina, or as conjoined with some other disease of the organ or general system. Among the local complications are to be noticed cataract, fungus hæmatodes of the eye, glaucosis, cirsophthalmia, hydrophthalmia, exophalmus, atrophy, paralysis of one or more muscles of the eyeball or lids, ophthalmitis, &c. The general complications especially meriting enumeration are, diseases of the nervous system, the debility from typhoid and other fevers, hydrocephalus, organic and functional diseases of the abdominal viscera, worms, pregnancy, and diseases of the brain and cranium.

Amaurosis is not restricted to any particular age or sex. Perhaps, on the whole, persons of middle age are most liable to it. Children are less liable to the disease than adults, but congenital cases are upon record. In Germany, an opinion prevails, that dark-coloured eyes are more frequently attacked by amaurosis than those of light colour. A tendency to the disorder is produced by pregnancy, by every kind of immoderate exertion of the eyes on small or shining objects, a full habit, and whatever has the effect of keeping up a great determination of blood to the head and eyes. Mr. Lawrence considers organic amaurosis as not essentially different from a very slow insidious inflammation of the retina, and not a disease of debility, as represented by numerous writers. His opinion on the pathology of amaurosis, of course, has great influence on the practice which he particularly inculcates ; and which, in the early stage, is generally antiphlogistic ; in the second, mercurial.—(See *Treatise on the Diseases of the Eye*, 8vo., 1833.)

The doctrine most usually adopted, however, refers a certain class of cases to debilitating causes ; as typhoid fevers, profuse discharges or evacuations, excessive venery, the suckling of infants, &c.

That particular articles of food or medicine will produce amaurosis sympathetically, is amply proved. It is true, that in some of the examples of this fact we are obliged to suppose the existence of an idiosyncrasy ; as when a person is affected with blindness whenever he takes chocolate or bitters, which have not the slightest effect upon the sight of other persons. The sympathy of the eyes with the stomach and intestines is often illustrated in cases of worms, which, according to the admission of every writer, are not an unfrequent occasion of amaurosis. A child has been known to become amaurotic from accidentally swallowing a bead, and to regain sight on the foreign body being voided by means of an emetic. In Germany and Italy, indeed, the opinion that amaurosis is very frequently prevalent on gastric disorder has been entertained to a great and perhaps an unwarrantable extent ; we say unwarrantable, because in this country, experience does not furnish evidence of the efficacy of the treatment which the doctrine naturally points out, and which, in the hands of Schmücker, Richter, and Scarpa, has proved remarkably successful. Beer himself had little faith in the opinion, except in relation to the amaurosis from worms ; and in this metropolis, repeated trials of the emetic practice have not created an impression in its favour.

The great influence of hereditary disposition in producing amaurosis has been remarked by all the most correct observers. Beer in particular adverts to the frequent examples of this fact, and mentions a certain family, in which all the females who had not had children became amaurotic about the period of the cessation of the menses ; and what is very remarkable, it is stated that this had been the case through three generations.

One form of imperfect amaurosis, named amblyopia senilis, is ascribed by Beer to deficiency of the pigmentum nigrum. This case is commonly attended with a tremulous or vibratory motion of the globe : the admission of light produces great uneasiness, and vision is seriously weakened. It is usually met with only in old persons ; but sometimes occurs in others after fevers, and in the last stage of consumption.—(*Vetch on Diseases of the Eye*, p. 144.) Although it is declared to be incurable, the power of vision may be very usefully assisted with cylindrical shades, goggles, and other contrivances calculated to absorb light.

An amaurosis rarely cured, is that arising from blows on the eyebrow, or injury of the frontal nerve. All cases, likewise, depending upon organic changes in the eye itself, optic nerve, brain, or orbit, do not admit of relief. The prognosis in every instance of complete amaurosis is unfavourable. The functional and sympathetic forms of the complaint are generally more easy of cure than the organic ; but whether they can be relieved or not, will depend upon the circumstance whether the original complaint in another part of the body, with which they are connected, can itself be removed or not. The length of time that the loss of sight has prevailed, will also materially influence the prognosis. Generally speaking, amaurosis that has been formed recently and suddenly, but without violence or immoderate previous inflammation of the eye, is more easily cured than that which has come on with great slowness. The disease is absolutely incurable, when accompanied by any change in the shape and dimensions of the eyeball. When amaurosis affects only one eye, unless it be from sympathy with a neighbouring part,* as a carious tooth, the other eye is in great danger of being also attacked. The occasional mobility of the iris in this disease, and a moderate dilatation of the pupil, are no proof that the amaurosis will be more easily cured ; for the iris often regains its mobility without the least im-

---

* See Wardrop's Essays on the Morbid Anatomy of the Eye ; and Frick on Diseases of the Eye by Welbank, p. 150, 2d edit.

provement in vision, and sometimes the eyesight may improve, though the iris continue sluggish or even motionless.

The treatment of amaurosis must of course be regulated by the view taken of the cause of the disease. Thus, notwithstanding the fact that emetics have not proved as successful in this country as they have abroad, they should be prescribed when bilious disorder of the gastric organs is evidently present, and unaccompanied with much determination of blood to the head. Richter has recorded the case of a priest who became suddenly blind in a fit of passion, but recovered his sight immediately after taking an emetic. Schmucker cured many cases by a combination of the emetic and antiphlogistic practice, and the evidence of Scarpa is strongly in favour of the same method. In general, it is to be taken into the account, that emetics and bleeding have been assisted with the simultaneous exhibition of purgatives, so that it would be assuming too much in numerous examples to refer the success of the practice altogether to the emetics. Purgatives are, on the whole, in far greater repute for their good effects on amaurotic disorders, than the free employment of tartarized antimony. They are particularly indicated when there is much disorder of the primæ viæ, when the disease is attended with habitual costiveness, and any manifestly increased determination of blood to the brain and eyes. This state may be presumed to exist whenever amaurosis is connected with the suppression of any accustomed discharge, as of the menses, bleeding from piles, secretion of matter from an old ulcer, &c. The origin of the greater number of cases of amaurosis, that is to say, of those which directly affect the retina or optic nerve, is ascribed by Mr. Lawrence to vascular excitement, to congestion, or even a slow inflammation of the nervous structure constituting the seat of vision. His practice, therefore, in such instances, is at first decidedly antiphlogistic, comprehending local and general bleeding, purgatives, low diet, &c., afterward followed up by the free use of mercury, aided with blisters and a seton.

This mode of treatment, however, he recommends to be graduated according to the violence of the attack, the constitution, age, and strength of the individual, and other circumstances. It must not be supposed, he observes, that all amaurotic patients require to be bled and salivated. When we meet with the affection in the form of active inflammation of the retina, more especially in young and vigorous individuals of full habit, where there are obvious marks of local vascular congestion and constitutional excitement, the antiphlogistic treatment cannot be too active or too quickly followed up. Amaurosis often comes on in a slow and very insidious manner in persons of enfeebled constitution: the organ suffers from habitual excessive exertion, at the same time that the constitution is depressed by residence in confined dwellings, bad air, by sedentary occupations, unwholesome diet, costiveness, and other hurtful influences. In the treatment of a thin, pallid, feeble woman, who had destroyed her health by close confinement to needlework, less active measures would be required. Emptying the alimentary canal, perhaps, taking away a little blood by cupping, or by leeches to the temples, and then using mercury in the alterative manner, with mild aperients, would here be the best plan. Mr. Lawrence recommends a few grains of Plummer's pill to be given every night or every second night, and the bowels to be kept open with occasional doses of electuary, castor-oil, or rhubarb and magnesia. The blue-pill, he says, may be taken in combination with aloes or the compound extract of colocynth. It may be necessary to persevere with the mercury, slowly increasing the dose until the mouth is slightly affected. A nutritious diet without stimuli, good air and exercise, and repose of the organ, Mr. Lawrence deems important auxiliaries. With these means may be joined a succession of moderate sized blisters. After mild antiphlogistic means, and the alimentary canal has been cleared, it may be expedient to combine tonics with aperients, as rhubarb with bark, columba, or cascarilla, and allow a generous diet, with a little porter and wine. Dr. Frick has seen much benefit from mercury or calomel in those cases of incipient amaurosis which come on with deep-seated pain in the head and orbit, more particularly when such pain is found to intermit.—(*On Diseases of the Eye*, 2d edit. by Welbank, p. 153.)

Although modern practitioners place little reliance on the real utility of various local stimulating applications in the treatment of amaurosis, and not much more on electricity, galvanism, and several internal medicines, once supposed to have a specific effect in removing blindness, the editor has considered it right not to suppress the following remarks delivered by the author, as they bring before us many plans which have occasionally been strongly recommended.]

Sternutatories demand attention: they are best formed of turbeth mineral, with about ten times its proportion of mild snuff, or any other light powder. The vapour of ammonia, ether, or camphire, mixed with hot water, has sometimes also afforded benefit; as has probably the use of moxa frequently repeated, so warmly recommended by Baron Larrey. "By this remedy," says he, "not only has the progress of amaurosis been arrested, but in some cases removed, even where the blindness was complete."—(*Rec. des Mém. de Chirurgie*, &c., Paris, 8vo., 1821.)

Professor Beer is minute in describing the modifications that proceed from plethora, and a morbid state of the digestive organs; but gives a still more copious detail of that which depends upon local rheumatism, and which he hence calls the rheumatic amaurosis. In this he remarks, that the pupil is perfectly clear, and the iris unalterable, slightly dilated, and thrust a little nearer the nose and the eyebrow than naturally, so as to be in a small degree displaced inwards and upwards. The tears flow on slight occasions, and the light is often troublesome, accompanied with an aching pain in the eyeball. The movement of the eye is impeded, and more in one direction than in others.

This modification rarely proceeds to perfect blindness.

The rheumatic form is frequently treated with success, and principally by diaphoretics. Beer employs guaiacum and camphire combined during the day, and Dover's powder at night ; and with these he has recourse also to blisters, placed in succession behind the ear, on the temple, and over the eyebrow, so as to maintain a catenation of counter-irritative actions. Both this and the plethoric modification, in which local bleeding is of the utmost benefit, are frequently hurried on to a complete development of disease and a total insensibility of the retina by stimulants, and particularly by galvanism and electricity.

Where it has followed repelled eruptions, it has also been occasionally found to yield to setons and blisters, or a restoration of the suppressed efflorescence ; and as in other diseases, what has sometimes proved the source of its production, has been found its best remedy ; so that the cause has become the cure. Thus, it has at times yielded to the violence of a fever, to that of a sudden blow on the head, to a strong light, to a paroxysm of convulsions. Electricity, and especially voltaism, has probably been serviceable in some instances ; at least, the assertions to this effect are very numerous, though in various cases both these have sometimes been altogether unsuccessful, and, as just observed, sometimes highly mischievous. Nor is the magnet without its recommendations, having been applied to the upper part of the spine, while minute bags filled with iron filings were placed on the eyes.—(Würkung des Kunstlischen Magnets, &c., pp. 24, 25 ; Hell. v. Nootnagel, 1, c., § 22 ; Eph. Nat. Cur. Dec., ii., ann. v., obs. 247.) The chief dependances, besides these, have been on camphire, cajeput, musk, mercury, iron, bark, arnica, and externally the pulsatilla nigra. Collier employed the flowers of arnica in decoction (Dr. Layard, Phil. Trans., 1757–8, vol. l., p. 747) in the proportion of about half an ounce to a pint of the strained liquid, which may be taken in a day or a day and a half. Richter, Schmücker, and other German writers, declare it to be of no avail. The pulsatilla is certainly better entitled to attention. "I would recommend it," says Dr. Cullen, with his usual liberality, "to the attention of my countrymen, and particularly to a repetition of trials on that disease, so frequently otherwise incurable, the amaurosis. The negative experiments of Bergius and others are not sufficient to discourage all trials, considering that the disease may depend upon different causes, some of which may yield to remedies, though others do not."—(Mat. Med., vol. ii., part ii., chap. v., p. 216.) When distilled with water, it gives forth a terebinthinate substance resembling camphire, which necessarily possesses a stimulant, and hence a medicinal power. Whence the euphrasia officinalis, or eye-bright, obtained the character it once possessed as a specific in this disease, it is difficult to say. By Hildanus and Lieutaud, however, it was chiefly confined, even in its zenith of popularity, to the amaurosis of old age. Its chief sensible quality is that of being a mild astringent. Rue, which rivalled it at one time, and by Milton is put upon a level with it, has far better pretensions when used externally in the form of a potent infusion ; for it unites the properties of volatile pungency and bitterness : both which, as concentrated in strong chamomile tea, I have occasionally found highly serviceable in an incipient state of this disease, produced by weakness ; though, as already remarked, none of these should be employed in several forms of the disease.

With respect to narcotics, the aconite has been chiefly popular in Germany : it has been strongly recommended by many writers of reputation, and has sometimes been given by gradual augmentation to the amount of a drachm daily.[*] Chevillard combined the use of antimonials with blisters ; but cold applied externally, and cold bathing, as recommended by Warner, is much entitled to our attention.

Dr. Powell relates a case of sudden loss of vision, preceded by an acute cephalæa, in which an emetic was found, during the act of vomiting, abruptly to restore sight to the right eye (for both were affected), with a sensation as if a flash of lightning had taken place, but the vision was soon again lost. More than a twelvemonth afterward, the patient returned to emetics ; when, after the use of the second, the pupils of the eyes recovered the power of dilating and contracting on exposure to light, and preserved it till death ; but the power of vision was not restored. During the whole of this case of blindness, the sense of hearing was peculiarly acute. —(Trans. Med., vol. v., p. 226.) The discovery of Dr. Bock, that a few nervous filaments, appertaining to the great sympathetic nerve, are thrown off while this nerve is within the cavernous sinus, and entering the orbit unite with the lenticular ganglion, may account for these remote influences ; the ear, as is frequently the case, sympathizing with the morbid state of the eye, either directly or reversely.[*]—(Beschreibung des fünften Nervenpaares und seiner Verbindungen mit anderen Nerven, &c., von D. A. Carl Bock, Leipsic, 1817.)

SPECIES XII.
PAROPSIS STRABISMUS.
SQUINTING.

OPTIC AXES OF THE EYE NOT COINCIDING ON AN OBJECT.

This disease, in colloquial language now called squinting, was formerly denominated goggle-eye, whence the word goggles is still applied to the glasses which are used by persons affected with the complaint. The French called

* Beobachtungen und Untersuchungen, &c., band ii., Nuremb., 1767. All faith in the virtue of these medicines against amaurosis, is at the present day totally abandoned.—Ed.

† Dr. Hays has published an extremely judicious article on amaurosis, in the American Cyclopedia of Practical Medicine, vol. i. See likewise Copland's Dictionary of Practical Medicine, p. 50.—D.

these glasses *masques à louchette*, literally *squint-ing-guards.* The technical term STRABISMUS, is derived from the Greek στραβὸς, "tortus oculis," or "sight-twisted."

The optic axis is 'an imaginary line passing from the centre of the vitreous humour, lens, and globe of the eye, to the object of vision. In perfect vision, the optic axis of the one eye is in unison with that of the other; and consequently, they converge or coincide at the same point; and the object which would otherwise appear double, as being seen by each eye, is contemplated as single. In order to this coincidence the muscles of each eye must constantly assume the same direction, their position and configuration be precisely alike, and the sight be of an equal power and focus: a deviation from each of which postulates must necessarily produce squinting, or an inaccordant action of one eye with the other. From common and early habit we acquire an equal command over the muscles of both, and are able to give them any direction, or power of direction, and to fix them upon any object we please. And such is the force of habit, that they at length involuntarily associate in the same action, and it is difficult for us to give to the one eye a different direction from that of the other; or in other words, to make their optic axes diverge instead of converge. In persons born blind no benefit can be derived from this unity of action, and hence it is never attempted; and the muscles being never subjected to discipline, the eyeballs roll at random, and wander in every direction. In consequence of which, one of the most difficult tasks to be acquired by such persons, after obtaining sight, is that of keeping their eyes fixed, and giving the same bearing or convergent line to each. And hence, again, they see things double at first, and in a state of great confusion.

When one eye is naturally stronger, or of a more favourable focus, or more frequently employed, than the other, as among watchmakers and jewellers, the latter, from comparative neglect, relapses into an undisciplined state, and less readily obeys the control of the will. Its muscles do not assume the same direction as those of the eye employed; and if they do, in the two former cases, the object still appears double; and hence the neglected or weaker eye wanders and stares at one or at various objects, while the eye relied upon is fixed upon some other. And it is this divergence of the optic axes, this inaccordance of direction, or looking at different objects at the same time, that constitutes the present disease.*

---

* When the axis of the eyes of persons who do not squint, and sometimes also of amaurotic individuals, are directed in different lines, objects are seen double: squinting persons, however, do not see objects double. Yet the principal reason assigned for the singular phenomenon, that the images impressed upon the two eyes excite only one image in the mind, is, that the two images fall upon corresponding points of the retina. The probability therefore is, that in a squinting person, both eyes do not see the object looked at. In many cases, as Sir Everard Home has remarked, " this is pretty evident to a by-stander, who is able

It is obvious, therefore, that strabismus may have three varieties :—

α Habitualis.	From a vitiated habit; or
Habitual squinting.	the custom of using one eye, and neglecting the other.
β Atonicus.	From debility of the affect-
Atonic squinting.	ed eye, whence the sound eye possesses a different focus and power of vision, and is alone trusted to: in consequence of which the weak or neglected eye insensibly wanders as already stated.*
γ Organicus.	From the eye being differ-
Organic squinting.	ently constructed in form or position.*

The FIRST of these VARIETIES constitutes the NYSTAGMUS of Dr. Plenck, and its cause is sufficiently obvious. In the SECOND, the sound eye is alone trusted to, because it is the only eye on which any dependance can be placed; and hence the weak eye, neglected by the will, wanders insensibly, as in the preceding order we have seen that any one of the mental faculties will wander in like manner under the same want of discipline. [It has been ascertained by experiment, that in individuals who have a confirmed squint of this kind, one of the eyes is too imperfect to see distinctly. Of this, however, the patient is not always conscious, as was evinced in a young lady whose case is re-

to determine that the direction of one of the eyes differs so much from that of the other, that it is impossible for the rays of light from any object to fall on the retina of both, and therefore that one eye does not see the object. The same thing may be proved in another way. For since a small deviation in the direction of either eye from the axis of vision produces double vision, any greater deviation must have the same effect, only increasing the distance between the two images, till it becomes so great that one eye only is directed to the object. In squinting, there is evidently a greater deviation from the axes of vision than in double vision, and the object does not appear double; it is therefore not seen by both eyes."—Phil. Trans., vol. lxxxvii., 1797.—ED.

* Besides the hypothesis here adopted in explanation of the manner in which strabismus is produced, others have been suggested. M. de la Hire conceived that the defect might arise from the more sensible part of the retina not being placed in the axis of the eye, but at some distance from it, on one side or the other; and that, consequently, not the axis, but this more sensible part of the retina, is turned towards the object on which the axis of the other eye is fixed, so that both axes are not directed to the same point. A case of this description would of course be absolutely incurable. Dr. Darwin's observations rather tend to show the possibility of such a form of strabismus; but both this hypothesis, and that of obliquity of the crystalline lens, are mostly considered to have been refuted by Dr. Jurin. Buffon refers the cause of squinting to an inequality in the goodness or in the limits of distinct vision in the two eyes; a doctrine, the truth of which is at present generally admitted. The exclusive adoption of any one hypothesis will obviously not explain all the varieties of strabismus,—ED.

lated by Sir Everard Home. Neither she herself nor her friends believed that any defect of
the eye existed ; and upon being asked if she
saw objects distinctly with her eyes, she said,
certainly, but that one was stronger than the
other. To ascertain the truth of this, he covered the strong eye, and gave her a book to read ;
when, to her astonishment, she found she could
not distinguish a letter, or any other near object.
More distant objects she could see, but not distinctly : when she looked at a bunch of keys in
the door of a bookcase about twelve feet from
her, she could see the bunch of keys, but could
not tell how many there were. The obscurity
of vision in one eye, then, is the cause of this
common species of squinting, and may occasion
this irregularity in the following way. The obscure image being so imperfectly formed in the
weak eye as to excite little attention in the
mind, the use of the eye, and its uniform direction to the same object with the other, may
have been neglected from the beginning; for
as distinct vision was obtained at once by the
perfect eye, the end was answered, and therefore there was no necessity for any exertion of
the other ; or, in the effort to get rid of the confused image, the muscles may have acquired an
irregular and unnatural action. Under either of
these circumstances the eye is directed towards
the nose, because, as Sir Everard Home remarks,
this direction is determined by the superior force
of the adductor muscle.] In the THIRD VARIETY,
the difference of form or position respects the
situation or figure of the one eye compared with
the other, or of the particular parts of the one
eye compared with those of the other : in consequence of which the one is favoured, and the
other thrown into disuse. [Dr. Porterfield has
pointed out two cases referrible to this variety,
or rather, constituting two distinct varieties
themselves. One depends upon an oblique position of the crystalline lens within the eye, by
which the image of an external object is refracted out of the line of the axis of the eye ; and
the other from an oblique position and greater
protuberance of the cornea, producing a similar
effect.*]

In this last variety a complete cure is hardly
to be expected. In the second it is attended
with considerable difficulty ; and in the first is
rather to be accomplished by what, in manner,
we have called *moral* treatment, than by medicine. A constant and resolute exertion on the
part of the patient to obtain a command over
the weak or irregular eye is of absolute necessity, while the neglected eye itself, if weak,

should be strengthened by tonics and gentle
stimulants. Goggles, though often recommended, are seldom serviceable, and especially to
children ; for although the sight must hereby be
restrained in each eye to a common line, the
child will still use the sound eye alone, and
leave the irregular eye unemployed. It is a
better plan to affix some object near the orbit
of the affected eye at such a distance, that it
may constantly catch and draw off the pupil from
the inner angle to the outer. [If squinting has
not been confirmed by long habit, and one eye
be not much worse than the other, Dr. Darwin
recommends a piece of gauze, stretched on a
circle of whalebone, to cover the best eye some
hours every day, so as to reduce distinctness of
vision in this eye to a similar degree of imperfection to what exists in the other eye.] But
the method that I have myself found by far the
most effectual, is to blindfold the sound eye
with a blink for a considerable part of every day,
and thus force the affected eye into use and a
subservience to the will. I recommend this
simple plan most strongly, and especially in the
case of children ; and may venture to predict
that it will be sure to succeed in the first variety of the disease, that of habit, and frequently
in both the others. [The same plan, which was
first suggested by Dr. Jurin (see *Smith's Optics, Rem.*, p. 30), is recommended by Mr. Lawrence, who mentions, however, that the squinting
eye has sometimes been cured by it, but the opposite one has then become affected. As strabismus, says he, occurs from so many causes, of
course, the treatment cannot be uniform. A
close investigation, with the view to discover
the particular cause, is a necessary preliminary
to any remedial measures. When this has been
accomplished, the course of treatment will be
obvious ; or we shall see, perhaps, that the de-
feet cannot be remedied. In the forms of strabismus arising from accidental irritation affecting the sensorium or alimentary canal, the treatment will of course turn upon the removal of the
cause. When strabismus and double vision occur in the commencement of amaurotic affection,
they will disappear if we succeed in removing
that disorder. The squinting which is produced
from change in the pupil and cornea, will hardly admit of relief:—(Op. cit., p. 575.)

Dr. Darwin mentions a singular case of
squinting, in which the patient was equally expert in the use of either eye, but viewed every
object presented to him with only one eye at a
time, and always with the eye on the side opposite the object. Thus, if the object was present-

---

* Edin. Essays, vol. iii., art. xii. "The eye
may be turned inwards or outwards, towards the
nose or towards the temple, the one case being
termed *strabismus convergens*, the other *strabismus
divergens.* The deviation is not always confined
to one eye ; in some cases both are affected, the
patient appearing sometimes to squint with the
right eye, and at other times with the left. If the
sound eye be covered, and the patient be directed
to look at any object, the squinting eye resumes
its proper position, and can be moved in any direction in obedience to the will ; but there are instances in which this cannot be done."—See

Lawrence on the Diseases of the Eye, p. 574. In
the junior school of the London University, there
is at the present time (May, 1834) a boy, who
squints with one eye when he looks at near objects, and with the other when he looks at distant
ones. Here it is manifest that the power of accommodation to distances is different in the two
eyes ; and consequently, that when this boy is looking at near objects, the eye adapted only to distant
objects cannot preserve any harmonious movement and position with respect to the other eye,
which alone is now employed.—ED.

ed on his right side, he viewed it with his left eye ; and when it was presented on his left side, he viewed it with his right eye. At the same time, Dr. Darwin found that he turned the pupil of that eye which was on the same side with the object in such a direction, that the image of the object might fall on that part of the bottom of the eye where the optic nerve enters it, and where it would of course excite no impression ; and this insensible portion of the retina Dr. Darwin ascertained, by some ingenious experiments, to be four times greater in this patient than in ordinary persons. When an object was held directly before the patient, he turned his head a little to one side, and observed it with but one eye ; viz., with that most distant from the object, turning away the other in the manner just mentioned ; and when he became tired of examining it with that eye, he turned his head the contrary way, and observed it with the other eye alone with equal facility ; but never turned the axis of both eyes on it at the same time.

For remedying this curious example, in which there was no defect in either eye, but merely a depraved habit of using both eyes separately, Dr. Darwin says, " a gnomon of thin brass was made to stand over his nose, with a half circle of the same metal to go round his temples ; these were covered with black silk ; and by means of a buckle behind his head, and a cross-piece over the crown of his head, this gnomon was managed so as to be worn without any inconvenience, and projected before his nose about two inches and a half. By the use of this gnomon, he soon found it less inconvenient to view all objects with the eye next to them, instead of the eye opposite to them.

" After this habit was weakened by a week's use of the gnomon, two bits of wood, about the size of a goose-quill, were blackened, all but a quarter of an inch at their summits. These were presented for him to look at, one being held on one side of the extremity of this black gnomon, and the other on the other side of it. As he viewed these, they were gradually brought forwards beyond the gnomon, and then one was concealed behind the other. By these means, in another week, he could bend both his eyes on the same object for half a minute together.

" By the practice of this exercise before a glass almost every hour in the day, he became in another week able to read for a minute together with his eyes both directed on the same objects : and I have no doubt, if he has patience enough to persevere in these efforts, he will in the course of some months overcome this unsightly habit.—(*Phil. Trans.*, vol. lxviii., pp. 86–89.)

GENUS II.
PARACUSIS.
MORBID HEARING.

SENSE OF HEARING VITIATED OR LOST.

Paracusis is a term of Hippocrates, derived from παρακούω, " perperàm, depravatè, vitiosè audio." The mechanism of the ear is as complicated as that of the eye, and is admirably adapted, in all its parts, to the perfection of the sense which constitutes its function. Its lobes, its entrances, its openings, its various drums, its minute and multiplied foramina, its delicate bones, all contribute to one common effect. Even the surrounding bones, and, still more than this, the teeth, are in no small degree auxiliary to the same object, as the experiments of M. Perolle, given in the fifth volume of the Turin Transactions, have abundantly established ; as they have also, that bone in general is a far better conductor of sound than air, alcohol, or water.

We may hence learn one very important use of the four minute bones deposited in the posterior chamber of the tympanum, the loss of any one of which impairs the hearing, and in some instances, has produced total deafness ; of which we have a striking proof in the case of a lad who had parted with the incus on one side, and both the incus and malleus on the other, by means of an ulcerated sore throat that opened a passage from the fauces into each ear, and through which the bones were discharged. The tympanum, on the boy's recovery, seems not to have lost its vibratory power ; for he was sensible of violent or sudden sounds, but altogether insensible to conversation, and apparently as deaf in the ear that had only parted with the incus, as in that which had parted with both bones.*

From the complicated organism of the ear, it follows necessarily that, like the eye, it must be subject to a great variety of diseases ; while many of the diseases of the one sense must bear a striking analogy to those of the other. Thus, painful and obtuse hearing and deafness may be well compared with painful and obtuse vision and blindness. As the eye is sometimes affected with illusory objects, so is the ear with illusory sounds ; and as, when the optic axes do not harmonize, as in strabismus, the same object may be seen double, so may the same sound be heard double when the action of the one ear is inaccordant with that of the other.

And hence it is not at all to be wondered at that a peculiar degree of sympathy should exist between these senses, and the state of the one be frequently affected by that of the other. Bartholine gives a case in which deafness and blindness alternated with each other (*Epist.*, cent. iv., No. xl.) ; and we shall presently have to observe, that a temporary affection of the eyes may sometimes be produced by particular noises.

As the organ of the ear, however, is less ex-

---

* Phil. Trans., vol. ii., No. 1., 1761. The editor has seen one case in which a boy who was reported to have lost all the ossicula of one ear, was not completely deaf from it ; though certainly his hearing on that side was dull. Sir Astley Cooper is acquainted with another example of the same kind. According to Mr. Mayo, the stapes is so strictly applied to the membrana fenestræ ovalis, that the loss of this bone necessarily produces incurable deafness by injuring the labyrinth.—Outlines of Human Physiology, 2d edit., p, 415, 8vo., Lond. 1828.

posed than that of the eye, we are far less acquainted with the immediate seat of its diseases, and even with the exact bearing which every particular part sustains in the general phenomenon of hearing. It was at one time supposed that the nicest power of discriminating sounds, or in other words, that accuracy of distinguishing which constitutes what is called a musical ear, is seated in the cochlea; birds, however, whose perception is exquisite, have no cochlea. It has since been conceived by Sir Everard Home, that it is the membrana tympani in which this fine feeling is peculiarly lodged (*Phil. Trans.*, year 1800), and that it depends upon the muscularity of this membrane; yet the same feeling has remained, and in a high degree, in persons whose membrana tympani has been ruptured. —(See *Bell's Anatomy*, vol. iii., p. 180, Lond., 1820; and *Buchanan's Physiological Illustrations of the Organ of Hearing*, p. 14, London, 1828.) [Sir Charles Bell does not conceive that the cochlea, or any part of the organ, particularly conduces to the bestowing of a musical ear, although it is by hearing that we are capable of the perceptions of melody and harmony, and of all the charms of music. It would seem, says he, that this *depends upon the mind,* and is not an operation confined to the organ. It is enjoyed in a very different degree by those whose simple faculty of hearing is equally perfect.]

Paracusis as a genus includes the following species:—

1. Paracusis Acris.   Acrid Hearing.
2. ————— Obtusa.   Hardness of Hearing.
3. ————— Perversa.   Perverse Hearing. ·
4. ————— Duplicata.   Double Hearing.
5. ————— Illusoria.   Imaginary Sounds.
6. ————— Surditas.   Deafness.

SPECIES I.
PARACUSIS ACRIS.
ACRID HEARING.
HEARING PAINFULLY ACUTE, AND INTOLERANT OF THE LOWEST SOUNDS.

THIS occurs occasionally as an idiopathic affection in nervous and highly irritable idiosyncrasies, and bears a striking analogy to that acritude of sight which we have noticed under *paropsis lucifuga.* It is the *hypercousis*, or, as it should rather be, the *hyperacusis*, of M. Itard, who also regards it as an idiopathic affection in various cases.—(*Traité des Maladies de l'Oreille et de l'Audition,* 2 tomes, 8vo., Paris, 1821.)

It depends upon a morbid excitement, sometimes of the whole of the auditory organs, but more generally of some particular part, as the tympanum or the labyrinth, and especially the cochlea, or some of the internal canals. In many instances it seems confined to the branches of the nerve; and Bonet gives an instance of it from the very singular cause of a triple auditory nerve formed on either side (*Sepulchr.,* lib. i., sect. xix., add. obs. 7), in which case there is sufficient ground for its idiopathic origin. It is found more frequently, however, as a

symptom of earache, headache, epilepsy, otitis, cephalitis, and fevers of various kinds.

The sensation is sometimes so keen as to render intolerable the whisperings of a mere current of air in a room, or the respirations of persons present, while noises before unperceived become highly distressing.

I have at this moment before me a most impressive description of this effect in a letter from a young lady of about twenty-eight years of age, of an irritable habit, great genius, and a highly cultivated mind, who about a twelvemonth ago was attacked with a cephalitis which proved severe and alarming. The mental powers are rendered more acute, and the external senses, especially those of hearing and seeing, strangely sympathize with each other. "You think me," says she in this letter, "unfit for study; but study I must, whether I am fit for it or not, otherwise my mind preys upon itself, and no power can prevent my thinking, which is almost as bad as reading. Last night I was kept awake for some hours by so powerful an excitement of the brain, that I really thought it would have taken away my senses. The pain is very acute, but I do not mind that so much as the distraction which accompanies it. It usually comes on with a most painfully quick hearing. I feel as if the tympanum was stretched so tight as to make the least sound appear almost as loud as thunder; and a loud noise is just as if I received a blow quite to the centre of the brain. This really is not imagination, but actual sensation. Moreover, a noise affects my eyes so much, that I am obliged to darken my room when at any time I am under the necessity of hearing any thing like a noise: *a loud sound affects my eyes, and a strong light my ears.* They seem to act reciprocally. My head is certainly not so bad, nor any thing like it, as it was at Clifton, but still the sudden attacks I have from over-exertion of the mental powers, or upon any other excitement, make me always fearful I shall lose my senses."

Injections of warm water, or a few drops of almond-oil dropped into the ear, will occasionally afford relief. But cold water, and cold applications about the ear, and even pounded ice where there is no tendency to a periodic rheumatism, by directly inducing torpitude, will at times have a better effect; laudanum may also be introduced into the ear, and a blister be applied to its immediate vicinity.

SPECIES II.
PARACUSIS OBTUS.
HARDNESS OF HEARING.
HEARING DULL AND CONFUSED, AND DEMANDING A CLEAR AND MODULATED ARTICULATION.

THIS may proceed from organic defect; from local debility, in which case it is called NERVOUS DEAFNESS; or from some accidental obstruction in the external tube or passage, as that of mucus, wax, sordes, or any other extrinsic body; or, in the internal or Eustachian tube, from mucus, inflammation, or ulceration and its consequences.* It is also found occasionally as a symptom or sequel in various fevers, in hemiplegia, apoplexy, otitis, lues, and polypous caruncles or concretions in the passage of the ear; and has followed on drinking cold water during great heat and perspiration of the body, of which several examples are given in the Ephemerides of Natural Curiosities. Among the cases of organic defect, one of the least common is atresia, or imperforation; yet Albucasis (vide Marcell. Donat., lib. vi., cap. ii., p. 619) gives us an instance of this, as does Bartholine† and Henckel.—(N. Anmerk., ii.) And among the more singular obstructions of an accidental kind may be mentioned insects and the grub of insects or worms. Bartholine mentions a leech which was once found to have burrowed in the ear; and Walker a small stone which had unaccountably become lodged there, and was discharged by a fit of sneezing.‡

The cure must depend upon the nature of the cause. All foreign bodies must be carefully removed or destroyed, and the cavity of the ear be washed by means of a syringe. Accumulations of wax may be softened by oil of almonds and alcohol, which will dissolve whatever resi-

---

* That hardness of hearing sometimes depends on deficiency of the ceruminous secretion within the meatus auditorius, is a fact of which most surgeons are perfectly aware. It is a cause, however, that does not appear to have received the author's notice. The ceruminous lining of the meatus auditorius is regarded by Mr. Buchanan as very essential to perfect hearing; and he has termed it the *ceruminous tubular circle.* "Without this provision," says he, "the undulations would affect or strike upon various parts of the membrana tympani irregularly, and produce confused vibratory action. And hence we find, in patients divested of this secretion, almost total inability to partake of the pleasure of a conversational party, where the news, politics, or other matters are discussed by the generality of the company; more especially if an argument ensue, in which a part of the discussion is taken by each individual." Mr. Buchanan compares the effect of the "ceruminous tubular circle," in absorbing what he calls the *resilient* pulsations of sound, to that of the pigmentum nigrum in the eye, which absorbs the superabundant rays of light, and prevents them from being reflected so as to injure the retina, or render vision indistinct.—See Buchanan's Physiological Illustrations of the Organ of Hearing, p. 21, 8vo., Lond., 1828.

† Hist. Anat., cent. vi., n. 36. The editor of this work has seen a child which was born entirely destitute of both auricles, and with the places of the meatus auditorii covered by the common integuments. In this case the hearing was dull, but not annihilated.

‡ Observ. Medico-Chirurg., xx., 8vo., 1718. I once removed two pebbles from the ears of a child after they had remained there a twelvemonth, having been introduced by another child in play. The little patient was, at the time of my seeing him, in considerable pain; inflammation had attacked each meatus auditorius, and there was complete deafness. I succeeded in bringing out the pebbles by throwing warm water into the meatus with some considerable force by means of a syringe. I recommend surgeons to prefer this simple expedient to more painful, and dangerous, and less efficacious measures.—Ed.

---

nous part it possesses; and a like inunction will be found the best means of destroying insects. Atonic or nervous deafness will often bid defiance to our utmost exertions, but it will sometimes yield to local stimulants and tonics: of the former are alcohol, ether, camphorated spirits, essential oil of turpentine combined with olive-oil; and the tinctures of the gum-resins, as myrrh, amber, kino, balsam of Tolu, and blisters about the ear; of the latter, cold water, and solutions of alum, sulphate of zinc, or other metallic salts.

[When, hardness of hearing depends upon a deficiency of cerumen, Mr. Buchanan recommends warmth and stimulant applications. Two drops of the subjoined formula* he advises to be applied to the interior parts of the tube every night at bedtime, and a table-spoonful of the mixture, the composition of which is given below,† to be taken at the same time. If the patient be costive, the pilulæ rhei comp. are also to be prescribed. When the wax is deficient in quality, or deficient both in quantity and quality, Mr. Buchanan, with the view of improving the state of the digestive organs, gives two table-spoonfuls of an infusion of quassia, with rhubarb and magnesia. The patient should reside in a dry airy place; take regular exercise; use the warm bath at bedtime once or twice a week; and immediately after getting into bed take pulv. ipecac. comp. ℈j. and hydrarg. submur. gr. ij. Mr. Buchanan directs the underwritten injection‡ to be used every second or third day. He speaks also favourably of bathing the feet in warm water, and a light nourishing diet, with a glass of port wine after dinner. Sometimes he applies blisters behind the auricle, or uses them and an antimonial embrocation§ alternately.—(See Th. Buchanan's Illustrations of Acoustic Surgery, p. 60 et seq., 8vo., Lond., 1825.)

Where hardness of hearing is habitual, and cannot be radically cured, we can only endeavour to diminish the evil by advising the use of a hearing-trumpet, which is, in fact, an instrument formed upon the principle of imitating the cavities of the labyrinth of the ear itself, and the object of which is to collect a large body of sonorous tremours, and send them to the tympanum in a concentrated state, by means of a convergent tube, or in other words, to increase as much as possible the vibratory power of the sound. Now sound is well known to be propagated in straight lines, and hence persons partially deaf will always hear most distinctly when directly opposite the speaker. For the same reason the trumpet itself should be formed as nearly as possible in a straight line; though we are sometimes, for the sake of convenience, obliged to deviate from this direction, and to bend the tube into the segment of a circle, by which

---

* ℞ Acid. Pyrolign., Sp. Æther. Sulph., Ol. Terebinth. ā ā M.
† ℞ Tinct. Colchici ʒiij., Aq. distillat. ʒvj.
‡ ℞ Acid. Pyrolign. ʒij., Aq. distillat. ʒvj., M. ft. injectio.
§ ℞ Ol. Sabinæ ʒss., Antim. Tart. ℈j., Ung. Cetacei ʒiij., Misce.

some degree of power is always lost. The metal of which the tube is made should be that which is found most sonorous, or, in other words, which most completely reflects instead of absorbing the sound; and while the funnel or large aperture is as wide as possible, the extreme end of the pipe cannot be too small. M. Itard has found that a parabolical figure has no advantage over a conical or pyramidal tube; but that the tube is assisted in producing distinctness of sounds by an insertion into it of slips of goldbeater's leaf, at proper distances, in the manner of partitions.—(*Traité de Maladies de l'Oreille et de l'Audition*, 2 tomes, Paris, 1821.)

SPECIES III.
PARACUSIS PERVERSA.
PERVERSE HEARING.

THE EAR ONLY SENSIBLE TO ARTICULATE SOUNDS WHEN EXCITED BY OTHER AND LOUDER SOUNDS INTERMIXED WITH THEM.

THIS is a very extraordinary hebetude of the organ, though it has occasionally been met with in most countries. Where it exists, the ear, as in other cases of imperfect hearing, requires to be roused in order to discriminate the articulate sounds addressed to it, but finds the best excitement to consist in a great and vehement noise of almost any kind.—(*Feiliz in Richter Chir. Bibl.*, band ix., p. 555.) It consists, according to Sauvages, who seems to judge rightly concerning it, in a torpitude or paresis of some parts of the external organ, which, in consequence of this additional stimulus, convey the proper sounds addressed to them beyond the membrane of the tympanum, in the same manner as the drowsy, or those who are sluggish in waking, do not open their eyes, or admit the light to the retina, unless a strong glare first stimulates the exterior tunics. It seems, however, sometimes to depend upon an obstruction of the Eustachian tubes.

Under the influence of this species, it occasionally happens that particular sounds or noises prove a better stimulus than others, though equally loud, or even louder; as the music of a pipe, of a drum, or of several bells ringing at the same time. Holder relates the case of a man who never heard but when he was beating a drum (*Phil. Trans.*, 1668, No. xxvi.); and Sauvages a similar case of a woman, who on this account always kept a drum in the house, which was constantly played upon while she was conversing with her husband. The latter gives another case of a person who was always deaf except when travelling in a carriage, during which time; from the rattling of the wheels, he was perfectly capable of hearing and engaging in conversation. And Stahl gives an instance of like benefit derived from the shrill tones of a pipe.—(*Colleg. Casual.*, N., lxxvi.)

In ordinary cases of practice, if we can once hit upon a stimulus that succeeds in giving temporary tone to a debilitated organ, we can often avail ourselves of it to produce a permanent benefit, and sometimes a complete restoration, by raising or lowering its power, continuing its power for a longer or shorter term of time, or modifying it in some other way, so as to adapt it to the particular exigency. And it is hence probable, that if any of these sonorous stimuli were to be employed medicinally, and with a due respect to length of time and acuteness of tone, they might in some instances be made the medium of obtaining perfect success. Dr. Birch, indeed, gives an instance of such success in a person who only heard during the ringing of bells; and who, by a permanent use of this stimulus, recovered his hearing altogether.—(*Hist.*, vol. iv.) Voltaism may here also be employed in many cases with a considerable promise of advantage; and especially in connexion with the ordinary routine of general and local tonics and stimulants, as cold, and cold bathing, pungent masticatories and injections, bark, valerian, alone or with ammonia, and a free use of the siliquose and coniferous plants as a part of the common diet.

SPECIES IV.
PARACUSIS DUPLICATA.
DOUBLE HEARING.

THE ACTION OF THE ONE EAR INACCORDANT WITH THAT OF THE OTHER; SOUNDS HEARD DOUBLY, AND IN DIFFERENT TONES OR KEYS.

THIS pravity of hearing depends upon an inaccordance of the auditory nerve on the one side with that on the other; so that the same sound produces on each side a very different effect, and is consequently heard, not homotonously, or in like tones, but heterotonously, or in separate and unlike. And hence this species of morbid hearing, as I have already observed, has a considerable parallelism with that of strabismus or squinting, in which the optic axis of the one eye is not accordant with that of the other, whence the same object is seen double, and often in a different position. Sauvages has given two or three very curious examples of this affection. A musician, while blowing his flute, heard two distinct sounds at every note. The sounds were in different keys, and consequently not in harmony; and as they were heard simultaneously, the one could not be an echo of the other. On another occasion he was consulted by a person who for several months had been troubled with a hearing of two distinct voices whenever he was spoken to; the one at least an octave higher than the other, but not in unison with it, and hence producing a harsh and insupportable discordance.

This affection is mostly temporary, and, as proceeding altogether from a morbid condition of the auditory nerve, has been cured by blisters and other local stimulants. From not being attended to, however, in due time, it has sometimes assumed a chronic character, when it is removed with great difficulty; and in a few instances it has been connected with a constitutional irritability of the nervous system, in which case a plan of general tonics must co-operate with local applications.

[Mr. Buchanan does not coincide with the author respecting the cause of *paracusis dupli-*

cata, but ascribes its symptoms to an imperfect secretion of cerumen in only one ear.—(See *Buchanan's Physiological Illustrations of the Organ of Hearing*, p. 24, ·Lond., 1828.) In this view of the case, nothing more need be said on the ·treatment than what ·has already been stated under the head of *paracusis obtusa*. If some observations published by Sir Everard Home be correct, double hearing ·may sometimes arise from another cause, not ad·verted to by Dr. Good. "An eminent music-master (says he), after catching cold, found a confusion of sounds in his ears. On strict attention, he discovered that the pitch of one ear was half a note lower than that of the other ; and that the perception of a single sound did not reach both ears at the same instant, but seemed as two distinct sounds following each other in quick succession, the last being the lower and weaker. This complaint distressed him for a long time, but he recovered from it without any medical aid. In this case (Sir Everard Home observes), the whole defect appears to have been in the action of the radiated muscle (of the tympanum), exerted neither with the same quickness nor force in one ear as in the other, so that the sound was half a note too low, as well as later in being impressed on the organ."—(*Phil. Trans.*, 1800.) This case seems to be very similar to those above cited from ·Sauvages. Mr. Buchanan expresses his doubts about the reality of the alleged cause, which he suspects might be a defective state of the ceruminous secretion.]

SPECIES V.

PARACUSIS ILLUSORIA.

IMAGINARY· SOUNDS.

INTERNAL SENSE OF SOUNDS WITHOUT EXTERNAL CAUSES.

THIS is in most instances strictly a nervous affection, and bears a striking analogy to *paropsis illusoria*, or that illusory or false sight in which unreal objects, of various forms, colours, and other sensible qualities, appear before the eyes. The morbid state is often confined to the auditory nerves, or some of the branches alone ; yet it is not unfrequently the result of a peculiar irritability that extends through the whole of the nervous system. And occasionally it proceeds from an obstruction of one or both the Eustachian tubes. M. Itard ascribes it to two other causes : a peculiar state of the blood-vessels, local or general, and an impeded motion of the air in the tympanal cavity (*Traité des Mal. de l'Oreille et de l'Audition*, 2 tomes, 8vo., Paris, 1821); [Mr. Buchanan, to the imperfect secretion ·of cerumen.—(*Physiological Illustrations of the Organ of Hearing*, p. 23.)] The sounds hereby produced differ greatly in different persons, and sometimes in the very same person at different periods ; but it is sufficient to contemplate them under the three following varieties, all which the French express by the term *bourdonnements* :—

α Syrigmus.	A sharp, shrill, successive
Ringing or tinkling.	sound.
β Susurrus.	An acute, continuous, his
Whizzing.	sing sound.
γ Bombus.	A dull, heavy, intermitting
Beating.	sound.

Heister recommends, in cases arising from a debility of the local nerves, to fumigate the ears with the vapour of a hot vinous infusion of rosemary and lavender ; and where a spasmodic affection of the inner membrane may be supposed to follow such debility, he advises a simultaneous use of diaphoretics internally. If it proceed from an obstruction of the Eustachian tubes, in consequence of spasm or inflammation, the fumes of tobacco drawn into the mouth, and forcibly pressed against these tubes by closing the lips and nostrils, and then urgently sniffing the vapours upwards to the palate, have often proved serviceable, by taking off the irritability on which the spasmodic or inflammatory action is dependant. Stimulating the external ear by blisters or aromatic injections has sometimes availed, though not often. Chronic cases are extremely difficult of cure ; though I had lately an elderly lady for a patient, who after having at different times suffered from each of these modifications of illusory sounds for several years, and tried every remedy that could be suggested in vain, at length lost the distressing sensation by degrees, and without the assistance of any medicine.*

SPECIES VI.

PARACUSIS SURDITAS.

DEAFNESS.

TOTAL INABILITY OF HEARING OR DISTINGUISHING SOUNDS.

IN the preceding species, the sense of hearing is in various ways depraved or impaired ; in the present, it is altogether abolished, and may proceed from causes which offer three distinct varieties of affection :

α Organica.	From organic defect or impediment.
Organic deafness.	
β Atonica.	From local debility or relaxation.
Atonic deafness.	
γ Paretica.	From nervous insensibility.
Paretic deafness.	

The ORGANIC DEFECT or impediment may exist in the outer or inner entrance, or in the cavity of the ear. The outer entrance has in a few instances been imperforate (*Cels de Medicin*, lib. vii., c. 8 ; *Büchner, Miscell. Phys. Med.*, p. 318, 1727), but far more generally blocked up with indurated wax, excrescences, concretions, or some other substance. The inner entrance or Eustachian tube has been sometimes also found imperforate on both sides, but more frequently obliterated by ulceration (*Haller, Elem. Phys.*, tom. v., p. 286), or

---

* The treatment suggested by Mr. Buchanan has already been briefly noticed under the head of *Paracusis Obtusa*.

closed by the mucous secretion of a catarrh, or the pressure of the tonsils, in whatever way morbidly enlarged. If the defect or impediment exist in the cavity of the ear, its precise nature can seldom be known during the life of the patient, and if known would rarely admit of a remedy. It often consists of a malformation of the helix ; and, as we have already seen under PAROTITIS, in a loss of the articulation or substance of one or more of the tympanal bones.

ATONIC DEAFNESS, or that dependant on local debility or relaxation, may be superinduced by a chronic cold, abruptly plunging the head into cold water in a heated state, a long exposure to loud and deafening noises, or the sudden and unexpected burst of some vehement sound upon the ears (*Schulze, Diss. de Auditûs Difficultate,* sect. 23), as that of a cannon or a thunderclap (*Borelli, Observ.,* cent. iv., Paris, 1656), where the constitution is in a state of great nervous irritability : in which state, moreover, it has in a few instances been produced by a violent fright.—(*Eph. Nat. Cur.,* cent. ix., obs. 6.) It has also proceeded from an atony of the excretories of the outer ear, in consequence of which there has been neither wax nor moisture of any kind. And it has followed as a sequel upon various fevers and inflammations, especially cephalitis and otitis, rheumatic hemicrania, and other nervous headaches, repelled gout, and repelled cutaneous eruptions.

PARETIC DEAFNESS may be regarded in many cases as nothing more than an extreme of atonic deafness ; and almost all the causes producing the one, when operating with greater violence or upon a feebler frame, may also produce the other. It has not only been induced suddenly by loud sounds and violent frights, but by a vehement fit of sneezing, and from sympathy, by the use of powerful sternutatories (*Eph. Nat. Cur.,* dec. ii., ann. ix., obs. 26); the olfactory nerve hereby becoming insentient through all its branches.

Deafness has often been transmitted hereditarily ; of which numerous instances are to be found in Hoffmann (*Consult. et Respons.,* cent. i., cas. 40), Morgagni (*De Sed. et Caus. Morb.,* epist. xlviii., art. 48), and other writers of established reputation.

The most usual causes of total deafness are beyond the power of the medical art to relieve ; and hence the disease runs very generally through the whole period of life. Where the cause is an imperforation of either of the passages, an opening has been often effected with success. Many other impediments, as of indurated wax, or infarction from inflammation, are in general removable still more easily ; and some obstructions have been suddenly carried off by a fall, or other violent concussion of the head. The great difficulty, however, is in getting at such impediments when they are formed in the tympanal cavity. The perforation of the mastoid process, recommended by Riolanus, has been practised occasionally with success, and especially by the Swedish anatomists, Jasser and Hagstrœm. But the difficulties are so considerable, that the plan has usually been superseded by a puncture of the membrane, or by injecting the Eustachian tube, as first proposed by an unprofessional artist, Guyot of Versailles, and since followed up successively by Cleland, Petit, Douglas, and Wathen. Of late, however, even this has been dropped ; though now once more revived in France by M. Itard, and in Great Britain by Mr. Buchanan.—(*Engraved Representation of the Anatomy of the Human Ear,* &c., Hull, 1823.)

In deafness from atonic relaxation, almost all the stimulant and tonic methods pointed out under the preceding species have been tried in turn, occasionally with palliative success, sometimes altogether in vain. The fumes of tobacco sniffed up the Eustachian tubes from the mouth, in the manner described under the last species, were recommended by Morgagni (*Epist. Anat.,* vii., art. 14 ; *Eph. Nat. Cur.,* dec. i., ann. vi., obs. 110) and many other writers of earlier times, and have occasionally been found beneficial in our own day ; the spasm or other obstruction of the fine tubes ceasing of a sudden, and with the sensation of a smart snap, that almost startles the patient. And as sight has sometimes been restored in amaurosis by a violent fever or a flash of lightning, so has deafness from atony, approaching to paralysis, been recovered by a like fever or a thunderclap (*Bresl. Samml.,* 1718, p. 1541) ; ordinary causes being thus transferred into extraordinary modes of cure.

Among the stimulants most useful, where the deafness is dependant upon debility of the membrane of the tympanum, or the nerve of hearing, have been the aura of voltaic electricity, applied two or three times a day for half an hour or longer each time, and persevered in for many weeks, a series of blisters continued for a long period, and a diluted solution of nitrate of silver. Yet a chronic ulcer forming in the ear, and discharging plentifully, has often proved still more effectual.

Mr. Gordon relates a case of total deafness, produced suddenly in a soldier in good health, by plunging overhead into the sea ; which, after a long routine of medicines had been tried in vain for three months, yielded to the use of mercury as soon as the mouth began to be affected. A gentle salivation supervened, his hearing was gradually restored, and in six weeks from its commencement, he returned to his duty perfectly cured.—(*Edin. Med. Comm.,* vol. iii., p. 80.) The excitement of the salivary glands seems in this case to have extended by sympathy to the Eustachian tubes, or whatever other parts of the organ of hearing were diseased.

When the Eustachian tubes are imperforate or irrecoverably closed, which may commonly be determined by an absence of that sense of swelling in the ears which otherwise takes place on blowing the nose violently, Riolanus, and afterward Cheselden, proposed a substitute for the canal by making a small perforation through the membrane of the tympanum ; and Sir Astley Cooper has boldly put their recommendation to the test. The artificial opening does not destroy the elasticity of the membrane, and it has hence been occasionally attended with success ; and perhaps would be always, if it were to be limited, as M. Itard (*Traité des Maladies de l'Oreille et de l'Audition,* &c., 2 tomes, Paris, 1821) has shown it ought to be, to a permanent obstruction of the Eustachian tube, unaccompanied with inflammation or any other cause of deafness. And it is from a wanton application of this remedy to other cases that it has so often been tried in vain since Sir Astley Cooper's successful sanction.

<hr>

GENUS III.
PAROSMIS.
MORBID SMELL.
SENSE OF SMELL VITIATED OR LOST.

THIS is the parosmia and anosmia of many writers ; from παρὰ, "malè," and ὄζω, "olfacio," analogous with PARACUSIS and PAROPSIS : anosmia, however, will not include one of its species, and the present termination is preferred on account of its analogy with that of the parallel terms.

Under this genus may be arranged the three following species :—

1. Parosmis Acris.   Acrid Smell.
2. ———— Obtusa.   Obtuse Smell.
3. ———— Expers,   Want of Smell.

SPECIES I.
PAROSMIS ACRIS.
ACRID SMELL.
SMELL PAINFULLY ACUTE OR SENSIBLE TO ODOURS NOT GENERALLY PERCEIVED.

GENERALLY speaking, the sense of smell in all animals is in proportion to the extent of the Schneiderian or olfactory membrane with which the nostrils are lined, and over which the branches of the olfactory nerves divaricate and ramify. And hence this membrane is much more extensive in quadrupeds and birds, which chiefly trust to the sense of smell in selecting their food, than in man ; for it ascends considerably higher, and is for the most part possessed of numerous folds or duplicatures. It is hereby the hound distinguishes the peculiar scent thrown

forth from the body of the hare, and the domestic dog recognises and identifies his master from all other individuals.

Yet the nerves of smell are not only spread in great abundance over the olfactory membrane of all animals possessing such an organ, but they are distributed so near the surface as to be almost naked ;* and hence in every class they are easily and hourly excited into action, being covered with little more than a layer of bland, insipid mucus, thin at its first separation, but gradually hardening by the access of air into viscid crusts, and which is expressly secreted for the purpose of defending them. From this nearly naked state it is, that they are stimulated by aromatics, however finely and impalpably divided ; whence the violent sneezings that take place in many persons in an atmosphere in which only a few particles of sternutatories or other acrid olfacients are floating : and hence also the rapidity with which a sympathetic action is excited in the neighbouring parts, or in the system at large, and the refreshment which is felt on scenting the pungent vapour of carbonate of ammonia, or vinegar, or the grateful perfume of violets or lavender, in nervous headaches or fainting-fits. The fetid odours are well known to affect the nostrils quite as poignantly as the pleasant, and to produce quite as extensive a sympathy ; and hence the nausea, and even intestinal looseness, which often follow on inhaling putrid and other offensive effluvia.

Under peculiar circumstances, however, the ordinary apparatus for smell possesses an activity, and sometimes even an intolerable keenness, which by no means belongs to it in its natural state. M. Virey, who has written a very learned treatise upon the subject of odours, asserts that the olfactory sense exists among savages in a far higher degree of activity than among civilized nations, whose faculty of smell is blunted by an habitual exposure to strong odours, or an intricate combination of odours, and by the use of high-flavoured foods. And he might have added, that this sense, like every other, is capable of cultivation, and of acquiring delicacy of discrimination by use ; that savages, many of whom make an approach to the life of quadrupeds, employ it, and trust to it in a similar manner ; and that this is perhaps the chief cause of the difference he has pointed

<hr>

* Over the whole of the Schneiderian membrane, branches of the fifth nerve are distributed. In the human subject, the first or olfactory nerve does not spread so extensively, but goes principally to the septum-narium and upper turbinated bone. M. Magendie has ascertained the effect of the separate division of the first and fifth nerves in animals ; and has thus more correctly demonstrated how much of the impression received by the nostrils belongs to smell, properly so called, and how much to touch. " It appears that upon the division of the first nerve, the animal remains as sensible as before to the disagreeable impression of odours which act pungently. A young dog thus mutilated, appeared conscious of an unpleasant impression when ammonia, acetic acid, oil of lavender, or Dippel's oil, was held to its nose. On the other hand, after the division of the fifth, the first nerve remaining entire, an animal is not affected by the presence of the substances above mentioned." But a dog that survived the division of the fifth nerve for a considerable period, would at times, when food was offered to it rolled up in paper, unrol the paper, and expose and eat the food although at other times he appeared to want the power of distinguishing by smelling the presence of objects placed near it. " Pungent odours seem to offend the nose upon the same principle that they irritate the conjunctiva of the eye ; their acrid impression, without their scent, being perceived when the influence of the first nerve is artificially destroyed." The first nerves, therefore, constitute the organ of smell.—See Mayo's Outlines of Physiology, p. 412, 2d edit. ; and Magendie's Journ. de Physiol. Exp., tom. iv., p. 173.—ED.

out. It is in like manner relied upon by persons who are deprived of one or two of the other external senses, as those of sight or hearing, or both : not merely in consequence of more frequent employment, but from the operation of the law we have already pointed out, that where one of the external senses is destroyed or constitutionally wanting, the rest, in most cases, are endowed with an extraordinary degree of energy ; as though the share of sensorial power naturally belonging to the defective organs were distributed among the rest, and modified to their respective uses. One of the most interesting examples that I am acquainted with of this transfer of sensorial power, is to be found in the history, first given to the public by Mr. Dugald Stewart, of James Mitchell, a boy born both blind and deaf ; and who, having no other senses by which to discover and keep up a connexion with an external world than those of smell, touch, and taste, chiefly depended for information on the first, employing it on all occasions, like a domestic dog, in distinguishing persons and things. By this sense he identified his friends and relatives ; and conceived a sudden attachment or dislike to strangers, according to the nature of the effluvium that escaped from their skin. "He appeared," says Mr. Wardrop, who has also published an account of him, "to know his relations and intimate friends by smelling them very slightly, and he at once detected strangers. It was difficult, however, to ascertain at what distance he could distinguish people by this sense ; but from what I could observe, he appeared to be able to do so at a considerable distance from the object. This was particularly striking when a person entered the room, as he seemed to be aware of such entrance before he could derive information from any other sense than that of smell. When a stranger approached him, he eagerly began to touch some part of the body, commonly taking hold of his arm, which he held near his nose ; and after two or three strong inspirations through the nostrils, he appeared to form a decided opinion concerning him. If it were favourable, he showed a disposition to become more intimate, examined more minutely his dress, and expressed, by his countenance, more or less satisfaction ; but if it happened to be unfavourable, he suddenly went off to a distance, with expressions of carelessness or disgust."[*]

The *Journal des Sçavans* for 1667 gives a curious history of a monk who pretended to be able to ascertain, by the difference of odour alone, the sex and age of a person, whether he were married or single, and the manner of life to which he was accustomed. This, as far as the fact extended, may possibly have been the result of observations grafted upon a stronger natural sense than belongs to mankind in general, and is scarcely to be ranked in the list of diseased actions. But among persons of a

highly nervous or irritable idiosyncrasy, I have met with numerous instances of an acuteness of smell almost intolerable and distracting to those who laboured under it ; which has fairly constituted an idiopathic affection, and sometimes nearly realized the description of the poet, in making its possessors ready at every moment to

"Die of a rose in aromatic pain."

Mr. Pope seems to have written this line as a play of fancy at the time, but the writings of various collectors of medical curiosities abundantly show that he has here described nothing more than an occasional and sober fact. Thus M. Orfila gives us an account of a celebrated painter of Paris, of the name of Vincent, who cannot remain in any room where there are roses without being in a short time attacked with a violent cephalæa, succeeded by fainting (*Sur les Poisons*, tom. ii., Cl. v., sect. 972) ; and M. Marrigues informs us that he once knew a surgeon who could not smell at a rose without a sense of suffocation, which subsided as soon as the rose was removed from him ; as he also knew a lady who lost her voice whenever an odoriferous nosegay was applied to her nostrils.—(*Journ. de Physique*, year 1780.)

We have observed that a keen stimulation of the olfactory nerves is often productive of a very powerful sympathetic action in other organs. There are few persons who, on inhaling the fine particles of black hellebore and colocynth while in the act of being pounded, would not feel their effect on the intestines by a copious diarrhœa ; but where the acuteness of smell exists which constitutes the present disease, whether limited to particular odours, or extending to all odours equally, the sympathetic action is sometimes of a very singular description. M. Valtain gives the history of an officer who was thrown into convulsions and lost his senses by having in his room a basket of pinks, of which, nevertheless, he was very fond. The flowers were removed, and the windows opened, and in the course of half an hour the convulsions ceased, and the patient recovered his speech. Yet, for twelve years afterward, he was never able to inhale the smell of pinks without fainting.—(*Hygiène Chirurgicale*, p. 26.) And M. Orfila relates the case of a lady, forty-six years of age, of a hale constitution, who could never be present where a decoction of linseed was preparing, without being troubled, in the course of a few minutes afterward, with a general swelling of the face, followed by fainting and a loss of the intellectual faculties ; which symptoms continued for four-and-twenty hours.—(*Sur les Poisons*, loc. cit.)

The predisponent cause of the species before us is a nervous or irritable habit. The occasional causes are, local irritation from a slight cold, in which the contact of the air alone, as inhaled, often produces sneezing ; or excoriation of the mucous membrane of the nostrils, from the use of sternutatories in those not accustomed to them. It is often the result of idiosyncrasy ; and perhaps at times, as in *paracusis acris*, of a superfluous distribution of olfactory

---

[*] History of James Mitchell, a boy born blind and deaf, &c. ; by James Wardrop, F. R. S., 4to. edit., 1813.

nerves. As a symptom, it is often found in ophthalmia and rheumatic hemicrania.

Where the disease is connected with the habit, the nervous excitement should be diminished by refrigerants and tonics, as the shower-bath, bark, acids, neutral and several of the metallic salts. And where it is chiefly local, we may often produce a transfer of action by blisters in the vicinity of the organ; or relax the Schneiderian membrane, and moisten its surface by the vapour of warm water. The sniffing up cold water will also prove serviceable in many instances, by inducing torpitude at first, and additional tone afterward. Dr. Darwin advises errhines for the first of these purposes, that of exhausting the excitability and blunting the sense.

SPECIES II.
PAROSMIS OBTUSA.
OBTUSE SMELL.
SMELL DULL AND IMPERFECTLY DISCRIMINATIVE.

THIS is often a natural defect, but more frequently a consequence of an habitual use of sternutatories, which exhaust, weaken, and torpify the nerves of smell, just as exposure to a strong light weakens and impairs the vision, and sometimes destroys it altogether. To those unaccustomed to sternutatories, the mildest snuffs will produce such an excitement as is marked by a long succession of sneezing, which is nothing more than an effort of the remedial power of nature to throw off the offending material; while those who have habituated themselves to snuff for years, can hardly be excited to sneeze by the most violent ptarmics.

The evil is here so small, that a remedy is seldom sought for in idiopathic cases; and in sympathetic affections, as when it proceeds from catarrhs or fevers, it usually, though not always, ceases with the cessation of the primary disease. It is found also as a symptom in hysteria, syncope, and several species of cephalæa, during which the nostrils are capable of inhaling very pungent, aromatic, and volatile errhines, with no other effect than that of a pleasing and refreshing excitement.

Where the sense of smell is naturally weak, or continues so after catarrhs or other acute diseases, many of our cephalic snuffs may be reasonably prescribed, and will often succeed in removing the hebetude. The best are those formed of the natural order verticillatæ, as rosemary, lavender, and marjoram: if a little more stimulus be wanted, these may be intermixed with a proportion of the *teucrium Marum*; to which, if necessary, a small quantity of asarum may also be added; but pungent errhines will be sure to increase instead of diminishing the defect.

SPECIES III.
PAROSMIS EXPERS.
WANT OF SMELL.
TOTAL INABILITY OF SMELLING OR DISTINGUISHING ODOURS.

THIS species is in many instances a sequel of the preceding; for whatever causes operate in producing the former, when carried to an extreme, or continued for a long period, may also lay a foundation for the latter. But as it often occurs by itself, and without any such introduction, it is entitled to be treated of separately. It offers us the two following varieties:—

α Organica.　　　　From natural defect, or
　Organic want of　　accidental lesion, injuri-
　smell.　　　　　　ous to the structure of
　　　　　　　　　　the organ.

β Paralytica.　　　From local palsy.
　Paralytic want of
　smell.

The FIRST VARIETY occurs from a connate destitution of olfactory nerves, or other structural defect; or from external injuries of various kinds; and is often found as a sequel in ozænas, fistula lachrymalis, syphilis, smallpox, and porphyra. The SECOND is produced by neglected and long-continued coryzas, and a persevering indulgence in highly acrid sternutatories.

The author once knew a very beautiful and elegant young lady, who had from birth so total a want of smell as not only to be incapable of perceiving any difference in the odours of different perfumes or flowers, but of sweet and corrupt meats, and who could inhale very powerful errhines without sneezing. Though this affection seemed to have been connate, and dependant upon a natural imperfection of the nerves of smell, the Schneiderian membrane had something of the thickening which is ordinarily produced by catarrhs, and the lady always spoke as though under the influence of a slight cold.

When this affection is a sequel of local irritation, as from a coryza or catarrh, warm stimulating vapours, as of vinegar or frankincense, are often useful. If produced by syphilis, the fumes of cinnabar may be inhaled by the nostrils, or a sternutatory may be used, composed of turbeth mineral and ten times the quantity of any mild and light powder, as orris-root.

GENUS IV.
PARAGEUSIS.
MORBID TASTE.
SENSE OF TASTE VITIATED OR LOST.

PARAGEUSIS is derived from παρὰ, "male," and γεύω, "gustum præbeo," whence παραγεύω, and consequently παραγεύσις. The author has preferred, with Vogel, the present termination to parageusia, as analogous to the names of the preceding genera of the order before us.

In the senses of taste and smell there is a considerable association. The young lady I have just noticed, who was destitute, or nearly so, of the sense of smell, was equally destitute of that of taste, and could not distinguish by this criterion between beef, veal, and pork; and consequently, in respect to all these, had no preference.

The chief organ of taste is the tongue; but this is not the only organ, nor is it absolutely necessary for an existence of the sense. The Philosophical Transactions give us examples of persons who possessed a perfect taste after the tongue had been wholly destroyed ; and Professor Blumenbach, in his Comparative Anatomy, affords us a similar example in an adult whom he visited, and who was born without a tongue. Consonant with which, many insects appear to have a faculty of taste, though they have no organ of a tongue ; and among these the gustatory function is supposed by Professor Knoch to be performed by the posterior pair of palpi or feelers ; while, on the other hand, there are many animals possessing a tongue who do not use it as an organ of taste. All birds possess a tongue, for even the pelican, which has been said to be tongueless, has a rudiment of this member ; yet there are but few birds, comparatively, that taste or are able to taste with this organ. Parrots, predaceous and swimming birds, are an exception to this remark ; for they possess a soft thick tongue, covered with papillæ, and moistened with a salivary fluid, and select that food which is the most agreeable. Yet, in by far the greater proportion of birds, we do not find the tongue appropriated to this purpose. In many of them, indeed, it is stiff, horny, and destitute of nerves. The tongue of the toucan, though sometimes several inches in length, is scarcely two lines broad at its root : it has throughout the appearance of whalebone, and its margins are fibrous. The tongues of the woodpecker and cock of the woods are equally hard and horny : in themselves they are short, and in a quiescent state he backward in the mouth, and are covered with a sort of sheath issuing from the os hyoides or the œsophagus : but they possess a mechanism which renders them extremely extensile, and capable of being thrust forward to a considerable distance. That of the woodpecker is sharp-pointed, with barbed sides, and is darted with great rapidity out of the mouth to an extent of some inches ; by which means it follows up such insects as the animal is in pursuit of through all their crannies in the bark of trees, sticks them through with its apex, and in this state drags them out for food. The chameleon has a tongue of a somewhat similar kind, which in like manner answers the purpose, not of taste, but of preying for food. It is contained in a sheath at the lower part of the mouth, and has its extremity covered with a glutinous secretion. It admits of being projected to the length of six inches ; and is used in this manner by the animal in catching its spoil, and especially in catching flies. It is darted from the mouth with wonderful celerity and precision ; and the viscous secretion on its extremity entangles minute animalcules, which constitute another portion of its food.

The tongue, when it forms an organ of taste, as in man, is studded, and especially on its upper surface and lateral edges, with innumerable nervous papillæ, issuing from a peculiar membrane that lies beneath, and has a near resemblance to the skin in other parts, but is softer and more spongy. Its external tunic or cuticle is an exquisitely fine epithelium, which is moistened, not by an oily fluid like that of the surface of the body, but a peculiar mucus.

We have here, therefore, a more exquisite sense of touch than on the general skin, whose papillæ are not only smaller but dry. There can be no question, also, that the sentient fluid with which they are supplied is differently modified from that of the skin ; and hence the provinces of the two senses, though they occasionally approach each other,—are still kept distinct ; and the tongue becomes a discerner of certain qualities which the skin cannot discriminate, as sour, sweet, rough, bitter, salt, and aromatic.*

Thus much we know ; but we do not know the cause of that different effect, or in other words, of that variety of tastes which different substances produce upon the papillæ of the tongue, and which constitute their respective flavours. It was supposed by the Epicureans, and the doctrine has descended to the present day, that all this depends upon the geometrical figure of the sapid corpuscles ; and particularly so with respect to saline bodies, which are cubic in sea-salt, prismatic in nitre, and equally diversified in vitriol, sugar, and other crystals. It is sufficient, however, to annul this explanation, to observe, that many crystals of very different forms are alike insipid ; while others of the same, or nearly the same shape, possess very different flavours ; as also that the flavour in any of them continues the same, even where we are able to change the figure ; as, for example, by rendering common nitre cubical. The cause of flavours, therefore, appears to reside in the ele-

---

* Instead of this hypothesis of a modification of the nervous fluid, modern discoveries teach us rather to seek in the different nerves with which the tongue is supplied for an explanation of the cause of the peculiar and diversified faculties which it enjoys ; as, for instance, the power of motion, the power of common sensation or touch, and the power of taste. "In man," as Mr. Mayo has observed, "the apparent sense of taste is the tongue and palate ; the same surfaces have an exquisite sense of touch ; and an attentive examination shows that the latter occupies a larger surface than the former, and is, indeed, the only sense with which the palate is endowed.

"Upon the surface of the tongue, again, the sense of taste is very partially distributed, being restricted to the papillæ fungiformes. The largest of these are found upon the dorsum of the tongue, while the smaller and more numerous are situated along the sides and towards the tip of the tongue. They are vascular and erectile, and shoot up when the tongue is touched by a sapid substance."— (See Outlines of Human Physiology, p. 406, 2d edit.) It is clear, however, that if some facts to which the author of the Study of Medicine has adverted be correct, either the sense of taste must be more extensive than here represented, or else that, under particular circumstances, other parts than those specified must acquire a gustatory power. The ninth pair of nerves, which are distributed to the muscles of the tongue, are merely the nerves of motion ; while those of taste and sensation appear to be, first, the gustatory branch of the ganglionic portion of the third division of the fifth, which is distributed not merely to the muscles of the tongue, but to its mucous surface and to two of the salivary glands ; and secondly, the glosso-pharyngeal nerve, which sends branches to the surface of the root of the tongue.—Ed.

mentary principles of substances that lie beyond the reach of our senses.

But the variable condition of the peculiar covering of the papillæ of the tongue, together with the condition of the adjoining organs which concur in the purpose of the tongue, as also the changeable nature of the saliva and of the substances lodged in the stomach, all concur in influencing the taste, and giving a character to the flavour. And hence the same flavours do not affect persons of all ages, nor of all temperaments ; nor even the same person at all times. In general, whatever contains less salt than the saliva, seems insipid. The spirituous parts of plants are received, in all probability, either into the papillæ themselves, or into the absorbing villi of the tongue ; and hence the rapid refreshment and renovation of strength, not easy to be accounted for otherwise, which these stimulating materials produce, even when they are not taken into the stomach.

It is from the diversity of flavours by which nature has distinguished different substances, that animals are taught instinctively what is proper for their food : for, speaking generally, no aliment is unhealthy that is of an agreeable taste ; nor is any thing ill-tasted that is fit for the food of man. We here take no notice of excess, by which the most healthy foods may be rendered prejudicial, nor of mineral preparations, which are not furnished by nature, but prepared by art. And hence the wisdom of Providence incites man to select the nutriment that is best fitted for his subsistence, equally by the pain of hunger and the pleasure of tasting. Man, however, is often guided by instruction and example, as well as by his own instinct : but animals, which are destitute of such collateral aids, and have to depend upon their instinct alone, distinguish flavours, as we have already observed they do smells, with a far nicer accuracy than mankind ; and, admonished by this correct and curious test, abstain more cautiously than man himself from eating what would be injurious. And hence herbivorous animals, whose vegetable food grows often intermixed with a great diversity of noxious plants, are furnished with much longer papillæ and a more delicate structure of the tongue than mankind, as they are endowed also with a more accurate sense of smell ; both which, indeed, they jointly rely upon for the same purpose.

The sense of taste, therefore, which possesses so close an analogy to that of smell, is subject to a similar train of specific diseases, and consequently the genus parageusis must contain the three following species :—

1. Parageusis Acuta.　　Acute Taste.
2. ————— Obtusa.　　Obtuse Taste.
3. ————— Expers.　　Want of Taste

SPECIES I.
PARAGEUSIS ACUTA.
ACUTE TASTE.

TASTE PAINFULLY ACUTE, OR SENSIBLE TO SAVOURS NOT GENERALLY PERCEIVED.

THE sense of taste, like that of sight, smell,

or hearing, is capable of acquiring a higher degree of accuracy by use : and hence those who are in the habit of tasting wines by this organ perceive a variety of flavours, or modifications of flavour, which another person, not versed in such trials, is insensible of. We also perceive that the nerves of taste, like those of every other sense, become exhausted, and consequently torpid, by much labour and fatigue. And hence the nicest discriminator, after having tried a variety of wines, spirits, or other pungent savours in quick succession, is far less capable of judging concerning them, and has at last little more than a confused perception of gustatory excitement.

Morbid acuteness of taste, however, varies essentially from accuracy of taste : for, under particular states of irritation, pungent savours, of whatever kind, give equal pain to the tongue, which at the same time is altogether incapable of distinguishing between them.

This painful acuteness may proceed from two causes : a morbid or excessive sensibility in the nerves of taste, or a deficient secretion of the peculiar mucus that lubricates the lingual papillæ ; in consequence of which the latter are exposed in a naked state to whatever stimuli are introduced into the mouth. The former is sometimes found, though for the most part only temporarily, in highly nervous and irritable constitutions, and especially during a state of pregnancy ; the latter in certain morbid conditions of the stomach, accompanied with great thirst and a parched tongue. Both these causes, however, very frequently coexist ; as in ulcerated sore throats, or other excoriations of the mouth, in which the papillæ are in a state of the keenest excitement, while the tongue is sore, either from a defective secretion of mucus, or from its being carried off by a morbid and augmented action of the absorbents as fast as it is formed.

In this state of diseased action, moreover, it not unfrequently happens that the mucus itself is secreted in a morbid condition ; and the palate, instead of being soft and smooth, becomes harsh and rugous or furrowed, exquisitely irritable, and intolerant of the slightest touch or the mildest savours. I have sometimes met with this distressing affection, apparently as an idiopathic ailment, or at least unconnected with any manifest disease of the stomach or any other organ ; and seemingly induced by a rheumatic pain from carious teeth. It is, however, far more frequently a symptom of dyspepsy, porphyra, and chronic syphilis.

In treating this affection, we should in the first instance direct our attention to the state of the stomach, and clear it of whatever sordes may probably be lodged there. This may sometimes be done by aperients, but it will be the surest way to commence with an emetic.

The local symptoms may, in the meanwhile, be relieved in two ways. First, by changing the nature of the morbid action, or exhausting the accumulated sentient power by acid or astringent gargles, or a free use of the coldest water alone ; for which purpose also sage leaves and acrid bitters have often been employed with advantage. And next, the naked and irritable tongue may be sheathed with mucilages of various kinds, and thus a substitute be obtained for its natural defence. And in many cases, both these classes of medicines may be conveniently united.

When the affection is a symptom of some other disease, as in the case of syphilis and scurvy, it can only be cured by curing the primary malady. Carious teeth, if such exist, should be extracted; and if the palate be rugous or spongy, scarification should be employed.

SPECIES II.
PARAGEUSIS OBTUSA.
OBTUSE TASTE.
TASTE DULL AND IMPERFECTLY DISCRIMINATIVE.

This species rarely calls for medical attention. It occurs sometimes idiopathically, and seems to be dependant on a defective supply of nerves, or nervous influence, subservient to the organ of taste. I have seen it under this form in various instances; and as already observed, have found it connected in a few cases with obtuseness of smell. The patient has not been altogether without taste or smell, but both have been extremely weak and incapable of discrimination. In the case alluded to at the commencement of this genus, the individual could distinguish the smell of a rose from that of garlic, and the flavour of port wine from that of mountain or madeira; but she could not discriminate between the odour of a rose and that of a lily, nor between the taste of beef, veal, or pork, and consequently gave no preference to either of these dishes.

As a symptom, this affection occurs in almost all the diseases that are accompanied with hebetude of smell, as catarrh, hysteria, and several species of cephalæa.

SPECIES III.
PARAGEUSIS EXPERS.
WANT OF TASTE.
TOTAL INABILITY OF TASTING OR DISTINGUISHING SAVOURS.

As an utter want of smell is sometimes a natural or congenital effect, so in a few instances is an utter want of taste; and unquestionably from the same cause, an absolute destitution of nerves or nervous power subservient to the gustatory organ. This default is altogether immedicable: as is also for the most part the same when a result of palsy, general or local; though here stimulant gargles or masticatories, as mustardseeds, horseradish, pyrethrum, and camphire, have sometimes succeeded in restoring action to the torpid nerves. When, however, it occurs, as it sometimes does, from a long use of tobacco, whether by smoking or chewing, or of other acrid narcotics, these stimulants will be of no use.

In fevers, various exanthems, and inflammations, this species exists temporarily, partly perhaps from a diminished or morbid production of sensorial power, but chiefly from a conversion of the mucus of the tongue into a dry, hard, or tough and viscid sheath. And where there is much increased heat and action, the epithelium or cuticle of the tongue itself becomes often peculiarly thickened and coriaceous or leathery. Acids, in the form of gargles, are the pleasantest means of removing this morbid substance, but they will often succeed best if rendered viscid and converted into a soap by mixing with them a little almond-oil, which may at the same time be sweetened with honey.

GENUS V.
PARAPSIS.
MORBID TOUCH.
SENSE OF TOUCH OR GENERAL FEELING VITIATED OR LOST.

Parapsis is derived from the Greek terms, παρὰ and ἅπτομαι, "perperam tango." The common technical name for the genus is dysæsthesia, but not quite correctly; since this word, as we have already had occasion to observe, is also employed to express morbid external sensation of any kind, whether of touch, taste, smell, sight, or hearing: while by Dr. Young it is equally applied to one at least of the faculties of the mind, as in dysæsthesia interna, which he characterizes as "a want of memory, or confusion of intellect."

This genus embraces three species as follow:—

1. Parapsis Acuta.   Acute Sense of Touch or General Feeling.
2. ———— Expers.   Insensibility of Touch or General Feeling.
3. ———— Illusoria.   Illusory Sense of Touch or General Feeling.

[The skin is the principal seat of touch; though modifications of this sense are said to reside in various mucous surfaces, and in the voluntary muscles. The power of distinguishing with the finest discrimination the tangible properties of bodies is certainly in the hand, and especially in the extremities of the fingers. "The nerves," says Mr. Mayo (Physiology, p. 402, 2d edit.), "which minister to the sense of touch, are the posterior roots of the spinal nerves, the large division of the fifth, the nervi vagi, and the glosso-pharyngeal nerves. The body, the neck and occiput, and the limbs, are supplied by the spinal nerves; the face, temples, and fauces, by the fifth; the pharynx and œsophagus by the nervi vagi and glosso-pharyngeal nerves. It is remarkable, that the nerves of touch have ganglions near their origin."]

SPECIES I.
PARAPSIS ACUTA.
ACUTE SENSE OF TOUCH.
THE SENSE OF TOUCH PAINFULLY ACUTE, OR SENSIBLE TO IMPRESSIONS NOT GENERALLY PERCEIVED.

This species of morbid sensibility shows itself under almost innumerable modifications; but the four following are the chief:—

α Teneritudo.	Soreness.
β Pruritus.	Itching.
γ Ardor.	Heat.
δ Algor.	Coldness.

In the first variety, or that of soreness, there is a feeling of painful uneasiness or tenderness, local or general, on being touched with a degree of pressure that is usually unaccompanied with any troublesome sensation. This is often an idiopathic affection ; but more generally a symptom or sequel of fevers in their accession or first stage, inflammations, or external or internal violence, as strains, bruises, and spasms.

It is not always easy to account for this feeling, and perhaps the cause is in every instance more complicated than we might at first be induced to suppose. It occurs where there is distention of the vessels, where there is contraction of them, and where there is neither. Wherever it exists, however, it is a concomitant of debility, and may in many instances be regarded as the simple pain of debility, the uneasiness of an organ thrown off from its balance of health. The general health of the body depends in a very considerable degree upon the harmonious co-operation of its respective organs ; insomuch, indeed, that this harmony of action, as we had occasion to observe in the Physiological Proem prefixed to the present class, was supposed, by a distinguished school of ancient philosophers, and is still supposed by many physiologists of the present day, to constitute the principle of life itself. Regarded as a universal principle, the hypothesis is unfounded, though in many respects beautiful and plausible. Yet, notwithstanding that the life of the animal frame does not altogether depend upon an harmonious co-operation of the whole of the organs that enter into its make, much of the comfort of life has such a dependance ; and we trace the same principle in the minutest and comparatively most trivial parts of the animal functions, as manifestly as in the largest and most complicated organs. Where every portion of a member, however subordinate in itself, as a toe or a finger, works well or healthily, there is a feeling of ease and comfort ; but wherever it works ill or with difficulty, there is a sense of disquiet, and, under peculiar circumstances, of tenderness or soreness. A change in the diameter of a vessel, whether by dilatation or contraction, provided it be moderate and gradual, is accompanied with no uneasy sensation whatever ; but if it either be violent or sudden, a feeling of soreness is a certain result.

Warmth, gentle friction, and stimulants, as spirits, balsams, and essential oils, are of general advantage, wherever the kind of tenderness we are now describing occurs, and is unconnected with inflammation.

The sense of itching, which may be defined a painful titillation, local or general, relieved by rubbing, is commonly a result of some mechanical or morbid irritant applied externally or internally to the part affected ; though sometimes, unquestionably, dependant upon a morbid sensibility of the nerves of feeling themselves. If the summit of the nerves or their extreme points

be alone touched, the effect is tickling or titillation, as in the vellication of the skin by a feather ; if it descend a little below the summit, it is accompanied with a vibratory feel which we call tingling, as when the beard of barley-corns creeps unobserved by us up the arms ; and if it reach still deeper, it is combined with a sense of piercing which we call pricking, as when the keen hairs of several species of dolichos or cowhage are handled or blown upon the skin by a light breeze.

In many cases all these modifications of itching are the effect of some acrimonious secretion on the surface of the body, or of an acrimonious change in the common matter of perspiration, in consequence of its lodging in the cutaneous follicles longer than it should do. The papulous efflorescences we shall have to treat of under the third order of the sixth class, will afford abundant examples of both these causes of itching, apparently produced by, or closely connected with, a morbid sensibility of the cutaneous nerves themselves. For the present we can do nothing more than refer generally to various species of exormia, as lichen and prurigo ; and of ecpyesis, as impetigo and scabies. It is, moreover, highly probable, that the disorder called fidgets is sometimes chiefly dependant on a morbid sensibility of the summits or extreme ends of the cutaneous nerves.

This affection is also found as a very troublesome symptom in pernio and other cutaneous inflammations, as likewise in urticaria and other rashes.

The sensations of heat and cold may be explained at the same time. An easy and pleasurable warmth depends, in a state of health, upon a moderate temperature of the atmosphere, which cannot be very accurately laid down, because, from habit or constitution, or some other circumstance, different persons enjoy very different temperatures. Now it is the well-known property of heat and cold to disturb the temperature, whatever it may be, that affords ease and comfort to the nerves of feeling ; and to produce disquiet as they either raise or depress it. And this both of them do in two distinct ways. Heat is a strong irritant, and even if it made no change in the bulk of a living organ, or the juxtaposition of its particles, like all other irritants, it would still excite a troublesome feeling, amounting at length to acute pain, if raised to a considerable range beyond the ordinary scale. But it does, in every instance, excite a change in the bulk of living organs and the juxtaposition of their particles ; for it enlarges the former in every direction, and only does this by separating the particles from each other ; in which forcible and sudden divellication we have a second source of the troublesome and acute sensation which so constantly accompanies a temperature when carried very considerably above the point of health.*

---

* The effects of heat upon the human body are partly influenced by the state of the innervation at the period of its application. This is illustrated by a fact mentioned in Mr. Earle's Essay on

Heat, as an idiopathic affection, occurs chiefly in plethoric and irritable habits. In the former it is relieved by bloodletting, and evacuants of neutral salts ; in the latter by mild diaphoretics, and afterward cold bathing and other tonics.

As a symptom it is found also in the second stage of fever, in inflammation, and entonic empathema.

COLD is also a strong irritation, though it acts by the opposite means of heat. When the atmospheric temperature is too high, it is a pleasant and reviving agent, inasmuch as it both reduces the heated medium, and restores the particles of the affected organ from a state of disquieting tenseness to their usual scale of approximation. If the cold be pushed farther, it may go a little beyond this, and still be pleasant and healthful ; for the organ or the general system may be in a state of morbid relaxation, and consequently, in their actual scale of approach, the living particles may be too remote for the purposes of high elasticity and vigour. And it is in such a condition as this that cold chiefly shows its stimulant power, and is so generally resorted to as a tonic. But if the agency of cold be carried farther than this, it produces uneasiness to the nerves of feeling by a process precisely the reverse of that we have just shown to be pursued by heat, and consequently in a twofold manner. First by sinking the warmth of the organ, or of the system, below its scale of ease and comfort ; and next, by forcing the living particles into too close and crowded a state, and not allowing them sufficient room for play.

Cold, as an idiopathic affection, is chiefly local, and most common to the head and feet. It is temporarily relieved by warmth and stimulants, and particularly by the friction of a warm hand ; and, where it can be used, the exercise of walking. It is permanently relieved by the warmer tonics, as sea-bathing and aromatic bitters.

Considerable mischief has often been produced by a sudden exposure of the feet to severe cold, and especially in delicate and irritable habits, unused to such applications : as colic, cephalæa, catarrh, fevers of various kinds, and, in a podagral diathesis, gout. But the application of severe and sudden cold to the head or stomach by drinking ice or cold water, and especially when the individual is heated and perspiring, has been followed with more alarming effects, and even with death itself. Mauriceau relates an instance of death produced during baptism, by applying to the head the water of the baptismal font.—(Tom. ii., 348.) But this must be a rare occurrence ; while the fatal effects of drinking ice or iced water in a state of heat are innumerable.

It is observed by Dr. Fordyce (On Simple Fever, p. 168), and the observation is quoted

Burns :—A lady met with a comminuted fracture of the clavicle, and severe injury of the shoulder, producing paralysis of the arm ; and it was noticed, after the accident, that she could not put her hand into moderately warm water without redness, vesication, and the other usual consequences of the application of high degrees of heat, being immediately excited.—ED.

and called curious by Dr. Darwin, " that those people who have been confined some time in a very warm atmosphere, as of 120 or 130 degrees of heat, do not feel cold, nor are subject to paleness of their skins, on coming into a temperature of 30 or 40 degrees ; which would produce great paleness and painful sensation of coldness in those who had been for some time confined in an atmosphere of only 86 or 90 degrees." The cause is not difficult of explanation. The sensorial power is exhausted, and the nerves of feeling rendered torpid, by a long exposure to the heat of 120 or 130 degrees, and the turgid capillaries, whose dilatation produces the general blush, lose their power of constriction or collapse ; while in a heat of 86 or 90 degrees neither of such effects takes place.

Cold, as a symptom, is found in the first stage of fever, in syncope, hysteric syspasia, nausea, and atonic empathema ; in all which the affection is general.

SPECIES II.

PARAPSIS EXPERS.

INSENSIBILITY OF TOUCH OR GENERAL FEELING.

THE ORGAN OF TOUCH TOTALLY IMPERCIPIENT OF OBJECTS APPLIED TO IT.

UNDER this species, by some writers denominated amblyaphia, we may mention the two following varieties :—

α Simplex. Numbness.	Confined locally or generally to the organ of touch : sometimes accompanied with uneasiness.
β Complicata. Complicated insensibility.	Complicated with insensibility in several of, or all the other senses.

Occasional and local NUMBNESS is common to most persons. A tight bandage, or accidental pressure of one limb upon another, by obstructing the communication or activity of the nervous influence, will often produce this, when the limb is commonly and emphatically asserted to be asleep. A very slight motion, however, takes it off, when the irregular transmission of the sensorial power, on its first return, produces a sense of pricking, as though a ball of needles were in the limb, and pushing in every direction. Where such numbnesses, however, occur without pressure or any manifest cause, they well deserve watching and resisting by tonics or stimulants, local or general ; for they clearly show a tendency to paresis, if not to paralysis.

But there are some persons who possess by nature a numbness, or privation of the sense of feeling, in particular organs or parts of the surface, which appears to depend on a natural destitution of the nerves of touch wherever such insensibility is to be found. And hence they are able, in such parts of the body, to prick or cut themselves, or to run pins to any depth below the skin, without pain. I have seen several striking examples of this peculiar affection. Sometimes the numbness has been limited to a single limb, but common to the whole of it, as the hand, for example, which at the same time has possessed a full power of motion. Sometimes the insensibility has been universal, or extended over the whole surface. Lamarck relates a case in which this want of feeling was confined to the arm ; but at the same time was so complete, that the man who laboured under it had no pain during the progress of a phlegmon ; and who, on another occasion in which he broke his arm, felt nothing more than a crash, and merely thought he had broken the spade he was at work with. Dr. Yelloly has described another interesting case in the third volume of the Medico-Chirurgical Transactions. The patient, aged 58, had been first affected in Jamaica about three years before, and the affection had become permanent. "The hands," says Dr. Yelloly, "up to the wrist, and the feet half way up the legs, are perfectly insensible to any species of injury, as cutting, pinching, scratching, or burning. The insensibility, however, does not suddenly terminate ; but exists to a certain degree nearly up to the elbow, and for some distance above the knee. He accidentally put one of his feet, some time ago, into boiling water, but was no otherwise aware of the high temperature, than by finding the whole surface a complete blister on removing it. The extremities are insensible to electrical sparks taken in every variety of mode."*

As an example of the SECOND MODIFICATION, or insensibility in the organ of touch, complicated with insensibility in several other senses, we may mention the following, which Sauvages has copied from the Academy Collections :—"The patient, a delicate young man, was suddenly in the morning deprived equally of speech and of the sense of touch, without any assignable cause or premonition. Punctured and pricked in different parts of his body, in his head, neck, back, shoulders, breast, arms, abdomen, he felt nothing whatever, and even laughed at the singularity of the phenomenon ; as, with the exception of numbness and cutaneous insensibility, he laboured under no kind of disease. The complaint continued two days, and seemed to have yielded to venesection."

Insensibility of touch, either simple or complicated, is also felt as a symptom in apoplexy, palsy, catalepsy, epilepsy, syspasia, and syncope.

Where the numbness is complete and constitutional, it lies beyond the reach of medicine ; where it is recent and less extreme, it will often yield to friction alone, or with camphorated oil or spirits ; to heat, especially that of the warm bath ; ether, ammonia, and water, and the voltaic stream, or small shocks of electricity.

SPECIES III.
PARAPSIS ILLUSORIA.
ILLUSORY SENSE OF TOUCH.

IMAGINARY SENSE OF TOUCH, OR GENERAL FEELING, IN ORGANS THAT HAVE NO EXISTENCE.

THIS is the pseudæsthesia of Ploucquet ; and

* In the case mentioned in the note to page 258 of the present volume, a paralytic state of the arm rendered it extraordinarily susceptible of the influence of heat.—ED.

is frequently found among persons that have suffered amputation ; who, for a long time after the loss of the separated limb, have still a sense of its forming a part of the body, and suffer in idea the same kind of pain, or other inconvenience, they endured before its removal.

It proceeds from the close sympathy which peculiarly prevails between the extremities of the living fibre in all organs whatever, and which, as we have already had occasion to show, extends also between the terminating links of various chains of action that run into organs at a considerable distance from each other. Of the first we have an example in the constrictive pain produced in the glans penis, when the neck of the bladder is irritated by the lodgment of a calculus upon it. So, if the fauces or upper end of the œsophagus be tickled by a feather, the stomach at the lower end will be excited to nausea and sickness ; and if the stomach itself feel suddenly faint and enfeebled, the rectum will at the same time give way, and involuntarily discharge its contents. Of the second kind of sympathy, or that which shows itself between remote organs engaged in a common chain of action, we have a striking instance in the swelling of the mammæ on the irritation of the uterus in pregnancy ; and we had occasion to point out another equally striking, when treating under the last class of several species of marasmus, in which the chylific and assimilating organs, constituting the two extremities of the great chain of the nutritive function, maintain, on various occasions, a wonderful harmony both of energy and weakness.*

And hence, in a diseased limb, the pain which originates in the part affected is often extended, or even transferred, by sympathy, to its tendinous extremities, where the morbid impression remains in many instances long after the diseased portion of it has been removed. Nor is this protraction of the impression to be wondered at ; for we are perpetually witnessing cases in which, when a morbid impression has once been established, it continues to manifest itself in the same manner. Thus, when dust has been blown into the eye, a sensation of pricking is just as much felt in the conjunctiva for some hours after the dust has been washed out, as when it was actually goading the tender tunic : and in like manner, when an ague has been once generated in the animal frame by an exposure to marsh miasm, the patient will be still subject for many weeks, or perhaps months, to the same return of febrile paroxysm, how widely soever he may remove from the tainted region, and thus free himself from the cause of the disease.

In the case before us, the illusory feeling becomes fainter by degrees, and as the affected fibres return to a healthy condition. And if in the meantime it be very troublesome, it may generally be relieved by a moderate use of narcotics.

A like imaginary sensation is occasionally felt

* Vol. ii., Cl. III., Ord. IV., Gen. III., Spe. 1, Marasmus Atrophia ; and Spe. 3, M. Climactericus.

R 2

as a symptom in hypochondrias, and various other mental affections; in which ideas of pain and distress are mistaken for realities, and produce as severe a suffering.*

GENUS VI.
NEURALGIA.
NERVE-ACHE..

ACUTE SENSIBILITY AND LANCINATING PAIN IN THE COURSE OF ONE OR MORE BRANCHES OF NERVES IN AN ORGAN; MOSTLY WITH AN IRREGULAR MOTION OF THE ADJOINING MUSCLES; RECURRENT IN SHORT PAROXYSMS, WITH INDETERMINATE INTERVALS OR REMISSIONS.

THE term NEURALGIA, from Νεῦρος, "nervus," and ἄλγος, "dolor," has been for many years employed with great accuracy to express a division of diseases which will probably hereafter be found to be peculiarly numerous, and in some modification or other, to appertain to most of the organs of the animal frame.

The term neuralgia has of late been employed by various nosologists to express this group of diseases, especially by Professor Chaussier of Paris, and Dr. Meglin of Strasburg. Yet, till of late, only the neuralgia of the face seems to have been known to any pathologist : M. Chaussier, however, has added the second of the present species, under the name of *neuralgia plantaris.*

Since the publication of the volume on Nosology, I have been consulted on a very striking disease of the same kind, occurring, with a few local peculiarities of feature, in the female breast ; and we are hence put into possession of another

---

* The history of Caspar Hauser, the individual who, as is well known, was kept in a dungeon, separated from all communication with the world, from early childhood till about the age of seventeen, and who was found at Nuremberg in 1828, presents a most wonderful instance of morbid exaltation of the senses of seeing, hearing, tasting, and feeling. His biographer, the eminent Feuerbach, remarks as follows :—

"As to his sight, there existed in respect to him no twilight, no night, no darkness. This was first noticed by remarking that at night he stepped everywhere with the greatest confidence ; and that in dark places he always refused a light when it was offered to him. He often looked with astonishment or laughed at persons, who in dark places, for instance, when entering a house or walking on a staircase by night, sought safety in groping their way or in laying hold on adjacent objects. In twilight, he even saw much better than in broad daylight. Thus, after sunset, he once read the number of a house at the distance of 180 paces, which in daylight he would not have been able to distinguish so far off. Towards the close of twilight, he once pointed out to his instructer a gnat that was hanging in a very distant spider's web. At a distance of certainly not less than sixty paces, he could distinguish the single berries in a cluster of elderberries from each other, and these berries from black currants. It has been proved by experiments carefully made, that in a perfectly dark night he could distinguish different dark colours, such as blue and green, from each other.

"When at the commencement of twilight a common eye could not yet distinguish more than three or four stars in the sky, he could already discern the different groups of stars, and he could distinguish the different single stars of which they were composed from each other, according to their magnitudes and the peculiarities of their coloured light. From the enclosure of the castle at Nuremberg, he could count a row of windows in the castle of Marloffstein ; and from the castle, a row of the windows of a house lying below the fortress of Rothenberg. His sight was as sharp in distinguishing objects near by, as it was penetrating in discerning them at a distance. In anatomizing plants, he noticed subtle distinctions and delicate particles which had entirely escaped the observation of others.

"Scarcely less sharp and penetrating than his sight was his hearing. When taking a walk in the fields, he once heard, at a distance comparatively very great, the footsteps of several persons, and he could distinguish these persons from each other by their walk. He had once an opportunity of comparing the acuteness of his hearing with the still greater acuteness of hearing evinced by a blind man, who could distinguish even the most gentle step of a man walking barefooted. On this occasion he observed that his hearing had formerly been much more acute ; but that its acuteness had been considerably diminished since he had begun to eat meat ; so that he could no longer distinguish sounds with so great a nicety as that blind man.

"Of all his senses, that which was the most troublesome to him, which occasioned him the most painful sensations, and which made his life in the world more disagreeable to him than any other, was the sense of smelling. What to us was entirely scentless, was not so to him.—The most delicate and delightful odours of flowers, for instance the rose, were perceived by him as insupportable stenches, which painfully affected his nerves.

"What announces itself by its smell to others only when very near, was scented by him at a very considerable distance. Excepting the smell of bread, of fennel, of anise, and of caraway, to which he says he had already been accustomed in his prison,—for his bread was seasoned with these condiments—all kinds of smells were more or less disagreeable to him. When he was once asked, which of all other smells was most agreeable to him ? he answered, none at all. His walks and rides were often rendered very unpleasant by leading him near to flower-gardens, tobacco-fields, nut-trees, and other plants which affected his olfactory nerves ; and he paid dearly for his recreations in the free air by suffering afterward from headaches, cold sweats, and attacks of fever. He smelt tobacco when in blossom in the fields at the distance of fifty paces, and at more than one hundred paces when it was hung up in bundles to dry, as is commonly the case about the houses in the villages near Nuremberg. He could distinguish apple, pear, and plum-trees from each other at a considerable distance, by the smell of their leaves. The different colouring materials used in the painting of walls and furniture, and in the dying of cloths, &c., the pigments with which he coloured his pictures, the ink or pencil with which he wrote, all things about him, wafted odours to his nostrils which were unpleasant or painful to him. If a chimney-sweeper walked the streets, though at the distance of several paces from him, he turned his face shuddering from his smell. The smell of an old cheese made him feel

species, making the entire number three that have now exhibited themselves under precise and determinate characters. These species, therefore, are as follow :—

1. Neuralgia Faciei.   Nerve-ache of the Face.
2. ———— Pedis.   Nerve-ache of the Foot.·
3. ————— Mammæ.   Nerve-ache of the Breast.

There can be little doubt that other organs besides these are subject to the same misaffection ; and it is not improbable that accident or a minuter investigation of the subject may show that almost every part of the body may become a seat of neuralgia.* M. Recamier has of late met with a painful and intractable disease of the

---

unwell, and affected him with vomiting. The smell of strong vinegar, though fully a yard distant from him, operated so powerfully upon the nerves of his sight and smell as to bring the water into his eyes. When a glass of wine was filled at table at a considerable distance from him, he complained of its disagreeable smell, and of a sensation of heat in his head. The opening of a bottle of champaign was sure to drive him from the table or to make him sick. What we call unpleasant smells were perceived by him with much less aversion than many of our perfumes. The smell of fresh meat was to him the most horrible of all smells. When Professor Daumer, in the autumn of 1828, walked with Caspar near to St. John's churchyard, in the vicinity of Nuremberg, the smell of the dead bodies, of which the professor had not the slightest perception, affected him so powerfully that he was immediately seized with an ague, and began to shudder. The ague was soon succeeded by a feverish heat, which at length broke out into a violent perspiration, by which his linen was thoroughly wet. He afterward said that he had never before experienced so great a heat. When on his return he came near to the city gate, he said that he felt better; yet he complained that his sight had been obscured thereby. Similar effects were once experienced by him (on the 28th of September, 1828), when he had been for a considerable time walking by the side of a tobacco-field.

"Professor Daumer first noticed the peculiar properties of Caspar's sense of feeling, and his susceptibility of metallic excitements, while he was yet at the tower. Here a stranger once made him a present of a little wooden horse and a small magnet, with which, as the forepart of the horse was furnished with iron, it could be made to swim about in different directions. When Caspar was going to use this toy according to the instructions he had received, he felt himself very disagreeably affected; and he immediately locked it up in the box belonging to it, without ever taking it out again, as he was accustomed to do with his other playthings, in order to show to his visiters. When he was afterward asked why he did so, he said that that horse had occasioned him a pain which he had felt in his whole body and in all its members. After he had removed to Professor Daumer's house, he kept the box with the magnet in a trunk ; from which, in clearing out his things, it was accidentally taken and brought into notice. The idea was suggested thereby to Professor Daumer, who recollected the occurrence that had formerly taken place, to make an experiment on Caspar with the magnet belonging to the little horse. Caspar very soon experienced the most surprising effects. When Professor Daumer held the north pole towards him, Caspar put his hand to the pit of his stomach, and drawing his waistcoat in an outward direction, said that it drew him thus; and that a current of air seemed to proceed from him. The south pole affected him less powerfully; and he said that it blew upon him. Professor Daumer and Professor Herrmann made afterward several other experiments similar to these, and calculated to deceive him ; but his feelings always told him very correctly, and even

though the magnet was held at a considerable distance from him, whether the north pole or the south pole was held towards him. Such experiments could not be continued long, because the perspiration soon appeared on his forehead, and he began to feel unwell.

"In respect to his sensibility of the presence of other metals, and his ability to distinguish them from each other by his feelings alone, Professor Daumer has selected a great number of facts, from which I shall select only a few. In autumn, 1828, he once accidentally entered a store filled with hardware, and particularly with brass wares. He had scarcely entered before he hurried out again, being affected with violent shuddering, and saying that he felt a drawing in his whole body in all directions.—A stranger who visited him, once slipped a piece of gold of the size of a kreutzer into his hand, without Caspar's being able to see it : he said immediately that he felt gold in his hand.—At a time when Caspar was absent, Professor Daumer placed a gold ring, a steel and brass compass, and a silver drawing-pen, under some paper, so that it was impossible for him to see what was concealed under it. Daumer directed him to move his finger over the paper without touching it ; he did so ; and by the difference of the sensation and strength of the attraction which these different metals caused him to feel at the points of his fingers, he accurately distinguished them all from each other, according to their respective matter and form.—Once, when the physician, Dr. Osterhausen, and the royal crownfiscal, Brunner, from Munchen, happened to be present, Mr. Daumer led Caspar, in order to try him, to a table covered with an oil cloth, upon which a sheet of paper lay, and desired him to say whether any metal was under it ; he moved his finger over it and then said, there it draws ! 'But this time,' replied Daumer, 'you are nevertheless mistaken; for,' withdrawing the paper, 'nothing lies under it.' Caspar seemed at first to be somewhat embarrassed ; but he put his finger again to the place where he thought he had felt the drawing, and assured them repeatedly that he there felt a drawing. The oil cloth was then removed, a stricter search was made, and a needle was actually found there.—He described the feeling which minerals occasioned him, a kind of drawing sensation which passed over him, accompanied at the same time with a chill, which ascended accordingly as the objects were different, more or less up the arm ; and which was also attended with other distinctive sensations. At the same time, the veins of the hand which had been exposed to the metallic excitative, were visibly swollen. Towards the end of December, 1828, when the morbid excitability of his nerves had been almost removed, his sensibility of the influence of metallic excitatives began gradually to disappear, and was at length totally lost."—D.

* The editor has seen several examples of neuralgia of the arm, which arose from injuries of the thumb or fingers. M. Ribes has recorded a case of neuralgia of the external sciatic popliteal nerve, which disorder gradually extended its paroxysms of violent pain, with convulsions of the muscles, over the greatest part of the body. It

uterus, which he has regarded as of this kind, and has denominated *uterine neuralgia*, though he does not speak of it with much decision.*

The corporeal senses which have hitherto passed within the range of our observations as the seats of different genera of diseases, are external, and serve to convey impressions peculiar to themselves. It is, however, sufficiently known to every one, that there is not an organ in the body but is possessed of nerves productive of a very different kind of sensibility from any of these; less distinct perhaps and elaborate, but the index of its weal or wear, its comfort or disquiet; and which may be sufficiently expressed by the name of *general feeling*. It is possible, indeed, that this general feeling may in some degree be differently modified in every organ; but as the distinctions, whatever they may be, are not nice enough for us to trace out and arrange, as they are in the local senses, it is sufficient for all the purposes of pathology to regard this feeling as common to all the sentient organs, and consequently as one and the same. We have already taken some notice of it in the proem to the present class, and have observed that it has been described by some pathologists under the name of cænesthesis, and by the Germans is denominated Gemeingefühl, or general-feeling. Dr. Hubner published an inaugural dissertation on this subject in 1794, in which he enumerates its properties at some length.—(*Commentatio de Cænesthesi Dissert. Inaug. Medica; Auctore C. F. Hubner*, 1794.) I have never seen this treatise, but Sir Alexander Crichton, who has, describes it as a very ingenious production.

It is these nerves of general sensibility that seem to constitute the seat of disease in the three species we are now about to enter upon, and consequently indicate that the present is their proper place in a system of physiological nosology.†

SPECIES I.
NEURALGIA FACIEI.
NERVE-ACHE OF THE FACE.

LANCINATING PAINS SHOOTING FROM THE REGION OF THE MOUTH TO THE ORBIT, OFTEN TO THE EAR, AND OVER THE CHEEK, PALATE, TEETH, AND FAUCES; WITH CONVULSIVE TWITCHINGS OF THE ADJOINING MUSCLES.

THIS is the *trismus maxillaris* or *t. dolorificus* of M. de Sauvages, for it is not necessary

to make a distinction between them, as Sauvages himself has done; by Dr. Fothergill it is denominated dolor crucians faciei. As the French give the name of tic to trismus or locked-jaw, they distinguish this first species of neuralgia, affecting the nerves about the jaw, by the name of tic doloureux, by which term the disease is, perhaps, chiefly known even in our own country in the present day. I shall have occasion to observe more at large, under the genus TRISMUS, that the word *tic* is commonly supposed to be an onomatopy, or a sound expressive of the action it imports; derived, according to some, from the pungent stroke with which the pain makes its assault, resembling the bite of an insect; but according to Sauvages and Soleysel, from the sound made by horses, that are perpetually biting the manger when labouring under this peculiar affection. We do not, however, appear to be acquainted with the real origin of the term.

From the symptoms by which this complaint is distinguished, it is not difficult to decide concerning both its seat and nature. The character of the pain is very peculiar, and its course corresponds exactly with that of the nerves. The second branch of the fifth pair is perhaps more frequently affected than either the first or the third. But the portia dura of the seventh pair, which is distributed more extensively upon the face, under the name of pes anserina, is more frequently the seat of affection than any of the branches of the fifth pair seem to be; which is a matter of no small regret, as it is difficult for any operation to reach this quarter effectually, although it is a difficulty which we shall presently find has, in one instance at least, been encountered and surmounted. When, however, the disease is seated in the seventh pair of nerves, we can be at no loss to decide concerning it, in consequence of the course and divarications of the pain, which commenees with great acuteness in the forepart of the cheek, towards the mouth and alæ of the nose, sometimes spreading as high as the forehead, and ramifying in the direction of the ears. At other times, the forehead, temple, and inner angle of the eye on the side affected, and even the ball of the eye itself, form the chief lines of pungent agony, while, from irritation of the lachrymal gland, the eye weeps involuntarily. In this case we may reasonably suspect the disease to be seated in some part of the superior maxillary nerve, constituting the second branch of the fifth pair. And it is hence obvious, that the radiation of the pain must vary according to the nerves or nervous twigs that are affected.*

---

arose from a gunshot wound of the upper third of the leg, and resisted various medicines, the moxa, &c.; but was very materially relieved, though not completely, by the division and excision of a portion of the above nerve.—See Magendie's Journ. Expér. de Physiol., tom· ii., p. 343. See also cases of neuralgia in various situations, by Dr. Evans, in Edin. Med. Journ., No. lxxix., p. 278.

* Tableau des Maladies observées à l'Hôtel-Dieu, dans les Salles de Cliniques, &c. Par L. Martinet, Révue Médicale, &c., 1824.

† Dr. Good's prophecy, "that accident or a minuter investigation of the subject may show that almost every part of the body may become a seat of neuralgia," is fully verified. In addition to those species of neuralgia mentioned by Dr. Good and the London editor, Itard has observed

neuralgia of the ear; Siebold that of the *intercostal* nerves; Chaussier and Jadelot in the first lumbar nerve; Francis and Barras in the spermatic nerve; and Cotugno and Chaussier in the anterior crural nerve. Boisseau has described a still greater number of neuralgic affections.—See his Nosographie Organique, vol. iv., p. 714.—D.

* Some practitioners, remembering that the portio dura is only a nerve of motion, consider it doubtful whether this nerve is ever truly the seat of neuralgia. One of Dr. Elliotson's patients,

The disease has been occasionally mistaken for rheumatism, hemicrania, and toothache: but the brevity of the paroxysm, the lancinating pungency of the pang, the absence of all intumescence or inflammation, the comparative shallowness, instead of depth, of its seat, and its invariable divarication in the course of the facial nerves or their offsets, will always be sufficient to distinguish it from every other kind of pain.

Of its exciting causes we know but little. It seems sometimes to have been produced by cold, and sometimes by mental agitation, in persons of an irritable temperament. But it has been found in the robust as well as in the delicate, in the middle-aged as well as in the old. In a few cases the irritation has been local, of which Mr. Jeffreys has given a very striking instance in a young woman, who, when only six years old, fell down with a teacup in her hand, which was hereby broken, one of the cheeks lacerated, and a fragment of the teacup imbedded under the skin. The wound healed, though slowly and with difficulty; the buried fragment of the teacup was not noticed, and consequently was not extracted. From an early period, a violent nervous pain returned nightly, and one side of the face was paralytic. These dreadful symptoms were endured for fourteen years: at the end of which time an incision was made through the cicatrix down upon what was then found to be the edge of a hard substance, and which appeared, when extracted, to be the piece of the teacup above noticed. From this time the neuralgia and paralysis ceased; the affected cheek recovered its proper plumpness, and the muscles their due power.[*]

It is possible, as suggested by M. Martinet, that as a symptom, it may sometimes occur in what he calls, and perhaps correctly, an inflammation of the nerves, or a thickening of the neurilemma in some particular organ, of which he has given various examples, accompanied with a reddish or even violet tinge, and studded with minute ecchymoses.[†] But that this is not

however, complained of the disorder not only in the cheek, but in the course of the portio dura from the stylo-mastoid foramen. Two, or even all the three branches of the fifth pair may be affected, and the pain may extend also to the other side of the face. Dr. Elliotson has known it extend down the neck to the shoulder, and along the inside of the arm to the ends of all the fingers and the thumb. Various nerves of the legs, arms, fingers, or toes, are occasionally the seat of the disease; and an intercostal, a lumbar, and even the spermatic nerve, have been attacked. The pain does not always shoot in the course of the nerve, but frequently in the opposite direction.—See Cyclop. of Pract. Med., art. NEURALGIA.—ED.

[*] Lond. Med. and Phys. Journ., March, 1823, p. 199. Sir Henry Halford mentions the case of a lady who suffered violent tic douloureux till an apparently sound tooth was extracted, on account of the attacks being frequently preceded by uneasiness in it: an exostosis was found at its root. Another case was relieved by an exfoliation of a portion of the antrum.—ED.

[†] Mémoire sur l'Inflammation des Nerfs, &c.

the only, or even the ordinary proximate cause, is clear, since, in the cases alluded to, pressure upon the part is intolerable, while in idiopathic neuralgia it is commonly consolatory, and considerably diminishes the agony.

André appears to have been the earliest writer who remarked this painful affection with accuracy; and he succeeded in removing it permanently by applying a caustic to the infra-orbitary or maxillary branch of nerves in one case in which a previous division of the nerve by the scalpel, as practised by Marechal, had produced only a temporary cure. André, who resided at Versailles, published his account in 1756, whimsically enough inserting it in a treatise on diseases of the urethra. A few unsatisfactory experiments and operations were given to the public in the course of the next fifteen years, chiefly by French practitioners, from which little of real value is deducible. In 1776, Dr. Fothergill, in the fifth volume of Medical Observations and Inquiries, communicated a very full and elaborate description and history of the disease: since which time M. Thouret and Pujol have each published a valuable paper on the same subject, in the Memoirs of the Society of Medicine of Paris, containing various cases collected and described with great minuteness; and we have already adverted to the more recent publications of Dr. Meglin and Professor Chaussier.

It has of late been suspected, that in some cases, at least, of this disease, the seat of irritation might be at the origin instead of at the extremity of the nerve; an idea that has arisen from the powerful sympathetic action manifested by the eye and the stomach[*] forming the boundaries of the chain, upon which subject we shall have to speak at large when treating the genus ENTASIA in the ensuing order "The nerves," remarks Dr. Parr, "that supply the eye externally, and the slight connexion of the intercostal with the brain, are nearly from the same spot in the cerebrum, and it did not seem improbable in the case alluded to, that the disease may have really been at the origin of the nerves, although felt as usual at its extremity." Dr. Parr was in consequence induced to try arsenic, and in one instance, he tells us, with a decidedly good effect. It is also said to have

1824. Also, cases by Evans in Edin. Med. Journ., No. lxxix., p. 282.

[*] Dr. Elliotson assures us that he has never seen one case of neuralgia referrible to disorder of the digestive organs.—(See Cyclop. of Pract. Med., art. NEURALGIA.). Where inflammation is obvious, whether rheumatic or not, he approves of local bleeding, mercury, colchicum, and antiphlogistic treatment in general. Should these means fail, he recommends anodynes to be added to them. When the complaint is rheumatic, but inflammatory, he approves of stimulants, internal and external, especially ammoniated tincture of guaiacum, a generous diet, tonics, mercury, and all modes of counter-irritation. In some cases, warm temperature and warm clothing seem essential; in some, the warm water or steam bath; and in others, the cold bath, followed by friction, answer best.—ED.

been since found serviceable in a few other cases. In Mr. Thomas's hands, however, we shall presently perceive that it completely failed. Mercury is also reported to have occasionally proved successful, and especially when carried to the extent of salivation; though in numerous instances it has been tried even to this last effect without any benefit whatever. [Some cases of facial neuralgia have been cured by applying a drop or two of the oil of croton to the tongue.—(*Med. Chir. Review*, Sept., 1821.) The effect on the nerve was almost instantaneous. Bark, and the sulphate of quinine,* have also been tried with various results.]

When, about thirty years ago, animal magnetism was a fashionable study in France, it was had recourse to for this disease among others, and had its day of favour as a popular remedy. —(*Edin. Med. and Surg. Journ.*, July, 1823.) Of late, however, neuralgia has been attempted to be cured in France by an external use of acetic ether; while in Germany Dr. Meglin has employed pills composed of the extract of henbane,† and sublimed oxyde of zinc, and according to his own statement, with great success. But, beyond controversy, one of the most valuable medicines that have hitherto been tried is the subcarbonate of iron, for the first use of which, so far as I know, we are indebted to the late Mr. Hutchison,‡ of Southwell, who commonly employed it in doses of a drachm three times a day.

[Dr. Borthwick, however, has found the last

---

* Obs. de Neuralgie sus-orbitaire droite, guérie par le Sulfate de Quinine, par M. Piedagnel. Magendie, Journ. de Physiologie Expér., tom. ii., p. 124.

† The best anodyne narcotics for trial in cases of neuralgia, are the acetate, muriate, or sulphate of morphine, and the extracts of stramonium and belladonna. The editor has known great relief produced by the application of a plaster to the integuments covering the painful nerves, which was composed of one or two drachms of the extract of belladonna and an ounce of soap cerate.—Ed.

‡ Cases of Neuralgia Spasmodica, &c., by B. Hutchison, &c., 8vo., Lond., 1825. Numerous examples of the utility of subcarbonate of iron are now on record, and Dr. Elliotson adduces his testimony in favour of its efficacy in chronic neuralgia. When there is debility, and especially paleness, iron in full quantities operates much more effectually, he says, than quinine. Should no structural nor mechanical cause, and no inflammation, be present, and should the disease be of the exquisite character, he deems iron the remedy most worthy of trial. Although the doses specified in the text sometimes succeed, it is found that children will often take an- ounce or six drachms every four hours. If given in twice its weight of treacle, Dr. Elliotson finds that it rarely constipates; but the bowels must always be kept open during its employment, for otherwise it is apt to accumulate in the intestinal canal in large masses.—(See Cyclop. of Pract. Med., art. Neuralgia.) Ice applied to the parts has sometimes been of service.—See Med. Chir. Trans., vol. xiii., p. 252; and Cyclop. of Pract. Med. Also, Crawford, in Med. Chir. Review; Dr. Belcher's case of neuralgic amaurosis, successfully treated by the carbonate of iron.—Edin. Med. Journ., No. lxxxvi., p. 37.—Ed.

plan so successful, and his confidence in it is such, that he regards the point now almost settled in practice, "that iron will relieve, if not cure, tic douloureux (neuralgic affections, generally speaking), as certainly and as speedily as quicksilver, in particular forms, will relieve and cure the lues venerea." The dose which he gives in severe cases, is one drachm and a half four times a day.—(See *Edin. Med. Journ.*, No. lxxxiii., p. 297.)]

The instances of success appear to be very numerous, though this also, like all other medicines, has often failed. But there is another energetic medicine, which has also a fair claim to attention from a very different property— that of subduing the sensibility; and this is *prussic acid*. Mr. Taylor, of Cricklade, Wilts, has made repeated trials of this powerful sedative in various cases, and apparently with more rapid relief than is afforded by the carbonate of iron. He commenced his career with a drop of Scheele's preparation, in twenty-four hours, in divided doses; but as he grew better acquainted with the effects of the medicine, he gave a drop for a dose at first, and then increased the dose to two drops, repeating it three times a day. In one or two instances he has carried the quantity, by a gradual augmentation, to twenty-four drops a day, in the course of a month's use; and very often to five and six drops a day, by adding a drop to every day's account.—(*Edin. Med. and Surg. Journ.*, July, 1823.) Time alone must determine whether the cures thus obtained will prove as permanent as those effected by the tonic power of the subcarbonate of iron. To induce ease, however, under any circumstances, and for any period of time, in the midst of so much torment, is an invaluable blessing.

In effect, neither narcotics nor tonics, nor any other class of medicines hitherto employed, can be in every case depended upon for a radical cure, though some of them, and particularly the subcarbonate of iron, are worthy of high commendation. "My father," says Dr. Perceval of Dublin, in his manuscript comment on the present author's Nosology, "was subject to *neuralgia faciei* for several years, and used a variety of medicines without relief. He was worse in close damp weather, and much worse when his mind was occupied. At length he had an issue inserted in the nucha, kept his bowels free with James's analeptic pills, and exchanged a town residence for the country. In this situation he soon threw off the disease, from which he was free for a considerable time before his death." Change of scene, a transfer of morbid action, and a recruited cheerfulness of spirits, are valuable auxiliaries in the present as in every other nervous affection; but I much question whether these alone have ever operated a cure. A spontaneous cure is the work of time alone; and time, though often a long and tedious period is requisite, will generally accomplish it, and probably did so in the case before us. The fact is, that the nervous system in every part, and every ramification, becomes gradually torpefied by excess of action; and as the eyes grow blind and the nostrils inolfacient by strong stimulants applied to them, so the nervous twigs of every kind, after a long series of irritation from the present disease, become exhausted of power and obtuse in feeling: and it is probably by hastening this state, that the most active stimulants and the warmer tonics produce whatever benefit is to be ascribed to them.

[In the treatment of various cases of neuralgia, Baron Larrey was very successful with the moxa, which he repeated the application of according to circumstances. Delpech used the actual cautery, and after the separation of the eschar, kept up a discharge for a long time.]

How far acupuncture or needle-pricking, the zin-king of the Chinese, which we have already described under chronic rheumatism, might be useful, has not yet been determined. It has at least a fair claim for experiment, before having recourse to a curative attempt by the knife.

This radical cure consists in a division of the affected branches, provided they can be followed home. Dr. Haighton completely succeeded, some years ago, in a case in which he divided the sub-orbital branch of the fifth pair; and Mr. Cruickshank and Mr. Thomas more recently in a case of considerable complication, and where the affection was evidently not confined to the different branches of any single nerve. This last case is given by Dr. Darwin, whom the patient had intermediately consulted, in the second part of his Zoonomia, and is one of the most interesting sections of the work. The patient, a Mr. Bosworth by name, was between thirty and forty years of age. When he first applied to Dr. Darwin, he complained of much pain about the left cheek-bone. Dr. Darwin suspected the antrum maxillare might be diseased; and as the second of the grinding teeth had been lately extracted, directed a perforation into the antrum, which was done, and the wound kept open for two or three days without advantage. Afterward, by friction about the head and neck with mercurial unguent, he was for a few days copiously salivated, and had another tooth extracted by his own desire, as also an incision made in such direction as to divide the artery near the centre of the ear next the cheek, which gave also a chance of dividing a branch of the affected nerve; but without success. When the pain was exceedingly violent, opiates were administered in large quantity; bark being used freely in the intervals, but without effect.

The pain spread in various directions from a point in the left cheek a little before the ear, sometimes to the nose, and forepart of the lower jaw, and sometimes to the orbit of the eye on the same side; the under part of the tongue being at times also affected. It returned on some days many times in an hour, and continued several minutes; during which period (it is well worth observing, as showing the connexion between an irregular sensitive and an irregular motive power in the same muscles) the patient, says Dr. Darwin, seemed to stretch and exert his arms, and appeared to have a tendency to epileptic actions, so that his life was rendered miserable. The complaint gradually grew worse, and Mr. Bosworth removed to London, for the purpose of again putting himself under Mr. Cruickshank's care, and of submitting to any operation he should recommend. The pain was now intolerably acute and almost unremitting; and opiates afforded him little or no relief, though taken to the quantity of six teaspoonfuls of laudanum at a time. The operation of dividing the diseased nerve was therefore determined upon.

"As the pain," says Mr. Thomas, in his letter to Dr. Darwin after its completion, "was felt more acute in the left ala of the nose and the upper lip of the same side, we were induced to divide the second branch of the fifth pair of nerves as it passes out at the infra-orbital foramen. He was instantly relieved in the nose and lip; but towards night the pain from the eye to the crown of the head became more acute than ever. Two days after, we were obliged to cut through the first branch passing out at the supra-orbital foramen: this afforded him like relief with the first. On the same day the pain attacked, with great violence, the lower lip on the left side, and the chin: this circumstance induced the necessity of dividing the third branch, passing out at the foramen mentale. During the whole period, from the first division of the nerves, he had frequent attacks of pain on the side of the tongue; these, however, disappeared on division of the last nerve.

"The patient was evidently bettered by each operation: still the pain was very severe, passing from the ear under the zygoma towards the nose and mouth, and upwards round the orbit. This route proved pretty clearly that the portio dura of the auditory nerve was also affected, at least the uppermost branch of the pes anserina. Before I proceeded," continues Mr. Thomas, "to divide this—Mr. Cruickshank had operated hitherto—I was willing to try the effect of arsenic internally; and he took it in sufficient quantity to excite nausea and vertigo, but without perceiving any good effect. I could now trust only to the knife to alleviate his misery, as the pain round the orbit was become most violent; and therefore intercepted the nerve by an incision across the side of the nose, and also made some smaller incisions about the ala nasi. To divide the great branch lying below the zygomatic process, I found it necessary to pass the scalpel through the masseter muscle till it came in contact with the jaw-bone, and then to cut upwards: this relieved him as usual. Then the lower branch was affected, and also divided: then the middle branch running under the parotid gland. In cutting this, the gland was consequently divided into two equal parts, and healed tolerably well after a copious discharge of saliva for several days.

"I hoped and expected that this last operation would have terminated his sufferings and my difficulties; but the pain still affected the lower lip and side of the nose, and upon coughing or swallowing his misery was dreadful. This pain could only arise from branches from the second of the fifth pair passing into the cheek, and lying between the pterygoideus internus muscle and the upper part of the lower jaw. The situation of this nerve rendered the operation hazardous, but, after some attempts, it was accomplished." This finished the series of operations, and restored the afflicted patient to perfect health.

I have dwelt the longer on this interesting case, because it seems to show, first, that there is occasionally no certain cure but in the use of the knife;* secondly, that a delay in performing the operation only affords time for the disease to spread from one branch of the affected nerve to another, and even to different branches of nerves in a state of contiguity ; and thirdly, that the disease betrays the spasmodic character of the diathesis when minutely watched, even in cases in which this character is most obscure. Dr. Darwin objects, properly enough, to arranging this disease as a trismus, "since no fixed spasm," says he, "like the locked-jaw, exists in this malady." He adds, indeed, that in the few cases he has witnessed, there has not been any convulsion of the muscles of the face ; but in Mr. Bosworth's case he has expressly noticed the morbid stretching of the arms, and the tendency to epileptic actions. Its proper place, however, seems to be where it is now arranged.

SPECIES II.
NEURALGIA PEDIS.
NERVE-ACHE OF THE FOOT.
RACKING AND LANCINATING PAINS RANGING ABOUT THE HEEL, AND TREMULOUSLY SHOOTING IN IRREGULAR DIRECTIONS TOWARDS THE ANKLE AND BONES OF THE TARSUS.

THIS is the *neuralgia plantaris* of Professor Chaussier; who mentions a very decided case of it, to which Dr. Marino, a physician of Piedmont, had been long subject. It commenced, he tells us, in early life; was relieved by the mineral waters of Vivadio, and still more by the pressure of a tight bandage. With advancing years it became less severe, the cause of which we have already explained in the preceding species, but never ceased altogether. It alternated with other nervous affections, and was at length complicated with convulsive asthma.

In calling the attention of the medical profession to this species, by introducing it into the volume of Nosology, so long ago as the beginning of 1817, I had my eye directed to a very marked case, which had then lately occurred to me in a clergyman of this metropolis, about forty-five years of age, but otherwise in firm health and cheerful spirits. He had for many years been a victim to it. The paroxysms were short, and of uncertain recurrence, but so acute as nearly to make him faint, and at length compelled him to relinquish the duties of the pulpit, for which, from his zeal and eloquence, he was admirably qualified, but where he had frequently been obliged to break off with great abruptness from the unexpected incursion of a

* As this expression may induce young practitioners to promise too much from the operation, the editor deems it right to mention that the knife has frequently failed.

fresh paroxysm. The pain usually extended up the calf of the leg towards the knee, and ramified towards the toes in an opposite direction ; and was usually compared by himself to that of scalding verjuice poured over a naked wound. The tibial branches of the popliteal nerve, and particularly the plantar twigs, seem in this species to have been the part chiefly affected, though it is probable that some of the offsets from the peroneal branch associated in some instances in the morbid action.

Every therapeutic process that the art of medicine in the hands of the most experienced physicians of this metropolis could devise, was in this case tried, in a long and tedious succession, in vain. Sometimes external and sometimes internal preparations, or a tight ligature, appeared to afford a temporary alleviation, and to protract the intervals : but never any thing more. It was in consequence proposed by a surgeon of great eminence to amputate the leg, which was at one time on the point of being submitted to, though protested against by the present author on two accounts. First, the uncertainty whether the morbid condition of the nerve might not be seated chiefly in its origin instead of in its extremity, in which case amputation could be of no avail ; and secondly, the chance, that in process of time the keen sensibility of the affected branches would be worn out and obtunded by the violence of the action. Such was the undecided and miserable condition of this patient at the time of noticing his case on the publication of the author's volume of Nosology. Since this period, the prediction that the disease would gradually wear itself out has been completed : the paroxysms are now slight and tolerable, and the intervals much longer : and the patient has for nearly a twelvemonth been able to resume the duties of his profession without any interruption.

SPECIES III.
NEURALGIA MAMMÆ.
NERVE-ACHE OF THE BREAST.
SHARP, LANCINATING PAINS, DIVARICATING FROM A FIXED POINT IN THE BREAST, AND SHOOTING EQUALLY DOWN THE COURSE OF THE RIBS AND OF THE ARM TO THE ELBOW ; THE BREAST RETAINING ITS NATURAL SIZE, COMPLEXION, AND SOFTNESS.

ABOUT the year 1820, I was requested by Mr. Blair to examine a young woman, then eighteen years of age, who for more than two years had been subject to a painful disorder of the breast, that seemed equally to defy all parallel and all modes of treatment. On examining into the nature of the symptoms, I found them as described in the preceding definition. The organ was full-formed, soft, and globular, without the slightest degree of inflammation or hardness. When the paroxysm of pain was not present, it would bear pressure without inconvenience ; but during the pain, the whole breast was acutely sensible. The paroxysms returned at first five or six times in the course of the day, and were short and transient : but as the disease became more fixed, it became also more severe and extensive ; for the agonizing fits at length recurred as often as once an hour, and sometimes more frequently ; and, from being comparatively concentrated, the lancinating shoots darted both downward in the course of the circumjacent ribs, and upwards to the axilla, whence they afterward descended to the elbow, below which I do not know that they proceeded at any time. These fits were at length so frequent and vehement as to imbitter her whole life, and incapacitate her from pursuing any employment ; for it frequently happened, that if she attempted needlework, her fingers abruptly dropped the needle a few minutes after taking hold of it, from a mixture of pungent pain and tremulous twitching. The twitching or snatches in the shoulder, for it at length reached to this height, were at one time so considerable as to give the patient an idea, to use her own words, that something was alive there ; while, though the lacinating pain did not descend below the elbow, a considerable degree of trepidation reached occasionally to her fingers' ends. Her general health was in the meantime unaffected, and she was regular in menstruation.*

I had no hesitation in regarding this as a nondescript species of neuralgia ; and as little in communicating my fears that no plan of medicine we could lay down would be more than palliative, even if it should prove thus far beneficial, and that we must trust to time alone for a cure, and that obtuseness of sensibility, which I have already noticed, as a common consequence of high nervous irritation, continued till the organ becomes exhausted and torpefied.

Every remedial process was nevertheless tried in series for the purpose of obtaining relief, if not full success. Bleeding, local and general, frequently and profusely repeated ; purgatives of all kinds ; tonics and antispasmodics of every sort ; the hot and cold bath ; electricity and galvanism in every form ; rubefacients, blisters, setons, issues, and whatever else could be suggested, were enlisted into service in succession. But every thing was equally without avail ; nor do I know that even a temporary relief was obtained by any of these. Narcotics of all kinds proved impotent : drowsiness, indeed, and a comatose stupor, were hereby in various instances obtained, but the interval of wakeful-

ness was as much as ever tormented with the same racking paroxysms. From the powerful influence of nux vomica in many cases of nervous affection, to some of which we shall have occasion to advert hereafter, I had some hope of producing a slight impression on the nerves affected ; but the hope proved illusory : the patient took it in infusion as far as to about eight grains at a dose three or four times a day, till her head was intolerably confused, and every other part became numb ; but the paroxysms were intractable.

The poor sufferer, whose relations were incapahle of affording the resources of private practice, tried one dispensary after another, and at length one of the largest hospitals of this metropolis, without the smallest benefit, and from each was discharged as incurable. About six months since, however, being nearly four years from the commencement of the disease at home, and having utterly relinquished all medical means, with the exception of a seton under the breast, which was not dried up, she began to think herself rather better, and has continued to improve ever since, till a week ago, when her mother came to inform me she was worse again. This intelligence greatly surprised me, till I learned that the seton was now quite healed. It has since been opened, and there is a hope of her again improving.*

---

* Since the time of Fothergill, neuralgia has been noticed by many physicians and surgeons in this country. Prof. James Jackson, of Boston, seems to have been the first who wrote at any length on the subject, and according to him, little attention was paid to it prior to his publication in 1813: the remarkable case of the late Dr. Jones of New-York, who died from neuralgia, had however already appeared in the Phil. Med. Museum of 1809, and Dr. Hosack remarks, that he had repeatedly encountered this disease many years before.—Am. Med. and Phil. Reg., vol. iv. At the present day it is unfortunately not uncommon, and seems to be more frequent in females than in males. In regard to treatment, although the division of the nerve may at times prove successful, yet surgery must surrender her claims to the physician in removing this calamity. From carefully examining the recorded cases of neuralgia, if we except those from mechanical injury, we are led to conclude that in many instances it is constitutional, and hence that the treatment must be conducted with reference to the whole system. Among particular remedies, the datura stramonium is in more repute among American physicians than conium or belladonna, and the arsenical solution is sometimes employed with success. Dr. Hosack has on several occasions prescribed the volatile tincture of guaiacum with good effect. Dr. James Jackson, pursuing the suggestions of Fothergill, has administered three hundred grains of conium in six hours: the patient was cured. The carbonate and phosphate of iron, so warmly recommended by Hutchison, are frequently given with it. Dr. Francis has found that sulphate of quinine relieved, in many cases, where the narcotics had failed: his practice is recommended by Roche and Sanson.—See their Nouveaux Pathol. Med. Chirurg., vol. ii. Veratria has been employed by Dr. Turnbull in many instances.—(See Turnbull on Veratria.) And recently some curious cases have been published in the London Lancet, show-

---

* Many good practical observations on this subject will be found in Sir Astley Cooper's Illustrations of the Diseases of the Breast, chap. ix., part i., 4to., Lond., 1829. "The breast," says he, "is liable to become irritable without any distinct or perceptible swelling, as well as to form an irritable tumour composed of a structure unlike that of the gland itself, and which, therefore, appears to be a specific growth. Both states of disease, in the greatest number of examples, occur in young persons from the age of 16 to 30 years. I have never witnessed it prior to the commencement of puberty."—(P. 76.) The suffering increases very much just as menstruation is about to take place ; it is somewhat relieved on the evacuation occurring, and decreases on its cessation. An operation, when there is no distinct tumour, must be entirely out of contemplation.—Ed.

Thus far was written in the first edition of this work. The patient, under the kindness of Sir William Blizard, obtained an entrance into the Margate Sea-bathing Infirmary, and, after five or six weeks' use of the marine bath, returned home—not indeed entirely free from pain, but in comfortable ease, and able to resume the use of her needle. About six months afterward, however, the complaint returned with as much violence as ever, and again the most powerful tonics and antispasmodics were tried in vain. The subcarbonate of iron, in the fullest doses employed by Mr. Hutchison, was had recourse to, and steadily persevered in, but to as little purpose as every other medicine. She has now again returned to the Margate Infirmary, where I hear she has again found benefit. In various cases, however, even in this species, I have reason to believe that the iron has proved as successful as in *neuralgia faciei.* And Dr. Alderson has given another example in a very striking instance of mammary neuralgia, but in an older and less irritable period of life.*

ORDER III.

CINETICA.

DISEASES AFFECTING THE MUS-CLES.

IRREGULAR ACTION OF THE MUSCLES OR MUS-CULAR FIBRES: COMMONLY DENOMINATED SPASMS.

HAVING, in the Physiological Proem to the present class, glanced, as far as our space would allow, at the disputed question concerning the nature of muscular irritability, or *contractility*, to adopt the language of Dr. Bostock, and its affinity with sensorial or nervous influence, it is only necessary at present to take a very brief view of the general character and mode of action of muscles, as they appear to the naked eye in a massive form, or in other words, as composed of an almost infinite variety of minute fibres.

A muscle, thrown into action, increases in absolute weight, in density, and in power of resistance. It is also said to increase in absolute bulk, but the experiments on this subject are contradictory; the middle or belly of the muscle, indeed, is at this time evidently enlarged, but then its length appears to be proportionally diminished. [The ventricular portion of the heart, removed from a large dog immediately after the animal had been hanged, was immersed in warm water, contained in a glass vessel which was closed below with a ground glass stopper, and terminated above in an open vertical tube one third of an inch in diameter. The ventricles continued alternately to contract and dilate for a considerable length of time, during which the water stood at the same level in the tube, totally unaffected by the varying condition of the muscular fibres.—(*Mayo's Anat. and Physiolog. Commentaries*, vol. i., p. 12.)] Muscles constitute the cords, as bones do the levers of the living frame; and in most cases the muscles

grow tendinous, as the bones do cartilaginous, towards their extremities, by which means the fleshy and the osseous parts of the organs of motion become assimilated, and fitted for that insertion of the one structure into the other upon which their mutual action depends: the extent and nature of the motion being determined by the nature of the articulation, which is varied with the nicest skill to answer the purpose intended. Whether, however, the substance of tendons consists of the same fibres as the belly of a muscle, but only in a state of closer approximation, and possessed of finer vessels, which do not admit the introduction of red blood, or whether they form a distinct system of fibres, merely attached to those of the muscles, is at present undecided. It is certain that tendons possess nothing of the peculiar structure of muscles, and seem to be more nearly allied to the simple solid. —(*Bostock's Physiology*, p. 67, 8vo., 1824.)

It appears singular, at first sight, that the tendinous fibres, which thus seem to be compacted into a firmer and more substantial cord than those of the muscles, should be sometimes broken by muscular exertion, while the muscular fibres remain uninjured; yet this unquestionably depends upon their greater rigidity, and, consequently, inability of yielding to the force by which they are opposed. And hence the bones themselves are sometimes broken in the same manner as by a violent jerk, or a sudden spasmodic contraction, of which we shall presently meet with examples, especially in the patella, the ribs, and the arms. The muscles themselves, however, are occasionally ruptured by a like irregular violence and excess of power, as the recti abdominis in tetanus, and the gastrocnemii in cramps.

Muscular action, then, consists in a mutual attraction and concentration of the constituent fibres and muscles, in a manner peculiar to liv-

---

ing that magnetism sometimes has a powerful effect.—D.

* Cases of Neuralgia Spasmodica, &c., by B. Hutchison, &c., 8vo., London, 1822. Sir Astley Cooper considers equal parts of soap cerate and extract of belladonna, or a poultice with solution of belladonna and bread, the best applications. Covering the breast with oil-silk, or hareskin, he has also found tranquillize the part, by exciting perspiration from it. "As constitutional remedies, the submuriate of mercury, with opium and conium, should be given for a time, with an occasional aperient; and then, the medicine which I have prescribed with most advantage in lessening the irritability of the part, is as follows :—℞. Extracti conii, extracti papaveris ā ā gr. ij.; extracti stramonii e seminibus gr. ss. M. ; ft. pil."

The above pill may be given twice or three times during the day ; but if the gr. ss of the extract of stramonium be found too powerful, half that quantity may be tried. When the menses are obstructed, Sir Astley Cooper prescribes the carbonas ferri, the ferrum ammoniatum, or the mist. ferri comp. combined with aloes. He also recommends a hip-bath of seawater.—See Illustrations of the Diseases of the Breast, pp. 79, 80.—ED.

ing matter; for we cannot imitate it by any combination or action of mechanical fibres. It is not, however, a contraction in every dimension, since in this case the muscular volume would be diminished; but in length only, attended with a proportional increase of bulk, so as to preserve the absolute volume unchanged, or nearly so.

It is easy to conceive, from these few remarks, that the force exerted by muscular contraction may be enormous; but by the mechanical physicians it was calculated in the most extravagant manner, from premises in many instances wholly chimerical. Thus Borelli estimated the force with which the heart contracts, in order to carry forward the circulation of the blood, to be equal to not less than 180,000 lbs. at each contraction; while Pitcairn, applying the same speculation to the function of digestion, conceived that this process is accomplished by a muscular exertion, divided equally between the stomach and the auxiliary muscles that surround it, amounting in the stomach alone to the force of 117,088 lbs., for which, "had he assigned five ounces," says Professor Monro, "he would have been nearer the truth."—(*Monro, Comp. Anat., Pref.,* p. 8.) Yet we do not want these visionary calculations to prove the wonderful power possessed by muscular fibres; the facts we have already adverted to, and others we shall have to notice in the course of the present order, are sufficient to establish their astonishing energy, without having recourse to unfounded hypotheses or exaggerated statements.

In general, says Dr. Parr, in a very excellent article upon this subject (*Med. Dict. in verb., Musculus*), it appears that the force with which a muscle contracts is in proportion to the number of its fleshy fibres, and the extent of the surface to which these fibres are attached; but its degree of contraction, or the extent of its motion, is in proportion to their length. The limits of contraction differ in the long and in the circular muscles: for the former do not contract more than one third of their length, but the circular fibres of the stomach, which in their utmost dilatation may be expanded to a foot in circumference, may, after much fasting, be reduced to the circle of an inch. It must, however, be added, that in circular muscles no fibres pass completely round; bundles of fibres are collected and end at different points, while some begin where others end. Each may therefore admit of only a limited contraction, while the dilatation just mentioned may be the sum of the whole.

The action of muscles never intermits, and is only diminished in the sleeping state; though, where the sleep is profound and lethargic, the diminution amounts to almost a cessation, except in the involuntary organs. When the muscles are not exercised (to use the words of Haller), "the vis insita is very slightly exerted;" but we can still trace its influence by the position which the limbs assume, and discover the relative strength of the antagonizing muscles. Thus we find the flexors stronger than the extensors; for, during sleep, the head falls forward, and the body, legs, arms, and fin-

gers, are slightly bent. The cause of this additional strength is easily explained: for the flexors have stronger and more numerous fibres, their insertion is farther from the centre of their motions, and under a larger angle, which must increase when flexion has begun. This superiority of the flexors bends the fœtus in the womb into a round ball. The same superiority of power continues, though in a less degree, after birth, and hence frequent pandiculations are required to give activity and energy to the extensors, which they again lose in advanced age. On awakening from a sound sleep, the same yawnings and stretchings occur from the same cause; and Bethel fancifully refers the crowing of the cock, and the fluttering of his wings, to a similar purpose. It is always useful in diseases to examine the position of the limbs during sleep, particularly the sleep of children. If they deviate from the ordinary degree of flexure to a more straight position, there is generally some irregularity in the state of tone, and of course in the vital influx.

The irritability or contractility of a muscle is a very different power from that of elasticity. The latter always depends upon simple reaction, and is never a source of actual energy: it merely restores, in a contrary direction, the force which had been impressed, and the effect which it produces can never be greater than the amount of the cause. But in muscular contraction, the mechanical effect produced is infinitely greater than the mechanical cause producing it, as, when the organ of the heart, recently detached from the body just dead, is slightly scratched in its inside by a needle, it will contract so strongly as to force the point of the needle into its substance.—(*Fordyce, Phil. Trans.,* 1788, p. 80.) But the chief proof of the difference between the two is, that the irritable power of a muscle is often excited without any mechanical cause at all, and from the mere influence of the will, which has no effect upon the simple elasticity of organs. Hence, while contractility belongs to the muscular structure alone, elasticity appertains to many other substances as well, whether animal, vegetable, or even metallic. Muscles also have their elasticity, but the principle is altogether of a different kind, though often confounded with the preceding by modern pathologists; and particularly in their use of the term *tonicity* (*Bostock, Physiology,* p. 168, 8vo., 1824), which is often employed with little precision, and frequently means nothing more than this common principle of elasticity, to which indeed it seems directly to be applied by Dr. Cullen.

The muscles of the body may be divided into two grand classes; voluntary or animal, and involuntary or automatic. In the former we meet with some that are peculiarly remarkable for strength and continuity of contraction, as the greater part of the round muscles; and others as remarkable for mobility and vacillation, among which we may place most of the long muscles. These properties are strikingly exemplified in a state of disease, and call for particular attention; the muscles characterized by mobility presenting examples of atonic or agitatory spasm; while those that are conspicuous for continuity of action, are chiefly subject to rigid or entastic spasm.

Continuity of exertion, however, is generally less evident in the voluntary than in the involuntary muscles, of which last some organs, as the heart, continue their efforts through life without intermission; though all of them relax, or remit, occasionally or periodically. For this greater permanency and regularity of action they are indebted to the peculiar provision which has been made for their supply of nervous power; for while the voluntary muscles are furnished in a direct line from the sensorium, whence indeed the close connexion they hold with it, the control the will exercises over them, and their catenation with the prevailing emotion of the moment, the involuntary muscles are dependant chiefly on the intermediate or ganglionic system described in the proem to the present class, and are more remotely connected with the sensorium: they are in consequence far less influenced by the variable impulses of the mental faculties, and are placed beyond the jurisdiction of the will. And hence the tenour of their action is more equable, more permanent, more uninterrupted, and less subject to fatigue or weariness.

But as these organs are by no means free from the power of injury or diseased action, they are also subject at times, in common with the voluntary organs, to those abnormal motions which are ordinarily denominated spasms: and it is not a little curious to observe the uniform tendency which different spasmodic affections manifest towards some organs or functions, rather than towards others. Thus the vital function, in which the heart and lungs are such prominent agents, is chiefly disturbed by palpitation and syncope; the natural, or that in which the abdominal organs so generally co-operate, by hysterics; and the animal, extending through the range of the voluntary organs, by tetanus and epilepsy. In the prosecution of the present order, indeed, we shall see that this does not hold universally; that epilepsy, for instance, is often a disease rather of the stomach or intestines than of any other organ, and that the heart is sometimes affected with rigid instead of with clonic spasm: but the rule holds generally, and is not essentially shaken by these casual exceptions.

Dr. Cullen has contended, that in all spasmodic affections the brain is the actual seat of disease, and that they consist in some morbid modifications of its energy. "The scope and purpose of all that he has said," he tells us, "is to establish the general proposition, that spasmodic affections, whether they arise primarily in the brain or in particular parts, do consist chiefly, and always in part, in an affection and particular state of the energy of the brain: and that the operation of antispasmodic medicmes must consist in their correcting this morbid or preternatural state in the energy of the brain, by their correcting either the state of preternatural excitement or collapse, or by obviating the too sudden alteration of these states."

This proposition seems rather to follow from Dr. Cullen's singular doctrine concerning the mutable condition of the energy of the brain, and the immutable nature of the nervous power, which is propagated from it by vibrations, than from the clear face of facts before us. Spasms, in many instances, are altogether local; they are confined to particular muscles, or particular sets of associate muscles, and have no effect on the brain whatever, so as to disturb its energy; of which we have examples in hiccough, priapism,* chorea, and often in palpitation. They depend upon some irritation existing not at the origin but at the extremity of the nerves: and where such is their source, even though the chain of morbid action should at length reach the brain and affect its energy, as in convulsions from teething, epilepsy from worms, or some palpitations from ossific or polypous concretions, all the antispasmodics in the world will afford no relief, so long as the local cause of irritation continues to operate; while, the moment this is removed, where it is capable of removal, as by the use of a gum-lancet or active anthelmintics, all the powers of the brain become instantly tranquillized; its faculties are rendered clear, its energy is re-invigorated, and its motive power or sensorial energy is distributed in an uninterrupted tenour. The greater number of spasmodic affections, therefore, do not so much depend upon the state of the brain as of the living fibres that issue from it, and maintain a correspondence with it; for the stream may be vitiated while the fountain is untouched. We have seen, indeed, in the proem to the present class, from the concurrent results of various physiological experimenters, that although, while the organ of a brain exists, it exerts a certain influence over the principle of muscular motion, this principle is far less dependant upon the encephalon than that of general feeling or of the local senses; that it is found abundantly in animals totally destitute of a brain; and that, hence, those possessing a brain may be excited not only into abnormal and spasmodic, but even into a continuation or reproduction of regular and natural motions of various muscular organs after the brain has been separated from the spinal chain, by stimuli applied to this chain, or even by the artificial breath of a pair of bellows.

We have seen, also, that the nervous filaments of the muscles are of two kinds, sensific and motific; the former proceeding from the cerebellum, or the posterior trunk of the spinal cord, to which it gives rise, and the latter from the cerebrum, or anterior trunk of the same double cord; and as these two sets of filaments do not necessarily concur in the same affection, it is obvious that the muscles of a limb, or of the whole body, may be thrown into the most violent agitation, or the firmest rigidity, without

---

* This cannot be explained by the action of any muscle, and consequently is not a spasmodic affection.—ED.

much, or perhaps any degree of painful emotion or increased sensibility. And we can hence readily account for the little complaint that is made by patients upon this subject, on their being freed from a severe paroxysm of tetanus, convulsion-fit, or hysterics.

The following are the genera of diseases which will be found to appertain to the present order:

I. Entasia.　　Constrictive Spasm.
II. Clonus.　　Clonic Spasm.
III. Synclonus.　Synclonic Spasm.

GENUS I.
ENTASIA.
CONSTRICTIVE SPASM.

IRREGULAR MUSCULAR ACTION, PRODUCING CONTRACTION, RIGIDITY, OR BOTH.

ENTASIA is derived from the Greek ἔντασις, "intentio," "vehementia," "rigor," from ἐντείνω, "intendo." By many nosologists the genus is called tonos, or tonus, which is here dropped in favour of the present term, because tonus or tone is employed by physiologists and pathologists, in direct opposition to irregular vehemence or rigidity, to import a healthy and perfect vigour, or energy of the muscles; and by therapeutists to signify medicines capable of producing such or similar effects.

The genus ENTASIA includes the following species:—

1. Entasia Priapismus.　Priapism.
2. ――――― Loxia.　Wry neck.
3. ――――― Rhachybia.　Muscular Distortion
　　　　　　　　　　　　of the Spine.
4. ――――― Articularis.　Muscular Stiff-joint.
5. ――――― Systremma.　Cramp.
6. ――――― Trismus.　Locked-jaw.
7. ――――― Tetanus.　Tetanus.
8. ――――― Lyssa.　Rabies. Canine Madness.
9. ――――― Acrotismus.　Suppressed Pulse.

SPECIES I.
ENTASIA PRIAPISMUS.
PRIAPISM.

PERMANENT RIGIDITY AND ERECTION OF THE PENIS WITHOUT CONCUPISCENCE.

THE specific term is derived from the name of Priapus, the son of Venus and Bacchus, who is usually thus represented in paintings and sculptures, but with a concupiscent feeling. Galen applies the term also to females, as importing a rigid elongation of the clitoris without concupiscence.

Spasm is, in all instances, a disease not of vigour, but of debility, with a high degree of irritability; and there is no case in which this is more striking than in the present species. It has been found occasionally in infancy; but it is far more frequently an attendant upon advanced years. It has sometimes also followed cold, and especially local cold, clap, dysury, and the use of cantharides. It has at times been a result of free living, and particularly hard drinking. The spasms consist in a stiff and perma-

nent contraction of the erectores penis,[*] unconnected with any stimulus arising from a fulness of the vesiculæ seminales.

Dr. Darwin says he had met with two cases where the erection, producing a horny hardness, continued two or three weeks, without any venereal desire, but not without pain. The easiest attitude was lying upon the back with the knees bent upward. The corpus cavernosum urethræ at length became soft, and in a day or two the whole rigidity subsided. One of these patients had been a free drinker, had a gutta rosacea on his face, and died suddenly a few months after his recovery from the present complaint. It is singular that this spasm should sometimes continue after death; at least we have accounts of such cases in Marcellus Donatus and other writers.[†]

As the disease is a case of both local and general debility, its cure is in most instances difficult. Antispasmodics and tonics are the only medicine that promise relief, as camphire, opium, bark, warm aromatics, warm bathing, cold bathing: but the whole are often tried without effect.

[In the case which surgeons most frequently meet with, namely, that excited by the irritation of ulcers and excoriations about the glans, or by gonorrhœa attended with chordee, the most effectual treatment is the antiphlogistic, combined with antispasmodics. This is quite inconsistent with the notion of the complaint being connected with debility, a notion that has no foundation, except the author's hypothesis of the cause of spasm.]

SPECIES II.
ENTASIA LOXIA.
WRY NECK.

PERMANENT CONTRACTION OF THE FLEXOR MUSCLES ON THE RIGHT OR LEFT SIDE OF THE

---

* That the author has fallen into an error in representing *priapismus* to be a species of constrictive spasm, cannot be doubted; because erection of the penis is not really produced by the action of the erectores muscles, as they are termed, but by the injection and distention of the glans, corpus spongiosum urethræ, and corpora cavernosa, with blood. "Each of the crura penis gives attachment at its origin to a tolerably strong muscle, named the erector penis, probably because, when a power capable of producing the effect indicated by that name was sought by anatomists, this muscle seemed to be their only resource. At present the name appears very ill adapted, since the muscles in question obviously draw the penis downward and backward, instead of upward and against the pubes. Those who explain the erection of the penis by the compression of its vein, should find out a power capable of elevating the organ against the bone, and of carrying it forward."—(See Rees's Cyclopædia, art. GENERATION.) In fact, mechanical pressure of the vein will not produce erection.—ED.

† Dr. Francis remarks, "that in cases of severe parturition, when the head has been greatly compressed, the child is often born with a strong erection of the penis." In instances of sudden death, where opium has been taken freely, the penis is sometimes found erect.—D.

NECK, DRAWING THE HEAD OBLIQUELY IN THE SAME DIRECTION.

THE term LOXIA is derived from the Greek, λοξός, "obliquus, tortus ;" whence loxarthrus in surgery, an obliquity of a joint of any kind, without spasm or luxation. By the Greeks, however, the term was specially applied to the joints or muscles of the neck.

This disease, in its genuine form, proceeds from an excess of muscular action, particularly of the mastoid muscle on the contracted side. But we frequently meet with a similar effect from two other causes : one in which there is a disparity in the length of the muscles opposed to each other, and consequently a permanent contraction on the side on which they are shortest ; and the other in which, from cold or a strain, there is great debility or atony on the side affected, and consequently an incurvation of the neck on the opposite side, not from a morbid excess, but an overbalance of action.

This species, therefore, offers us the three following varieties :—

α Dispars. Natural wry neck.	From disparity in the length of the muscles opposed to each other.	
β Irritata. Spastic wry neck.	From excess of muscular action on the contracted side.	
γ Atonica. Atonic wry neck.	From direct atony of the muscles on the yielding side.	

The FIRST VARIETY is mostly congenital, though sometimes produced by severe burns or other injuries. And a like effect occasionally issues from a cause that may be noticed in the present place, though not connected with a morbid state of the muscles,—a displacement of the muscles, from an incurvation in the vertebræ of the neck ;* by which, though the antagonist muscles be of equal length and power, those on the receding side of the neck are kept on a perpetual stretch, while those on the protruding side are in a state of constant relaxation. The other TWO VARIETIES are commonly the result of cold, or inflammation, or a strain ; often by carrying too heavy loads on the head. M. Boyer gives instances of the disease produced by moral causes : and Wepfer relates the case of a man who had a wry neck, occasioned by a convulsive action of the muscles on one side of the neck, which appeared whenever he was tormented by chagrin, but ceased as soon as he was restored to a state of mental tranquillity.—(Traité de Maladies Chirurgicales, &c., tom. vii., 8vo., Paris, 1821.)

The cure must depend upon the nature of the cause: In colds and strains, warmth, the friction of flannel, and the stimulus of the ammonia or camphire liniment combined with opium, will be found most serviceable, as tending to diminish pain, and restore action to the weakened

* In almost every instance, the change in the bones is the consequence of the long-continued action of the preponderating muscle. This doctrine, which is maintained by Jörg, is now generally admitted.—ED.

organ. In direct spasms the same process will also frequently be found useful ; but the application of cold water will often answer better. [About four years ago the editor was consulted by a gentleman at Clapham, whose right sterno-cleido mastoideus muscle was not only affected with permanent and rigid spasm, but had attained a vast increase of bulk and force. Under the direction of Dr. Babington, Mr. Brodie, and Sir Charles Bell, the patient had tried various narcotics, ammoniated copper, and different local applications, without benefit. A seton in the nape of the neck, and friction over the muscle with camphorated mercurial ointment, was now suggested, with a course of the compound calomel pill, combined with hyosciamus and conium, and occasional purgatives ; but the patient had not courage to begin the plan. In this case, the wry neck was evidently associated with considerable disorder of the nervous system ; and the patient could only lift a glass to his mouth by using both hands for the purpose.] Where the antagonist muscles are of unequal length, the case lies beyond the reach of medical practice ; and if relieved at all, can only be so by a surgical operation. If the cervical vertebræ be incurvated, but the bones sound, the disease may not unfrequently be made to yield to a skilful application of machinery by the hands of an ingenious surgeon. It sometimes happens, however, that the bones in this case are soft and occasionally carious, and the slightest motion of the head is attended with intolerable pain. Setons have here been found serviceable, with an artificial support of the head ; but this kind of affection is often connected with a constitutional softness of the bones, of which we shall have to treat in the first order of the sixth class, under the head PAROSTIA flexilis.

SPECIES III.
ENTASIA RHACHYBIA.
MUSCULAR DISTORTION OF THE SPINE.

PERMANENT AND LATERAL CURVATURE OF THE SPINE, WITHOUT PARALYSIS OF THE LOWER LIMBS : MUSCLES OF THE BACK EMACIATED ; MOSTLY WITHOUT SORENESS UPON PRESSURE.

DISTORTION of the spine is produced in various ways ; and it is chiefly owing to a want of due attention to this fact, that so much confusion has of late prevailed respecting the real nature of the particular case to be treated, and the particular treatment that ought to be adopted.

The disease, under this general name, was first introduced before the public with any considerable degree of notoriety by Mr. Pott, as connected with a palsy of the lower extremities, and as dependant upon a scrofulous diathesis ; which at length fixed itself upon some part of the vertebral column, softened or rendered carious the bones that became affected, and hereby necessarily produced crookedness, and a morbid pressure upon the right line of the spinal marrow.

This is a case that often happens, and a like effect occasionally occurs in a very early period of life from a rachitic instead of a scrofulous diathesis ; though from the greater facility with which the principle of life is able to adapt itself to deviations from the ordinary laws of health at this latter period than afterward, a paralysis of the lower extremities is less common,[*] and even the mischiefs incidental to a misformation of the chest less fatal. So that, while the disease of a humpback can rarely take place in puberty or later life without a serious injury to almost every function, we often find it occur in infancy without making much encroachment on the general health.

In all cases of this kind, the malady is primarily and idiopathically an affection of the vertebral *bones;* and there is always to the touch a mollescence in their structure, or a manifest soreness and ulceration. And from the peculiar contour of the vertebral column, the distortion is always from within outwards, forming what has been called an *angular,* in contradistinction, to a *lateral* curvature. So that the characters of the osseous gibbosity are sufficiently clear and specific.

But the muscles of the vertebral column and their appendages, the ligaments and cartilages into which the latter are inserted, are of as much importance to its healthy contour as its bones. And hence any morbid affection of these several structures may as essentially interfere with the natural curve of the spine, and the wellbeing of the constitution, as a disease of the vertebral bones.

It is possible that these are all affected in particular instances, sometimes separately, sometimes jointly (*Copeland on the Spine,* p. 15) ; but there can be no doubt that the muscular fibres of the neck, back, and loins, those on which all the complicated movements of the vertebral column depend, and which compose more than three hundred distinct muscles in the

whole, are most frequently thus enfeebled, either in part or in their entire range ; though an enfeebled state of any of these organs must produce an inability of preserving the spine in its natural sweep and equilibrium. And where distortion proceeds from this cause, the indications are in most cases as clear as where it is the result of a diseased condition of the bony structure ; for first the morbid curvature, instead of being *from within outwards,* takes place *laterally,* the crookedness being manifestly on the right or the left side, according as the muscles on the one side or the other overpower the action of their antagonists ; there is little or no soreness upon pressure, unless indeed the bones or their cartilages should ultimately become affected from the protracted state of the disease ; and the distortion being less abrupt or angular than in the ossific gibbosity, the lower limbs are not affected with paralysis.

The distinction, therefore, between the osseous and the muscular distortion of the spine, is clear and definite ; and so far as regards the peculiar character of the curvature, was minutely noticed by the Greek writers, who identified the first by the name of LORDOSIS or CYRTOSIS, according as this curvature was anterior or posterior, and the second or the lateral curvature by the term HYBOSIS, from ὕβος (*hybos*), incurvus. It is from this term that the author has derived the name which he has ventured to assign to the present species—RHACHYBIA—as an allowable contraction of *rhachyhybia,* literally SPINAL INFLECTION. Swediaur has denominated it, from the same source, *hyboma Scoliosis.*—(Tom. ii., p. 740.)

The distinction is very accurately pointed out by Mr. Pott, who,—while he affirms that " the ligaments and cartilages of the spine may become the seat of the disorder (scrofula) without

---

[*] Scrofulous caries of the corpora vertebrarum, whether in adults or children, most frequently after a time causes paralysis of the lower extremities, though exceptions are met with. In rickets, where the spine may be said to be deformed rather from imperfect development of the bones than from disease of them, palsy of the legs is not produced, however great the lateral curvature of the back. Cruveilhier, in his Anatomie Pathologique, livr. iv., gives us the particulars of a case in which no paraplegia existed, though not less than five of the dorsal vertebræ had been totally annihilated by disease, and the alteration in the shape of the vertebral column was such, that the upper half formed over the lower an extremely acute angle, which, from what is demonstrated in the engraving, would have been still more acute if it had not been prevented by the eleventh and fifth dorsal vertebræ touching each other. The intervertebral foramina were all preserved, though more or less deformed, contracted, or displaced backwards. In those which were most diminished the corresponding intercostal nerves must have been compressed, and consequently, the action of the intercostal muscles impaired, and an asthmatic affection been the result. The engraving shows how nature in this instance contrived to maintain the integrity of the vertebral canal, and the spinal cord uncompressed, in the midst of such a deviation of the spine from its normal shape. Although five of the vertebræ were de-

molished, anchylosis took place, and the medulla suffered no pressure adequate to the production of paralysis of the lower parts of the body. A beautiful preparation, illustrative of an equally extensive destruction of the bodies of the vertebræ, and of as sudden a bend of the spine, may be seen in the anatomical museum of the London University. Cruveilhier also gives the particulars of the body of a child ten years old that was brought to his dissecting-room, in which only a few vestiges of the third, fourth, fifth, sixth, seventh, eighth, ninth, tenth, and eleventh dorsal vertebræ were left. According to this pathologist, diseases of the vertebral column, like those of every other part of the osseous system, are seated, not in the osseous tissue itself, but in the adipose cellular or medullary tissue occupying its interstices. When this cellular tissue inflames, sometimes it pours out pus in abundance, constituting an abscess; sometimes in scanty quantity, which admits of being entirely absorbed. The cells of the osseous tissue being distended by the development of the cellular tissue, and deprived of the materials of nutrition, may be completely absorbed; and thus Cruveilhier accounts for the total disappearance of the texture of bone, without a vestige of it being left. The reader is probably aware, that Cruveilhier's doctrine is, that all disease is seated in the cellular tissue of organs, the other tissues being only liable to atrophy and hypertrophy.—ED.

any affection of the vertebræ," in which case "it sometimes happens that the whole spine, from the lowest vertebra of the neck downwards, gives way laterally, forming sometimes one great curve to one side, and sometimes a more irregular figure, producing general crookedness and deformity of the whole trunk of the body, attended with many marks of ill health ;" —yet admits that paralysis of the lower limbs never accompanies cases of this sort, so far as his experience had extended, nor even that untempered and misshapen structure of the spine which occurs at birth or during infancy from a rachitic softness of the bony material. "I have never," says he, "seen paralytic effect on the legs from a malformation of the spine, however crooked such a malformation might have rendered it, whether such crookedness had been from the time of birth, or had come on at any time afterward during infancy.—None of those strange twists and deviations which the majority of European women get in their shapes from the very absurd custom of dressing them in stays during their infancy, and which put them in all directions but the right, ever caused any thing of this kind, however great the deformity might be. The curvature of the spine which is accompanied by *this affection of the limbs* (i. e. that which takes place from a diseased condition of the bones themselves subsequently to childhood, and from a supposed scrofulous diathesis), whatever may be its degree or extent, is at first almost always the same ; that is, it is always from within outwards, and seldom or never to either side."

Now it has unfortunately happened, that as Mr. Pott's remarks were written chiefly to explain this last form of spinal distortion, and addressed to the single cause of scrofula, the hints he has given respecting distortions from every other cause have been too often forgotten ; and the moment a young female is found to have a tendency to a vertebral distortion of any kind, it has too generally been taken for granted that the bones were in a diseased state, or on the point of becoming so ; that the patient was labouring under the influence of a strumous diathesis, which was manifesting itself in this quarter ; and all the severe measures of caustics or setons, with an undeviating permanent confinement to a hard mattress, or inclined plane, for many weeks or months, which a strumous affection of this kind calls for and fully justifies, has been improvidently had recourse to, with a great addition to the sufferings of the patient, and, in many instances, no small addition to the actual disease which has been so unhappily misunderstood.

Mr. Baynton seems justly chargeable with having adopted this general view of the subject, and extending it indiscriminately to every case. Mr. Wilson, who, though he conceived the disease to originate in a rachitic rather than a strumous diathesis, and had recourse, as we shall observe presently, to a different mode of treatment, seems to have stretched his parallel hypothesis over the same extent of ground. And Mr. Lloyd, who has lately favoured the profession with a valuable work on the same subject, in like manner contemplates every case of spinal distortion as issuing from a common, and that a strumous cause ; to which cause also it has since as uniformly been assigned by Dr. Jarrold. —(*Inquiry into the Curvature of the Spine*, &c., 8vo., 1824.) Mr. Lloyd, correctly indeed, distinguishes between the angular and the lateral curvature ; and with equal correctness observes, that "in the former there is always some destruction of some portion of the vertebral column, and often, for a considerable time, progressive destruction of bone, cartilage, and ligament ; and the vertebræ undergo precisely the same changes as the extremities of other bones in scrofulous diseases of the joints :" while he adds that "in the latter there is no destruction of parts, but merely an alteration of structure ;" that "a wasting of the muscles always attends it in a greater or less degree ;" and that "it has been supposed by some authors that the cause of the curvature is entirely in the action of the muscles. But although," he continues, "this may be and most probably is the *immediate* cause, I am much more inclined to believe that the *primary* cause is in the vertebræ ; that scrofulous action is set up in them, which increases their vascularity, and softens their texture."

Here, then, is a distinct recognition of the two forms of morbid distortion of the spine to which I am anxious to direct the attention of the reader : and each of them is allotted its peculiar seat and diacritical signs ; the bones with manifest injury of the bones, and the muscles with manifest injury of the muscles. The rest is matter of mere hypothesis, and needs not urge us into a discussion.

So obvious and so much more common indeed is muscular than osseous distortion of the spine, that other pathologists, from this fact chiefly, have contended that this is the only form of the disease in its commencement. Such was the opinion of the late Mr. Grant, of Bath, and such is the opinion of Dr. Dods, of the same city, in an interesting tract he has lately published on this subject (*Path. Obs. on the Rotated or Contorted Spine*, 8vo., L_{ond}., 1824); while Dr. Harrison refers its origin to "the connecting ligaments of the vertebræ." "These," he observes, "get relaxed, and suffer a single vertebra to become slightly displaced ;" in consequence of which, he adds, "the column loses its natural firmness, other bones begin to press unduly upon the surrounding ligaments ; they in turn get relaxed and elongated, by which the dislocation is increased, and the distortion permanently established. The direction becomes *lateral, anterior,* or *posterior,* according to circumstances ; but the malady has in every instance the same origin, and requires the same mode of cure."—(*Lond. Med. and Phys. Journ.*, No. cclxiv.)

There is much ingenuity in this explanation, and I have no doubt that it is a correct expression of various cases of vertebral distortion. It chiefly fails, like the osseous hypothesis, in too wide a spirit of simplification, and in allowing no other origin in any instance, than that which forms the keystone of its own pretensions. Admitting the disease to commence in the connecting ligaments, the associating muscles must soon be involved in the mischief; while, if it commence in the latter, the ligaments which unite them to the bones cannot long continue unaffected. So that the question is merely one of primogeniture, and imposes little or no difference in the mode of treatment. Nay, even the bones themselves, by being irregularly pressed upon, may at length suffer in such parts from increased absorption, become thinner and more spongy, or even ulcerate and grow carious; so as in process of time to give a direct proof of osseous or angular contortion, though induced instead of taking the lead.

One of the chief difficulties, in cases where we have no reason to apprehend a morbid state of the bones, consists in accounting for the change that seems to take place in the relative position of several of the vertebræ or their processes; and especially in the greater elevation or prominence of their transverse processes on one side, while those on the other are scarcely perceptible. And it is in truth chiefly to solve this question, that most of the hypotheses of the present day are started in opposition to each other. The idea of an actual dislocation of the vertebral bones, which enters into that of Dr. Harrison, would sufficiently account for the fact, if such a dislocation could be unequivocally shown. But while the change of position does not seem in any instance to amount to a complete extrusion of a vertebra from its seat of articulation, the ease and quietude with which, under judicious management, it often seems to recover its proper position, and to evince its proper shapes, are inconsistent with the phenomena that accompany a reduction of luxated bones in every other part of the body.

The explanation, therefore, has not been felt satisfactory to a numerous body of pathologists; and Dr. Dods has hence offered us another solution, which is also highly ingenious, and may perhaps in the end be found correct in those cases in which the miscurvature is very considerable, and especially where it becomes double or assumes a sigmoid figure. He supposes, in the first place, that the whole disease in its origin is seated in the extensor muscles of the back, or that part of them to which it is confined: more especially in the quadratus lumborum, sacro-lumbalis, and longissimus dorsi. He supposes next that the right hand being habitually more exerted than the left, the effect of such surplus of force, in consequence of our throwing the body towards the left to preserve its centre of gravity, and hence strongly contracting the muscles of this side of the spine, must fall in a greater degree upon those muscles, and more dispose them " to suffer disorganization and become contracted;" and he hence accounts for the greater frequency of contortion on the right side than on its opposite. He then proceeds to account for the single or double curvature which the contortion effects, by remarking that the morbidly contracted muscles of the left side, in

overcoming the action of the muscles of the right, do not drag the vertebræ forward towards themselves in a direct line, but rotate the vertebræ to which they are attached, because of the angles formed relatively between the vertebræ and the pelvis (the points of origin and insertion of these muscles), and the force of their contraction acting upon moveable, horizontal, or transverse levers, namely, the transverse processes of the vertebræ.—(Op. cit., p. 93.)

Morbid curvature of the spine, therefore, in the opinion of Dr. Dods, does not consist in an evulsion of separate vertebræ from their natural course and position, but in a twist of a great part of the entire column, by which means the morbid lateral flexure is nothing more than the natural sigmoid sweep of the vertebral chain, wrested more or less round to one side, as by the turning of a corkscrew.

Whatever displacement is met with in the ribs, or the other bones of the chest, is necessarily a result of the first deviation from the line of health. " All the ribs," he observes, " have a double attachment to the vertebræ : one, by their heads to the bodies of them; and the other, by their tubercles to the transverse processes. When the vertebræ, then, are made to rotate upon each other in the manner described, by the permanent contraction, and this, for example, to the right side, which is the more frequent direction they take, from the causes noticed, they by this movement push out or backward the heads of the ribs of the left side, and force their sternal extremities considerably forward, because of the quick circular turn which the ribs make between their angles and their points of attachment to the vertebræ, and the very small motion, from such a formation of them, requisite here to produce them. Together with this movement of the ribs, which produces the projection of the left side of the chest in front, they are also made, from their double attachment to the vertebræ, to fall down and approximate, or, as it were, overlap each other at their angles. This causes that hollowness or sinking in of the left side of the chest behind. The falling down of the ribs here described appears to me to be in part owing, also, to the permanent contraction of the sacro-lumbalis muscle, which is inserted into all their angles. While these movements take place with the ribs on the left side of the body, the very opposite, of necessity, happens to those on the right. By the rotatory movement of the vertebræ, the ribs on the right side have their heads, contrary to those on the left, drawn inward, and their sternal extremities made to recede backward, while their double connexion with the vertebræ causes them, contrary also to those of the left side, to be raised up and separated from each other at their angles. This rising up and separation of the ribs at their angles is what produces the projection of the right side of the chest behind."

From this general change of position, and particularly the twist of the ribs, Dr. Dods accounts for the unnatural situation of the scapulæ, and in many instances, of the clavicles and the sternum, with the falling down of the right shoulder. He observes, moreover, that though the contortion of the spine most frequently takes place to the right side, yet that it occasionally takes place to the left; that the whole column is not always moved round, but only a part of it; and that hence, instead of a profile of three morbid flexures brought into view, which invariably follows in the former case, we have often a profile of only two: and that where the muscles of both sides of the column become contracted from position, which sometimes takes place, the greater number of the vertebral joints acquire an anhylosis, and the body is arched backwards.

There is much ingenuity through the whole of this explanation, which plausibly accounts for that ridgy line of projection so frequently felt on the left side of the loins when the morbid curvature is on the right, ascending nearly to a level with the spinous processes, while there is not only no such ridge on the opposite side, but even no appearances of the transverse processes. Upon the hypothesis before us, these processes are conceived to be equally elevated on the one side and depressed on the other, which gives us the two phenomena of an unnatural and ridgy prominence in the former line, and of an unnatural disappearance in the latter. The hypothesis nevertheless (for at present it cannot be entitled to a higher appellation) requires further elucidation and support; and after all, can never altogether reach the precise object at which it aims,—that of establishing itself at the expense of every other view, and especially of subverting the doctrines of a diseased action of the other moving powers or their appendages, the ligaments of the spinal muscles, or the cartilages into which they are inserted; a morbid condition of which is often capable of proof from the very limited area of pain and tenderness to which, on pressure, the disease seems to be confined: to say nothing of the affection of the vertebral bones themselves, in which, as already observed, spinous distortion sometimes commences, though from a very different source, and in which, even when derived from the source now contemplated, it sometimes terminates.

There can be no doubt, however, that the spinal distortion of the present day is a disease far more frequently of the muscles and their appendages than of the bones, and is the result of a want of equilibrium between the antagonist forces on the one side and on the other of the vertebral column, as well those of the trunk as of the back; in consequence of which this column is deranged in its natural sweep, and either twisted or deflected in particular parts, or in its whole length: all the other changes in the general figure, and deviations from the general health, being dependant upon this primary aberration.

It is hence a disease of muscular debility, or irregular, and hence clonic, action in the fibres of the yielding muscles, and an inability to resist the encroachment that is made on them by their more powerful antagonists.

The complaint almost invariably shows itself from the age of puberty to that of mature life, though sometimes later; and is nearly limited to females, and, among females, to those of delicate habits, and who are especially disciplined in the false and foolish rules for obtaining a fine figure. It is hence a perpetual inmate in our public female schools, and is by no means an unfrequent attendant upon domestic education.

The progress of the disease may be so easily collected from the physiological survey we have already taken, that only a few words in addition will be necessary.

The complaint first shows itself by a general listlessness and aversion to muscular exertion of any kind, and an unwonted desire to lounge and loll about. No signs of constitutional disease, however, are as yet manifest; the nights are not disturbed, the appetite does not fail, the evacuations are regular, and the pulse unaffected. There is soon after a sense of weariness, and even at times uneasiness, about the back, and especially the loins; and if the muscles of these parts be minutely examined, several of them will give proof of flaccidity and emaciation. If no steps be taken at this time to arrest the disease in its march, or if the steps taken be injudicious or inadequate, the vertebral column will soon be involved in the morbid action; and especially, as Mr. Ward observes, "on the occurrence of any particular disturbance to the constitution" (*Pract. Obs. on Distortions of the Spine, Chest, and Limbs,* p. 36, 8vo., 1822): its numerous joints will lose their nicely-adjusted poise; they will in various parts be left too loose on the one side, and dragged too rigidly on the other; and the elegant contour of the spinal chain will progressively be broken in upon. All the other changes, whether upon the general form or the general health, which progressively take place in the advance of the disease, are entirely consecutive upon the symptoms before us, and may be anticipated by any one. From the morbid contest which is thus continually going on between the antagonist muscles, their internal organization must necessarily become greatly affected, and the growing debility, which is manifest in the contractile and extensile power of their aggregate fibre, will enter into every part of every separate fibril, and affect their vis insita. The debility and irregular action of one muscle will spread by sympathy or association to various others; and from the derangement of the bones of the spine and the chest, the functions of respiration and digestion, and consequently, in a greater or less degree, all the other functions of the body, must be interfered with in their respective powers, so that there is scarcely any other disease but may follow; and the frame will become generally emaciated.

As the proximate cause is debility of the extensor muscles of the back or loins on either side, the occasional cause will consist in whatever has a tendency to produce such debility. Too rapid growth is a frequent source of this complaint; a casual strain of the muscles on either side is a source not less common; chlorosis, or any other constitutional weakness, may lead to the same effect; and assuredly the use of stiff and girding stays, or any other part of that fashionable compression which is designed, in the school-discipline of the present day, to mould the form into a somewhat different and more graceful shape than perhaps the niggard hand of nature has intended—such as back-boards, braces, steel bodices or steel crutches, spiked collars, neck-swings, and even education-chairs. The tendency of all these to produce deformity where it does not exist, and to aggravate it where it does, is forcibly pointed out by Dr. Dods; who nevertheless seems to censure, with rather more acrimony than needful, the whole system of school-drilling education, as practised in many of our most fashionable establishments. A course of discipline for giving grace and elegance to the growing form, if conducted with judgment, devoid of rigorous compression to the expanding organs, and allowing a sufficient alternation of relaxation and ease, so far from being injurious to the health and strength of the general frame, has a natural tendency to invigorate it. But the greater frequency of the lateral distortion of the spine in our own day compared with its apparent range in former times, together with the increased coercion and complication of the plan laid down in many of our fashionable schools for young ladies, seems clearly to indicate that some part at least of its increased inroad is chargeable to this source : and the following remarks of Mr. Pott upon the various instruments applied to a growing girl in order to prevent a crooked shape, have a wider claim to attention in the present day than when they were first given to the world. "These," says he, "are used with design to prevent growing children from becoming crooked or misshapen; and this they are supposed to do by supporting the backbone, and by forcing the shoulders unnaturally backward. The former they cannot do; and in all cases *where the spine is weak, and therefore inclined to deviate from* a right figure, the latter action of these instruments must contribute to, rather than prevent, such deviations, as will appear to whoever will with attention examine the matter. If, instead of adding to the embarrassment of children's dress by such iron restraints, parents would throw off all of every kind, and thereby give nature an opportunity of exerting her own powers ; and if, in all cases of manifest debility, recourse were had to friction, bark, and cold bathing, with due attention to air, diet, exercise, and rest ; the children of the opulent would perhaps stand a chance of being as stout, as straight, and as well-shapen, as those of the laborious poor."

The simple fact is, that the system of discipline is carried too far, and rendered much too complicated ; and ART, which should never be more than a handmaid of NATURE, is elevated into her tyrant. In rustic life we have health and vigour, and a pretty free use of the limbs and the muscles, because all are left to the impulse of the moment to be exercised without restraint. The country girl rests when she is weary, and in whatever position she chooses or finds easiest ; and walks, hops, or runs, as her fancy may direct, when she has recovered her-

self ; she bends her body and erects it as she lists, and the flexor and extensor muscles are called into an equal and harmonious play. There may be some degree of awkwardness, and there generally will be, in her attitudes and movements ; and the great scope of female discipline should consist in correcting this. With this it should begin, and with this it should terminate, whether our object be directed to giving grace to the uncultivated human figure or the uncultivated brute. We may modify the action of muscles in common use, or even call more into play than are ordinarily exercised, as in various kinds of dancing ; but the moment we employ one set of muscles at the expense of another, keep the extensors on a full stretch from day to day, by forbidding the head to stoop, or the back to be bent, and throw the flexors of these organs into disuse and neglect, we destroy the harmony of the frame instead of adding to its elegance, weaken the muscles that have the disproportionate load cast upon them, render the dejected muscles torpid and unpliant, sap the foundation of the general health, and introduce a crookedness of the spine instead of guarding against it. The child of the opulent, while too young to be fettered with a fashionable dress, or drilled into the discipline of our female schools, has usually as much health and as little tendency to distortion as the child of the peasant : but let these two, for the ensuing eight or ten years, change places with each other ; let the young heiress of opulence be left at liberty, and let the peasant-girl be restrained from her freedom of muscular exertion in play and exercise of every kind ; and instead of this, let her be compelled to sit bolt upright in a high narrow chair with a straight back, that hardly allows of any flexion to the sitting muscles, or of any recurvation to the spine ; and let the whole of her exercise, instead of irregular play and frolic gayety, be limited to the staid and measured march of Melancholy in the Penseroso of Milton—

" With even step and musing gait ;"

to be regularly performed for an hour or two every day, and to constitute the whole of her corporeal relaxation from month to month, girded moreover, all the while, with the paraphernalia of braces, bodiced stays, and a spiked collar ; and there can be little doubt that, while the child of opulence shall be acquiring all the health and vigour her parents could wish for, though it may be with a colour somewhat too shaded and brown, and an air somewhat less elegant than might be desired, the transplanted child of the cottage will exhibit a shape as fine, a demeanour as elegant, as fashion can communicate ; but at the heavy expense of a languor and relaxation of fibre that no stays or props can compensate, and no improvement of figure can atone for.

Surely it is not necessary, in order to acquire all the air and gracefulness of fashionable life, to banish from the hours of recreation the old rational amusements of battledoor and shuttlecock, of tennis, trap-ball, or any other game that calls into action the bending as well as the extending muscles, gives firmness to every organ, and the glow of health to the entire surface.

Such, and a thousand similar recreations, varied according to the fancy, should enter into the school-drilling of the day, and alternate with the grave procession and the measured dance, for there is no occasion to banish either; although many of the more intricate and venturous opera dances, as the Bolero, should be but occasionally and moderately indulged in; since, as has been sufficiently shown by Mr. Shaw, " we have daily opportunities of observing, not only the good effects of well-regulated exercise, but also the actual deformity which arises from the disproportionate development that is produced by the undue exertion of particular classes of muscles.—(*On the Nature and Treatment of Distortions*, &c., p. 15, Lond., 8vo., 1823.) It may be observed," continues the same excellent writer, "that the ligaments of the ankles of some of the most admired dancers are so unnaturally stretched, that in certain postures, as in the Bolero dance, the tibia nearly touches the floor. So bad, indeed, is the effect occasionally produced by a frequent stretching of the ligaments, that the feet of many of them are deformed; for the ligaments which bind the tarsal and metatarsal bones together become so much lengthened by dancing and standing on the tips of the toes, that the natural arch of the foot is at length destroyed."—(*Inquiry into the Causes of the Curvature of the Spine*, &c., ut suprà, p. 119.)

Such, then, are the best preventive means against muscular or ligamentous distortion of the young female frame, and especially of the vertebral column, in conjunction with pure air, plain diet, and well-regulated hours of rest.

If, notwithstanding such means, a tendency to crookedness on either side should manifest itself, evidenced by the symptoms already pointed out, no time should be lost in making an accurate examination of the spinal chain: and if such tendency should be accompanied with pains about the pelvis and lower extremities, our attention should be particularly directed to the state of the vertebræ seated in the centre of the different flexures of the column, but especially of the lumbar, for it is probable, in this case, that one or more of them may be in a state of inflammation.

Where this is the case, the usual means of taking off inflammatory action, and especially depletion by cupping-glasses, should be instantly had recourse to. But where the cause is debility alone, and a want of equilibrium between antagonist sets of muscles, rest, reclination, general tonics, especially myrrh, steel, and in many cases the sulphate of quinine, sea-bathing, and, in effect, whatever may tend to introduce a greater firmness of fibre and general vigour of constitution, constitute the best plan of treatment.

To these should be added a series of friction, and especially of shampooing or manipulation, applied down the whole course of the spine, and particularly that part of it where the distortion is most evident; and it may be of advantage, as proposed by Dr. Dods, to direct the course of the manipulation in a particular manner to such transverse processes of the vertebræ as appear peculiarly elevated, so as artfully, and by insinuation, to assist in restoring them to their proper position. It will also be found expedient in most cases to smear the hand with oil, or some other unctuous substance, in order to prevent the friction from irritating or excoriating the skin.

Those who ascribe the disease to a strumous diathesis in every instance, have of course a medical treatment of their own adapted to this view of the case. Such is the practice of Dr. Jarrold, who has lately written a treatise upon this subject containing many valuable hints, but who limits the seat of the malady to the intervertebral cartilages, as he does its cause to a strumous taint. His Materia Medica, therefore, for the present purpose, is nearly restricted to burnt sponge and carbonate of soda. " Conceiving," says he, that " there might be some relation between it and bronchocele, I have made use of similar remedies."—(*Inquiry into the Causes of the Curvature of the Spine*, &c., ut suprà, p. 119.) To which he occasionally adds, when the debility is considerable, twenty drops of nitric acid daily. And with this simple process he tells us that he has been so successful in a restoration of health, strength, plumpness, and uprightness, that " medical treatment is seldom further required, unless the appetite and digestion be impaired."

Not acceding to this causation, I have not tried the plan; which seems here to have been far more successful than in bronchocele itself; even when the more powerful aid of iodine is called into co-operation, which it is singular that Dr. Jarrold does not appear to have had recourse to. To all the confederate means, however, of recumbency, friction, shampooing, pure air, and occasional exercise, he is peculiarly friendly: and as these have of themselves effected a cure in the hands of various other practitioners, it is not improbable that Dr. Jarrold is far more indebted to such confederates than he is aware of, and that his auxiliaries have been of more service to him than his main force.

It has been made a question of some importance, which is the best position for a patient to rest in who is labouring under the complaint before us, or has a striking tendency to it; as also what is the best formed couch for him to recline upon?

All seem to agree that the couch should be incompressible, or nearly so, in order that the weight of the body may be equally instead of unequally sustained, and not one part elevated and another depressed; and hence a mattress is judged preferable to a bed, and a plain board is by many esteemed preferable to a mattress. It is also very generally agreed, that the board or mattress should form an inclining plane, so that the body, placed directly on the back, may be kept perpetually on the stretch: while Dr. Dods maintains, in opposition to this general opinion, that the line should be horizontal, or even curved; that a position on the back is by no means necessary; and that a posture of extension cannot fail of being injurious, and adding to the strength or extent of the disease.

Either of these opinions may be right or wrong, according to the nature of the case; and hence neither of them can be correct as a universal proposition. Ease and refreshment are the great points to be obtained; and whatever couch or whatever position will give the largest proportion of these, is the couch or the position to be recommended, whether that of supine extension or relaxed flexure.*

Dr. Dods, who refers all kinds of lateral distortion to debility of the fibres of the extensor muscles, prescribes an extended position in every instance; and as already observed, recommends a curved relaxing couch in its stead, so that the patient may sink into it at his ease, instead of being put upon the stretch. The advice is good so far as the opinion is correct, and the disease is dependant upon debility of the extensor muscles alone; for here nothing can afford so much ease to the patient as such an indulgence. But it is not to be conceded that the fibrous structure of these muscles forms the seat of the disease in every case, and consequently the recommendation will not always apply; for the flexor muscles may be affected, or the debility be seated in the extensor ligaments, or the vertebral cartilages with which they are connected. I have at this moment under my care a lady just of age, who for four years past has been labouring under a slight affection of lateral distortion, feeling much more of it whenever she suffers fatigue, or is affected in her spirits. A position strictly supine, and somewhat extended, upon a hard mattress or a level floor, is the only posture that affords her ease, and takes off the sense of weight on the spine and oppression on the chest. She has often tried other positions, but in vain. To this, therefore, she has uniformly recourse after dinner, and occasionally, at other times in the day as well. Pure country air has also been of great service; but above all things, sea bathing. She has just returned from an excursion around the Devonshire coast. The first day's journey, though in a reclined position in an open landaulet, with every attention that could afford ease and accommodation, proved so fatiguing, and produced so much pain in the spine, that it was doubtful whether she would be able to proceed. A better night, however, than was expected, capacitated her for another trial, and the fatigue was considerably less: on the third or fourth day she had an opportunity of beginning to bathe; and by a daily perseverance in the same, was enabled, soon after reaching Teignmouth, to engage in long walks, climb its loftiest hills, and enjoy the entire scenery: her appetite became almost unbounded, and her flagging spirits were restored to vivacity.

It is hence perfectly clear, that while that position and that mode of dress are most to be

recommended which afford the highest degree of ease and comfort, gestation, pure air, sea-bathing, and every other kind of tonic, whether external or internal, are also of the utmost importance; and that perfect and continued rest, in whatever position it be tried, is far less efficacious than when interrupted by such motion as can be borne, though with some degree of fatigue, and the other tonic auxiliaries just adverted to. In extreme cases, indeed, such exercise as is here adverted to should be postponed till the debilitated and, most probably, irritable organs, have lost some part of their disease; yet the motion of friction or manipulation by a skilful and dexterous hand may still be adverted to, and should supply its place: and although the use of tight and girding stays cannot be too much reprobated as applied to growing girls in the full bloom and health of nature, and may well be accused as an occasional cause of the deformity before us; yet there is much soundness of judgment in Mr. Shaw's recommendation of a dress of this kind, capable of giving support without cramping the form by too close a lacing, in cases where the complaint has in any considerable degree established itself, and the mischief is not now to be warded off, but to be prevented from becoming worse. In this case stays may not only be allowed, but "they should be made sufficiently stiff and strong to sustain the weight, which the muscles that have been deteriorated by want of action are unable to support."—(*Further Illustrations on the Lateral or Serpentine Curvature of the Spine, &c.,* 8vo., 1825.) This, indeed, is the only mechanical aid that should be allowed; and if applied with caution, and without an uneasy restraint, they will often be found an auxiliary of great value.

SPECIES IV.
ENTASIA ARTICULARIS.
MUSCULAR STIFF-JOINT.

PERMANENT AND RIGID CONTRACTION OF ONE OR MORE ARTICULAR MUSCLES OR THEIR TENDONS.

THE joints of the limbs are as subject to muscular contractions as the neck, and in many instances from like causes: the following are the varieties of affection hereby produced:—

α Irritata.	From excess of action in
Spastic stiff-joint.	the muscles contracted.
β Atonica.	From direct atony in the
Atonic stiff-joint.	yielding muscles.
γ Inusitata.	From long confinement
Chronic stiff-joint.	or neglect of use.

Besides the ordinary causes of cold, inflammation, and strains, by which the first and second variety are produced, the former has sometimes followed a sudden fright.—(*Starke, Klin. Instit.,* p. 32.) Freind, also, mentions a case in which it has been cured by a fright (*Vit. Gabriel*); and Baldinger one in which it disappeared on the revival of a suppressed eruption which had given rise to it.—(*N. Magazin.,* band

---

* The figures of several machines, invented by Dr. Wm. Grigg, and which have proved extremely useful in treating distortions of the spine, may be seen in the Boston Med. and Surg. Journal, vol. xi., p. 228.—D.

xi., 78.) Rheumatism has often produced it, and particularly the second variety, in the joint of the knee and thigh-bone.

In a case of the latter kind, it was successfully attacked by Richter (*Chir. Bibl.*, band x., 219) with a cautery of a cylinder of cotton. In this and the third variety, much benefit is often derived from repeated and long-continued friction with a warm hand, or with some stimulant balsam or liniment. In an obstinate contraction of the fingers succeeding to a fractured arm, Dr. Eason relates an instance, in which the rigidity suddenly gave way to a pretty smart stroke of electricity after every other means had failed; and the patient had the use of his fingers from this time.—(*Edin. Med. Comment.*, v., p. 84.) Such exercise, moreover, or exertion of the limb, should be recommended, as it may bear without fatigue. The cold bath, as an antispasmodic, has sometimes been serviceable in the FIRST VARIETY,* and more frequently, as a tonic, in the SECOND.

Most men exhibit proofs of the THIRD VARIETY, or chronic stiff-joint, from a neglect of using many of their muscular powers: for nearly a fourth part of the voluntary muscles, from being seldom called into full and active exertion, acquire a stiffness which does not naturally belong to them; while many that by exercise might have been rendered perfectly pliant and obedient to the will, have lost all mobility, and are of no avail. Tumblers and buffoons are well aware of this fact, and it is principally by a cultivation of these neglected muscles that they are able to assume those outrageous postures and grimaces, and exhibit those feats of agility, which so often amuse and surprise us. It is a like cultivation that gives that measured grace and firmness, as well as erect position in walking, by which the soldier is distinguished from the clown; and that enables the musician to run with rapid execution, and the most delicate touch, over keys or finger-holes that call thousands of muscular fibres into play or into quick combinations of action, which in the untutored are stiff and immoveable, and cannot be forced into an imitation without the utmost awkwardness and fatigue.

SPECIES V.
ENTASIA SYSTREMMA:
CRAMP.

SUDDEN AND RIGID CONTRACTION AND CONVOLUTION OF ONE OR MORE MUSCLES OF THE BODY, MOSTLY OF THE STOMACH AND EXTREMITIES: VEHEMENTLY PAINFUL, BUT OF SHORT DURATION.

SYSTREMMA, literally "contortio, convolutio," "globus," is derived from συστρέφω, "contor-queo," "convolvo in fascem." Stremma, the

primary noun, is an established technical term for "strain, twist, wrench;" and the author has hence been induced to add the present term to the medical vocabulary in the sense now offered, for the purpose of superseding and getting rid of *crampus*, which has hitherto been commonly employed, though at the same time commonly reprobated, as a term intolerably barbarous, derived from the German krampf. The proper Latin term is, perhaps, "raptus nervorum;" whence opisthotonia or opisthotonos is denominated by the Latin writers "raptus supinus." But raptus is upon the whole of too general a meaning to be employed on the present occasion, unless with the inconvenience of another term combined with it.

The parts chiefly attacked with cramp are the calves of the legs, the neck, and the stomach. The common causes are sudden exposure to cold, drinking cold liquids during great heat and perspiration, eating cold cucurbitaceous fruits when the stomach is infirm and incapable of digesting them, the excitement of transferred gout, and overstretching the muscles of the limbs; in which last case it is an excess of reaction produced by the stimulus of too great an extension. Hence many persons are subject to it, and especially those of irritable habits, during the warmth and relaxation of a bed, and particularly towards the morning, when the relaxation is greatest, the accumulation of muscular or irritable power most considerable, and the extensor muscles of the legs are strained to their utmost length, to balance the action which the flexor muscles have gained over them during sleep. Cold night-air is also a common cause of cramp, and it is a still more frequent attendant upon swimming, in which we have the two causes united of cold and great muscular extension. An uneasy position of the muscles is also in many cases a sufficient cause of irritation; and hence we often meet with very painful cases of cramp in pregnant women, down the legs, or about the sides, or the hypogastrium.

When the hollow or membranous muscles are affected, they feel as though they were puckered and drawn to a point; the pain is agonizing, and generally produces a violent perspiration; and if the stomach be the affected organ, the diaphragm associates in the constriction, and the breathing is short and distressing. If the cramp be seated in the more fleshy muscles, they seem to be writhed and twisted into a hard knot; and a knotty induration is perceivable to the touch, accompanied with great soreness, which continues for a long time after the balance of power has been restored.

In common cases where the calves of the legs are affected, an excitement of the distressed muscles into their usual train of exertion is found sufficient; and hence most people cure themselves by suddenly rising into an erect position. I have often produced the same effect, and overcome the reaction without rising, by forcibly stretching out the affected leg by means of other muscles, whose united power overmatches that of the muscle that is contracted. Warm friction with the naked hand, or with

---

* In an example of this kind, brought on by a wound of one of the fingers, the editor applied a succession of blisters to the back of the hand and wrist; and the patient, a woman residing at Weybridge, was very soon enabled to extend her fingers again.

camphorated oil or alcohol, will also generally be found to succeed. A forcible exertion of some remote muscles, which thus collects and concentrates the irritable power in another quarter, will also frequently effect a cure ; and it is to this principle alone, I suppose, we are to refer the benefit which is said to arise from squeezing strenuously a roll of brimstone, which suddenly snaps beneath the hold. The brimstone snaps from the warmth of the hand applied to it ; but its only remedial power consists in affording a something for the hand to grasp vehemently, and thus excite a sudden change of action.

Where the stomach is affected, brandy, usquebaugh, ether, or laudanum, affords the speediest means of cure ; and it is often necessary to combine the laudanum with one or other of the preceding stimulants. Here also the external application of warmth, and diffusable irritants, as hot flannels moistened with the compound camphire liniment, are found in most cases peculiarly beneficial. Exciting a transfer of action to the extremities, as by bathing the feet in hot water, or applying mustard sinapisms to them, is frequently of great advantage ; as is the use of hot, emollient, and anodyne injections, whose palliative power reaches the seat of spasm by sympathetic diffusion, and often affords considerable quiet. Here, also, the patient should be particularly attentive to his diet and regimen, confining himself to such viands as are most easy of digestion, and least disposed to rouse the stomach to a return of these morbid and anomalous actions ; for a habit of recurrence is soon established, which it is difficult to break off.

In pregnancy, where the crampy spasms are often migratory and fugitive, the position should frequently be changed, so as to remove the stimulus of uneasiness by throwing the pressure upon some other set of muscles ; and if the stomach be affected with gout, opium, rhubarb, chalk, or aromatics, should be taken on going to rest.

The best preventives when the cause is constitutional, are warm tonics, and habituating the affected muscles to as much exercise as their strength will bear : and hence the same forcible extension used in swimming which produces cramp the first or second time of trial, will rarely do so afterward.

Cramp is also found as a symptom, and as one of the severest symptoms of the disease, in various species of colic and cholera ; in which cases it must be treated according to the methods already pointed out under those respective heads.

SPECIES VI.
ENTASIA TRISMUS.
LOCKED-JAW.

PERMANENT AND RIGID FIXATION OF THE MUSCLES OF THE LOWER JAW.

This disease is by the French writers called *tic*. The technical term is derived from the Greek τρίζω, "to gnash or grind the teeth ;" which, like the French synonyme, is supposed by the lexicographers to be an onomatopy, or a word formed from the sound that takes place in the act of gnashing.

In truth, it was to a disease in which morbid gnashing formed a symptom, that both the Greek and French term were originally applied ; for the trismus of the old writers consisted, not of a rigid, but convulsive or agitatory spasm of the lower jaw ; an affection comparatively trifling, and rarely to be met with, and when it does occur, appertaining to the CLONUS of the present system of nosology, the clonic spasm of authors in general. And the use of trismus or tic to import a state of muscle directly opposed to that which it first indicated, is another striking proof of the incongruous change which is perpetually occurring in the nomenclature of medicine, for the want of established rules and principles to give fixation and a definite sense to its respective terms.

Dr. Akerman is the only writer of reputation I am acquainted with in recent times who has used trismus in its original intention, or rather, who has united its original with its modern meaning. For he employs the term generically ; and arranges under it the two species of *trismus tonicus*, being that now under consideration, and *trismus clonicus*, or the disease it originally denoted. But this arrangement is uncalled for and inconvenient, and has not been received into general use ; the term trismus being, with every writer of the present day, limited to the first of these two species alone, notwithstanding the origin of the word. And hence, as it is so generally and completely understood, there would be an affectation in changing it for any other. The Germans call it kinnbakkenzwange, which is precisely parallel with the LOCKED-JAW of our own tongue.

Dr. Cullen, in the first edition of his Nosology, made trismus and tetanus, our next species, distinct genera ; but he altered his opinion before the publication of his First Lines, and regarded them as nothing more than degrees or varieties even of the same species. "From the history of the disease," says he, "it will be evident, that there is no room for distinguishing the tetanus, opisthotonos, and trismus or locked-jaw, as different *species* of this disease, since they all arise from the same causes, and are almost constantly conjoined in the same person." —(*Pract.*, *of Phys.*, book iii., sect. i., chap. i., § 1267.) In consequence of which, in the later editions of Dr. Cullen's Synopsis, in which the supposed error is attempted to be corrected, the disease is introduced with a very singular departure from nosological method : for first, tetanus is employed as the term for a distinct genus, defined " a spastic rigidity of many muscles ;" and next, under this generic division are given no species whatever, but two varieties of degree alone ; to the first of which is again applied the name of TETANUS, defined "the half or whole of the body affected with spasms," and to the second that of TRISMUS, defined "spastic rigidity, chiefly of the lower jaw."

Passing by this irregularity of method, the proper view of the subject seems to lie in a middle course; in contemplating trismus and tetanus, not as distinct genera, or mere varieties of a single disease, but as distinct species of a common genus; and under this view it is contemplated in the present arrangement. Trismus bears the same relation to tetanus as synochus does to typhus: the two former, like the two latter, may proceed from a common cause and require a similar treatment; and the first may terminate in the last. But trismus, like synochus, may run its course alone, and continue limited to its specific symptoms. And as Dr. Cullen has thought proper to make synochus and typhus distinct genera, he ought at least to have ranked trismus and tetanus as distinct species.

Trismus is found in all ages, sexes, temperaments, and climates. In warm climates, however, it occurs far more frequently than in cold; and chiefly in the hottest of warm climates. Dr. Cullen observes, that the middle-aged are most susceptible of the disease, men more so than women, and the robust and vigorous than the weakly. Other animals are subject to this complaint as well as man, particularly parrots; and from many of the causes (*Bajon. Abhandlungen von Krankheit. auf der Insel Cayenne,* &c.) that affect the human race.

These causes, for the most part, are chilliness and damp operating upon the body when heated, and hence sudden vicissitudes of heat and cold; wounds, punctures, lacerations, or other irritations of nerves in any part of the body; whence it has not unfrequently followed venesection when unskilfully performed (*Delaroche, Journ. de Med.,* tom. xv., p. 213; *Forestus,* lib. x., obs. iii.; *Schenck,* obs. 1., i., N. 250), and still more frequently amputation, worms, or irritation in the stomach and bowels, especially in those of infants. We have thus the three following varieties offered to us, which, however, chiefly differ in symptoms peculiar to the period of life in which the disease is most disposed to show itself, or in the interval between the casual excitement and the spastic action:—

a Nascentium. Locked-jaw of infancy. — Attacking infants during the first fortnight after birth.

β Algidus. Catarrhal locked-jaw. — Occurring at all ages, after exposure to cold and damp, especially the dew of the evening, the symptoms usually appearing within two or three days.

γ Traumaticus. Traumatic locked-jaw. — Occurring as the consequence of a wound, pnucture, or ulcer, with particular frequency in hot climates; and rarely appearing till ten days or a fortnight after local affection.

The pathology is highly difficult, if not mysterious, and has hence been purposely avoided by most preceding writers. Dr. Cullen expressly avows that he "cannot in any measure attempt it."—(*Pract. of Phys.,* book iii., sect. i., chap. i., § 1269.) There is one principle, however, to which I have frequently had occasion to direct the reader's attention, which will help us in a considerable degree to develop something of its obscurity, and to account more especially for so remote a separation between the seat of primary irritation and that of spasmodic excitement, which constitutes, perhaps, its most embarrassing feature. The principle I allude to is the sympathy that prevails throughout the whole of any chain of organs, whether continuous or distinct, engaged in a common function, and which is particularly manifest at its extremities; so that let a morbid action commence in whatever part of the chain it may, the extremities in many instances become the chief seat of distress, and even of danger. We had occasion to notice this law of the animal economy when treating of PARAPSIS ILLUSORIA, or that imaginary sense of feeling and of acute pain in a limb that has been amputated and is no longer a part of the body, which we referred to the principle before us; and farther noticed, by way of illustration, the pain often suffered at the glans penis from the mechanical irritation of the neck of the bladder by a calculus. So, irritating the fauces with a feather excites the stomach, and even the diaphragm, to a spasmodic action, and the contents of the organ are rejected. Irritating the ileum, as in ileac passion, produces the same effect upon the stomach and œsophagus; at the same time that the other extremity of the canal is attacked with rigid spasm, and consequently with obstinate costiveness: while in cholera both extremities are affected in a like way, and we have hence both purging and vomiting. It is to the same principle we are to ascribe it, that when the surface of the body is suddenly chilled, as on plunging into a cold bath, the bladder becomes irritated, and evacuates the contained urine: and in treating of MARASMUS we had occasion to show, that while in one of its species the disease seems to commence in the digestive, and in another in the assimilating organs, constituting the extreme ends of a very long and complicated chain of action, it very generally happens, that at which end soever the decay commences, the opposite end is very soon affected equally.

In a continued chain of nervous fibres, however, this principle of sympathy, which induces remote parts, and particularly remote extremities, to associate in the same morbid action, is peculiarly conspicuous. Hence, if a long muscle be lacerated in any part of its belly, the tendinous terminations are often the chief seat of suffering. As the ulnar nerve sends off twigs from the elbow to supply the forearm and fingers, a blow on the internal condyle of the humerus gives a tremulous sensation through the forearm and hand: and as the ulnar nerve itself is only an offset from a plexus or commissure of the cervical nerves, which also give a large branch to the scapula, a paralysis of the ring or little finger has sometimes been removed by stimulating the scapular extremity by a caustic applied at the internal angle of the scapula. In inflammation of the liver, a severe pain is often felt at the top of the shoulder; and in palpitation of the heart, at the left orifice of the stomach.

Both these are to be accounted for by recollect-ing that the radiations of the phrenic nerve ex-tend in an upper line to the shoulder, and in a lower to the diaphragm, which constitutes its extreme points; and that one of its branches passes over the apex of the heart. Now as the under surface of the diaphragm participates, from its contiguity, in an inflammation of the liver, the top of the shoulder suffers, as forming the extreme point of the phrenic chain by which these organs are connected; and as the upper surface of the diaphragm is in direct contact with the left and very sensible orifice of the stomach, an uneasiness at the apex of the heart becomes the cause of irritation to this orifice in consequence of its connexion with the dia-phragm, and hence, of necessity, with the lower branch of the phrenic nerve at its extreme dis-tribution.

These remarks apply with particular force to the disease before us, and many others of the same class with which it has a close analogy, as tetanus, lyssa, and hemicrania. And although, from the intricacy of the intersections and decus-sations with which various nerves pursue their radiating courses, it is impossible for us, in many instances, to determine why one line of connex-ion suffers while another remains unaffected; yet in most instances we may be able, by an accurate survey, to trace the catenation, and hence to obtain some insight into the physiology of these exquisitely curious and complicated dis-orders.

In mapping the nervous ramifications which give rise to trismus or locked-jaw, we must re-gard the ganglionic system, consisting of the various branches of the intercostal trunk, and the numerous branches which unite with it from the whole line of the spinal marrow, as consti-tuting the centre; and as from this centre we perceive ramifications radiating in every direc-tion to the face, the entire length of the back, the upper and lower limbs, and the thoracic and abdominal viscera, we see a foundation laid, even by a continuous chain, for an association of re-mote parts and even extreme points in morbid changes, though we may not be able, satisfacto-rily perhaps, in any instance, to trace out the in-dividual line by which the diseased action is carried forward, and to separate it from other lines with which it is inextricably interwo-ven. Thus, in the case of *trismus nascen-tium*, forming the first variety under the present species, the irritation of the nerves of the stom-ach, which is very clearly the primary seat of disease in most cases, is propagated directly to the central branches of the ganglionic system by the tributary offsets which the stomach receives from it. But we have already observed, that the chief contribution to this grand junction canal is derived from the intercostal nerve itself. In the first instance, an arm from the trigeminus or fifth pair of nerves, two branch-es of which radiate upwards, constitute the maxillaris superior and maxillaris inferior, and are lost in the muscles of the jaws: so that the upper extremity of the nervous line distribu-ted over the stomach is the nerves of the jaws

themselves; while various branches of the fifth occasionally unite with the portio dura, or respi-ratory trunk of the seventh pair, which divari-cates not only to the diaphragm, but over all the muscles that have the remotest connexion with the respiratory system. And hence, agreeably to the law of the animal economy we have just pointed out, the muscles of the jaws, forming this extremity in the chain of morbid action, are the organs in which we may expect an irritation of the nerves of the stomach in various instances to manifest itself most strikingly.

In like manner we may account for the second and third varieties of trismus, or that produced by a chilly dampness or irritative vio-lence applied to the upper or lower extremities: for as these are all supplied by nerves from the vertebral source, which, we have already re-marked, gives off branches from every aperture in the spine to the ganglionic system, and as this system, at its upper end, terminates in the maxillary branches of the fifth pair of nerves, the muscles into which these nerves are distrib-uted constitute one extreme point of a long chain of nervous action, while those of the up-per and lower limbs constitute the other. And hence the same law which produces a spastic fixation of these muscles in certain irritations of the stomach, may reasonably be expected to operate with like effect in certain irritations of the upper and lower limbs. And as the inter-costal nerve, at its first rise from the common source of itself and the maxillary branches, re-ceives also, in its progress, offsets from the sixth, seventh, eighth, and ninth pairs of cere-bral nerves, as well as from all the vertebral, and as all these, in consequence of such an in-terunion and decussation, are sending forth branches over the muscles of the back, the chest, and the thorax, there is no difficulty in conceiving, when a rigid spasm has once commenced in the lower jaw, why it should be propagated through any of the muscles apper-taining to these parts of the system, or even originate in them from any of the causes that excite locked-jaw, and hence lay a foundation for tetanus as well as trismus, both as a primary and a secondary disease. And I have touched upon this subject now, that we may not have to repeat the present explanation when treating of tetanus in its proper place.[*]

---

* See Cloquet, Traité d'Anatomie Descriptive. Bock Beschreibung des fünften Nervenpaares und seiner Verbindungen mit anderen Nerven, vorzug-lich mit dem Ganglien Systeme, Leips., 1817. The whole of the above hypothesis is only an at-tempt to explain the origin and extension of teta-nic disorders, by the intricate communications of the nerves of different parts of the body. The view of the pathology of tetanic affections enter-tained by Dr. Elliotson is, that they depend upon a peculiar state of that part of the brain, or spinal marrow, which is immediately connected with the nerves of the voluntary muscles. The mind is unaffected, and so is sensibility. The disorder appears to be an affection of the voluntary mus-cles through the medium of the voluntary nerves, and those parts of the brain and spinal marrow with which they are connected.—See Dr. Elliot-

In the simplest state of trismus, indeed, there is some degree of stiffness found at the back of the neck, and even in the sternum. The disease, in some cases, shows itself with sudden violence, but more usually advances gradually; till at length the muscles that pull up the jaw become so rigid, and set the teeth so closely together, that they do not admit of the smallest opening.

In tropical climates, for Dr. Cullen's remark that it is most common to the middle-aged, only applies to the temperate regions of Europe, children are particularly subject to this complaint, and with a few peculiarities, which, though producing no specific difference, are sufficient to establish a variety. The disease in this case is vulgarly known by the absurd name of FALLING OF THE JAW. It occurs chiefly between the ninth and fourteenth day from birth; seldom after the latter period. Without any febrile accession, and often without any perceptible cause whatever, the infant sinks into an unnatural weariness and drowsiness, attended with frequent yawnings, and with a difficulty, at first slight, of moving the lower jaw, which last symptom takes place in some instances sooner, in others later. Even while the infant is yet able to open its mouth, there is, occasionally, an inability to suck or swallow. By degrees, the lower jaw becomes rigid, and totally resists the introduction of food. There is no painful sensation; but the skin assumes a yellow hue, the eyes appear dull, the spasms often extend over the body, and in two or three days the disease proves mortal.

The ordinary cause is irritation in the intestinal canal. Hence viscid and acrimonious meconium frequently produces it; as worms are said also to do some months after birth. It seems, moreover, in some instances, to have followed from irritation in tying the navel-string,[*] its not being properly attended to afterward, in which case, though the stomach may be affected by contiguous sympathy, the disease makes a near approach to the third or traumatic variety. Yet the appearance of the spastic action is as early as where the stomach is primarily affected.

In cold and even mountainous countries, this variety is also sometimes found. " I am informed," says Dr. Cullen, " of its frequently occurring in the Highlands of Scotland; but I never met with any instance of it in the low country."—(Loc. citat., § 1281.) Whether, according to the conjecture of this celebrated writer, it is more common to some districts than to others, has not been sufficiently determined. "It seems," says he, "to be more frequent in Switzerland than in France." Hot climates, however, constitute its principal domain; and hence it is not very surprising, that

Bajon should place one of its chief residences at Cayenne (Bajon, Abhandlung von Krankheit. auf der Insel Cayenne, &c., Erp. 1781), or that Akerman should assert it to be endemic in Guinea.

In the SECOND VARIETY of the disease, or that proceeding from cold or night dew, the symptoms often appear within a day or two after exposure to the exciting cause. It is not common that the spasm extends to the muscles of the chest or back, so as to produce tetanus, though there is often an uneasy sensation at the root of the tongue, with some difficulty in swallowing liquids after their introduction into the mouth; the disease thus making an approach towards lyssa, or canine madness, in its symptoms, as we have just endeavoured to show that it does in its physiology. According to the observations of Baron Larrey, indeed, this approach is in many instances very considerable; for he informs us, that on post-obituary examinations he has often found the pharynx and œsophagus much contracted, and their internal membranes red, inflamed, and covered with a viscid reddish mucus. Dr. Hennen, however, does not place much dependance upon any such appearances: he admits, nevertheless, that they are to be traced occasionally, though he ascribes them more to an increased flow of blood, consequent on increased action, than to any other cause.—(Principles of Military Surgery, 246.)

In this variety, from the slighter nature of its attack, the patient not unfrequently recovers by skilful medical treatment, and there are unquestionably instances of spontaneous recovery (Briot, Hist. de la Chirurgie Militaire en France, &c., 8vo., Besançon, 1817), though cases of this kind are very rare. The intellect remains unaffected, there is little quickness of the pulse, sometimes none whatever, and little or no disorder of any kind, though the bowels are usually very costive. If the patient pass the fourth or fifth day, we may begin to have hopes of him; for the spasmodic constriction will then frequently remit or intermit; but as, even in the last case, it is apt to return at uncertain intervals, there is still a considerable danger for many days longer.

When, as in the THIRD VARIETY, the disease proceeds from a nerve irritated by a wound[*] or

---

son's Lectures on Medicine, as delivered at the Univ. of London, and reported in Med. Gaz. for 1832–3, p. 470.—ED.

* Two cases of trismus, arising from this cause, have occurred in the practice of Dr. Francis; in one of these there was considerable hemorrhage from the cord.—D.

* Trismus traumaticus sometimes follows surgical operations, and very frequently lacerated wounds of the fingers, toes, and other tendinous parts. The editor has seen several cases of it brought on by gunshot injuries, amputation, castration; and he knew of one instance in which it was induced by the amputation of a cancerous breast. In warm climates it occurs from very slight causes, and hence is much more frequent in them than in temperate and cold countries. A wound will sometimes not produce the disease till the person is suddenly exposed to cold, and then he will have it immediately. Last autumn, the editor saw an example of this in a farmer, who had met with a lacerated wound of the scalp, by being thrown from his horse: from this accident he was recovering in the most favourable way; but on going out into the cold air, at the end of a

sore, the spasmodic symptoms are much later in showing themselves; and sometimes do not make their appearance till eight or nine days afterward, occasionally, indeed, not at all till the wound is healed.. The disease is more dangerous in proportion to the delay; the adjoining muscles of the face become more affected, and, as is already observed, the spasms often shoot downward into the back or chest, and trismus is complicated with tetanus. The breathing is nasal and abrupt, the accents are interrupted and slow, and uttered by the same avenue; the muscles of the nose, lips, mouth, and the whole of the face, are violently dragged and distorted, and the patient sinks from nervous exhaustion and want of nutriment, the jawbone being set so fast that it will often break rather than give way to mechanical force.

The disease, from this cause, is generally fatal; and we are indebted to the ingeniousness of Sir James M'Grigor and Dr. Hennen for a confession that, whatever remedies were employed in the British army, whether in India or in Spain, the mortality was nearly the same. But as the treatment of the present variety and the ensuing species should be founded on a like principle, we shall reserve this subject till we have entered upon a distinct history of the latter.

SPECIES VII.
ENTASIA TETANUS.
TETANUS.

PERMANENT AND RIGID FIXATION OF MANY OR ALL THE VOLUNTARY MUSCLES; WITH INCURVATION OF THE BODY, AND DYSPNŒA.

TETANUS is derived from τεταίνω, which itself is a derivative from τείνω, "tendo, extendo." Like trismus, it is a term common to the early Greek writers, among whom it was used synonymously with opisthotonos and emprosthotonos, though the two latter were afterward employed to express two distinct modifications of the disease.

From peculiarities in the seat or mode of its attack, this species offers us the four following varieties :—

---

fortnight, when the wound was nearly healed, he was attacked with trismus, which soon assumed the form of universal tetanus, and he died in about six or seven days from the commencement of the disorder. Tetanus occurs in all conditions of wounds; in some of a healthy, and others of an unhealing appearance: sometimes also when they are almost, or even entirely, healed up. It occurs, too, whether the wound be large or small. Dr. Elliotson had a case of tetanus, as severe as any he ever saw, where there had been merely a contusion of the thumb. There was no pain, no irritation; the nail was separated and loose, but under it all was dry, and no secretion was going on. A case is mentioned in the Trans. of the Lond. Med. Society, in which the disease occurred after a burn, at the time when there was merely a dry scab on the leg, and no inflammation around it; nay, as Dr. Elliotson observes, the disease has sometimes declined and ceased, while the wound every day grew worse and worse. In Egypt, the wounded of the French army were

a Anticus. Tetanic procurvation.	Tetanus of the flexor muscles. The body rigidly bent forwards.
β Dorsalis. Tetanic recurvation.	Tetanus of the extensor muscles. The body rigidly bent backward.
γ Lateralis. Tetanic transcurvation.	Tetanus of the lateral muscles. The body rigidly bent laterally.
δ Erectus. Tetanic inflexibility of the body.	Tetanus of both the posterior and anterior muscles. The body rigidly erect.

The FIRST of these VARIETIES is the emprosthotonos of early writers; the SECOND the opisthotonos; the THIRD the pleurosthotonos of authors of a later date; the FOURTH the proper tetanus of Dr. Lionel Clarke and a few others. To these varieties it has been usual to add the singular disease called catochus; which by Sauvages, Cullen, and various other authorities, is regarded as closely connected with this species. It has a near affinity to it unquestionably, and hence, out of deference to concurrent opinions, it was suffered to stand as a variety of tetanus in the first edition of the author's Nosology; but with a note intimating that it seems rather to belong to the genus CARUS of the fourth order of the present class, and to be a modification of the species ECSTASIS, under that genus: and as this appears to be its proper place, it will now be found arranged there accordingly.

The general physiology, so far as it seems capable of elucidation, has been already given under the preceding species; the proximate cause being that of a peculiar irritation of a certain chain or association of nerves, chiefly operating with the greatest violence at the two extremities of the morbid line. This irritation seems, in many instances, to consist in inflammation; and hence is made a common cause by many of the most valuable writers of the present day. Professor Frank seems first to have started the idea, and he has been followed in succession by Dr. Saunders of Edinburgh, Dr. Chisholm, Dr. James Thomson, and Dr. Abercrombie, who have been upheld in Italy by MM. Brera, Rachetti, and Bergamaschi, and in France by M. Esquirol. Bergamaschi* advances, indeed, so far as to maintain, that where

---

found by Larrey to be safe from traumatic tetanus, if they were not attacked by it before the sixteenth day. Sir Gilbert Blane has known the disease commence at all periods of a wound between the second day and the end of the fourth week. In Spain and Portugal, Sir James M'Grigor found the twenty-second day the limit. Dr. Murray relates an instance in which a midshipman trod on a rusty nail one evening at nine o'clock; and, after exposing himself to the cold night air in keeping watch, had tetanic symptoms on the following morning at eight o'clock.—(See Lond. Med. Gaz. for 1832-3, p. 623.) In hot countries the disease has been known to follow a local injury directly after its occurrence.—ED.

* Osservazioni Medico-pratiche sul Tetano. Giornale di Medicina practica del Sig. Cons. e Prof. Cav. V. L. Brera.

wounds themselves, of whatever form, are the remote cause, a neurostenia,' as he calls it, or inflammatory affection of the nerves, is still the proximate cause; extending itself from the wounded part, by the nervous extremities, to the spinal marrow and the brain, or, *vice versâ*, from the brain to the spinal marrow and principal nerves, and thence to the parts that are subservient to locomotion. Dissection, however, is very far from giving proofs of such inflammatory change in every instance; while in many cases the disease is of too fugitive a character, and makes its seizure or its disappearance too rapidly, for the more measured progress of inflammation.*

The exciting causes are also for the most part those of TRISMUS; though it appears in infancy far less frequently, unless as a concomitant of that disease. Damp and cold, therefore, and simple nervous irritation from wounds† or sores in hot climates and crowded hospitals, are the chief sources of its production; and where these accessories exist, terror seems to be a powerful auxiliary, and has alone, in some instances, been sufficient for its production. "Passion or terror," says Dr. Hennen, "after wounds and operations, has been known to produce the disease in some; and sympathy, though a rare cause, in others." It is said also to have been produced by insolation or exposure to the direct rays of the sun (*Pathol.*, lib. v., p. 372); and has unquestionably followed, as M. Magendie and numerous other French authors (*Desportes, Raffenean, Fonquier, Dupuy*) have abundantly shown, from various irritant narcotics, as strychnine, or the active principle of nux vomica, as

---

* Dissections reveal no appearance of any regular or constant description in the bodies of persons who die of tetanus. In most cases nothing remarkable is met with; and hence the best modern pathologists all agree, that when morbid changes are noticed, they are not essential, but incidental. Sometimes there are traces of inflammation of the spinal marrow; though if the weather be hot and the body not examined promptly, the coverings of the spinal marrow will look red, though no inflammation may have existed in it.—ED.

† Dr. Armstrong mentions that one of his friends, who had had extensive experience in hot climates, never knew a case of tetanus occur without local injury; and he was led to believe that such was the fact by a careful examination of the whole surface of the body.—(See Lectures on the Morbid Anatomy, Nature, and Treatment of Acute and Chronic Diseases, p. 742, 8vo., Lond, 1834.) There can be no doubt, however, that many cases of tetanus are idiopathic, and not traumatic, and that we know that the latter are infinitely more difficult to control, and more frequently fatal. Dr. Armstrong states that the local injuries which most frequently produce tetanus are those which are accompanied with friction. Lacerated or punctured wounds of tendinous parts, injuries of the fingers, thumb, or toes; dislocations, especially compound ones; burns, scalds, and ulcers, may be exciting causes of traumatic tetanus; and what is remarkable, the disorder may come on, as already noticed, when the wound or sore is healing, or nearly healed. It may be produced by the irritation of a seton, an issue, the partial division of a nerve or the inclusion of it in a ligature.—ED.

also from galvanism, when raised to a sufficient power for the purpose.

LATERAL TETANUS is very rarely to be met with, and seems to be rather a chronic than an acute malady. Fernelius, who first described it (*Med. Obs. and Inq.*, vol. vi.), gives a case in which it occurred annually, but only in the winter, during which season the patient had two or three paroxysms daily: the head was first attacked with a peculiar vibratory feeling, which gradually descended to the neck, with a sensation of cold; and by the time it reached the scapula was immediately succeeded by symptoms of opisthotonos, and afterward of lateral contraction; during which the mind and external senses were unaffected, but the flexor muscles were so firmly fixed, that no antagonist force of the bystanders was able to overpower the contortion.

Nor are the other varieties nearly so frequent as trismus, except where they form a subsequent part of the general chain of morbid action. My observant friend, Dr. Hennen, confesses that, during the whole period of his superintending the British hospitals in Spain, he never met with but one case of emprosthotonos, and even this he describes as an incurvation that rather approached it than constituted the disease itself. "It was observed," says he, "at the same time and in the same hospital, with the various degrees of trismus: rigid spasms of almost every muscle of the body, and violent periodical convulsions, all from similar injuries to that in which it was produced."—(*Military Surgery*, p. 247, 8vo., Edin., 1820.)

From the complicated manner, indeed, in which tetanus shows itself, and its anomalous attack upon different sets of muscles at the same time, it seems in many instances to put all the subordinate divisions of classification at defiance. It is, in truth, for the most part, a mixed disease, affecting various and opposite sets of muscles; and this in many cases so equally, that the spastic action of the flexors just balancing that of the extensors, "the patient," to adopt the language of Dr. Lionel Clarke, "seems often to be braced between opposite contractions." It is to this form, indeed, that this last very intelligent writer has limited the name of tetanus, as that to which it applies most emphatically. Like Dr. Hennen, he asserts that he had never seen a single case of genuine emprosthotonos; and that of the other two varieties of which he treats, the opisthotonos and proper tetanus, the former occurs most frequently.*

In opisthotonos, or TETANIC RECURVATION, the symptoms sometimes show themselves suddenly, but more commonly advance slowly and

---

* According to Baron Larrey, who had extensive opportunities of seeing tetanus while he was serving with the French army in Egypt, it appears that in that country, when the wound was in the back, tetanus commonly assumed the form of opisthotonos; but if the wound happened to be in the anterior part of the trunk, and tetanus followed, the latter was generally in the shape of emprosthotonos. Sir Gilbert Blane published two cases, where the side of the body on which the local injury was situated became the seat of tetanic disorder.—ED.

imperceptibly, the patient mistaking the uneasy stiffness which he feels about the shoulders and cervical region for a crick in the neck, produced by cold and rheumatism. The. stiffness, however, increasing, he finds it impossible to turn his head on either side without turning his body : he cannot open his jaws without pain, and he has some difficulty in swallowing. A spastic and aching traction now suddenly darts at times towards the ensiform cartilage, and thence strikes through to the back, augmenting all the previous symptoms to such a degree, that the patient is no longer able to support himself, and is compelled to take to his bed. The pathognomonic symptom in this variety is the spasm under the sternum, which is perpetually increasing in vehemence ; and instead of returning, as at first, once in two or three hours, returns now every ten or fifteen minutes. Immediately after which all the host of concomitant contractions renew their violence, and with additional severity : the head is forcibly retracted, and the jaws snap with a fixation that rarely allows them to be afterward opened wide enough to admit the little finger. This vehemence of paroxysm may not, perhaps, last longer than for a few minutes or even seconds ; but the spastic action prevails so considerably, even through the intervals, that it is difficult for an attendant to bend the contorted limbs into any thing like an easy or reclined position.* The breathing is quick and laborious ; and the pulse, though calm and less hurried, small and irregular. The face is sometimes pale, but oftener flushed ; the tongue stiff and torpid, but not much furred ; the whole countenance evinces the most marked signs of deep distress ; and swallowing is pertinaciously abstained from, as accompanied with great difficulty, and often producing a sudden renewal of the paroxysms. The last stage of the disease is truly pitiable. The spasms return every minute, and scarcely allow a moment's remission. The anterior muscles join in the spastic action, but the power of the posterior is still dominant ; and hence, while every organ is literally on the rack from the severity of the antagonism, the spine is more strongly recurvated than ever, and forms an arch over the bed, so that the patient rests only on the back part of the head and on the heels. During the exacer-

batlon of the spasms, the lower extremities, even while they continue rigid, are so violently jerked that the utmost attention is necessary to prevent the patient from being projected from his bed : and Desportes gives a case, in which both the thigh bones were broken from the violent contraction of the flexor muscles during a momentary remission of the extensors (*Hist. des Maladies de .St. Domingue*, ii., p. 171) ; similar results to which we shall have occasion to notice hereafter.

The tongue is in like manner darted spasmodically out of the mouth, and the teeth snapped suddenly and with great force ; so that unless a spoon covered with soft rags, or some other intervening substance, is introduced between the teeth at such periods, the tongue must be miserably bitten and lacerated.* The exertion is so laborious, that the patient sweats as in a hot bath ; and the heat has in some instances been raised to 110° Fahrenheit. The pulse is at this time small and irregular ; the heart throbs so violently that its palpitations may be seen ; the eyes are sometimes watery and languid, but more commonly rigid and immoveable in their sockets ; the nostrils are drawn upward, and the cheeks backward towards the ears, so that the whole countenance assumes the air of a cynic spasm or sardonic grin, while a limpid or bloody froth bubbles from the lips. There is sometimes delirium, but this is not common : the patient is worn out under this laborious agony in a few hours ; though more usually a general convulsion comes to his relief, and he sinks suddenly under its assault.

In the ERECT TETANUS, in which there is a balance of spastic action between the anterior and posterior sets of muscles, the progress of the disease is not essentially different. The march of the spastic action, however, varies in some degree, as we have already observed, in almost every instance, from trismus to tetanus, and from one modification of tetanus to another : yet the course we have now described is that which chiefly takes place where the disease advances in something of a regular and uninterrupted progress. Its danger and duration are commonly to be estimated from the degree of violence of the incursion. Where this is very severe, the patient rarely survives the third day, and is sometimes cut off on the second, or even in six-and-thirty or four-and-twenty hours. But where the attack is less acute, the patient may continue to suffer for a week before he reaches his tragic termination. If he have strength enough to survive the ninth day, he commonly recovers ; for the paroxysms diminish in violence, the intervals of remission are longer, and the muscles being generally more relaxed, he is able to take a little nourishment. Through the whole period there is an obstinate costiveness ; partly from want of food in the stomach, but chiefly from an association of the mouths of the

---

* One symptom, very characteristic of the disease, is the pain at the scrobiculus cordis. As Dr. Elliotson observes in his invaluable Lectures on the Practice of Medicine, it is a pain not increased pressure, but a sudden, violent, sharp, stabbing ~~pain~~ ; it may be more or less constant, but at periods ~~it~~ is exceedingly severe. Then the spasmodic rigidity of the muscles is constant, not convulsive ; not a spasm alternating with relaxation. The peculiar posture into which the body is drawn in opisthotonos, emprosthotonos, and pleurosthotonos, and the closed or nearly closed state of the jaw in trismus, without any inflammation, or any organic disease near the part to account for such closure, are all so many circumstances throwing light on the diagnosis. There is no terror in this disease, no excitement of mind, no morbid corporeal sensibility, no fear of noise, light, a current of air, &c., as in hydrophobia.—Ed.

* The muscles of the fingers are observed to remain unaffected, even in the latest stage of the disorder. Sometimes, but not invariably, the sphincter ani is so violently contracted that it is difficult to administer a clyster.—Ed.

intestinal excernents in the spasmodic constriction.*

The general principle of cure is far more easily expressed than carried into execution. It is that of taking off the local irritation, wherever such exists, and of tranquillizing the nervous erethism of the entire system. The first of these two objects is of great importance in the locked-jaw or trismus of infants ; for by removing the viscid and acrimonious meconium, or whatever other irritant is lodged in the stomach or bowels, we can sometimes effect a speedy cure without any other medicine. Castor-oil is by far the best aperient on this occasion, and it may be given both by the mouth and in injections. But if this do not succeed, we should have recourse to powerful anodynes ; and of these the best by far is opium, which should be administered from three to five drops in a dose, according to the age of the patient. Musk and the host of antispasmodics have been tried so often with so little succes, that it is not worth while to put the smallest dependance upon them; nor has the warm or cold bath produced effects sufficiently general or decisive to allow us to lose any time in trusting to their operation. They may be employed, however, as auxiliaries ; but our sheet-anchor must be opium ; which, if the spastic action have made much advance when we first see the patient, should instantly be employed in conjunction with the prescribed aperient. By taking off the constriction from the intestinal canal, and thus restoring and quickening the peristaltic motion, it may even expedite the dejections.

In trismus or tetanus from wounds or sores, the local irritation is not so easily subdued ; nor is its removal of so much importance, though in no case of small moment. But generally speaking, the spastic action is in these instances as much dependant upon constitutional as upon topical irritability ; and when it has been once excited it will run through its career, whether the local cause continue or not. It is owing chiefly to this fact, that the best and most active plan of cure so often fails of success ; and the most cautious practitioners hesitate in their prognostications, whatever be the march of symptoms, for the first four or five days. "From the state of the pulse," says Dr. Hennen, "I have derived no clew to either the proper treatment or the probable event : it has, in the cases I have met with, been astonishingly unaffected. From the state of the skin, I have been left equally in the dark. Sweating, which some have imagined critical, I have seen during the whole course of the disease, and attended with the most pungent and peculiar smell ; while in others it has never appeared

at all : and suppuration, which is generally interrupted, I have seen continue unaffected by the spasms. Even the process of healing, which, it would be reasonable to conclude, should be altogether put a stop to, has gone on apparently uninfluenced by the disease : and in the most severe case I ever saw, which occurred after a shoulder-joint amputation, sent into Elvas from before the lines of Badajos, the life of the patient and the perfect healing of the wound were terminated on the same day." So powerfully does the constitutional irritability operate in many cases after the disease has once displayed its hideous features, and render the local treatment of subordinate importance.

In numerous instances, however, a change in the condition of the wound has produced a beneficial result ; and hence various means have been resorted to for the purpose of effecting such a change, as local bleeding, anodyne applications to allay the morbid sensibility, resinous, terebinthinate, or mercurial stimulants to excite a new action, and amputation of the diseased limb. The first of these three plans is the ordinary mode of practice, and in full plethoric habits it has sometimes proved favourable ; the second plan seems to have been very generally employed by Baron Larrey, who occasionally used stimulants of a far higher power, as pencilling the wound with lunar caustic, or an application of the actual cautery. It is upon this principle of counter-irritation that advantage has sometimes been derived from needle-puncturing, of which the periodical journals have lately furnished us with various examples (London Med. Repos., vol. xx., p. 403, case furnished by Mr. Finch) ; and, by the French pathologists, from an employment of strychnine or the active alkaline part of nux vomica, where the disease has not been primarily induced by this irritant.—(M. Coze, Remarques sur la Nux Vomique, &c.) Amputation seems to have answered in a few cases, if we may give full credit to those who have chiefly tried and recommended it ;* but it is at best a clumsy and desperate kind of remedy ; and for reasons already assigned, must be often altogether inefficient if it do not add to the constitutional erethism.

The general treatment has consisted in a free use of opium, salivation, the bot or cold bath, and wine or ardent spirits, in some instances so far as to produce intoxication. Dr. Cross gives a case in which, after other medicines had been used in vain, and every hope seemed to fail, the patient was inebriated with spirits, and kept in this state for ten days, with

---

* If tetanus arise from a wound, the result is generally fatal. It is an observation made by Dr. Parry, that in tetanus, if the pulse be not above 100 or 110 on the fourth or fifth day of the attack, the patient mostly recovers; but that when the pulse is quicker than this in the early stages, the issue is commonly unfortunate. The danger generally lessens in proportion to the protracted duration of the disorder.—ED.

* Silvester, Med. Obs. and Inq., i., art. i. White, Med. Obs. and Inq., ii., art. xxxiv. Mr. Liston amputated in a case of tetanus from laceration of a branch of the median nerve distributed to the thumb; but though partial relief followed, the patient died. After the operation, it was wished to let the stump bleed for a time ; but not more than eight ounces of blood could be thus obtained, and only one vessel was tied. "Could this arise," says Mr. Liston, "from the coats of the vessels partaking in some measure of the general rigidity and contraction ?"—See Edin. Med. Journ., No. lxxix., p. 292.—ED.

the result of a perfect recovery.—(*Thomson's Annals of Philosophy.*) A generous use of wine appears to be almost indispensable,* and considering the ordinary constitution in which the disease occurs, the difficulty of supporting the system by common means, and the great sensorial exhaustion which is perpetually taking place, it is far from difficult to explain in what manner it operates beneficially; but intoxication is a frantic experiment, and where it succeeds once, we have reason to apprehend it would kill in a hundred instances.

The warm and the cold bath have each of them a much better claim to attention; and their votaries are so equally divided, that it is no easy matter to say which is most strongly recommended. The latter demands more general strength in the system than the former; but neither of them is to be depended upon except as an auxiliary. The cold bath has the authority of Dr. Lind in its favour (*Essay on Diseases in Hot Climates*, p. 257), and has in some instances been tried with success in America.— (*Tallman, Amer. Phil. Trans.*, i., xxi.; *Cochran, Edin. Med. Comm.*, vol. iii., p. 183.)

Mercury, in various forms, has been had recourse to from a very early period; and on the authority of Dr. Stoll, has occasionally been used for the purpose of exciting salivation. On what ground it has been carried to this extent I do not know, except it be that a pretty free flow of saliva from the mouth spontaneously has, by many persons, been regarded as a favourable sign. The disease, however, does not seem to be accompanied with any symptom that can be called critical; and it is hence probable, that this spontaneous flow of saliva is nothing more than a result of the violent action and alternating relaxation of all the parts about the fauces. Nevertheless, salivation, where it has been accomplished, is said by many writers to have been serviceable, though I know of no practitioner who has relied on it alone. And, in reality, such is the rapidity with which both trismus and tetanus usually march forward, where they have once taken a hold on the system, that we have seldom time to avail ourselves of this mode of cure, were its pretensions still more decisive than they seem to be. It is most successfully employed after copious venesection, and in conjunction with opium.

Opium, indeed, in every stage and every variety of both tetanus and locked-jaw, is the remedy on which we are to place our chief, if not our only dependance; but to give it a full chance of success it should be administered in very free doses, and it is not easy for us to be too free in its use. In the Edinburgh Medical Commentaries (vol. i., p. 88) we have a case, in which five hundred grains were taken within seventeen days, which is about thirty grains a day: and in the Edinburgh Journal (*Edin. Med. and Surg. Journ.*, No. lxxi.; Mr. Barr's case) an-

other case, in which, after smaller doses along with calomel, the practitioner at last gave a drachm of solid opium at one time. This, however, proved too high a dose; for the induced stupor was accompanied with very laborious respiration, and nearly an extinction of the pulse; and the patient was obliged to be roused by stimulants. He recovered ultimately. Yet, in the West Indies, opium is often carried, with the most beneficial effects, to as great an extent as this, though not at once. Thus Dr. Gloster of St. John's, Antigua, gave to a negro, labouring under tetanus from an exposure to the night air, not less than twenty grains every three hours, in conjunction with musk, cinnabar, and other medicines; and continued it with but little abatement for a term of seventeen days, in the course of which the patient took five hundred grains of this narcotic. For the first six days, little benefit seemed to be effected; but after this period the symptoms gradually declined under the same perseverance in the medicine, and in thirteen days more, they were so much diminished that no further assistance was thought necessary.*

If there be any thing which adds to the sedative power of opium in this disease, it is sudorifics, and particularly ipecacuanha. And upon this subject Dr. Latham has given a valuable paper in the Medical Transactions, in which he offers examples of failure in the use of James's powder, when used either alone or in alternation with opium; but of full success by uniting the two powers of the narcotic and the sudorific, though he afterward preferred ipecacuanha to James's powder, and prescribed it in the form of the compound powder of this name. He gives cases in which he employed this compound in very severe attacks, and sometimes in what seemed to be its last stage of the disease, with an immediate arrest of its symptoms, and progressively a perfect restoration to health. His doses consisted of ten grains, repeated every three or four hours. In no instance was there any unusual inclination to sleep, how long soever this treatment was continued, which, in one case, was for a fortnight; nor was there any degree of sickness, nor any other inconvenience, except that of a perspiration, troublesome from its excess.—(*Med. Trans.*, vol. iv., art. iv.)

It is only necessary to observe further, that, during the treatment either of trismus or tetanus, a very particular attention should be paid to ventilate the chamber with pure air; and especially to purify the air of close and crowded hospitals, without which no plan of treatment in the world can be of any avail. We should also remove, if possible, the costiveness, to

---

* In Hosack's Essays, vol. ii., reference is made to a number of instances of tetanus cured by the use of wine. Dr. H. gives also the details of a case treated by himself, and with success, in which the quantity of wine used was three gallons.—D.

* In the West Indies one hundred drops of laudanum are sometimes given as the first dose, and repeated every two hours, with an addition of one third to every succeeding dose. This plan is combined with the free use of mercury, an allowance of wine and ardent spirits, the employment of the warm bath; and attention to remove constipation. Dr. Morrison has given a favourable report of the effect of this practice, even in traumatic tetanus.—Ed.

which the bowels are so peculiarly subject, by some gentle aperient : for it sometimes happens, not only in infantile trismus or tetanus, but in that from obstructed perspiration, or cold and dampness, that the primary cause of irritation is seated in the bowels ; while, whatever accumulation takes place in this quarter during the course of the disease, may add to and exacerbate the general erethism. At the same time, nothing can be more mischievous than the drastic purges which practitioners are apt to give at the commencement of this disease, consisting of jalap, scammony, and aloes. We have already seen, that the general excitement is so extreme, that the slightest occasional irritation, even that of changing the position of the head, is sometimes sufficient to produce a return of the spasms ; and hence there can be nothing more likely to do it than the griping effects of such medicines. And it will be far safer to pass by the constipation altogether, than to attempt to remove it by such dangerous means. The best medicine is castor-oil, which may be given either by the mouth or in the form of injections ; and if this do not succeed, we may employ calomel. But the action of the bowels must only be solicited, and by no means violently excited.*

---

* The editor freely confesses that he does not participate in the author's aversion to the employment of strong purgatives in tetanus. While Dr. Good condemns them, we find some other physicians prescribing them in extraordinary doses, and with decided success. Thus, in an example under Mr. Manifold, of Liverpool, on which Dr. Briggs has offered some reflections, half a drachm of calomel, as much scammony, and fifteen grains of gamboge, were given in one dose, followed by a clyster of half an ounce of turpentine and two drachms of aloes. As these powerful means had produced no effect, two drops of the oil of croton in a little treacle were given in the evening, and at the same time a clyster of four ounces of the sulphate of magnesia in a pint of infusion of senna. In less than an hour afterward a black stool was voided, and relief immediately experienced from the evacuation. By continuing the same active remedies, a cure was effected.—(See Edin. Med. Journ., No. lxxxv., p. 277.) Indeed, the oil of croton, owing to its great efficiency in procuring stools, promises to be a most valuable medicine in tetanus. Dr. Briggs even maintains, in direct opposition to Dr. Good, that the principle on which the utility of purgatives rests in this disorder, is that of *counter-irritation* on the bowels ; a theory which we need not investigate too deeply, provided the practice be found to answer.

Dr. Good describes opium as the sheet-anchor in the treatment ; yet, in almost every case in which the editor has seen this medicine used as the chief or only one, the disease proved fatal.

Our author has not delivered any opinion with regard to venesection as a means of relieving tetanus. Sir Astley Cooper has found it hurtful ; and the editor of this work has seen some cases in which he thought that the patient's chances of recovery were rendered worse by it. Dr. Elliotson states that the bleeding is not at all useful unless the wound is inflamed, or there is some decided internal inflammation present, or the patient is in a state of plethora.

In consequence of many practitioners suspecting tetanus to be dependant upon inflammation of the spinal marrow or its coverings, they have had recourse to blistering the skin in the track of the vertebral column. The efficiency of the plan is far from being well proved.

One remedy for tetanus, in favour of which we have now many facts recorded, is tobacco.† Two examples of its efficiency are detailed by Dr. Anderson, of Port Spain, Trinidad. He fomented the jaws, throat, and chest frequently with a strong decoction of this plant, and applied cataplasms of the boiled leaves to the lower jaw and throat. The patient was also put into a warm bath, impregnated with tobacco, every three hours, and had a clyster of the decoction administered to him twice in twenty-four hours. Purgatives, consisting of. gamboge, calomel, and of ricini, were likewise employed.—(See Ed. Med. Chir. Trans., vol. i., p. 187.) An earlier paper, particularly in recommendation of tobacco and the purgative practice, is that of Mr. O'Beirne, who adverts to various opinions and facts communicated on this subject by other previous writers.—(See Dublin Hospital Reports, vol. iii., p. 343, &c.) From the share which the state of the medulla spinalis is sometimes conceived to have in the production of the disease, the practice of applying a blister the whole length of the spine has been derived. Dr. Reid is an advocate for this practice and powerful cathartics.—(See Trans. of Physicians of King's and Queen's College, vol. i., p. 122.) Oil of turpentine is another valuable medicine in tetanus. It is given by the mouth, and in clysters. The facts in its favour are numerous. It operates with excellent effect on the bowels. Prussic acid and belladonna have been tried in tetanus, and found to do no good.

In consequence of the benefit which Dr. Elliotson had seen the carbonate of iron produce in some examples of St. Vitus's dance, another spasmodic disease, he determined to try it in tetanus ; and the account which he has published of the results of some cases which fell under his own observation, and of others which occurred in the West Indies, certainly encourages the hope that this medicine will be a valuable one in the present disorder. The editor has tried it only in one case of traumatic tetanus, but in that it did not succeed ; indeed, the trial was not a fair one, because commenced in too advanced a stage of the disease.

Whether veratria would prove serviceable, as a means of relieving tetanus, is a point which may deserve further investigation. Its external use seems to have great power in mitigating and curing neuralgia, and other nervous affections. From Əj. to Əij. of it may be blended with ointment, and rubbed on the painful or disordered parts. Dr. Turnbull, some months ago, mentioned to the editor several very extraordinary proofs of the power of veratria, employed in this way, in curing neuralgic diseases.

In traumatic tetanus, amputation has sometimes been practised, with the view of stopping the disorder ; but the most experienced surgeons disapprove of the proceeding as useless. The plan of dividing the nerve distributed to the wounded part, has also been done with various results. One of the strongest facts in support of this practice was published a little while ago by Dr. Murray, assistant surgeon in the Honourable East In-

---

† Dr. Skinner, of N. Carolina, has communicated a case of tetanus treated successfully by tobacco injections.—See the Phil. Journ. of Med. and Phys. Sc., May, 1827. Arsenic, also, has been found efficacious by Dr. Holcombe of Virginia.—D.

SPECIES VIII.
ENTASIA LYSSA.
RABIES.

SPASMODIC CONSTRICTION OF THE MUSCLES OF THE CHEST ; SUPERVENING TO THE BITE OF A RABID ANIMAL ; USUALLY PRECEDED BY A RETURN OF PAIN AND INFLAMMATION IN THE BITTEN PART: GREAT RESTLESSNESS, HORROR, AND HURRY OF MIND.

THE Greek term for rabies was LYSSA : and the antiquity of the disease is sufficiently established from its being referred to several times under this name by Homer in his Iliad, who is perpetually making his Grecian heroes compare Hector to a mad dog, κύνα λυσσητῆρα, which is the term used by Teucer ; while Ulysses, speaking of him to Achilles, says,

————κρατερὴ δέ ἑ ΛΥΣΣΑ δέδυκεν.*

" So with a furious LYSSA was he stung."

The author has ventured to restore the Greek term, not only as being more classical, but as being far more correct than the technical term of the present day, which is *hydrophobia*, or *water-dread ;* since this is by no means a pathognomonic symptom ; being sometimes found in other diseases ; occasionally ceasing in the present towards the close of the career ; and though almost always observable among mankind, in numerous instances wanting, even from the commencement, in rabid dogs, wolves, and other animals. " Constat repetitâ," says Sauvages, " apud Gallo-provinciales experientiâ, canes luposque rabidos bibisse, manducasse, flumen transisse, ut olim Marologii, et bis Forolivii observatum, adeoque nec cibum nec potum aversari." The same fact is affirmed of rabid wolves, in a case given by Trecourt in his Chirurgical Memoirs and Observations. Dr. James in like manner relates the case of a mad dog, that both drank milk and swam through a piece of water (*On Canine Madness,* p. 10) ; and one or two similar cases are said to have occurred among mankind ;† though even here a

dia Company's service.—(See Med. Gaz., 1832-3, p. 623.) A midshipman in the ship " James Pattison," aged fifteen, trod upon a rusty nail, which penetrated the left foot, between the metatarsal bones of the great toe and the adjoining one. After the accident the patient kept his watch, and was exposed to cold. At eight o'clock on the following morning, the symptoms of locked-jaw had commenced. Under the administration of opium the disorder gained ground ; Dr. Murray therefore cut down to and divided the posterior tibial nerve, about an inch behind the malleolus internus. Although the patient had not been able to speak before the operation, he immediately opened his mouth with an exclamation, and expressed that he felt himself already greatly relieved. The original wound was then dilated, and covered with a poultice containing laudanum, and the case had a favourable termination.—ED.

* Iliad, ix., 239.

† Fehr. Nachricht von einer tödslichen Krankheit nach dem tollen Hundsbisse, Gött., 1790, 8vo. In a case published by Dr. Satterley, the patient had fits of biting, and between these he was perfectly well—even took warm fluids, and had a sound sleep. It seems, then, as if the disease may

spasmodic constriction of the muscles of the chest, and sometimes of the throat, seems to have been present. Dr. Vaughan, indeed, gives the case of a patient who called for drink through the whole course of the disease, and only ceased to ask for it a short time before his death.

I have occasionally met, on the contrary, with a few obstinate cases of hydrophobia, or waterdread, without any connexion with rabies : one especially in a young lady of nineteen years of age, of a highly nervous temperament, which was preceded by a very severe toothache and catarrh. The muscles of the throat had no constriction, except on the approach of liquids, and the patient, through the whole of the disease, which lasted a week, was able to swallow solids without difficulty ; but the moment any kind of liquid was brought to her, a strong spastic action took place, and all the muscles about the throat were violently convulsed if she attempted to swallow.

Similar examples are to be found in Battini, Dumas, Alibert, and several of the medical records, and particularly one of great obstinacy in the Edinburgh Medical Essays, which was chiefly relieved by repeated venesections (*Inflammation of the Stomach, with Hydrophobia,* &c., by Dr. J. Innes ; Ed. Med. Ess., i., p. 227), as the preceding case was by large doses of opium. Hydrophobia is therefore too general and indefinite a term to characterize the genus before us, unless we mean to include under it diseases to which it is by no means commonly applied, and which, in truth, have little connexion with rabies. Hunauld has, indeed, employed it in this extensive signification, and has hence made it embrace no less than seven distinct species, of which two only are irremediable (*Discours sur la Rage, et ses Remèdes, Chateau-Gontier,* 1714, 12mo.) ; and Swediaur has followed his example.—(*Nov. Nosol. Meth. Syst.,* vol. i., p. 511.)

There is, even in the present day, so little satisfactorily known, and so few opportunities of acquiring any practical knowledge concerning the general nature and pathology of rabies, that it might, perhaps, be most prudent to imitate the example of modesty which Dr. Cullen has set us upon this subject, and to let it pass without a single remark. Yet the following hints, derived from the only three cases in which the author has ever been consulted, compared with the larger range of observation and practice of a few other physicians, and especially the valuable work of Professor Trolliet of Lyons, together with the reflections to which they have given rise in his own mind, may afford a little glimmering light into the principle of the dis-

be attended with a decided remission. Dr. Elliotson had a patient with this disorder, who, to please him, would wash his hands, stir the water about, and play with it. In the Medical and Surgical Journal, vol. v., p. 497, is a case related by Dr. Macrorie of Liverpool, in which so marked an amendment took place, that the patient became almost free from the dread of swallowing liquids, and took coffee without difficulty.—ED.

ease, and give an opportunity to succeeding pathologists of describing it more perspicuously.

The symptoms enumerated in the definition, and especially the constrictive spasm that oppresses the muscles of deglutition and of the chest generally, sufficiently show that the present species of disease bears a very close analogy to the two preceding, in the mischief which it excites; and as by far the most frequent cause of the two preceding species is the irritation of a wound or puncture on the surface of the body, it bears quite as close an analogy to them in the nature of its cause as in that of its effects.

We have seen it to be a law, operating throughout the animal system, that if a morbid action commence in any part whatever of a continuous chain of functions or of fibres, it often produces a peculiar impression upon its extremities; so that the extremities themselves form, in many instances, the chief seat of distress, and even of danger; and this more especially when the one extremity of the chain becomes affected in consequence of the primary affection of the other. And we have also endeavoured to show, from the general course and intermediate connexion of the nerves which supply the surface of the body, and particularly the extremities, that they constitute a direct fibrous chain, of which those that are, in all common cases, primarily irritated by wounds or punctures in the spastic diseases before us, form the one extremity, and those which enter into the muscles of the upper regions of the chest and the cheeks the other. It is not necessary, therefore, to travel over the same ground again; the reader may turn to it at his leisure: and he will find that we have hence endeavoured to trace out something of the means by which trismus and tetanus are produced by simple wounds or punctures in the limbs, and especially in an irritable habit.

Now, if the reasoning be sound, as applied to trismus and tetanus, it must be equally good as applied to lyssa; and will induce us to expect a more complicated disease, and a still more severe and desperate result: as we have, in the present instance, not merely an ordinary and mechanical, but a specific and chymical source of irritation to encounter, and so indecomposable in its nature, that it is capable of lurking in the system, and apparently in the part where it may chance to be deposited, for weeks or even months, without losing its activity; of continuing dormant, if there be no sufficient irritability of constitution or nervous fibre for it to operate upon, and of operating as soon as such a condition may arrive: for that some exciting cause is usually necessary to rouse it into action, will sufficiently appear in the sequel of this inquiry. Sir Lucas Pepys, however, Dr. Bardsley, and various other writers, have made it a question, whether the virus of rabies is ever originated or produced spontaneously, or in any other way maintained, than by a direct communication from one animal to another; while M. Girard of Lyons has denied that there is any such thing at all, and contended that ra-

bies consists in nothing more than an acute degree of local irritation, and its effects on a highly mobile and excitable constitution. We have long, however, had various examples on record, and have recently been furnished with another by Mr. Gillman, in which a dog, chained up in a yard, and cut off from all medium of contamination with other animals, has occasionally been attacked with genuine lyssa, and exhibited its most decisive characters. Professor Trolliet, whose extensive experience I shall soon have occasion to advert to more minutely, while he has no doubt of its occasional spontaneous origin, limits its appearance in this form to the dog, the wolf, the fox, and the cat, believing that all other animals only receive it from the one or the other of these by inoculation.*

Nevertheless, while we are thus establishing that the symptoms of rabies are dependant upon a specific virus, it may not be foreign to remark, that most animals, when roused to a high degree of rage, inflict a wound of a much more irritable kind than when in a state of tranquillity: and we have numerous examples in which such wound has been very difficult of cure, and not a few in which it has proved fatal; as though at all times, under such a state of excitement, some peculiar acrimony were secreted with the saliva. In the Ephemera of Natural Curiosities is an example of symptoms of hydrophobia or water-dread, produced by the bite of a man worked up into fury (Ann. ix., x., App., p. 249); and in the Leipsic Acta Eruditorum is another instance of the same kind (Ann. 1702, p. 147), though neither of them seems to have been fatal. Meekren (Observ., cap. lxvii.), however, Wolff (Observ. Med. Chir., lib. ii., N. 5.), and Zacutus Lusitanus (Prax. Admir., lib. iii., obs. 84, 88), have each an instance of such a bite terminating in death, yet without hydrophobia. Le Cat gives a case of death produced by the bite of an enraged duck (Recueil Périodique, ii., p. 90); and, in a German miscellany of deserved repute, we have another of the same kind.—(Samml. Med. Wahrnehm., b. ii., p. 98.) The instances, indeed, are innumerable; but it may be sufficient to observe further, that Thiermayer gives us two cases; one in which the bite of a hen, and another in which that of a goose, proved fatal on or about the third day (In Goekelii Consil. et Obs., N. 19), without hydrophobia; and that Camerarius has an instance of epilepsy produced by the bite of a horse.†

---

* Nouveau Traité de la Rage; Observations Cliniques, Recherches d'Anatomie Pathologique, et Doctrine de cette Maladie, 8vo., Lyon, 1820.

† Diss. de Epileps. freq., p. 15. No doubt many of the cases here adverted to were of the nature of traumatic tetanus. At the present day, medical practitioners are less likely to confound other nervous diseases with hydrophobia. If the case be a spurious one, the difficulty in swallowing generally comes on too early after the bite. In true hydrophobia, a certain period, usually some weeks, elapses between the bite and the commencement of the disease. One great feature of the complaint is a sudden and deep inspiration

Marvellous as these facts may appear, it is more consistent with reason to accredit them, than to impugn the host of authorities to whose testimony they appeal. And unless tetanus were mistaken for hydrophobia, an error that no doubt has frequently happened, it follows, that the passion of rage, whose influence is always considerable on the salivary glands, has often a power of stimulating them, among most animals, to the secretion of a malignant virus with which the saliva becomes tainted.

Rabies, however, has sufficiently shown itself to be dependant upon a peculiar virus, and capable of producing specific effects; to be sometimes originated, and sometimes received by communication. Now the only animals which have hitherto been ascertained to have a power of originating it are, as just observed, several species of the genus canis, as the dog, fox, and wolf, and one species of the genus felis, which is the domestic cat. It is probable, however, that there are others belonging to different classes endowed with a like power; and some writers have attempted to bring instances from the horse, mule, ass, ox, and hog, yet they are not instances to be depended upon. In like manner, Plater, Doppert, and even Sauvages himself, have asserted the same of mankind, and have brought forward a few casual cases in support of such assertion. These, however, are in every instance modifications of empathema, and especially of rage or fright, grafted on a highly irritable temperament, and hence associated with hysterical or some other spasmodic motions.

Of the remote or predisposing causes of this disease, we know nothing. The excitement of vehement rage, putrid food, long-continued thirst from a want of water to quench it, severe and pinching hunger, a hot and sultry state, or some other intemperament of the atmosphere, have been in turn appealed to as probable predisponents; but the appeal in no instance rests upon any authority. That the stimulus of vehement rage will often produce a peculiar influence affecting the saliva, and rendering it capable by a bite of exciting the most alarming symptoms of nervous irritation, may not be impossible; but these symptoms are not those of lyssa; and the virus, whatever it consists in, appears to be of a different kind. Putridity is, perhaps, the ordinary state in which dogs and cats obtain the offal, on which for the most part they feed: they show no disgust to it, and it offers a cause far too general for the purpose. In long voyages, again, when a crew has been without water, and reduced to short provisions, dogs have been in innumerable instances known to die

with which the patient is frequently affected, the diaphragm all at once descending, as it does when a person first enters a cold bath. The patient also generally sighs a good deal, and is severely agitated by the impression of cold air, the glare of a mirror, the noise of a pump, the sound of water, and other circumstances which do not commonly disturb, in any remarkable degree, persons who are labouring under some tetanic or nervous difficulty of swallowing.—Ed.

both of thirst and hunger, without betraying any signs of genuine rabies. That a peculiar intemperament of the atmosphere may at times be a cause, it is impossible to deny; but the disease, even when of spontaneous origin, has appeared under perhaps every variety of meteorological change, and seems to be far less common in hot and tropical regions, than in those of a more moderate temperature; for it is not known except by report in South America, though it is said to have occasionally appeared in the West Indies, as I have been repeatedly informed by intelligent residents in those quarters; while M. Volney tells us that it is equally uncommon in Egypt and Syria, and Mr. Barrow, at the Cape of Good Hope and in the interior of the country, where the Caffrés feed their dogs on nothing but putrid meat, and this often in the highest degree of offensiveness.

It is not improbable, that several of these may occasionally become exciting causes; but it is obvious, that they are not competent of themselves to produce the disease. Some of them, indeed, have been put to a direct test, and have explicitly proved their incompetency. Thus, in the wards of the Veterinary School at Alfort, three dogs were shut up and made the subjects of express experiments. One was fed with salted meats, and totally restrained from drinking; the second was allowed nothing but water; and the third allowed neither food nor drink of any kind. The first died on the forty-first day of the experiment, the second on the thirty-third day, and the third on the twenty-fifth: not one of them evincing the slightest symptom of rabies.

That the specific virus of rabies is less volatile and active than many other kinds of morbid poisons, is clear, from the fact that it is never found diffused in the atmosphere, so as to produce an epidemy; that it never operates on those who are most susceptible of its influence, except when accompanied with a wound or inserted into the cutis; and that, even in this case, it usually requires in mankind, and probably also in other animals, some auxiliary excitement to enable it to carry forward the process of assimilation: for it rarely happens, that all the men or quadrupeds that are bitten by a rabid dog suffer from the inoculation. Mr. Hunter, indeed, gives an instance, in which out of twenty persons who were bitten by the same dog, only one received the disease. This want of activity is a happy circumstance, as it affords an important interval for medical treatment, if we should ever be so fortunate as to hit upon any curative process that may be depended upon. At the same time I cannot avoid again to observe, that as this virus is less volatile than most others, it is perhaps less indecomposible than any of them; and hence is capable of remaining in a dormant and unaffected state in any part of the system into which it has been received by insertion, for a far longer period than any other known contagion whatever.* It is generally calculated, but

* According to Sir David Barry, "The notion that the hydrophobic poison is absorbed, after the

I do not know upon what data, that of those who are exposed to the venom, about one in four matures the complaint, and the rest escape.

When the disease has once fixed itself among a large establishment of hounds, it has been said that the poison becomes more concentrated and active, operates through an unbroken skin, and even taints the atmosphere. There is, however, no solid foundation for such an opinion; and, though the disease runs rapidly from one dog to another, and it may be difficult in many cases to trace the marks of a bite, yet, considering that the smallest and most imperceptible scratch of a tooth may be a sufficient medium of infection, and that every inoculated dog adds to the sources from which it may be derived, there is no difficulty in accounting for such rapidity of spread, without ascribing anomalies to the laws by which it is regulated. Heister, indeed, has given a case of lyssa in one of the foreign colleetions, produced in a man by his having merely put into his mouth the cord by which the mad dog had been confined : but, as in this instance there was probably some ulceration in the mouth at the time, there is nothing marvellous in its production. Palmarius, in like manner, relates the case of a peasant

---

manner of other substances similarly circumstanced, but that it does not produce its peculiar effects until it has wandered through the *penetralia* of the animal for forty days or longer, is in direct opposition to all analogy. The experiments which we have witnessed with the vegetable, mineral, and reptile poisons, applied to animals externally, prove that the commencement of the symptoms is synchronous with the consummation of absorption, and that their repetition is dependant upon its renewal."—(Experimental Researches on the Influence of Atmospheric Pressure upon the Blood in the Veins, &c., p. 151.) However, although the hypothesis rejected by Sir David Barry is said by him to be contrary to all analogy, a somewhat similar one was adopted by John Hunter, and even now generally prevails in relation to syphilis, the constitutional effects of which follow absorption of the virus at very indeterminate periods, and in a great diversity of forms. Now this absorption is not a conjecture, but often actually proved by the occurrence of a bubo. The editor, however, merely adverts to those circumstances, in order to remind the reader that analogy is not entirely against the hypothesis of the hydrophobic poison being absorbed some time previously to the commencement of the symptoms; and not with the view of denying the correctness of Sir David Barry's conclusion. In hydrophobia it is not improbable, as this gentleman's arguments maintain, that the poison which is afterward to affect the constitution, is generated in the wounded part from the germ first deposited there by the tooth of the rabid animal, just as we see happen in variola, vaccinia, and lues itself. But, if the commonly received opinions of syphilis be well founded, its virus is generally absorbed, without giving rise to any immediate constitutional effects, and even is sometimes expelled again without such effects ever taking place at all. The assertion of Dr. Marochetti, that the hydrophobic poison is translated to the place on each side of the frænum of the tongue, where the submaxillary salivary ducts terminate, and where it produces vesicles or pustules, will be presently noticed.—ED.

---

who, in the last stage of the disease, communicated it to his children in kissing them and taking leave of them.—(*De Morb. Contagios.*, p. 266, Paris, 4to., 1518.) Yet, unless we could be certain that there were no cracks or other sores on the lips, and no eruption on the checks of these children, the example affords no proof.

I can distinctly state, that I have seen the same intercommunication successively repeated between a rabid young man and a young woman to whom he was betrothed, and who could not be restrained from such a token of affection, without any evil consequences; notwithstanding that the patient was labouring at that time under hydrophobia and all the severest marks of the disease, which destroyed him in a few hours afterward, and had also a perpetual desire to spit his saliva about the room. M. Trolliet asserts, not only that the virus will not permeate a sound skin, but that it is only contained in the frothy matter communicated from the lips ; and that neither the blood nor the secretions of any kind are tainted with it, or give rise to the disease, whatever scratch or other injury may be received during dissection.

It has still farther been doubted whether the virus itself is capable of propagation from the human subject to any animal, even by inoculation : but a bold experiment of M. Magendie and M. Breschet has completely settled this question ; for on June 19, 1813, having collected upon a piece of linen a portion of the saliva of a rabid man in the last stage of the disease, they inserted it under the skin of two dogs that were in waiting, both of them in good health ; of which one became rabid on the 27th of July, and bit two others, one of which also fell a victim to the disease just a month afterward.*

---

* The experiments made on rabid animals at the veterinary school at Berlin, by Dr. Hertwich, are curious and valuable. The results he has obtained are as follows : of 59 dogs inoculated, 14 became affected with lyssa canina. In those cases where the inoculation failed, no assignable cause for failure could be discovered. There exists, accordingly, a peculiar disposition for the virus of rabies, as for that of other contagious diseases—(a mastiff, 4 years old, went through several regular series of experiments, but without effect, while several other dogs who were inoculated with him and in the same manner became rabid. Several dogs were inoculated several times before any contagion took place : in others the effect was observed after the first experiment). It appears accordingly, that in cases of doubtful rabies, one or two accidental inoculations are not sufficient to serve as negative proofs of the existence of rabies. No communication of rabies ever took place by the perspiration ; the contagious matter of rabies cannot therefore be of a volatile nature. Its vehicle is saliva, the mucus of the mouth, the blood, and the substance of the salivary glands. It does not appear to exist in the nervous pulp. The power of infecting exists at every period of the confirmed disease, and even for about twenty-four hours after the death of the animal. The virus of rabies appears to be inactive if administered internally : of 22 dogs which were made to swallow it, none took the disease. The application of saliva to fresh wounds appears to be as often followed by rabies as the bites of rabid animals. Hence the dis-

The general aggregate to the symptoms point forcibly to the nervous system as the immediate quarter of disturbance. Such was the opinion of Morgagni, Cullen, Percival, and Marcet; and such indeed is the common opinion of the present day. By many writers, however, the effects have been rather referred to the sanguiferous system, and regarded as a fever; Mangor describes it as a continued fever (*Act. Hafn.*, ii.), and Rush and many others as an inflammatory affection; Bader as a fever *sui generis.*—(*Versuch einer neuen Theorie*, &c.) Nor is the difficulty in the least degree removed by dissection, for nothing can be more at variance than the appearances in different cases. Generally speaking, the fauces and parts adjoining exhibit redness and inflammatory characters. But while in some instances these are so considerable as to be on the point of gangrene, in others there is no inflammatory appearance whatever. Morgagni has examined and described bodies in both these states. Rolfinc gives one or two decided cases of the latter sort (*Dissert. Anat.*, lib. i., cap. xii.); while Ferriar notices examples, in which the inflammation of the fauces had spread over the whole œsophagus, and even the stomach (*Medic. Facts and Observations*, vol. i.); and another writer has recorded an instance, in which it had descended to the ileum, which was in a state of gangrene.—(*N. Act. Nat. Cur.*, vol. iv., obs. 20.) In some cases, the encephalon, and even the spinal marrow, have appeared to be as much diseased as the fauces: the vessels turgid; the plexus choroides blackish; the ventricles loaded with water: though, in the cases examined by M. Magendie, which were confined to dogs, there was no appearance of inflammation either in the brain or spine. Sometimes the lungs have been inflamed; sometimes the liver; sometimes the vagina; while the blood, according to Sauvages, has been also found in a dissolved state, and, according to Morgagni, in a state highly tenacious and coagulable. From all which we can only conclude, that owing to the violence of the disease, every organ is greatly disturbed, and those the most so that in particular cases are most severely

ease is produced neither by the lesion, as Gerard thinks, nor by the fear of the patient. The opinion of Bader and Capello, that in dogs who had become rabid from the bite of an animal primarily affected with the disease, the saliva did not contain the contagion, and thinks it existed only in primary rabies, has been proved by several experiments to be erroneous. During the period of the inactivity of the virus, there is no morbid alteration observable either locally or in the general health of the dog thus infected, nor does the lower surface of the tongue ever exhibit vesicles. The disease generally breaks out within fifty days after the inoculation or the infliction of the wound: inoculation or infection from animals afflicted with fierce rabies, very often produces the other modification of the disease, and vice versâ; they are consequently only different forms of one and the same disease. Healthy dogs are unable to distinguish those affected with rabies by the smell; nor do they abhor food mixed with the secreta or excreta of rabid dogs."—See Am. Journ. of Med. Sc., vol. v., p. 485.—D.

affected. Riedel asserts, that among dogs, a highly offensive fetor of a peculiar character is thrown forth from every part of the body (*Act. Acad. Mogunt.*, Erf., 1757): but I have not found this remark confirmed by the veterinary practitioners of our own country; and it certainly does not apply to mankind, with an exception or two that seem to depend upon some accidental circumstances; for Wolf informs us, that in one of his patients, and a patient that ultimately recovered, the blood stunk intolerably as it was drawn from a vein; and a patient of Dr. Vaughan's complained of a most offensive smell that issued from the original wound, but of which no one was sensible except himself. In like manner, the patient described by Dr. Marcet, towards the close of the disease, complained loudly of an intolerable stench that issued from his body generally, but without being perceived by any other person.—(*Medico-Chir. Trans.*, i., 132.) Dissection in this case produced nothing striking.

Desault, in his treatise on rabies, tells us that he has often met with numerous minute worms in the heads of those who have died of this disease; and he hence regards such animalcules as its cause. But this writer was a slave to the Linnéan hypothesis of invermination, and applied the same cause to syphilis, which he also supposed to be maintained by a transfer of vermicules from one individual to another: and hence proposed to treat syphilis, lyssa, and itch, as diseases of a like origin, with the common antidote of mercury; and gives instances of a success which no one has met with out of his own practice. The cases, however, which he describes, had not advanced to the stage of water-dread; and, in all of them, he thought it prudent to combine with his mercurial inunction, cold bathing and Palmarius's antilyssic powder.

Vander Brock, and after him Rahn, maintain that the return of pain and inflammation to the bitten part, on the onset of the disease, does not occur from any virus which has hitherto been lying dormant there, but from the universal excitement alone. It may be observed, however, in opposition to such an opinion, that this local affection is in most instances a prelude to the general disease, and forms the punctum saliens from which it issues; as though the contagious ferment had remained dormant there, and was at length called into action by some exciting cause.

There seems, nevertheless, to be a slight departure from the general character of the disease in a few cases, and particularly in those that are produced by the bite of a rabid cat, whether the latter have originated it, or received it from a rabid dog, as though by a passage through the domestic cat the virus undergoes a similar change to that which takes place in the virus of smallpox, when passing through the system of an individual who has previously submitted to the influence of cowpox: for, upon the whole, the disease appears to evince somewhat less malignity, to be more disposed to intermit, and its spastic symptoms, and especially that of water-dread, to be both less frequent and less violent: so that in respect to symptoms we may perhaps mark out the two following varieties:—

| *α* Felina. Feline rabies. | The spastic symptoms less acute and frequently intermitting; produced by the bite of a rabid cat. |
| *β* Canina. Canine rabies. | The spastic constriction, for the most part, extending to the muscles of deglutition, which are violently convulsed at the appearance or idea of liquids: produced by the bite of a rabid dog, wolf, or fox. |

There is a case of FELINE RABIES, if it be rabies, in Morgagni, and which is copied from him into Sauvages' Nosology, in which the above distinction is so strongly marked, that the author, in the first edition of his own Nosology, was induced to follow M. de Sauvages' mode of classifying it, and made it, after him, a distinct species, though he deviated from the name under which it occurs in this justly celebrated writer, which is that of Anxietas à Morsu.—(Classis vii., Ord. i., v., 6.) The history of the enraged cat is not given, nor is it certain that the rage was that of rabies. The master of the animal was attacked and wounded both by its teeth and claws. The symptoms took place four days after the bite, and were confined to spasms of the chest without hydrophobia; nor do these seem to have been of great violence, for they are described as " magna præcordiorum anxietas." Local and general bleedings were useless: a frequent repetition of the warm bath afforded relief; but it only yielded to an ephemera with copious sweat. The intervals were lunar: for it returned with the full moon for two years; the bitten part, as usual, first becoming highly irritable, and the spasms or vehement anxiety of the præcordia supervening, which were now relieved by bleeding. After this period, it returned with every fourth full moon for two years more, and then appears to have ceased:

A few instances of intermission, with a return of periodical paroxysms, produced by the bite of a rabid dog, are also to be found in the medical collections: of which Dr. Peters' case (*Phil. Trans.*, 1745, No. cccclxxv.) affords a striking example, the paroxysm returning for many months afterward, severely, once a fortnight, or at every new and full moon, and slightly at the quarters, or in the intervening weeks. Selle, indeed, asserts that he has met with an instance of the same kind of intermission among dogs; and hence, where the individual recovers, both varieties seem occasionally to subside in this manner.—(*Neue Beiträge zur Natur und Arzney-wissenschaft*, b. iii., 118.)

Dr. Fothergill has given two cases of unquestionable affection from feline rabies, produced by the same animal. The cat first bit the maid-servant, and afterward the master of the house, about the middle of February. The wound inflicted on the maid-servant remained open and irritable from the first, and continued to resist every application for many months; it healed, however, at length, and no constitutional symptoms supervened. The wound inflicted on the master healed easily and in a short time, but in the middle of the ensuing June, being four months afterward, the usual symptoms of lyssa appeared, yet with comparatively slight and occasional water-dread; insomuch that the patient, far from resisting the use of the warm bath, sometimes called for it, expressed a high sense of the comfort it afforded him, and was able at times to dash the water over his head with his own hands. It terminated, however, fatally, and with the usual symptoms of distress.*

In the Transactions of the Medical Society of London we have a highly interesting case of the same kind, which proved equally fatal, in seventy-four days from the time of receiving the injury, and fifty-eight hours. from the commencement of the disease; all the symptoms, moreover, exhibiting less violence than usually occurs in canine madness, with little or no water-dread, and consequently an ability to drink fluids to the close of the disease, though the muscles of deglutition, as well as those of the chest, evinced always some degree of constriction, with occasional exacerbations.—(Vol. i., art. iv., p. 78, 8vo., 1810.) The patient was a young lady of eighteen years of age; the attack was made in the month of January, with both claws and teeth, by a domestic cat that was lurking under the bed, and which, though not known to be ill, had for some time before been observed to be wild, and had been roving in the woods. The fate of the animal is not mentioned. The lacerated parts were incised and purposely inflamed by the application of spirit of turpentine. The wounds healed, and the general health of the patient continued perfect till the beginning of the ensuing April, when she was suddenly frightened by looking out of a window, and seeing a mad dog pursued by a crowding populace. This proved an exciting cause. She instantly expressed alarm, anxiety, and dejection of mind. In the afternoon she complained of an unusual stiffness in moving her left arm, and its sense of feeling was impaired; she discovered an aversion to company; the irritations of noise, heat, and light were offensive to her; she avoided the fire, and forbade a candle to be brought near her. The rigidity and insensibility of the affected arm seemed to shoot in a line from the middle finger which had been lacerated, and was accompanied with an acute pain which termi-

* Med. Observ. and Inquir., vol. v. On the other hand, Dr. A. Thomson has recorded, in the Medico-Chir. Trans:, an instance, proving that when the disease arises from the bite of a rabid cat, the dread of swallowing fluids may be as strongly marked as in examples proceeding from the bites of rabid dogs. What was noticed by Dr. Fothergill is not a constant feature in the disorder as it appears after the bite of a rabid cat.—EDd

uated in the, glands, of the axilla, where she complained of a considerable swelling. Yet neither of the hands (for both had been injured) was affected with discoloration, tension, tumefaction, or any other mark of local injury, though a degree of lividity had been observed upon the lacerated part of the finger a short time before the disease made its appearance. She had a painful constrictive sensation in her chest, and the respiration was interrupted by frequent sighings. The spasmodic symptoms increased, and at length the whole system, but especially the lungs, was affected with violent convulsions: the breathing was exquisitely laborious, but the paroxysm subsided in about two minutes. Frequent sickness and vomiting followed: the convulsive spasms about the throat obliged her to gulp what she swallowed, and she showed a slight reluctance, but nothing more, to handling a glass goblet. The pulse was 132 strokes in a minute; the skin was cool, the tongue moist, the bowels open, the thirst urgent, without any tendency to delirium. She was worn out, however, by sensorial exhaustion and distress, and at last expired calmly, at the distance of time from the attack already stated.

In the general progress of CANINE RABIES, all the above indications are greatly aggravated, and the mind often participates in the disease, and becomes incoherent. Whatever be the exciting cause, the wounded part almost always, though not universally so, takes the lead in the train of symptoms, and becomes uneasy; the cicatrix looking red or livid, often opening afresh, and oozing forth a little coloured serum, while the limb feels stiff and numb. The patient is next oppressed with anxiety and depression, and sometimes sinks into a melancholy from which nothing can rouse him. The pulse and general temperature of the skin do not at this time vary much from their natural state. A stiffness and painful constriction are, however, felt about the chest and throat; the breathing becomes difficult, and is interrupted by sobs and deep sighs, as the sleep is, if any be obtained, by starts and frightful dreams. Bright colours, a strong light, acute sounds, particularly the sound of water poured from basin to basin, even a simple agitation of the air by a movement of the bed-curtains, are sources of great disturbance, and will often bring on a paroxysm of general convulsions, or aggravate the tetanic constriction. The patient is tormented with thirst, but dares not drink; the sight, or even idea of liquids, making him shudder: his eye is haggard, glassy, fixed, and turgid with blood from the violence of the struggle; his mouth filled with a tenacious saliva, in which, we have already shown, lurks the secreted and poisonous miasm, and he is perpetually endeavouring to hawk it up, and spit it away from him in every direction; often desiring those around him to stand aside, as conscious that he might hereby injure them. The sound which is thus made, from the great oppression he labours under, and from his vehement effort to excrete the tough and adhesive phlegm, is often of a very singular kind; and

being sometimes more acute than at others, as well as quick and sudden, and also, frequently repeated, like every other motion of the body, has occasionally, to a warm and prepossessed imagination, seemed to be a kind of barking or yelping. And hence, probably, the vulgar idea that a barking, like that of a dog, is a common symptom of the disease. The restlessness is extreme, and if the patient attempt to lie down and compose himself, he instantly starts up again, and looks wildly round him in unutterable anguish: "On going into the room," says Dr. Munckley, describing the case of a patient to whom he had been called, and the author can bear witness to the accuracy of his very forcible delineation, "we found him sitting up in his bed, with an attendant on each side of him: he was in violent agitation of body.: moving himself about with great vehemence as he sat in the bed, and tossing his arms from side to side. On seeing us, he bared one of his arms, and striking it with all his force, he cried out to us with the greatest eagerness, to order him to be let blood. His eyes were redder than the day before; and there was added to the whole look an appearance of horror and despair, greatly beyond what I had ever seen, either in madness or in any other kind of delirium." The patient was, nevertheless, "perfectly in his senses at this time, and there was not the least appearance of danger of his biting any person near him; nor, among the variety of motions which he made, was there any which looked like attempting to snap or bite at any thing within his reach: and they who were about him had no apprehension of his doing this."—(*Med. Trans.*, vol. ii., art. v., p. 53.) The patient had at this time reached the third day of the disease, and expired about two hours after Dr. Munckley had left him.

There is, however, a considerable difference in many of the symptoms which characterize the progress of this malady, derived from difference of age, idiosyncrasy, or some other casualty, so that it is possible no two cases are in every respect precisely parallel. The volume of the Medical Transactions, from which I have just quoted, contains three instances of lyssa, communicated by different practitioners. In the first, which is Dr. Munckley's, no notice whatever is taken of the original bite, which was both in the hand and cheek, from a favourite lapdog, and the patient does not seem to have had any return of pain or irritation in these organs. In the second case, which is that of a lad of fifteen years of age, the bite, which was in the leg, was so small that it was scarcely perceptible at the time, and from first to last never gave the least uneasiness.—(Op. cit., vol. ii., art. xii., p. 192.) In the third case, which is that of an adult woman, the disease was preceded by the ordinary prelude of torpor, stiffness, and tingling in the bitten part, shooting upwards to the trunk.—(Id., art. xv., p. 222.) In the first case, the patient's mind never wandered, to the last moment of life, which is a common character of the disease; in the second and third, both were furiously mad, bit themselves, the bedclothes, and whatever else fell in their way. In all of them, however, there was a severe hydrophobia, and in all of them the pulse did not essentially vary from its common standard. The first died on the third day; the two last recovered; the one under a treatment which consisted principally of opium, and the other under that of salivation; leaving it therefore doubtful how far the recovery may be ascribed to the natural powers of the constitution, and how far to remedies so widely different in their nature. Dr. Marcet's patient did not expire till the sixth day after the appearance of water-dread, and without any affection in the bitten part (*Medico-Chir. Trans.*, i., p. 157); and, towards the close of the disease, he sometimes suddenly gulped half a pint of water, or splashed it over his body.

There is, also, in these three cases, an equal and most singular discrepancy in the interval between the infliction of the wound and the incursion of the disease, or, in the language of Professor Trolliet, its period of incubation. The first interval was about six weeks, which may be regarded as the ordinary term: the second was only five days: the third is not set down with any degree of precision; the patient is only stated to have been seized "about the time that the second horse died" that had been bitten by the same rabid dog; and hence this interval consisted probably of about a fortnight.

A like variation in the course of morbid symptoms, distinguished the series of cases published by Professor Brera, and which took place in the month of November, 1804, on the incursion of a wolf sufficiently proved to be rabid. Generally the patients showed no desire to bite or otherwise injure persons about them; but, in one instance, such a desire was strikingly prominent. In another case, also, though there was a fatal water-dread, there was no flow of saliva. In some, the horror extended to liquids of every kind; in others, water alone produced it, while wine was drank with ease.* '

This discrepance seems to depend entirely upon the nature or presence of the predisponent or exciting cause that gives energy to the virus, and without which it may lie, as we have already observed, for an almost indeterminable period dormant, but undecomposed, and therefore as malignant as when first generated.† In the

three cases just quoted from the Medical Transactions, the lad who was soonest affected seems to have had a strong predisposition to the disease from the first moment, and which alone became an exciting cause; in the woman, who suffered about a fortnight afterward, there was probably some degree of predisposition, but the immediate exciting cause appears to have been over-exertion in walking, for we are told that "she was seized as she was going on an errand on foot, and had walked about two miles."

There is a like uncertainty among quadrupeds. We have just taken the interval of ten or twelve days as the common term; but, in the instance just referred to, it may have been considerably longer. According to Meynall, the disease among dogs appears from ten days to eight months after the bite. In Earl Fitzwilliam's hounds, which were bitten June 8, 1791, the interval varied from six weeks to more than six months; and not much less in Mr. Floyer's hounds, as described by Mr. James. It is not therefore to be wondered at, that there should be a great uncertainty among mankind. And hence we find it has occurred a week or a fortnight after the bite, three weeks, a month, and sometimes six weeks, and even three months: after which last period, however, notwithstanding occasional instances to the contrary, the patient is generally considered safe. There are two cases published by Dr. Thacher (*Hosack and Francis' Amer. Med. and Phil. Reg.*, vol. i., p. 457), in which the injury inflicted by the same dog, August 16, 1810, did not produce hydrophobia in either instance till nearly three months afterward, namely, November 3, and November 14, ensuing: and it is the more remarkable, that the first case was that of a child under four years of age, the second that of an old man of seventy-three. Both terminated fatally; the former case in six days, the latter in seven, from the onset of the disease. Upon the whole, we may calculate the interval as varying from five or six days to as many months, the usual period being about the same number of weeks.*

The academical journals and monographic writers, nevertheless, have numerous instances of the malady appearing after a bite of many years standing; sometimes twelve, eighteen, twenty, and even thirty years; but the evidence is mostly imperfect. I shall presently, however, have occasion to notice one, in which it occurred

---

* Commentario Clinico per la cura dell' Idrofobia, &c. Mem. Soc. Ital. Scienz., tom. xvii., Modena.

† If this doctrine were positively proved, the information would be of high importance in practice, as justifying the excision of the parts at a very late period after they had been healed up, when this measure, so indisputably prudent in an early stage, has been neglected. However, whether the virus first inserted lie dormant in the part or not, if the bite be known with certainty to have been inflicted by a rabid animal, the extirpation of the bitten parts is advisable also on the other hypothesis, that the virus, though not now actually present itself, may have communicated to the parts a disposition to assume at a subsequent period a specific action, by which the hydrophobic poison will be regenerated, and subjected to absorption, with all its horrible consequences.—ED.

* Dr. Ramsay mentions a case in which fifteen months elapsed before the disease appeared. The late Duke of Richmond, Governor of Lower Canada, presents a similar instance. Having cut himself while shaving, the duke lifted a small dog to lick off the blood, and received a bite on his chin. Five months afterward he was suddenly attacked with hydrophobia; venesection gave temporary relief, but he died three days after the accident.— (Thacher on Hydrophobia.) In the fifth volume of the New York Medical Repository, Dr. Mease has communicated a case "where this destructive virus lay dormant four years and three months before it began to operate." In the same volume may be seen some valuable remarks by Physick, Mease, Coxe, and others.—D.

and proved fatal more than nine months afterward : and there is another, communicated by Dr. Bardsley to the Manchester Society, strongly entitled to credit, however difficult it may be to account for the fact, in which the attack did not commence till twelve years after the bite of a dog supposed to be mad. The patient died in the Manchester Infirmary, with decided symptoms of the disease. He had been for some time antecedently labouring under great nervous agitation and considerable depression of spirits.; and Dr. Bardsley inclined to ascribe it to this cause rather than to any specific poison lurking in the system. But this is to suppose that lyssa is capable, under particular circumstances, of being generated spontaneously* in the human frame, while Dr. Bardsley, as we have already observed, contends that it cannot exist, even among dogs, except by contact.†

There are few physicians, whose experience seems to have been so extensive upon this melancholy subject, and so actively followed up by judicious and even original views, and post-obit examinations, as that of Professor Trolliet, to whom I have already adverted. Independently of a variety of single and unconnected cases that had fallen under his care, he gives an account of a ravage committed on not less than twenty-three persons; besides cattle and dogs, in the department of the Isère in 1807, twelve of whom, for the most part, terribly bitten in the face, were conveyed to the Hôtel Dieu at Lyons, in which he was clinical professor, and as such, were placed under his immediate care.‡

The general train of symptoms, as the patients became successively affected and died, after an active and judicious treatment of preventive as well as curative means, did not essentially vary from those just related. The local indications mostly, but not always, preceded. The interval between the bite inflicted by the rabid wolf and the access of disease, varied from a fortnight to five weeks, and the patients uniformly sank on

* The doctrine that lyssa may be generated spontaneously is adopted by some approved physicians, among others by Dr. Francis, who remarks (Facts relating to Med. Jurisprudence), " that the causes by which spontaneous rabies may be induced are the violent emotions of the mind, sorrow, fear, rage, fright, the want of food, extreme fatigue, and the like." Dr. F. describes a case of spontaneous rabies which he attended in company with Dr. Hosack.—(See N. York Med. and Phys. Journal, vol. ii., p. 29.) Dr. Thacher has recorded a case of inflammation of the stomach, attended with spontaneous hydrophobia (see N. Y. Med. and Phys. Journal, vol. ii.), and Dr. Rush appears to have thought that many causes, independent of the bite of a rabid animal, are capable of producing it, and refers to the researches of Audry, " Sur la Rage."—D.

† The author overlooks the possibility of mistaking a tetanic affection for lyssa ; yet the close approximation, which one disease frequently makes to the other, is acknowledged by all men of experience and observation.—Ed.

‡ Nouvean Traité de la Rage, Observations cliniques, Récherches d'Anatomie pathologique, et Doctrine de cette Maladie, &c., 8vo., Lyon, 1820.

the second or third day after a clear development of the symptoms. In the preceding year, however, M. Trolliet had a case, produced by the bite of a mad dog, in which the disease did not show itself till *five months and a half after* the infliction of the wound. The patient was a strong, robust man, of thirty years of age, and the dog had died mad in the veterinary school at Lyons soon after the injury. The first symptoms in this case were the usual ones of pain in the bitten part, which gradually extended to the arm and neck. Two days afterward, the patient was sensible of a vapour or aura, which ascended from the abdomen to the head, accompanied with a general uneasiness. The symptom of hydrophobia was manifested on the day ensuing; the depleting plan was, in this instance, followed up with a daring urgency, and the man expired on *the evening of the same day.*

M. Trolliet's post-obit examinations are numerous, and they uniformly give proof, like the dissections already noticed, of extensive mischief in various organs remotely situated from each other; the chief of which, however, were the mucous membrane of the trachea and bronchiæ, and the membranes of the brain, especially the pia mater ; all which, in direct repugnance to M. Magendie's observations, were infiltrated with red blood, and gave evident proofs of inflammatory action ; while the mucous membrane of the bronchiæ and trachea were covered over with a frothy material of a peculiar kind, which M. Trolliet supposes to be the seat or vehicle of the specific virus, and which, in his opinion, is driven forward into the fauces, and intermixed with the saliva by each spastic expiration from the chest. The other organs he found affected as follows : the capillary vessels of the lungs were penetrated with a larger quantity of blood than ordinarily ; their substance was emphysematous, or contained an accumulation of air, as did also the heart and large bloodvessels in some instances. The blood itself was black, uncoagulating, and of an oily appearance. That taken from the veins during the disease, coagulated into an entire cake, without any separation of serum. The mucous membranes of the mouth and pharynx were of a pale gray, and lubricated by a gentle moisture ; they contained no saliva, nor any frothy material. The most singular fact of the whole is, that " the salivary glands, and the cellular substance which envelops them, afforded not the least vestige of inflammation, nor the slightest alteration in their volume, their colour, or their texture."

It is this last circumstance that seems chiefly to have induced M. Trolliet to venture upon a new hypothesis, and to suppose, that the actual seat of the specific virus is the mucous membrane of the bronchiæ or lower part of the trachea, rather than the fauces or the salivary glands ; and had these last in every instance been discovered as clear of any manifest morbid appearance as in the dissections of this ingenious pathologist, there would be strong ground for his conjecture : but as we have already seen, that in some cases, there have been found only slight marks of inflammatory action in the bronchiæ, while the fauces and œsophagus, and occasionally the stomach and even the ileum, have been so inflamed as to approach a state of gangrene, much further investigation is necessary before the old doctrine should fall a sacrifice to the new.* The only fact we are at present able to collect from dissections, is a very extensive and violent disturbance throughout the entire frame; sometimes fastening chiefly on one set of organs, and sometimes on another.

The mode of TREATMENT is a field still perfectly open for trial; for, at this moment, we have no specific remedy, nor any plan that can be depended upon, after the disease shows itself. Antecedently, indeed, to this period, our course is obvious, and particularly if we should be so fortunate as to be consulted at the time of the bite: it should consist in endeavouring, by the promptest and most efficacious means, to prevent the spread of the disease, by washing the part well and thoroughly at the nearest spring or river at hand, and by extirpating the virus before absorption has taken place. This has been done in various ways; for the lacerated part has been sometimes amputated or dissected out, and at other times totally destroyed by the actual or potential cautery. The actual cautery, by the means of irons heated to whiteness, was first adopted and recommended by Dioscorides (Lib. vi.), and afterward by Van Helmont, Morgagni (*De Sed. et Caus. Morb.*, ep. viii., art. 26), and Stahl: the potential cautery seems to have been proposed as a less terrific mode of operation, and has usually been accomplished by the means of lapis infernalis or decarbonated soda. It is recommended by Schenck, Pouteau, and Dr. Moseley. A notion, however, has obtained, from a very early period, that the irritation produced by a cautery, whether actual or potential, only increases the tendency to absorption; and Trampel has endeavoured to prove this (*Beobach. und Erfahr.*, &c., band ii., passim): on which account Hildanus and Morgagni have advised excision in combination with the cautery: the former proposing to cut out the eschar as soon as it is formed, without letting it remain for a spontaneous separation; and the latter, far more effectually, recommending that inustion should follow the application of the knife, instead of preceding it.

Of these three modes of operating, the potential cautery is least to be depended upon; for it is not sufficiently rapid in its action. Of the other two it is, perhaps, of little consequence which is selected, and either of them will generally prove sufficiently efficacious alone, if employed early enough to anticipate absorption, and

extensively enough to make sure of extirpating or destroying every portion of the bitten part. There is reason to believe that, in many instances, this has not been done; so that Camerarius places as little confidence in the actual cautery as in the potential, and Dr. Hamilton almost as little in excision: And hence another reason for employing both means in the manner recommended by Morgagni; and in which case we shall find it unnecessary to superadd any of those irritant, exulcerant, or suppurative applications which have been employed by many practitioners with a view of introducing a fresh local action, and maintaining a fresh local discharge, and which have chiefly consisted of cantharides, camphire, alliaceous cataplasms, resins, turpentine, or, as Celsus recommends, culinary salt.—(*De Medicinâ*, lib. v., cap. xxvii., § 1.) It may likewise be advisable, as proposed by Sir Kenelm Digby, and since his time by Dr. Haygarth, to wash the wound again thoroughly with tepid water, or tepid wine and water, before the excision is commenced. M. Portal, however, thinks the application of the cautery, whether actual or potential, may be serviceable long after the wound has been inflicted, and even after it has healed, though he advises its use as early as possible.—(*Mém. sur la Nature et le Traitement de plusieurs Maladies*, tom. iv., 8vo., Paris, 1819.)

There is also another, and a very easy, and perhaps a very salutary operation, which I would strenuously recommend from the first, even before the process of ablution. I mean that of applying a tight ligature to the affected part, wherever it will admit of such an application, at a short distance above the laceration. I have never had any opportunity of trying the benefit of such a measure in my own practice; but analogy is altogether in its favour, for it is well known to be one of the most important steps we can take in confining the poisonous effects of the rattlesnake and other venomous animals, and of mitigating its violence by the torpor which follows; and it has the sanction of many authorities of deserved credit, as Hacquet, Percival, Vater, Wedel, and Trolliet.*

* As the editor has already noticed, it is proved, by the ingenious experiments of Sir David Barry, that the commencement of the symptoms produced by vegetable, mineral, and reptile poisons, is synchronous with the consummation of absorption, and that their repetition is dependant upon its renewal. The same gentleman has also satisfactorily proved that absorption does not proceed under a vacuum. In the treatment of the recent bite of a rabid animal, therefore, he recommends, 1. The application of a powerful cupping-glass over the wound. This measure, he says, supersedes at once the ligature, ablution, excision, &c. during the period of its application, and for a certain time after its removal.—(See Exp. 5 and 7.) 2. After the cupping-glass has been applied for an hour *at least*, the whole of the parts wounded or abraded should be freely dissected out. 3. The cupping-glass should then be immediately reapplied. 4. Sir David Barry recommends the hermetical sealing of the vessels (as his expression is) with the actual cautery. 5. The part should be as little exposed to the contact of the air after the slough

* Trolliet's belief that the hydrophobic poison is formed with and contained in the mucous secretion of the respiratory organs, never gained many partisans; for the traces of inflammation noticed by Trolliet in those organs, and adopted as the ground of his doctrine, are well known not to be constant. M. Magendie dissected several rabid sheep, in which no marks of inflammation in any part of the lungs or air-passages could be perceived.—Ed.

If, however, the local plan should prove ineffectual, our curative practice, as already observed, is still unfortunately all afloat, and we have neither helm to steer by, nor compass to direct our course. There is indeed no disease for which so many remedies have been devised, and none in which the mortifying character of vanity of vanities has been so strikingly written on all of them. In the loose and heterogeneous manner in which they have descended to us, they seem indeed to have followed one another with-

---

comes away, and as soon healed up as possible.—(See Exper. Researches, &c., p. 149, et seq.) If the bite of a decidedly rabid animal were to be in one of the fingers, to which a cupping-glass could not be effectually applied, immediate amputation of the part would be prudent. The performance of this operation, previously to the commencement of the symptoms, is a very different practice froin that of amputating parts after the symptoms have begun. A few years ago a limb was amputated in Guy's Hospital under the latter circumstances, without the least check being put to the disorder. Unless, however, a limb were bitten in many places, or very deeply in parts not adᵣ mititng of excision, as through the tarsus or carpus, the editor conceives that amputation would not be warrantable, either before or after the accession of the symptoms; 1st, because the severity of the mutilation is too great to be encountered for the prevention of a disorder that is not certain of coming on at all; 2d, because the above mentioned proceedings would supersede the necessity for so severe a measure. According to Dr. Marochetti (Magendie, Journ. de Physiol., tom. v., p. 279), there is only one means of preventing the development of hydrophobia, viz. that of discharging the hydrophobic poison as soon as it is formed; and he asserts that the situation where this takes place is on each side of the frænum of the tongue, where one or two little vesicles or tubercles present themselves. The period when they become manifest, he says, cannot be stated with precision; but, when they occur, it is commonly between the the third and ninth day from the bite. When they are examined with a probe, he remarks, that a fluctuating liquid may be perceived in them which is, in fact, the hydrophobic poison, and which, if not discharged in twenty-four hours, is generally absorbed, and no vestiges of it remain. When a person has been bit by a rabid animal, Dr. Marochetti examines the frænum once or twice every day for forty-two days, and if the vesicles or tubercles do not appear in that time, he considers it certain that the patient has not been infected. When, however, they are seen, he opens them freely, directs the patient to wash the mouth with a gargle, and applies caustic to the cuts or incisions. Afterward, he prescribes genista in the form of decoction or powder. With respect to the vesicles or tubercles on each side of the frænum, M. Magendie apprehends that Dr. Marochetti may have mistaken the natural appearances of the orifices of Warton's ducts for the vesicles supposed to contain the hydrophobic virus. Here we see also, that Marochetti starts an hypothesis which interferes very much with prevailing opinions, already noticed, concerning the long dormant state of the poison in the bitten part, or the production of a similar poison by the vessels in this part at a late period after the bite, in consequence of the influence of a germ of the virus supposed still to continue there. Dr. Marochetti's assertions, however, require confirmation.—Ed.

out rational aim or intention of any kind. Yet, if we nicely criticise and arrange them, we shall find that this is not the case.

There are four principles by which physicians appear to have been guided in their respective attentions to this disease. That of stimulating and supporting the vital power, so as to enable it to obtain a triumph in the severe conflict to which it is exposed; that of suddenly exhausting the system by severe bleedings and purgatives, as believing the disease to be of a highly inflammatory character; that opposing the poison by the usual antidotes and specifics to which other animal-poisons were supposed to yield; and that of regarding the disease as a nervous or spasmodic, instead of an inflammatory affection, and, consequently, as most successfully to be attacked by an antispasmodic course of medicines and regimen.

The very popular use of ammonia and camphire may, by some, be ascribed to the first of these views, as being powerful stimulants; yet, in fact, they were rather employed from different motives, and fall within one or two of the principles of action which yet remain to be considered. But to this class of medicines, designed expressly to support the vital power, and enable nature herself to triumph in so severe a struggle, belong expressly the warm and cordial confections and theriacas that were at one time in almost universal estimation; as also various kinds of pepper given in great abundance, oil of cajeput, different preparations of tin, copper, and iron, and, in later periods, bark.

In direct opposition to this stimulating and tonic plan, was that of suddenly debilitating and exhausting the system, upon the hypothesis that the symptoms of canine rabies were those of violent and rapid inflammation. The practice of applying ice or the coldest water to the head, and of submersion in cold water, belongs mostly to this view of the subject, as used a century ago, though in the time of Celsus it was employed in a much slighter degree to take off the spasm of hydrophobia, and to quench the thirst that accompanied it. "Miserrimum genus morbi; in quo simul æger, et siti et aquæ metu cruciatur: quo oppressis in angusto spes est."—(*De Medicinâ*, lib. v., cap. xxvii., sect. 2.) In this almost hopeless state, the only remedy (unicum remedium), Celsus continues, is to throw the patient instantly, and without warning, into a fishpond; alternately, if he have no knowledge of swimming, plunging him under the water that he may drink, then raising his head; or forcing him under it if he can swim, and keeping him below till he is filled with the water; so that the thirst and water-dread may be extinguished at the same time. But there is here, continues our author, another danger, lest the body of the patient, exhansted and worn out by the submersion as well as by the disease, be thrown into convulsions: to prevent which, as soon as he is taken out of the pond, he is to be put into warm oil.—(*Cels.*, loco citato.)

The bolder practitioners of subsequent times, in pursuing the refrigerating plan, were regardless of convulsions, and persevered at all hazards in reducing the living power to its last ebb; believing that the nearer they suffocated the patient without actually killing him, the greater their chance of success. Hence Van Helmont kept the wretched sufferer under water till the psalm "*Miserere*" was sung throughout, which, under some choristers, occupied a much longer time than under others; and, in the experiments of the Members of the Académie Royale, we meet with instances of a still more dangerous pertinacity, though success is said to have accompanied one or two of them. Thus, M. Morin relates the case of a young woman, twenty years old, who, labouring under symptoms of hydrophobia, was plunged into a tub of water with a bushel of salt dissolved in it, and was harassed with repeated dippings till she became insensible and was at the point of death, when she was still left in the tub, sitting against its sides. In this state we are told, she was at length fortunate enough to recover her senses; when, much to her own astonishment, as well as to that of the by-standers, she found herself capable of looking at the water, and even of drinking it without choking. —(*Hist. de l'Académie Royale*, Ann. 1709.)

With respect to the warm oil-bath, which Celsus recommends in succession to that of cold water, the present author can say, that, in a single instance to which he was a witness when a young man, it produced no benefit whatever. It was prescribed by a physician in consequence of the recommendation of Celsus, but who certainly had not read him attentively, nor was acquainted with the scope of his reasoning. For, in this case, cold bathing had not been tried antecedently, and consequently there was no danger of those convulsions for which alone the Roman physician enjoins the use of the oil. The experiment, however, was so far perfect, that the tub was full of oil, and deep enough to reach the patient's chin.

In connexion with the cold bath thus persevered in to suffocation, the reducent or antiphlogistic plan was still farther forwarded, at one time, by the use of strong drastic purgatives, of which colocynth was, for a long period, the favourite (*Hellot, An de Morsis à Rabido Colocynthis?* Paris, 1676); and at other times by a very bold and perilous use of the lancet.

Bleeding has lately been revived, and carried to the extent of deliquium by large and rapid depletions, and the operation has been repeated almost as long as the powers of life would allow. Dr. Nugent employed it at Bath, in 1753, in one case, and the patient was restored, but musk and other antispasmodics were largely employed at the same time: and Dr. Schoolbred of Bengal has since had two patients who recovered under this process; but he employed mercury at the same time, and it is by no means certain, either from the history of the patients, or of the dog by which they were bitten, that the disease was a genuine lyssa.

Yet, whatever benefit this practice may possess, it has no pretensions to novelty; for there is not a single course of treatment ever invented for this intractable disease, that has been for upwards of a century more extensively tried and re-tried, both moderately and profusely, or excited a warmer controversy upon its merits. Poupart, in 1699, espoused the practice, and gives the case of a woman, who perfectly recovered by bleeding her to deliquium, and afterward confining her for a year to bread and water.—(*Hist. de l'Acad. des Sc.*, An. 1709.)

Berger, in the same year, recommended bleeding, but advised that the blood should be taken from the forehead. In the Breslaw Collections for 1719, is the case of a cow supposed to be rabid, and said to be cured by profuse bleeding. And the Philosophical Transactions abound with similar histories, some of them purporting to have been attended with similar success, derived from human subjects; but most of them too loosely given, or too undecided in their symptoms, to be in any measure entitled to reliance. That of Dr. Hartley and Mr. Sandys was, at one time, appealed to as demonstrative. It is the case of a groom who was bitten by a dog, supposed to be mad, towards the end of November, and who sickened about the middle of January ensuing; he had an aversion to drink, and was conjectured to be labouring under rabies. Venesection was here trusted to almost entirely, and every repetition of the lancet seemed serviceable: in consequence of which he lost a hundred and twenty ounces of blood in the course of a week, by different depletions, which consisted of sixteen or twenty ounces at each time. The man recovered: but few readers will believe him to have been really rabid, when they learn that, although he had an aversion to drink, he swallowed liquids; that his chief symptoms were sickness, trepidation, a faltering speech and memory; and that, through the whole course of the disease, he attended, though with some difficulty, to his duty in the stable.—(*Phil. Trans.*, year 1737–8.)

The Edinburgh Medical Commentaries are equally replete with cases in which the same plan of evacuation had been tried; but they are also equally unsatisfactory. Thus, Dr. Tilton informs us, that having heard of the recovery of a patient from the disease before us, who had bled profusely and almost to death, by an accidental fall from a high place, and a division of the temporal artery, he employed venesection freely in a case of his own, drawing off from twenty to thirty ounces at a time, and occasionally bleeding to deliquium.—(Vol. vi., p. 432.) But the symptoms are here also so doubtful, that the result is of no importance.

The practice, therefore, has been not uncommon for at least a century and a half; and had it proved as specific as some late reports would induce us to believe, it must have descended to us with a wider and more confirmed reputation, and formed the only course to be relied on. But the misfortune is, that however salutary at times, it has often completely failed in the hands of unprejudiced and judicious practitioners; and where it has succeeded, it has generally been combined with other means that have been resorted to at the same time. There is a case of failure related by Dr. Plummer in the Edinburgh

Medical Essays (vol. v., part ii.) ; but it is not much to be relied on, as not more than twenty ounces of blood was lost at a second and accidental bleeding, and only ten a day or two before by a prescribed venesection. Mr. Peters however, who employed profuse and repeated bleedings, sometimes even to deliquium, had in his day so little dependance on them alone, that he uniformly combined this remedy with opium and mithridate, or other cordials ; and in the case which he has introduced into the Philosophical Transactions, he ascribes the success which accompanied his plan to this combined mode of treatment.—(*Phil. Trans.*, 1745, No. 475.) In like manner, Mauchart, as quoted by Bühlmeier, while he advises bleeding, and to an extent proportioned to the length of the interval between the infliction of the wound and the attack of the paroxysm (and where the patient is of a melancholy temperament, even to deliquium), advises at the same time, that the bitten part be scarified ; and when this also has bled till nothing but serum escapes, that the wound be dressed with mithridate, theriaca, or rue, and a defensive plaster put over it, and that the patient take pills, compounded of mithridate and other materials, to the number of nine every day, for nine months, keeping himself in a free perspiration, and cautiously changing his linen.

In the case of dogs, venesection, how liberally soever made use of, does not seem to be of much benefit. It has lately been the subject of a series of experiments at Paris, under the superintendence of MM. Magendie, Dupuytren, and Breschet, who have carried it to deliquium, but without any success whatever. And hence, though it has unquestionably been serviceable, in many cases, the practice cannot be regarded as a specific.

To close the whole, Professor Trolliet has employed venesection so extensively, and in such variable proportions, from single or double bleedings of sixteen ounces each to not less than *seven pounds*, by different bleedings in the course of a few hours, and in every instance so entirely without effect, as reasonably to put the question at rest for ever. And the more so as, in his hands, the bolder the practice, the sooner the patient fell a sacrifice to it. We have a striking example of this in the case of the patient just referred to, whose interval between the infliction of the wound and the signs of the disease extended to upwards of five months. Early on the morning in which the hydrophobia first appeared, bloodletting to syncope was prescribed, and five pounds were drawn off before this effect was produced. The water-dread returned with the return of recollection ; and, at eleven o'clock on the same morning, he was again blooded to the amount of eighteen ounces, when he again fainted. The spasms of the chest and throat became more permanent. At three o'clock, fourteen ounces more were taken away, when deliquium followed, succeeded by a considerable augmentation of the spasms, in extent as well as in violence. At seven in the evening, the respiration became frothy as well as difficult, the difficulty increased, and the patient expired in a

few minutes, about twelve hours only after the commencement of the hydrophobia.

The poison of rabies has, by a numerous body of pathologists, been contemplated as of a nature akin to the poison of other venomous animals, and particularly serpents, and consequently best to be opposed by the usual remedies and specifics, to which these are found most effectually to yield. And hence in the first place, the use of the *radix Mungo* of Kœmpfer (*ophiorrhiza Mungos*, Linn.), still supposed to be a specific for the bite of the cobra di capello and the rattlesnake. In India and Ceylon, it is used to the present day as an antidote against the bite of the mad dog : Kœmpfer highly extols it, and Gremmius, who practised with great reputation at Columbo, employed it very largely.

Acids and alkalis belong to the same class of antilyssics. Of the former, Agricola, who was hostile to the depleting system, preferred the muriatic acid, and regarded this as a specific (*Chirurg.*, p. 391) even when restrained to a topical application. Poppius preferred the sulphuric ; but, by far the greater number of practitioners, the acetous was held in most esteem. Many combined this last with butter, and used it both internally and externally : Wedel, with other materials ; "as a cure," says he, "for the bite of a mad dog, let the patient drink vinegar, theriaca, and rue."—(*Exerc. Semiot. Pathol.*, cap. 8.)

The general suffrage, however, was far more considerable in favour of the alkalis, and especially of ammonia. There is some reason for this preference. It is well known that ammonia is a valuable medicine, whether applied externally or internally, against a variety of animal poisons. I have successfully used it more or less diluted, in various instances, as a lotion against the sting of wasps and bees, and the bites of gnats and vipers ; and I have seen it of great service in checking the poison of the rattlesnake, and restraining the extent of the inflammation. On the continent, and especially in France, the usual form in which ammonia was formerly employed in cases of lyssa, was that of the eau de luce, a caustic spirit of ammonia, prepared with quicklime combined with rectified oil of amber, rendered more easily miscible by being rubbed into half its weight of soap. This was in general employed both externally and internally,[*] though we have several reports of a successful use of it when confined to an internal trial alone ; especially one related by M. Hervet (*Journ. de Médecine*, tom. lxii.), and another by M. Rubiere.—(Id., tom. lxiv.)

Mercury, from its proving a specific in syphilis, and more especially from its specific action on the salivary glands, the immediate outlet of the poison of rabies, has had a strong claim to general attention ; and has been very extensively tried in various forms. It was first recommended by Desault of Bordeaux, in 1736, and afterward very confidently by Dr. James, in our own

---

[*] Sage, Erfahrungen, &c., p. 49 ; Guettard, Mémoires sur différentes Parties des Sciences et des Arts, p. 122, Paris, 1768.

country, as a certain cure for man and other animals. He used it both as a prophylactic at the time of the bite, and an antidote at the commencement of the disease. He employed it as well externally as internally ; but his favourite form was that of the turbeth mineral, in the shape of pills. He has published a full account of his success with this medicine on Mr. Floyer's hounds, after they had made a trial of every other favourite and fashionable remedy in vain. These dogs, as we have already observed, were affected with a severe hydrophobia, which has been denied by some writers to be a symptom of the disease as appertaining to quadrupeds. All the hounds, we are told, that were salivated with the mercury, in whatever stage of the malady, recovered, and the rest died.—(*Phil. Trans.*, vol. xxxix., year 1735-6.) His experiments on mankind are less complete : for they amount to not more than three, and in each of these the medicine was employed as a preventive, shortly after the affliction of the bite ; and hence, as the patients never became rabid, we cannot be sure that they had received the contagion, or would have had the disease had the mercury never been employed. The muriate of the metal was another favourite form, which, by Loisy, was used together with inunction.

The grand object was to excite a speedy salivation, and maintain it so long as there was supposed to be any danger ; and especially where the administration had been delayed till the paroxysm had shown itself. Frank, Girtanner, De Moneta, Raymond, and a host of writers upon the subject, deny not only that mercury is a specific, but that it has ever produced a cure, in whatever way it may have been employed. Kaltschmid, on the contrary, with an unjustifiable confidence, calls it *remedium indubium,** and De Choiseul a *méthode sure et facile.*† In the fortieth volume of the Journal de Médecine, there is a relation in which mercurial inunction seems to have been successful in a genuine case, and I have heard of one or two other instances that have occurred in our own country.

As diuretics were supposed to possess a strong alexipharmic power, or that of expurgating the system from animal poisons in general, these have also had their votaries, and been in high reputation as a remedy for lyssa. Cantharides were at one time the favourite medicine under this head, or some other stimulant insect of the coleopterous order, as the meloe, lytta, or one or two species of scarabæus ; which, like mercury and ammonia, were sometimes taken internally alone, and sometimes applied topically also, to keep up a perpetual irritation. Bohadsch tells us gravely, that the disease will always yield to ten cantharides powdered and introduced into the stomach.—(*Posit. Zoolog. in Klinkosch. Diss. Select.*) Monconys, that the

powder should be continued from the bite to the time in which we may reasonably expect the symptom of hydrophobia ; and adds, that this medicine, which was regarded as an arcanum in his day, was a remedy of publicity over all Greece. —(*Voyages,* i., p. 406.) He might have extended his theatre ; for Egypt was as well acquainted with the general principle of this practice as Greece or Hungary ; and it is a positive exhortation of Avicenna, that whatever diuretic may be employed should be carried to its utmost acrimony, even to the discharge of bloody urine.—(Lib. iv., Fen. vi., Tr. iv.) M. Axter of Vienna has of late revived the use of cantharides, and tells us, that he has for thirty years employed this medicine with far more success than any other, after having previously made experiments with and been disappointed in the use of all other remedies, as musk, camphire, belladonna, opium, or oil, used internally and externally, and water bathing. But it does not seem that he can speak further than to its supposed prophylactic powers, as he does not appear to have tried it in the acute stage of the disease.—(*Nouv. Biblioth. Germ. Medico-Chir.,* Paris, 1821.)

The ash-coloured liverwort (*lichen terrestris cinereus Raii*) was another diuretic of great popularity, and which seems at length to have triumphed over the stimulant insects, and to have superseded their use ; on which account Linnéus changed its trivial name from *cinereus* to *caninus*. In our own country, this medicine was at one time peculiarly in vogue. It was given in powder, with an equal quantity of black pepper, a drachm and a half of the two forming the dose for an adult, which was taken for four mornings, fasting, in half a pint of warm cow's milk ; the patient, however, was first to lose nine or ten ounces of blood, and afterward to be dipped in cold water for a month together, early in the morning. And such was the general confidence in this plan, or rather in the antilyssic power of which the lichen was supposed to be the most active principle, that its virtues formed one of the most common subjects of eulogy in the Philosophical Transactions at the time when Mr. Dampier introduced it to public notice at an early period of the history of the Royal Society (*Mechanical Account of Poisons,* art. 3) ; while, at the earnest solicitation of Dr. Mead, the powder was admitted in the year 1721 into the London Pharmacopœia, under the title of pulvis antilyssus ; who declares that, "when united with the previous venesection and subsequent cold bathing, he had never known it fail of a cure (*Chirurg. parv. Nurüb.,* &c., 8vo., 1643), though he had used it a thensand times in the course of thirty years practice."

How far emetics may be serviceable, general trial has not perhaps been sufficient to determine. They have often been found capable of relieving spasms of the throat, and enabling the patient to swallow liquids, when every other plan has failed. They were hence recommended by Agricola, but only perhaps on account of their violence upon a weakened frame, as a sort of forlorn hope, for he does not advise them till

---

* Dissertatio de Salivatione Mercuriali, ceu indubio præservationis et curationis remedio adversus rabiem caninam, Jan., 1760.

† Nouvelle Méthode, sure et facile, pour le Traitement des Personnes attaquées de la Rage, Paris, 1756.

after the third day. Dr. Satterley, however, has given a case in the Medical Transactions which he regards as rabies, in which vomiting was employed from an early period of the disease, and with very decided advantage.—(Vol. iv., p. 343.) But there seems to be a doubt whether the patient here referred to laboured under genuine lyssa. He had been bitten three months before by a dog, but the fate of the dog was not known ; the cicatrix betrayed no uneasiness or irritation precursive to the disease, or during its course ; the hydrophobia was remittent or intermittent, so that the patient drank liquids at times with tolerable ease ; the spastic action ran to a greater extent over the muscular system than usual, so as at one time to produce emprosthotonos ; and the patient did not expire till at least a week after the attack : all which are very unusual symptoms in lyssa, and have seldom if ever been combined in the same individual.

In lyssa, however, the nervous system appears to be that which is by far the most severely tried, and to which the disease may be most distinctly referred. And hence it is not to be wondered at that antispasmodics and sedatives should also have been had recourse to very extensively, and obtained a very general suffrage. In effect, whatever benefit in this disease has at any time been derived from ammonia, camphire, or cold bathing, it is more easy to resolve their palliative or remedial power into the principle of their being active antispasmodics, than to any other mode of action. The more direct antispasmodics and sedatives, however, employed in this malady, were musk, opium, belladonna, nux vomica, tobacco, and stramonium. The last has been chiefly tried in India, where three drachms and a half of the leaves, infused in a very large portion of water or other common drink, and swallowed daily for three days in succession after the bite, was at one time a very approved and popular remedy.

Musk, opium, and belladonna, however, are the antispasmodics which have been chiefly depended upon in Europe. They have sometimes been given in very large doses alone, but more generally in union with other medicines. Cullen seems doubtful of the powers of either, apparently from not having had sufficient opportunities of witnessing the disease and their effects upon it, and hence refers us, in both instances, without venturing upon any decisive opinion of his own, " to the labours of the learned industrious Société Royale of Paris, who have taken much pains and employed the most proper means for ascertaining the practice in this disease."— (*Materia Medica*, vol. ii., pp. 252, 380.) With respect to musk, he admits, however, that Dr. Johnston has given us two facts that are very much in favour of its power : and " I have," says he, " been informed of an instance in this country of some large doses of musk having proved a cure after symptoms of hydrophobia had come on."—(Ibid.) Hilary says, " in these cases it acts as a sudorific ;" and Gmelin regarded it as a specific antidote.—(*Diss. de specifico antidoto novo adversus effectus morsû canis rabidi*, Tub., 1750.)

Vol. II.—U

Opium, in like manner, when employed alone, was given in large doses, and we have numerous cases on record in which this, like the preceding medicines, is said to have operated a cure.—(*Dantzic, Gazette de Santé*, 1777, p. 51.) But, unfortunately, neither musk nor opium, in whatever quantity employed, has been found successful in general practice. Tode more especially has pointed out the inefficiency of the latter, in the largest doses referred to (*Annalen*, ix., p. 33), and Raymond has confirmed his remarks.—(*Med. Observ. and Inquiries*, vol. v.) But a late experiment of Professor Dupuytren, of the Hôtel Dieu, has given a still more striking and incontrovertible proof of its utter inefficacy, if not in all cases of the disease, in certain states and circumstances. Surlu, a man aged twenty-four, who had been bitten by a dog sufficiently proved to be mad, had been cauterized immediately afterward, and been discharged as supposed to be cured. In about a month from the time of the bite, he was attacked with rabies in its severest symptoms, and conveyed to the hospital. Opium was the medicine determined upon, and as the constriction of the throat prevented it from being given by the mouth, a gummy solution was injected into the veins, for which the saphæna and cephalic were alternately made use of. Two grains of the extract were in this manner thrown in, and the patient was in some degree tranquillized for an hour or two : the dose was doubled towards the evening of the same day. It was repeated at intervals, and at length increased to eight grains at a time. The relief it afforded, however, was never more than temporary, and he expired on the fifth day from the incursion.[*] M. Trolliet used it freely in the form of pills, in combination with belladonna ; but in no instance had he reason to boast of his success, though he gave in some cases twenty-seven grains of opium, and nine of the extract of belladonna, in the course of twenty-four hours. Professor Brera employed the belladonna, but united it with mercury instead of with opium : his doses were carried gradually to a great extent, insomuch that the patients at length took the powdered root of the belladonna to the amount of three drachms a day ; and in about forty-four or forty-six days swallowed seven ounces and a half of this drug, and ten grains of corrosive sublimate, besides rubbing in some ounces of mercurial ointment.—(*Mem. Soc. Ital. Scienz.*, tom. xvii., Modena.) The object was to keep the system as much as possible under the influence of mercury, evidenced by ptyalism, and of the narcotic effects of belladonna, so long as the combination was continued. As a preventive, it seems to have been successful ; though several of the patients appear to have advanced to the first symptoms of acute affection, having had some degree of water-dread, and recurring irritation in the bitten parts, the disease did not proceed beyond these initiary steps. But we have no proof of success from this plan after the

* Orfila, Traité des Poisons, &c. The extract of belladonna in solution and other narcotics, have likewise been injected into the veins without success.—ED.

pathognomonic signs had shown themselves. The warm bath was also combined with the above practice. In like manner, musk, opium, and belladonna have been all united; and sometimes combined with camphire, oil of amber, inunction with olive oil,* or bleeding. Musk was also at one time very generally combined with cinnabar, and in this form supposed to be peculiarly efficacious. The famous powder employed by the natives of Tonquin, and introduced into this country by Mr. Cobb, on which account it was called pulvis Cobbii, or Tunguinensis, consisted of sixteen grains of musk with forty-eight grains of cinnabar, mixed in a gill of arrack. This, taken at a dose, is said to have thrown the patient into a sound sleep and perspiration in the course of two or three hours: and where it did not, the dose was repeated till such effect was produced. And this medicine also was regarded as a specific during the short career of its triumph, and a cure was commonly supposed to follow the administration of the medicine.

The sedative power of several of the preparations of arsenic, however, had perhaps a fairer pretension than any of these, and especially as, like mercury, it has for ages been employed with decided benefit in Asia in the case of syphilis. Agricola mentions its use in his day (*Comment. in Popp.*, p. 54), but the forms in which it was then employed were rude and incommodious, and they do not appear to have been followed with much success. It is to be regretted, however, that even in the elegant and manageable form of Dr. Fowler's solution, it has not been found to be more efficacious. It has of late years been tried internally in various cases, and particularly, with great skill and in full doses, by Dr. Marcet; but in every trial it has disappointed our hopes. Applied externally, as a preventive to the bitten part, Dr. Linke of Jena thinks it has succeeded; but as his trials were made on dogs inoculated from the froth of rabid animals after death, no dependance can be placed on them.

Under this head I may also observe, that the Prussic acid has occasionally been had recourse to, but without any apparent benefit. In the form of the distilled water of the *prunus Laurocerasus*, it was not long since made a subject of experiment at Paris by Baron Dupuytren, who injected this fluid into the veins of various dogs, and appears to have done so in one instance into those of a man: but in every case without effecting a cure.

There are two or three other remedies, which it is difficult to arrange, but which have also acquired a considerable celebrity in the cure of lyssa; and hence it is necessary to notice them.

The first is the Ormskirk medicine, so called from its preparer, Mr. Hill of Ormskirk, supposed, for the inventor could not be prevailed upon to publish his secret, to consist of the following materials: powder of chalk, half an ounce; ar-

menian bole, three drachms; alum, ten grains; powder of elecampane root, one drachm; oil of anise, six drops. The single dose, thus compounded, is to be taken every morning for six times in a glass of water, with a small proportion of fresh milk. If this be the real formula, and the analysis of Dr. Black concurred with that of Dr. Heysham in determining it to be so, the inventor seems to have contemplated the specific virus to be an acid, for the basis of this preparation is unquestionably an alkaline earth. And with regard to its occasional efficacy, the latter writer, following the general current of opinion of the day, informs us, that this has been so thoroughly established by experience, that there can be no room to doubt it. Dr. Heysham himself, however, admits of various cases in which it failed, while in many instances his successful ones do not afford proofs of an existence of the genuine disease.—(*Diss. Med. Rabie Caninâ*, 8vo.)

The second of the anomalous remedies I have just referred to, might possibly have been introduced under the head of the common antidotes for the bites of venomous animals; but as it has reputed powers in some degree peculiar to itself, it is best to notice it separately. This is the alyssum, or *alysma Plantago* (madwort plantain), of established reputation in America as a specific for the bite of the rattlesnake, where it seems to rival the imprescriptible claims of the *ophiorrhiza Mungos*, though its juice is generally given in combination with that of the common horehound—an addition that certainly does not promise much accession to its strength.

This species of alyssum has for some ages been a popular remedy for canine madness, especially in the north of Europe: and in a late communication to Sir Walter Farquhar in the Russian tongue, translated and published in Mr. Brande's Journal (*Jour. of Sciences and the Arts*, No. ix., p. 142), we are told that it still retains its popular sway and reputation over a great part of the Russian empire, and that in the government of Isola it has never failed of effecting a cure in a single instance for the last five-and-twenty years. The preparation is simple: the root is reduced to a powder, and the powder is to be eaten by being spread over bread and butter. Two or three doses are said to be sufficient in the worst cases, and will be found to cure mad dogs themselves.

The butcher's broom (*genista tinctoria*), and side-leaved scull-cap (*scutellaria laterifolia*), have however rivalled the reputation of the plantago; and, in our own day, the first is powerfully recommended by M. Marochetti of Moscow, in the St. Petersburgh Miscellanies of Medical Science, as employed with great success in the Ukraine; and the second by Dr. S. Spalding of New-York, who tells us that it has been successful in America in upwards of a thousand cases, not only in men, but in dogs, swine, and oxen.*

---

* Vater, Pr. de Olei Olivarum efficaciâ contra morsum canis rabiosi, experimento Dresdæ facto, adstructâ, Viteb., 1750.

* Chymical analyses have shown this plant to be nearly inert.—See N. York Med. Repository, vol. xiv.— D.

The next remedy I have to notice is also of extensive use in the present day, and comes before ' us with no mean authority. While the medical practitioners of the east are pursuing their plan of abstracting rabid blood from the system, as the surest means of curing canine madness, the physicians of Finland have undertaken to accomplish the same effect, by introducing rabid blood into the morbid frame. In the second number of the Hamburgh Medical Repository, Dr. W. Rithmeister, of Powlowsk in Finland, has given an article, in which he has collected a multiplicity of striking cases, and various authorities in proof that the blood of a rabid animal, when drunk, is a specific against the canine hydrophobia, even where the symptoms are most strongly marked. The rabid wolf-dog, or other quadruped, is for this purpose killed, and its blood drawn off and collected as an antilyssic ptisan. Dr. Rithmeister's communication contains a letter to himself from Dr. Stockmann of White Russia, confirming this account, and stating the practice to be equally common and successful in his own country.

I will only add, that a discussion has lately taken place between two Italian physicians of distinguished reputation, Professor Brugnatelli of Pavia, and Professor Valetta of Milan, upon the virtues of chlorine as an antidote for the disease in question. The former has strongly recommended it (*Giornale di Fisica*, &c., Pavia, Dec., 1816), and the latter has denied that it is of any use (*Biblioteca Italiana*, Gennaj., 1817): in answer, however, to which denial, Professor Brugnatelli has adduced various authenticated facts, by which what he calls the *specific* powers of the chlorine have been established and verified.—(*Giornale di Fisica*, &c., Pavia, Febbraj., 1817.*)

I have thus endeavoured, upon a subject of so much interest and importance, to put the reader into possession of the general history of the practice that has hitherto prevailed; and he

---

* M. Magendie (Journ. de Physiol. Expér., tom. i., p. 44, &c.) conceived, that the sudden production of an artificial plethora might have the effect of arresting this ungovernable disease, and with this view he injected about a pint of warm water into the veins of a hydrophobia patient; but though the operation relieved for a time the violence of the symptoms, death took place nine days after the experiment. The patient having lived, however, much beyond the usual period after the dread of water had commenced, hopes were entertained that this plan might prove more successful in subsequent cases; but experience has now fully shown, that the injection of water into the venous system, is of as little use as every thing else that has hitherto been suggested for the purpose of curing the disorder, after it has been decidedly formed. The guaco, a vegetable matter employed in South America as an antidote for the bites of serpents, has been strongly recommended as a remedy for hydrophobia. It has been tried in this country by Dr. Roots, Dr. Elliotson, and others; and though in one or two instances a temporary amendment followed its exhibition, the patients all died about the usual period, namely, on the third or fourth day from the commencement of decided hydrophobia.—Ed.

---

will at least allow, that if the result be highly unsatisfactory—as most unsatisfactory it is—such conclusion does not result from idleness on the part of the medical profession.*

But how are we to reconcile the clashing and contradictory statements which the present analysis unfolds to us? This is a question of no easy solution. Yet there are many circumstances which ought to be borne in memory, and will, in a certain degree, account for such opposite views and decisions, without rudely impeaching the veracity of any of the experimenters.

In the first place, it is possible, that the morbid poison itself, like that of plague or intermitting fever may vary in its degree of virulence, in certain idiosyncrasies, certain countries, or certain seasons of the year; and hence that a medicine which has proved useless in general practice, may succeed in particular persons, particular places, or at particular periods; or if inactive in itself, may be employed in so much milder a degree of the disease, that the constitution may be able, in most or many instances, to triumph over it by its own powers alone.

It is a just remark of Celsus, that omnis ferè morsus habet quoddam virus (*De Medicinâ*, lib. v., x.); and we have already given proof, that this is particularly the case when the animal that bites is labouring under the influence of violent rage or other sensorial excitement; the symptoms incident upon which produce a severe effect upon the nervous system, and often stimulate those of the genuine lyssa. And hence there can be little doubt, that these symptoms have often been mistaken for lyssa, and have given celebrity to the medicines employed for their cure, to which they were never entitled. In various cases, as we have already seen, the disease commences almost coetaneously with the external injury, or inoculation; in others, not till months or even years afterward. In some instances, the first symptoms of the disease show themselves in the bitten part, and even this in a very different manner; for there may be a troublesome sense of numbness, or of irritation; and this irritation may be confined to the cicatrix, or travel up the limb, and produce acute pain or spastic action: while, in other instances, there is no local affection whatever through the entire progress of the malady. Ordinarily speaking, hydrophobia or waterdread is one of the most common as well as one

---

* According to Roche and Sanson, no less than 300 medicines have been proposed as specifics for hydrophobia. The American editor, however, would add but few remedial agents to those already mentioned: Dr. Ramsay of South Carolina recommended the treatment by alkalis, as alluded to in a previous page. The *sapo* or contrecu-libri, another American remedy, has been sometimes employed; the seeds of this plant are preferred, but if these cannot be obtained, the leaves may be used. Dr. Becariè of New-Spain, speaks warmly of its efficacy.—See Med. Repository, vol. xvii. The vapour bath has been introduced into practice lately by M. Brisson. He has succeeded in curing upwards of 80 patients with it. It is employed at a temperature of 108° F.—D.

of the severest symptoms of the disease; yet there are instances, even where the rabies has terminated fatally, in which water-dread has not been once complained of. Most commonly again, on an early examination after death, the fauces and parts adjoining are found red and inflamed; but we have already observed, that Morgagni dissected patients in whom there was no such appearance whatever: and in two bodies, examined after death by Dr. Vaughan, the fauces, œsophagus, stomach, diaphragm, and intestines, were all in a natural state.

There can be little or no doubt, moreover, where many persons are bitten in quick succession by the same rabid animal, that the poison is not equally introduced into all of them. In some cases it may be expended entirely upon the earlier victims, and hence the rest, though bitten, may be free from the virus; while in others, where the teeth have to pass through various foldings of clothes, it is possible that the virus which still remains may be wiped off in its passage, and the larceration be nothing more than a clean wound from the first. And in all such cases a sanguine experimenter, without allowing for these circumstances, will be apt to persuade himself, whatever medicine he makes use of, that the absence of the disease is owing to the efficacy of the plan or the medicine he has prescribed, and which he is hence tempted to hold up to the world as an antidote or specific.

Some of these remarks will best explain the very different results of the same mode of treatment, in the eleven patients intrusted in 1775 to the care of M. Blaise of Cluny, after having been dreadfully bitten and torn by a mad wolf. The principal remedy was mercurial inunction, though combined with antispasmodics. The mercury was carried on in all of them to salivation, and the treatment continued for above a month, in those that lived long enough for this purpose. One died with great horror and water-dread about the twelfth day from the injury, and after the mercury had begun to act. A second perished under hydrophobia, furious, and at length comatose, just at the close of a mouth, his mouth and gums being slightly affected by the mercury. A third died nearly six weeks after the commencement of the mercurial plan, having been taken away by his friends on the eighteenth day, apparently in a state of doing well. The remaining eight, after having exhibited greater or less symptoms of spasmodic affection, but never amounting to hydrophobia, are said to have recovered, and were discharged accordingly (*Méthode éprouvée pour le Traitement de la Rage*); but, in a subsequent work, M. Blaise informs us, that even one of these died in a paroxysm of hydrophobia six weeks after his discharge and supposed restoration to health.*

* Hist. de la Société de Medecine, tom. ii. Dr. Elliotson saw two little girls, sisters, who were bitten at the same moment by a dog, and in the same part, namely, the face. One of them died, and the sister had the symptoms which commonly usher in hydrophobia; but, after lasting four or five days, they ceased, and she recovered. Facts

In all these cases, the success is ascribed to the action of the mercury, and the want of success to some irregularity or other, committed by the patient while under medical care. The enormities, however, are in general rather far fetched, and not very convincing. Thus, in the last of the above cases, it is ingeniously observed, that the man who had been so long discharged as well, *four* days only before the symptoms of hydrophobia appeared on him, had thrust his arm down the throat of an ox which was said to be mad; though no proof is offered that the ox was really mad, nor is it pretended that even this reputed mad ox inflicted any bite upon the arm whatever. Who does not see, that in all these cases, the mercury may have been guiltless of exercising any control! that those who died may have died in consequence of an effective lodgment of the virus in the wound inflicted, and that those who survived may have survived because it obtained no admission to the bitten part?

It is moreover highly probable, that a spontaneous cure is occasionally effected by the strength of the constitution, or the remedial power of nature alone. The fact appears to be, that the disease requires about six or seven days to run through its course, at the expiration of which period the system seems to be exonerated, by the outlet of the salivary glands, of the poison with which it is infested. And hence, if by any means it be able to sustain and carry itself through this period, without being totally exhausted of nervous power in the course of so protracted and prostrating a conflict, it will obtain a triumph over the disease; and any prescribed medicine made use of on the occasion, will seem to have effected the cure, and will run away with the credit of having done so, till subsequent instances dissolve the charm, and prove beyond contradiction the utter futility of its pretensions. I have already had to observe, that the contagion of lyssa, though highly malignant, is neither remarkably volatile nor very active, and in every instance perhaps, requires some exciting or predisponent cause to enable it to take effect: but, as it seems to be more indecomposible than any other contagion we are acquainted with, it is capable of lying latent and undissolved for months, if not years, till it meets with a cause of this kind. And hence the very long and uncertain interval, which sometimes occurs between the attack of the rabid animal and the appearance of rabid symptoms, has often proved another source of deception; of which we have a singular example in Mr. Nourse's case, related in an early volume of the Philosophical Transactions (No. 445), which states, that a lad, who had been bitten in the thumb by a mad dog, took morning and evening for forty days a drachm of the pulvis antilyssus already described, and bathed in the sea for ten days in succession. He was in due time reported to be

of this kind prove, at all events, that the constitutional disturbance, preceding the occurrence of actual hydrophobia, is not absolutely irremediable, and that in this stage, the patient may be saved. —ED.

well, and the cure was altogether ascribed to the specific virtues of the antilyssic powder. He was shortly afterward cut for the stone, from which also he recovered : NINETEEN MONTHS after which operation, however, he was attacked with hydrophobia and the other symptoms of canine madness, and fell a victim to their violence. Had this patient died under the operation of lithotomy, or from any other circumstance in the interval, the virtues of the antilyssic powder would have obtained a complete, and indeed a rational triumph in this instance : and even now, there may be a question whether the appearance of the disease was not retarded by the plan pursued, though its specific power can no longer be maintained for a moment. The occasional exciting cause which, in this instance, at length gave activity to the dormant virus, is not pointed out to us. But it is difficult, if not impossible, to account without such a cause for the quickening of the lurking seminium of the poison at this time rather than at any other.* And the following valuable remarks of Dr. Percival, occurring in his manuscript comment on the author's volume of Nosology, in relation to this subject, are in full illustration of the same opinion. ?

" A wine porter was attended, in Dispensary practice, for a low fever : after a time appeared symptoms of lyssa ; and much inquiry elicited the recollection of his having been slightly bitten by a dog six weeks before. In the interval he was convicted of some fraudulent practice in the cellar of his master, to whom he owed great obligation, and was dismissed with disgrace. Anxiety on this event seemed to produce the fever, which terminated in lyssa.

" Lately, an officer in our barracks was bitten by a dog, whose madness being recognised, the bitten part was excised immediately. After an undisturbed interval of two months, he was advised to go to England to dissipate the recollection of the accident : there he exercised himself violently in hewing wood ; felt pain in the hand which had been bitten ; embarked for Ireland ; had symptoms of hydrophobia on board the packet, and died soon after his arrival.

" I have lately seen a case of hydrophobia treated ineffectually by most profuse bleeding and large doses of opium. Here too, the bitten part was extirpated by caustic within an hour. The patient was a man of steady mind, nor could any occasional cause be assigned for bringing the poison into action, except that a bilious diarrhœa was suddenly checked.

" From the varying period of attack we might infer, that the influence of occasional causes is very considerable. In the last patient hydrophobia supervened exactly five weeks from the time of the bite ; he lost a hundred and eight ounces of blood in twelve hours, which sunk

him much ; violent perspiration, and at length delirium, attended the water-dread : during the last twenty-four hours he swallowed, and recovered his senses ; and died slightly convulsed while cutting an egg. These cases seem to point out agitation of mind and feverish excitation as powerful occasional causes."

In a disease so intricate as lyssa, a very complex treatment is by no means unpardonable ; but it may fairly, I think, be questioned, whether the complexity and the energy of the means employed to produce a cure may not rather, in some instances, have had an opposite effect, and have hastened and confirmed a fatal issue. A patient bitten by a mad dog, having in vain tried and persevered in the use of the Ormskirk medicine, was next put under the joint care of Dr. Watson and Dr. Fothergill. Having been bled standing, as long as he could stand, he was next immersed in a warm bath, where he was ordered to remain till he again became faint ; a clyster of milk and water, with a drachm of Dover's powder dissolved in it, was injected as soon as he was removed from the bath ; half an ounce of mercurial ointment was at the same time rubbed into the legs and thighs, and three grains of thebaic extract given in the form of pills, two grains being ordered to be continued every hour till he became sleepy.

To stand the brunt of a treatment thus vigorous, would demand no ordinary constitution, even without the co-operation of any disease. But that the wretched sufferer should sink (as he did, in a few hours) under the assault of such a malady and such a mode of cure, cannot be matter of surprise.

The whole subject is afflictive, as well in respect to its treatment as its progress. But how, after all, is a young practitioner to proceed when he meets with a case of rabies ? This is a most important question ; and the following remarks, submitted with great deference as the result of some little personal experience and no small degree of reflection, are meant to meet it, and to point out the path which, in the present unsettled state of the subject, it may perhaps be most expedient to adopt.

From the whole of the preceding survey it is sufficiently clear that we have no direct specific for the cure of the disease ; and hence, whatever plan we employ, must be palliative only. It appears also, that the disease consists in a poison of a peculiar kind, capable of assimilating some of the animal secretions to its own nature, and that the new matter, or contagion, hereby produced, continues to be eliminated for five or six days, principally, if not entirely, from the excretories of the salivary glands, as the inflammation of gout unloads itself on the extremities, and the specific matter of exanthems on the surface generally ; and that at the expiration of this period, or as soon as such depuration has been effected, the disease abates, and the patient is restored. It appears also, that the disease is one of the most dangerous in the whole catalogue of nosology, and that few patients recover from it under any plan of medicine that has ever been devised ; but that nevertheless,

---

* It deserves to be recollected, however, that modern practitioners do not puzzle themselves about the exciting cause, in cases where the syphilitic poison first produces constitutional symptoms several weeks or months after the application of the virus, and the formation of a chancre.—ED.

some patients have recovered under almost every mode of treatment, however incongruous and contradictory to other modes ; and hence, that many cases of restoration must be rather referred to a natural or spontaneous cure than to the virtue of medicines.

In this state of things, it seems reasonable that our first intention should consist, as in various other kinds of animal poisons communicated in the same manner, in supporting the system generally, and the nervous part of it more particularly, so that it may not sink under the violent excitement and augmented secretion which the organ of the nerves has to encounter during so perilous a struggle. And it is to this principle we have to resolve all the benefit which has at any time been found to result from the use of the stimulant theriacas and other cordials of the old practitioners. On this account, ether, ammonia, and camphire have a strong claim on our attention, and especially the two last, as they may be given in a solid form. All the pungent spices belong to the same class, as cardamomseeds and capsicum, and may be adverted to as auxiliaries ; nor should wine or even ardent spirits be refrained from, if the patient can be induced to swallow them ; moderately through the entire course of the disease, but liberally and profusely as his strength declines. Our grand object must be to keep him alive, and prevent a fatal torpitude in the sensorium for a certain number of days, at any expense of stimulants, or of subsequent debility. Wine is profusely given with great success in the bite of the most venomous serpents of the East, and analogy justifies us in proposing it in the present instance.

Our next intention should be to diminish, as much as possible, the spastic action of the chest and fauces, and to prevent a return of the exacerbations. And to this end as much quiet and composure as we can possibly procure, under so restless a state of body, seems imperatively called for, and is far more likely to be serviceable than the fatigue of taking the patient repeatedly out of bed for the purpose of plunging him either into a hot or cold bath. And though opium has never of itself, perhaps, produced a cure, it seems advisable to try it in liberal doses ; and the more so, as several of the cases already adverted to afford a direct proof, that it is capable occasionally of producing some degree of tranquillity for a short period. In employing it, however, it seems most reasonable, from analogy, to combine it with some diaphoretic, and particularly with ipecacuanha in the form of Dover's powder, since at all times the animal frame is most disposed to be quiet and free from irregular actions when there is a general moisture upon the surface. In many cases of rabies, such a state of body has been found unquestionably favourable ; and in one of the instances already quoted from the Medical Transactions, the benefit was so striking, that the practitioner could not avoid regarding it as critical. It is possible, also, though no great stress can be laid upon this remark, that a part of the virus itself may be hereby eliminated, as in various other cases of animal poisons.

To obtain and encourage such elimination should indeed be our first object, if we had any means of accomplishing it upon which we could fully depend. This, however, we have not ; but as the quarter to which the virus is directed is the salivary glands, of which, indeed, we have full proof in consequence of the saliva being the fomes of the poison apparently as soon as it becomes elaborated, and as we have a medicine which possesses a specific influence on this organ, and is capable of augmenting its secretion to almost any extent, it seems of the utmost importance that, while we endeavour to support the system, and to allay the nervous irritation, we should endeavour at the same time to quicken the elimination of the morbid matter, by exciting the salivary emunctories, and thus probably also carrying it off in a diluter and less irritant form. It is difficult to withhold one's assent to all the numerous instances of cure which are so confidently asserted to have followed the use of mercury carried to the point of free salivation. And hence, without allowing this medicine to be a specific more than any other, we may indulge a reasonable hope of its forming a good auxiliary, and should employ it freely, either externally, internally, or in both modes simultaneously, but with as little disturbance to the patient as possible, till a copious ptyalism is the result.

Fever, or inflammatory action, does not necessarily belong to lyssa in any stage ; and the present mode of treatment is altogether grounded upon this principle. Either, however, may become incidentally connected with it, from the peculiar state of the habit or some other cause. Hence, as a preventive, the bowels should be kept moderately open ; and when there is any just apprehension of plethora, or a turgid state of the vessels, and particularly of the brain, blood should be drawn freely from the arm, and, if necessary, be repeated. We have already seen that such a state of congestion is sometimes produced even at the onset of the disease, and is so forcibly felt by the patient himself, that he earnestly entreats the medical attendant to bleed him. Such entreaty should, perhaps, never be urged in vain ; but the bleedings to deliquium, which have of late years been so strongly recommended, are a rash and dangerous practice. *

Such, in the doubt and darkness that at present beset us concerning the real physiology of lyssa, seems to be the safest and most promising path we can pursue. Our best time for action, however, and almost the only time we can improve, is immediately on the infliction of the wound : a tight ligature above which, with the

* Instead of persevering in these and other plans, which, when allowance is made for the ambiguous nature of many imperfectly reported recoveries, and the influence of the remedial powers of nature, cannot be said positively to have done effectual good in a single example, practitioners ought undoubtedly to make new experiments on the subject. If we always continue in the same path, we shall never discover the long desired object, namely, a method of treatment which can be depended upon.—ED.

treble precaution of the cupping-glass, excision and cauterization,' may in general be regarded as an effectual preventive. I do not know, indeed, that the profession is acquainted with any other.* It has, however, been proposed in France, to fight off the poison of lyssa by preoccupying the ground with the poison of a viper, upon the principle of combating variolous with vaccine matter : and for this purpose it has been suggested, that the part bitten by a mad dog should be again bitten, a little below the wound, as soon as may be, by a venomous serpent, whose virus, from its greater activity, will, in most cases, be certain of taking the lead, and may, it is presumed, guard the constitution against any subsequent effects from the wound of the mad dog. I have not, however, heard that this proposal has ever been carried into effect, and the claim of ingenuity is, most probably, the whole it will ever have to receive.†

I ought not, however, to conclude without noticing one very extraordinary fact in the economy of morbid poisons, and especially of that before us, which I have had confirmed by the testimony of several veterinary practitioners entitled to credit. It is, that no dog which has ever had the *distemper*, as it is called, which is the canine catarrh or influenza, has been known to become rabid spontaneously, though he is capable of receiving the disease by the bite of another dog. If this be true, for which however, I cannot fully vouch, we have certainly another instance of morbid poisons mortally conflicting with each other ; and it might be worth trying how far inoculation with the matter of canine catarrh might succeed in protecting a human subject after the infliction of a rabid bite ; though in the dog, perhaps from a stronger predisposition to rabies, it seems to be impotent. In South America, rabies, as already observed, has been altogether unknown, and I have hence been anxious to learn, whether the distemper be unknown there also ; and in answer to this inquiry, it has been told me, by several intelligent residents in that quarter, that this last disorder is so common and so fatal, that two thirds of the dogs littered there perish of it while pups ; a remark which still further confirms the home-report concerning its influence on rabies, and may partly explain the non-existence of the latter on the shores of the Plata.

SPECIES IX.
ENTASIA ACROTISMUS.
PULSELESSNESS.

FAILURE OR CESSATION OF THE PULSE, OFTEN ACCOMPANIED WITH PAIN IN THE EPIGASTRIUM ; THE PERCEPTION AND THE VOLUNTARY MUSCLES REMAINING UNDISTURBED.

ACROTISMUS is literally " defect of pulse," from κρότος, " pulsus," with a privitive *a* prefixed ; whence the technical term *crotophus* or *crotophium*, importing "painful pulsation or throbbing in the temple." Asphyxia is the term employed for this disease by Ploucquet, and, would have been used in the present arrangement, but that it has been long appropriated to import suspended animation or apparent death ; a total cessation, not of the pulse only, but of sense and voluntary motion.

This failure or cessation of pulsation sometimes extends over the whole system, and is sometimes confined to particular parts. In every case, it imports an irregularity in the action of the heart, or of the vessels that issue from it, and, in most cases, an irregularity proceeding from local or general weakness, and dependant upon a spasmodic disposition hereby produced in the muscular tunic of the vessels. Of this last cause, we have a clear proof in the universal chill and paleness that spread over the entire surface in the act of fainting or of death, to which fainting bears so striking a resemblance. Except, however, in the agony of dying, the spasmodic constriction for the most part soon subsides, and the arteries recover their proper freedom and diameter. Yet this is by no means the case always, for in violent hemorrhages, and especially hemorrhages of the womb, the rigidity has sometimes continued for several days, during the whole of which time the heart has seemed merely to palpitate, and there has been no pulse whatever. Morgagni relates, from Ramazzini, a case of this kind which extended to four days. The patient was a young man of great strength and activity, even during this suppression. The arteries were as pulseless as the heart ; and through the whole period he was quite cold to the touch, and without micturition. On the fourth day he died suddenly.—(*De Sed. et Causis Morb.*, ep. xlviii., Lugd. Bat., 4to., 1767.) Examples, indeed, are by no means uncommon, in which the spasm has existed for three (*Pathology*, p. 25), four, or even five days (*Pelargus, Med. Jahngänge.*, band v., p. 23) before death.

Other irritations besides that of weakness, have occasionally led to a like spastic state of the arteries. The stimulus of aneurism of the aorta has produced it in the brachial arteries, so that there has been no pulse in the wrists ;* and gout or some irritation in the stomach has operated in like manner on the arterial system to a much greater extent ; as has likewise general

---

* Dr. Marochetti's prophylactic treatment has already been mentioned.—ED.

† By referring to the article "hydrophobia" in the Dictionary of Practical Surgery, the reader will perceive that this expedient has really been tried.—ED.

* The hypothesis of such a degree of spasm as is here referred to, and supposed to be capable of rendering the large arteries impervious, is one that would not be generally adopted by modern practitioners. Many physiologists, perhaps all the most eminent ones, consider the small arteries as possessing the power of becoming completely constricted by a kind of action that may be sometimes spastic, but a contraction of the arterial trunks in this degree is a position that could not be so well established. In aneurisms of the arch of the aorta, the occasional interruption of the pulse can be explained on a better principle, and one confirmed by dissection ; namely, the manner in which the disease obstructs or breaks the impetus of the blood destined for the upper extremities.—ED.

pressure on the larger thoracic or abdominal organs, from water in the chest or cavity of the peritoneum. The cause however, is not always to be traced, and hence Marcellus Donatus has given an instance, which he tells us was unaccompanied with any disease whatever (Lib. vi., cap. ii., p. 620), the irritation probably having subsided. Berryatt, in the History of the Academy of Sciences, has furnished us with a very singular example of this disease, which was general as well as chronic, and continued through the whole· term of life. In all which cases, however, though the heart itself should seem to participate in the pulselessness, we are not to suppose that it is entirely without any alternation of systole and diastole, but only that its action is indistinct from weakness or irregularity. In treating of the nature of the pulse in. the Physiological Proem to the third class, we observed, that it is in some persons unusually slow, and has been found, as measured by the finger, not more than ten strokes in a minute: and that, in many of these cases, the cause of retardation seems to be a spasticity or want of pliancy in the muscular fibres of the heart or arteries, or both, rather than an actual torpor, which is also an occasional cause. I have never met with any case in which the ordinary standard of the pulse was not more than ten strokes in a minute; but I have at this time a patient, of about thirty-six years of age, whose pulse has not exceeded twenty-four or twenty-six strokes, and has often been below these numbers. He is a captain in the Royal Navy, of a sallow complexion and bilious temperament; till of late he enjoyed good health, but about three years since was attacked with a fit of atonic apoplexy, from which he recovered with difficulty. At an interval of a few weeks from each other, he had several other fits; on recovering from the last of which he instantly married a young lady to whom he had for some time been engaged. · He has now been married about fifteen months, has a healthy infant just born, and has had no fit whatever. His spirits are good, and he is residing by the seaside, which situation he finds agree with him best.

Dr. Latham gives a similar example in a merchant whose pulse, though never intermissive, seldom, for ten or twelve years that he had known him, exceeded thirty-two beats in a minute; occasionally was as slow as twenty-two, and at one time only seventeen. "I once," says Dr. Latham, "attended him through a regular fever, when his pulse was not more than sixty, notwithstanding the disease ran on for at least a fortnight with a hot and dry skin, white and furred and parched tongue, and occasional delirium."—(Med. Trans., vol. iv., art. xx.)

In many of these anomalies there is not only no perceptible pulse, or a very retarded one, but often intermissions more or less regular, and occasionally a want of harmony between the stroke in some of the arteries compared with that in others. Reil gives a case in which the heart, the carotids, and the radial arteries all pulsated differently (Memorabilia Clinica, vol. ii., fasc. i., 6, Hall., 1792); and Beggi another, in which the acrotism, or want of pulsation, extended over the entire frame, with the exception of the heart, which pulsated violently. —(Opp. Pacchioni, Rom., 4to., 1741.)

This species is strikingly exemplified in the biographical sketch of Mr. J. Hunter, drawn up and prefixed to his volume on Blood and Inflammation by Sir Everard Home. Mr. Hunter, for the four preceding years, had annually suffered from a fit of the gout in the spring. In the year 1773, this did not return, and having on a particular occasion been greatly affected in his mind, "he was attacked," says Sir Everard Home, "at ten o'clock in the forenoon, with a pain in the stomach, about the pylorus: it was the sensation peculiar to those parts, and became so violent that he tried change of position to procure ease; he sat down, then walked, laid himself down on the carpet, then upon chairs, but could find no relief: he took a spoonful of tincture of rhubarb, with thirty drops of laudanum, but without the smallest benefit. While he was walking about the room, he cast his eyes on the looking-glass, and observed his countenance to be pale, and his lips white, giving the appearance of a dead man. This alarmed him, and led him to feel for his pulse, but he found none in either arm. He now thought his complaint serious. Several physicians of his acquaintance, Dr. William Hunter, Sir George Baker, Dr. Huck Saunders, and Sir William Fordyce, all came, but could find no pulse: the pain still continued, and he found himself, at times, not breathing. Being afraid of death soon taking place if he did not breathe, he produced the voluntary act of breathing, his working his lungs by the power of the will, the sensitive principle with all its effect on the machine not being in the least affected by the complaint. In this state he continued for three quarters of an hour, in which time frequent attempts were made to feel the pulse, but in vain. However, at last the pain lessened, and the pulse returned, although at first but faintly, and the involuntary breathing began to take place. While in this state, he took Madeira, brandy, ginger, &c., but did not believe them of any service, as the return of health was very gradual. In two hours he was perfectly recovered."—(Sir E. Home's Life of Mr. Hunter, prefixed to the Treatise on Blood, &c., p. 46.)

This is one of the most extraordinary cases on record, considering the extensive group of important functions that were jointly affected, and the total freedom of the rest; and nothing can more strikingly prove how close is the sympathy that in many instances prevails between discontinuous organs, the chief disease having prevailed in the heart, and the chief pain in the stomach or its upper side.

The nature of the pain and the collateral symptoms seem sufficiently to show that this disease was of a spasmodic kind; for the deficiency of pulse was subsequent to the pain, and ceased upon its removal, while the deadly paleness of the face gave proof of a constriction of the capillaries.

So far as my own experience has extended,

such failures of the pulse, whether consisting in a total suspension or a preternatural retardation, and attended with acute or with very little pain, are dependant upon the diseased state of the larger arteries, or the larger viscera of the thorax or abdomen, and generally lead to sudden death. The case of the captain of the navy which I have just related, and which was drawn up while the first edition of this work was in the press, I may now apply to in illustration of this remark ; for I have since been informed by his sister, that while at Swansea, apparently in as good health as he had ordinarily enjoyed for several years, he was attacked with a fit of apoplexy, which carried him off in less than an hour. Such, too, was the fate of Dr. Latham's patient, for we are told, that " one day, when in complete health, as he then considered himself, he dropped down in the street and expired." And so sudden was the decease of Mr. J. Hunter, that feeling himself unwell while in the course of his professional attendance at St. George's Hospital, he went into an adjoining room, gave a deep groan, and dropped down dead.

In all cases of this kind, therefore, the mode of treatment must depend upon the nature of the exciting or predisponent cause, as far as we are able to ascertain it. Where the cause is constitutional, a sober, quiet, and regular habit of life, with a due attention to the ingesta and egesta, and particularly to a tranquillized state of mind, will often enable the valetudinarian to reach his threescore and tenth year with cheerfulness and comfort ; but he must content himself with

"——the cool sequestered vale of life,"

and not form a party in its contentions and its glitter, its bustle and " busy hum."

Where the affection appears to be dependant upon a particular state of any one of the larger thoracic or abdominal organs, as the heart itself, the lungs, the stomach, or the liver, our attention must be specially directed to the nature of the primary disease. And, in these cases, it is often essentially relieved by some vicarious irritation, as a seton or issue, a regular fit of the gout, a cutaneous eruption, or a painful attack of piles. During the paroxysm itself, the most powerful and diffusive stimulants should be had recourse to, as brandy, the aromatic spirit of ammonia, or of ether, which is still better, and opium in any of its forms.

Some persons are said to possess a natural power of thus keeping the heart upon a full stretch, and hereby producing a universal deficiency of pulsation, and of simulating death. Of this Dr. Cleghorn and Dr. Cheyne both give an instance. It should be observed, however, that the individuals died suddenly ; and one of them, Col. Townshend, within a few hours, after having maintained this rigidity of the heart for half an hour, at the expiration of which time he consented to resuscitate himself, and awoke from the apparent sleep of death. It should hence seem, that the natural energy of the heart sinks gradually, or abruptly, beneath the mischievous exertion, wherever such a power is found to exist.

GENUS II.
CLONUS.
CLONIC SPASM.

FORCIBLE AGITATION OF ONE OR MORE MUSCLES IN SUDDEN AND IRREGULAR SNATCHES.

THE Greek terms κλόνος and κλόνησις import " agitation, commotion, concussion." The clonic or agitatory spasms form two distinct orders in Sauvages, and a single genus in Parr. The first is unnecessarily diffuse ; the second is too restricted. The two orders of Sauvages are in the present arrangement reduced to two genera, and constitute that immediately before us, and SYNCLONUS, or that which immediately follows. Dr. Cullen seems at one time to have had a desire of distinguishing the diseases of both these genera by the name of convulsions ; and of limiting the name of spasm to the permanent contractions, or rigidities of the muscular fibres, produced by spastic action, constituting the different species of the preceding genus. " I think it convenient," says he, in his First Lines, " to distinguish the terms of spasm and convulsion by applying the former strictly to what has been called the tonic, and the latter to what has been called the clonic spasm." Yet the whole are treated of in his nosological arrangement under the common name of SPASMI, and even in his First Lines, notwithstanding this distinction, under that of " spasmodic affections without fever." These spasmodic affections are, indeed, subsequently divided into a new arrangement of " spasmodic affections of the animal functions ; of the vital ; and of the natural :" throughout which an attempt is still made to separate the term convulsion from that of spasm, and apply it to all clonic or agitatory motion of the muscles, while CONVULSIO is nevertheless retained in the Synopsis, as the technical name of that single species of disease, which is colloquially called convulsion-fit, and not extended to any others. There is doubtless a difficulty in drawing the line between entastic and clonic spasm in many cases, from the mixed nature of the symptoms ; but if it be felt of importance to take terms out of their general meaning, and tie them down to a stricter interpretation, such interpretation should be rigidly adhered to, or some degree of confusion must necessarily ensue.

To understand the real nature of the spasms we are now entering upon, it may be expedient to recollect, that the nervous power appears to be naturally communicated to parts by minute jets, as it were, or in an undulatory course, like the vibrations of a musical cord. But the movement is so uniform, and the supply so regular in a state of health and where there is no fatigue, that we are not conscious of any discontinuity of tenour, and can grasp as rigidly and as permanently with a muscle as if there were no relaxation in its supply of power. To prove the nature of the influx, however, nothing more is necessary than to reduce the muscle from a state of healthy tone to a state of languor, or to wear it down by fatigue ; for, in this condition, all the muscles tremble, and the stoutest man is incapable of extending his arm with a small weight in his hand, or even of raising a glass of wine slowly to the mouth, without a manifest and even a painful oscillation.

The flow of the nervous power, in a state of health, is augmented by the application of various stimulants, both mental and corporeal. The ordinary mental stimulus is the will, but any other mental faculty, when violently excited, will answer the same purpose, though the action which takes place in consequence hereof will in some degree be irregular, as proceeding from an irregular source, and will in consequence make an approach to the character of spasms ; of which a violent excitement of almost any of the passions affords examples sufficiently evident, and especially the passions of fear and anger, under the influence of which it is sometimes found impossible to keep a single limb still.

The ordinary corporeal stimulants are the fluids, which are naturally applied to the motory organs themselves. Thus the air which we breathe becomes a sufficient excitement to the action of the lungs ; the flow of the blood from the veins a sufficient excitement to that of the heart ; while the descent of the feces maintains the peristaltic motion of the intestinal canal.

Where these stimulants are regularly administered, and the organs to which they are applied are in a state of health, the alternations of jets and pauses in the flow of the nervous energy, as we have already remarked, are uniform. But in a state of diseased action, this uniformity is destroyed, and in two very different ways; for, first, the nervous energy may rush forward with a force that prohibits all pause or relaxation whatever, and this too in spite of all the power of the will ; and we have then a production of rigid or entastic spasms, or those abnormal contractions in different parts of the body of which the preceding genus furnishes us with abundant examples: and, next, the pauses or relaxations may be too protracted ; and, in this case, every movement will be performed with a manifest tremour. Where this last is the case, moreover, the succeeding jet from the accumulation of nervous power that necessarily follows upon such a retardation, must at length take place with an inordinate force and hurry; and the movement in the voluntary muscles, when attempted to be controlled by the will, must be irregular, and often strongly marked with agitation, giving us examples of convulsive or clonic spasm. And as, moreover, in such a state of the nervous system or of any part of it, there will often be found a contest between the retarding and the impelling powers, the spasm will not unfrequently partake of the nature of the two ; the nervous energy, after having been irregularly restrained in its course, will rush forward too impetuously, and for a few moments without any pause : and we shall have either a succession of constrictive and clonic spasms in the same muscle or sets of muscles, or a constrictive spasm in some parts, while we have a clonic spasm in others : and hence those violent and ramifying convulsions which we shall have more particularly to notice under the ensuing genus.

A sudden and incidental application of any irritant power whatever to any of the muscular fibres, will throw them into an irregular action, not only in a morbid state when they are most prone to such irregularities, but even in a state of health. Hence the involuntary jerk that takes place in all the limbs when a boat in which we are sailing at full speed gets aground without our expecting it, or we are assailed unawares with a smart stroke of electricity.

Now, whenever a forcible and anomalous movement of this kind has once been excited in any chain of muscular fibres whatever, there is a strong tendency in them to repeat the same movement even from the first ; and when from accident, or a continuance of the exciting cause, it has actually been repeated, it forms a habit of recurrence that is often broken off with great difficulty. Hence the convulsive spasm of the hooping-cough always outlasts the disease itself for some weeks, and is best removed by the introduction of some counter-habit obtained by a change of residence, atmosphere, and even hours. A palpitation of the heart, first occasioned by fright in an irritable frame, has in some cases continued for many days afterward, and in a few instances become chronic.

A habit of sneezing has sometimes been produced in the same manner, and followed an obstinate catarrh ; after which the slightest stimulants, even the sneezing of another person, have been sufficient to call up fresh paroxysms, and, in some cases which I have seen, of very long and troublesome continuance.

Hiccough affords us another example of the same tendency to a recurrence of muscular abnormities. This is usually produced by some irritation in the stomach, not unfrequently that of fulness alone: the irritation is by sympathy communicated to the diaphragm, which is thrown into a clonic spasm, and the spasm being a few times repeated, the habit becomes so established as in many instances to be broken through with considerable difficulty.

It is to these physiological laws that most of the affections we are now about to enter upon are referrible ; and the concentrated view we have thus taken of their operation, will render it less necessary for us to dwell at much length upon any of them.

The genus CLONUS comprises the six following species :—

1. Clonus Singultus. Hiccough.
2. ———— Sternutatio. Sneezing.
3. ———— Palpitatio. Palpitation.
4. ———— Nictitatio. Twinkling of the Eyelids.
5. ———— Subsultus. Twitching of the Tendons.
6. ———— Pandiculatio. Stretching.

SPECIES I.
CLONUS SINGULTUS.
HICCOUGH.

CONVULSIVE CATCH OF THE RESPIRATORY MUS-CLES, WITH SONOROUS INSPIRATION ; ITERATED AT SHORT INTERVALS.

THOUGH the spasmodic action in this affection exists chiefly in the diaphragm, the principal seat of the disease is the stomach, when strictly idiopathic ; an observation which was long ago made by Hippocrates, and has in recent times been more copiously dwelt upon by Hoffmann, but which Sir Charles Bell has been the first to establish by experiments on the nervous system. "Vomiting," says he, "and hiccough, are actions of the respiratory muscles, excited by irritation of the stomach.—(*Experiments on the Structure and Functions of the Nerves ; Phil. Trans.*, 1821, p. 406.)

Debility is perhaps the ordinary remote cause, and irritability, or some accidental stimulus, the exciting. Thus excess of food, and especially in a weak stomach, is often a sufficient stimulus : and hence the frequency of this complaint among infants.*

For the same reason, it is occasionally produced by worms, acidity, or bile in the stomach. External pressure on the stomach is another exciting cause ; and hence it has sometimes followed an incurvation of one or more of the ribs (*Schenck*, lib. iii., obs. 49, *ex Fernelio*), or of the ensiform cartilage (*Bonet. Sepulchr.*, lib. iii., sect. v., obs. 8., Appex.) of the sternum, produced by violence, and pressing on the coats of this organ. The stomach, however, is not at all times the only organ in which the morbid cause is seated, that excites the diaphragm to the spasmodic action. The liver is frequently to be suspected. "I have often," says Dr. Percival, in his manuscript notes on the volume of Nosology, "found hiccough symptomatic of an enlargement or inflammation of the liver on the upper convex side." It also frequently follows strangulated hernia ; and, according to Mr. John Hunter, in numerous instances accompanies local irritation after operations of various kinds. It has sometimes attended the passage of a stone in one of the ureters.—(*Darwin, Zoonom.*, iv., i., i., 7.)

The affection is often very troublesome, but it cures itself in ordinary cases, and where the exciting cause is lodged in the stomach ; for the spasmodic action very generally removes the accidental irritant ; and if not, the disorder usually yields to very simple antispasmodics, as a draught of cold water, or a dose of camphire or volatile spirits. Where these have failed, a nervous action of a different kind, and which seems to operate by revulsion, has often been found to succeed, such as holding the breath, and thus producing a voluntary spasm of a rigid and opposite kind in the diaphragm ; or a violent fit of sneezing. An emetic (*Rigaud, Ergo solvunt Singultum Vomitus et Sternutatio?* Paris, 1601) will sometimes answer the purpose ; and, still more effectually, a sudden fright, or other emotion of the mind.—(*Riedlin, Lin. Med.*, 1696, p. 276.). If these do not prove sufficient, we must call in the aid of opium ; and, in the intervals, have recourse to tonics internal and external, the warm bitters, bark, pure air, exercise, and cold bathing.

---

* It is very frequent in drunkards when the stomach is overloaded with spirituous drink.—D.

We have already pointed out the tendency which these irregular actions have to form a habit, and the more so in proportion to the general weakness and irritability of the frame ; and hence, indeed, their arising so readily in the later stages of typhus and other low fevers, and their continuing to the last ebb of the living power.

Even where the constitution is possessed of a tolerable share of vigour, hiccough is too apt to become a chronic and periodical affection ; and as the frequency of the spasm is also usually increased with the frequency of the series, it has sometimes become almost incessant, and defied every kind of medical treatment that could be devised. As a chronic affection, it has been known to return at irregular periods from four (*Bartholin, Hist. Nat.*, cent. ii., hist. 4,) to four-and-twenty years (*Alberti, Diss. Casus Singultûs chronici viginti quatuor annorum,* Hal., 1743) ; and as a permanent attack, to continue without ceasing for eight (*Riedlin*, cent. i., obs. 15), nine (*Act. Nat. Cur.*, vol. v., obs. 108), twelve days (*Tulpius*, lib. iv., cap. 25), and even three months.—(*Schenck*, lib. iii., obs. 49, *ex Fernelio*.) Dr. Parr tell us, that he once knew it continue for a month with scarcely any intermission even at night. "The sleep," says he, "was at last so profound, that the convulsion scarcely awoke the patient." In a few instances it has proved fatal. Poterius mentions one (Cent. ii., obs. xxvii.) ; and another, produced by cold beverage, occurs in the Ephemerides of Natural Curiosities.—(*Eph. Nat. Cur.*, dec. iii., an. i., obs. 48.)

In the Gazette de Santé for 1817 is the case of a young girl, who had been tormented for six months with an almost incessant hiccough. It ceased during deglutition, but re-appeared immediately afterward. The sleep was frequently disturbed. Baron Dupuytren, on being consulted, after antispasmodics and the warm bath had failed, applied an actual cautery to the region of the diaphragm, and the hiccough immediately ceased ; but perhaps terror operated in no slight degree in this mode of cure.

SPECIES II.

CLONUS STERNUTATIO.

SNEEZING.

ɪʀʀɪᴛᴀᴛɪᴏɴ ᴏꜰ ᴛʜᴇ ɴᴏsᴛʀɪʟs, ᴘʀᴏᴅᴜᴄɪɴɢ sᴜᴅ-
ᴅᴇɴ, ᴠɪᴏʟᴇɴᴛ, ᴀɴᴅ sᴏɴᴏʀᴏᴜs ᴇxᴘɪʀᴀᴛɪᴏɴ
ᴛʜʀᴏᴜɢʜ ᴛʜᴇɪʀ ᴄʜᴀɴɴᴇʟ.

Sɴᴇᴇᴢɪɴɢ is a convulsive motion of the respiratory muscles, commonly excited into action by some irritant applied to the inner membrane of the nose, and not unfrequently, when so applied, to an extremity of almost any one of the respiratory nerves ; in the course of which the air from the lungs is sonorously forced forward in this direction as the lower jaw is closed at the time. "In sneezing," says Dr. Young, "the soft palate seems to be the valve, which, like the glottis in coughing, is suddenly opened, and allows the air to rush on with a greater velocity than it could have acquired without such an obstruction."—(*Med. Literat.*, p. 107.)

It is a common and rarely a severe affection in its ordinary course. But, from the habit which irregular actions of the irritable fibres are perpetually apt to assume, as we have already explained, and particularly in a relaxed and mobile state of them, sneezing has occasionally become a serious complaint. Forestus, Horstius, Lancini, and many of the German medical miscellaneous collections, give instances of its having been sometimes both permanent and violent, sometimes periodical, and a few cases wherein it proved fatal; which last termination is confirmed by Morgagni. The Ephemerides Naturæ Curiosorum contain one instance, in which the sneezings continued for three hundred times in a single paroxysm.

The ordinary irritants, operating immediately on the membrane which lines the interior of the nostrils, are sternutatories, a sharp pungent atmosphere, indurated mucus, the acrimonious fluid secreted in a catarrh or measles, or a morbid sensibility of the Schneiderian membrane itself. But the severest cases have usually been produced by sympathy with some remote organ, as an irritable state of the lungs, stomach, or bowels. For the same reason, sneezing often accompanies pregnancy and injuries on the head, and sometimes the last stages of low fevers. The benediction, formerly bestowed with so much courtesy on the act of sneezing, is said to have been congratulatory, on account of its frequent violence; but we do not seem to be acquainted with the real origin of this custom.

As sneezing is a symptom of catarrh, if it be repeated for some time with quick succession in an irritable habit that has been frequently affected with catarrh, it will sometimes, in the most singular manner, call sympathetically into action the whole circle of symptoms with which it has formerly been associated, and the patient will seem at once to be labouring under a very severe cold. An instance of this singular sympathy has occurred to me while writing. The patient is a lady of about fifty years of age, in good health, but of a highly nervous temperament. She began to sneeze from some trifling and transient cause, and having continued to sneeze for five, or six times in rapid succession, her eyelids became swollen, her eyes bloodshot and full of tears, her nostrils discharged a large quantity of acrid serum, her fauces were swollen and irritable, and a tickling and irrepressible cough completed the chain of morbid action. The sneezing at length ceased, and, within a quarter of an hour afterward, the whole tribe of sympathetic symptoms ceased also.

Sneezing, in its ordinary production, though a convulsive, is a natural and healthy action, intended to throw off instinctively from the delicate membrane of the nostrils whatever irritable or offensive material may chance to be lodged there. But when it proceeds from a morbid cause, or becomes troublesome from habit, we should use our endeavours to remove it. That there is nothing of proper convulsion in sneezing is shown, as Sir Charles Bell has justly observed,

by the admirable adjustment of the muscles to the object. A body irritating the glottis will call into simultaneous action the muscles of respiration, so as to throw out the air with a force capable of removing the offending body; but if the irritation be on the membrane of the nose, the stream of air is directed differently, and by the action of sneezing, the irritating particles are removed from these surfaces. By the consideration of how many muscles require the adjustment to produce this change in the direction of the stream of air, we may know that the action is instinctive, ordered with the utmost accuracy, and very different from convulsion.— (*Of the Nerves which associate the muscles of the Chest in the Actions of Breathing*, &c.; *Phil. Trans.*, 1822, p. 305.)

When the complaint is idiopathic and acute, or, in other words, when the Schneiderian membrane is morbidly sensible, or stung with some irritant material, it may be relieved by copiously sniffing warm water up the nostrils, or throwing it up gently with a syringe, or forcing up pellets of lint moistened with opium dissolved in warm water, the pressure of which is sometimes of as much service as the sedative power of the fluid itself. If this do not succeed, leeches or cold epithems should be applied to the nose externally. But a free and spontaneous epistaxis, or hemorrhage from the nostrils, effects the best and speediest cure, of which Riedlin has given an instructive instance.—(*Lin. Med.*, 1695, p. 148.) Its return has been prevented by blisters to the temples and behind the ears, and frequently sniffing up cold water. It has also been attempted to be cured by pungent sternutatories, so that the olfactory nerves may be rendered torpid and even paralyzed by over-exertion; but this has rarely answered; for when once a morbid habit is established, it does not require the primary cause or stimulus for its continuance.

When the complaint proceeds from sympathy, the most effectual mean of removing it is by ascertaining the state of the remote organ with which it associates, and removing the stimulus that gives rise to it. This, however, cannot always be done; and, in such cases, camphire in free doses will often prove a good palliative, and if this do not succeed, we must have recourse to opium.

SPECIES III.

CLONUS PALPITATIO.

PALPITATION.

SUBSULTORY VIBRATION OF THE HEART OR ARTERIES.

Palmus or palpitatio is used in very different senses by different writers. By Cullen and Parr it is limited to a vehement and irregular motion of the heart alone. By Sauvages and Sagar it is applied to an irregular motion "in the region of the heart." By Linnéus it is denominated "a subsultory motion of the heart or a bowel—cordis viscerisve;" and by Vogel is defined "a temporary agitation of the heart, a bowel, a muscle, a tendon, or an artery." The first of these views is too contracted, for palpitations, or quick abnormal beats, are felt almost as frequently in many other organs, and particularly those of the epigastric region. Yet, as in these, it seems in every instance, however complicated with - other symptoms, to depend upon a morbid state of the heart itself, or of the arteries which supply them, or are in their vicinity ; the definitions that extend palpitations to other organs than the heart and arteries, as separate from these, appear to be as much too loose and out of bounds as the first definition is too limited.

The view now offered takes a middle course : it contemplates palpitation as dependant on a diseased action of the heart alone, or of the larger arteries alone, or of the one or the other associating with some organ more or less remote ; and hence lays a foundation for the three following varieties :—

a Cordis.　　　Palpitation of the heart.
β Arteriosa.　　Palpitation of the arteries.
γ Complicata.　Complicated or visceral palpitation.

The vibratory and irregular action, which we denominate PALPITATION OF THE HEART, is sometimes sharp and strong, in which case it is called a THROBBING OF THE HEART, and sometimes soft and feeble, when it is called a FLUTTERING of this organ. Both may possibly proceed from two distinct causes ; the one a morbid irritability of its muscular fibres, or some sudden stimulus applied to it, either external or internal, by which its systole becomes harsh and unpliant, and evinces a tendency to a spastic fixation ; and the other an irregular motion of the entire organ of the heart in the pericardium, by which it literally strikes against the chest : the cause of which we do not always know, though we see it very frequently occasioned by a sudden and violent emotion of the mind, and have reason to believe, that it is often a result of the spastic systole or contraction of the heart which we have just noticed. When, however, the substance of the heart is thus irregularly acted upon, and jerked backward and forward from a cause extrinsic to itself, the palpitation is confined to the pericardium, and the pulse does not partake of the abnormity.

The last is, perhaps, the most common proximate cause of the palpitation of this organ, and we are indebted to Dr. William Hunter for having first pointed it out to us. The heart, in its natural state, lies loose and pendulous in the pericardium ; and when the blood which it receives is, from an irritation of any kind, thrown with a peculiar jerk into the aorta, the moment it reaches the curvature of this trunk, it encounters so strong a resistance as to produce a very powerful rebound in consequence of the aorta being the first point against the spine : the influence of the heart's own action is now, therefore, thrown back upon itself, and this organ, as a result of its being loose and pendulous, is tilted forward against the inside of the chest, between the fifth and sixth ribs on the left.— (See *J. Hunter on Blood*, p. 146, note.)

The rebound of so strong a muscle as the heart against the inside of the chest, must de-

pend for its violence, upon the violence of the jerk with which the blood is spasmodically thrown into the aorta : and this has often been so powerful as to be distinctly heard by bystanders.[*] Castellus has given an example of this sonorous effect : and Mr. Dundas has observed it in various cases. " The action of the heart," says the latter, " is sometimes so very strong as to be distinctly heard, and to agitate the bed the patient is in so violently, that his pulse has been counted by looking at the motions of the curtain of the bed."—(*Trans. Medico-Chirurg. Soc.*, i., 27.) The heart has sometimes palpitated with a force so violent as to dislocate (*Horstii*, ii., 137–139) or break the ribs (*Schenck*, obs. 215, *ex Fernelio*), for both are stated to have occurred on respectable authorities,[†] and, in one instance, to rupture its own ventricles.[‡]—(*Portal, Mémoires de Paris*, 1784.) Upon the wonderful power of the soft parts, or rather of the muscles over the bones, when thrown into vehement spasmodic action, we had occasion to observe in the Physiological Proem to the present order : and hence we have sometimes had examples of the humerus, and other long bones, being broken by a convulsion-fit. A contraction of the left auriculo-ventricular opening is sometimes found to produce the phenomenon of a double pulse.— (*Hodgson on the Diseases of Arteries and Veins*.)

I have said, that we are not always acquainted with the remote or exciting causes of the palpitation of the heart. Violent emotion of the mind, as already observed, is a frequent excitement, and one or two others have been already indicated. The first of these, is perhaps the most frequent cause ; and hence we can readily admit with M. Corvisart, that palpitation, together with many other diseases of the heart, have been far more frequent in France since the commencement of its late horrible revolution. M. Portal has, indeed, proved this fact by various interesting examples, from which the following may be selected, as it is short :—A young lady, who had suddenly learned that her husband had been cruelly murdered by a band of the popular ruffians, was instantly seized with a violent palpitation that terminated in a syncope so extreme, that she was supposed to be dead. This apprehension, however, was erroneous. She recovered ; but the palpitation continued for many years ; and she at length died of water in her chest.—(*Mem. sur la Nature et le Traitement de plusieurs Maladies*, tome iv., 8vo., Paris, 1819.)

The remote causes are rarely to be discovered till after death, and for the most part seem to consist in a morbid structure of the heart itself, or the pericardium, by which last the muscular

---

[*] Castellus, P. Vascus. Exercitat. ad affectus Thoracis, tr. ix., Toloso, 1614, 4to. Lettsom, Med. Soc. Lond., vol. i. A Vega, De Art. Med., lib. iii., cap. 8.
[†] The editor has no doubt of the incorrectness of such reports.
[‡] Another case of spontaneous rupture of the heart is recorded by Dr. Valentine Mott, in the New-York Medical Magazine.—D.

walls of the heart have either been obstructed in their play, or have had too much liberty of action. The heart has sometimes been found ossified in its general substance, as in the case of Pope Urban the Eighth; and more frequently in its valves or in its connexion with the aorta. It has sometimes been thickened, and has grown to an enormous size, which change of structure has lately been distinguished by the name of hypertrophy, and has been found in one instance of a weight of not less than fourteen pounds.— (*Eph. Nat. Cur.*, dec. iii., ann. iii., obs. 166.) A case occurred to the present author not long ago in a young lady of fourteen, in whom it reached half this weight, as well as of a general dropsy. By close confinement and quiet, and the use of elaterium and scarification to carry off the water, she recovered an apparently good share of health; but the exercise of dancing, a few months afterward, produced a recurrence of all the symptoms in a more violent and obstinate degree, and she gradually fell a sacrifice to them.

In other cases, the heart has been peculiarly small and contracted, chiefly, perhaps, in the disease of tabes or marasmus; and consequently there has not been a sufficient capacity for the regular influx of venous blood.

The space of the pericardium has often been morbidly diminished by inflammation, or an undue growth of fat; and hence, again, the heart has been impeded in its proper action; while occasionally it seems to have been filled, or nearly so, with a dropsical fluid.

Organic injury from external violence, is also a frequent cause of palpitation. Yet it is singular to observe the severity of lesion which the heart and its appendages will sometimes undergo, when the constitution is sound, without affecting the life. M. Latour, who during the French war was first physician to the Grand Duke of Berg, attended a soldier who laboured under a tremendous hemorrhage from the breast, produced by a wound from a musket that had penetrated this organ. The hemorrhage, however, ceased on the third day, the patient's strength gradually recruited, and suppuration proceeded kindly. It was nevertheless necessary to cut several pieces of fractured rib away; yet the wound cicatrized at the end of three months, and the only inconvenience that remained was a very troublesome palpitation of the breast, that annoyed him for three years. Six years after the accident, he died of a complaint totally unconnected with the wound. His body was opened by M. Mansion, chief surgeon of the hospital at Orleans; and the ball, which had entered his breast, was found lodging in the right ventricle of the heart, covered over in a great measure by the pericardium, and resting on the septum medium.*

To these causes may be added a scirrhous or other morbid structure of the lungs, and perhaps of the spleen, liver, stomach, or intestinal canal; for it is a frequent accompaniment upon most species of parabysma: and, in these cases, appears as a symptomatic affection alone. For reasons already assigned, it is also an occasional symptom in hydrothorax; during which it shows itself in a very violent degree upon mental agitation, especially that produced by fright or vehement rage.

We should not, however, be hasty in deciding upon any structural affection of the heart, or of any of the larger organs that closely associate with it, nor, in reality, upon any incurable cause whatever. For it has not unfrequently happened, that a palpitation of long standing, and which has been regarded as of a dangerous kind, has gradually gone away of its own accord, and left us altogether in the dark. Dr. Cullen gives a confirmation of this remark in the following very instructive case:—"A gentleman, pretty well advanced in life, was frequently attacked with palpitations of his heart, which, by degrees, increased both in frequency and violence, and thus continued for two or three years. As the patient was a man of the profession, he was visited by many physicians, who were very unanimously of opinion, that the disease depended upon an organic affection of the heart, and considered it as absolutely incurable. The disease, however, after some years, gradually abated both in its frequency and violence, and at length ceased altogether; and since that time, for the space of seven or eight years, the gentleman has remained in perfect health, without the slightest symptom of his former complaint."— *Mat. Med.*, part ii., chap. viii., p. 357.) A case precisely similar, and in a professional gentleman somewhat beyond the middle of life also,

---

* Dict. des Sciences Médicales, Art. Cas. Rares. The following causes of palpitation are specified by Dr. Hope as inherent in the heart itself:—1. Hypertrophy, and hypertrophy with dilatation. In these affections, palpitation consists in an increase both of the force and of the frequency of the heart's action. 2. Dilatation with attenuation. Palpitation in this case consists in an increase of the frequency, but often not of the strength of the beats, though the patient may experience the *sensation* of an increased impulse. 3. Disease of the valves. Palpitation from this cause varies in its characters, according to its nature, situation, and extent of the valvular affection, and according to the presence or absence of hypertrophy, dilatation, or both. 4. Pericarditis, carditis, and inflammation of the internal membrane. 5. Adhesion of the pericardium. Palpitation from this cause is violent, and of an abrupt kind. As physical causes of palpitation, exterior to the heart, Dr. Hope specifies, 1. Acceleration of the circulation by muscular efforts. 2. Plethora. 3. Anæmia. 4. Convulsive, epileptic, and hysteric fits. 5. Obesity. 6. Obstructions in the lungs from hydrothorax, empyema, pneumothorax, hepatization, bronchitis, &c. 7. Asthmatic bronchial constriction. 8. Acute Laryngitis. 9. Abdominal infarction from enlarged liver or spleen, ovarian dropsy, utero-gestation, &c. Afterward Dr. Hope adverts to palpitation from causes operating entirely through the nervous system.—(See Cyclop. of Pract. Med., art. PALPITATION.) Nervous palpitations, as this writer correctly observes, are *intermittent*, their causes being only occasional, whereas those from organic diseases are *continued*, their causes being incessant.—ED.

has occurred to the present author, with a spontaneous termination equally as favourable. M. Laennec's ingenious method of MEDIATE AUSCULTATION by the stethoscope, as we have already explained, will often be found of great importance in the different forms of this species of disease.*

The same alternating spasmodic motion, into which the muscular substance of the heart is occasionally thrown by one or other of the causes thus glanced at, seems, at times, to take place in some of the LARGER ARTERIES, and extends to a greater or less length in proportion to the nature of the cause, or the extent of the morbid irritability by which they are affected, producing the SECOND VARIETY before us. That a morbid irritability may exist in a part of an artery while the rest is free from any such condi-

* See Cl. III., Ord. IV., Gen. III., Spe. 5. In nervous palpitations, it was remarked by Laennec, that "the first impression which the application of the stethoscope to the region of the heart produces on the ear, shows at once that this organ has not great dimensions. The sound, although clear, is not loud over a great extent ; and the shock, even when it at first appears strong, has little real impulsive force, for it does not sensibly elevate the head of the observer. This last sign," says Laennec, "appears to me the most important and the most certain of all, when we add to it the frequency of the pulsations—most commonly from 84 to 96 in a minute."

It is stated by Dr. Hope (Cyclop. of Pract. Med., art. PALPITATION), that in dilatation of the heart, dulness on percussion indicates enlargement of the organ, further evidence of which is derived from the impulse being situated lower down than natural. The first sound is short, smart, and clear, resembling, and in dilatation with attenuation, becoming identical with the second.

In hypertrophy with dilatation, the dulness on percussion is increased over a still greater extent, and the dulness and impulse are also lower down than natural. Both sounds are very loud, and the impulse is much more forcible than in nervous palpitation, very frequently raising the head of the auscultator.

In simple hypertrophy the impulse is a slow, gradual, and powerful heaving, very sensibly elevating the head. Both sounds are diminished, and in extreme cases almost suppressed. In disease of the valves there is a permanent bellows sawing, or rasping murmur ; whereas the murmur in nervous palpitation is only occasional, and of a soft character. If the valvular contraction be great, the action of the heart is irregular. It is further observed by Dr. Hope, that irregularity also occurs in nervous palpitation, but it is not accompanied by those symptoms of an embarrassed circulation, which invariably attend valvular disease. Should hypertrophy, dilatation, or both, coexist with valvular disease, their signs will likewise be present. In nervous palpitation, Dr. Hope finds the pulse to be jerking, but with little fulness, strength, and incompressibility. In dilatation it is full and soft ; in hypertrophy with dilatation, it is full, strong, and sustained ; and in simple hypertrophy, though less full, it is strong, sustained, and even hard. These and other observations on the diagnosis of palpitation from various causes, as delivered by Dr. Hope, are replete with practical instruction, whose Treatise on the Diseases of the Heart is a valuable contribution to medical literature.—ED

tion, is easily conceived, since a like partial irritability is often found to exist in organs, in which we are capable of tracing it in the most manifest manner. Yet, even in arteries themselves, we can sometimes ascertain the same to the conviction of our senses ; as, for example, in the case of phlegmonous inflammation ; in which also we find it accompanied with the throb, or alternating spasm and relaxation, which constitute what is meant by palpitation. In a healthy and ordinary flow of the blood through the arteries, it is very well known, that there is no sensible series of contractions and dilatations whatever ; and we have already observed in the Physiological Proem to the third class, that there is no actual change of bulk of any kind, and that it is the pressure of the finger or of some other substance against the side of an artery that alone produces a feeling of pulsation. In a phlegmonous inflammation, however, every one is sensible of a considerable change in this respect ; for there is often a very smart and vibratory pulsation while the affected part is in perfect freedom, and no finger is applied to it : and that this is a pulsation, unconnected with the regular pulsation of the heart, is perfectly clear, because it is frequently less uniform, rarely if ever synchronous with it, and, in most instances, twice as rapid. We have here, therefore, a full proof of a local excess of irritability in an arterial tube, and of a palpitation, or alternating spasm and relaxation, as its effect.*

Yet inflammation is but one cause of this subsultory action, or of the irritability which gives rise to it. With other causes we are not much acquainted ; but we have reason to believe them very numerous, and wherever they exist, the artery operated upon will evince the same kind of vibratory throb, though, in general, the stroke will not be found quite so smart as that which takes place in the pulse of a phlegmon. It may appear singular, that this abnormal action, whether of the heart or arteries, should evince so much punctuality in its vibrations ; but there is often a wonderful tendency to punctuality in all intermissive affections whatever. We see it in hemorrhoidal discharges, in gout, and above all, in intermitting fevers : and, till the cause of such punctuality is explained in this last instance, it will be in vain to expect an explanation in the case before us.

In very irritable habits, or perhaps where there is a morbid sensibility through the whole of the sanguiferous system, the palpitation will not, unfrequently shoot from one artery to another ; and one or two cases are given in the Ephemerides of Natural Curiosities (Eph. Nat. Cur., dec. i., ann. vi., vii.), in which it appears

* The tenour of some of these observations disagrees with the results of certain microscopical observations made on parts in a state of inflammation. Thus Dr. Thomson of Edinburgh, in his experiments, was unable to discern any alternate expansion and contraction of the arteries. The statement about the pulse in an inflamed part not usually coinciding in number and time to the pulse of the left ventricle, is also at variance with other observations.—ED.

to have been universal. It was so, indeed, in the very irritable organization of that singularly constituted character, J. J. Rousseau, if we may credit the account he gives of himself in relation to this subject : for he tells us, that after a peculiar paroxysm of high corporeal excitement, he became, all of a sudden, sensible of a pulsation in every part of his body, which from this time accompanied him without intermission : and he adds, that the throbbing was so distinct and strong, that he was often capable of hearing as well as feeling it.

The temporal arteries are peculiarly apt to concur in this migratory throbbing, and occasionally the carotid : and the throbbing of both is sometimes synchronous with that of the heart, and sometimes successive to it. Mr. Dundas has observed, that this affection of the carotids is most common to persons in the prime of life ; and that, on dissection, the heart is often found enlarged in its size, but without any increase of muscular power ; an assertion collaterally supported by the case of a young lady described under the preceding variety. We here also sometimes meet with polypous concretions, and very generally adhesions to the pericardium.

And it is highly curious and interesting to notice the ramifying chain of morbid action, of which the heart sometimes forms the first link. I had lately a lady under my care, of delicate constitution and highly nervous habit, in the third month of pregnancy, who had for several weeks been uniformly attacked in the evening with a violent palpitation of the heart, that continued for nearly an hour or upwards ; it was then transferred to the temples, which throbbed with as much violence and for as long a period of time ; vertigo followed, with a tendency to deliquium, immediately after which there was a general reaction in the system ; the skin became heated, and at first very dry ; but the dryness at length yielded to a gentle diaphoresis, which concluded the morbid series ; for the patient at that time becoming tranquil, dropped into a sound and refreshing sleep, and woke free from all these symptoms in the morning.

In this case, also, there was a considerable tendency to that universal subsultus or alternating spasm of the arterial system to which we have just adverted : for all the arteries of the extremities pulsated or palpitated whenever accidentally pressed upon by any substance, though it required this additional stimulus to excite spasmodic action.

Arterial palpitation, however, is to be found, though not more frequently, still far more alarmingly, in the epigastric region, than in the head ; and appears to proceed from some particular excitement of the aorta, the superior mesenteric, or some branch of the cœliac artery. Its beat has here some resemblance to that of an aneurism of these vessels, and has often been pronounced to be such without the slightest foundation, to the great terror of the patient, and consequently to a considerable exacerbation of the disease. It may, for the most part, be easily distinguished from an aneurism by being destitute of any circumscribed pulsatory tumour

that can be ascertained by a pressure of the finger ; by a smarter vibration in the arterial stroke ; and by that degree of irregularity in the return of the stroke by which palpitation is distinguished from pulsation. In some cases, indeed, the line of the affected artery can be distinctly felt and followed up to a considerable length ; and the vibration has occasionally been so strong as to be visible to the eye, even at some distance, when the surface of the epigastric region has been exposed to view. "From a good deal of experience upon this subject," says Dr. Baillie, " I am enabled to say, that the increased pulsation of the aorta in the epigastric region very rarely depends upon any disease of the aorta itself, or of its large branches in that place ; and that this occurrence is almost constantly of very little importance."—(Med. Trans., iv., xix.) This distinguished physiologist tells us further, that he has had an opportunity of examining the state of the arteries in the epigastric region after death, in two persons who had this pulsation very strongly marked, and who died from other diseases. In both cases all the arteries were perfectly free from every appearance of diseased structure. He was also some years ago consulted by an old man upon a paralytic affection ; who afterward spoke to him incidentally concerning a palpitation of the kind before us, to which he had been subject for upwards of twenty-five years. The throb, on examination, was distinctly to be felt ; and on the patient's first perceiving it, and applying to Sir Cesar Hawkins, Mr. Bromfield, and Dr. Hunter, the two former had declared it to be an aneurism, while the latter, more modestly, confessed that he did not know what it was.

Dr. Baillie, in the article now alluded to, has imitated the modesty of Dr. Hunter. "It is perhaps difficult," says he, " to ascertain, in many instances, the causes of the increased pulsation of the aorta in the epigastric region : but, in most cases, it will be found to be connected with an imperfect digestion and an irritable constitution.* And hence, whatever may improve the digestion and render the constitution less irritable, will be of use in mitigating the complaint : and, above all, will be found highly serviceable to remove the patient's anxiety on the subject, whenever it can fairly be done.† It is here that M. Laennec's stethoscope may be employed as a valuable diagnostic, and will often enable us, better than any other means, to ascertain the real nature of the malady ; for an account of which the reader may turn to the remarks on Phthisis.—(Cl. III., Ord. IV., Gen. III., Spe. 5.)

* Dr. Valentine Mott has written an interesting paper on pulsation in epigastrio, which may be found in the Transact. of the New-York Physico-Med. Society, vol. i.—D.

† With respect to pulsation in the epigastrium, useful information will be found in A. Burn's work on Diseases of the Heart, Edin., 1809 ; and in a publication by the late Dr. Albers, of Bremen, entitled Uber Pulsationem im Unterleibe, 8vo., Bremen, 1803. The subject is also introduced into the editor's Dictionary of Practical Surgery, under the Head of Abdominal Pulsations.—ED.

But the throbbing or pulsatory motion is often communicated to other organs than the sanguiferous vessels, and forms that variety of affection, to which we have given the name of COM-PLICATED PALPITATION. This is clearly dependant, in many cases, upon the vicinity or close connexion of such organs with the heart or arteries that form the seat of disease ; and it may also in other cases be produced, as ingeniously conjectured by Dr. Young, by an accumulation of fluid in the pericardium or thorax, which transmits a pulsatory motion from the heart itself to whatever other organ or surface of a cavity such fluid may reach ; in the same manner as the fluctuation, produced by a slight blow given to one side of the abdomen when distended with water, is distinctly propagated to the opposite side. In the case of a middle-aged woman, of a rheumatic habit, labouring under symptoms of general dropsy (*Med. Trans.*, vol. v., art. xvii.), "a palpitation," he tells us, "was observed in the right hypochondriac region, and on the right side of the neck, which exhibited a vibratory motion more rapid and less regular than that of the pulse felt at the wrist ; and a similar vibration was observable in the heart itself : the pulsation of the neck was not confined to the jugular veins ; it was more forcible and extensive than it could have been if it had originated from those vessels ; and it had more the appearance of a violent throbbing of the carotid artery ; although, in the axillary artery, the pulse was comparatively regular and natural." Dr. Young found, nevertheless, upon making a strong pressure on the right side of the neck with a single finger, that the motion of the carotid artery was very perceptible, and totally independent of that of the superficial parts, being precisely synchronous with the pulse at the wrist, although it required considerable attention to distinguish it from the more irregular palpitation. The symptoms, however, of a dropsy of the chest or pericardium in this patient appear to have been obscure ; and at the time when the general hydropic enlargement, which had been much reduced in the course of the autumn, began to increase towards the end of October, the palpitation was considerably less, as well as the pulsations in the abdomen and neck, though the motion of the heart was still fluttering, the pulse at eighty, intermitting and very irregular. On the death of the patient, which occurred soon afterward, a considerable quantity of fluid was found in the pericardium, in the right cavity of the thorax, and in the ventricles of the brain, but little or none on the left side of the chest : the heart was inconsiderably enlarged, and some of its valves, as also those of the pulmonary artery, which were much ossified, so that a free passage of the blood was impeded.

I have said, that palpitation is sometimes dependant upon a morbid irritability of the sanguiferous system in general. In some instances, however, we find it rather dependant upon a morbid irritation and debility of the entire frame, and consequently connected with a very irregular performance of many, or all the func-

tions of the body. Of this highly complicated state of the disease we have a striking example in Dr. Bateman's history of himself (*Med. Chir. Trans.*, vol. ix., p. 227), which he ascribes to a poisonous action of mercury, employed on his own person copiously, in the form of an unguent, to relieve an amaurosis of the right eye, and which seems to have produced something of the mercurial erethism described by Mr. John Pearson (*Obs. on the Effects of various Articles of the Materia Medica in Lues Venerea*, ch. xii.) as taking place in some singular idiosyncrasies, already noticed by us under the head of Syphilis.—(Cl. III., Ord. IV., Gen. VII., Spe. 1.) In this case, the heart and arteries were equally subject to subsultory and violent motions, sometimes separately, and sometimes synchronously, but inaccordantly as to the number of the throbs in a given time, and almost perpetually accompanied with a most distressing sense of languor and sinking. There was also a very irksome cough, an occasional sense of constriction across the region of the diaphragm, and such a difficulty of respiration as to render an erect position at night imperatively necessary. Life was, in this case, unquestionably a forced state of being, and all the stimuli of the external senses and of the will seemed necessary to excite the sensorial organ to produce a sufficiency of nervous energy for the mere preservation of life. And hence, during sleep, or as soon as these stimuli were cut off, there was such an increase of languor, irregular action of the heart, and sinking as though in the act of dying, that it was at times necessary, notwithstanding the extreme drowsiness of the patient from a previous and long-continued watchfulness, to interrupt the sleep every two minutes ; since by this time or even sooner, the failure of the pulse and the appearance of the countenance indicated a supervening deliquium. The powers of the stomach, from the repeated paroxysms of the disease, seem to have declined rapidly. Frequent supplies of food and cordials, as spiced wine, appeared at first serviceable in warding off the languor ; but, at length, nothing but fluids could be taken and retained, without increasing the disturbed action of the heart. Yet so extreme was the sense of sinking and immediate dissolution, that, on one occasion, after a quarter of an hour's sleep, air was importunately demanded, and three glasses of undiluted brandy were drank in five minutes, without much relief : and afterward ammonia and ether repeated every ten minutes for two hours ; when the paroxysm rapidly declined after a copious discharge of limpid urine. The disease continued a twelvemonth before the patient felt, in any essential degree, amended : and little benefit was derived from medicines of any kind. It is well known, however, that this acute pathologist and excellent man has since fallen a sacrifice to a return of the complaint.

In a disease produced by so great a diversity of causes, often obscure, and very generally complicated with other affections, it is impossible to lay down any one plan of treatment that will apply to every case. Our first endeavour should be to ascertain, as far as we may be able, whether the palpitation be idiopathic or symptomatic ; and if the last, while we endeavour to palliate the present distress, our attention should chiefly be directed to the primary malady. If any other morbid state of the stomach or bowels be suspected, this, as far as possible, should be removed ; and if we have reason to suppose hydrothorax, or any other kind of dropsy to be present, the means hereafter to be recommended for this tribe of complaints should be resorted to from the first. In pregnancy, the disease will most probably cease upon a cessation of this state of body, and usually, indeed, ceases during the latter months, or after the period of quickening. And, if it seem to be chiefly dependant upon a general irritability of the sanguiferous system, or of the whole constitution, the sedative antispasmodics, tonics, and especially the metallic, quiet of mind as well as of body, regular hours, light meals, pure air, and such exercise as agrees best with the individual, will often prove of essential service, and sometimes effect a radical cure.

Much of this plan will also be requisite where we have reason to apprehend some structural affection of the heart or larger bloodvessels : and when, from any incidental excitement, the irritation is here more than ordinarily troublesome, recourse must be had to narcotics. Opium is by far the best where it agrees with the system : but its secondary effects are often very distressing, and we cannot employ it. In such cases, we must find out, by trial, what is its best succedaneum : the hop, henbane, hemlock, and prussic acid, have all been essayed in their turn, and sometimes one has succeeded where the rest have all failed. But, upon the whole, the henbane has answered far better and more generally under the author's own hands : and, in one or two instances of great obstinacy, he has known it effect a perfect cure, when all the rest had been tried in succession and had totally failed.

In Dr. Bateman's case, however, which was peculiarly severe and complicated, the henbane, though it seemed serviceable at first, taken in doses of from three to five grains of the extract every night, gradually lost its effect even when repeated three times a night in doses of five grains at a time. The tincture of hop, in doses of thirty drops every six hours, was next tried, but produced no other effect than a slight drowsiness. Musk seemed most successful in draughts of ten grains each ; yet even this was of transient duration, and was abandoned as of no use. Where the palpitation is accompanied with a distressing tendency to deliquium, I have occasionally relieved it by camphire pills, with the ammoniated tincture of valerian or the aromatic spirit of ether.

The disease has occasionally been carried off by a sudden attack of some other complaint, as gout, herpes, diuresis, or the formation of an abscess : and hence, setons and issues have been recommended, and have occasionally proved serviceable. Zacutus Lusitanus found the lat-

ter produced a radical cure in palpitation of the heart, which he ascribed to the rapid healing of some chronic ulcers.—(*Prax. Hist.*, lib. viii., obs. 30.) Schenck advises the wearing a bag of aromatics at the pit of the stomach (Lib. ii., obs. 216) ; and hence, perhaps, the origin of camphire-bags as a specific for irregularities of the heart of another kind.*

SPECIES IV.
CLONUS NICTITATIO.
TWINKLING OF THE EYELIDS.

RAPID AND VIBRATORY MOTION OF THE EYELIDS.

To a certain extent, twinkling or winking of the eyes is performed every minute without our thinking of it. It is a natural and instinctive action for the purpose of cleansing and moistening the eyeball, and rendering it better fitted for vision. Dr. Darwin has some ingenious remarks upon this subject. "When the cornea," says he, " becomes too dry, it becomes at the same time less transparent, which is owing to the pores of it being then too large ; so that the particles of light are refracted by the edges

---

* Our author speaks of *idiopathic* palpitation ; but, according to the editor's view, such a disease has no real existence, palpitation being only a symptom of some other primary affection, either organic or nervous. Thus, it may depend upon organic disease of the heart, aneurism of the aorta, hysteria, chlorosis, indigestion, plethora, uterogestation, anæmia, or nervous disorder, which primary affections, while they continue, prohibit all effectual relief of the palpitations dependant on them. Hence, inasmuch as several of the primary complaints are incurable, the palpitations themselves must also be incurable. On the mode of treating palpitations arising from plethora we need not here dwell. With regard to those occurring in early pregnancy, if they are connected with plethora, the treatment should consist in bleeding the patient, giving her gentle aperient medicines, and making her observe a diet without stimulants. In palpitations from anæmia, Dr. Hope (Cyclop. of Pract. Med.) recommends the exhibition of the preparations of iron with aloes, and especially the pills employed by Dr. Abercrombie, consisting of two grains of the sulphate of iron, two of aloes, and five of the compound cinnamon powder, in two pills, taken at dinner, and, if necessary, at bedtime also. Dr. Hope speaks favourably likewise of the carbonate of iron, in doses of from one to three drachms thrice a day, and of small doses of the pil. aloes c' myrrha, and pil. galban. comp. at bedtime. A nutritious animal diet, pure air, gentle exercise, the flesh-brush, salt water sponging, and the shower bath, are likewise commended.

For nervous palpitation, Dr. Hope recommends, at first, the lightest bitters, then bark and mineral acids, and afterward, metallic tonics, one of the best of which is the sulphate of zinc in the dose of one grain, with extract of gentian, in the form of a pill, twice or thrice a day. At the same time it is admitted that, in the first instance, a bracing air by the seaside, seabathing, a nutritious unstimulating diet, and a good regimen in general, are of more importance than medicine ; and that after the continuance of such means for a few weeks, chalybeates will often become extremely serviceable.—ED.

of each pore instead of passing through it; in the same manner as light is refracted by passing near the edge of a knife. When these pores are filled with water, the cornea becomes again transparent."—(*Zoonom.*, cl. i., i., 4, 2.) Moisture is indeed a frequent cause of transparency in various bodies; and hence, in dying people, whose eyelids are become torpid and do not nictitate, the cornea is sometimes so dry that its want of transparency is visible to by-standers. So when white paper is soaked in oil, and its pores filled with this fluid, from an opaque body it becomes transparent, and radiates the light that is thrown upon it; air itself is most transparent when as much moisture is dissolved in it as it will hold; when void of moisture, indeed, it forms a dry mist, which is occasionally met with in the morning, and through which distant objects are seen indistinctly; while, on the contrary, when distant objects are seen with perfect clearness, it is a sign of rain. In a mist, distant objects are also seen indistinctly; yet here the moisture is not dissolved in the atmosphere, but merely suspended, and formed by the attraction of cohesion into collected spherules. We may hence account for the want of transparency in the air, which is seen in tremulous motions over cornfields on hot summer days, and over brick-kilns, after the flame is extinguished, while the furnace still remains light. It is this dryness and want of transparency in the atmosphere over the summits of hot and arid hills, in a bright unclouded sky, as in Italy, which constitute what is called by the painters the blue shade of light, and which is copied in most pictures of Italian scenery.

The ordinary use of nictitation is therefore obvious: but there are many persons who wink or twinkle their eyes far more frequently than is necessary for the purpose of moistening the cornea, and in whom it forms an unsightly habit. This has usually been produced at first by some local irritation, as inflammation or dust in the eyes, which quickens the natural action, and, where the stimulus is considerable, renders it irregular and convulsive. If indeed the stimulus be very vehement, the nature of the spasm is changed, and the eyelids, instead of irregularly opening and shutting with great rapidity, become rigidly closed.

We have seen, in many of the preceding species of diseases, with what ease morbid actions are continued when once introduced into an organ: and hence, when any permanent irritation of the eye has excited and maintained for some days or weeks a quick repetition of twinkling, this iterative action will often be found to become habitual, and remain after the irritation has subsided.

This morbid habit has been sometimes cured by a powerful exertion of the will; but more generally by using one eye only at a time, and closing the other; the open eye being employed in examining an object for a considerable period with great attention and steadiness. A minute examination of the stars at night through a telescope has a like corrective tendency, and may be employed for the same purpose.

X 2

SPECIES V.
CLONUS SUBSULTUS.
TWITCHINGS.

SUDDEN AND IRREGULAR SNATCHES OF THE TENDONS.

This affection is to the tendinous extremities of the muscles in which the principle of irritation is often apt to accumulate, what palpitation is to the irritative fibres of the heart and arteries: and hence, as we have already seen, it is included under the general term of palpitation by Vogel.

We witness these starts or twitchings most frequently in extreme stages of debility produced by atonic fevers, and especially just before the act of dying. They are in such cases weak convulsions interruptedly undulating from one limb or part of a limb to another, too feeble to raise the limb itself, although sufficiently powerful to give slight but transient swellings to the belly of a muscle, and consequently a slight involuntary flickering to its tendons. In the ordinary close of life, they are the precursors of the fatal scene, the harbingers of the dying struggle, and generally indicate that the will has lost its hold, and the power of sensation is rapidly ceasing: thus affording another proof, if other proofs were wanting, to those adverted to in the Proem to the present class, that the irritative fibres are capable of maintaining their function, under particular circumstances, for a much later period than the organs of perception and sensation, occasionally, indeed, for some hours after the death of every other part of the body. And as debility and irritability often exhibit a joint march, the subsultory motions are apt to become stronger as the regular motion of the pulse becomes weaker, and at length work up those agonizing convulsions under which the little and loitering flame of life is sometimes extinguished instantaneously. Such twitchings of the tendons, however, do not always prove fatal, for they often show themselves where the case is not so extreme; and hence they may occasionally be allayed by cordials, antispasmodics, and warmer sedatives, and are altogether lost in a favourable turn of the disease.

It occasionally happens, that the debility producing these weak convulsive actions is local and habitual: and in such cases they may be seen to agitate and play over a limb, without any influence on the system generally, and without much injury to the limb itself. Such a state of nervous constitution may be produced by accident, but it is for the most part strictly idiopathic; and there are few practitioners perhaps who have not met with examples of it. Dr. Darwin gives us an instance in the following words: "A young lady, about eleven years old, had for five days had a contraction of one muscle in her forearm, and another in her arm, which occurred four or five times every minute; the muscles were seen to leap, but without bending the arm. To counteract this new morbid habit, an issue was placed over the convulsed muscle of her arm, and an adhesive plaster wrapped tight like a bandage over the whole forearm, by which the new motions were immediately destroyed, but the means were continued for some weeks to prevent a return."—(*Zoonomia, Catenation*, sect. xvii., i., 8.) The author has sometimes seen it about one of the shoulders, but the extremities are its most usual seat; and he was lately consulted by a lady of a strikingly irritable habit, who was suddenly attacked with it both in her hands and feet, so as to throw her into a considerable degree of alarm. Upon inquiring into the patient's age and state of health, he was informed, that she was between forty and fifty, that menstruation was on the point of leaving her, and had of late appeared very irregularly, and that she had a considerable oppression in her head. The cause was therefore obvious, and the cure was not difficult: for it yielded to a moderate venesection, and an habitual attention to the state of the bowels.*

SPECIES VI.
CLONUS PANDICULATIO.
PANDICULATION.

TRANSIENT ELONGATION OF THE EXTENSOR MUSCLES, USUALLY WITH DEEP INSPIRATION AND A SENSE OF LASSITUDE.

This is perhaps the slightest modification of spasmodic actions; but as it often occurs, as in nausea on the first stage of a febrile paroxysm, whether the will consents or not, and is frequently and irregularly repeated, it cannot but be regarded as belonging to the present family on many occasions. The muscles chiefly concerned are the extensors of the lower jaw and of the limbs: the particular kind of pandiculation to which the first of these movements gives rise being called OSCITANCY, YAWNING, or GAPING; and that produced by the second, STRETCHING. The muscles are excited to this peculiar action by a general feeling of restlessness or disquiet: and the spread of the action from one muscle or set of muscles to another, is from that striking sympathy or tendency to catenate in like movements which we so often behold in different parts of the body, without being able to explain. It is possible, however, that the synchronous motion of the muscles of the lower jaw and of the limbs, for it is rarely that yawning and stretching do not accompany each other, may be dependant upon the same line of intercourse, by which trismus so often accompanies a wound in one of the extremities, and which we have already attempted to illustrate; the irritant power, in the one case, leading to a fixed or entastic, and in the other to a transient and clonic spasm.

Pandiculation, considered physiologically, is an instinctive exertion to recover a balance of power between the extensor and flexor muscles, in cases in which the former have been encroached upon and held in subjection by the latter.

A very slight survey of the animal frame will

* There is some reason to think that clonus subsultus occurs more frequently from affections of the knee-joint than from any other local disturbance.—D.

show us that the flexor muscles have in every part some preponderance over the extensors; and that this preponderancy is perpetually counteracted by the stimulus of the instinct or of the will. We see it from the first stage of life to the last, and most distinctly in those states in which there is most feebleness, and consequently in which the controlling powers are least capable of exercising and maintaining a balance. In the fetus, therefore, in which the weakness is most pressing, the power of instinct is merely rising into existence, and no habit of counterpoise established in the nascent fabric, every limb, and part of every limb capable of bending, undergoes some degree of flexure, and the entire figure is rolled into a ball, as the hedgehog habitually rolls himself even after birth. As the fetus, however, increases in size and age, and the powers of instinct, sensation, and volition become more perfect, this general conflexure produces occasionally a sense of uneasiness; and hence every parturient mother is sensible of frequent internal movements and stretchings of the little limbs of the fetus to take off the uneasiness by restoring some degree of balance to the antagonist powers. After birth, and during wakefulness, the stimulus of the will, directed rather to the extensor than the flexor muscles, renders the counterpoise complete for all the purposes for which it may be necessary. But the moment we repose ourselves in sleep, and the will becomes inactive and withdraws its control, the flexor muscles exercise their preponderancy afresh, though in a less degree than in fetal life, since the extensors, from habitual use, have acquired a more than proportionate increase of power. The preponderance, however, when long exerted, still produces some degree of disquiet, and hence occasionally during sleep, and still more vigorously the moment we begin to awake, we instinctively rouse the extensor muscles into action; or in other words, yawn, stretch the limbs, and breathe deeply, to restore the equipoise that has been lost during unconsciousness.

In all these cases, pandiculation is a natural action; it is an effect produced by the will when it is called to the particular state of these two sets of muscles, or by the instinctive or remedial power of nature, which supplies its place when it is dormant or inattentive, to restore ease to a disquieted organ. But, in an infirm or debilitated condition of the system, it evinces a morbid and convulsive character, and takes place without our being able to prevent it, even when the will uses its utmost effort to resist instead of to encourage it.

How far its repetition may be of use in the shivering fit of an ague, or in a nauseating deliquium of the stomach, it is difficult to say. Yet we are at no loss to account for its frequency of recurrence; for as the whole system is, in such circumstances, thrown into a sudden prostration of strength, the extensor muscles, in consequence of being naturally weaker than their antagonists, must become soonest exhausted, and give way with a more than ordinary submission to their power. And hence we behold a painful retraction over the whole system, and the preponderance assumes a rigid and spastic character ; and we may fairly conclude, that much of the yawning and stretching which ensue, is for the purpose of getting rid of the constrictive spasm, though these counteractions themselves often run in the attempt into a spasm of another kind, and become convulsive.

Yawning and stretching, then, are among the signs of debility and lassitude. And hence, every one who resigns himself ingloriously to a life of lassitude and indolence, will be sure to catch these motions as a part of that general idleness which he covets. And, in this manner, a natural and useful action is converted into a morbid habit ; and there are loungers to be found in the world, who, though in the prime of life, spend their days as well as their nights in a perpetual routine of these convulsive movements over which they have no power ; who cannot rise from the sofa without stretching their limbs, nor open their mouths to answer a plain question without gaping in one's face. The disease is here idiopathic and chronic : it may perhaps be cured by a permanent exertion of the will, and ridicule and hard labour will generally be found the best remedies for calling the will into action.

GENUS III.
SYNCLONUS.
SYNCLONIC SPASM.

TREMULOUS, SIMULTANEOUS, AND CHRONIC AGITATION OF VARIOUS MUSCLES, ESPECIALLY WHEN EXCITED BY THE WILL.

WE have already observed, that clonus imports " agitative," or " tremulous motion of the muscles ;" and hence, SYNCLONUS means necessarily their " multiplied, conjunctive, or compound agitation, or tremulous motion." The term is therefore intended to denote a group of diseases more complicated in form, of more extensive range, or more connected with the general state of the constitution than those of the preceding genus ; and it runs parallel with the *clonici universales* of Sauvages, as far as they can be said correctly to belong to this family. The species included under this genus will be found to be the following :

1. Synclonus Tremor.   Trembling.
2. ———— Chorea.   St. Vitus's Dance.
3. ———— Balismus.   Shaking Palsy.
4. ———— Raphania.   Raphania.
5. ———— Beriberia.   Barbiers.

SPECIES I.
SYNCLONUS TREMOR.
TREMBLING.

SIMPLE TREMULOUS AGITATION OF THE HEAD, LIMBS, OR BOTH; MOSTLY ON SOME VOLUNTARY EXERTION.

THE proximate cause of this disease is an irregular transmission of irritable power to the motory fibres of the muscles that constitute its seat. It is strictly a disease of nervous debility, either general or local : debility produced by sudden exhaustion, as in the case of great muscular fatigue from violent exercise, severe cold, or a vehement exertion of the passions, and particularly of the passions of fear and rage ; or debility produced slowly and insensibly by causes of tardy operation, as an injudicious use of mercury, lead, opium, or other mineral and narcotic poisons ; an habitual excess in hard drinking or sexual commerce ; and, in some idiosyncrasies, an immoderate indulgence in tea.* And, as this disease is a result of debility, it necessarily occurs as a symptom on the general spasm and prostration of strength that so peculiarly distinguish the accession of an ague-fit, and the interruption of sensorial power that takes place in paralysis.

There are some persons, however, in whom the same convulsive action exists habitually, without any morbid state of other organs, or any other inroad upon the general health. I once knew a lady considerably beyond the middle of life, who was strikingly affected with this complaint, insomuch that the slightest voluntary exertion of any of the muscles threw the head and arms into as great a tremour as if they had been hung upon wires, but who enjoyed at the time, and had for a long term of years continued to enjoy, as perfect health as possible in every other respect ; was lively, cheerful, animated, possessed of brilliant powers of conversation, and able to use a more than ordinary portion of exercise without fatigue.

The earlier part of her life had been passed in India, but her constitution did not appear to have suffered from this circumstance ; and so gradual was the attack of the affection, that though she had laboured under it for many years, she could not date its commencement from any given point of time. She at length died at the age of seventy-two or seventy-three, her corporeal powers progressively declining, and laying a foundation for a general dropsy, while her mind continued firm to the last.

In all cases of this kind, the supply of nervous energy to the motory fibres of the affected muscles takes place interruptedly, and where the organ or the constitution is in a state of debility, it is also less abundant as well as less uniform. We have already observed, that the nervous energy (or fluid, as the author preferred calling it), in its natural course is transmitted only by waves or vibrations, and consequently with an interposing pause or relaxation after every efflux ; but that the pause is instantaneous, and the supply so regular as to answer the purpose of a permanent and continuous tenour. In clonic tremour, the pauses are, however, prolonged, and for the most part irregular, or untrue to themselves ; and the greater the retardation and irregularity, the more marked and alarming the spasmodic shake.

In the case just adverted to, there was no other diseased action whatever ; the nervous power was unquestionably supplied in sufficient

* It arises also from long indulgence in tobacco, particularly in the form of snuff ; it will occasionally be caused by the loss of sleep, and is sometimes seen in persons of a sanguineous temperament after severe seasickness.—D.

abundance, and the pauses, though prolonged, were uniform; and it was singular to observe the influence the will possessed over the affected muscles under these circumstances, and how completely they were still under its control: for, in consequence of the uniformity of the morbid interruptions, and from the force of habit, I have seen this patient, in the midst of a shaking that threatened every moment to overturn whatever she took hold of, raise a cup brimful of tea, or a glass brimful of wine to her lips by way of experiment, without spilling a single drop.

Where the corporeal health is so little interfered with as in the present case, a course of medical treatment might perhaps do more mischief than benefit. But where the constitution is generally affected, or the muscles that form the seat of the convulsion are manifestly debilitated, general and local tonics and stimulants may sometimes be tried with advantage, though they frequently fail of producing any good effects. Sea bathing and horse exercise, a generous diet, change of air and scene, may be found useful auxiliaries in the general treatment; and long-continued and daily friction by a skilful rubber, ammoniacal embrocations, blisters, setons, and a course of voltaism or electricity, offer the best promise as topical means of relief. The affected limbs may also be put into a train of gradual exertion, for the purpose of obtaining both strength and steadiness: and, to this end, the head or shoulders may be occasionally made to balance an easy weight for a given period of time, and the hands to suspend, or carry a wineglass or tumbler brimful of water.

Here also may be recommended the kneading friction, or shampooing of the Egyptians and Turks, which has of late become a fashionable refreshment in the watering-places of our own country; and there can be no question, that the pungent and exhilarating essential oils which are applied to and absorbed by the skin afterward, add considerably to the general efficacy. Something like this the French have long been in the habit of employing under the name of *frictions sèches*.—(*Ardouin, Essai sur l'Usage des Frictions Sèches,* &c.) The horse-hair shirts, and periodical flagellations of the old Franciscan friars, would probably be found to answer the same purpose. But this is a remedy which is not likely to be revived in the present day, whether from a medical or a moral call.

SPECIES II.
SYNCLONUS CHOREA.
ST. VITUS'S DANCE.

ALTERNATELY TREMULOUS AND JERKING MOTION OF THE FACE, LEGS, AND ARMS, ESPECIALLY WHEN VOLUNTARILY CALLED INTO ACTION; RESEMBLING THE GRIMACES AND GESTURES OF BUFFOONS; USUALLY APPEARING BEFORE PUBERTY.

THE term CHOREA, from χορὸς, "chorus," "cœtus saltantium," is comparatively of modern date in its application to the present disease; nor is it easy to determine satisfactorily who

originally employed it. It was first more limitedly denominated CHOREA SANCTI VITI, under which limitation it occurs in Sydenham, and is still known in popular language, being called in colloquial English, St. Vitus's Dance, and in colloquial French, Dance de St. Guy. According to Horstius, the name of St. Vitus's Dance was given to this disease, or perhaps more probably to a disease possessing some resemblance to it, in consequence of the cure produced on certain women of disordered mind, upon their paying a visit to the chapel of St. Vitus, near Ulm, and exercising themselves in dancing from morning to night, or till they became exhausted. He adds, that the disease returned annually, and was annually cured by the same means.

The marvellous accounts of this dance, as related by old writers, are amusing from their extravagance.* The paroxysm of dancing, we are told, must be kept up, whatever be the length of the time, till the patient is either cured or killed; and this also, whether she be young or old, in a state of virginity or of parturition; and, in the growing energy of the action, we are further told, that stools, forms, and tables are leaped over without difficulty if they happen to be in the way. Felix Plater gravely tells us, that he knew a woman of Basle, afflicted with this complaint, who on one occasion danced for a month together;† and the writers add generally, that it was hence necessary to hire musicians to play in rotation, as well as various strong, sturdy companions to dance with the patients, till they could stir neither hand nor foot.—(*Paracels. De Morb. Amentium,* tract. i.; *Schenck, de Maniâ,* lib. i.)

The nearest approach to this kind of gymnastic medicine which I am acquainted with in modern times, is a singular case of the same disease, described by Mr. Wood in the seventh volume of the Medico-Chirurgical Transactions. The morbid movements were in measured time, and constituted a sort of regular dance as soon as music was struck up, but ceased instantly upon a change of one time to another, or upon a more rapid roll of the drum, which was the instrument employed on the occasion, than the morbid movements could keep up with. Advantage was taken of the last part of this very singular influence, and the disease was cured by a perseverance in discordant or too rapid time. This form of the disease appears to have a near relation to the tarantismus of Sauvages, which is the carnevaletto delle donne of Baglivi, all of them probably nothing more than modifications of the present. Linnéus, and after him

* The best history of the dancing mania is that written by Prof. Hecker, which has been translated into English by Dr. B. G. Babington, London, 1835.—D.

† De Mentis Alienat., cap. iii. A case in which a girl, ten years of age, kept up the most extraordinary movements and exercises for five weeks, sometimes for fifteen hours a day, is related by Dr. Watt.—(See Med. Chir. Trans., vol. v.) As Mr. Hunter of Glasgow has truly remarked, it is perhaps the most extraordinary case of the kind on record.—(See Edin. Med. Journ., No. lxxxiii., p. 268.)—ED.

Macbride, from the epithet of *sanctus*, as applied to chorea, or a belief that such affections are induced by the immediate agency of a superior order of beings, have applied to it the name of hieronosos, or "morbus sacer"—a name, however, which by earlier writers was appropriated to convulsion-fits.

In Galen, chorea seems to be included under a disease which he calls scelotyrbe, literally, "cruris turba or perturbatio,"—"commotion of the leg;" and his description, which is as follows, is extremely accurate. "It is a species of atony or paralysis, in which a man is incapable of walking straight on, and is turned round to the left when the right leg is put forward, and to the right when the left is put forward, or alternately. Sometimes he is incapable of raising the foot, and hence drags it awkwardly, as those that are climbing up steep cliffs."

One of the best general descriptions which have been given us of chorea, is the following of Dr. Hamilton, contained in his valuable treatise on the utility of purgatives : "Chorea Sancti Viti attacks boys and girls indiscriminately ;* and those chiefly who are of a weak constitution, or whose natural good health and vigour have been impaired by confinement, or by the use of scanty or impropet nourishment. It appears most commonly from the eighth to the fourteenth year. I saw it in two young women, who were from sixteen to eighteen years of age. The approaches of chorea are slow. A variable and often a ravenous appetite, loss of usual vivacity and playfulness, a swelling and hardness of the lower belly, and in general, a constipated state of the bowels, aggravated as the disease advances, and slight, irregular, involuntary motions of different muscles, particularly those of the face, which are thought to be the effect of irritation, precede the more violent convulsive motions which now attract the attention of the friends of the patient.

"These convulsive motions vary. The muscles of the extremities and of the face, those moving the lower jaw, the head, and the trunk of the body, are at different times, and in different instances, affected by it. In this state the patient does not walk steadily ; his gait resembles a jumping or starting ; he sometimes cannot walk at all,† and seems palsied : he cannot perform the common and necessary motions with the affected arms. This convulsive motion is more or less violent ; and is constant, except during sleep, when in most instances it ceases altogether. ‡ Although different muscles are

sometimes successively convulsed, yet in general the muscles affected in the early part of the disease remain so during the course of it. Articulation is now impeded, and is frequently completely suspended. Deglutition is also occasionally performed with difficulty.* The eye loses its lustre and intelligence ; the countenance is pale, and expressive of vacancy and languor. These circumstances give the patient a fatuous appearance. Indeed, there is every reason to believe, that when the complaint has subsisted for some time, fatuity to a certain extent interrupts the exercise of the mental faculties."

Thermaier gives a case in which it was connected with a deeply melancholic temperament, and the limbs were in a state of constant snatching and trepidation (*Consil,* lib. ii., cap. xi.) : but this is a rare concomitant ; nor is fatuity a constant sequel of it, even in its most obstinate and chronic form. The present author has met with various instances in which the disease has continued with considerable violence from an early period to old age, without making any inroad whatever on the mind, or even spreading to any other joints, limbs, or muscles than those at first affected. He once knew a man under the habitual influence of this complaint, who was a good orator, always reasoning with great clearness, and delivering himself with much animation. The movements of his arms were indeed in ungraceful snatches, and the muscles of the neck frequently evinced a like convulsive start, yet not so as to interrupt the flow of his periods, or to abridge his popularity. He knew another person, for many years severely afflicted with the same complaint, who was an excellent musician, public singer, and composer of music ; and this, too, notwithstanding that he was blind from birth. The person alluded to, is the late Mr. John Printer, of the Foundling hospital. In walking he was always led, on account of his blindness, and used a staff on account of the unsteadiness of his steps ; but, notwithstanding every exertion, his gesticulation was extreme, and so nearly approaching the antics of a buffoon, that it was often difficult for a spectator to suppress laughter. Yet, in singing and playing, he had a perfect command over the muscles of the larynx and of the fingers ; his tones were exquisitely clear and finely modulated ; but his neck and head curvetted a little occasionally. He died when about sixty years of age, without ever exhibiting any debility of intellect.†

---

* Dr. Heberden states, that only one fourth of his patients were males ; which agrees with the result of Dr. Elliotson's experience. The latter physician considers the period of life most subject to chorea to be from three or four years to fourteen.—Ed.

† It is observed, that the patients generally walk quickly better than slowly ; Dr. Heberden adverts to one individual who could not walk, though he could run.—Ed.

‡ Dr. Elliotson has seen the skin of the chin and breast rubbed off by the perpetual scraping of one on the other. He has known the patient unable to lie on the bed, rolling off it, so that it was

necessary to strap him down. These, however, were very severe cases. Except in extreme instances, the movements are suspended during sleep.—Lect. on Med. at Lond. Univ., as reported in Med. Gaz. for 1832–33, p. 533 —Ed.

* As to feeding patients, Dr. Elliotson observes, that is often very difficult ; and it will sometimes require the aid of two or three persons to give them their meals—two to hold them still, and one to catch the favourable opportunity of putting the spoon into their mouths.—Op. cit.

† According to Dr. Elliotson, one leg and one foot generally first show the disease. The first symptom usually observed is that of one foot being dragged after the other. The arms are generally more affected than the legs. The face has

There is a singular form of this disease, which has been called by some writers MALLEATIO, consisting in a convulsive action of one or both hands, which strike the knee like a hammer. In this case the hands are usually open, but sometimes clinched. Morgagni (*De Sedibus*, &c., x., 16) relates a case in which it came on even in the sound hand, if the finger of the affected one were extended. If the motion be forcibly stopped, the convulsion becomes afterward still more violent and general.

Where the system is disposed to hysteria, the paroxysm is sometimes extremely vehement, and partakes of the constitutional diathesis, making an approach to epilepsy, but distinguished from it by a continuance of consciousness and sensibility. Dr. White of York has given us a striking example of this mixed affection in a lady forty-two years of age, who "had always a very weak system of nerves," and was rendered speechless for an hour or two upon any sudden surprise. In November, he tells us, she was affected with a fresh paroxysm, which, upon being sent for, he describes as follows:—"She complained of a violent pain in the right side of her face, and of universal erratic aches and soreness. There is a scorching heat all over the skin, except from the feet up to the ankles, which are as cold as marble. Pulse not quickened, but full; mouth dry, but no great thirst; body costive, which is indeed her natural habit, so as to oblige her to the frequent use of magnesia. She is regular as to the menses, the return of which she expects in five or six days. Appetite good, rather voracious; but her spirits always low after a full meal, especially dinner. Has a violent pain in the loins, which often shifts from hip to hip; the leg of the aching side being so much affected with stupor and numbness, that she drags it after her in walking. She falters in her speech at times, but this does not continue long. All the muscles of the body evince convulsive motions; not simultaneously, but successively: thus, her face is first violently affected, then her nose, eyelids, and whole head, which is thrown forcibly backward, and often twitched from one side to the other with exquisite pain. From this quarter the convulsive action removes first into one arm, and then into the other; after which both legs immediately became convulsed with violent and incessant motions, and in this manner all the external parts of her body are affected by turns. She is all the time perfectly sensible, and knows what limb is going to be attacked next, by a sensation of something running into it from the part already convulsed, which she cannot describe in words; but the foretoken has always been found to be true, though the transition is surprisingly quick. She is easiest in a prone posture. Such," continues Dr. White, "has been her situation upwards of forty-eight hours, with scarce a moment's remission, by which she complains of

very frequently a fatuitous appearance; the mind is apparently a little affected; and *certainly persons are somewhat childish* in this disease.—Lect. on Medicine at the Lond. Univ., op. cit.

great and universal soreness. No words can convey an adequate idea of her odd appearance: and I do not in the least wonder, that in the times of ignorance and superstition, such diseases were ascribed to supernatural causes and the agency of demons."—(*Edin. Med. Comment.*, vol. iv., p. 326.) Even Dr. White himself applies to it, perhaps in imitation of Sauvages, the name of hieronosos.

The predisponent cause of this disease is an irritability of the nervous system, chiefly dependant upon debility, and particularly a debility of the stomach and its collatitious organs. Most of the diseases of children are seated in this quarter; and it is from it that chorea commonly takes its rise, and shows itself in an early period of life; the ordinary occasional causes being bad nursing, innutritious diet, accumulated feces, worms, or some other intestinal irritant.*

About the age of puberty, there is another kind of general irritation that pervades the system: and where this change does not take place kindly, which is frequently the case in weakly habits, the irritation assumes a morbid character, and is exacerbated by a congestive state of the vessels that constitute its more immediate seat: and chorea takes its rise from this cause.†

In effect, where the predisponent cause of an irritable state of the nervous system is very active and predominant, a local or temporary excitement of any organ, and almost at any period of life, will give rise to the convulsive movements of chorea: and hence we find it so frequently united with an hysteric diathesis. It has been produced by a fright (*Stoll, Rat. Med.*, part iii., p. 405), by a wound penetrating the brain through the orbit of the eye (*Geash, Phil. Trans.*, vol. liii., 1763), by an improper use of lead, mercury, and some other metals (*De Haen, Rat. Med.*, part iii., p. 202), and by suppressed cutaneous eruptions.‡

---

* Chorea, says Dr. Armstrong, is always preceded by some disorder of the stomach, liver, or bowels; and the affection which takes place in the brain and spinal cord (for both of them are affected) seems to be secondary. "You may always trace its rise to some improper diet. It is very common in children who eat many vegetables, and are subject to worms." After adverting to its occasional production by the irritation of dentition, Dr. Armstrong mentions the case of a pregnant lady who laboured under chorea; she had a tapeworm, which the doctor dislodged by means of a dose of turpentine, and the chorea ceased.—See Armstrong's Lectures on the Morbid Anatomy, Nature, and Treatment of Acute and Chronic Diseases, 8vo., Lond., 1834, p. 733.

† According to Lisfranc and Serres, this disease depends on an affection and even an inflammation of the tubercula quadrigemina.—D.

‡ Wendt, Nachricht von dem Krankeninstitut zu Erlangen, 1783. What myriads of different diseases are referred to debility, disorder of the stomach and bowels, suppressed eruptions, discharges, &c.! Yet we remain quite in the dark how the effect is produced; why it should happen in one individual and not in another; and why, apparently, the same alleged cause should produce in different persons consequences entirely different? The clew to an explanation of these

From this view of the general nature and origin of the disease, we can be at no loss to account for the great benefit which has been derived from a steady course of brisk purging in recent cases, or those of early life; for this, while it carries off the casual irritation, or unloads the infarcted viscera, seems at the same time to act the part of a revellent, and to prohibit the return of the paroxysm by a new excitement. It may appear, perhaps, strange to those who have not thought upon the subject, that where the disease has proceeded from intestinal irritation, it should also be carried off by intestinal irritation. But the irritations are of very different kinds: and it is so far from following of necessity, that, because one kind of irritation, applied to a particular organ, excites a particular effect in a remote part, another will do the same, that the converse is more commonly true, and that any other kind of irritation, applied to the same organ, by exciting a new action, will be the most effectual way of taking off or preventing such effect. And it is upon this ground alone that we often endeavour to cure rabies, trismus, and tetanus, by laying open the original wound to a considerable extent, or the application of some new stimulus that may answer the same purpose.

The principle being a general one, it does not seem of much consequence what purgative is employed, provided it be sufficiently powerful; though, where worms are suspected, the essential oil of turpentine, from its being a good an-

thelmintic, as well as a good cathartic, will be found one of the best. It seems, indeed, to have been occasionally serviceable where worms have not been the cause, for Dr. Powell relates a case in which he completely effected a cure in a girl of seventeen, by a single dose of a fluid ounce (*Transact. Medico-Chir. Soc.*, vol., v., p. 358): and hence its antispasmodic power may at times co-operate with its purgative quality as well as its vermifuge power.

Sydenham, who recommended an alternation of bleeding and purging, probably derived far more advantage from the latter than the former part of his plan:[*] it has been found peculiarly advantageous in the hands of Dr. Hamilton: and Dr. Parr, who ascribes to Sydenham the first hint he obtained upon this subject, affirms, that having pursued the purgative plan with great activity through sixty cases of the disease, which occurred to him in a course of twenty years' practice, he was successful in the whole of these cases except one; and that in all but this one, he found the disease yield, not only soon, but with few instances of a relapse.[†]

There is, therefore, no malady whatever perhaps that calls so peremptorily for stimulating the abdominal viscera into increased action; and as chorea often precedes puberty, or occurs about this period of life, we have another reason for directing an augmented stimulus to the lower regions of the living frame, and rousing into energy the tardy development of the sexual organs. Even blistering the sacrum at this period of life is often attended with success. Dr. Chisholm (*On the Climate and Diseases of Tropical Countries*, p. 97, 8vo., 1822) affirms, that he found it so after a total failure of antispasmodics and the purgative plan: and as his patients were all eighteen years of age or below, the success

---

points would convey more information than the often repeated allusion to debility, disordered stomach, &c. Dr. Armstrong's pathological view of chorea is, that the disorder first commences in the primæ viæ; and that the brain is next affected, as seems to be proved by the countenance and by the state of the intellect, which, however be it remembered, is not always weakened. Dr. Armstrong believed the spinal cord to be implicated, because the upper and lower extremities are both affected. "Probably," he says, "the cerebrum, the cerebellum, and the spinal cord, are all affected."—(On the Morbid Anatomy, Nature, and Treatment of Acute and Chronic Diseases, p. 734.) M. Magendie details an extraordinary case, in which the power of the will over the muscular motions was at intervals entirely lost; but instead of the muscles being paralyzed, or remaining at rest, they were seized with the most irregular and indescribable movements for hours together. Some light has been thrown on the cause of such anomalous cases by the experiments which this distinguished physiologist made on some of the lower animals, rendering it probable that the *will* is more particularly seated in the cerebral hemispheres, while the direct cause of motion is in the spinal marrow. Hence, he observes, it is readily conceived why, in certain cases, these motions are not produced, though commanded by the will; and why, in certain circumstances of a contrary nature, very extensive and energetic motions are developed without any participation of the will.—(Compendium of Physiology, vol. i., p. 201. On these principles, explanations are attempted of the irresistible propensity to move forward and backward, and of the quick and continuous rotations to the right or left, &c., occasionally noticed in patients labouring under chorea.—Ed.

* "If large quantities of blood be drawn, especially in delicate habits, the disease will be invariably increased."—Armstrong, op. cit., p. 735.

† According to the experience of the late Dr. Armstrong, a due attention to the secretions of the liver, and to the alvine discharges and a regulated diet, with an occasional shower bath, will almost invariably cure chorea, provided the plan be followed up for six weeks, or two or three months. "The best diet for children in chorea is bread and milk in the morning and evening, and a small quantity of animal food with bread in the day. This diet is the best if there be no inflammation in the stomach or small intestines, and then the diet should be very bland, as milk, with some farinaceous food, arrow-root, or thin gruel. Get rid of acidity by an occasional dose of magnesia, or of the carbonate of an alkali. Give calomel every night, in conjunction with rhubarb or jalap; and sulphate of magnesia with infusion of senna, or compound decoction of aloes, or cold-drawn castor oil in the morning. As an alterative, give small doses of blue pill occasionally, not oftener than every second night. When the patient loathes food, but there is no pain on pressure, and the head is not affected, a mild emetic may be administered. If there be inflammation of the stomach or small intestines, apply leeches as long as the tip of the tongue is red, and there is obscure pain on pressure."—See Armstrong on the Morbid Anatomy, Nature, and Treatment of Acute and Chronic Diseases, p. 735.—Ed.

was probably dependant upon the principle here pointed out.

But it is necessary to attend to the state of the system generally as well as locally, to take off the constitutional weakness and irritability, as well as the topical irritation, and especially where the disorder has acquired a chronic character. And hence other remedies must be had recourse to as well as purgatives. The German physicians have strongly recommended the use of antispasmodics and sedatives, and especially musk, belladonna, and foxglove, with a view of allaying the irregular action, and Dr. Cullen speaks as decidedly of the benefit of opium.— (*Mat. Med.*, part ii., chap. vi., p. 246.) But the advantage derivable from these seems to be merely palliative ; and the stimulant tonics and alterants promise a better success.

The cuckoo-flower or lady's-smock, *cardamine pratensis*, so common to the meadows of our own country, was at one time supposed to be of essential service in the cure of this and various other spasmodic affections. Michaëlis, who is a great advocate for its use, employed it in the proportion of a drachm every six hours.— (*Richter, Chirurg. Bibl.*, b. v., p. 120.) But it owed of late its reputation in this country chiefly to the recommendation of Sir George Baker, who published five cases of spasmodic diseases, two of them instances of chorea, in which he conceived a most decided benefit was obtained from the use of these flowers. In the hands of later practitioners, however, they have not supported their credit, and have consequently sunk into disuse. The leaves of the Spanish or Seville orange-tree, as a stimulant and tonic bitter, are far more entitled to attention, not only in this, but in various other cases of convulsive spasm. They were first recommended to De Haen by Westerhoef, who, as well as Werlhoff, employed them with considerable success : and they were afterward introduced by Hoffmann as a valuable ingredient into his celebrated stomachic elixir ; and for the same reason formed a part in the composition of Whyt's stomachic tincture. They were given in the form of decoction, and in that of powder ; in the last case the dose is from half a drachm to a drachm, three or four times a day. The metallic salts and oxydes have been tried in every form. At one time, the most popular of these were the flowers of zinc. Dr. Gaubius first brought them into reputation, and gave to the metal the name of CADMIA ; and, according to his statement, they worked wonders in all clonic affections whatever, chorea, hooping-cough, hysteria, convulsion, and epilepsy ; on which account they were afterward employed upon a still larger and more popular scale by the famous empiric Luddemann, under the name of LUNA FIXATA.—(*Dissertatio Medica inaug. de Zinco, Aut. Jacob. Hart*, Lugd. Bat., 4to.) This medicine has, however, by no means been able to maintain its high character ; and even Stoll, who once employed it as a favourite, at length abandoned it as good for nothing,* and

returned to the belladonna in its stead, which he employed in the form of an extract from the juice of the root ; giving it from a sixth to a quarter of a grain every quarter of an hour, and, as he affirms, with very great advantage.

For the information of practitioners in general, however, it should be noticed that when the stomach has reached its full dose of the oxyde of zinc, it will still bear a full dose of ammoniated copper in conjunction with it, by which means the metallic power may be very much increased. Thus a delicate stomach will rarely bear more than two grains of either of these without nausea ; yet it has been found that the same stomach will continue at ease under a mixed powder of two grains of the former and two and a half of the latter at a dose.*

The nitrate of silver seems to have been radically successful in various well-established cases. It has commonly been given in the guise of pills, from one to five or six grains to a dose.

[In one interesting example recorded by Dr. Crampton (*Trans. of the King's and Queen's College of Physicians*, vol. iv., p. 111), purgatives were extensively tried, with various other remedies ; but the disorder scarcely remitted under any mode of treatment, until the nitrate of silver was prescribed.

Iron had been recommended in chorea, among a multitude of vegetable and mineral tonics ; but until Dr. Elliotson published the results of his experience with it, its powers were not appreciated, nor the possibility contemplated of giving it with advantage when the disorder was accompanied with headache, vertigo, and a $_{\text{degree}}$ of paralysis. The facts which this physician has published in favour of the efficacy of the sub-carbonate of iron, given every six hours in doses of two scruples and sometimes even of half an ounce, blended with gruel, mucilage, or treacle, are calculated to recommend it strongly to the notice of medical practitioners as a remedy of the highest value in chorea. When the bowels were confined, Dr. Elliotson sometimes gave his patients scammony, calomel, and other purgatives ; but, in some of the instances, they were rarely used.—(*Med. Chir. Trans.*, vol. xiii., p. 232, et seq.)]

Another remedy entitled to credit in the present day, is arsenic ; for it is difficult to resist

---

* The oxyde of zinc is still in great favour with some practitioners, being regarded by them

as a more manageable preparation than the sulphate. It may at first be given in doses of five grains, and gradually increased. According to Mr. Bedingfield, it was so successful in the Bristol Infirmary that he considers it as a specific. Upwards of forty cases occurring there, were, with one exception, cured by it.—See compendium of Med. Practice, p. 51 ; and Cyclop. of Pract. Med., art. CHOREA.—ED.

* Letter from Dr. Odier to Dr. A. Duncan, Edin. Med. Com., iii., p. 191. The sulphate of zinc is a medicine in high repute at the present time for the cure of chorea. Many practitioners prefer its exhibition to that of purgatives. With the exception of two cases, however, the late Dr. Armstrong never saw the purgative treatment fail. Sulphate of zinc may be given three times a day, in five-grain doses, gradually increased, and the bowels should of course be regulated.—ED.

the evidence from various quarters in which it seems not only to have produced benefit, but to have established a perfect cure. [Mr. Martin prescribed it in one case with success; and Mr. Salter, of Poole, found it answer in an instance in which the nitrate of silver, and many other medicines had failed. It has also been given with advantage by Dr. G. Gregory.] It is commonly given in the form of the solution of the London College, in doses of ten drops to a youth of twelve or fourteen years of age three times a day, increasing the dose as there may be occasion.*

In this disease, however, as in various others, it will often be found, and the remark is well worth attending to, that different remedies are required for different individuals, even where the cause is obviously the same; and that what produces no benefit in one case, is highly advantageous in another. Camphire in large doses has succeeded where turpentine or the nitrate of silver has completely failed; and a brisk purgative plan has sometimes answered where all the preceding have proved of no use whatever. It is hence we are to account for Dr. Cullen's peculiar attachment to the bark, which he tells us he has found "remarkably useful," and prefers to any of the preparations of copper, zinc, or iron (*Mat. Med.*, part ii., ch. ii., p. 112) while Dr. Powell informs us, that in a lady of *seventy* years of age, of a very irritable habit, attacked for the first time with this complaint in severe paroxysms at night, he found musk, in doses of ten grains every six hours, succeed and produce a cure, when purging, blistering, the ammoniated spirit of amber, nitrate of silver, ammoniated tincture of valerian, castor, muriated tincture of iron, bark, and opium had all failed.—(*Med. Trans.*, vol. v., p. 192; also *Maton's Case cured by Musk*, p. 188.)†

[In a severe example successfully treated by

* It would be imprudent to commence with this quantity. It is best to begin with one or two drops for a child six or eight years of age, three times a day, always taking care to administer it after a meal and very gradually increasing the dose according to its effects. In some of the cases alluded to in the text, it was the only medicine prescribed; in others, it had been preceded by purgatives.—ED.

† According to Dr. Eberle (Practice of Medicine, vol. ii., p. 91), the principal exciting causes of chorea are mental emotions, gastro-intestinal irritation, repelled, chronic, and acute cutaneous eruptions; the suppression of habitual discharges, and unsatisfied or over-excited sexual propensities. Vegetable and mineral poisons, as stramonium, mercury, and lead, have also been known to produce this affection.
In the treatment, it is highly important to regulate the alimentary canal by the judicious use of purgatives; and the state of the vascular system will sometimes require moderate and repeated venesection. This being done, the nitrate of silver will sometimes succeed when other remedies have failed; and more is accomplished by the continuance of this remedy for several weeks than by giving larger doses for a few days.
On the principle inculcated by Dr. Jenner for the use of the tartar-emetic ointment, Dr. Wharton of Virginia has lately employed it in a case

Dr. Crampton (*Trans. of the King's and Queen's College of Physicians*, vol. iv., p. 120), where headache was a prominent symptom, leeches were repeatedly applied to the temples, neck, and along the spine, in succession; the head shaved; the shower bath employed; and the action of the bowels regulated. In another case treated by Mr. Hunter of Glasgow, a cure was accomplished by rubbing antimonial ointment into the scalp, and along the course of the vertebral column.—(*Edin. Med. Journ.*, No. lxxxiii., p. 261.) In an instance recorded by Mr. Stuart, the patient was cured by the prussic or hydrocyanic acid, preceded by purgatives.—(Op. cit., No. xciii., p. 271.)]

Voltaism or electricity was warmly recommended by De Haen. Like the preceding remedies, either appears to have been serviceable in some cases; but they are far outbalanced by the instances in which they have failed. It is very possible, that in some instances, a long and punctual discipline of the affected limbs, where the disease is not very severe, to regular and measured movements, may progressively recall them to their wonted order and firmness, as a like discipline of the vocal organs in stammering has not unfrequently been found to restore them to a regularity of utterance: and, with this view, the gymnastic exercise of dancing, whose movements are all measured with the greatest nicety, and which was so much depended upon in former times, and asserted to have been so successful, may be well worthy of attention in the present day, provided it be kept within due bounds, and be not carried to the ridiculous extreme we had occasion to notice a few pages above.*

SPECIES III.
SYNCLONUS BALLISMUS.
SHAKING PALSY.

PERMANENT AGITATION OF THE HEAD OR LIMBS WITHOUT VOLUNTARY EXCITEMENT; BODY BENT FORWARD, WITH A PROPENSITY TO RUN AND FALL HEADLONG; USUALLY APPEARING AFTER MATURITY.

THIS is the SCELOTYRBE FESTINANS of Professor de Sauvages, and the SHAKING PALSY of Mr. Parkinson.—(*Essay on the Shaking Palsy*, 8vo., 1817.) The genus Tantarismus of Baligvi seems to hold an equal point between BALLISMUS and CHOREA, and the species usually arranged

of chorea with success.—See Am. Med. Recorder, vol. ix.—D.

* Dr. Armstrong saw one case where a strictly regulated diet and every other plan had failed, and which was cured by music. A travelling musician passed by the house, and, while he was playing, the child's parents noticed that its motions were remarkably still; they took the hint, and procured sleep regularly every night by means of music; and the child ultimately recovered.—See Lectures on the Morbid Anatomy, Nature, and Treatment of Acute and Chronic Diseases, p. 736.
Iodine has been successfully employed by Dr. Manson and others as a remedy for chorea. It was given in combination with mild cathartics.—Med. Researches, &c., p. 187, &c.—ED.

under it may be resolved into the one or the other, and are done so under the present arrangement.

The term Ballismus (βαλλισμὸς) is not used in a medical sense by the Greek writers, but occurs in Athenæus and various other authors in the literal sense of tripudiatio, or " tripping, capering, curvelling on the toes ;" from βαλλίζω, "tripudio, pedibus plaudo ;" and is hence well designed to express the characteristic feature of the patient's being thrown involuntarily, when he attempts to walk, "on the toes and forepart of his feet," to employ the language of Mr. Parkinson, " and impelled, unwillingly, to adopt a running pace :" or, as Dr. Cullen, who has indiscriminately blended this species with the preceding, expresses it, to " various fits of leaping and running."—(*Pract. of Phys.*, part ii., book iii., ch. iii., 1353.)

Ballismus, however, though not found in the writings of the Greek physicians, has been long established as a technical term in the medical nomenclature of later times, in which it has been used, with little discrimination, to import almost all or any of the species that belong to the present genus.

Sauvages observes, that while chorea or *scelotyrbe Sancti Viti* attacks the young, ballismus or *scelotyrbe festinans* attacks those in advancing life ; and the remark is founded on a just distinction of the characters of the two diseases ; though there are other features also of as striking a peculiarity, and which are here introduced into their respective definitions. SHAKING PALSY, as it is called by Mr. Parkinson, who has adopted the colloquial name, is by no means a correct designation ; for though in the disease before us there is a weakness of muscular fibre, and a diminution of voluntary power in the parts affected, there is none of that diminution of sensation by which PALSY is generally characterized. Mr. Parkinson's description of the disease, however, is the best we have hitherto had, and is as follows :—

" So imperceptible is the approach of this malady, that the precise period of its commencement is seldom recollected by the patient. A slight sense of weakness, with a proneness to trembling, sometimes in the head, but most commonly in the hands or arms, are the first symptoms noticed. These affections gradually increase, and at the period perhaps of twelve months from their first being observed, the patient, particularly while walking, bends himself forward. Soon after this, his legs suffer similar agitations and loss of power with the hands and arms.

" As the disease advances, the limbs become less and less capable of executing the dictates of the will, while the unhappy sufferer seldom experiences even a few minutes' suspension of the tremulous agitation : and should it be stopped in one limb by a sudden change of posture, it soon makes its appearance in another. Walking, as it diverts his attention from unpleasant reflections, is a mode of exercise to which the patient is in general very partial. Of this temporary mitigation of suffering, however, he is now deprived. When he attempts to advance,

he is thrown on the toes and forepart of his feet, and impelled unwillingly to adopt a running pace, in danger of falling on his face at every step. In the more advanced stage of the disease, the tremulous motions of the limbs occur during sleep, and augment in violence till they awaken the patient in much agitation and alarm. The power of conveying the food to the mouth is impeded, so that he must submit to be fed by others. The torpid bowels require stimulating medicines to excite them into action. Mechanical aid is often necessary to remove the feces from the rectum. The trunk is permanently bowed ; muscular power diminished ; mastication and deglutition difficult ; and the saliva constantly dribbles from the mouth. The agitation now becomes more vehement and constant ; and when exhausted nature seizes a small portion of sleep, its violence is such as to shake the whole room. The chin is almost immoveably bent down upon the sternum ; the power of articulation is lost ; the urine and feces are discharged involuntarily, and coma with slight delirium closes the scene."

The remote cause is involved in some obscurity. Long exposure to damp vapour, by lying from night to night on the bare earth, in a close unventilated prison, seems to have produced it ; and possibly other causes of chronic rheumatism : and hence it has frequently supervened on chronic rheumatism itself. Long indulgence in spirituous potation has often given rise to it ; and probably any thing that debilitates the nervous power.*

And on this account miners, and others exposed to the daily exhalation of metallic vapours, and especially those of mercury, are frequent and severe sufferers ; of which Hornung has adduced many interesting examples from the quarrymen in Carniola.—(*Cista*, p. 280.) It has also followed worms in the intestines (*Commerc. Liter. Nor.*, 1743, p. 55) ; and, in this case, has sometimes assumed a periodical type.—(*Act. Nat. Cur.*, vol. ii., obs. 143.)

The part of the nervous organ more immediately affected has also afforded some ground for controversy. Bonet ascribes it to a diseased state of some portion of the cerebrum, and has given examples of its being found, on dissection, to contain, in various quarters, proofs of serum, sanies, and other morbid secretions.—(*Sepul.*, lib. i., sect. xiv., obs. 7 ; 9.) But the misfortune is here, as we have already observed in similar appearances after mania, that it is impossible for us to determine whether these diseased fluids give rise to the disease, or the disease to them. And

---

* Modern writers distinguish the true paralysis agitans from the description of cases here adverted to. It certainly possesses many points of similarity to chorea and mercurial palsy ; yet differences are noticed not only from these affections, but from the trembling brought on by the abuse of spirituous liquors, strong tea or coffee, or by mere old age. In these examples the agitation stops if the limb be supported, and none of its muscles put in action ; whereas, in the real shaking palsy, the reverse takes place. The gait is also peculiar ; the patient, when he attempts to walk, being impelled unwillingly to adopt a running pace.—ED.

hence Mr. Parkinson seems to pay no attention to them, at least as a cause, and fixes the seat of the affection in the cervical of the spinal marrow, from which he supposes it to shoot up by degrees to the medulla oblongata. We have already shown sufficiently in the Physiological Proem to the present class, that the nervous fibres which ramify over the extremities, whether sensific or motific, originate from the chain of the spinal marrow; and we have also shown, in discussing the diseases of trismus, tetanus, and lyssa, how acutely one extremity of a chain of any kind, and particularly of a continuous fibrous chain, sympathizes with another: and there can be no difficulty, therefore, in conceiving, that wherever the cutaneous ends of the nerves of motion are torpified, or otherwise affected by any of the causes just adverted to, the vertebral column must itself very seriously participate in the mischief, and consequently the upper or cervical part of this column; and that from this point the disease must ramify to the brain before the general functions of the system become affected, as in its latter stages.

The remedial process is not very plainly indicated. Vesicatories and other stimulants applied to the neck, or even the dorsal vertebræ, have appeared useful. A seton or caustic, and especially the actual cautery, as practised so generally in France, might possibly be of more avail applied to different parts of the spine. Beyond this an active purgative system, as strongly recommended by Riedlin, has certainly been found efficacious (*Lin. Med.*, 4695, p. 101); and the subcarbonate of iron, the prussic acid, and solution of arsenic, bid as fair for a favourable result here as in the preceding species.* Starck tried musk, and carried it to very large doses frequently repeated every day (*Klin. und Anat. Bemerkungen*); but it does not seem to have produced any decisive success.

Friction of the affected extremities, resolutely persevered in by a skilful rubber, with stimulant embrocations of camphire or ammonia, should also be tried in an early stage of the disease, and be alternated with the use of the voltaic trough. Here, too, we may expect to derive advantage from a free use of diaphoretic and alterant apozems, as the decoction of the woods, and especially where the disease is suspected to be of a rheumatic origin:—to which may be added a regular course of bathing in the Bath springs.

* This statement is far too promising; for the disease does not, like chorea, take place in young, but generally old persons, and is commonly believed to be connected with organic disease of some part of the nervous system. Dr. Elliotson informs us, that he has never been able to cure but one case, and this was a patient not more than thirty-five. As there was pain in the head and giddiness, copious bleeding, blisters, mercury, low diet, and setons were first tried, but without any benefit. Zinc was next prescribed, and, as that did not answer, the subcarbonate of iron was given, which effected a cure. Dr. Elliotson has since tried the latter medicine in four or five other cases of shaking palsy, but without the least benefit.—Lectures at the Lond. Univ.—See Med. Gaz. 1832–33, p. 533.—ED.

SPECIES IV.
SYNCLONUS RAPHANIA.
RAPHANIA.

SPASTIC CONTRACTION OF THE JOINTS: WITH TREMBLING AND PERIODICAL PAINS.

OF this species we know little or nothing in our own country. It was first described by Linnéus, who called it Raphania, from his supposing it to be produced by eating the seeds of the *raphania raphanistrum*, a wild radish or sharlock that grows indigenously in our native cornfields, as well as in the cornfields of most parts of Europe. By other writers, as Herrmann and Camerarius, it has been ascribed to the use of darnel or rye* infested with the spur, or ergot, or some other parasitic plant, which, as we have already observed, is a frequent cause of other very severe complaints, as MILDEW MORTIFICATION (*gangræna ustalaginea*), and ERYTHEMATOUS PLAGUE (*pestis erythematica*). All these diseases, however, are so distinct from each other, that though there can be little doubt of their being severally produced by some poisonous material contained in the patient's food, the poison must be of different kinds, and we do not seem to be acquainted with the cause of this difference; and hence the question has given rise to much controversy, and been discussed with some warmth on the continent; for, while the greater number of writers refer the disease to raphania, or spurred rye (*secale cornutum*), many deny that it is produced by either of these (*Wichmann, Beyträg. zur Geschichte der Kricbelkrankheit*, Leips., 1771–8), and Lentin ascribes it to the honeydew of various plants, concerning which we shall have to speak further under PARURIA *mellita.* That it is a vegetable poison, however, seems to be admitted by common consent, and it is possible that the poison is not confined to a single plant.†

* Abhandlung von der Kriebelkrankheit, &c., Cassell, 177–8. De Lall. Lolio. temulento, Tubing., 1710.

† The pernicious effects of blighted rye, when used as an article of food, have been observed ever since the time of Duhamel. Mann, in his Medical Sketches, has attributed much of the sickness of the Northern army in the war of 1812–14 to this cause; and we think that sufficient evidence has been adduced by writers to place its noxious effects beyond dispute. Messrs. Wood and Bache (U. S. Dispensatory, 2d edition, 1834) speak thus confidently on the subject:—" Terrible and devastating epidemics in different parts of the continent of Europe, particularly in certain provinces of France, have long been ascribed to the use of bread made from rye contaminated with the degenerate grain. Dry gangrene, typhus fever, *and disorders of the nervous system attended with convulsions*, are the forms of disease which have been observed to follow the use of this unwholesome food. It is true that ergot has been deemed to be the cause, but accurate investigations made by competent men on the spot where the epidemics have prevailed, together with the results of experiments made upon inferior animals, leave no room for reasonable doubt upon the subject."—D.

That many poisonous plants have a direct tendeney to affect the nervous system, and excite entastic or clonic spasm, or a mixture of the two, according to the peculiarity of the poison itself, or of the habit into which it is introduced, we have frequently had occasion to notice already, and particularly under the head of ERUPTIVE SURFEIT (*colica cibaria efflorescens*). This is particularly the case with several of the deleterious agarics or funguses, some of which seem to operate chiefly on the sensific nerves, and produce a general stupor : and others on the motory, and produce palpitations, cramps, or convulsions over the whole system.—(*Heberden, Med. Trans.*, ii., 218.) It is very probable, therefore, that the cause ordinarily assigned for the present species of disease is the true one.

There is an excellent paper upon this subject in the Amœnitates Academicæ (Tom. vi., art. cxxiii., 1763), furnished by Dr. Rothman, a pupil of Linnéus, from which the disease seems to be not unfrequently epidemical, and always to commence in the autumn. It is found, however, only among the lower orders of the people, and, in the epidemic referred to, is sufficiently traced to impure admixtures with their grain, and the employment of this vitiated grain in too new a state. Dr. Rothman delineates the disease from actual observation, and does not believe it to be a new malady, as generally supposed, but thinks he has traced it in the writings of various authors from the year 1596 to 1727 ; which would establish, moreover, that it has been common to other parts of Europe as well as to Sweden. And in confirmation of this we may observe, that Dr. Mercard (*Medicinische, Versüche. Zweyter Theile.*, 8vo., Leipzig) describes a disease very much resembling raphania, that appeared at Stade in the winters of 1771, 1772, which was evidently epidemic, and accompanied with symptoms of fatuity, or that narcotic effect which many deleterious plants are sure to produce.

Dr. Cullen, who has generalized far too much his description of chorea in his Practice of Physic, seems to have imbodied this species, as well as the preceding, in the common delineation, and hence, when he tells us that "there have been instances of this disease (chorea) appearing as an epidemic in a certain corner of the country" (Part ii., book iii., chap. iii., 1353), there can be little doubt that he alludes to the species before us originating from the cause now assigned, although without some such interpretation as the present, the passage is not very intelligible.

The disease commences with cold chills and lassitude, pain in the head, and anxiety about the præcordia. These symptoms are followed by spasmodic twitchings, and afterward rigid contractions of the limbs or joints, with excruciating pains, often accompanied with fever, coma, or delirium, sense of suffocation, and a difficulty of articulating distinctly. It continues from eleven days to three or four weeks ; and those who die generally sink under a diarrhœa or a paroxysm of convulsions.

The warm antispasmodics, as valerian, cas-

tor, and camphire, appear to have been employed with decisive success. An emetic, however, given at the onset of the symptoms, as recommended by Henman, would probably cut short the course of the disease and mitigate its violence. This writer advises also blistering or bathing with Dippell's animal oil.—(*Abhandl. von der Kriebelkrankheit.*) Camphorated vinegar, as employed by other practitioners, would probably be found a more useful embrocation.—(*Nachricht. von der Kriebelkrankheit.*)

Towards the close of the disease, purple exanthems or vesications are said to be sometimes thrown out, which approximate it to mildew-mortification and the erythematic pestis, both which, as we have already observed, have been traced to a similar cause.

SPECIES V.
SYNCLONUS BERIBERIA.
BERIBERY. BARBIERS.

SPASMODIC RIGIDITY OF THE LOWER LIMBS, IMPEDING LOCOMOTION ; OFTEN SHOOTING TO THE CHEST, AND OBSTRUCTING THE RESPIRATION AND THE VOICE ; TREMBLING AND PAINFUL STUPOR OF THE EXTREMITIES ; GENERAL ŒDEMATOUS INTUMESCENCE.

BONTIUS seems first to have introduced the term BERIBERI or BERIBERIA into medical nomenclature, and tells us it is of oriental origin (*De Medicinâ Indorum*, cap. i.) ; and Sauvages has hence copied it into his list of "nomina barbara, seu nec Græca, nec Latina." Mangetus affirms, that the disease was known to Erasistratus, but certainly not under this name. Eustathius, however, has βίρβερι, but in the sense of "concha or ostreum," "conch or shell,"— and tells us that it is a term of Indian origin. He might have said, with more propriety, of oriental origin, for it is common both in its primary and duplicate form בֵּר or בָּרָא, בֶּרֶר or בְּרָבִים to the Hebrew, Chaldee, Syriac, and Arabic, in which last it is برابر (berabir), and in all of them is a nomadic term, importing tillage and its production, which is grain, or pasturage and its production, which is sheep, or other cattle ; and hence, probably, the origin of *brebis* or sheep in the French tongue. The term is said to be applied to this disease in India from the patient's exhibiting, in walking, the weak and tottering step of a sheep that has been ever-driven.

This disease, though common to various parts of India, is chiefly to be met with in Ceylon and on the Malabar coast [especially in that tract of country reaching from Madras as far north as Ganjam].—(*Hamilton in Edin. Med. Chir. Trans.*, vol. ii., p. 13.) It seems to be produced by sudden transitions of the atmosphere from dry to damp, and from sultry calms to chilling breezes. In these countries it attacks both natives and strangers, but particularly the latter during the rainy season, which commences in November and terminates in March ; through a great part of which, also, the land-winds blow from the neighbouring mountains every morn. ing, about sunrise with great coolness; and hence, those who sleep abroad, or without suffi. cient shelter, are equally exposed to the influence of a penetrating chill and damp.* [The instances are comparatively rare in which it has occurred at a distance from the sea exceeding sixty or seventy miles.]

Fresh troops, partly from their being new to the climate, but chiefly from their want of a sufficient degree of caution, very frequently suffer severely from this complaint so long as the rainy season continues. Thus we learn from Mr. Christie, that the 72d regiment was severely attacked with it in the autumn of 1797, not many months after its arrival, and continued to suffer from it till the ensuing spring; and that the 80th regiment, which relieved the 72d in March, 1797, was equally attacked with it in the ensuing November.† It is, however, in all such cases, most frequently to be found among those who have previously weakened their constitutions by sedentary habits or a life of debauchery; and particularly where too free an indulgence in spirits has co-operated with sedentary habits, as among the tailors and shoemakers of a battalion; who, in order to give them time to work at their respective trades, are often excused from the duties of the field, and, by their double earnings, are enabled to procure a larger quantity of spirits than other men. And we may hence, in some degree, account for Mr. Christie's remark, that during his stay at Ceylon, he never met with an instance of this complaint in a woman, an officer, or a boy under twenty.‡

The disease commences with a lassitude and painful numbness of the whole body, the pain sometimes resembling that of formication. The legs and thighs become stiff, the knees are spasmodically retracted, so that the legs are straightened with great difficulty, and instantly relapse into the retracted state, whence the patient is apt to fall if he attempt to walk. In some cases, indeed, the motory and sensific power, instead of being distributed to the muscles of locomotion irregularly, is not distributed at all, and the limbs become paralytic. And even where the spasmodic action exists, it often travels or extends to those parts of the body, and particularly to the chest and the larynx, so that speak-

ing and respiration are conducted with great difficulty.

At the same time, the whole of the absorbent system exhibits equal proofs of torpitude, the legs first, and afterward the entire surface of the body becomes bloated and œdematous, and all the cavities, particularly those of the chest, are progressively loaded with fluid: and hence, towards the close of the disease, where it terminates fatally, the dyspnœa is extreme, and accompanied with an intolerable restlessness and anxiety, and constant vomiting; the muscles are convulsed generally; while the pulse gradually sinks, the countenance becomes livid, and the extremities cold.

Such is the course of the disease as it shows itself at Ceylon, where it seems to rage more severely than on the Malabar coast, and where we are told by Mr. Christie, whose account is confirmed by Mr. Colhoun,* that its progress is so rapid, that the patient is often carried off in six, twelve, twenty-four, or thirty-six hours from its onset, though it ordinarily runs on for several weeks.†

Since the first edition of the present work, various important communications have been made to the Army Medical Board upon the subject before us. These, by the kindness of my eminent friend the director-general, I have been enabled to examine, and they concur in supporting the general character of the disorder as given above; as they do also in affirming, that neither women, officers, nor persons under twenty years of age become the subjects of beribery; evidently because such individuals are rarely called upon to expose themselves at night, or sleep in the open air.

From the complicated nature of the disease, however, and the variety of organs that are linked in the general chain of morbid action, suggestions have often occurred, whether beribery be not rather a modification of some other malady than an idiopathic affection; and especially whether it be not a peculiar form of anasarca, deflected from its common course by

---

* According to Mr. Wright, who had opportunities of making remarks on the disease, as it presents itself on the Malabar coast, it was most prevalent towards the end of the rainy season, when the night temperature was many degrees lower than that of the day.—See Edin. Med. and Surgical Journal, vol. xli., p. 235.—Ed.

† "So far as I know," says Mr. Hamilton, "there is no instance on record of an individual being attacked with the disease immediately upon his arrival in India."—Edin. Med. Chir. Trans., vol. ii., p. 21.—Ed.

‡ This agrees with Mr. W. P. Wright's statement, that "the periods of infancy and boyhood are exempt; and females are seldom attacked."—See Edin. Med. and Surgical Journal, vol. xli., p. 323.—Ed.

* Essay on the Diseases incident to Indian Seamen or Lascars on long Voyages, by W. Hunter, A. M., &c.

† On the Malabar coast the disease appears in different forms. The first of these is named by Mr. Wright the severe, or inflammatory, which is generally a first attack, the patient being robust, and dropsical symptoms present, of the kind termed by pathologists acute or arterial. The second is the asthenic, when the patient has been reduced by some previous disease, or by a relapse of it; then the dropsical symptoms resemble those observed after protracted fevers or other debilitating causes. The third is the local variety, the disease seeming to be confined to the lower extremities, with merely œdema and paralysis of them, unaccompanied by constitutional irritation. —(See Edin. Med. and Surgical Journal, vol. xli., p. 324.) It is admitted, however, that the cases sometimes vary, according to the constitution of the patient and the effect of noxious influences; so that, though he has at first only local symptoms, he may be suddenly attacked by general acute anasarca.—Ed.

accidental circumstances. The last is more especially the opinion of Mr. Collier, a staff-surgeon of considerable talents and authority ; and to the same opinion I find Dr. Dwyer inclining, physician to the forces at Kandy in Ceylon. Yet, after having, in his manuscript report, which is a very valuable document, called it incidentally by the name of *acute anasarca*, he tells us that, from the great diversity of its symptoms, many cases have been referred to apoplexy, carditis, aneurism, gastritis, which were purely examples of beribery : and he then proceeds as follows :— " Although allied in many of the symptoms to dropsical affections, IT IS TO BE CONSIDERED DISTINCT BOTH IN SYMPTOMS AND TREATMENT." —(*Lord Valentia's Travels*, vol. i., p, 318.) And to the same effect, a very able inspector of hospitals in the same quarter, Dr. Farrell, who observes as follows :—" I cannot help thinking still, notwithstanding the weight of his (Mr. Collier's) authority, that the affection commonly called beri-beri is a disease of exhaustion and debility, occurring chiefly in persons of intemperate habits, and labouring under other maladies." In effect, it is not only a disease of exhaustion and debility, but of these properties peculiarly applied to the nervous system ; the dropsical and apoplectic symptoms only taking place secondarily, and as a result of the general weakness. " The more prominent symptoms," observes Dr. Dwyer, " were numbness of the extremities, muscular power greatly impaired, walking attended with a considerable degree of unsteadiness, pain, tottering, and weakness of the joints ; such instability of gait as resembles a person walking on his heels ; sometimes paralysis. *In the latter stages of the disease, when the thorax becomes affected*, increased uneasiness of the epigastrium and vomiting succeed ; dyspnœa and all the symptoms of hydrothorax."

At times the spasmodic action spreads, even from the first, to other organs than the limbs, and produces a very striking effect. A sergeant of the 45th regiment, of sober habits, who seems to have nearly recovered from two previous attacks at Kandy about a year before, and had left the hospital, was suddenly seized, April 1, 1822, with " an extreme difficulty of breathing, inability to walk or speak much. The muscles of the forehead, face, and nose were in motion at the exertion made to speak or breathe. The corrugations of the latter gave a sharpness of countenance very peculiar, but indicative of great distress and anxiety. The countenance soon became livid ; the pulsations of the heart were loud and fluttering ; its strokes against the side could not be distinctly counted. He was bled two pounds without much relief. The appearance of this poor man was very affecting. The blood drawn was sizy ; and, upon re-opening a vein from a large orifice, he again bled freely ; but, becoming exhausted, it was thought prudent to stop it again. His legs were much swelled, and pitted on pressure. They were covered with small livid spots, as well as other parts of his body, like fleabites, but much larger. *He died in half an hour afterward.* The thighs

and abdomen were but little swelled in proportion to his legs, but evidently larger than natural. His arms were emaciated, and no part œdematous. He appeared of stout make."

The intumescence of the legs seems to have been a result of debility from the two prior attacks ; but it was nevertheless expected, that most of the cavities of the body would have given proof of an hydropic affection ; and I have selected this case as one of the strongest in support of such an opinion : for, in general, though water is traced, sometimes in one cavity and sometimes in another, yet there is seldom much accumulation, and still more seldom such as to produce oppression. Dr. Dwyer took a minute of sixteen cases ; and his remark upon the whole of these is, "water is *usually* found in some of the cavities, but the organs vary :" and such an observation is alone sufficient to take beribery out of the list of proper dropsies, whatever other place we may assign to it.

An early post-obit examination, however, of the case before us, showed as follows :—"About an ounce of serous straw-coloured fluid escaped in various ways on opening the dura mater. Filling up the gyri on the surface of the brain, we observed a gelatinous transparent matter of some tenacity and consistence ; it looked like a coating of isinglass. *In the ventricles there was but very little fluid ;* in no other part of the cranium were indications of pre-existing disease observed." In the thorax there were various adhesions, especially within the pericardium, on opening which seven ounces of a straw-coloured serum were found in it, yet warm. *No fluid in the thoracic cavity.*—In the abdomen there were few morbid appearances, except in regard to the spleen, which was as large as an ordinary sized liver, and weighed three pounds ten ounces. The liver of its usual size, but had a mottled appearance. *Only eleven ounces of serous or dropsical fluid were found in this cavity.**

---

* The morbid appearances observed by Mr. Hamilton, materially differed from those above described. Upwards of an ounce of serum was effused between the pia mater and tunica arachnoidea ; and, in two or three places, there were dark red-coloured patches, one of which was exceedingly vascular, and extended into the substance of the brain from a quarter to half an inch. *There was likewise found considerable effusion in all the ventricles except the fourth.* In the base of the cranium, four ounces of fluid tinged with blood were contained. The lungs were much loaded with dark-coloured blood, and *in both cavities of the thorax there was extensive effusion.* The heart was healthy, nor did the pericardium contain more fluid than usual. Both its external and internal surface, however, exhibited evident marks of inflammation. The diaphragm was also much inflamed, particularly its right portion. The stomach was healthy. The liver was larger than natural, and gorged with blood, as were also the mesentery and pancreas. The intestines presented nothing remarkable. Traces of congestion were remarked in the spinal marrow. From three to four pounds of fluid were found in the cavity of the abdomen, and the cellular texture, nearly all over the body, was anasarcous.—(Edin. Med. Chir. Trans., vol. ii., p. 18.) **Mr.**

The curative intention is to re-excite the absorbent system and the affected branches of the nerves to a discharge of their proper functions, by a process of diaphoretics and stimulants. Squill pills and calomel are chiefly depended on for the latter, and James's powder for the former; though the compound powder of ipecacuanha seems better calculated for the purpose, as containing a sedative admirably adapted for allaying nervous irregularities.

On the Malabar coast, it is no uncommon practice to excite perspiration in this complaint by burying the patient in a sand bath; for which purpose a hole is dug in the sandy soil, into which he is plunged as deep as to his neck, and confined there as long as he can bear the heat of the sand that surrounds him. The strength, throughout the whole, is supported by cordials, and in many instances even by ardent spirits diluted for the purpose; punch is a common drink on this occasion, and the refreshing and sedative power of the acid entitles it to a preference. To remove the numbness and pricking or formicative pain from the limbs, friction and stimulant liniments are applied locally, and not unfrequently the legs are plunged into a pediluvium. And where the disease assumes an alarming appearance, and the spasmodic symptoms are very violent, recourse is had to a hot bath, and the strongest cordials and antispasmodics, as brandy, sulphuric ether, or its aromatic spirit, and laudanum, which it is sometimes found necessary to continue for several weeks.

In convalescence, the patients should be removed, as soon as may be, to a drier and more equable temperature, and be put upon the ordinary plan of tonics, regular exercise, and nutritive diet. In milder cases, they generally recover with the shifting of the monsoon, which carries off the remote cause of the disease, and brings a change of temperature home to them.

[The evident congestion, noticed by Mr. Hamilton in his dissections, made him resolve to try the effects of bloodletting. This was practised freely and repeatedly, after which twenty grains of calomel and thirty drops of laudanum were exhibited, and the patient's body fumigated with the hydrargyri oxydum cinereum. In an hour and ten minutes, the calomel and laudanum were repeated. In three hours more, the calomel was given again with six

grains of gamboge, and the body was exposed again to the fumigation, "which, together with the scruple doses of calomel, and friction over the surface of the abdomen and thighs with the unguentum hydrargyri fortius and liquor ammoniæ, was repeated every three or four hours, until ptyalism was fully established. Every unfavourable symptom then speedily disappeared. Three other cases treated in the same way, proved equally successful."[*]]

Beriberi has not been hitherto described as existing in any other part of the world; and if it should be found, it will probably exhibit a modification of some of the symptoms, according to the quarter in which it appears. I am induced to make this remark from observing an account (*Med. Chir. Trans.*, vol. ix., art. i., p. 1) of a very singular spasmodic disease by Dr. Bostock, which evidently belongs to the present genus, and seems to be a variety of the present species, assuming a chronic form. The patient, who was in the middle of life, was first attacked with achings in the lower limb on one side, accompanied with a difficulty and irregularity of motion, which soon spread to the other side, and then gradually to the throat, so as to hinder deglutition, except with great pain and severe exertion: the larynx next became affected, so as to prevent speech, and afterward the back of the neck, the muscles affected being the voluntary alone. From the spastic rigidity of the limbs, they were both bent and straightened with a like difficulty. The pricking pain, like that of pins, or of a limb awaking from stupor, common to the extremities in beribery, was present here also, though apparently without stupor or œdematous swellings. Yet the intellectual powers were at length affected and weakened; the failure of understanding gradually increasing, but principally showing itself in paroxysms, during one of which the patient died. No cause of the disease could be traced before death, or by dissection afterward.

---

* Hamilton in Edin. Med. Chir. Trans., vol. ii., p. 23. Those practitioners who regard beriberia as a disease of debility, prefer stimulants, deobstruents, and antimonials; while others, who look upon it as an inflammatory complaint, recommend bloodletting and evacuants. Mr. Wright is of opinion, that both methods are applicable, if varied according to the peculiar form of the disease, which seems to him to be in many instances of the tribe of idiopathic dropsies, such as, according to Drs. Parry, Blackall, and other modern writers, are originally caused by increased momentum and disorder of the sanguiferous system, and have a general alliance with inflammation, whatever appearance they may afterward present. In other instances in which the patient has long suffered from this disease, compheated with abdominal dropsy, Mr. Wright is in favour of supporting the patients with cordials, wine, bark, and nourishing diet.—See Edin. Med. and Surgical Journ., vol. xli., p. 328.—Ed

---

Hamilton notices, that the *post-mortem* appearances described by Mr. Ridley (Dublin Hospital Reports, vol. ii.), mark the existence, not only of internal congestion, but of visceral inflammation, in beribery still more decidedly. " Dissections show," says Mr. Wright, "that the patient is at times killed by suffocation from the increased pressure of accumulated fluid in the lungs, and, at others, by apoplexy." His other remarks on this subject generally confirm those of Mr Hamilton.—Ed.

ORDER IV.

SYSTATICA.

DISEASES AFFECTING SEVERAL OR ALL THE SENSORIAL POWERS SIMULTANEOUSLY.

IRRITATION OR INERTNESS OF THE MIND, EXTENDING TO THE CORPOREAL SENSES, OR THE MUSCLES; OR OF THE CORPOREAL SENSES, OR THE MUSCLES, EXTENDING TO THE MIND.

THE sensorial powers are those which are dependant on the sensorium or brain as their instrument or origin; and are three in number, —the intellectual, the sensific, and the motory. Thus far we have only contemplated these as they are affected singly, or, where more are affected than one, as influencing the rest only secondarily or sympathetically. The diseases of the present order are of a more complicated origin and nature, and affect several or all the sensorial powers conjointly from the first. The order is hence denominated SYSTATICA, a Greek compound, from συνίστημι, "congredior, consocio." *Syncoptica* might have been employed, and upon as large a scale, so as to denote increased, as well as diminished action, *impellentia* as well as *concidentia*; but this term is usually limited to express maladies of the latter kind; and, consequently, might have produced confusion, since the present order, like all the preceding, includes diseases evincing different, and even opposite states of action.

The genera appertaining to it are the following :

I. Agrypnia.	Sleeplessness.
II. Dysphoria.	Restlessness.
III. Antipathia.	Antipathy.
IV. Cephalæa.	Headache.
V. Dinus.	Dizziness.
VI. Syncope.	Syncope.
VII. Syspasia.	Comatose Spasm.
VIII. Carus.	Torpor.

GENUS I.

AGRYPNIA.

SLEEPLESSNESS.

DIFFICULTY OR INABILITY OF OBTAINING SLEEP.

AGRYPNIA (ἀγρυπνία) is a Greek term significant of the English SLEEPLESSNESS, by which it is here rendered. The affection is not introduced into Dr. Cullen's nosological arrangement, and has consequently been omitted by most nosological writers since his time; but it occurs in the greater number of those who preceded him; and its claim to be considered as an idiopathic affection is as clear as that of most diseases concerning which there is no dispute.

The two following species are embraced by this genus :—

1. Agrypnia Excitata. Irritative Wakefulness.
2. ——— Pertæsa. Chronic Wakefulness.

SPECIES I.

AGRYPNIA EXCITATA.

IRRITATIVE WAKEFULNESS.

SLEEP RETARDED BY MENTAL EXCITEMENT; LISTLESSNESS TO SURROUNDING OBJECTS.

ON the physiology of sleep and dreaming, we briefly touched under the genus PARONIRIA, or SLEEP DISTURBANCE, in the first order of the present class ; but the subject is of great extent and complexity, and cannot be followed up into any detailed explanation in a work on pathology. At present, therefore, I can only observe, that natural sleep is a natural torpitude of the voluntary organs of the animal frame, produced by a general exhaustion of sensorial power, in consequence of an exposure to the common stimulants or exertions of the day. And hence, if such exhaustion do not take place, natural sleep cannot possibly ensue, though morbid sleep undoubtedly may, as produced by other causes.

Now it often happens, that from an energetic bent of the mind to a particular subject, the sensorial power continues to be produced, not only in a more than usual quantity, but for a more than usual term of time ; and, in consequence of this additional supply, there is no exhaustion at the ordinary period, and therefore no sleep. Severe grief is often a stimulus of this kind ; during which a morbid redundancy of sensorial power continues, followed by a morbid excitement of the system generally from day to day, and from night to night, till the frame is worn out by the protracted watchfulness or sensorial erethism. And it is astonishing to witness, in various instances, how long the frame will support itself before it is worn out, or the irritation that prevents sleep sufficiently subsides for its return, and particularly where the mind is labouring under the influence of the depressing passions, or of depressing pain. A hemicrania has kept a person awake for three months ;[*] and a melancholy or gloom on the spirits for fourteen months. Overwhelming joy has often a similar effect, though seldom in an equal degree, or for so long a period of time. The mind may also be intensely directed to some peculiar object of study, and the energy of the will becomes in this case a like stimulus to the production of a fresh or protracted supply of sensorial power, so that the usual exhaustion of the nervous system does not take place at the accustomed period. This is peculiarly the case in a pursuit of the abstract sciences, or those of a more strictly intellectual nature, as the higher branches of the mathematics.

* Bartholin, Hist. Anat., cent. i., hist. 64 ; Schenck, lib. i., obs. 256. The editor once attended a young lady, whose complaints consisted in violent palpitations of the heart, cough, and difficulty of breathing, and who was kept almost constantly awake by her distressing sensations for nearly three months. As sitting up or the least exertion aggravated the palpitations, she continually kept her bed. This patient was one of the last visited by Dr. Good, who recommended a trial of hyoscyamus. This medicine, and many others, were tried in vain ; but under Dr. Oke, now of Southampton, and Mr. Taylor, of Farnham, a complete recovery gradually took place.—ED.

Where the determination of the mind to a particular subject is exquisitely intense, whether that subject be a passion or a problem, by far the greater part of the sensorial power is expended at this particular outlet; and consequently the frame at large, with the exception of those organs to which such outlet peculiarly appertains, is so far drawn upon, as a common bank, for a contribution of sensorial power, that it labours under a certain degree of deficiency, and hence a certain degree of torpitude, so as to become insensible to the world around it; making, in this respect, an approach to the state of mind we have already described under the name of APHELXIA *intenta*, or *mental* ABSTRACTION.

The cure of this species of sleeplessness is to be accomplished by allaying the mental excitement by which it is produced. This is best done by recalling the mind from the pursuit that leads it astray, and a free surrender of the will to listlessness and quiet. The perturbation will then subside, the sensorial organs become tranquillized and inactive, and the habit of refreshing slumber resume its influence. But where this cannot be obtained by the mere exercise of the will, we must call opium or some other narcotic to our aid, which, by its revellent stimulus, may coincide with the consent of the will, and produce the exhaustion, and consequently the quiet, that is requisite for sleep.

SPECIES II.
AGRYPNIA PERTÆSA.
CHRONIC WAKEFULNESS.
SLEEP RETARDED BY BODILY DISQUIET; ATTENTION ALIVE TO SURROUNDING OBJECTS.

THE exhaustion, in which the very essence of natural sleep consists, supposes a perfect quiescence and inactivity of the sensorial powers. Uneasiness of any kind will become an obstacle; and hence, an aching coldness of the extremities or of any other part will prevent it; an uneasy sensation of the stomach or any other part will prevent it; an absence of the common pleasurable feeling with which we ordinarily prepare ourselves for sleep will prevent it: "And, on this account," as Darwin observes, "if those who are accustomed to wine at night take tea instead, they cannot sleep." And the same evil happens from a want of solid food for supper to those who are accustomed to use it; as, in these cases, there is an irksome or dissatisfied feeling in the stomach. And hence, also, too great an anxiety or desire to sleep is another cause of its suspension; for this, as a mental disquiet, will only add to the corporeal disquiet which has produced it; and, as already observed, the emotions of the mind must be as quiescent as those of the body, and the will, instead of commanding or interfering, must tranquilly resign itself to the general intention.

Where uneasiness of this kind has been permitted to continue for several nights in succession, the sleeplessness is apt to become chronic, and to be converted into a habit. We have hence had examples, as noticed with their appropriate references in the volume of Nosology, in

which vigilance or sleeplessness has continued for a month without intermission (*Grüling*, cent. iv., obs. 90), for six months (*Panarol, Pentecost*, v., obs. 4), and even for three years.—(*Plinii*, lib. v., vii., cap. 51.)

Mr. Gooch gives us a singular case of a man who never slept, and yet enjoyed a very good state of health till his death, which happened in the seventy-third year of his age. He had a kind of dozing for about a quarter of an hour once a day, but even that was not sound, though it was all the slumber he was ever known to take.—(*Med. and Chir. Observations*, &c., 8vo.)

The cure of this disease demands a particular attention to its cause; for if we can get rid of the organic disquiet on which it depends, we shall be pretty sure to succeed in obtaining our object. All irksome chills, and especially those of the feet, should be taken off by a sufficient warmth of clothing; and the habitual supper, or other indulgence which has hitherto preceded and introduced sleep, should be freely allowed.

The lulling sounds of soft and agreeable music, or agreeable reading, have been tried as concomitants, and not unfrequently with success. And narcotic aromas have at times been had recourse to, especially that of the hop, heaped into pillows; but, so far as I have seen, and I have once or twice witnessed the experiment, with as little efficacy as the pillows of the male fern in cases of rickets, which were once, according to Van Swieten, in equal estimation for this last complaint. A pediluvium, as recommended by Lang (*Epist.*, xlv.), will often be found a much better prescription, or any means which will excite that breathing moisture which is indicative of general ease. Soft, gentle, and general friction, and especially where there is any chill or rigidity upon the limbs, will frequently produce the same effect in a very agreeable way; and this, too, without combining it with the external use of opiates, as proposed by De la Prada (*Journ. de Médecine*, tom. xxxvi.) and various other writers.—(*Anscrt. Abhandl.*, b. i., iv., st. 45.)

Mosch was the favourite medicine of Thilenius (*Medicinische und Chirurgische Bemerkungen*, &c.), and hyoscyamus of Stoerck (*Libellulus quo continuantur Experimenta*, &c.), but a free and exhilarating glass of wine, as proposed by Fordyce, will often answer much better than either of them. In many cases of disquiet, and particularly in the stomach and præcordia, it might be well to try the hypnotic powers of the nutmeg, as warmly recommended by Dr. Cullen. We have already noticed this reputed effect in the East Indies, which Bontius confirmed by his own experience, and which has since been confirmed by practitioners in Europe: and when taken in a large dose, there can be little doubt of its somnolent virtue. In the case recited by Dr. Cullen in proof of this, the person had swallowed more than two drachms by mistake, and the effect was a drowsiness, commencing an hour afterward, which gradually increased to a complete stupor and insensibility. After this he was delirious, and continued to be alternately stupid and delirious for several hours : but, in six hours from the attack, he was pretty well recovered from every symptom.—(*Mat. Med.*, part ii., ch. v.)

Where, however, the morbid habit is too rigidly established to give way to any of these means, we must forcibly break through it by the use of opium, till the habit itself be overcome, when all narcotics should be gradually omitted.

The wakefulness so common to old people is hardly a disease. They use but little exertion, and hence require but little sleep ; and the internal inactivity is upon a par with the external. A third part of the vessels, perhaps, that took a share in the general energy of the middle of life, is obliterated, and the wear and tear of those that remain are much less. The pulse beats feebly ; the muscles of respiration are less forcibly distended ; the stomach digests a smaller portion of food, for only a smaller portion is required ; the intellect is less active, the corporeal senses less lively, and a minuter quantity of nervous energy produced by the brain and its dependencies. And hence, though there is far more weakness than in earlier life, there is a less proportionate demand for exertion, and consequently a far smaller necessity for sleep.

From such a line of reasoning may we see why sleeplessness should be found as a symptom in excessive fatigue, violent pain of any kind, inflammation, fevers, and various affections of the brain.

GENUS II.
DYSPHORIA.
RESTLESSNESS.

TROUBLESOME AND RESTLESS UNEASINESS OF THE MUSCLES ; INCREASED SENSIBILITY ; INABILITY OF FIXING THE ATTENTION.

THIS is the *inquietudo* of many authors, which the Greeks expressed by the generic term now chosen, importing, literally, " tolerandi difficultas," " a difficulty of enduring one's self." It does not expressly enter into the classification of Sauvages, nor that of Cullen, but is nearly synonymous with the *anxietas* of the former, which in the present system becomes a species of this genus. " *Molesta sensatio*," says Sauvages, " quæ ad jactitationem cogit, sed quomodo ab affinibus morbis discrepet, dicant qui experti sunt."

The genus embraces two species, as exhibiting restlessness or inquietude, chiefly confined to the sensific or the irritable fibres ; or as dependant upon the state of mind.

   1. Dysphoria Simplex.   Fidgets.
   2. ———— Anxietas.   Anxiety.

SPECIES I.
DYSPHORIA SIMPLEX.
FIDGETS.

RESTLESSNESS GENERAL, AND ACCOMPANIED WITH A PERPETUAL DESIRE OF CHANGING THE POSITION.

THIS is what we mean by the English colloquial term *Fidgets*, from *fidgety*, most probably a corruption of *fugitive*, though the lexicographers have given us no origin of the term. Both import restlessness, unsteadiness, and per-

petual change of place. The proper Latin term is *titubatio ;* and, indeed, most languages have some peculiar term to express this troublesome and irritable sensation, though it has been rarely introduced as a disease into the nosological catalogue.

The actual cause seems to consist in an undue accumulation of sensorial power, which seeks an outlet, so to speak, at every pore, for want of a proper channel of expenditure. Thus every one becomes fidgety who is obliged to sit motionless beneath a long-drawn and tedious story of commonplace facts totally destitute of interest : and still more so when he is eagerly waiting, and fully bottled up as it were, to reply to an argument loaded with sophisms, absurdities, or untruths, and over which he feels to have a complete mastery. So the high-mettled horse is fidgety that, called out, in full caparison, and still restrained in his career, is panting for the race or the battle. " So the squirrel, when confined in a cage, feels," as Dr. Darwin has ingeniously observed on this disease, which he calls jactitatio, " a restless uneasiness from the accumulation of irritative power in his muscles, which were before in continual and violent exertion from his habit of life ; and, in this situation, finds relief by perpetually jumping about his cage to expend a part of his redundant energy. For the same reason, children that are constrained to sit in the same place at school for hours together, are liable to acquire a habit of playing with some of the muscles of their face, or hands, or feet, in irregular movements, which are called tricks, to exhaust a part of the accumulated irritability by which they are goaded."

In the two last instances, this irritability is simply accumulated for want of a proper outlet, and not from inordinate secretion. In the two preceding cases, of the restrained horse and the restrained orator, there is added to this simple accumulation, for want of disbursement, an accumulation also from inordinate excitement.

It is this last source alone that can give the present affection any thing of a morbid character : and in irritable temperaments this is often the case ; for there is a diseased excess of sensorial power produced constitutionally, which is apt, on various occasions, to show itself by a perpetual restlessness or jactitation, as troublesome to those who are of the company as to those who are afflicted with it.

Paulini (*Lanx. Sat.*, dec. ii., obs. 10) observes that worms, and Lentin (*Beobacht. der Epidemischen Krankheiten*, p. 47) that atony alone is a cause ; and hundreds of other sources of irksome irritation may be added to these ; one of the most common of which is an obstinate and unconquerable itching, like that of *prurigo senilis*, and especially in a part of the body that we cannot conveniently get at to scratch : and hence ascarides in the rectum or pudendum, into which last organ they have been sometimes found to creep, is a most distressing, and, in some cases, a maddening cause.

A course of cooling purgatives, warm bathing, or increased exercise, will probably be found most serviceable in this harassing complaint; with an attention to the primary disease, where it is sympathetic.

SPECIES II.
DYSPHORIA ANXIETAS.
ANXIETY.

THE RESTLESSNESS CHIEFLY AFFECTING THE PRÆCORDIA; WITH DEPRESSION OF SPIRITS, AND A PERPETUAL DESIRE OF LOCOMOTION.

THIS species, in persons of an irritable or highly nervous temperament, and especially among those inclined to hysteria or hypochondriacal symptoms, is occasionally to be met with as an idiopathic affection, to which such a temperament gives a peculiar predisposition. But we see it more frequently as a feature in the first attack of fevers, in nausea, in various affections of the præcordia, and most powerfully and most distressingly in lyssa or canine madness. It has been ascribed to the want of a free passage for the blood through the heart, in consequence of a polypus concretion, or some other obstruction; to a similar difficulty of its passage through the lungs; and to a constriction of the vena portæ, producing a like impediment in the lower belly; and the anxiety has been denominated præcordial, pulmonary, or epigastric, according to the part affected, which, however, we cannot always trace out. The complaint is particularly noticed by Hippocrates, who distinguishes it by the name of alysmus (ἀλυσμὸς), literally, restlessness or inquietude.

It has sometimes, and especially in persons of an acutely irritable habit, been accompanied with great excitement of the nervous system generally, and spasmodic action of some or even all the muscles, displaying, according to the idiosyncrasy, the symptoms of chorea, hypochondrias, or lyssa; and has occasionally, as I have reason to believe, been mistaken for lyssa, where the morbid mind has pored incessantly on the recollection of some former scratch or bite of a dog or cat; and, like lyssa, it has sometimes terminated fatally, though by no means with a like rapidity.

Where the affection is idiopathic, an emetic will be generally found to produce the readiest assistance; after this, the warmer antispasmodics, and, if necessary, narcotics may be successfully employed, with gentle exercise and a light diet.

GENUS III.
ANTIPATHIA.
ANTIPATHY.

INTERNAL HORROR AT THE PRESENCE OF PARTICULAR OBJECTS OR SUBJECTS; WITH GREAT RESTLESSNESS OR DELIQUIUM.

ANTIPATHIA (ἀντιπαθὴς, from ἀντιπαθέω, "naturalem repuguantiam habeo") does not occur in Swediaur, nor in Dr. Cullen's classification; but enters into his supplementary catalogue, "Morborum à nobis omissorum quos omisisse fortassis non oportebat;" or, as he expresses it, in another place, or diseases which were either forgotten when the arrangement was settled, or for which no fit place could be found within its limits. It occurs, however, in Sauvages, Linnéus, Vogel, and Ploucquet, and seems to comprise two species:—

1. Antipathia Sensilis.   Sensile Antipathy.
2. ———— Insensilis.   Insensile Antipathy.

SPECIES I.
ANTIPATHIA SENSILIS.
SENSILE ANTIPATHY.

ANTIPATHY PRODUCED THROUGH THE MEDIUM OF THE EXTERNAL SENSES.

VERY singular examples of both species belonging to this genus are recorded by the collectors of medical curiosities; while others are of everyday occurrence. Some may be accounted for from early fright, stories told in the nursery, or that incongruous association of ideas in early life, which we had occasion to notice in the Proem to the present class. But many are of difficult solution, and others altogether inexplicable.

Under the species before us, we may mention an antipathy produced by the smell of roses, of strawberries, of mint, and some other herbs; by the sound of music; or the sight of a drawn sword, which is said to have existed in King James I.; or the rattling of a carriage over a bridge, which continued for some years after mature life in Peter the Great of Russia, who was frightened, while an infant, by a fall from a bridge into the water, and who only overcame the antipathy by resolutely accustoming himself to the object of disgust.

The sight of crabs and lobsters, and, still more frequently, of toads and vipers, has produced the same effect; and we have a few instances of its being occasioned by what we should much less expect as a cause, the appearance of bread and cheese, or even bread alone.—(*Eph. Nat. Cur.*, dec. i., ann. i., obs. 144, *et in Schol.*, dec. iii., ann. iii., obs. 149.) The object itself, however, seems to be of little or no importance; the feeling in most of these cases results from an association of such object, whatever it may be, with some painful occurrence in early life, of which it continues to be as much the symbol or expression as letters are of ideas. In many instances, the original occurrence is forgotten; but the impression indelibly remains, and the object recalls the mind to its influence. There is reason to believe, however, that the antipathy is often the result of idiosyncrasy, or something peculiar in the framework of the individual constitution.

SPECIES II.
ANTIPATHIA INSENSILIS.
INSENSILE ANTIPATHY.

THE ANTIPATHY PRODUCED THROUGH AN UNKNOWN MEDIUM.

IN the preceding species the feeling of antipathy is excited through the medium of one of the external senses, to which the object of antipathy presents itself, or with which it is associated on recollection; for it is the sight, or taste, or smell, or touch, or hearing of such object, or the idea of such sensible impressions, that alone calls the antipathy into action.

There are some persons, however, that are struck with a peculiar and indescribable kind of horror at the presence of an object, which is unperceived by any of these senses, as soon as it comes within the atmosphere of some unknown influence. The presence of a cat has been often known to produce this effect under the circumstances now, adverted to; or when the animal, though present, has been concealed, and not one of the senses has been alive to its presence. Instances of this kind are to be found in most of the collections of medical curiosities, as well as in various other works;* and I have met with several decided instances in the course of my own practice. The affection, in this case, depends unquestionably upon an extraordinary idiosyncrasy; but by what means such an idiosyncrasy is influenced we know not. Sauvages inquires whether the effluvium thrown from the object of aversion into the atmosphere may not, in combining with the fluids of the affected person, produce an irritating and distressing tertium quid, as corrosive sublimate is produced by a combination of mercury with oxymuriatic acid. The fact, at present, appears inexplicable; but it is not more singular than the wonderful power so well known to be possessed by the *viverra noctula* (common or great bat), which renders it conscious of the presence and position of objects when all its senses are muffled, and which enables it, when flying in this state, to avoid them. This extraordinary faculty, to which we adverted in the Proem to the present class, has been called a sixth sense by several naturalists.

In all these cases, whether of the preceding or of the present species, the only means in our power of destroying the anomalous or morbid impression is by introducing a counter-habit; or, in other words, by gradually inuring the sensorium to the influence of the disgustful object. By being familiarized with what at first we most shrunk from, our courage becomes hardened, and the painful impression blunted; and sights, and sounds, and smells, and the most imminent dangers, that could not at one time be encountered, or even contemplated without fainting, in process of time no more affect us than the roar of a cannon affects the war-horse, or the mountain-tempest the mariner.

GENUS IV.
CEPHALÆA.
HEADACHE.

ACHING PAIN IN THE HEAD; INTOLERANCE OF LIGHT AND SOUND; DIFFICULTY OF BENDING THE MIND TO MENTAL OPERATIONS.

CEPHALÆA (κεφαλαία, from κεφαλή, "caput") is employed by Galen chiefly in the sense of chron-

* Eph. Nat. Cur., dec. ii., ann. ii., obs. 50. Borelli, cent· iv., obs. 61. Emercetanus, Diætet. Polyhistor., p. 82.

ic headache; whence the term *cephalalgia* has been invented in later times to express affections of shorter duration. Headaches of all kinds, however, form a natural group, and should be described under a common genus, which is here named after the oldest and most authorized term. Sauvages has particularly remarked the symptom of disability of the mental powers in the first species we are about to notice, and the remark may be applied to all the others: "difficultas cogitandi, distinctè ratiocinandi, reminiscendi." The species which may be enumerated under this genus are the following:—

1. Cephalæa Gravans. Stupid Headache.
2. ————— Intensa. Chronic Headache.
3. ————— Hemicrania. Megrim.
4. ————— Pulsatilis. Throbbing Headache.
5. ————— Nauseosa. Sick Headache.

SPECIES I.
CEPHALÆA GRAVANS.
STUPID HEADACHE.

PAIN OBTUSE; WITH A SENSE OF HEAVINESS EXTENDING OVER THE WHOLE HEAD; SOMETIMES INTERMITTENT.

THE remote causes of headache are so numerous and so complicated, that it is difficult to catch or arrange them; and many of them are so completely concealed from view, by a confinement to the brain itself, that we vainly endeavour to discover and analyze them. Repelled discharges from the hemorrhoidal vessels, repelled or retarded catamenia, repelled fluids from the surface, are very frequent causes of one or other of the species of cephalæa now enumerated. Whatever retards the current of the blood in the sinuses of the brain, or the veins which convey the blood from the head, will produce it. Of this kind are various tumours, particularly of the conglobate glands, polypi, exostoses, or bony fragments separated by some violence from the internal table of the scull, not producing irritation, perhaps, till the accident that gave rise to them has long passed by and been forgotten. Hence some part of the brain has often, on dissection, been found diseased in its structure, producing, occasionally, an abscess with a considerable lodgment of pus. And, in some cases, the disease has been cured by the pus making its way through the frontal sinuses (*Nicolai, Decad. Observationum Illustr. Anat.*; *Schrader, Obs. Anat. Med.*; *Lentilius, Miscel.*, i., 599), or through the ears (*Gockell, Gallicin. Med. Pract.*; *Trecourt, Mém. et Obs. de Chirurgie*, No. 5), and escaping externally. It has, in every age, been produced by a decayed tooth, and has ceased on its removal: a profusion of hair on the head has been also an occasional cause, in which case it has yielded to shaving or merely thinning the hair. It has often followed a neglected catarrh or neglected rheumatism, and still oftener has resulted from some morbid irritation of the stomach, and especially from worms.—(*Walther, Thes.*, obs. 17; *Blumenbach, Med. Bibl.*, b. ii., p. 434.) So again, whatever prevents a free evacuation of the right auricle and ventricle of the heart, and contributes to retard the motion of the blood in the veins which discharge their contents on this side of the heart, has a tendency to lay a foundation for this complaint.

Under these circumstances, nothing is more difficult than to determine, in many instances, whether a headache of any kind be an idiopathic or a symptomatic affection, and on this account Dr. Cullen, deviating from the general opinion of the nosologists who preceded him, has regarded it as a symptom in every instance. This, however, is to suppose, that the encephalon, which, from its magnitude and complexity, seems to open a theatre for more intrinsic disquietudes than all other organs whatever, is exempted beyond any of them.

The species immediately before us, emphatically distinguished by the name of stupid head-ache, seems, when idiopathic, to be strictly a nervous affection of the organ, originating from nervous debility or exhaustion; or, in other words, from the want of a proper supply of that kind of sensorial energy on which the organic feeling of comfort and refreshment depends. It is hence peculiarly marked by a general disquiet and confusion, rather than by acute pain; by a general hebetude of sensorial power, which disqualifies the person labouring under it for a continuance of mental labour; and in which the sight is dim, and the hearing dull, and the memory vacant. On which account it is frequently experienced by hard students, who have sat up through the whole of the night in pursuit of some abstruse and difficult subject, or who have laboured upon the same from week to week, with too small an allowance of time for sleep or exercise: in all which cases it is often relieved by surrounding the temples with a bandage steeped in cold water, which acts as a tonic upon the spent and enfeebled brain, and once more excites it to a little temporary energy. A sudden blow of severe grief often produces the same kind of exhaustion, and is accompanied with the same symptoms, during which the sufferer is equally incapable of thinking, sleeping, or attending to external objects.

A similar effect is produced by whatever else has a tendency to induce debility and torpitude in the nervous structure of the brain, as a profuse diarrhœa, repeated and immoderate venesections, and particularly any sudden faintness or debility of the stomach. The last acts, indeed, in a double way; directly, as withholding the means of sensorial recruit; and indirectly, from the close sympathy that, on all occasions, exists between the two organs. And hence, wherever we meet with *cephalæa gravans* as a sympathetic affection, and are doubtful to what particular organ to ascribe it, we shall, in most cases, find the stomach affected, and may venture to treat it accordingly.

As much as the remedial process, however, which may be serviceable in any one of the species of headache before us, may be useful in the rest, it will be most expedient to reserve this subject for the close of the entire genus.

SPECIES II.
CEPHALÆA INTENSA.
CHRONIC HEADACHE.

PAIN VEHEMENT, WITH A SENSE OF TENSION OVER THE WHOLE HEAD: PERIODIC; OFTEN CHRONIC.

This species is, perhaps, always dependant upon some local irritation, and may be produced by many, probably most of the irritants noticed at the opening of the preceding species: and as not a few of these have a seat in the brain itself, and must remain concealed till disclosed to us by dissection, and would be still beyond our reach if we could ascertain them from the first attack, there is no difficulty in conceiving why this form of headache should often defy all medical aid whatever, and run parallel with life itself.

Among the external causes, those productive of rheumatism are perhaps the most frequent, as exposing the feet for a long time to cold and damp, or lying in a damp bed with a small quantity of covering. And as all rheumatic affections, when they become chronic, have a tendency to intermit, and return periodically, we may easily see why the disease before us should do so in many instances.

The species may therefore be distinguished by its being rather limited to some particular part of the head than extending over the whole organ; by its remissions or intermissions; by the acuteness of the pain during the return of the paroxysm; by an intolerance of all motion of the head, far more than of light or sound, both of which, however, are sometimes highly irksome; and by a peculiar feeling of tenseness or constriction over the encephalon, as though its membranes were muscles, and spasmodically contracted.

This last symptom rarely takes place till the disease has established itself for some time, and seems to indicate a thickening of one or more of the tunics of the brain from increased action, produced by a long course of irritation; a result which has frequently been discovered on dissection. Where the affection is entirely rheumatic, the local pain in the head ceases as soon as a rheumatic pain takes place in any other part of the body. There is, indeed, no great difficulty in accounting for a cessation of pain in this case, upon the principle of a transfer of action. But we find it cease also, or very much remit, not unfrequently in other cases, in which post-obit examinations have proved the disease to be dependant on local irritation, as some bony protuberance from the interior of the scull, ossification, or calcareous concretions in some part of the substance of the brain, a tumour in the pineal gland, or some other portion of the cerebral mass, or an aneurism of the carotid artery; the two last of which are particularly described by Sir Gilbert Blane, as having been detected, after death, in persons who had been long and severely troubled with this modification of cephalæa. To account for the intervals of ease experienced, as in the foregoing instances, while the cause of irritation is permanent and perpetually acting, we must call to our recollection that most organs, when they have been long exposed to a more than ordinary stimulus, become gradually exhausted and blunted in their sensibility in consequence of such exposure. And hence the pain they are occasionally sensible of, and which returns in irregular paroxysms, is produced by fresh causes of excitement, periodical or incidental, or a serious aggravation of the disease itself.

In a few instances, an obstructing material, forming the exciting cause, appears to have been carried off, and, in one or two very rare cases, by channels whose communication it is peculiarly difficult to account for. A caries, or some other disease, affecting a small part of the bony substance of one of the sutures, is a cause noticed by many pathologists; and this cause has, in some instances, been so obvious, that while the patient has been able to point out the precise spot of pain with his finger, the practitioner has been able to discover a considerable indentation or vacuity, proving that a part of the suture had been absorbed or detached.* A case of this kind is related by Mr. Henry of Manchester. —(*Mem. Med. Soc. of Lond.*, vol. i.)

For the few remarks we shall have to make under the head of medical treatment, it will be most convenient, as already observed under the preceding species, to refer to the close of the genus, in order that the plan proper to be pursued under one species may be compared with that under another. At present it is only necessary to add further, that the irritating causes of chronic headache we have thus noticed, excite occasionally other symptoms than acute pain, and particularly clonic agitations of the muscular fibres adjoining the seat of pain, not unlike those of neuralgia and severe and irremediable hemiplegia.

SPECIES III.
CEPHALÆA HEMICRANIA.
MEGRIM.

PAIN VEHEMENT : CONFINED TO THE FOREHEAD, OR ONE SIDE OF THE HEAD : OFTEN PERIODICAL.

THIS is, in most cases, a disease of far less importance than the preceding. Its seat seems to be chiefly in the integuments of the head, and its principal symptoms are tenderness on pressure, an obscure redness of the skin, and a suffusion of the eyes. And with these there is frequently a nauseating uneasiness at the stomach, but whether as a cause or a consequence of hemicrania, it is not easy to determine; it is most probable, indeed, that in some instances it is the one, and in others the other.

The disease is most common to persons of delicate health or relaxed habits, and an irritable temperament, and particularly when subject to dyspepsy and hypochondriacism. In such persons, all the causes of catarrh and rheuma-

tism are sufficient for its production, as is any thing that disturbs the balance of the circulation. And hence it is often a result of cold feet, or the chill that follows a dinner not comfortably digested.

Hemicrania frequently assumes a periodical character, in which case, the pain mostly fixes itself on the same side or the same part of the head, in some cases being limited to a small disk of the integuments, with little affection of the encephalon, and in others striking deeply into the interior of the head, and down towards the the eye, which cannot endure the least glimmer of light. In many instances, its intermissions are perfectly regular, and the paroxysm returns daily at the hour of noon (*Schenck*, libr. obs. 78, 79; *Zecchii, Consult. Med.*, 90, 98, Franc. 1650); but more commonly its attacks are produced by some incidental excitement, and are consequently of uncertain recurrence. Yet it is more frequently found in the afternoon than in the morning. So far as I have observed, indeed, it usually takes place in the evening, during, or soon after the digestion of the dinner, and in persons of the middle age of life who live temperately. In one instance, in which the disease is still very obstinate, it returns at this hour after an interval of two or three weeks, continues through the whole of the night and the ensuing day, and subsides towards the evening; the paroxysm thus lasting about twenty-four hours. In a very active and otherwise healthy man, however, about thirty years of age, who has no apparent disorder of the stomach or bowels, it commences uniformly before breakfast, continues with great violence about six hours, and then subsides, leaving intervals of about six weeks or a month.

SPECIES IV.
CEPHALÆA PULSATILIS.
THROBBING HEADACHE.

PAIN PULSATORY, CHIEFLY AT THE TEMPLES ; OFTEN WITH SLEEPLESSNESS, AND A SENSE OF DRUMMING IN THE EARS.

IN discussing the genus PALPITATION (CLONUS PALPITATIO), we entered into an explanation of the very curious phenomenon of the throbbing or beating of the heart, or of a particular artery, or part of an artery, which frequently takes place without any connexion with the regular systole of the circulation, often, indeed, discordantly with it both in time and force : and we endeavoured to show that these anomalies, for the most part, depend upon a peculiarly nervous irritability, and spastic tendency of the muscular fibres of the arterial fabric, sometimes limited to the artery, or portion of an artery in which the palpitation occurs, and sometimes common to the whole arterial system.

Whenever any of the preceding species of the present genus are grafted upon a constitution of this kind, or at least upon an idiosyncrasy in which one or both the temporal arteries are possessed of this spastic tendency, and are consequently disposed to run into this anomalous contraction and relaxation, we shall have an in-

---

* Bonet, Sepulchr., lib. i., sec. i., obs. 92. Morgagni, De Sed. et Caus. Morb., epist. iii., art. 8. Stalpart, Van der Weil, cent. i., N. l.

stance of the species before us, which commonly originates in this manner. The consequence of which is, that a regular arterial stroke, as though influenced by the systole and diastole of the heart, is often feigned, which has no existence : and a pulsation is produced, which is in no respect synchronous with the movements of the heart, and is often half as rapid again. It occurs, not unfrequently, however, that the morbid beat is in perfect accordance with that of the heart ; but it is not less a spasmodic action on this account, for, in the discussion already adverted to, as well as in the Proem to the third class, we have observed that the arteries, when in a state of health, suffer no alteration in their diameter during the passage of the blood through them, and that their ordinary pulsation is only produced by the pressure of the finger or of some other hard substance against their sides.*

The species of headache before us, therefore, is to be regarded as something of a more compound kind than the rest, in consequence of the peculiarity of the constitution in which it occurs ; with the exception of which, its causes and history, and, as we shall presently show, mode of treatment, do not essentially differ.

SPECIES V.
CEPHALÆA NAUSEOSA.
SICK HEADACHE.

THIS is the spasmodic affection of Dr. Fothergill, who has described it at great length and with much accuracy. As the last species consists of almost any of the preceding, set down upon a constitution peculiarly predisposed to irregularity of arterial action, the present consists of the same set down upon a constitution peculiarly predisposed to irregular action of the intestinal canal. In its general symptoms, however, it is chiefly related to the stupid headache and the hemicrania, particularly to the last ; only, that while proper hemicrania most frequently makes its attack in the afternoon, sick headache

---

* If the doctrine inculcated by the author and some other eminent medical writers were unequivocally correct, that an artery can really both dilate and contract itself in an extraordinary degree, and this sometimes without any accordance to the action of the heart, all the doubt entertained by some distinguished physiologists in relation to the muscularity, not only of the small but of the large arteries, would be removed. That the arteries can undergo a dilatation is certain, for the change is visible in various circumstances, and particularly in inflammation. But Mr. Hunter, Dr. Thompson, and others, could never discern in this state any movements consisting of an alternate dilatation and contraction. At all events, if a power of alternate relaxation and constriction exist in any arteries, there is reason to believe that it is restricted to the capillaries, the state of which is not particularly a question in the consideration of the present disorder. The editor has seen the carotids in several instances affected with extraordinary pulsation ; but this accorded in time to that of the heart, and the greater determination of blood into them might have depended simply upon an increase of their diameter.

usually shows itself in the morning ; though the latter, like the former, occasionally varies its hour, as it does also its length of intermission.

The patient, observes Dr. Fothergill (*Fothergill's Works*, p. 597, 4to. ; *Med. Obs. and Inq.*, vol. vi., p. 103), commonly awakes early in the morning with a headache that rarely affects the whole head, but only some particular part of it, most frequently the forehead, extending over one or both eyes. Sometimes it is fixed about the upper part of the parietal bone of one side only, sometimes the occiput is the part affected ; or it darts from one place to another, and equally varies during its continuance in its degree of intensity. There is some degree of sickness usually connected with it, mostly limited to nausea, but occasionally amounting to vomiting. If the pain commence in the morning before any meal is taken, phlegm only is thrown up, unless the straining be severe, in which case bile is intermixed with it. After this the pain soon begins to abate, leaving a soreness about the head, a squeamishness at the stomach, and a general uneasiness which induces the patient to wish for repose. Perhaps, after a short sleep, he recovers perfectly, only a little weakened by his sufferings. The duration of this species of headache differs, however, in different persons : in some it subsides in two or three hours ; in others it extends to twenty-four hours or longer, and with a violence scarcely to be endured, the smallest light or noise rendering the pain intolerable. In young persons the paroxysm goes off soon ; but after the disease has been a companion for years, it is of longer duration, and the system becomes extremely debilitated. Its returns are very irregular : some persons suffer from it every two or three days, some every two or three weeks, and others have still longer intervals. Those who use but little exercise, and are inattentive to their diet, are afflicted most severely : costiveness, when habitual, is a frequent predisposing cause ; and hence a protracted laxity of the bowels, supervening on habitual constipation, has removed the complaint altogether.

Dr. P. Warren, in a very valuable paper on this subject, seems to think that a line of distinction may be drawn between the disease as produced by a morbid state of the stomach, and of the collatitious viscera, or, in other words, as it makes an approach to the first or to the third species before us. "Upon the whole," says Dr. Warren, " that form of headache which is attended more with confusion than pain, and in which there is a temporary dimness of sight, appears to depend chiefly upon a defective action or secretion of the STOMACH ; the other (that in which the pain is acute, or exceeds the confusion), which is the most prevalent form, more particularly upon inactivity of the upper bowels, from whatever cause it may be produced, and an imperfection of that part of digestion in which the bile is concerned.*

---

* On Headaches which arise from a defective Action of the Digestive Organs; Med. Trans., iv., art. xviii.

The connexion between all these species of headache is so close, and several of them are so apt to run into the others, that the author has reserved the few remarks he will have to make upon the remedial treatment till the whole have, as now, passed under review, and have furnished us with an opportunity of concluding how far any thing like a common plan of treatment may be advantageous, and upon what points it ought to vary.

A very slight recurrence to the preceding history will show us, that the chief causes of headache are local irritations, suddenly checked perspiration, or exposure to cold and damp; a peculiar irritability of the nervous system, and particularly a spastic idiosyncrasy of the temporal arteries, and a morbid condition of the chylopoetic viscera.

The last is, perhaps, the most common cause; and hence, whenever there is any doubt as to the specific character of the disease, we can never do better than treat it as chiefly appertaining to the fifth species, and implicated with a diseased action of the stomach or its collatitious organs.

It is on this account that emetics, with an anodyne given afterward, have been so generally found serviceable, and have often effected a cure in a few hours. And hence also the great advantage of keeping the bowels not only free from costiveness, but with some kind of warm irritant, slightly, though constantly acting upon them, of which one of the best is aloes, where there is no tendency to piles, and copayva, or the extracts of rhubarb and colocynth, where there is. Piles, however, are not an affection to be much regarded in cephalæa, for it is probable, that they may often become a useful revellent : and Dr. Arbuthnot was so firmly of

we have a clear proof of great irritability of the nervous system, the prussic or hydrocyanic acid may be had recourse to with considerable advantage, in moderate doses of a drop or two, three times a day, in a little cinnamon water, gradually increasing the power, and uniting the acid with full doses of subcarbonate of iron, as in the case of neuralgia.

In some instances, thinning the hair where it is profuse, has also been found serviceable, but in others it has failed ; and the following remarks of the author's late valued friend, Dr. Parr, upon the subject of shaving, are well entitled to attention. "This practice," says he, "has not the sanction of long experience, nor is it supported by reason. Each hair is a vegetable, nourished by a bulbous root, supplied by numerous bloodvessels. These, though small from their number, convey no inconsiderable quantity of fluids; and, as the external and internal carotids arise from a common trunk, and anastomose in some of their branches, whatever cause increases the circulation in the former must lessen it in the latter." He adds, that he himself was for many years a sufferer from an irregular returning paroxysm of headache, for which he could assign no cause, but at last discovered, that it frequently returned after shaving the head : he consequently suffered his hair to grow, and from that time the disease gradually lessened in violence, in duration, and in frequency of its recurrence. "From being a complaint," says he, "highly serious, and beginning to affect the memory, its returns are now rare, and never so violent as to unfit the frame for any exertion of body or mind."

Temporary relief has also, in many cases, been obtained by the external application of volatiles and aromatics, as ammonia, camphire,

of exercise and early hours should combine, or little advantage will be gained by any plan. Linnéus is said to have cured himself of a severe and obstinate hemicrania, which returned at the interval of a week, and continued for twenty-four hours, by merely drinking a draught of cold water early in the morning, and then walking himself into a glowing heat.

The verticillated stimulant plants have, in many instances, also been found serviceable in most of the species thus far considered, whether the disease originate in the head or in the stomach; and of these the most active, as well as the most pleasant, are lavender, rosemary, and marjoram.

There is one species of headache, however, to which but little of what we have thus far recommended will in all cases apply, and that is, the second or chronic cephalæa: and, on this account, it is of great importance that we endeavour to distinguish it from the rest; or rather that we endeavour to distinguish those causes of it, under the operation of which it is necessary to pursue a different plan; for, in many instances, even here the cause of irritation may be palliated, or destroyed, by some part of the process already recommended. But we have stated, that this form of the disease is often dependant upon some structural irritation within the cavity of the scull, such as a node or toph, or caries of the interior table of the cranium, a scirrhous or other tumour in some part of the brain, or a thickening of the membranes that surround it.

And here, in conjunction with the aperient plan, or even a brisker plan of this kind than has yet been recommended, local bleeding by cupping or leeches should be had recourse to without delay. Free venesection, indeed, has often been of great service in diminishing the inflammatory action, and taking off the topical irritability for many weeks or even months. And hence the temporal artery has often been opened on the continent, and with very good effect: and we may see why a vicarious hemorrhage from the nose, the mouth, the liver, or some other organ, has been followed, in various cases, by a perfect cure.—(*Heister, Wahrnemungen*, i., p. 70; *Abhandl. der Königl. Schwed. Acad. der Wissenchaft.*, xiii., 39.) And, where some other obstruction has been the cause, it has occasionally yielded to a severe fright (*Reidlin*, cent. ii., obs. 55), or a fortunate concussion of the brain (*Ephem. Nat. Cur.*, cent. ix., obs. 6), or a wound on the head.—(*Desgranges, Journ. de Méd.*, tom. lxii., p. 360.) Hildanus refers to several inveterate cases effectually overcome by accidents of this kind.—(Cent. ii., obs. 8.)

Here also, if anywhere, we may possibly expect advantage from a long-continued use of mercury as an alterant and absorbent, in connexion with apozems of sarsa, bardana, or some other warm diluent. In organic enlargements and obstructions in other parts of the body, such a plan has often answered, and analogy will therefore lead us to expect some benefit in the present disease. Velschius describes a case of a most obstinate cephalæa, in which it completely succeeded.—(*Hecatost.*, ii., 67.)

But where every other mean has failed, and the symptoms are violent, and the painful spot is clearly definable, and we have strong reason to apprehend some local organic irritation, it may become a question how far the use of the trepan has a chance of being serviceable. Vogel gives a case, in which the pain was hereby considerably mitigated (*Chirurg. und Medic. Beobachtungen*, p. 410), and Baglivi another, in which a radical cure was effected.—(*Specim. Quatuor Librorum de fibrâ motrice et morbosâ.*) But, in this instance, a portion of the brain was found in a state of suppuration, and the confined pus hereby obtained a way of escape. Marchetti gives an example of a temporary cure, the headache being suspended so long as the wound was open, but returning after it was healed.—(*Observ.*, 36, 38.) And hence, even where no structural cause of irritation has been reached, this operation has sometimes proved serviceable as a revellent. It must, however, be admitted, that it has often been performed without any benefit whatever.*

It is hardly needful to observe, that where cephalæa is evidently a secondary disease, as in plethora, chlorosis, gout, or neuralgia, our attention must be chiefly directed to the malady on which it is dependant. Where it appears as a sequel to any suppressed and habitual evacuation or repelled eruption, the best means of obtaining relief will always be found in restoring the system to its former state; and, where this cannot be done, we must furnish the best substitute we can by some temporary irritation or drain.

As a general palliative, strong coffee has often proved serviceable; and, where its own sedative virtue is not sufficient, it forms one of the best vehicles for the administration of laudanum, in doses of eighteen or twenty drops. It diminishes, in some degree, the hypnotic power of the latter, but it counteracts its distressing secondary effects. When laudanum is intermixed with strong coffee for the cure of many modifications of headache, tranquillity and ease are produced, though there may be no sleep; when laudanum, on the contrary, is taken alone, sleep will perhaps follow, but is mostly succeeded by nausea and a return of the pain. Hence the Turks and Arabians make strong coffee their common vehicle for opium, from its tendency to counteract the narcotic principle of the latter.—(*Phil. Med. and Exp. Essays, by Thomas Percival, M. D.*, vol. iii.)†

---

* The editor has seen two cases, in which the patients lost their lives by submitting to such treatment.

† A paper on the sick headache, by Dr. James Mease of Philadelphia (Philadelphia Journ. of the Med. and Phys. Sc., vol. v.), contains many important practical remarks. Dr. M. considers this disease to result from our advanced state of civilization, the increase of wealth and of enjoyments, as it is unknown among the natives of our forests, and those of the frontier inhabitants who are obliged from their necessitous circumstances to live frugally. He regards the stomach as the seat

GENUS V.
DINUS.
DIZZINESS.

ILLUSORY GYRATION OF THE PERSON WHILE AT REST, OR OF OBJECTS AROUND THE PERSON, WITH HEBETUDE OF THE SENSORIAL POWERS.

THE distressing sensation of DINUS, a strictly Greek term, occurs, in different persons and different circumstances under very different modifications, or is connected with very different symptoms. It is often united with cephalæa, and hence, by some nosologists, it is made a mere species of this last genus; but there are few practitioners who have not witnessed instances of both, that have commenced, continued, and terminated their career without any interference with each other: and hence Linnéus has not only separated them from each other, and regarded them as distinct genera, but has even made scotoma, or dizziness with blindness and a tendency to swoon, a distinct genus also.

In the author's volume of Nosology, scotoma, with two other forms of dinus, were regarded as separate species. But, as on a fuller consideration of the subject, I am induced to think, that all these diversities originate from the particular habit or temperament of the individual, or the nature of the exciting cause, it will be more correct to reduce them to a single species, and to contemplate the diversities of symptoms and sensations they produce as varieties or modifications alone: and hence, adopting the common name for this purpose, we shall denominate this species

1. Dinus Vertigo.   Vertigo.

SPECIES I.
DINUS VERTIGO.
VERTIGO.

DIZZINESS, WITH A FEAR OF FALLING.

COMMON as this complaint is, I have not hitherto met with any satisfactory explanation of its cause. Sauvages (*Nosol. Method.*, class viii., Vesaniæ), indeed, has entered upon the subject pretty fully, as has Darwin (*Zoonom.*, class iv., ii., i., 10) since his time, and Crichton (*Of Mental Derangement*, vol. i., p. 324) since the time of Darwin; while, on the continent, it has been investigated with much patience and ingenuity by Dr. Herz of Berlin.—(*Versuch über der Schwindel.*, Berlin, 1791.) For the most part, it has been ascribed to a morbid excitement, or increased action in the organ of

---

of the disease, which affects the head by means of sympathy, and hence the remedies should be directed to the stomach and to the restoration of the nervous function. In commencing the treatment, a laxative should be the first remedy. After the digestive tube is regulated, Dr. Mease recommends the use of tonics, for instance, carbonate of iron, columbo, and orange-peel, and strict attention to diet and regimen; ample directions for which may be seen in the paper referred to above.—D.

vision, which is the view taken of it by Sauvages and Darwin, or to "a state of mental confusion arising from too rapid a succession of representations," which is the explanation of Herz and Crichton.

That there is, in all instances, some degree of mental confusion may perhaps be allowed, and that there is often too rapid a succession of representations with a morbid increase of sensorial action, may be allowed as readily: but if the following remarks be found entitled to attention, and succeed in delineating the real nature of vertigo, it will appear, that the external senses are only indirectly, if at all, the seat of the morbid action; that the energy of these is far more frequently in a state of diseased diminution than of diseased increase; and that even a rapid succession of representations is not essential to the sensation.

We have had frequent occasions of showing, that the nervous power, which supplies the muscular fibres, is communicated, not strictly speaking in a continuous tenour, but in minute and successive jets, so that the course of it is alternately broken and renewed by a series of fine and imperceptible oscillations. In a state of health and vigour, this succession of influx and pause is perfectly regular and uniform, and hence, whatever movements result from it will partake of the same uniformity, and appear to be one continued line of action instead of a successive series. But as soon as ever the harmonious alternation through which the nervous power is thus supplied, is interfered with, the oscillations become manifest, the apparently uniform current is converted into a tremulous undulation, and the muscular exertion to which it gives rise, instead of being seemingly one and undivided, is sensibly multiplied into hundreds: of which any person may convince himself on observing a strong and healthy arm extended for a few minutes with a small weight at the end of the fingers, and an arm reduced in strength by a fever, or any previous labour; for, while the first maintains an even and uniform line, in the second this line is broken into perpetual tremours and undulations.

That the nervous power, which supplies the muscular fibres, is communicated in this way, there is no doubt; and, as it is highly probable that all the different kinds of nervous fibres are fed by a like process, there can be little doubt, also, that those which maintain an intercourse between the brain and the external senses, and even those which belong to the external senses themselves, are supplied by the same kind of alternating pause and flow. And consequently, that as a perfect regularity and uniformity in this alternation is the means of conveying from the organ of vision to the sensorium one undivided perception of every single object presented to it, so, an irregularity and want of uniformity in the alternating series must confuse and complicate the perceptions, and multiply them into as many as the series of jets themselves consist of, though each perception may, perhaps, be less distinct and perfect than the single perception conveyed in the ordinary course. Thus, in looking through a window or an eyeglass, the objects that pass before us in regular order, pass singly without confusion ; but, if this order be interrupted by movements we are not accustomed to, or the objects jerked about, as in a magic lantern, they make us dizzy with their motion, and we see them confusedly and in delusive numbers.

In this manner then, it appears to me, that the increased motion and apparently rapid succession of representations, is produced in the affection we call vertigo ; which, under this explanation, is a clonic action of the nervous fibres subservient to perception, in the same manner as the rapid and tumultuous agitation of the muscles in tremour, shaking palsy, or epilepsy, is a clonic action of the fibres subservient to voluntary motion. In the last of these affections, we find a considerable difference in the nature and intervals of the clonic movements ; for these must depend upon the greater or less degree of interruption which the nervous power sustains in its flow, or upon the peculiarly relaxed or spastic state of the nervous fibres themselves, and probably, at times, upon some other cause, of which we are totally ignorant. And we have, hence, reason to expect, and do in fact perceive, an equal diversity in the clonic and illusory motions of vertigo ; for the objects, or their representations presented to the perception, appear sometimes to circumvolve horizontally from right to left, or perpendicularly from above downwards, or from below upwards, or to be very whimsically changed in their form. And not unfrequently the patient himself seems to be moving as well, and commonly in a contrary direction to the apparent motion of the objects : and, as the intermediate nerves between the other external senses and the brain seem occasionally to coincide in the same morbid agitation, we can easily conceive how that very common modification of the disease may be produced, in which the dizziness is combined with illusory sounds, as of whispering or murmuring, the ringing of bells or beating of drums, or even the roar of cannon ; for as single objects may, under the influence we are now contemplating, be prodigiously multiplied or magnified, so may single and otherwise almost imperceptible sounds ; and especially where the auditory nerve is itself in a state of high morbid acuteness, during which we have already had occasion to remark, that the gentlest and lightest tones, even the whisperings of a mere current of air in a room, or the breathing of persons present, is intolerable, while sounds before unperceived become highly distressing.— (See *Paracusis acris*, p. 246, Cl. IV., Ord. II , Gen. II., Spe. 1.) And in like manner, by an equal irregularity in the supply of the nervous energy, subservient to the perceptions of smell and taste, we may account for similar illusions upon these faculties.

In many instances, we find the vertigo equally present, whether the patient be in the dark or light, whether the eyes be closed or open ; and we have hence a full proof, that it is not dependant, as Dr. Darwin conceives, upon an increased energy in the irritative motions of the organs of vision. In some cases, the representations of objects are very numerous and rapid, but in others far less so, and particularly where the affection is severe from the first, or the patient is in a state of constitutional debility ; under which circumstances we may conceive the pauses in the flow of the nervous power to be more irregular, or of longer duration than they otherwise would be. In many cases, indeed, the only sensation is that of a buoyant undulation or swimming, without any succession of representations whatever ; affording us a proof, that the rapid succession of representations described by Dr. Herz, is not more essential to vertigo than the increased energy of Dr. Darwin.

But as the disease advances, or, in other words, as the transmission of the nervous power becomes still more interrupted, the representations are confused, indistinct, and rapid in succession, often conjoined with a sense of dimness or darkness, existing equally whether the eyes be shut or open, forming a state by Hippocrates and the Greek writers generally called scotoma or scotodinus : and as the disease makes a further progress by a further interruption of the sensorial principle, every power of body and mind augments in languor, till at length sensation, both external and internal, fails altogether, the action of the heart and the other involuntary organs is enfeebled, and the patient swoons away.

The great predisponent cause in all these cases, whether of muscular agitation or of vertigo, is nervous debility or exhaustion : the exciting causes are whatever has a tendency to disturb the uniformity with which the nervous power is supplied. And hence, those persons are most subject to both kinds of affection whose nervous system is constitutionally weak and mobile, or has become debilitated by disease or accident. Hence dyspeptic patients are peculiarly subject to both these affections ; as are those who are faint from sudden and violent evacuations, want of food, or a long course of labour. Hence we meet with it as a frequent and distressing attendant upon those who have too freely indulged in the pleasures of the table, in those of sexual intercourse, and particularly the gross gratification of self-pollution. And hence, too, we may see why it is so often an accompaniment of cephalæa, as the nervous fibres subservient to the organs of perception are here influenced from contiguous, in some cases from continuous, sympathy.

The exciting causes we have stated to be whatever has a tendency to disturb the uniformity with which the nervous power is supplied. Of these the chief are, motion or exertion to which the strength is not equal, motion to which the system has not been accustomed, or hurried motion, whether external or internal.

In a state of great weakness, whether from hunger, hard labour, hemorrhage, or a protracted fever, even the ordinary motion of gentle walking is more than the little remaining strength can support ; and the man who tries it trembles in every limb, and becomes immediately vertiginous. In like manner, whatever be his degree of strength, he will feel vertiginous by exchanging the motion to which he has been uniformly accustomed, for one of a different kind, and which he has seldom or never engaged in ; and hence, the reason of the vertigo that accompanies swinging, sailing in a ship walking in a circle, sitting backward in a carriage, or standing on one's head ; for the uniformity of the external habit has by length of time associated itself with the uniform production of the sensorial power, and the one cannot be interfered with without interfering with the other. And that this is the cause of the dizziness hereby produced is obvious, since, as soon as the old habit is overpowered by a new one, or, in other words, as soon as the man has accustomed himself to the new action, it may be persevered in without any vertiginous sensation whatever. In some persons, this sympathy of association is not so strong as in others, and hence they are not so soon affected : in infants and young children, such a kind of sympathy has rarely commenced ; for while their age has not given time for it, they have had so little walking in a straight line, and been accustomed to so much swinging and tossing about in the arms, in every direction, that they are equally prepared for all ; and hence can run round a circle, or even circumvolve on their heel, without any feeling of giddiness whatever.

For the same reason, hurried, tumultuous, or confused motion of any kind, whether external or internal, has a tendency to produce the same effect ; for the current of the nervous supply will partake of the agitation, and dizziness be a necessary result. Hence the vertigo that accompanies intoxication, in which, from the inordinate excitement that prevails throughout the system, the regular and uniform supply of the sensorial power is quickened into a confused and disorderly rush. And hence the same effect from congestion, or compression of any kind, as also from a sudden influence of mental emotion, and particularly of the depressing passions ; though, in such cases, the uniformity of the sensorial principle is interfered with by a check, instead of by a rapidity of action ; and where the check is considerable, as in cases of sudden fright or apprehension, a fainting-fit is at once produced without the preceding stages.

It is to this cause, exercised indeed in a less degree, that we are to ascribe the dizziness which is felt in looking down a precipice, climbing a tall ladder, or walking over a very narrow bridge, with a roaring torrent below ; for, in all these cases, we are conscious of danger, and lose our firmness in our fear. And that such is the real cause is quite obvious from the fact, that those who possess their firmness, and have no apprehension or trembling whatever, have no dizziness ; and that we ourselves are able to endure an exposure to the same scenes and the same motion with as great a freedom from it, when habit has given us calmness, and we have no longer any apprehension. So the sleepwalker has been known to tread firmly and fearlessly over planks and precipices, the sight of which has whirled all his brains when awake.

Vertigo then, as thus explained, consists in a clonic action of the nervous fibres subservient to the faculty of perception, and lays open to us the three following varieties :—

a Undulans. Swimming of the head.	Dizziness, with a sense of swimming or undulatory motion.
β Illusoria. Illusory vertigo.	Dizziness, with dimness of sight, and imaginary objects before the external senses.
γ Scotoma. Blind headache. Nervous fainting-fit.	Dizziness, with blindness and tendency to swoon ; often succeeded by headache.

Vertigo is not generally an alarming affection, but it is only to be remedied by a partienlar attention to its cause, and especially the predisposition of the system to a relapse.

If we have reason to suspect congestion or extravasation in the head, bleeding, and especially from the temporal artery, will often afford effectual relief. I have seen a very severe attack of vertigo cease instantly, as by magic, on opening this artery, although not more than a teacupful of blood was drawn from it. Where the stomach has been gorged, an emetic, and afterward a purgative, will prove most effectual ; where the cause, on the contrary, is debility or exhaustion, it is best relieved by cordials and a generous diet ; and where it is an idiopathic affection of the nervous system, the warm antispasmodics and tonics, with a tonic regimen, will bid fair to succeed. Such persons will derive great benefit by a change of air, of scene, and of company ; by visiting the most quiet of our watering-places, cold bathing, and a cold ablution of the head, or the whole body every morning. Here also a particular attention should be paid to the state of the bowels, as costiveness is always an exciting cause. During the paroxysm, perfect rest and a reclined position will be always found necessary ; and where there is a tendency to fainting, stimulant odours may be applied to the nostrils, and ether, ammonia, and the volatile fetids to the stomach, in draughts of cold spring water.

GENUS VI.

SYNCOPE.

SYNCOPE.

MOTION OF THE HEART AND LUNGS FEEBLE OR IMPERFECT : DIMINISHED SENSIBILITY : INABILITY OF UTTERANCE.

SYNCOPE, from συγκόπτω, "concido," "to fell or cut down," is a neoteric rather than an antique term. It occurs, indeed, among the Greek writers, but rather in the description of battles than of diseases. I cannot find who first introduced it into the medical nomenclature. In Hippocrates, the common synonyme is leipopsychia, and in Galen apopsychia: but it answers its purpose, and is, in the present day, so generally established, that there is no kind of necessity for exchanging it.

Dr. Cullen's definition of the genus is "motus cordis imminutus vel aliquamdiu quiescens." But this is by no means sufficient; for the heart has been sometimes totally void of motion without syncope, as in acrotismus, and especially in the well-known case of Mr. John Hunter, which we have noticed under that division. The leipothymia of Sauvages and other nosologists is only syncope in its first attack or mildest degree. Its character is "subitanea et brevis virium dejectio, superstite pulsûs vigore, et cognoscendi facultate." The pulse is, perhaps, always affected in some measure; but in slight cases it still retains a certain degree of power: the perception rarely fails altogether; but the voice seems to be uniformly lost.

The species in some systems of nosology are very numerous, and unnecessarily multiplied. Out of deference to high and established authorities, the author was induced, in his volume of Nosology, to offer five; but as several of these differ only in cause or some accidental symptom, they may be reduced to the two following, and the accidental differences be regarded as constituting varieties or modifications alone :—

1. Syncope Simplex.   Swooning.
2. ——— Recurrens.   Fainting-fit.

SPECIES I.
SYNCOPE SIMPLEX.
SWOONING.

OCCURRING SUDDENLY AND ACCIDENTALLY, AND CEASING WITHOUT ANY TENDENCY TO A RECURRENCE.

In vertigo, the defective or irregular action is chiefly confined to the nerves, and particularly to those of perception: in swooning it is sometimes the result of nervous exhaustion, as in cases of exquisite pain or torture, whether of body or of mind, but it more commonly originates in the sanguific or digestive organs, though the sentient participate in the affection. Vertigo, as we have already observed, occasionally terminates in swooning; and in like manner, swooning is not unfrequently succeeded by vertigo.

To maintain the faculty of perception clear and true to the impressions that are made on the external senses, we endeavoured to show, under the preceding genus, that the motion of the nervous power which connects it with those senses, must be equable and uniform; and, to maintain the action of the heart in a firm and regular order, it is necessary that the blood should flow into it in an equal and uniform stream: for if its volume be altered from any canse, whether of obstruction, surcharge, or deficiency, its motion will be checked and enfeebled, the brain and respiratory organs will participate in the debility, and syncope be a frequent result. And hence we may account for the fainting that frequently takes place on the commencement, and sometimes on the close of venesection. On tying the arm for this purpose, a considerable stream of supply is cut off, and ten ounces of blood flow, in perhaps five minutes, into a basin, which would otherwise have flowed into the heart in the same period of time. The volume of blood is hence diminished, and the heart must collapse or contract itself in proportion. In many habits, this is done with great facility; but in others, and particularly where there is a feeble supply of motific or irritative power, the contraction takes place slowly and irregularly, and with a considerable degree of flutter, or, as we have already explained it, clonic spasm; and fainting or a temporary failure of sensation is the necessary consequence; during which the alternating systole is very feeble, and the blood ceases to flow at the puncture. This effect is ordinarily ascribed to a loss of the stimulus of distention; and there may be some degree of truth in such an explanation. But that there is a something beyond this is certain, because, on removing the ligature from the arm, this stimulus is once more obtained; for the blood, instead of flowing away at the venous orifice, now takes its proper course, and flows back to the heart. Yet we see almost as often a syncope produced at this moment, and consequently by a renewal of the distention, as by an interruption of it. The fact is, that the heart, which by this time has accommodated itself to the diminished volume of the returning current, has now once more to change its diameter, and to expand itself in proportion to the increased measure and momentum of the returning tide. And as a change in its diameter produced a syncope in the former case, a change in its diameter in like manner produces it in the latter.*

For the same reason, we may see swooning take place when any extensive range of bloodvessels, that have been pressed upon by any other means, suddenly acquire a power of dilatation, as when a large cavity is formed in the abdomen by the process of tapping for an ascites, or on opening an extensive abscess in any other quarter.—(*Meckel, Epist. ad Haller, Script.*, vol. iii. ; *Eph. Nat. Cur.*, dec. ii., ann. v., obs. 53.)

But the flow of sensorial power from the brain may also be suddenly exhausted or checked; and syncope may ensue from this source, the action of the heart being diminished, not primarily, but secondarily, or by sympathy with the state of the sensorium. In fainting, from entonic passions or emotions, as a sudden shock of vehement joy, the sensorial power is perhaps abruptly expended, as also in severe pain.—(*Amat. Lusitan.*, cent. ii., cur. i. ; *Plater*, observ. ii., p: 431.) In fainting, under the influence of the atonic passions, as fear or heartsick grief, this power is unquestionably checked in its regular flow, and probably checked also in its production ; as we have reason to believe it is where

* The explanation here given seems very doubtful. The patient often faints about the time when the ligature is loosened, or immediately afterward; but this is in consequence of the blood already lost.—ED.

fainting occurs from a repulsion or retrocession of gout, exanthems, or various other diseases. And to the same cause may be referred those cases of swooning which, in some idiosyncrasies or indisposition of body, are well known to take place on exposure to particular odours, as those of cheese, apples, or, as we have already had occasion to observe, of roses, lilies, and other fragrant plants.

Syncope then, in its simple state, as unconnected with any structural disease of the heart or its adjoining vessels, seems to appear under the following modified forms or varieties :—

a Inanitionis. Swooning from inanition.	The swooning produced by fatigue, long fasting, or a sudden and excessive discharge of any fluid, whether natural or morbid, accompanied with a sense of inanition, and great prostration of strength.
β Doloris. Swooning from acute pain.	Preceded by severe pain or irritation of body, internal, as from poisons, flatulency, or worms ; or external, as from wounds or other injuries.
γ Pathematica. Swooning from mental emotion.	Preceded by an exercise of some sudden and overwhelming passion or emotion.
δ Metastatica. Swooning from metastasis.	Accompanied with a retrocession or repulsion of gout, exanthems, or other diseases.

The degree and duration of the paroxysm depend upon the peculiarity or the violence of the cause, the extent of the sensorial exhaustion, or the nature of the constitution, and hence must greatly differ in different individuals. In some cases it ceases in a few minutes, and the patient, though incapable of speaking, retains enough perception and sensation to be conscious of his own disorder, and to understand what is passing around him. The pressure and irritation of flatulency in dyspeptic and hypocondriacal habits are often sufficient of themselves to produce a fainting of this kind. In other cases the general feeling and understanding fail totally, and the pulse is scarcely perceptible. Occasionally, the sensorial power has been totally as well as suddenly exhausted, and the syncope has run into asphyxy, and even proved fatal.

Hence, Portal has justly remarked that " we may have apparent death from syncope as well as from asphyxy, and that, from not attending to this, we may mistake, and bury the living with the dead. I have seen," he adds, " a man who, after a violent fit of colic, remained for many hours in a state of syncope, without pulse, with the colour and coldness of death, and without any respiratory motion of the chest whatever. After some hours of such apparent death, he passed a bilious concretion, and the fainting vanished."—(*Mémoires sur la Nature et le Traitement de plusieurs Maladies*, tom. iv., 8vo., Paris, 1819.)

When not assisted by medicine, the system recovers itself by the gradual accumulation of sensorial energy that must necessarily take place, so long as the living principle continues, during such a state of quietism ; aided, unquestionably, by the continual action of the instinctive, or remedial power of nature, which is always aiming to repair what is amiss. The process of recovery, however, varies almost as much as that of sinking. Some revive almost immediately, without any inconvenience or sense of weakness whatever ; while others improve slowly and almost imperceptibly, and require many hours before they fully regain their self-possession. In various cases, the head becomes clear as soon as the pulse becomes regular : while, not unfrequently, the recovery is accompanied with a confusion of ideas, vertigo, and headache.

As this disease is always attended with an irregularity in the flow of nervous power, and some degree of spasmodic action, entastic or clonic, about the heart, the best remedies we can have recourse to, during the paroxysm, are antispasmodics and stimulants ; and those which are the most volatile are the most useful. Hence the advantage of admitting a free current of cold air, sprinkling cold water over the face, and pouring a little of it, if possible, down the throat. And hence also the advantage of holding ammonia, the strongest vinegar, or any other pungent odours, to the nostrils. A recumbent position is always advisable, as most favourable to an equable circulation of the blood ; and irritating and warming the extremities by the friction of the hand, or the application of rubefacients, will commonly be found to expedite the recovery, upon the principle we often had occasion to advert to, that, in a chain of organs united by sympathy or continuity, an impression produced on the one extremity is sure to operate on the other. As soon as the patient is capable of swallowing, some spirituous cordial, a glass of wine, brandy and water, fetid tincture, or the aromatic spirit of ammonia or of ether, should be administered ; and the occasional cause should be sedulously avoided in future.

SPECIES II.
SYNCOPE RECURRENS.
FAINTING-FIT.

RECURRING AT PERIODS MORE OR LESS REGULAR ; OCCASIONAL PALPITATION OF THE HEART DURING THE INTERVALS ; AND UNQUIET RESPIRATION DURING THE PAROXYSM.

THIS is, in most cases, a far more serious form of syncope than the preceding, and is commonly ascribed to some structural disease of the heart or the large arteries that immediately issue from it, as an ossification of the valves, polypus concretions, an enlargement or thickening of the substance of the heart, an accumulation of water in the pericardium, or an aneurism.

Each of these may possibly be a cause in some instance or other ; and where, during the paroxysm, the breathing, though feeble, is anxious and obstructed, the face livid, and the patient in the midst of the swoon shows a tendency to jactitation, or an uneasiness on one side or on the other; and, more especially still, where no ordinary exciting cause can be assigned, and it has commonly followed some unusual exertion or hurry of the blood through the lungs, it would be imprudent not to suspect such mischief.

But there are causes of a different and much slighter kind that I cannot avoid believing frequently operate in the production of recurrent syncope, and that too with many of the peculiar symptoms just enumerated. And I now allude to any of the ordinary causes of syncope, as set down under the first species, or any other incidental irritation whatever, occurring in a constitution of great mobility and excitability, or where the heart alone, or in conjunction with the whole arterial system, is peculiarly disposed to that irregular and clonic action which we have noticed under the species PALPITATION, and particularly under the first and second varieties.

In such a frame of body, any sudden alarm, a longer abstinence than usual, a fuller dinner than common, unwonted exercise, and a thousand minute excitements of daily occurrence, will often succeed in producing a fainting-fit; and especially where a morbid habit of recurrence has been once established, and there is a predisposition to return. Atonic plethora is another frequent cause in the peculiar constitution we are now considering, and a cause far too liable itself to establish a circle of recurrence, and consequently to give recurrence to the form of syncope before us. There is a singular example of periodic swooning in the Ephemera of Natural Curiosities (Dec. ii., ann. i., obs. 10), which seems to have been dependant upon this state of body; and another example, in which it was evidently produced by a return of the term of menstruation, and became its regular harbinger.—(Id., dec. ii., ann. v., obs. 53.)

In all cases of this kind, therefore, it is of the utmost importance to study minutely the character of the patient's idiosyncrasy and habit, and not to excite any alarm concerning organic mischief, and thus add another excitement to those which already exist, while there is a probability that the affection may be owing to one or other of these lighter and more manageable causes.

In the latter case, tonics, cold bathing, equitation, regular hours, and light meals, will form the best prescription. Where we are compelled to suspect some organic impediment, or other mischief about the heart, small bleedings, that may anticipate the usual time of the return, camphire, nitre, hyoscyamus, and whatever other sedative may be found best to agree with the patient and diminish the rapidity of the cirenlation, will form the most rational medical plan we can devise; while tranquillity of body and mind, an abstinence from all stimulant foods, and a regular attention to the state of the bowels, should form a standard rule for the whole tenour of his life.*

---

* In the treatment of syncope, we should remember that it may arise from two opposite states of the system, from plethora and exsanguinity: the

GENUS VII.
SYSPASIA:
COMATOSE SPASM.

CLONIC SPASM; DIMINISHED SENSIBILITY; INABILITY OF UTTERANCE.

SYSPASIA or SYSPASIS, from συσπάω, "contraho, convello," literally imports convulsion, in the popular sense of the term, or, in other words, clonus or agitatory spasm, in combination with a greater or less degree of failure of the sensation and the understanding. The term seems wanted as a generic name for the three following diseases, whose symptoms and, for the most part, mode of treatment, are so discordant, as to establish the propriety of linking them under a common division:—

1. Syspasia Convulsio.		Convulsion.
2. ———— Hysteria.		Hysterics.
3. ———— Epilepsia.		Epilepsy.

The author has entered so fully into the nature and principle of clonic or agitatory spasm under the genus CLONUS, that a very few remarks will be necessary in explaining the pathology of these three species. They are all of them clonic spasms, as expressed in the definition, but complicated with other morbid affections, and particularly with those of the two preceding genera: for if we combine clonic or synclonic spasm with different modifications of vertigo or syncope, we shall produce the three species now before us. In explaining the nature of clonic spasm, we noticed the tendency there frequently exists, when the uniformity of the flow of the sensorial power is once-interfered with, to alternations of a hurried and excessive, as well as of a restrained and deficient supply, and consequently to an intermixture of constrictive or entastic spasm with clonic or agitatory, of which palpitation, and various other affections of this kind, afford perspicuous examples. In the diseases immediately before us, the proofs of such an intermixture are still more striking; for there is not one of them but evinces a union of both descriptions of spasmodic action, in a high, though not an equal degree of véhemence. In convulsion-fit the two kinds of spasm are nearly upon a balance, commonly with a retention of some share of both sentient and percipient power. In hysteria, the spastic or entastic action, in its sudden and transient irruptions, is more violent than the clonic; the force exercised at this time is enormous, and there is also, in many cases, a small retention of sensation and understanding. In epilepsy, the clonic action is most conspicuous, and the failure of the mental and sentient faculties generally complete.

Of the essence of the nervous power, we have repeatedly stated that we know nothing; for we can trace it, only by its effects: but we are compelled to conceive it to be formed by some particular organ within the animal system, which organ there can be no difficulty in con-

---

former is often the immediate cause when syncope occurs in advanced life, and then moderate blood-letting may judiciously precede or accompany our other remedies.—D.

templating as the brain singly, or the brain and nerves jointly, which constitute only different parts of one common apparatus. Admitting this, the nervous power may be produced in excess or in deficiency, or be imperfectly elaborated, and, however produced, it may be irregularly transmitted, as well by precipitation as by interruption. The means by which these diseased actions take place we have already touched upon; and have shown that the common causes are sometimes mental, sometimes mechanical, sometimes sympathetic, and sometimes chymical, as narcotics and other poisons, and repelled eruptions.

Now it is in persons of relaxed or debilitated fibres that we find these exciting causes chiefly operative. For in those of high health, full vessels, and a firm constitution, however the circulation may be accelerated, or the nervous power excited, it is rarely that we meet with clonic spasms, or, indeed, spasms of any kind: or, at least, we meet with a far less tendency to such abnormities, than in persons of lax and debilitated fibres, possessing necessarily more mobility or facility of being put into new actions, from the very quality of debility itself.

The common predisponent, then, is weakness, particularly of the nervous system; and the common excitement, irritation. The peculiar effect must, however, be modified by the idiosyncrasy or peculiarity of the constitution, or of collateral circumstances, by which it may be influenced at the time. And hence the very exciting cause that in one individual may produce hysteria, in another may produce epilepsy, and in a third the more fugitive and less impressive attack of syspasia, as convulsion.—(*Pritchard, on Nervous Diseases,* p. 139.)

The nature of the idiosyncrasy, or, more particularly, of the individual constitution, is rarely within our control; but the collateral circumstances are often before us: they constitute the occasional cause of the disease, and should form a prominent point in our attention to its progress.

There are, perhaps, few more common causes of weakness than over-distended vessels; and hence plethora is a frequent occasional cause of each of the diseases belonging to the genus before us, the species actually produced depending, as just observed, upon the influence of other circumstances. Thus, if such plethora take place in a young woman of eighteen or nineteen, whose menstrual flux has been accidentally suppressed or retarded, it is most probable, if an irregularity in the nervous system be hereby excited, that such an irregularity will lead to a fit of hysterics rather than to one of convulsion or epilepsy, since we shall find, as we proceed, that this species of spasm is peculiarly connected with an irritable and especially an orgastic state of the genital organs.

On the contrary, if the plethora produce chiefly a distension of the vessels of the brain, epilepsy is more likely to be the result; in other words, that form of spasmodic action, in which the sensation and the intellect suffer more severely than in either of the others. While, if the plethora be general, we have reason to expect that the spasmodic effect will be general also, or, in other words, take the form of convulsion in which no single organ is tried more than another. Yet plethora, in a firm and vigorous frame, is seldom found to produce either of these affections, for the resistance of the coats of the bloodvessels is here sufficient to counterbalance the impetus of the sanguineous fluid, and, consequently, to prevent an over-distention. And hence, again we see in what manner debility becomes a remote or predisponent cause of the diseases under our consideration.

Plethora, thus acting by over-distention, may be regarded as a mechanical stimulus, upon the removal of which, as upon the removal of other mechanical stimuli, the disease will cease. Venesection is the most direct means of such removal; but it labours under the inconvenience of being only a temporary remedy. It takes off the occasional cause; but, by adding to the general debility, it gives strength to the predisposing cause.

The more direct mechanical stimulants are sharp-pointed ossifications formed in the membranes of the brain, or arising from the internal surface of the cranium; splinters of a fractured cranium, or the introduction of some wounding instrument. The occasional causes resulting from mental emotions, we have already been called to notice more than once; as also to show that, while some of these appear to act by instantaneously exhausting the sensorial organ of its living principle, others operate by giving a check to the production of the sensorial power. These modes of action are indeed opposite, but the result, which is a depletion of the nervous apparatus, is the same. And as, in weakly or relaxed habits, there is in every organ a greater mobility or facility of passing from one state of action to another than in the firm and robust, we see also why the former should be not only more subject to spasmodic actions from mental emotion, but to sudden changes of mental emotion, and consequently, to caprice and fickleness of temper.

SPECIES I.
SYSPASIA CONVULSIO.
CONVULSION.

MUSCULAR AGITATION VIOLENT; TEETH GNASHING; HANDS FORCIBLY CLINCHED: TRANSIENT.

In defining CONVULSION, most of the nosologists represent the faculties of the mind and the external senses as still sound and unaffected. Sauvages says, "superstite in paroxysmis animæ functionem exercitio." Vogel distinguishes it, "cum integritate sensuum." Dr. Cullen is more exact than either of these. His words are, "musculorum contractio clonica abnormis, *citra soporem;*" "an irregular clonic contraction of the muscles, bordering on but short of lethargy." The influence of the disease on the sensation and perception varies considerably in different cases, but, so far as I have seen, the sensibility is always in some degree diminished, and I have hence ventured to introduce this feature into the generic definition as a pathognomonic symptom.

There are also some other-differences that occur in the character of the disease in its different attacks, and which have been laid hold of as the groundwork of very numerous subdivisions by many nosologists. For these differences we cannot always account: but in general they will be found to depend upon the idiosyncrasy, habit, or stage of life in which the disease makes its appearance, and to give rise to the following varieties :—

α Erratica. Migratory convulsion.	The convulsion shifting irregularly from one part to another.
β Universalis. General convulsion.	The convulsion attacking every part simultaneously; occasionally protracted in its stay.
γ Recurrens. Recurrent convulsion.	The convulsive paroxysm returning after intervals more or less regular.
δ Ejulans. Shrieking convulsion.	The convulsion accompanied with shrieks or yells, but without pain.
ε Puerperalis. Puerperal convulsion.	Occurring during pregnancy or labour, usually with coma, and stertorous breathing.
ζ Infantilis. Infantile convulsion.	Occurring during infancy; preceded by twitchings or startings, and accompanied with a blueness about the eyes and upper lip.

In the FIRST or MIGRATORY VARIETY, the convulsion travels, in some instances, so completely from organ to organ, and from one set of muscles to another, as to make an entire circle.

In the SECOND or UNIVERSAL VARIETY, the convulsion is often accompanied with a peculiar kind of percussion or hammering of one limb against another, or against some other part of the body, resembling the malleation we have already had occasion to describe, and constituting the MALLEATIO of some authors.

In the RECURRENT VARIETY, the intervals are often very irregular; but the ordinary return, where any thing like a regular period is established, is menstrual or lunary. To this, as also to the preceding, many writers have applied the name of HIERONOSUS or MORBUS SACER; which by others, as we have above observed, has been limited to some modifications of chorea.

In the FOURTH or SHRIEKING VARIETY, the muscles of respiration, and especially those of the larynx, appear to be chiefly affected; and the shrill sounds, or yelling to which it gives rise, proceed rather from an involuntary motion of these organs, than from any greater degree of pain that is suffered under this form than under any other.

In PUERPERAL CONVULSION, the irritation is supposed by Dr. Bland to derive no peculiar character from the state of the body at the time. But it is impossible to shut our eyes

Z 2

to the close and active sympathy which exists between the sexual organs and the sensorium, and which is peculiarly striking in hysteria; nor to the distinctive symptoms which take place in convulsion from this cause; in which there is a greater tendency to oppression in the head than in any other modification whatever; the breathing is stertorous, and the spastic action particularly violent. Convulsions of this kind occur during pregnancy, in the midst of labour, or immediately afterward: they rarely, however, take place before the sixth month. Yet, if the irritation were not of a particular kind, we might rather expect it on the first turgescence of the uterus. But we shall have occasion to recur to this subject under the ensuing class.*

In INFANTILE CONVULSION, the mobility of the frame is impressively conspicuous. The clonic motions are exquisitely rapid, and the fingers work and the eyelids nictitate with a quiver that is often difficult to follow up. This constitutes the ecclampsia of Sauvages. In the subsequent stage of teething, as the irritative fibre is somewhat firmer, the clonic vibration is rarely so rapid. Antecedently to the time of teething, the usual causes of excitement are retained meconium, flatulency, and acrimonious food.†

---

* With regard to the treatment of puerperal convulsions, it seems to be settled by the most experienced practitioners in midwifery, that, when the pulse is strong and full, and the frame robust, the copious abstraction of blood in a large stream is the most efficient means of shortening the attack. Active purgatives may be given, and if there be difficulty of swallowing, one or two drops of croton-oil may be smeared on the tongue. Dr. Locock also recommends a stimulating purgative injection to be thrown into the rectum, particularly one containing turpentine. For the comatose or chronic stage, he advises blisters to the head or back of the neck, and the bowels to be kept freely open, turpentine clysters being now of great service. In cases where the patient has been much reduced by previous illness, Dr. Locock recommends bleeding, if employed at all, to be so only with great circumspection; and when admissible, he prefers local bleeding to general. He has a favourable opinion of opium and camphire in the latter class of cases, and prescribes it, in the dose of one or two grains with five of camphire, every hour or two, till the proper effect is produced. Dr. Locock approves of emetics only where the attack has arisen from a loaded stomach or indigestible food.—(See Cyclop. of Pract. Med., art. CONVULSIONS.) Respecting the question of delivering females in all cases where the child or placenta still remains in the uterus, the reader should consult the best authorities on midwifery.—ED.

† Beaumes, Des Convulsions de l'Enfance, et leur Cause, et de leur Traitement, &c., 8vo., Paris, 1805. In the majority of examples, the convulsions of young children are symptomatic of some other disease. According to Mr. North, who has written an able work on the convulsions of infants, an impending attack is indicated by various symptoms, independently of the existence of any particular disease, and all of which show an increased irritability of the system; such are, starting at very slight noises, a disturbed sleep, frequent fits of crying from trifling causes, and great

The ordinary excitements of convulsion, however, operate at all periods of life. Though often concealed, they are generally those of clonic spasm. They consist not unfrequently, as we have already observed, in pressure or other irritation, from a deformity or some spicular node within the cranium ; and are said by Desessarts (*Journ. de Méd.*, xlvii., 114), to occur most frequently in those whose sculls are peculiarly large, or in the language of Morgagni (*De Sed. et Caus. Morb.*, ep. ix., 9), nearly cubical in the occipital region. Pressure, however, or congestion in the brain, from whatever cause, is an occasional source of this complaint. And hence convulsion is a frequent result of severe fright, or any other violent agitation of the mind ; and, like several of the species we have just noticed, it is a frequent result of some suddenly-suppressed natural or morbid discharge, or suddenly repelled complaint affecting a remote organ. It has hence appeared on suppressed menstruation, suppressed flow of milk, leucorrhœa, or lochia, suppressed dysentery (*Hoefner, Baldinger N. Mag.*, b. vi., p. 323), the suppressed discharge from an old ulcer (*Gruellmann, Diss. Observ. de usu cicutæ*, Goett., 1782 ; *Ephem. Nat. Cur.*, dec. iii., ann. ii., obs. 74), repelled gout, exanthems, and cutaneous eruptions. The usual causes in pregnancy and infancy have been already noticed.

Convulsions are also frequently produced by many of the narcotic poisons in a certain degree of strength or activity, and a certain state of the constitution. For, if the dose be very large, or the system much debilitated at the time, the irritability will be entirely destroyed, and death will often ensue instantaneously, without any struggle whatever. Thus the distilled water of the leaves or kernels of the *prunus lauro-cerasus*, under different circumstances, will produce both these effects ; as will also the distilled water of the kernels of various other fruits possessing prussic acid, as those of the black-cherry and bitter-almond-tree ; and hence the prussic acid itself. And we may hereby understand the remark of Sir Hercules Langrishe, that one

peevishness : there is also a frequent fixing of the eyes, an oscillatory motion of the pupils, a momentary contraction, and again a sudden dilatation of them, or a want of consent between them, so that one will contract while the other dilates. The countenance is alternately flushed and pale ; sudden animation is followed by as sudden a fit of languor, and irregularity in the breathing. Hiccough is not unfrequent, and, in many instances, a peculiar blueness about the mouth.—(See North on the Convulsions of Infants, 8vo., Lond., 1826 ; and Locock in Cyc. of Pract. Med., art. CONVULSIONS.) It was inculcated by Dr. John Clarke, that " in every case of convulsion, the brain is at the time organically affected, either directly or indirectly."—(See Commentaries on the Dis. of Children.) This doctrine is criticised by Mr. North, who points out the mistakes into which it has led practitioners. So far from admitting that the brain is organically affected in every case, he does not allow that its vessels are even congested, as a matter of course ; and he argues that, when they are so, it is often only a temporary condition, existing merely during the attack.—ED.

ounce of laurel water will occasion more violent and stronger convulsions than five or six ounces. The dose of this water, given by way of poison, to Sir Theodosius Boughton, was a draught-vial full, and consequently about an ounce and a half. The struggling-fit in this case began in a minute and a half, or two minutes after it was swallowed (*Gurney's Trial of John Donellan, Esq.*, folio, pp. 18, 19) ; it continued for about ten minutes, when he expired.

The spasmodic action produced by these plants is chiefly clonic, which, in effect, is the ordinary action with which life ceases : but there are others that render it of a mixed character, the entastic alternating with the clonic ; and some, in which the rigid or entastic power considerably predominates, as in the poisonous juice of the upas tiente, which, though with occasional relaxations, fixes the muscles as rigidly as in tetanus, and continues the rigidity till the patient dies.

In ordinary cases, however, the mode of attack and the progress of the paroxysm exhibit a considerable variation. Sometimes the assault is sudden and without any warning ; but, more generally, there are a few precursive indications, and especially in patients who are subject to returns of it ; such as coldness in the extremities, with a dizziness in the head, and floating spectra before the eyes, or a flatulent uneasiness in the bowels, and a tenseness in the left hypochondrium. In other cases, the patient complains of tremours in different muscles, and a cold aura creeping up the back, which makes him shiver.

The struggle itself, I have already said, varies equally in its extent and violence, and I may add, in its duration. The muscles are alternately rigid and relaxed, the teeth gnash, and often bite the tongue, the mouth foams, the eyelids open and shut in perpetual motion, or are stretched upon a full stare, while the protuberant balls roll rapidly in every direction : the whole face is hideously distorted. The force exerted is enormous, so as frequently to shake the entire room, and overpower the strength of six or eight attendants. In some instances, it has been so violent as to break a tooth, and even fracture a bone.—(*Ephem. Nat. Cur.*, dec. ii., ann. vii.) When the lungs are much oppressed in the course of the contest, the lips, cheeks, and indeed the entire surface, is died with a dark or purple hue.

The paroxysm will sometimes cease in a few minutes, but occasionally lasts for hours, and, after a short and uncertain period of rest, returns again with as much violence as before ; a fact peculiarly common to puerperal and infantile convulsions. Great languor commonly succeeds ; sometimes headache, vertigo, and vomiting, occasionally delirium : but not unfrequently, and especially in infants, there are no secondary symptoms whatever.

The treatment of convulsion must apply to the paroxysm itself, and to the state of the constitution which gives a tendency to its recurrence.

If it proceed from a narcotic or any other poison introduced into the stomach, much benefit may often be obtained from the stomach pump. ' If the poison be in a liquid form, most of it may hereby be withdrawn, while the remainder, or the whole, if it be a powder, may be diluted and pumped up afterward.

As there is danger from congestion in the brain, venesection is, in most cases, a good measure of caution, and in many instances is absolutely necessary : and hence, where plethora has preceded, and has threatened to become a cause, the disease has often been prevented, and sometimes effectually cured, by a spontaneous hemorrhage from the nose, the ears, or some other organ.' But we have often had occasion to observe, that in weak and relaxed habits, bleeding, if frequently repeated, increases the tendency to plethora ; and, on this account, how necessary soever at the time, it should be employed with caution, and persevered in with reluctance.

Brisk cathartics, introduced into the stomach if possible, and where this cannot be accomplished, in the form of an injection, lower the morbid distension almost as effectually, and in some instances directly remove from the system the principal fomes of the complaint. Emetics are of more doubtful effect : they also may occasionally carry off the actual cause of irritation, and by powerfully determining to the surface, make a favourable diversion of action. But, in many cases of debility, they have evidently increased the violence and prolonged the duration of the fit. In puerperal convulsions, they are strongly disapproved by Dr. Miguel.—(*Traité des Convulsions chez les Femmes Enceintes*, &c., Paris, 1824.) The authorities, however, in their favour are numerous and highly respectable. Le Preux (*Diss. An Convulsionibus recens natorum Vomitoria?* Paris, 1765), strongly recommends them in early infancy : and Hoeffner asserts, that he has found them highly serviceable where the irritation proceeded from dysentery.—(*Balding. N. Mag.*, b. vi., 323.) Schenck employed them generally with considerable success, and preferred the preparations of copper, and particularly the verdigris, to any other emetic, from their rapidity of action.—(Lib. i., obs. 244.) Antispasmodics are certainly entitled to our attention, and often succeed in allaying the irregular commotion. Those most commonly resorted to are ammonia, ether, musk, camphire, and valerian. The empyreumatic oils, both animal and vegetable, seem to have fallen as much below their proper value in the present day as they were once prized above it. And the same may be observed of the volatile fetids generally, as fuligo, assafœtida, and *chenopodium Vulvaria*, or stinking arach : the last of which, however, under the older name of *atriplex fœtida*, seems to have been a favourite with Dr. Cullen.

It is not very easy to explain the operation of antispasmodics of this kind. Dr. Cullen refers it to their volatility alone, and hence concludes, that they are useful in proportion as they are volatile ; which is, in fact, to regard them in the light of stimulants. But, beyond this, they seem to possess a sedative power, which probably resides in their fetor. Where flatulency or some other misaffection of the stomach is the exciting cause, as is frequently the case in infancy, after

opening the bowels, the warmer carminatives of anise, mint, ginger, and cardamoms will often be found sufficient ; and where these fail, recourse has been had to opium, hyoscyamus, belladonna, and sometimes St. Ignatius's bean, or M. Wedenberg's favourite medicine in this disease, the extract of stramonium.—(*Dissertatio Medica de Stramonii Usu in Morbis Convulsivis*, 4to., Upsaliæ.)

Cold and heat have also been very frequently resorted to as powerful antispasmodics, and in many cases with considerable success. Heat appears to act by a double power, and especially when combined with moisture, with which it is always most effectual. It both relaxes and stimulates ; and hence is admirably calculated to harmonize two alternating and contending states of a morbid rigidity and a morbid mobility, on which the disease depends, and consequently, to restore a healthy equipoise of action. On this account we find warm bathing, and especially in infantile convulsions, of great benefit. It ought not to be forgotten, however, that both effects, as well the stimulating as the relaxing, have a considerable tendency to exhaust and debilitate, and hence the warm bath must not be frequently repeated.

The immediate effect of a sudden application of cold, whether by a blast of air or by an affusion of water, is a general shuddering, a spasmodic contraction of the entire skin. And hence, where cold, applied in this manner, takes off either clonic or entastic spasm, it is by a revulsive power ; by a transfer of the spasmodic action from a particular organ or set of organs, to the surface of the body generally ; in the same way as blistering the neighbourhood of an inflamed organ takes off the primary inflammation, by a transfer of the inflammatory action to the part where the blister is applied. If the cold excite a general reaction, and the shuddering be succeeded by a glow, it becomes a direct and very powerful tonic ; and, in both these accounts, is a remedy highly worth trying in hysterics, convulsions, and even those cases of epilepsy in which a suspicion of some structural cause of irritation within the cranium does not form a bar, by prohibiting every thing that may increase the impetus of the blood.

In the convulsion fit of infancy the affusion of cold water, so far as I have seen, may be much oftener resorted to with perfect safety, than the fears of mothers will allow ; and be found much more successful in a hot, close, unventilated nursery, than the more popular prescription of a warm bath. And where I have not been able to proceed thus far, and the warm bath has been tried repeatedly in vain, I have frequently succeeded by taking the little infant in my arms, and exposing him naked, or nearly naked, for a few moments, to the air of the window, thrown open to allow it to blow upon him.* The great

---

* Other means specified for the relief of infantile convulsions, are wet cloths, or bladders filled with snow or powdered ice, and constantly applied to the scalp; clysters of assafœtida, combined with castor-oil or neutral salts ; and chafing the hands and feet with brandy or ether. Should the abdo-

diminution of sensibility which prevails at such a time, prevents all danger of catching cold ; while, on the contrary, the little patient is usually revived by the sudden rush of the external air, and the fit in many cases, ceases instantly.

Cold bathing, when not prohibited by any other complaint, will also be found a useful tonic in the intervals of the attacks, and may conveniently be employed in conjunction with internal medicines of the same character.—(*Y. W. Wedel, Liber de Morbis Infantum*, cap. xiii.) Of these the metallic salts and oxydes are chiefly to be depended upon, and especially those of iron, copper, arsenic, silver, and zinc. Zinc has had by far the greatest number of advocates, and is generally supposed to have succeeded best in the form of its white oxyde, ten or twelve grains of which are usually given to an adult in the course of twenty-four hours. Mr. Dugaud increased the proportion to fifteen grains (*Edin. Med. Comment.*, v., 89) ; and Mr. Bell, at length, prescribed not less than ten grains at a time, repeated three times a day.—(*Edin. Med. Comment.*, i., 120.) [Dr. Brachet joins the extract of henbane with the oxyde of zinc, giving to children four grains of the former and two of the latter, in divided doses, one of which is taken every three or four hours.] In the hands of the present author, zinc has proved more salutary in the form of its sulphate, which has not unfrequently succeeded where the oxyde has failed ; the usual proportion which he has employed being a grain three times a day, given in the emulsion of bitter almonds. Where silver has been made choice of, the usual preparation has been its nitrate, and the dose has begun with a grain given four or five times a-day in the shape of a pill, and gradually increased to eight or ten grains, or as much as the patient's stomach will bear.*

---

men be distended with air, a few drops of sal volatile may be given in peppermint water, and the belly rubbed freely with the hand, or with any gently stimulating liniment. A purgative of calomel and jalap, or scammony, may be given, if the child can swallow ; or an emetic, if any improper article of food has been recently taken. Bleeding is not always right, as a matter of course, though proper when the vessels of the brain are in a plethoric state. The jugular vein may be opened, or leeches applied to the temples or behind the ears. Should the child be of an age when dentition is going on, the gums ought to be freely scarified. If the case were one of great irritability of the nervous system, without plethora, we should first endeavour to remove the exciting cause, and when the convulsions still continue, have recourse to antispasmodics, assafœtida mixture, ammonia, camphire, ether, and musk, and even opium, with caution. When the bowels are very irritable, the pulvis cretæ comp. cum opio, in doses of from one to ten grains, according to the child's age, and repeated every hour or two, until relief is obtained, is an excellent medicine. In some cases, and those not always in very weak children, there is constitutionally an exceedingly irritable state of the nervous system, leading to convulsions resembling those of an epileptic nature. Here the carbonate of iron, in doses of five grains, mixed with honey, has sometimes proved beneficial.—See Locock in Cyclop. of Pract. Med., art. CONVULSIONS.—ED.

* In particular cases, iron has the advantage of

The virtue of all these, however, seems considerably improved by a combination with camphire, which has often been found to be advantageous even alone. " In spasmodic or convulsive affections," says Dr. Cullen, " it has been of service, and even in epilepsy it has been useful. I have not, indeed, known an epilepsy entirely cured by camphire alone ; but I have had several instances of a paroxysm, which was expected in the course of a night, prevented by a dose of camphire exhibited at bedtime ; and even this, when the camphire was given alone ; but it has been especially useful when given with a dose of cuprum ammoniatum, or the sulphate or the flowers of zinc."-(*Med. Transactions*, vol. i., art. 19.)

The vegetable tonics are little to be depended upon. The bark recommended by Dr. Home, Sumeire, and many other distinguished writers, is rarely of use, except where the paroxysm is periodical : and the *cardamine pratensis* (ladysmock), *sempervivum tectorum* (house-leek), and *viscus quercus* (mistletoe), are hardly worthy of notice in the present day, notwithstanding the specific virtues they were supposed to possess formerly. The cardamine, the εισύμβριον ἕτερον of Dioscorides, is of ancient celebrity, and in modern times has been warmly extolled by the commanding authorities of Mr. Ray, Sir George Baker, and Dr. Home ; the second of whom, as was noticed under the head of chorea, declares himself to have succeeded in its use, not only in cases of convulsion, but of all clonic spasms whatever, and this too when almost every other medicine had failed.—(*Auserl. Abhandl. für Pract. Aerzte.*, b. x., 13.)

The house-leek was employed in the form of an expressed juice intermixed with an equal quantity of spirit of wine, which gives a white coagulum, resembling cream of fine pomatum, that has a weak but penetrating taste, and was supposed, from its ready evaporation, to contain a considerable portion of volatile alkaline salt. The mistletoe has rarely been employed in our own country, except by Dr. Home, who thought he found it serviceable : though it is chiefly indebted for its fame as a specific in convulsions, to the practice and writings of Colbatch.—(See also *Diss. sur le Gui de Chène, Remède Spé-*

---

acting as an emmenagogue, and correcting that deficiency and irregularity in the functions of the uterus which are so often the sole cause of the disordered state of the health. Dr. Abercrombie gives a remarkable instance of this power of the sulphate of iron, which, in the dose of three grains thrice a day, combined with a sufficient quantity of aloes to regulate the bowels, effected the cure of a most anomalous convulsive disease, that had been treated ineffectually for six years on the plan of copious depletion and counter-irritation. This case would be considered by many, however, rather as one of chorea. In similar cases, Dr. Adair Crawford has prescribed with considerable advantage the carbonate of iron, combined with a mixture of carbonate of ammonia and tincture of aloes : he recommends it to be given to the extent of one or two drachms in the twenty-four hours, but not more freely, as then it remains accumulated and inert in the bowels,—ED.

cifique pour les Maladies Convulsives, Paris, 1719.) It has been given in powder, infusion and extract.

SPECIES II.
SYSPASIA HYSTERIA.
HYSTERICS.

CONVULSIVE STRUGGLING, ALTERNATELY REMITTING AND EXACERBATING; RUMBLING IN THE BOWELS; SENSE OF SUFFOCATION; DROWSINESS; URINE COPIOUS AND LIMPID; TEMPER FICKLE.

HYSTERIA, from ὑστέρα, "the uterus or vulva," or, more correctly, "viscus posterius vel inferius," evidently imported in an early period of medical science, some misaffection of the womb or other sexual organ: and hence -hysteria, among the Greeks and Romans, was also a term by which female midwives were denominated, or those who especially attended to affections of the hysteria or womb. The Latin term uterus, although it approaches it in sense and sound, is altogether of a different origin. For this has a direct reference to the use and figure of the uterus as a single organ, and is an immediate derivation from *uter*, a bag or bottle.

With a morbid condition of this organ, indeed, hysteria is in many instances very closely connected, though it is going too far to say, that it is always dependant upon such condition: for we meet with instances occasionally, in which no possible connexion can be traced between the disease and the organ; and sometimes witness it in males as decidedly as in females. It has been contended by various writers, that in this last case, the disease ought to be called hypochondrism, the HYPOCHONDRIAS of the present work; and that hysteria and hypochondrias are merely modifications of a common complaint. Nothing, however, can be more erroneous. These two diseases have often a few similar symptoms, and more particularly those of dyspepsy; but they are strictly distinct maladies, and are characterized by signs that are peculiarly their own. The convulsive struggling paroxysms; the sense of a suffocating ball in the throat, the fickleness of temper, and the copious and limpid urine, which are pathognomonic of hysteria, have no necessary connexion with hypochondrias, and are never found in this disease when strictly simple and idiopathic. While, on the contrary, the sad and sullen countenance, the dejected spirits and gloomy ideas that characteristically mark hypochondrias, have as little necessary connexion with hysteria, and are in direct opposition to its ordinary course. Hysteria is strictly a corporeal disease, hypochondrias a mental, though it commonly originates in corporeal organs, but organs that have a peculiar influence upon the mental faculties, and has not established itself till these participate in the morbid action. Hysteria is a disease of the irritative fibres, hypochondrias of the sentient; hysteria is a disease of early life, hypochondrias of a later period. Both, however, are diseases of a highly nervous or excitable temperament,

and, as such, may coexist in the same individual: but so also may vertigo or cephalæa with either of them; which would nevertheless continue to be regarded as distinct diseases, notwithstanding such an incidental conjunction. And hence Mieg (*Epistolæ ad Hallerum scriptæ,* No. v.) and various other established writers[*] upon the subject, have not incorrectly, though perhaps unnecessarily, treated of the disorder before us under the two divisions of male and female hysteria, *hysteria virorum* or *masculina,* and *hysteria fœminina.* Swediaur, who affirms that men may labour under the hysteric passion as well as women, arranges this and hypochondrism as distinct species of a common genus, to which, with his extravagant fondness for long Greek terms, he has given the name of *hyperkinesia.*

Hysteria, like all other clonic affections, shows itself most frequently in mobile and irritable temperaments, and particularly during that period of life in which irritability is at its highest tide, as from the age of puberty to that of thirty-five years, seldom appearing before the former, and rarely after the latter of these terms.[†] The common occasional causes of convulsion, which we have already described, are also those of hysteria; and hence, disorder of the stomach, or other abdominal organs, mental emotions,[‡] plethora, and particularly turgescence of the sexual region, are among the most frequent; on which account we are told by Forestus (*Observ. et Curat. Medic.,* lib. xxviii., obs. 29, 33) and Zacutus Lusitanus (*De Praxi Admiranda,* lib. ii., obs. 85) that one of the most common causes of hysteria in males is a retention of semen, as one of its surest cures is an excretion.

As every thing, moreover, that disturbs the uniform transmission of the nervous energy, or the other ordinary diameter of the bloodvessels or cavity of the heart, becomes a powerful irritant, we may also see why this disease should occur on debilitating, and especially sudden evacuations, and be at no loss to account for its appearing on excessive as well as on suppressed menstruation, and consequently in leucorrhœa. And as the sexual organs lose much of their orgasm during the period of parturition, we may

---

[*] Eph. Nat. Cur., dec. ii., ann. iv., obs. 1861; Traité Nouveau de Médecine, &c., Lyons, 1684.

[†] The menstrual period of life, or that between the ages of fifteen and forty-five, may be stated to be the time when this disorder is most disposed to show itself. If it appear at any other age, it is more frequently earlier than later; it is more common to meet with hysterical girls who have not menstruated, than with old women who have done menstruating.—See Elliotson's Lect. at Lond. Univ., as reported in Med. Gaz. for 1832-3, p. 642. —ED.

[‡] "Any woman may have hysteria, if she can have but emotion of mind strong enough." Anger or grief, especially grief for ungratified desire, or, to use a more elegant expression, "disappointed love," is the most common cause. It is during the period of menstruation that all the feelings of women are most active; it is then that they are most likely to fall in love, and to experience sorrows of all sorts, whether real or imaginary.—See Elliotson's Lectures.—ED.

also see why the disease should attack barren rather than breeding women, particularly young widows, who are cut off from the means of exhaustion they formerly enjoyed ; and, more especially still, those who are constitutionally inclined to that morbid salacity, which has often been called nymphomania, and in the present work, will be found under the genus LAGNESIS..

I have already endeavoured to show by what means, in a habit of great nervous irritability, both clonic and entastic or rigid spasms are produced, and the disposition there frequently exists for them to pass into each other, or to alternate in rapid succession. And we have also seen that the former is most predominant in laxer and more mobile, and the latter in firmer and more vigorous constitutions. There is no frame, however, that may not become a prey to spasmodic action of some kind or other, and hence, there is no frame that may not become a prey, under particular circumstances, to the species of spasmodic action we are now describing. These circumstances are very generally concealed from us ; but we uniformly perceive, that the rule we have now adverted to holds true , and that the hysteric spasms will assume more or less of a clonic or of a spastic character, in proportion as the individual is of a more relaxed or of a more vigorous make. And hence the most violent, though the least common instances of hysteric struggle that occur to us, are in young women of the most robust and masculine constitution.

The paroxysm often takes place without any previous warning or manifest excitement whatever, and especially where it has established itself by a frequency of recurrence. Occasionally, however, we have a few precursive signs, which rarely show themselves in vain : as a sense of nausea or sickness, flatulency, palpitation of the heart, depression of spirits, and sudden bursts of tears without any assignable cause. The fit soon succeeds, with a coldness and shivering over the whole body, a quick fluttering pulse, and an acute feeling of pain in the head, as though a nail were driven into it. The flatulency from the stomach or colon rises in the sensation of a suffocating ball into the throat, and forms what is known by the name of globus hystericus. The convulsive struggle now commenees, which in women of very mobile fibres is sometimes very feeble, the relaxant alternations prevailing over the contractile ; but in other cases, is prodigiously violent, evincing during the contractions a rigidity as firm as in tetanus, and a force that overcomes all opposition. The trunk of the body is twisted backward and forward, the limbs are variously agitated, and the fists are closed so firmly that it is difficult, if not impossible, to open the fingers ; and the breast is violently and spasmodically beaten. An equal spasm takes place in the sphincter ani, so that it is often found impracticable to introduce a clyster pipe ; and the urine discharged, though copious, is colourless. The muscles of the chest and trachea are agitated in every way, and hence there is an involuntary utterance of shrieks, screams, laughing, and crying, according to the

direction the spasm takes, sometimes accompanied with or succeeded by a most obstinate and distressing fit of hiccough. When the fit ceases, the patient appears to be quite spent, and lies stupid and apparently lifeless. Yet, in an hour or two, or often much less, she perfectly recovers her strength, and has no other feeling than that of a general soreness, and perhaps some degree of pain in the head. It is rarely indeed that an hysteric fit becomes dangerous ; though it has in a few instances terminated in epilepsy or insanity.*

The temper is fickle, and the mind is as unsteady as the muscles : " and from hence," observes the sagacious Burton, who has painted strongly, but from the life, " proceed a brutish kind of dotage, troublesome sleep, terrible dreams, a foolish kind of bashfulness in some, perverse conceits and opinions, dejection of mind, much discontent, preposterous judgment. They are apt to loathe, dislike, disdain, to be weary of every object. Each thing almost is tedious to them. They pine away, void of counsel, apt to weep and tremble, timorous, fearful, sad, and out of all hopes of better fortunes. They take delight in doing nothing for the time, but love to be alone and solitary, though that does them more harm. And thus they are affected as long as this vapour lasteth ; but by-and-by they are as pleasant and merry as ever the were in their lives ; they sing, discourse, and laugh in any good company upon all occasions. And so by fits it takes them now and then, except the malady be inveterate, and then it is more frequent, vehement, and continuate. Many of them cannot tell how to express themselves in words, how it holds them, what ails them. You cannot understand them, or well tell what to make of their sayings."—(*Anat. of Melancholy,* part i., sect. iii.)

The mode of treatment bears so close a resemblance to that of the preceding species, that it will be unnecessary to enlarge upon it.† Pungent applications may be applied to the nostrils,

---

* In hysteria there are fits of general convulsions and insensibility, as in epilepsy ; but not a continuance of the insensibility after the convulsions are over. For the most part, the convulsions are renewed in the midst of the insensibility. Sometimes, but not always, there is a regular collection of sobbing, crying, laughing, and shrieking in the midst of the convulsions. The insensibility is generally incomplete ; the patient has some knowledge of what is going on around, or, if she have not all the time, yet she has more or less of the time.—See Elliotson's Lectures delivered at the Lond. Univ. as reported in Med. Gaz. for 1832–3, p. 641.—ED.

† Hysteria, like the other species of clonus, is most common in the plethoric, or in persons of a nervous character. Next to derangement in the uterine system, or in the uterus, one of its most frequent causes is a torpid state of the alimentary canal. Hence bloodletting, and active cathartics continued for some time, are among the most efficacious remedies. Croton-oil and spirits of turpentine have recently gained some reputation, and when a tonic plan is thought expedient, the sulphate of iron has proved efficacious where the carbonate has failed.—D.

or round the temples, or the face and neck may be sprinkled or dashed with cold water during the paroxysm,* and warmth and the friction of the hand be applied to the feet. The peristaltic action of the bowels should be increased, which can only be done by stimulant and cathartic injections, if the contraction of the sphincter ani will allow them to pass.

Our chief attention, however, should be directed to the intervals. And here the first recommendation is, sedulously to avoid every remote or exciting cause. If the menstruation be in a morbid state, this must be corrected as soon as may be, concerning which, however, we shall have to speak in the ensuing class. If plethora be a striking symptom, the lancet should be employed. In robust and vigorous habits, we may bleed freely and have nothing to fear ;† but in loose and relaxed constitutions, far more caution is necessary, as has been already explained under CONVULSIO.

In this last state of body, tonics should also be had recourse to, and many of the warmer sedatives and antispasmodics, as assafœtida, camphire, most of the verticillate plants, and cajeput, which was a favourite remedy with Mieg.—(*Epist. ad Haller.*, ut suprà, No. 5.) Valerian has often proved serviceable, but is rarely prescribed in sufficient quantity to produce any good effect."—" It seems," says Dr. Cullen, "to be most useful when given in substance and in larger doses. I have never found much benefit from the infusion in water."— (*Mat. Med.*, part ii., ch. viii.) The ammoniated tincture of the London College, however, is an excellent form ; but even here the quantity of the root employed should be double what is prescribed. The cinchona may be usefully united with valerian, but does not seem to be of much benefit in this disease by itself.‡

---

* The water should be thrown with considerable force, and in plentiful quantities. Dr. Elliotson mentions, that filling the mouth with salt generally succeeds in stopping the fit. If the patient is able at intervals to swallow, we may give her from half a drachm to a drachm of the spiritus ammoniæ aromaticus, or of the spiritus ætheris aromaticus, or fœtidus, or of the spiritus æther. sulph. comp., or nitrici, blended with water.—Ed.

† When, in such patients, there is pain in the head, that part should be cupped, and active purgatives prescribed. Hysteria seems frequently to be combined with habitual constipation.—Ed.

‡ When a tonic plan is judged advisable, Dr. Elliotson considers iron, with cold affusion and cold bathing, the best means of relief. For the extreme languor the patient feels, and the sense of sinking experienced in the epigastrium, he prefers the ferrum ammoniatum. When the disorder is attended with trismus, he recommends two or three ounces of oil of turpentine to be thrown up the rectum ; there is usually difficulty in getting a patient in this state to swallow turpentine, and hence the injection is best. As chalybeate tonics, Dr. Conolly prefers to the carbonate half a grain or a grain of the sulphate of iron in a draught with a few drops of diluted sulphuric acid. If more of the sulphate is deemed necessary, he gives it in a pill with the extractum anthemidis, vel gentianæ, night and morning. If the tinctura ferri muriatis can be taken without inconvenience, he prescribes

Opium is a doubtful remedy : where the precursive signs are clear, it will often allay the irritation, and thus prove of great value. But it so frequently produces headache, and adds to the constipation, that it is rarely trusted to in the present day. When resorted to, it is best combined with camphire.* ·

· Where the disease occurs in the bloom of life, and there is reason to apprehend the ordinary orgasm of this age to be in excess, the surest remedy is a happy marriage.†

---

it in doses of from seven to ten drops twice a day. He adds, that he has generally found these forms of medicine less objected to by patients than the mistura ferri composita, although the compound iron pill is taken without complaint, and, in doses of eight or ten grains twice a day, is a valuable tonic. The vinum ferri, or the mistura ferri, with the decoct. aloës comp., is mentioned as a useful combination, when it is desired to promote the activity of the bowels, or the periodical functions of the uterus.—See Cyclop. of Pract. Med., art. HYSTERIA.—ED.

* Sydenham has given a description of a cough dependant on hysteria. In its treatment, he chiefly depended upon opium ; but, in a case recorded by Dr. Sinclair, powerful cathartics effected a cure, after the failure of bleeding, opium, antispasmodics, and various other means.—Edin. Med. Journ., No. lxxxii. p. 38.—ED.

† M. Pinel, on instituting an examination of the patients detained in the Salpêtrière as epileptic, found a great number of women, several of them young women, who were only hysterical, and yet who were separated from their families and from society.—(Traité des Maladies Nerveuses, tom. i., p. 117.) In referring to this circumstance, Dr. Conolly introduces the following just observations : —" To pronounce a young female patient epileptic, is often in its consequences only second to pronouncing her insane : the disease is considered to be incurable, to have a tendency to destroy the understanding, and to be transmissible to offspring ; none of which terrible evils are associated with the name of hysteria. The attack of hysteria is commonly less sudden and less violent than an attack of epilepsy. Epilepsy is often ushered in by a loud cry ; the patient falls violently to the ground ; the muscles of the face are severely convulsed ; the eyes are distorted ; the tongue is protruded and bitten, and frothy saliva forced out of the mouth. In hysteria there is seldom any incipient cry, although the patient may cry or laugh during the paroxysm ; the patient, except in the comatose variety, does not fall suddenly, but feeling the approach of the fit, is usually attacked after sitting or lying down ; the muscles of the face and the eyes are usually tranquil, and the face is generally flushed ; whereas in epilepsy it often has a ghastly paleness. The hysteric patient does not obtrude or bite the tongue, nor is there a discharge of frothy saliva. The epileptic patient does not laugh or shed tears, but is in a state of fixed and intense agony ; neither is globus a sensation known to him. During the paroxysm of hysteria, the pupils of the eyes are commonly sensible to light, which is not the case in epilepsy. After the paroxysm, the hysteric patient often remembers all that has passed, which the epileptic patient does not. It may be added, that epilepsy is most common in men, in whom hysteria is rare ; and that the character, habit of body, and history of the cases will frequently afford instructive circumstances of difference."—See Cyclop. of Pract. Med., art. HYSTERIA.—ED.

SPECIES III.
SYSPASIA EPILEPSIA.
EPILEPSY. FALLING-SICKNESS.

SPASMODIC AGITATION AND DISTORTION, CHIEFLY OF THE MUSCLES OF THE FACE, WITHOUT SENSATION OR CONSCIOUSNESS; RECURRING AT PERIODS MORE OR LESS REGULAR.*

THE Greek physicians gave the name of EPILEPSY, from ἐπιλαμβάνομαι, to the present disease, from its "sudden seizure or invasion," which is its direct import : and as the violence of passion or mental emotion to which the Roman people were accustomed to be worked up in their COMITIA, or popular assemblies, from the harangues of their demagogues, was one of the most common exciting causes, it was among the latter denominated MORBUS COMITIALIS, in the popular language of our own day, "electioneering disease," in reference to the time and occasion in which it most frequently occurred ; or, according to Seneca, because, whenever the disease appeared, the comitia were instantly broken up.—(*De Irâ*, iii., 7.) There are many other names also by which epilepsy was distinguished in former times ; but it is unnecessary to recount them.

The general pathology of the two preceding species, and which has been given at some length under the genus CLONUS, will apply to the present : but it is obvious from the symptoms, that the muscular power, commonly speaking, though not always, is affected to a less extent, and the sentient and intellectual to a much greater, and consequently that the irritative fibres suffer in a smaller degree than the sensific and percipient.

Before we enter upon the history of the disease, it will be convenient to remark, that from the different modifications under which it shows itself, it has been subdivided by many nosologists into very numerous varieties, but that the whole may be reduced to the following :—

a Cerebralis. Attacking abruptly, without
Cerebral epilepsy. any evident excitement, except in a few instances a slight giddiness. In this case, the predisposing cause is external violence or some internal injury, misformation, or disease of the head.

β Comitata. Catenating with some mor-
Catenating epi- bid action of a remote
lepsy. part, with the sense of a cold vapour ascending from it to the head, or

some other precursive sign.

γ Complicata. The limbs fixed and rigid,
Complicate epi- with clonic agitation of
lepsy. particular organs.

The causes of epilepsy, like those of the two preceding species, may be mental or corporeal : but to produce this, rather than either of the others, there must be a peculiar diathesis, which seems to depend upon the state of the nervous system. Where this exists, almost any of the passions or mental emotions, when violent, have been found sufficient to occasion a paroxysm, as anger, grief, fright, consternation ; of all which the records of medicine afford abundant examples. In a like diathesis, any kind of corporeal irritability will often become an exciting cause, whether more or less remote from the head itself ; and particularly where it is productive of a preternatural flow of blood into the vessels of the brain. Thus, an irritability in the ear from an inflammation, abscess, or some insect or other foreign substance that has accidentally entered into it, or the sudden suppression of a discharge to which it has been subject, has in various instances produced epilepsy. Hildanus (Cent. i., obs. 4) mentions a case, in which it followed a considerable degree of irritation, excited in the same organ by the accidental introduction of a small piece of glass. In like manner, an irritable state of the stomach, or intestines, or the liver, from chronic inflammation, debility, worms, or the presence of substances that do not naturally belong to it, has proved a frequent origin. Bartholine gives an instance, in which it supervened upon swallowing pieces of glass (*Hist. Anat.*, cent. v., hist. 66), and Widenfield another upon swallowing a needle.—(*Diss. Obs. Med. Triga*, Goett., 1768.) Confirmed drunkards are peculiarly subject to this complaint.

Particular affections of the uterus are, in like manner, an occasional source of epilepsy as well as of hysteria : and sometimes the latter has run into the former, where the epileptic diathesis has predominated. What this diathesis consists in, it is difficult to determine, for it gives no external signs : and hence Dr. Pritchard seems to doubt its existence (*On Nervous Diseases*, p. 95, 1822) ; but it is otherwise no easy matter to determine why a like irritation in the uterus should in one woman produce hysteria or convulsions, and in another epilepsy ; examples of which last occur very numerously in all the medical collections of cases.* Menostation, or a suppression or retention of the menstrual flux, is perhaps the most common of this class of causes ; and we may hence see why it should occasionally be excited by a suppression of the lochial discharge. A sudden suppression, indeed, of discharges of almost every kind, natural or morbid, of long continuance in an irritable habit, has occasionally proved a sufficient source of excitement.

* "In epilepsy there are fits of a sudden loss of sense, with convulsions of the voluntary muscles ; and the loss of sense continues after the convulsions have ceased, so that the person is said to go to sleep after the fit. The fact is, the convulsions cease before the loss of sense terminates."—(Elliotson.) Generally, says Dr. Armstrong, epilepsy may be defined to be clonic convulsions, followed by stupor, which after a time return.—See Lectures on the Morbid Anatomy, Nature, and Treatment of Acute and Chronic Diseases, p. 750, 8vo., Lond., 1834.—ED.

* Moranus, Apologia de Epilepsiâ Hystericâ, Orthes., 1626, 4to. Schulze, Diss. Casûs Hysterico-epileptici Resilutió, Hal., 1736. Eickmeyer, Diss. de Epilepsiâ Uterinâ, Ultraj., 1638.

Hence, also, repelled gout has been a cause, and still more generally repelled eruptions and exanthems, as itch, various species of ecpyesis, smallpox, and in one instance miliaria.* Sometimes it has occurred with the regular flow of the menses, and been re-excited by every periodical return; for where the peculiar diathesis exists, the slightest stimulus is often sufficient to call forth the disease. In the case before us, however, the periodical discharge is usually accompanied with pain iu the loins, or other local distress, as has been justly observed by Professor Osiander.†

Yet the most frequent cause of epilepsy is seated in the head itself; and has been found, on post-obit examinations, to consist in some morbid structure or secretion in the bones, tunics, or substance of this organ, as tubercles, exostoses, caries, apostemes, natural misconstruction of the whole or of particular parts, injuries from external violence,‡ loose calcareous earth, hydatids, pus, ichor, and other diseased fluids.§ Of these, some are predisponent, others occasional causes; the former of which will often continue inactive for a long period of time, and, as we have already observed, appertain chiefly to the first or cerebral variety. It has been observed, also, that in this modification the disease often makes its attack suddenly, and without any manifest exciting cause. Yet there can be little doubt that, in every instance, some occasional cause does exist, though, from its acting upon a morbid part of an organ that lies beyond our research, it entirely eludes all notice.

*. Baraillon, Hist. de l'Acad. Royale de Méd., an. 1776, p. 220. Inflammation of the membranes of the brain; certain poisons, as those of lead and the vegetable narcotics; acute hydrocephalus; the stage of smallpox in which the eruption is coming out; and profuse hemorrhage; may all prove so many exciting causes of epilepsy.—Ed.

† Uber die Entwicklungs-krankheiten in den Blüthen jahren des weiblichen Geschlechts, theil. i., 58, Götting., 1817.

‡ Several cases of epilepsy, caused by injury of the head, and relieved by trepanning, are detailed by Professor Dudley in the Transylvania Journal of Medicine.—D.

§ Epilepsy is frequently attended with a curious form of the head; it is very often united with deficiency of intellect, with a deficiency of brain, and of course fatuity, or idiocy. Many epileptic patients have a narrow forehead, a low forehead, sloping back. Many persons are idiots, not from there being a deficiency of brain, but the brain is of bad quality. However, there is one kind of idiocy which depends entirely upon a deficiency of the anterior part of the brain. Where such is the case, it is common for epilepsy to be united with it. It is very common to find a sugar-loaf form of head in epileptic patients. Epilepsy is sometimes united with a large head. A man with hydrocephalus, who had ten pints of water in his head, was epileptic. Sometimes the magnitude of the head arises from a preternaturally thick bone. Epilepsy may also occur in a person that has a most beautifully formed head, simply from some accidental disease in the head.—(See Professor Elliotson's Lectures, as delivered at the London University, Med. Gaz. for 1832-3, p. 582.) Very often, he adds, you will find the predisposition inexplicable.—(P. 609.)—Ed.

tice. The organ chiefly affected, as appears from the numerous and delicate dissections of M. Wenzel, is the cerebellum. He tells us, indeed, that he never opened the body of a single epileptic patient, in which he did not find the cerebellum diseased in some way or other.* But then Dr. Prout, who examined the bodies of numerous epileptics in the hospitals of Paris, tells us the same respecting the existence of worms in the intestines (Médecine éclatrée par l'Observation et l'Ouverture du Corps, Paris, 1804); while "it is proper to remark," observes Dr. Cook, in his essay on Epilepsy, "that in some instances after this disorder, no marks of disease whatever could be found within the cranium, the thorax, the abdomen, or any other part of the body."—(On Nervous Diseases, vol. ii., part 41.) So that, however curious in themselves, it is only in a few cases such morbid appearances can be turned to any account; while some of them may occasionally, perhaps, be effects of the disease rather than its causes. Dr. Löbenstein-Löbel, however, thinks that there ought always to be found some marks of disease or other within the cranium; and there is something humorous in his mode of accounting for their absence. "This is owing," says he, "to an injudicious treatment on the part of the practitioner, or neglect of the patient, by means of which the disease, instead of confining itself to a particular organ, is thrown over the nervous system at large."—(Weser und Heilung der Epilepsie, &c., 8vo., Leipsig, 1818.)†

The paroxysm in most cases occurs suddenly, and the patient is, so to speak, cut down at once, and loses all sense of perception and power of motion; so that if he be standing he falls to the ground with a greater or less degree of convulsion.‡ . There are a few rare instances of some degree of consciousness and perception throughout the paroxysm (Bresl. Sammlung, 1724, band i., p. 436); but the exceptions are few,

* Obs. sur le Cervelet, et sur les diverses Parties du Cerveau dans les Épileptiques, &c., Mentz. Dr. Elliotson, however, has opened persons who died of epilepsy, and nothing wrong was noticed in the cerebellum, or anywhere else.—(See his Lectures as delivered at London University.) In Dr. Carter's account of a lunatic hospital in France, it is stated that one of the physicians of the institution, found no disease of the brain, but of the medulla spinalis; which observations would agree with the view taken of this disease by Dr. Reid. —Ed.

† Dr. Otto (N. A. Med. and Surg. Journal) takes the same view of the subject, and prescribes accordingly.—D.

‡ The scream with which epilepsy usually commences, is described as one of the most startling sounds that can be uttered. "A young lady, while in the drawing-room of an eminent physician, waiting the assembling of a consultation summoned to consider her case, was suddenly attacked with epilepsy. She uttered a scream so piercing, that a parrot, himself no mean performer in discords, dropped from his perch, seemingly frightened to death by the appalling sound."—Dr. Cheyne in Cyclop. of Pract. Med., art, Epilepsy.—Ed,

and by no means enough to disturb the general rule. Commonly, the limbs on one side are more agitated than those on the other. The muscles of the face and eyes are always much affected, and throw the countenance into various and violent distortions. The tongue is thrust out of the mouth, which discharges a frothy saliva; the lower jaw is strongly convulsed; the teeth gnash violently upon each other; and as this occurs while the tongue is protruded, it is often most grievously wounded.*,

During the continuance of the fit, there is generally an alternate remission and exacerbation of the symptoms; though the whole does not usually last long, and is often of shorter duration than hysteria. On the cessation of the paroxysm, the patient remains for some time motionless, quite insensible, and apparently in a profound sleep or lethargy. He recovers from this attack sometimes suddenly, but more generally by degrees, and without any recollection of the sufferings he has undergone.†

---

* Dr. Cheyne states, that the patient is often found labouring under a general spasm, more especially of the extensor muscles. In a girl under this physician's care, the muscular contractions were so violent, that her arm was observed to be dislocated after every fit.—(Cyclop. of Pract. Med., art. EPILEPSY.) Burserius describes a similar case, and another in which the lower jaw was found dislocated after each attack.—ED.

† Portal, Mémoires sur la Nature et le Traitement des plusieurs Maladies, tom. ii., p. 229. Sometimes the urine and feces are discharged involuntarily; and occasionally there is a discharge of the semen. The hands are generally clinched, and the heart palpitates strongly. The pulse is quick, and respiration short, deep, and irregular. "When the patient wakes from the state of sopor, he has generally no recollection of what has passed, and perhaps, therefore, there is no suffering. The want of recollection of suffering is no proof that there has been no suffering; for we have all suffered enough in cutting our teeth, and we know nothing of it now, and so it may happen respecting more recent events: the fit may be attended with more or less suffering, and yet the individual not be aware of it afterward; but," says Dr. Elliotson, "I should think there is no suffering, and for this reason, persons do not suffer in general when they are hung. There is an account in Lord Bacon's works of a person who was hung, and all but killed, and yet he did not suffer. There is a short account of Cowley the poet (which is very scarce), from which it appears that he three times attempted to commit suicide, and one of these attempts was by suspension. The account was written by himself, and found among his manuscripts. He there mentions, that be suspended himself over his chamber door in the Temple, and became perfectly insensible. He only recollected a flash of light appearing before his eyes. His weight at last caused him to drop on the floor; there he was found, and after a time he recovered. He says, that although he was thus in the jaws of death, and had become perfectly insensible, yet he had no previous suffering; and therefore, as there was no previous suffering in that state, it is probable that there is no suffering in epilepsy. I should suppose that in drowning there is no suffering, if it occur at once. Shakspeare's expression is, 'Oh, Lord! methought what pain it was

[In one example, recorded by Dr. Burnet (Med. Chir. Trans., vol. xiii.), there was considerable dyspnœa, and a remarkable slowness of the pulse, which at times did not exceed fourteen strokes a minute.]

Under the first or CEREBRAL VARIETY, or where there is little or no appearance of an occasional cause, and the predisponent cause is supposed to exist in the head, the comatose symptoms, and, indeed, the general mischief to the external as well as to the internal senses, are most striking. Yet the effect is even here very different in different individuals. The optic nerve affords severe proofs of this. Sometimes surrounding objects appear brighter or larger than natural, or both.—(Bartholin, Hist. Anat., cent. iii., hist. 45; N. Samml. Med. Wahrnem., b. iv., p. 229.) Yet, in many cases, the irritability of the nerve or its adjoining muscles has been destroyed, and a paresis, more or less general, has been the result. Hence a perpetual nictitation, strabismus, or blindness, is no unfrequent consequence. Yet, in one instance, a most fortunate and directly opposite effect was produced, for an habitual blindness was removed.—(Ephem. Nat. Cur., cent. i., ii., obs. 130.) Where the muscles of speech have suffered in an equal degree, speechlessness has in like manner followed (Hagendorn, cent. i., obs. 14; Act. Nat. Cur., vol. i., obs. 71); and for the same reason, where the joints have been violently affected with a predominance of rigid over clonic action, they have sunk into an insuperable contraction.—(Horstius, ii., p. 90.) It is hence not to be wondered at, that the whole system should occasionally be nearly exhausted of its entire stock of sensorial power, and that the paroxysm, as observed by Aretæus, should terminate in mania, idiocy, or even death itself; sometimes instantaneously, and at other times through the medium of a fit of apoplexy.*

---

to drown;' but there is no reason to suppose there is pain, if the individual go down and do not come up again; but if he come out of the water, the suffering is dreadful."—See Elliotson's Lectures, as delivered at the Lond. Univ.—ED.

* Aretæus, de Caus. et Sign. Morb., cent. i., 4. The following observations by Dr. Cheyne are replete with practical instruction :—"In our endeavour to determine the species to which a case of epilepsy belongs, we may proceed as follows :— first, we may inquire into the state of the natural functions, the state of the appetite, digestion, and nutrition, and into the condition of the secretions and excretions; then into the state of the nervous system; and lastly, if the patient is a female, into the functions of the uterus, especially with respect to menstruation. If we are unable to detect any affection of the nerves, any local irritation, or disorder of a remote part of the brain, we may with probability consider the case as a specimen of the epilepsia cerebralis. In this conclusion we may repose with more confidence, if we discover that the disease is inherited; that the patient has been liable to vascular congestion in the brain from determination of blood to the head, increased action in the arterial system within the cranium, &c., flushing in the face, throbbing in the temples, epistaxis, vertigo, dulness or weakness of intellect, tightness across the forehead, headache, false perceptions; that there is any

The warning or precursive symptoms by which epilepsy is sometimes ushered, have been most common to the second or CATENATING VARIETY. The most usual sensation is that of the ascent of a cold creeping vapour from some particular part of the body, of the nature and cause of which we know nothing, but which has often been called an *aura epileptica*. This halitus usually ascends from the extremities, but there is no organ from which it has not issued in different individuals, according to examples accumulated by the collectors of medical curiosities; as the feet, the hands, the fingers, the thumb, the great toe, the legs, the arms, the hypochondria, the crown of the head. And, in various instances, spots on the face or feet have preceded, and at other times accompanied the paroxysm.

We sometimes meet, however, with other harbingers, of quite as singular a character, in the other varieties; as a heaviness of the eyes, pain, heat, and sparkling, which, by Sir Clifton Wintringham, were regarded as signs that peculiarly distinguish the idiopathic from the symptomatic disease.—(*Ricardi Mead Monita et Præcepta, permultis notationibus et observationibus illustrata*, tom. i., 8vo.) Sometimes there has been a wild play of phantasms or illusive objects before the sight:* and Portius relates the case of a woman, who was always warned of an approaching fit by the appearance, as it were, of her own image in a mirror.—(*Medicæ Considerationes Variæ.*) On many occasions, indeed, as Paulini has rightly observed, there is a peculiar overflow of spirits, and a tendency to merriment, as though the mind were entirely thrown off its balance.—(Cent. ii., obs. 13; *Bresl. Samml.*, 1724, band. ii., p. 434.) Sometimes the patient exhibits sudden starts of run-

thing peculiar in the form of the head or expression of the countenance; and that the habits of the patient have been such as to produce considerable or long-continued excitement of the brain. Paroxysms of epilepsy, which occur late in life in persons who have had apoplexy, or whose diathesis is apoplectie, rank under the epilepsia cerebralis; as also do those cases of not unfrequent occurrence, in which epilepsy almost invariably leads to an attack of insanity."—See Cyclop. of Pract. Med. art. EPILEPSY.—ED.

* Bartholin, Hist. Anat., cent. i., hist. 81, cent. ii., hist. 72. Hagendorn, cent. iii., obs. 12. Also Armstrong's Lectures on the Morbid Anatomy, Nature, and Treatment of Acute and Chronic Diseases, p. 747, 8vo., Lond., 1834. This latter physician knew a patient who married, and then became remarkably dissipated, and used to go to bed intoxicated every night. As he was sitting one day after dinner, he suddenly started from the table in great alarm, and asked his friends if they did not see any writing on the wall. In a few hours he had his first attack of epilepsy, of which disease he ultimately died. Dr. Gregory, of Edinburgh, used to mention the case of an officer, who, before a fit occurred, always saw an old woman in a blue coat, who approached him, and with a stick which she held in her hand, knocked him down. Such spectral illusions denote the cerebral variety of the disease. Dr. Armstrong knew a lady who always squinted a day or two before the attack.—Op. cit. —ED.

ning. (*Boot. De Affectionibus Omissis*, cap. vi.; *Schenck*, obs. i., lib. ii., p. 202) or dancing (*Chesneau*, lib. i., cap. iv., obs. 4; *Eph. Nat. Cur.*, passim); occasionally he is strangely talkative (*Eph. Nat. Cur.*, dec. ii., ann. 6, obs. 229); and, in one instance, exhibited a new and peculiar talent for singing.—(*Act. Nat. Cur.*, vol. v.) Vic-D'Azyr relates the case of a woman who had been subject to epileptic fits for twelve years, and which at length became as frequent as four or five times a day. They always commenced with a peculiar sensation in one leg, near the lower part of the gastrocnemius muscle. A surgeon present on one of these accessions, plunged a scalpel into the part affected, which came in contact with a hard body, that he soon cut out, and found to be a dense cartilaginous ganglion, of the size of a very large pea, that pressed upon the nerve which he divided. The woman had no return of epilepsy.* We have already noticed a similar cause of irritation and mode of cure in a case of *neuralgia faciei*; and it is highly probable, that under a slight variation of the nervous erethism in either instance, the one disease would have been substituted for the other.

Under the third or COMPLICATED VARIETY, while many of the limbs are rigidly fixed, almost without relaxation, the muscles of other parts are thrown into the most grotesque and ludicrous gesticulations of chorea; and, if the muscles of the chest be affected in this way, the patient appears in some cases to burst into involuntary fits of laughter from their irregular and clonic action.—(*Eph. Nat. Cur.*, dec. i., ann. iii., obs. 304.) At the same time, such has been the force of the spastic muscles, as to break one or more teeth, to rupture an artery, or render a vein varicose; and in one case, at least, to burst the left ventricle of the heart itself.—(*Johnston, Med. Remarks*, &c., vol. ii.)

It has been observed, that the epileptic paroxysm occurs chiefly at irregular periods, and is for the most part of short duration. There are, however, some instances on record of a singular exception to this rule in both cases: for it has occasionally lasted for two or three days, with little or no remission. It has also returned at stated times, and with great frequency; with the revolution of the morning, or even of the night; in one instance six times in a single day (*Tulpius*, lib. i., cap. xi.); and in another, on the revolution of the birthday of each of the patient's parents (*Eph. Nat. Cur.*, dec. iii., ann. iv., app. 193): and hence it may occasionally have obeyed lunations, and appeared to be in-

* Dict. des Sciences Médicales, art. CAS RARES. In the Edinburgh Med. Essays, there is likewise an instance of the disease being produced by a small hard body in a nerve, at the lower part of the gastrocnemius muscle. The disease had existed twelve years; but, on this body being removed, it entirely ceased. Dr. Curry, of Guy's Hospital, has mentioned an instance, in which the aura epileptica rose from the extremities; yet, after death, a little tumour was found in the head. The case was referred to by Dr. Elliotson, in his Clinical Lectures at St. Thomas's Hospital, in Dec., 1830.—ED.

fluenced by the phases of the moon (*Forest.*, lib. x., obs. 60), while running a regular course from some other cause. In a highly nervous temperament it is not difficult to account for such returns; since the dread of its return alone, when it has once established a circle of action, will form a sufficient source of irritation. In a few instances, it seems to have been hereditary,* and perhaps in an equal number congenial, appearing soon after birth, and mostly produced by a fright of the mother during pregnancy. Hildanus gives an example, in which a fright of this kind was occasioned by the presence of an epileptic patient when suddenly attacked with a paroxysm (Cent. iii., obs. 8.): and other medical records contain instances of a like effect on the sudden rush of a hare, or some other animal against a pregnant woman.

Many persons, habitually disposed to epilepsy, are attacked immediately on waking in the morning from a sound sleep, when we may be inclined to think they would be least liable to such a surprise. Dr. Cullen finds a difficulty in explaining this curious fact. But when we reflect that epilepsy is a disease of irregular action, chiefly in a debilitated system, depending, where there is a confirmed diathesis, upon whatever may disturb the balance of perhaps any of the circulating fluids—and that this balance may be disturbed either by too much as well as too little excitement ;—when we reflect, moreover, that during sound sleep there is always taking place a considerable accumulation of sensorial power, and may at times be an excess of it—we shall no longer, I think, be at a loss to account for an adequate cause of this very singular phenomenon.†

The general mode of treatment proposed for the last two diseases, will apply to the present. The twofold intention is to remove, as far as we

are able, the exciting cause,* and to allay the habitual irritation of the nervous system.

Where plethora manifestly exists, we may use venesection with great hope of success, and, generally speaking, more freely than in hysteria.† But here also cathartics will be of considerable avail, and, in the hands of Dr. Hamilton, have been found sufficient alone to produce a cure.‡ To effect this, they should be used freely and maintained steadily, so as to keep up a perpetual counter-irritation in the bowels, which may act as a revellent against the morbid irritation in any other part, and directly carry off whatever irritating matter may exist in the bowels themselves.

Provided this be accomplished, the particular medicine employed does not appear to be a matter of great moment. Colocynth, gamboge, sulphate of magnesia, and calomel, seem to have been used with almost equally good effects ; though in visceral congestion the last should never be omitted. If worms be suspected, and especially the vermicular ascaris, the rectified oil of turpentine should undoubtedly be allowed a preference. Even where worms are not found to exist, this has often proved highly successful, apparently by the revulsive action it excites. As a purgative, it should be given in ounce or ounce and a half doses to an adult ; but as an alterant, in smaller doses repeated daily.—(See *Dr. Latham, Med. Trans.*, vol. v., art. xxiii., *and compare with his Treatise on Diabetes.*)

Cold affusion, whether general or confined to the head, has been rarely tried in our own country ; but is strenuously recommended by many foreign authorities, as well during the paroxysm as in the intervals ; particularly by Dr. Löbenstein-Löbel. He employs it, indeed, both in an entonic and atonic state of the frame, only in the former case premising venesection. Under

---

* Frid. Hoffm. Diss. de Affectibus hæreditariis eorumque Origine, Hal., 1699. App. Suppl., ii., l., p. 523. Abhandlung über die erblichen Krankheiten, &c., von J. Clund. Rongemont, Frankf., 1794, 8vo. In speaking of a certain hereditary predisposition to epilepsy, Dr. Elliotson observes, " you will find this shown, perhaps, not by brothers and sisters, fathers and mothers, grandfathers and grandmothers having had the disease, but by their having had other affections of the nervous system. The same state of the nervous system will frequently not produce the same disease ; one shall have epilepsy, and another some other nervous affection. When, however, you see these things in different generations, you may class them together, and consider them as the development of an hereditary predisposition."—Lectures delivered at the London Univ., as reported in Med. Gaz. for 1832–3, p. 582.—Ed.

† On the cause of epilepsy, Dr. Jackson of Philadelphia remarks (Philadelphia Journal of the Med. and Phys. Sc., vol. xiv., p. 209) :—" If direct deductions from the symptoms, which are derangements of function, will lead us to a knowledge of the organ affected in any disease, and the nature of the organic lesion, we must conclude that the brain is indubitably the seat of epilepsy, and sanguine congestion, suddenly and periodically induced, the character of the morbid lesion." Dr. J. H. Wright, of Balt., states as follows :—" From the result of all the dissections I have hitherto

prosecuted, to discover the cause or condition predisposing to epilepsy, or the tenour of lesion by which that form of disease had involved a fatal issue, I infer that the sensorial irritations exciting epileptic phenomena, depend on organic degenerations of the brain or membranes more frequently than is generally admitted."—(Am. Journ. of Med. Sc., vol. ii., p. 45.) Prof. Chapman also contends for its cerebral character.—See his Materia Medica.—D.

* Dr. Armstrong saw more benefit derived from removing the exciting cause, than from any thing else. As to diet, he says, simplicity in the kind of food, and moderation in its quantity, is the golden rule. He knew of several cases which were cured by adopting this rule, and avoiding all circumstances which act on the mind and circulation. " A regulated diet," he observes, " occasional bloodletting, if the patient be of a full habit, and purgative medicines, are the remedies upon which I have the most reliance."—See Lectures on the Morbid Anatomy, Nature, and Treatment of Acute and Chronic Diseases, p. 754, 8vo., Lond., 1834.—Ed.

† " If there be an inflammatory state within the head, or the patient be plethoric without inflammation, then, certainly, blood should be taken away."—Elliotson.

‡ With the purgative plan, free bleeding and a blister to the nape of the neck may often be usefully combined, as in the case related by Mr. Gunn. See Edin. Med. Journ., No. xc., p. 78.—Ed.

particular circumstances it may be useful, but it requires great caution; for even this writer prohibits it where the patient is subject to gout, rheumatism, diarrhœa, or nervous trepidations; at the period of menstruation, or any other expected discharge; or on repelled eruptions.—(*Wesen und Heilung der Epilepsie*, &c., 8vo., 1818.)

De Haen often employed emetics, and chiefly for the purpose of exciting and maintaining a new action, for which purpose he continued them daily for a week or two. His example was followed at one time, but has long been relinquished.—(*Rat. Med.*, part v., cap. iv., § 1; *Eph. Nat. Cur.*, cent. vi., obs. 58.)

Externally, stimulants have also been tried, and, in various instances, seem to have been attended with good success. The spine has been rubbed night and morning with different preparations of ammonia, camphire, cantharides, and the antimonial ointment;[*] and setons and issues have been applied to different parts of the body, as have also the actual and potential cautery (*Ab. Heers, Observ. Var. Locher, Observ. Pract.; Roekard, Journ. de Méd.*, tom. xxv., p. 46), and the moxa. Where the cause of the disease has been suspected to be seated in the head,[†] they have been chiefly confined to this organ, but where there has been a manifest aura epileptica to the limb or other part of the body from which the vapour has seemed to ascend. And there can be no question that these means have frequently proved serviceable, especially in prevent-

ing the recurrence of subsequent fits, where a habit of return has been established. The practice is of considerable antiquity, for, under some modification or other, it is recommended by Galen, and many other Greek writers. In later times, it has been chiefly employed by Baron Percy (*Pyrotechnie*, passim) and by M. Gondret. Schenck has examined, at considerable length, the successful and unsuccessful cases which, in his day, had been published upon the use of cauteries.—(*Observ.*, lib. i., No. ccxxxiii.) In several instances, an accidental burn has answered the purpose of a surgical escharotic, and fortunately proved a radical cure.—(*Eph. Nat. Cur.*, dec. i., ann. ii., obs. 9.) Professor Zoeffler, of Altona, instead of cauterizing the limb from which the epileptic halitus seems to ascend, has ingeniously tied a tight ligature above the part whence the vapour issues, probably upon the ground of the success with which it is often attended in the bite of the rattlesnake and other venomous animals, and, in one or two cases, the ligature seems to have proved quite as favourable in the present disease.[*]

The general irritability of the nervous system has been attempted to be overcome by sedatives and tonics. Of the former, the chief have been camphire, cajeput, valerian, hyoscyamus, stramonium, opium, and digitalis. *Stramonium*, like many other medicines, has had a strange alternation of fortune. About a century ago it was esteemed every thing, half a century ago it declined greatly in its reputation, and has of late been once more rising into esteem. Fourteen epileptic patients in the royal hospital at Stockholm were, many years since, treated with pills of stramonium.[†] Of these, eight are declared by Dr. Odhelius, in the official report upon this subject, to have been entirely cured, five had their symptoms mitigated, and only one received no relief. The greater number, on first using this remedy, were affected with confusion in their heads, dimness in their eyes, and thirst; but these symptoms gradually diminished.

Where hyoscyamus has been given, it has been employed both in the leaves and seeds: Dr. Parr preferred the latter, and usually combined the seeds with some aromatics, commencing with doses of a grain, and advancing them to four or five grains. [One or two cases in favour of the utility of digitalis are recorded (See *Edin. Med. Journ.*, No. xc., p. 19) by Mr. Scott of Liverpool.]

The tonics employed have been both vegetable and metallic. Among the former, the mistletoe of the oak stood at one time at the head

---

* See Creighton on the use of Tartar Emetic Ointment in Epilepsy.—(Trans. of the Assoc. of Physicians, Ireland, vol. iv., p. 332.) This gentleman applied it also to different parts of the body; and he noticed that the eruption produced by it is not confined to the spot on which the ointment is rubbed, but mostly appears in very remote parts; thus proving that its action is in some degree on the constitution.—Ed.

† It is seldom that the seat of the local mischief, which causes epilepsy, in those cases which arise from organic derangements within the head, can be exactly ascertained; and it is not always that, when ascertained, they are within the reach of a surgical operation; yet such cases are on record, and one remarkable instance is related by Dr. Rogers of New-York. It was a protracted epilepsy, cured by elevating a portion of the os frontis, which had been depressed upon the brain fourteen years. —(See New-York Med. and Physical Journ., 1826.) Facts of this kind, and others in which strabismus and other unequivocal signs of affection of the brain take place, are decidedly adverse to Dr. Reid's theory, that epilepsy should be ranked among those diseases to which, what he terms, the spinal system is liable.—(Trans. of Assoc. of Physicians, Ireland, vol. iv., p. 355.) That epilepsy does not always depend upon the state of the spinal cord, is also proved by the morbid changes in the head, frequently revealed by dissections as the cause of the disease. That they are not merely consequences, is shown by the fact, that when removable, as in the case adverted to, the cure follows. At the same time, what is here stated is by no means intended to controvert Dr. Reid's position, that in epilepsy the medulla spinalis is sometimes found in a morbid state, and may be concerned in the production of the disease.—Ed.

* Speaking of the aura epileptica, Dr. Armstrong confirms the statement of many other writers, that if a tourniquet be applied above the part, the fit will frequently be prevented. He adds, "Sometimes, when this has occurred, tumours have been found in the course of the nerves."—See Lectures on the Morbid Anatomy, Nature, and Treatment of Acute and Chronic Diseases, p. 748, 8vo., Lond., 1834.—Ed.

† Mém. de l'Acad. Royale des Sciences de Stockholme, traduit par M. Keralio, tom. iii.; Razoux, Diss. Epist. de Stramonio, &c.

of the remedies for epilepsy. It was regarded as a specific by Colbatsch (see also *Abhandlung von dem Missel, und dessen kraft wieder die Epilepsie,* Altenb., 1776), and most warmly recommended by Haller and De Haen.—(*Rat. Med. Pract.,* part vi., p. 317.). It appears, however, of no importance from what tree it is taken, for, as a parasite, it flourishes equally on many, and preserves its own peculiarities on all; and from every tree, so far as late experiments have been made, it is equally inefficacious and futile.

In plethoric habits, cinchona will generally do mischief; in the cerebral variety, it can do little or no good; and it is only in a relaxed and mobile state of the animal frame that any benefit can be expected from it.

Mercury has been tried in almost every form and to almost every extent; sometimes indeed to that of salivation, in which state some practitioners pretend to have found it highly useful. As a general plan, however, this can never be advisable: and Muralt admits that, in most cases, where it has seemed to answer, it has only restrained the disease, or prolonged the interval, but not effected a radical cure.*

Of the preparations of zinc we took notice under CONVULSION, and the remarks there offered are equally applicable to epilepsy. Such, however, has been the state of exhausted irritability produced by this disease in some instances, that the patient would bear almost any quantity of them. Mr. Johnson of Lancaster gave the sulphate of zinc in doses of five grains twice a day at first, and increased the dose gradually to twelve grains. Thelenius had previously given eight grains of the same daily.—(*Medicinische und Chirurgische Bemerkungen,* Franc., 1789.) Arsenic has of late been chiefly employed in the form of the common solution, and, as united with nickel, in the compound of an arseniate.† But the preparations of copper and silver have met with more success than any of the preceding. The best form of the first is that of the cuprum ammoniatum; and the Edinburgh Medical Commentaries are full of cases that afford proof of its remedial power. The simplest mode of exhibiting this medicine is that of pills, as the *pilulæ cæruleæ* of the Edinburgh Pharmacopœia, which is nothing more than ammoniated

copper made into a pilular consistence by means of crumbs of bread. The patient should begin with half a grain of the metallic salt every night, and increase it to double the quantity if his stomach will bear it.

The best, and indeed the common preparation of silver for the purpose before us, is its nitrate. Under a more operose and unscientific form, it was employed as early as the beginning of the seventeenth century by Angelus Sala, and afterward by Boyle and Geoffrey, though for other complaints rather than the present. Dr. Albers of Bremen has observed, and the remark has since been confirmed by Dr. Roget (*Trans. Medico-Chir. Soc.,* vol. vii., p. 290), Dr. Badeley (see *Epichrosis Pæcilia of this Work,* Cl. VI., Ord. III., Gen. X., Spe. 6), and numerous other practitioners, that the use of this medicine, if persevered in, gives a peculiar darkness to the colour of the skin, which remains for many months after its discontinuance, in some cases for upwards of two years.—(*On the Effect of Nitrate of Silver, Trans. Medico-Chir. Soc.,* vol. ix., p. 234.)

Dr. Powell tried the nitrate of silver in St. Bartholomew's Hospital upon a large scale, and in two forms, that of pills and that of solution, the solvent being mint-water, which seems best to cover its unpleasant taste. Many of the cases seem to have been strongly marked, and they are given in a communication to the London College.* They relate chiefly to young persons of both sexes from nine to fifteen years of age; in all of whom the medicine proved successful, and is said to have operated a perfect cure. The dose consisted at first of not more than half a grain or a grain of the metallic salt, whether in the form of pill or of solution, given usually every four hours, but this was gradually increased to doses of three or four grains taken at the same distance of time: and the increase was still continued till sickness or some other inconvenience forbade. It is singular, that while the earlier writers complain very generally of the purgative powers of this medicine, and the griping it produces, the modern preparation excites no such effects; not even when it has been carried, as it has occasionally been, to the amount of fifteen grains to a single dose in the shape of pills; though it should be remembered, that few stomachs will bear more than five grains in a dissolved state. Dr. M'Ginnis of Portsmouth affirms, that he has employed it repeatedly both in recent and chronic cases, without any perceptible effect, in doses of twelve grains; and M. Georget, who, however, does not seem to be much acquainted with its use, has condemned it as a medicine dangerous to the coats of the stomach.†

---

* Hippocr. Helvet., p. 247. Dr. Elliotson is of opinion that there can be no harm in trying mercury and iodine, because there may be some disease in the head which these will remove. He is not aware that they do good, except in removing the effects of chronic inflammation.—See his Lectures, delivered at the London Univ.—Ed.

† See a valuable article on this and similar medicines in the Edin. Med. and Surg. Journ., No. xix., p. 374. The following are Dr. Elliotson's observations on zinc, tin, and arsenic:—" The sulphate of zinc has been much praised, as well as the oxyde. I have given it in St. Vitus's dance: you may exhibit it in large quantities (sometimes twenty or twenty-four grains), but I never saw it do good in epilepsy. The oxyde of tin has been much praised, and so has arsenic; but I have seen persons from taking the latter become epileptic. I do not believe these things are to be depended upon.—Ed.

* Med. Trans., vol. iv., art. viii. A case in favour of the nitrate of silver is related by Dr. Williams of Liverpool, though many other potent remedies were also employed, as oil of turpentine, blisters, cold washes to the head, sulphate of zinc, issues, and mercury.—Edin. Med. Journ., No. lxxxv., p. 297.—Ed.

† Phys. de Syst. Nerv., tom. ii., p. 401. According to Dr. Armstrong, the nitrate of silver some-

Iron, in all its preparations, offers a far less hazardous remedy, and in some instances, appears to have been attended with considerable success. The best form perhaps is that of the subcarbonate, in the proportion of a drachm three times a day, as already recommended in the case of Nᴇᴜʀᴀʟɢɪᴀ ; and thus administered, it has occasionally produced a radical cure.*

All these tonics seem to operate by taking off the tendency to irregular nervous action, and, consequently, the tendency to a return of the paroxysm, where a habit of recurrence has once been established ; for in many instances, such habit alone appears to be as much an adequate stimulus as a similar habit in intermittents : and hence, whatever has a tendency to break through such a habit must have a beneficial effect ; fevers themselves of various kinds have often done this,† and especially quartans, the most obstinate of the whole tribe of fevers ; and the above remark explains their mode of operation in this respect : it is that of introducing a new circle of actions.

But the exciting causes of epilepsy are so numerous, and the disease itself so complicated, that it would be in vain to expect success in every instance from metallic tonics, or any one description of medicines whatever.‡ The rem-

times stops epilepsy, but most frequently fails.—(On the Morbid Anatomy, Nature, &c., of Acute and Chronic Diseases, p. 755.) Dr. Elliotson seldom prescribes it : "if it be not given for a long time," says he, "you will not do good ; and if it be given for a long time, you run the chance of blackening the patient." He considers it as a medicine calculated to bring on gastritis and diarrhœa ; points on which he disagrees with the author's statements.—Eᴅ.

* Dr. Elliotson has never seen iron do good in epilepsy, execpt as a tonic, when the patient has been improperly lowered.—Eᴅ.

† Hornung, Cista Medica, Norih., 1625, 4to. Augzüge aus dem Tagebuche eines ausübenden Arztes, &c., 1 Samml., Berl., 1791.

‡ This is a truth which the practitioner should never lose sight of; for while he is guided by it, he will know what degree of value ought to be attached to various alleged remedies for epilepsy. Professor Elliotson, in his Lectures, after adverting to preparations of copper, iron, lead, zinc, tin, and arsenic, and to narcotics, cold affusion, oil of turpentine, &c., as means for the cure of epilepsy, very properly remarks :—"Now all these things may fail, entirely through our not attending to the antiphlogistic regimen. It is possible that cases happen now and then that would yield to some of these remedies ; but we neglect to lower the patient. I am quite sure that remedies are completely prevented from doing good, because we do not remove a plethoric state of the system. In some local inflammations, and in many cases of various diseases, it is necessary to lower the system to a certain point, and then remedies, which would not otherwise be useful, become so. The reason that the disease is so generally intractable, —the reason that so many remedies are so uncertain and unsatisfactory,—is very evident. This is a disease which arises from every sort of irritation in every part of the body ; and the irritation may be structural, may be slow inflammation, or something we cannot remove. If it arose from one cause, it would be a different thing ; but it will

Vᴏʟ. II.—A ᴀ

edies must often be varied to meet the varying case. And on this account, it is by no means uncommon to find epilepsy removed by oil of turpentine or some other purgative, that had obstinately resisted the most powerful doses of the metallic salts ; while, in some instances, the disease is altogether irremediable.*

GENUS VIII.
CARUS.
TORPOR.

MUSCULAR IMMOBILITY ; MENTAL OR CORPOREAL TORPITUDE, OR BOTH.

Cᴀʀᴜs or κάρος, "sopor cum gravedine," is derived from κάπα, "the head," being the organ in which the disease is chiefly seated. As employed in the present arrangement, the genus signified by this term will readily include the following species :—

1. Carus Asphyxia.	Asphyxy. Suspended Animation.
2. —— Ecstasis.	Ecstasy.
3. —— Catalepsia.	Catalepsy.
4. —— Lethargus.	Lethargy.
5. —— Apoplexia.	Apoplexy.
6. —— Paralysis.	Palsy.

Carus, therefore, will be found to embrace, under the present arrangement, a field somewhat more extensive than that allotted to it by most other writers, so as to include several of the species arranged by Sauvages under his two orders Leipopsychiæ and Comata ; to be nearly synonymous with the Defectivi and Soporosi of Linnéus ; and still more so with the Adynamiæ of Macbride.

As a generic sign, the author has preferred the term torpor or torpitude to stupor or sopor, which have hitherto been chiefly made use of for the same purpose ; and this on two accounts. First, as being of wider signification, since it includes the general idea furnished by both the arise from any cause whatever, physical or mental, organic or inorganic, and situated in any part of the body. You will see, therefore, not only that it must be usually an incurable disease, but you will see that there can be no remedy for it."—See Elliotson's Lectures, as delivered at the London University, Med. Gaz. for 1832-3, p. 614.—Eᴅ.

* Dr. Reid mentions two modes in which the convulsions of epilepsy may be stopped. "During the inordinate struggle," says he, "to perform respiration, the practitioner may abstract some of the force applied to the respiratory organs by attracting the exertion in another direction. Thus, while the hands and arms are violently contracted, if the attendants forcibly extend them, and open the fingers, so much exertion is involuntarily made by the patient to oppose this, that the violent operation of the respiratory muscles subsides, the organs fall into their natural train of action, the patient draws a heavy sigh, and the paroxysm is at an end. Any unusual irritation," Dr. Reid adds, "may have this effect." The other mode is to let an assistant press forcibly the soft parts of the abdomen towards the spine with his closed hand. The theoretical explanation of the practice we need not examine, if the plan answer, as Dr. Reid has found it do.—See Trans. of Assoc. of Physicians, Ireland, vol. iv., pp. 363–365.—Eᴅ.

others: and secondly, because neither stupor nor sopor has been uniformly employed in a determinate sense of any kind. Thus stupor is often, perhaps usually, restrained to mental insensibility or morbid sleep; while Sauvages has explained it as meaning hebetude of the sense of touch, "molestia quæ sensum tactûs obscurat;" and Linnéus, transient sleep of any part with a sense of formication, "*sopor* transitorius partis alicujus cum sensû formicationis." In this place, and indeed generally, Linnéus makes *sopor* combine the two ideas of a cessation of motivity and of feeling; or of irritability and sensibility; while Cullen objects, and correctly, to this strained extent of the term, and limits it to the ordinary signification of "sleep, or a sleep-like state." Torpor, or torpitude, in the definition of carus now offered, imports insensibility, mental or corporeal, in a frame still alive, and actuated, though often imperceptibly, by the vital principle. The term insensibility would not so well answer the purpose; it is of too wide a range and too loose a meaning, being often predicated of insentient, unorganized matter, that never possessed the principle of life.

'Carus or torpor, thus explained, will equally apply to all the species we have just enumerated, some of which are very uncommon, and a few of which have been supposed doubtful; though, upon the whole, the authorities are in their favour, and they ought neither to be omitted nor merged, as they seem to be by Cullen, in the sweeping name of apoplexy: constituting in his hands a genus that includes a variety of distinct, and in some instances, very different diseases, but which, under his own classification, Dr. Cullen found it difficult to distinguish or place separately.

SPECIES I.
CARUS ASPHYXIA.
ASPHYXY. SUSPENDED ANIMA-TION.[*]

TOTAL SUSPENSION OF ALL THE MENTAL AND CORPOREAL FUNCTIONS.

Asphyxy, from *a* privative, and σφύξις, "pulsus," is here used in the general sense of the term, though it has occasionally been employed to import mere failure or cessation of the action of the heart and arteries, which, in the present classification, is made a species of entasia under the name of ACROTISMUS; and has already passed in review as belonging to the second order of the present class.

---

[*] The meaning of the term *asphyxia* is often more limited than what Dr. Good has assigned to it; being applied only to cases in which the cessation of the heart's action proceeds from a particular cause, namely, the interruption of respiration, or, to speak more correctly, the interruption of the effect produced by that function on the blood. In this sense, then, asphyxia is the condition of the body consequent to the interruption of the arterialization of the blood, and attended with a suspension of all the powers of sensation and voluntary motion.—See Dr. Roget's Obs. in Cyclop. of Pract. Med., art. ASPHYXIA.—ED.

Asphyxy offers us several varieties, from a difference of occasional cause, which produces a like diversity in a few of its symptoms. Sauvages, who has made the disease a genus, gives us no fewer than seventeen species or subdivisions; Dr. Goodwin contents himself with three, and denominating the disease *melanæma*, from the black colour which the blood ordinarily assumes under its influence, distinguishes them by the names of melanæma from hanging, from drowning, and from inspiration of fixed air.

Of these, the first arrangement is unnecessarily diffuse and complicated; and the second too limited and not quite correct, since it will presently appear, that the direct cause of asphyxy in hanging and drowning is one and the same.

The author has, in consequence, been induced to divide the species into the following table of varieties, forming a middle line between the two preceding arrangements, and including, as he hopes, every modification with which it is of importance to become acquainted:—

α Suffocationis. Asphyxy from suffocation.	Produced by hanging or drowning: countenance turgid and livid.
β Mephytica. Choke-damp.	Produced by inhaling carbonic acid or some other irrespirable exhalation: countenance pallid.
γ Electrica. Electrical asphyxy.	Produced by a stroke of lightning or electricity. Limbs flexible; countenance pale; blood uncoagulable.
δ Algida. Frostbitten asphyxy.	Produced by intense cold. Limbs rigid: countenance pale and shrivelled.

In the first variety, or ASPHYXY FROM HANGING or DROWNING, the immediate cause is suffocation, or a total obstruction to the respiration, and is so explained by Bonet, Haller, Lancisi, Petit, and De Haen.

The face, as we have just noticed, is turgid and suffused with livid blood; and the general symptoms are given with so much truth and emphasis by Shakspeare, in Suffolk's description of the body of Henry VI., that I copy them as a guide to the medical student:—

"See how the blood is settled in his face!
Oft have I seen a timely parted ghost
Of ashy semblance, meager, pale, and bloodless;
Being all descended to the labouring heart:
Who, in the conflict that it holds with death,
Attracts the same for aidance 'gainst the enemy,
Which, with the heart, there cools, and ne'er returneth
To blush and beautify the cheek again.
But see! his face is black and full of blood;
His eyeballs further out than when he lived,
Staring full ghastly, like a strangled man,
His hair up-rear'd, his nostrils stretch'd with struggling;
His hands abroad display'd as one that grasp'd
And tugg'd for life, and was by strength subdued."[*]

This description, however, applies more fully to asphyxy from hanging than to that from drown-

---

[*] Henry VI., Second Part, Act. III.

ing, in which last there is more flaccidity of the limbs, and consequently less of "struggle and grasp, and tug for life." In both cases, nevertheless, the countenance has a semblance of apoplexy, as though there was a congestion of blood in the head, to which the application of the rope to the neck, in the case of hanging, affords some countenance. And hence many eminent writers of earlier times, as Boerhaave, Wapfer, and Alberti, referred suffocation from both the causes before us to apoplexy; while Cullen made it a subdivision of this last disease: and M. Portal has, still more lately, entered into the same view.—(*Observations sur les Effets des Vapeurs Méphytiques*, Nouv. edit., Paris, 1774.) But in apoplexy there is always oppressive, generally stertorous sleep, which never exists in asphyxy, unless, indeed, the exciting cause has only partially operated, and produced a different disease, or apoplexy instead of asphyxy; affording us a proof of what in fact we have noticed in the same view, that different maladies may issue from the same cause; according to the degree of its violence, or perhaps the accidental condition or constitution of the patient. In asphyxy, wherever we can trace any sign of diseased action, the lungs are chiefly affected; in apoplexy, the brain. In the first, the irritability of the system is sudden and total; in the second, it is progressive and partial. In the former, the patient is often restored after all the common symptoms of death have for some minutes, perhaps for nearly an hour, fixed upon him: in genuine apoplexy, this is never the case. The appearances on the dissection of drowned animals are very accurately given by Dr. Curry, and precisely coincide with the distinction here offered. The vessels of the brain were found in every instance free from distention or any other morbid condition, while the lungs were overloaded.

The author has observed that the immediate cause of asphyxy, or, in other words, an occlusion of the larynx, may be partial, and, in such case, give a tendency to apoplectic symptoms. And in effect, wherever the larynx or glottis is only imperfectly closed, we meet with such a tendency; and it is on this account that the face of those who die by hanging is more generally turgid, and the muscles give proof of more convulsive action than the face of those who die by drowning; for in the former case, either from a rigidity in the coats of the larynx, or from the rope not being properly applied, a small current of air is often capable of moving backward and forward for some time, and particularly in suicides, many of whom suffer much before they die, in consequence of applying the rope very bunglingly, and whose cheeks, lips, eyes, and tongue, are peculiarly turgid and prominent. The reason of this may be partly collected from the history already given, in the Physiological Proem to the third class, of the state of the heart in the act of dying. The immediate cause of the contraction or systole of the heart, we observed, has not been satisfactorily settled: but we may safely affirm, that a part of this cause, if not the whole, depends on the change, whatever that change consists in, which takes place in the blood during its ventilation in the lungs, by which it is rendered more active and stimulant; for as this change gradually subsides in those who are in the act of dying, the heart contracts more feebly; and when, with the last expiration of air, it ceases altogether, the heart as instantly contracts no more: the consequence of which is, that the lungs, the heart, and the larger vessels in the vicinity of the heart, are usually found filled with blood, the smaller vessels empty, and the general surface of the body pale. Now whatever has a power of instantaneously cutting off inspiration must necessarily produce the same effect: and hence, as we have already observed, the gorged state of the lungs, and the livid hue of the countenance, in most cases of suffocation by drowning; and, consequently, the only reason why the lungs are not quite so full, and the countenance more turgid, in most cases of suffocation by hanging, is that, from the inexpert manner in which the rope is usually applied, and the necessary admission of a certain portion of air to the lungs, the heart is for some time able to contract feebly, and to keep up a feeble circulation, while the pressure of the rope on the jugulars prevents a ready return of the blood from the head, and consequently accumulates it in all the vessels of the face; and hence, the more inexpertly this operation is performed, the more turgid these vessels must become, and the more apoplectic the general appearance.

It is the same, as we shall presently have occasion to notice more fully, with persons who are exposed to the action of carbonic acid gas or other mephitic vapours, so far lowered or intermixed with respirable air as to render them incapable of destroying life instantly; in which cases there has not only been sometimes a feeble prolongation of the circulation, but even a stertorous breathing, and many other symptoms of apoplexy, of which we shall have to speak further under the next variety.

There are some of the narcotic poisons that seem to act in the same manner. Given in a full dose, they destroy life instantly; but in an under-dose the circulation is continued feebly, and apoplectic symptoms ensue. Thus, according to Mr. Brodie's experiments, infusion of tobacco, when *injected into the intestines*, and the upas antiar, when applied to a wound, have a power of rendering the heart insensible to the stimulus of the blood, and thus suddenly stopping the circulation; while alcohol, the juice of the leaves of aconite, the woorara, essential oil of almonds, whether applied to wounded surfaces or taken internally, produce death by destroying the functions of the brain, while they act only indirectly on the circulation.

In like manner, De Haen gives one instance of apoplectic signs discovered on the dissection of a criminal who had been publicly executed by hanging; in which the pia mater was found unusually florid, the vessels of the brain turgid, and some degree of serous effusion had taken place under the tunica arachnoides: but in this case he found, also, that the lungs were equally

A a 2

overloaded, and that the rope had not pressed upon the trachea, but upon the part lying between the scutiform cartilage and the os hyoides, and consequently that the compression had been imperfect.—(*Rat. Med., continuat.*, tom. i., part ii., 8vo.)

But, except in cases where the occlusion of the trachea has not been entire, the patient who suffers from asphyxy produced by hanging is as void of apoplectic symptoms as he who suffers the same disease from drowning. In the dogs hanged by way of experiment by De Haen (*Abhandlung über die art. des Todes der Ertrunkenen, Ernheukten, und Erstikten*, Wien, 1772), and cut down as soon as they were dead, and in those drowned by Dr. Goodwin,* there was an equal absence of apoplectic signs; and, in truth, wherever an executioner does his duty completely, the death is too sudden to allow of accumulation as its cause. By the double effect, however, of stopping the circulation and obstructing the passage of the air, the public punishment of hanging, when dexterously conducted, is probably attended with very little pain. It has been said of late, that another, and indeed a chief cause of the suddenness of the death hereby produced, is to be found in a luxation of one of the upper vertebræ. Such an effect may take place at times upon our public scaffolds, on which the hardened criminal jumps from the gallows to produce a rapid result, but it is rarely met with in the private retreat of the more timid suicide.†

That a total obstruction to the respiration, moreover, is the chief cause of death in hanging, is clear from the cases in which the asphyxy has been cured by inflation of the lungs after the unhappy wretch has been cut down; and from one or two instances, in which the individual has escaped death from an ossification of the trachea; of which we have a few curious examples in Bonet and Fallopius (*Bonet.*, lib. vii., sect. xii., obs. ii.; *Fallop.*, tom. i., obs. vi.); and more particularly from the case of Inetta de Balsham, stated by Dr. Plott in his Natural History of Staffordshire; who having been hung, in the reign of Henry VI., according to the due form of law, was cut down alive, after suspension from nine o'clock on Monday till later than sunrise on the ensuing Tuesday; in consequence of which she received the king's

pardon. Dr. Plott ascribes this extraordinary escape to an ossification of the larynx. "She could not," says he, "be hanged, upon account that the larynx or upper part of her windpipe was turned to bone."—(*Hist.*, p. 292.)

It has hence been occasionally proposed to save a criminal condemned to the gallows by introducing a silver cannula into the trachea. It is commouly reported that such an attempt was in agitation among the friends of the unfortunate Dr. Dodd, but we have no reason to believe it was actually tried.

The following experiment, however, as related by Dr. Curry, is also demonstrative as to the immediate organ through which the attack of death is received in hanging. It was performed at Edinburgh, many years ago, by the senior Dr. Monro, and, in the language of Dr. Curry, "clearly proves that the exclusion of air from the lungs is the immediate cause of death. A dog was suspended by the neck with a cord, an opening having been previously made in the windpipe below the place where the cord was applied, so as to admit air into the lungs. In this state he was allowed to hang for three quarters of an hour, during which time both the circulation and breathing went on. He was then taken down without appearing to have suffered much from the experiment.* The cord was now shifted from above to below the opening made into the windpipe, so as to prevent the ingress of air into the lungs, and the animal being again suspended, he was completely dead in a few minutes."†

---

* A case is recorded by Dr. Mahon, in which this expedient was tried by a criminal for preventing the fatal interruption of respiration by the cord.—(*Méd. Légale et Police Méd.*, tom. iii., p. 62.) In the beginning of the last century, a butcher, named Gordon, was condemned to be hanged at the Old Bailey for highway robbery. Having amassed a great deal of money by his dishonest practices, he tempted a young surgeon, by the offer of very high remuneration, to make an opening low down in the trachea, and then pass a small cannula into it. This was secretly accomplished p   to the execution. After the body had been suspended the usual time, it was taken down, consigned to the relations, and quickly removed to a neighbouring house. The surgeon immediately took some blood from the jugular vein, and tried every means calculated to restore animation. Gordon opened his eyes, gave a deep sigh, but expired a few minutes afterward. The failure was attributed to the great weight of the body, which increased the violence done to the parts compressed by the rope.—Ed.

† Observations, p. 71. It was first clearly proved by Bichat, that the primary effect of the circulation of venous blood is on the brain, and that this effect extends, through the medium of the same organ, to the whole nervous system. On this subject the following reflections by Dr. Roget are judicious:—" The first, in point of time, in the series of phenomena consequent upon the suspension of the arterializing process, is the affection of the brain. Were this the sole effect directly produced by the want of oxygen, or superabundance of carbon in the blood, then might asphyxia be ranged under the head of apoplexy ; and the subsequent failure of the circulation would be

---

* Connexion of Life with Respiration, or an experimental Inquiry into the Effects of Submersion, Strangling, &c., Lond., 1788.

† The dislocation spoken of is asserted to have happened in certain executions formerly at Lyons, where the executioner used to communicate to the body of the criminal a particular rotary motion, or twist, at the moment of the fall; but at St. Bartholomew's hospital, the bodies of numerous criminals executed at Newgate have been dissected, and though the state of the cervical vertebræ was particularly examined, no luxation was found to have taken place. Respecting the degree of pain experienced by persons who die by hanging or drowning, an interesting quotation from Dr. Elliotson's lectures has been inserted in the form of a note to Dr. Good's observations on epilepsy in the present volume, p. 364.—Ed.

Asphyxy from submersion has been very generally accounted for, even by many who have regarded it as an effect of suffocation, by supposing the suffocation produced by a rush of the water into the cavity of the lungs, which prevents the access of air, and consequently of respiration. This idea, first, perhaps, advanced by Galen, has been in modern times adopted by Haller, Goodwin, Pouteau, and indeed most physiologists, and attempted to be supported by various experiments on drowned cats. It is now well ascertained, however, that, in many cases from drowning, not a drop of water enters into the lungs; that where it does enter, the quantity is, for the most part, very small; and that, whether small or large, it passes the trachea after death instead of before it, and consequently cannot be a cause of death.

The immediate cause, as in the case of suspension, is suffocation. The glottis is extremely irritable: the access of the surrounding water produces a rigid or entastic spasm upon its muscles; and the rima is as completely closed against the entrance of air as in the case of a cord round the throat. And hence, the suffocation often produced by a very small substance of any other kind accidentally thrust into or stimulating its aperture, as a minute crust of bread, a hair or blade of grass, a peach, or even a grape-stone; to which last Anacreon is well known to have fallen a victim.

How long the living principle may, under these circumstances, remain attached to the animal frame, and afford a chance of recovery, is not ascertained, with any degree of accuracy, even in the present day; and the answer to the question

must, in a considerable measure, depend upon the degree of irritability, or perhaps the idiosyncrasy, of the individual. M. Brodie is reported to have asserted in his Lectures before the College of Surgeons, that "when the action of the heart has ceased after the suspension of the breathing, or even has become so feeble as no longer to be able to maintain the circulation, it can never be restored by *artificially* inflating the lungs." This may be true: but we have innumerable proofs of a *natural* restoration of both these organs to healthy action after such action has ceased for many minutes, perhaps for many hours, in *Catalepsia* or *Trance.*

It has been known, however, from a very early age, that torpitude from drowning may be induced and continue for some minutes, without much danger: since this, as we have already observed, was a common practice among the Greeks and Romans for the cure of lyssa; and was carried by Van Helmont so far, that he would not suffer the individual to be raised from under the water till the psalm *Miserere* had been solemnly chanted, which was the measure of time he allowed. If the submersion have not exceeded five minutes, and no blow against a stone or other violence have coincided, persons will usually be found to recover without much difficulty. After a quarter of an hour, recovery is not common; and after twenty minutes or half an hour, it is nearly hopeless. Divers, from habit, are able to remain under water for three minutes; but, according to Dr. Edwards of Paris, this is the longest period.—(*De l'Influence des Agens Physiques sur la Vie,* &c., Paris, 8vo. 1824.) Young animals require less change of

---

a consequence of the impaired energy of the nervous powers which maintain the energy of the heart. But this can scarcely be admitted to be the sole cause of death; because the motion of the heart in asphyxia is arrested much sooner than it ever is in simple apoplexy. We find, indeed, that in the latter disease the heart continues to beat for many hours, or even days, after the destruction of the faculties of sensation and consciousness; and it appears at length to stop principally in consequence of the cessation of breathing, which always takes place when the abolition of the powers of voluntary motion has proceeded a certain length. So that, in fact, it may more properly be said, that apoplexy proves fatal by inducing a state of asphyxia, than that asphyxia is merely a species of apoplexy, as it has been erroneously classed in some systems of nosology."—(Dr. Roget in Cyclop. of Practical Med., art. Asphyxia.) While this physician admits that a paralytic affection of the pulmonary capillaries, rendering them incapable of transmitting blood through them, is one of the principal causes of the cessation of the heart's action, he considers it very probable that the diminution of its energy, occasioned by the circulation of venous blood through its substance, contributes in a great degree to the same effect. Dr. Roget does not, however, entirely adopt Bichat's views of the latter point. "The cessation of the action of the heart," says he, "was accounted for by Bichat on the supposition that it was itself paralyzed by the deleterious qualities of the venous blood, which, by entering the coronary arteries, penetrated its muscular substance, and destroyed its irritability. If we were to admit this doctrine,

however, this obvious difficulty would present itself in accounting for the renewal of the contractions of that organ in the re-establishment of respiration; namely, that the very power to which it must owe the restoration of its irritability, by the propulsion of fresh arterial blood through its vessels, has, on this hypothesis, been itself destroyed; and, therefore, the means of recovering it do not exist. Resuscitation from asphyxia would, if this were true, be impossible. But, since daily experience shows us that the heart may be made to renew its contractions even some time after they have ceased, we are forced to conclude that the organ still retains, under these circumstances, a considerable share of irritability, ready to be called into action when a proper stimulus is applied. On the renewal of the action of the pulmonary capillaries, by which means a fresh supply of arterial blood is poured into the left auricle and ventricle, these cavities are urged by their appropriate stimulus again to contract and renew the circulation. Arterial blood being thus again diffused over the system, imparts its vivifying influence to all the organs; their suspended functions are resumed, and animation is restored."—See Cyclop. of Pract. Med., art. Asphyxia.) In confirmation of these views, Dr. Roget refers to the experiments of Dr. Kay (Edin. Med. and Surg. Journ., vol. xxix.), and of Dr. Edwards (De l'Influence des Agens Physiques sur la Vie, part i., chap. i., and part iv., chap. iv.), which tend to prove, that when venous blood is made to circulate through the substance of muscles, it contributes to support their irritability in a certain degree, although less effectually than arterial blood.—Ed.

respirable air than those that are old. Dr. Edwards has known puppies live under water fifty-four minutes, though their voluntary motions had ceased in four minutes alone.

The first report of the establishment for the recovery of drowned persons at Paris, divides the cases that had occurred to it into three classes, the first of which includes those that were restored to life, and comprehends twenty-three instances. Of these one recovered after having been three quarters of an hour under water ; four after having been half an hour, and three after a quarter of an hour ; the rest after a still shorter period.—(*Détail des Succès de l'Etablissement que la Ville de Paris a faite en faveur des Personnes Noyées*, &c., Paris, 1773.) Of twelve dogs drowned by De Haen for the purpose of experiment, not a single one was recovered, though only confined under water for a few minutes. It is very possible, however, that in these cases, the force necessary to keep them submerged may have considerably added to the extent of the mortality. Among mankind, where no such force is applied, this eminent physiologist conceives, that one in sixteen is no unfavourable average of the portion that recover.—(*Rat. Med. Cont.*, tom. i., part ii.)

There are cases, indeed, of recovery from drowning after a submersion of some hours ; but these are rare and wonderful, and some of them altogether incredible : for we have histories of recovery after eighteen hours (*Pechlin, De Aëris et Alimentorum Defectu et Vita sub Aquis*, Kiel, 1676, 8vo.), four-and-twenty hours (*Lepi, Submersos per 24 horas vitam protrahere posse*, Rom., 1670), and even three days (*Eph. Nat. Cur.*, dec. i., ann. vi., vii., obs. 20), while some of the retailers of the marvellous have stated intervals of fifteen days, and in one instance, related with much gravity, not less than seven weeks.—(Id., obs. 125, 130, 192.) From all which, however, we may at least learn the useful lesson of the necessity of redoubling our exertions when called upon for medical aid, and not of despairing very early.

Dr. Edwards of Paris instituted some singular experiments on the Batrachian amphibials (*reptiles* of the Linnéan system), and especially on frogs and salamanders, to determine how long the living principle may continue in a state of asphyxy, which afford some light on the subject before us in at least two important points. He has first clearly ascertained, that the rapidity of death depends very considerably upon the temperature of the water in which the experiments are made, compared with the actual temperature of the medium in which the animal has been living for some time antecedently : for that frogs, taken in November from an atmospheric temperature of 50° and immersed in water of the same temperature, lived from five hours and ten minutes to eleven hours and forty minutes, being double the length of time they lived in water of the same temperature in summer. Whence it is probable, that the relative speed or tardiness with which a man dies in submersion, depends partly upon the temperature of the atmosphere in which he has lived for several preceding days,

compared with that of the water at the time of the accident. And secondly, he has satisfactorily established, that frogs and salamanders, deprived of the heart, continue to live for a longer period in the air, than in water whose air has been withdrawn from it. At the end of four hours, the salamanders which were in the water appeared to be dead, though they manifested some degree of activity on being pinched or agitated. At the end of nine hours, however, they were all entirely void of living power ; while those which were retained in the air lived for twenty-four or twenty-six hours. The frogs lived four hours under the water, and five out of it. The experiment was varied by suffocating other reptiles of the same kind, their heads being closely tied up in a piece of bladder, instead of cutting out their hearts ; and the result was in every instance consentaneous. Dr. Edwards hence concludes, and the conclusion seems well supported, that air has an influence on the economy of animals, independently of its action through respiration ; and that this influence is probably exerted through the medium of the skin.[*] And we may hence see why recovery from hanging is more frequent than from drowning, under like intervals of protraction.

Unfortunately, we have no means of determining whether the vital principle lies latent in the body or has utterly dropped its connexion. Want of heat is no more to be relied on than cessation of the pulse or of breathing : for while in submersion, heat, in consequence of its rapid absorption by the surrounding elements, is one of the first properties of life that disappears, whether the patient recover or not ; in death from convulsions and various other sudden causes, it often continues for hours, and sometimes even for days after the event, cheating the by-standers with an empty and unfounded hope of a restoration never to take place. The present author was a few years since sent for in haste to a female domestic of Mr. Salmon of Mecklenburgh-square, who however died under a convulsion-fit before his arrival. In the evening, nearly twelve hours afterward, he was again requested to attend, as, notwithstanding the body had been laid out from the first and merely covered with a sheet, it still possessed a considerable degree of warmth. He was sorry to repress a hope which he found fondly and highly cherished, but the symptom was illusive, and the heat gradually disappeared. On the decease of a robust and corpulent lady, whom he also attended in Bedford-row, and who died of a spasmodic asthma, this symptom continued, or rather showed itself afresh, eight-and-forty hours after death, so that the author was requested to attend at the time the body was on the point of being put into the coffin. In this case, the heat was produced by putrefaction ; for the body was livid and offensive. Bartholine has an example or two of the same kind ; and the Ephemerides, among other cases less marvellous, one in which

[*] Mémoires sur l'Asphyxie considerée dans les Batraciens. Paris, 1817 ; also, De l'Influence des Agens Physiques sur la Vie, &c. Paris, 8vo., 1824.

the heat is said to have continued till the fourth day after death : and which should no doubt fall within the solution just given.—(*Ephem. Nat. Cur.*, dec. ii., ann. iv., obs. 18.)

As heat has occasionally maintained itself for hours after death, so also has perspiration. Paullini mentions a case in which tears flowed from the eyes (Cent. iii., obs. 10, Franc., 1698, 8vo.) ; Riedlin another, in which the eyes themselves recovered their brightness (*Lin. Med.*, 1696, p. 203) ; and Hagendorn a third, in which the face swelled and looked red.—(Cent. iii., obs. 46.) In all these cases, we have proofs of a lingering of the irritable principle in particular parts after the sentient principle has totally disappeared. And hence, in a few instances, some of the muscles have been thrown into irregular action, the penis has become erect (*Eph. Nat. Cur.*, dec. i., ann. ix., x., obs. 34, 158), the jaws have opened and shut, as though masticating (*Commerc. Nor.*, 1732, pp. 82, 90, 173) ; and, as is well known, the heart, when dissected from the pericardium, has leaped from the table.*

In attempting a CURE of suffocation BY SUBMERSION, the two grand means by which we are to operate are those of warmth and inflation of the lungs. The body should be quietly conveyed to a warm and dry situation, and rubbed all over with moderate stimulants, as diluted flower of mustard, or the warmer balsams ; while the nostrils are plied with ammonia, and the eyes exposed to a strong light.† But a restoration of the action of the lungs is chiefly to

---

* The post mortem appearances of drowned persons, as stated by different writers, vary. " Upon dissection" says a distinguished authority in medical jurisprudence (Paris and Fonblanque, vol. ii., p. 36), " we shall perceive the vessels of the brain more or less gorged with blood ; in the trachea, a watery and bloody froth will be found ; the lungs will appear expanded, full of frothy mucus, and generally livid ; the right cavities of the heart gorged with blood, the left nearly empty ; and it has been sometimes noticed that the blood remains fluid, and follows after every incision by the scalpel." Orfila believes that a greater or less quantity of water is generally inspired during the agony of drowning : he remarks (Dict. de Méd., tome xx., p. 25), " I have examined at La Morgue the bodies of many who have been drowned, which had been in the water for a few hours only, and I have frequently found a froth or frothy fluid in the trachea and bronchi." Dr. E. J. Cox has rendered it very probable (N. A. Med. and Surg. Journal, Oct., 1826), that water seldom enters into the lungs before the last moments of life, when the glottis loses that organic sensibility which generally prevents the entrance of a foreign fluid into the trachea.—D.

† The Humane Society, in their Report for 1831, very properly recommend the wet clothes to be immediately taken off, and the body to be wiped, cleaned, and wrapped in dry clothes or blankets, so as to prevent evaporation, and the effects of exposure to a cold medium. The body should then be carried in the recumbent posture on the back, with the head and breast raised. As soon as it has arrived in the room for its reception, it should be stripped and covered with warm blankets. If the mouth and nostrils be obstructed, they must be thoroughly cleansed. The lungs are then to be

---

be aimed at ; and for this purpose, a full expiration of warm air from the lips of a by-stander should be repeatedly forced into the patient's mouth, and his nostrils held close to prevent its escape by that channel. Inflation may also be attempted by a pair of common bellows ; or, which is far better, if it can be readily procured, by a pair of bellows communicating with a pipe introduced into the larynx, or, as some have recommended, into an aperture made between the rings of the trachea. Stimulating injections of acrid purgatives, or camphire, ammonia, and brandy, or other spirits, have often been introduced with success into the rectum, and sometimes injections of warm air alone ; and it would be better that the air introduced into the lungs should be also moderately warm. Besides this active process, it may be possible to convey some warm and cordial stimulant, as ammonia, or the compound spirit of lavender, into the stomach by means of a syringe ; or what may probably in this case answer better, by a piece of sponge, impregnated with one of these, fixed to the end of a small rod of whalebone. In the Berlin Transactions is recommended the use of a *ventriculi excutia*, or stomach-brush, to produce internal friction in the same manner.

There is no family of diseases in which the internal use of phosphorus seems to promise more success. The German physicians have employed it very generally in the last ebb of typhus fevers, in apparent death from convulsion (*De Phosphori, loco Medicamenti ad sumpti, virtute medicâ*, &c., *Anat. J. Gabi*, Mentz), and in most cases in which the nervous power has been suddenly annihilated. It is one of the most powerful stimulants we know, and in asphyxy should be given to the amount of two or three grains for a dose, dissolved in ether.*

Venesection, and especially that of the jugular vein (*Jo. Wences Nachtigal, Dissertatio de Submersis*, Vindobon, 8vo.), has been strenuously recommended by physicians of high authority ; and wherever there is reason to believe that the drowning has followed a sudden fit of apoplexy, the recommendation is rational enough ; provided it can be practised with effect. But, commonly speaking, it is advice to no purpose, for the blood will not flow ; and in other cases, if it would, such depletion, we have reason to believe, would do more injury by weakening, than good by removing what is erroneously supposed to be congestion. It may occasionally, perhaps, be serviceable as soon as the living powers begin

inflated, and dry warm flannels, bags of warm grains, or bottles or bladders of warm water, applied to the epigastric region, the soles of the feet, and other parts of the body. Bleeding ought never to be employed in this stage of the process ; though it may become necessary when the circulation has returned, and reaction has taken place.—Ed.

* With regard to stomach-brushes and stomach-mops, the editor coincides with Dr. Roget in thinking the proposal of them altogether extravagant.—(See Cyclop. of Pract. Med., art. ASPHYXIA.) The commendations also bestowed on the virtues of phosphorus in asphyxy are not entitled to any confidence.—ED.

to show themselves, but it is rarely to be tried in the first instance.

Returning life is first usually discoverable by the symptoms of sighing, gasping, twitching, or subsultus, slight palpitation, or pulsation of the heart ; in effect, by a weak or clonic action in most of the organs. Our efforts should here be redoubled, for the feeble spark still requires to be solicited, and nourished into a permanent flame—and has often disappeared from a relaxation of labour. A spoonful or two of warm wine, or wine and water, should now be given by the mouth as soon as the power of swallowing is sufficiently restored ; which should, be shortly succeeded by a little light, warm, and nourishing food of any kind, with gently laxative clysters, a well-heated bed, and perfect tranquillity.

I have dwelt the longer upon this subject, because the general principles of the remedial treatment here recommended apply to most of the other varieties under which asphyxy or suspended animation is to be traced ; and the reader who is desirous of following the operative plan into a still minuter detail, will do well to consult Dr. Cullen's letter to Lord Cathcart, the president of the Board of P$_{olice}$ in Scotland, concerning the recovery of persons drowned and seemingly dead, an able extract of which is given in the Medical Commentaries of Edinburgh.— (Vol. iii., p. 243.) We may observe, however, that in attempting the recovery of those who have been hung, and particularly who have inexpertly hung themselves, bleeding from the jugulars may be more frequently found necessary than in attending the drowned, since in the former, as we have very fully observed above, there is a greater tendency to apoplectic symptoms than in the latter : yet, even here, the quantity abstracted needs not be large.

In the SECOND VARIETY of asphyxy, or that from an inhalation of irrespirable auras, death in many cases takes place instantaneously ; and consequently, for reasons already advanced, the general surface of the body, and even the countenance itself, is pale.—(*Brukser von den Ungewissheit der Kennzeichen des Todes.*) Yet as the gas is often in some degree diluted with atmospheric air, the circulation, and even the breathing, are occasionally continued for some time in a feeble and imperfect state, and the asphyxy is united with symptoms of apoplexy, or genuine apoplexy takes place in its stead. In Cornwall and other mining regions, these gases are vulgarly called *damps*, from the German *dampff*, " a vapour or exhalation."

The direct effect of such gases, when in a concentrated state, is utterly and instantaneously to destroy the irritability and sensibility of the nervous system, of which we have examples perpetually occurring in persons who incautiously descend foul beer-casks or the shafts of mines. By what means, however, such exhalations, when they have penetrated the lungs, become so rapidly communicated to the nervous system as to prove instantly destructive, we do not seem to be very well informed. Absorption would be the most ready way of accounting for it ; but, till the objections thrown out by Mr.

Ellis against an absorption of oxygen or any other gas by the lungs, and which we have noticed in the Physiological Proem to our second class, are more satisfactorily replied to than they appear to have been, it is an hypothesis that can hardly be allowed. In the case of hanging or drowning, it does not seem to be owing to a direct want of irritability that the heart ceases instantly to contract, but as we have already remarked, to its being deprived of the necessary stimulus, which is no longer afforded by the lungs, however they may act, in providing it. Yet, in the present case, there seems to be not only a cessation of action for want of a proper stimulus, but a total abstraction of both sensific and motific power ; and this as completely in one part of the frame as in another.

The gases of the description before us that are found most fatal, are the carbonic acid, hydrogen, nitrogen,[*] and several of a more compound kind, which are thrown forth from putrefying animal and vegetable substances, and especially from cemeteries, on opening fresh graves, in which the process of decomposition is proceeding rapidly, and the concentrated effluvium bursts forth with an intolerable stench. Of the powerful effects of this last exhalation, Fourcroy has furnished us with a very particular and striking account from the narration of grave-diggers examined for the purpose : from which it appears that those who are immediately hanging over a corpse whose abdomen is accidentally penetrated with a pickaxe, often fall down in a state of senselessness and apparent death, while persons who happen to be at a little distance, and receive the exhalation in a form diluted with atmospheric air, are attacked with nausea, vertigo, faintness, and tremours, which continue for some hours.

The most common of these gases is the carbonic acid, which is chiefly found in the guise of a torpefying vapour in close rooms where charcoal has been burnt; at the bottom of large beer-casks, or of wells, and in many natural caverns in the earth's surface. Its weight prevents it from escaping readily, even where there is an accession of atmospheric air ; and its want of smell, when pure, prevents it from being detected otherwise than by its effects. As it will not support flame, the common and easiest test, where it is supposed to exist, is that of a lighted candle, which is well known to be extinguished immediately, if this gas be present in a quantity sufficient to be injurious to respiration.

---

[*] From the experiments of Sir Humphrey Davy, it would seem that hydrogen and azotic gases have no positively injurious operation on the system. The voluntary respiration of them for a short time is unattended with danger. The deviations from this result, occasionally noticed, are ascribable to an admixture of other gases, particularly that of carbonic acid. The phenomena exhibited by animals confined in hydrogen or azotic gas are those of simple asphyxia. They are not killed at once by any actively deleterious principle of such gases, as they are when carbonic acid gas, carburetted hydrogen, and certain other kinds of air enter the lungs.—ED.

Nitrogen and hydrogen, when pure, have probably as little smell as carbonic acid gas ; but they are generally combined with other gases, sulphur, carbon, or phosphorus. The first, formerly denominated phlogistic air, and sometimes mofette, is thrown forth largely during the decomposition of animal matter, and in a small degree during that of vegetable matter. Combined with hydrogen, it forms ammonia ; with oxygen, nitric acid. Fourcroy asserts that it possesses a peculiar and distinct odour, resembling that of fishes just beginning to putrefy ; but this is probably at all times produced by its combination with other materials. It seems chiefly concerned in giving the greenish colour to parts, and especially muscular parts, in a putrid state. In some gases of this kind, a candle will burn freely.

Hydrogen issues also from fecal matter, and in combination with sulphur, phosphorus, and carbon, produces the chief part of the nauseating and putrid stench thrown forth from decomposing animal and vegetable substances. It is emitted in a much purer state from the sides of coal and metallic mines, and often exists in considerable abundance without being perceived by the nostrils. If mixed with an equal proportion of oxygen, it may be breathed for about an hour without any great inconvenience. If inhaled beyond this time, or in a more concentrated form, it has a great tendency to occasion the effects we have just noticed, lower the irritability of the animal frame, and induce stupor or an inclination to sleep.

The fumes of mercury, lead, and some other metallic substances, when highly concentrated, seem to operate not very dissimilarly to those of charcoal, and give a check to the mobility of the nervous power at once.

The fumes of charcoal are generally inhaled in a diluted form, but they are still highly deleterious, and produce asphyxy more or less complete, according to the degree of concentration, and in some cases according to the strength or weakness of frame of those who are exposed to them. We have a striking illustration of this in the case of two persons communicated by Dr. Babington to the Medico-Chirurgical Society, who had gone to bed in a room in which a charcoal fire was kept up through the whole of the night, with the gas of which the surrounding atmosphere was strongly impregnated. According to the principle we have endeavoured to establish, we ought here, from the dilution of the vapour, to expect, that whatever tendency there might be to asphyxy would be united with a tendency to apoplexy. And such we find to have been the fact ; for, of these two persons, the younger and less vigorous, a boy of thirteen, died apparently during his sleep, and without commotion ; while the elder and more robust, a man of thirty-eight, was found, upon being called in the morning between six and seven, in an apoplectic state, with a swollen, projecting tongue, suffused and prominent eyes, and laborious breathing.[*]

---

[*] The power of resisting the effects of carbon-

The patient, if any degree of sensibility remain, should in this variety be freely exposed to the open air, instead of to a heated atmosphere, as in the preceding : and if he can swallow, acidulated liquids should be given him. If insensible, cold water should be dashed on his face ; strong vinegar, and especially aromatic vinegar, be rubbed about his nostrils, and held under them, and stimulating clysters be injected, as recommended under the first variety. The lungs should be inflated with the warm breath of a healthy man, or, which is better, with oxygen gas.

A proper use of voltaic electricity is also in many instances found highly serviceable. No advantage, however, is likely to accrue from passing the electric aura across the chest, directly through the heart and lungs, which is a common practice. The fluid should be transmitted along the channel of the nerves, from the seat of the phrenic nerve in the neck, to the seat of the diaphragm, or that of the par vagum immediately under the sterno-mastoid muscles, and that of the great sympathetic nerve, which send forth branches to the heart.[*] In Dr. Babington's case, the application of voltaic electricity surprisingly increased the power of the muscles of respiration, but appeared rather to diminish the action of the heart. It was hence used alternately with a forcible inhalation of oxygen gas, and various external stimulants. Venesection was tried, but does not seem to have been beneficial. The man recovered in a few days.[†]

M. Portal recommends opening the external jugular vein ; but the blood will rarely flow from any vein, and is still more rarely succeeded by any advantage, even where it is obtained. And if every other remedy fail, he advises bronchotomy, and a scarification of the feet and hands.[‡]

---

ic acid gas is supposed to be less in youth than in more mature age. The boy referred to in the text was found completely dead ; but the man eventually recovered. A similar case is reported by Bourdon, of a woman thirty-five years of age, who resolved to destroy her own life and that of her daughter, a child five years old.—(Principes de Physiologie Médicale, partie ii., p. 650.) Having shut herself up with the little girl in a closet, with a large brasier of burning charcoal, the bodies were afterward found extended on the floor. The mother was soon restored ; but no means were of any avail for the recovery of the child.—En.

[*] Greg. Consp. Med. Theor. Hüfeland, Diss. usus Ver. Elect. in Asphyxiâ, Goet., 1783.

[†] Notwithstanding the text maintains the inutility of bloodletting in cases of asphyxia from carbonic acid gas, the abstraction of a few ounces of blood has in some cases been found useful, co-operating with other means in relieving the oppressed state of the lungs. Even the instructive case of Dr. Babington (Medico-Chirurg. Trans., vol. i.) proves the value of the practice. In most cases, however, the operation is impracticable. In Russia, where from the mode of burning fuel asphyxia from irrespirable gases is not unfrequent, the common mode of treatment is to rub the bodies with snow ; a practice followed, it is said, with the happiest results.—D.

[‡] Obs. sur les Effets des Vapeurs Méphytiques

' The sprinkling or dashing of water upon the body seems to be useful, by having a tendency to rouse the vessels on the surface to contract.*

In the THIRD or ELECTRIC VARIETY, the whole system appears to be not so much rendered inirritable to stimulants, as to be suddenly exhansted of its entire stock of nervous power, like a Leyden vial upon an application of the discharging rod; in consequence of which the limbs are flexible, the countenance pale, and the blood uncoagulable. The mode in which the electricity is communicated is of little importance; for, if sufficiently powerful for the purpose, real or apparent death is instantaneously produced, whether the stroke flow from lightning, an electric battery, or a voltaic trough.

Upon plants, on the contrary, we often find a stroke of lightning of the same intensity occasion very different effects in different kinds or branches of the same plant, in consequence of the variety they exhibit as conducting powers. Upon some, it descends without mischief; in others, it exhausts itself on particular parts, which are withered, as though attacked by a hemiplegia. In the *betula alba*, or common birch, it never runs along the stem, but confines its stroke to the top alone, beating off the boughs in every direction.

In animal life, however, there is also a difference of effect, but only in proportion to the degree of intensity of the electric power that attacks the system; and it is curious to observe the nature of this effect. Small doses of electricity prove a powerful stimulus to the nervous function, increase the flow of sensorial energy, and augment the irritability of the muscles: while a violent shock, as we have just seen, exhausts the nervous system instantaneously, carries off the entire stock from the animal fabric, and leaves the muscular fibres flaccid and flagging. This singular result is extended to the blood, and extended to it in both cases; for its coagulability, or the firmness of its texture, is increased by the application of small doses of electricity; while the shock of lightning, which renders the muscles lax and uncontracted, renders the blood loose and uncoagulable. It is to this variety of effect that Mr. John Hunter makes a powerful, and certainly a very impressive appeal, in proof that the blood, though a fluid, is actuated by the same living principle as the muscular fibres.†

The general principle of medical treatment has been laid down under the first variety. Stimulants of the most active kind should be resorted to without loss of time : but of all stimulants, that of electricity, or voltaism, seems to be especially called for in the present modification of asphyxy. I do not know that it has ever been tried to any great extent in the variety before us, on the human subject, but M. Abildgaard has related a few experiments on other animals that are well worthy of attention. The animals chiefly selected were from the poultry-yard, and consisted of cocks and hens. These the action of the heart. Death took place precisely in the same manner as from a severe injury of the head, and the animal died manifestly from the destruction of the functions of the brain. The facts, that the muscles are relaxed and incapable of contraction, that the limbs do not stiffen as in other cases of death, that the blood does not coagulate, and that the body runs rapidly into a state of putrefaction, are well established : yet exceptions occur. Beccaria mentions a case of death by lightning where the body became exceedingly stiff soon after, and in one of Mr. Brodie's experiments the same occurred in the muscles of a guinea-pig. " Dr. Francis," says Dr. T. R. Beck (Med. Jurisprudence, vol. ii.), " mentions that he has seen a case where the muscles immediately became extremely rigid." "The morbid evidences of death by lightning vary exceedingly," says Dr. Francis. " Death may follow from the force of the electric fluid, and no disorganized appearances externally be observed. The electric fluid may have nearly expended its force, and occasioned partial vesications on the surface of the body; these vesications will sometimes exhibit results like those produced by scalding water; sometimes the surface will present groups of vesicular patches, or the epidermis will be destroyed; the hair of the body may be scorched. In one case I observed, the common integuments about the anterior and superior parts of the chest were raised; the lesions appeared like the cortical desquamation of a tree, and several fissures or streaks extended to the pubes. In another instance where the individual was destroyed by a vivid stroke of lightning, which entored the crown of his hat, the scalp was torn from its bony attachment, the left eye rooted out, the upper lip torn off, and the left side of the body denuded to the heel of the left foot; the abdomen swelled to an enormous extent, and the tongue protruded. In two cases the brain internally appeared overloaded and turgid; the meningeal covering was surcharged with dark blood; there was arachnitic effusion under the arachnoid membrane; and about an ounce and a half of serous effusion in the two lateral ventricles. In a third case, the brain exhibited no disorganization. In one instance the right side of the heart was surcharged, while the left was nearly empty, and there was a slight degree of effusion in the pericardium; the lungs presented many of the appearances seen in asphyxia from charcoal. In one case I have found the bladder considerably distended with urine; in another, quite empty. In four of the cases I have examined, the bodies remained flaccid, and ran speedily into incipient decomposition; the blood seemed dissolved, and would not coagulate, and the cadaverous exhalation was very conspicuous; in one, however, an adult black aged about thirty-six, the body stiffened."—D.

---

sur les Corps de l'Homme, &c., nouv. edit., Paris, 1774

* Throwing cold water on the face and breast is well known to have considerable influence in dispelling syncope. The dogs which are made the subject of experiment at the Grotto del Cane, are usually plunged into a neighbouring lake, as a means of promoting their recovery.—ED.

† But few cases of the effects of lightning on the human body are recorded. Paris and Fonblanque refer to the dissection of a man killed by lightning in the London Philosoph. Transactions, but it contains nothing remarkable. Mr. Brodie concluded from an experiment on a guinea-pig which was killed by repeated strokes of electricity, that the electric shock did not destroy the irritability of the muscular fibre, nor did it affect

were first rendered asphyctic, or apparently dead, by a strong shock of electricity passed through the head ; and afterward recovered by another shock passed through from the chest to the back, the animal instantly walking about as if nothing had happened. M. Abildgaard does not say what interval he allowed between the shocks thus administered : but he observed, that where no second shock was employed, the apparent was converted into real death ; for the animal, in no instance, showed any tokens of resuscitation : and he observed farther, that if the second shock were thrown through the head like the first, instead of from the chest to the back, the same lifelessness continued, and no benefit whatever was produced.—(*Societatis Med. Havniensis Collectanea*, &c., vol. ii., art. *Tentamina Electrica in Animalibus*.)*

In FROSTBITTEN ASPHYXY, or that produced by intense cold, the limbs are rigid, and the countenance pale and shrivelled.† This variety is always preceded by an insurmountable desire to sleep, which the utmost exertion of the will is unable to overpower. The sleep is, in most cases, fatal, and becomes the sleep of death.— (*Rhazes ad. Almans.*, tract. vi., cap. v., vii.)

---

* Dr. A. H. Stevens of New-York has recorded a case of injury by lightning successfully treated by copious venesection : the amount of blood drawn within ten days was about one hundred and twenty ounces.—(See the Medical and Surg. Register, p. 55.) In the case of Frances Gray, detailed by Dr. Paul of Kingston, Jamaica, venesection was employed three times during the treatment, and with the happiest results.—(See the Jamaica Physical Journal, vol. i., p. 354.) The public journals recently contained the case of a person struck by lightning who was restored by pouring cold water on the head for several hours. —D.

† Dr. Kellie of Leith, when speaking of the external appearance and pathological condition of two persons perishing from cold, remarks: " In reviewing the appearances observed in the dissection of these two bodies, our attention cannot fail to be arrested by the striking resemblance which the one, in almost every particular, bears to the other; in both we observed the same soundness and freshness of the bodies, in the abdomen the same congestions of the viscera, especially the same remarkable redness of the small intestines from the turgescence of their bloodvessels, the same absence of fetor, putrescence, and tympanites, the same perfection of the other viscera, with the exception of the pancreas in the woman ; in the head, the same bloodless state of the scalp, the same turgidity of the vessels on the surface of the brain, the same congestion of the sinuses, the same soundness of the cerebral texture, and the same serous effusion, *amounting in the one to nearly four ounces, in the other, to about three*." Similar appearances have been described by Quelmalz (Progr. *quo frig. acrieris in corp. human. affectus expedit*, Lipsiæ, 1755.) Rosen (Anat., p. 142) found the vessels within the cranium were much distended with blood, and Cappel (Obs. Anat.) observed great congestion of the internal viscera. Dr. Kay remarks (Treatise on Asphyxia, London, 1834, p. 309), " perhaps the most remarkable circumstance observed in these post mortem examinations is, the great effusion of serum into the ventricles of the brain."—D.

Captain Cook, in the account he has given of his first voyage round the world, has strikingly exemplified this remark in the case of Dr. Solander and Mr. (afterward Sir Joseph) Banks. " Dr. Solander," says he, " who had more than once crossed the mountains which divide Sweden from Norway, well knew that extreme cold, especially when joined with fatigue, produces a torpor and sleepiness that are almost irresistible ; he therefore conjured the company to keep moving, whatever pain it might cost them. ' Whoever sits down,' said he, ' will sleep, and whoever sleeps, will wake no more.' Dr. Solander was the first who found the inclination, against which he had warned others, irresistible, and insisted upon being suffered to lie down. He soon fell into a profound sleep, from which, however, by the exertion of Mr. Banks, he was awakened. Several others of the party very narrowly escaped ; and two of them slept, and perished from the cold."—(*Hawkesworth's Account of Voyages*, vol. ii., p. 46.)

For these symptoms, and their effects, it is easy to account. Cold, so long as the living power is capable of producing a reaction, is one of the most strenuous tonics we are possessed of, and the glow that accompanies the reaction is felt to be peculiarly vigorous and elastic. But if it exceed this proportion, and no reaction ensue, the contraction of the vessels on the surface is converted into a rigid spasm, the blood is driven into the interior, and the surface must necessarily be pale. In this extremity of temperature, moreover, cold, instead of being a tonic, is one of the most formidable sedatives in animal chymistry : it carries off the heat of the body far more rapidly than it can be recruited, and as effectually exhausts it of all its irritable and sensible power. But such exhaustion, as we have already shown under the genus PARONIRIA, is a cause of stupor or sleep, and a cause so cogent that the will is, in many cases, incapable of resisting it, and falls a prey to its power.

In applying remedial means to this modification of asphyxy, great caution is necessary respecting the employment of warmth ; and particularly where the limbs are peculiarly rigid, and under the influence of frost.* In this last case it will be generally found most advisable in the first instance, as in frostbitten limbs, to plunge the body for a few minutes into a bath

---

* " In Siberia," says Gmelin (Voyage in Siber., trad. en Fr. par Keralio, Paris, 1767, Journ., p. 381), " the frozen, pale, and insensible limbs are first rubbed with snow ; as soon as they begin to regain their sensibility, the snow is replaced by warm water. If they have been frozen a short time, the most prompt remedy is to rub them with wool. The Jakrouts employ another process, which the Russians have *also* adopted ; they cover the frozen limb with mud or clay, or with both, to bring back sensation. These substances are used also as prophylactics, and when about to travel in the cold, they cover the hands and face with a layer of them. It would seem too that turpentine, applied to a frozen limb, and then gradually exposed to heat, so to be melted in as warmly as possible, is useful."—D.

of cold seawater or salted water, at the same time that warm air may be breathed into the lungs, and the stomach and rectum gently excited by moderate stimulants : for it does not follow that, because the limbs and surface of the body are frozen from frostbite, the central parts have suffered to the same extent. After a short immersion in seawater, the body should be taken out, wiped perfectly dry, laid in flannel in a moderately warm room, and submitted to the friction of warm hands, several persons being engaged in this process simultaneously.*

SPECIES II.
CARUS ECSTASIS.
ECSTASY.

TOTAL SUSPENSION OF SENSIBILITY AND VOLUNTARY MOTION ; MOSTLY OF MENTAL POWER ; PULSATION AND BREATHING CONTINUING : MUSCLES RIGID : BODY ERECT AND INFLEXIBLE.

THERE is so close a connexion between the present and the ensuing, and, in truth, most of the ensuing species of the order before us, that they are occasionally apt to run into each other, or to exhibit a few aggregate symptoms. And on this account, they have been very differently arranged by different writers. Sauvages, and most of the continental nosologists, have regarded them as distinct genera. Dr. Mead and Dr. Cullen, as species or subdivisions of apoplexy, and Dr. Cheyne, as the same of lethargy. Dr. Cooke has treated of them more cursorily than those who are acquainted with his talents and learning could wish ; and has so far followed Dr. Cullen as to place them conjointly in a chapter under the head of apoplexy.: while Dr. Young, coinciding with the view taken in the present work, has arranged the whole as a species, under the generic name of CARUS.

To understand the nature of their distinctive symptoms, and the reason of their occasional combination, it is necessary to bear in mind the remarks offered in the Physiological Proem to the present class respecting the natural division of the nervous ramifications into sensific and motific fibres ; since it happens that some of these diseases are confined to one set, and others to another, while other diseases again extend equally to both. And hence we are able to account for disorders in which the perception or sensibility is abolished, while the irritability continues without much interference : or in which there is

* Baron Larrey, in his account of the sufferings of the French army in the Russian campaign, refers to numerous examples of soldiers, who were under the influence of exposure to intense cold, falling down completely dead on their entering warm rooms, or approaching too near to the fires of the bivouacs.—(See Campagnes ou Mém. de Chir. Militaire, t. iv.) Caloric should be communicated in the most gradual manner, and this principle is essentially requisite, not only with the view of restoring animation suspended by cold, but for the purpose of preventing the attack of chilblains, and of a rapid and uncontrollable species of gangrene, in cases where the effects of intense cold are chiefly restricted to the extreme parts of the body, the feet, hands, nose, ears, &c.—ED.

a disturbed flow or total cessation of the irritable power, with little interference with the percipient, and sometimes also with the sentient, as in some cases of paralysis : or in which there is a disturbance or cessation of all these, with the exception of a partial supply of irritative power to the involuntary organs. It will also be necessary to recollect, as we have endeavoured to show in many of the preceding pages, and particularly under the genus CLONUS, that, where there is a disturbance of the motific or irritative power, this disturbance is of two kinds, one from excess, and one from deficiency ; and that, in both cases, there is a great irregularity of action, and consequently entastic or rigid, and clonic or agitatory spasms, exhibiting by their continuation innumerable modifications.

All the divisions of the nervous system, moreover, have a natural tendency to sympathize in the same action, however combined or interchanging ; and hence, in whatever division of it a disease commences, one or more of the other divisions are peculiarly apt to participate in the affection ; and the more so, as it is not very common for abnormal actions, when once communicated, to proceed with much order or regularity ; for if trismus and tremour give us examples of such order, tetanus very generally, convulsion-fit, epilepsy, and hysteria, furnish proofs of the most capricious alternations of spastic and clonic action, or of their existing in different trains of muscles simultaneously.

These remarks peculiarly apply to ECSTASY, the species immediately before us, compared with CATALEPSY or TRANCE, the species that immediately follows. In both, the nervous influence contributory to sensibility and irritability is disturbed in its transmission or regularity of action, but not equally, nor in the same manner ; for while the transmission of the sensific principle seems to be totally suspended, that of the irritable principle continues, though with a striking deviation from the uniform tenour of health. Thus far the two diseases agree. They differ in the nature of the disturbance of the motific principle. In ecstasy, this seems to be produced in excess, and irregularly accumulated ; in consequence of which the muscles are thrown into a rigid and permanent spasm, not incurvating the body, as in the different modifications of tetanus, but maintaining it erect from an equal excess of supply to the extensor and flexor muscles. In catalepsy, on the contrary, the motific principle seems to be in deficiency rather than in excess, though it is often irregularly distributed ; and hence, while some muscles appear sufficiently supplied, the action of others, even the involuntary ones, is often peculiarly weak. Whence also the limbs, instead of resisting external force, yield to it with readiness, and assume any position that may be given to them.

In both cases, the torpitude of the external senses appears to extend to those of the mind ; for the patient, on returning to himself, has no recollection of any train of ideas that occurred to him during the fit. Yet we shall find presently, that in a few instances, the power of sight and of judging, and perhaps some other powers, do not seem completely to have failed. It deserves, however, especially to be remarked, that both these diseases are most common to persons constitutionally disposed to some mental estrangement, as melancholy or revery, hypochondriacism, or morbid elevation of mind; thus pointing out to us the outlet at which the sensorial power is carried off: for we have already seen, that under intense revery, the external senses are for the most part inactive or torpid to the impressions of surrounding objects during wakefulness; while the mind is alike dead to every thing but the train of ideas which immediately constitutes the subject of the revery. The same tendency to abstraction, though not carried so completely into effect, is often to be found in Melancholy, and still more so in that species of alusia which, in the present work, is denominated elatio, mental elevation or extravagance, and particularly the variety called elatio ecstatica, false inspiration, visionary conceits. If the person labouring under any of these be attacked at the same time with a general entasia, or rigid tetanus, erecting instead of incurvating the body, he will be thrown into an ecstasy, constituting the present species. And if instead of an excessive there be a deficient supply of irritable power, and consequently a flaccidity or flexibility of the muscles instead of a rigidity, his disease will be a catalepsy, constituting the ensuing species, with this difference alone, that in most cases of the two diseases before us, the faculties of the mind unite in the torpitude of the senses, instead of giving rise to it.

I say in most cases, and have kept to the same limitation in the specific definition: for if it be true that one of the causes of both these affections is profound contemplation or attention of mind, or some overwhelming passion, as we are told by many writers, the mind does not seem in such cases to be without ideas, nor without them in a very energetic degree. And it is to ecstasis under this modification that I am inclined to think we should refer the catochus of most of the nosologists, which they arrange in the same order as, and next to tetanus, and define a "general spastic rigidity without sensibility."

Ecstasis is of rare occurrence; its predisponent cause is unquestionably a highly nervous or irritable temperament; the exciting or occasional causes it is not easy at all times to determine. For the greater part, they seem to be of a mental character, as profound and long-continned meditation upon subjects of great interest and excitement; and terror or other violent emotions of the mind. It seems also to have proceeded, like most of the spasmodic affections already treated of, from various corporeal irritations, and particularly those of the stomach and liver, suppressed menstruation, repelled chronic eruptions, and plethora; and perhaps occasionally, as hinted by the younger M. Pinel, from an inflammation of the spinal marrow.—(*Journ. de Phys. Expér., par F. Magendie, D. M.*, &c., tom. i., Janv., 1821.) The duration of the fit varies from a few hours to two or three days. The patient rouses as from a sleep, seems languid, and complains of nausea and vertigo; evidently showing that the morbid supply of sensorial power is exhausted, and that the spasm has ceased in consequence of such exhaustion.

As the disease evidently consists in a disturbance of the balance of the sensorial power, or in an excessive production of the irritable, but a deficient or suspended production of the sensific principle, the curative intention should lead us to aim at a restoration of this balance; and hence the remedial process will run so nearly parallel with that for tetanus, that it is only necessary to refer the reader to the treatment already laid down for that disease.

Where catalepsy is connected with a morbid state of the liver, mercury given to ptyalism has often proved highly successful. Dr. Chisholm has given a very interesting case of this kind in a young lady of eighteen, of an hysterical diathesis, and in whom the ecstasy, or paroxysm of rigidity, was alternated with paroxysms of mania. "At the end of ten minutes the patient suddenly started up in bed, the muscles became at once relaxed, but maniacal distraction of mind instantly succeeded. During the maniacal state, now, it was particularly singular that, although she could not articulate a single word, and was evidently unconscious of what she did, yet she sung some very beautiful airs with a sweetness of tone and correctness of measure extremely interesting and affecting: at the end of ten minutes, her head suddenly and unexpectedly dropped, and she fell back into the state of rigidity."—(*Of the Climate and Diseases of Tropical Countries*, p. 160, 8vo., Lond., 1822.) She finally recovered by the use of mercury.

SPECIES III.

CARUS CATALEPSIA.

CATALEPSY. TRANCE.

TOTAL SUSPENSION OF SENSIBILITY AND VOLUNTARY MOTION; MOSTLY OF MENTAL POWER; PULSATION AND BREATHING CONTINUING; MUSCLES FLEXIBLE; BODY YIELDING TO AND RETAINING ANY GIVEN POSITION.

This species is chiefly distinguished from the preceding by the flexibility instead of the inflexibility of the muscles. The cause of this difference has been explained under the preceding species, and needs not to be repeated in the present place. The specific term common to the Greek writers is derived from καταλαμβάνομαι, "deprehendor," "to be seized or laid hold of," and alludes to the suddenness of its attack.

The predisponent and exciting causes are the same as those of ecstasis; and the state of the habit or idiosyncrasy alone produces the difference of effect. The countenance is commonly florid, and the eyes open, and apparently fixed intently upon an object, but in most cases without perception. Yet here, as in ecstasis, we sometimes meet with examples in which one or more of the senses, mental as well as corporeal, do not associate in the general torpitude. So in paroniria, the sight or hearing continues awake, while the other external senses are plunged into a deep sleep, and in some cases of paralysis, the sentient fibres retain their activity, while those of motion are torpid.

The paroxysm commonly attacks without any previous warning, and closes with sighing, or a clonic effort of the nervous power to re-establish its regular flow. Its duration is from a few hours or minutes to two or three days ; and, according to well-established authorities, sometimes for a much longer period. And so completely exhausted of irritable power are some of the organs, and even those of involuntary action, that we have one example in a foreign journal of forty grains of emetic tartar having been given without any effect.—(*Behrends, Baldingers N. Magazin*, b. ix., 199.)

The disease, like the last, is not common. Dr. Cullen never saw an instance of it, except where it was altogether counterfeited, and asserts the same of other practitioners ; which, in fact, he offers as an apology for not knowing exactly where to arrange it. "Therefore," says he, "from the disease being seldom, differently described, and almost always feigned, I can scarcely tell where to place it with certainty ; but I am well persuaded that it does not at all differ from the genus apoplexy, and I have hence arranged it as a species of this division." Plethora or pressure of the brain may perhaps be an occasional cause of this, as of most other nervous diseases, in some habits ; but the greater number of cases that have occurred show very clearly that this disease in its genuine form is as distinct from apoplexy as from epilepsy.

We have said that both catalepsy and ecstasy are most frequently found in constitutions disposed to mental estrangements. Dr. Gooch has given a very interesting case in illustration of this remark, in his paper on puerperal insanity, published in the Medical Transactions. The patient was twenty-nine years of age, had been often pregnant, but had only borne one living child ; and was now confined after delivery of a dead child in her seventh month of gestation. "A few days after our first visit," says Dr. Gooch, "we were summoned to observe a remarkable change in her symptoms. The attendants said she was dying, or in a trance. She was lying in bed motionless, and apparently senseless. It had been said that the pupils were dilated and motionless, and some apprehensions of effusion on the brain had been entertained. But, on coming to examine them closely, it was found that they readily contracted when the light fell upon them ; her eyes were open, but no rising of the chest, no movement of the nostrils, could be seen ; the only signs of life were her warmth and pulse : the latter was, as we had hitherto observed it, weak, and about 120 ; her feces and urine were voided in bed.

"The trunk of the body was now lifted, so as to form rather an obtuse angle with the limbs (a most uncomfortable posture), and there left with nothing to support it. Thus she continued sitting while we were asking questions and conversing, so that many minutes must have passed.

"One arm was now raised, then the other, and where they were left, there they remained : it was now a curious sight to see her, sitting up in bed, her eyes open, staring lifelessly, her arms outstretched, yet without any visible sign of animation ; she was very thin and pallid, and looked like a corpse that had been propped up, and had stiffened in this attitude. We now took her out of bed, placed her upright, and endeavoured to rouse her by calling loudly in her ears, but in vain ; she stood up, but as inanimate as a statue ; the slightest push put her off her balance ; no exertion was made to regain it ; she would have fallen if I had not caught her.

"She went into this state three several times : the first time it lasted fourteen hours ; the second time, twelve hours ; and the third time, nine hours, with waking intervals of two days after the first fit, and one day after the second. After this, the disease resumed the ordinary form of melancholia ; and three months from the time of her delivery, she was well enough to resume her domestic duties."

From the rarity of the complaint and the singularity of several of its symptoms, many physicians, who have never witnessed an example of it, are too much disposed, like Dr. Cullen, to regard it in every case as an imposture. The instance just given is sufficient to clear it from this charge ; yet the following, from Bonet, is added in confirmation. George Grokatski, a Polish soldier, deserted from his regiment in the harvest of the year 1677. He was discovered a few days afterward, drinking and making merry in a common alehouse. The moment he was apprehended he was so much terrified, that he gave a loud shriek, and was immediately deprived of the power of speech. When brought to a court-martial, it was impossible to make him articulate a word : he was as immoveable as a statue, and appeared not to be conscious of any thing that was going forward. In the prison to which he was conducted, he neither ate nor drank, nor emptied the bowels and the bladder. The officers and the priest at first threatened him, but afterward endeavoured to sooth and calm him ; but all their efforts were in vain. He remained senseless and immoveable. His irons were struck off, and he was taken out of the prison, but he did not move. Twenty days and nights were passed in this way, during which he took no kind of nourishment, nor had any natural evacuation. He then gradually sunk and died.—(*Medic. Septentrion.*, lib. i. sect. xvi., cap. 6.)

The pliability of the muscles to any stimulus that acts upon them is sufficiently evident from both these cases : but it has not been generally observed by pathologists, that the force of the stimulus which is acting upon them at the time of the attack continues afterward, so that the same state of motion or rest is still maintained. In the case of a schoolboy aged eleven years, related by Dr. Stearns (*Hosack & Francis's American Med. Register*, vol. i., art. viii.), the paroxysms returned ten times in twenty-four hours, and never exceeded three minutes at a time. And if it commenced while the patient was walking, the same pace was maintained, though without the direction of the mind. The present author was consulted a few years ago on a similar case by a student of Gray's Inn, about nineteen years of age. Having been attacked with a fit of catalepsy while walking, within a few minutes after having left his chambers, he continued his pace insensibly, and without the slightest knowledge of the course he took. As far as he could judge, the paroxysm continued for nearly an hour, through the whole of which time his involuntary walking continued ; at the end of this period he began a little to recover his recollection and the general use of his external senses. He then found himself in a large street, but did not know how he got there, nor what was its name. Upon inquiry, he learned that he was at the further end of Piccadilly, near Hyde Park Corner, to which, when he left his chambers, he had no intention of going. He was extremely frightened, very much exhausted, and returned home in a coach. He was not conscious of any particular train of ideas that had passed in his mind during the fit ; but if such there had been, there can be little doubt that, like the visions of a dream, the reminiscence of them would have been completely banished by the terror he felt on first recovering his recollection, and finding himself in a strange place, to which he had been irregularly wandering through a great number of streets, without consciousness. He had several slighter attacks antecedently, shorter in duration, and, from his being at rest at the time, unaccompanied with a tendency to perambulate.

In this case, and in all of a similar kind, from the power which the patient seems to possess of avoiding danger, the faculty of the will and of sight must be in some degree of activity, however obtuned : bearing a near resemblance to *paroniria ambulans*, or sleep-walking, with the exception of the suddenness of the attack. Some pathologists, indeed, have noticed a modification in which the powers of deglutition and digestion continue, as well as those of pulsation and breathing, provided the food be thrust into the mouth. If we were right in ascribing the CATOCHUS of the ancients to that form of ecstasy in which the mind retains some train of ideas, we shall probably be right also in referring their CATOCHE to this modification of catalepsy ; though Galen seems to have regarded the term as a mere synonyme of catalepsy, and Ætius adopted his opinion.

Instead, however, of most of the involuntary organs being in a joint state of activity, instances have occasionally been known of an apparent cessation of activity in all of them. A critical examination of the region of the heart will mostly, indeed, give proof of a very feeble flutter, and if a clear mirror be applied to the mouth and nostrils, it will generally be found to have a thin vapour on its face. But even these signs have not always been given : insomuch that the disease has been mistaken for real death : and in countries where the rite of sepulture takes place speedily, it is much to be feared that the unfortunate sufferer has in a few instances been buried alive.—(*Pineau sur le Danger des Inhumations precipiteés*, Paris, 1776.) In a case of asphyxy of a singular kind, related by M. Pew, the patient, a female, was peculiarly fortunate in having had her interment postponed for the purpose of ascertaining the cause of her supposed death by dissection : for on being submitted to the scalpel, its first touch brought her to her senses, and threw her into a state of violent agitation, the anatomists being almost as much frightened as herself.* So Diemerbroeck relates the case of a rustic, who was supposed to be dead of the plague, and was laid out for interment. It was by accident three days before he could be carried to the grave, when, in the act of being buried, he showed signs of life, recovered, and lived many years.—(*Tractat. de Peste*, lib. iv., hist. 85.) Mathæus, Hildanus, and the collectors of medical curiosities, are full of stories of this kind ; many of them, indeed, loosely related ; but many also possessing every requisite authority for belief ; and urging the necessity of waiting for signs of putrefaction before the lid of the coffin is screwed down, or, I should rather say, before the body is removed from its deathbed.

We have already observed, that the predisposing and exciting causes are the same as those of ecstasy, and that the state of the habit or idiosyncrasy alone produces the difference of effect. This distinction has not been sufficiently attended to by pathologists in their mode of treatment : and hence one common plan has been too generally laid down and pursued in ecstasy, catalepsy, lethargy, and even apoplexy, the general treatment being as much confounded as the diseases themselves.

Commonly speaking, copious bleedings and purgings have been chiefly trusted to in all of them : and as the present disease, in some cases, arises from plethora, or obstruction, or some irritation of the stomach, it is not to be wondered at that this process should sometimes succeed. But if we have been correct in our pathology, if catalepsy be not only a nervous disease, but a disease of nervous debility, in which the sensorial power is distributed with enfeebled and clonic irregularity, and consequently with a necessary disturbance of the balance of the nervous system, it is perfectly clear that a reducent treatment, however serviceable in a few cases, cannot be laid down as the proper plan to be pursued in general, nor even in any case as an advisable practice, further than it may be called for by the contingency of the exciting cause. Stimulants of most kinds will usually be found far more serviceable, particularly in the form of blisters to the head and heart, sinapisms and other rubefacients to the extremities, and injections to the rectum.

It is now well known that the simplest substances, as a solution of gumarabic, or merely

* Pratique des Accouchemens, &c. Tozzetti's Raccolta de Teorie, Osservazioni e Regole per distinguere e promptemente dissipare le Asphyssie, o Morte apparente, Fiorenza, 8vo., 1772.

warm water, infused, to the amount of not more than an ounce or two, into the current of the blood, by opening a vein, will not only excite the heart to a more violent action, but affect the stomach and intestinal canal with a like increased action by sympathy, producing sickness in the former, and looseness in the latter : and hence Dr. Regnaudot, in an ingenious inaugural dissertation, has thrown out a hint well worthy of being followed up, that such a stimulus may probably succeed in rousing the system generally in the present and most of the preceding species.

Electricity or voltaism, in the manner already recommended, may also be tried with a hope of success : and if it be possible to introduce any thing into the stomach by means •of a syringe, brandy, ether, ammonia, camphire, or even phosphorus, in the form and dose already recommended, may be attempted in rotation. The body in the meanwhile should be kept warm, with a free influx of pure air, and general and persevering friction should often be had recourse to. A steady use of the metallic tonics should be chiefly confided in after the paroxysm is over.

SPECIES IV.

CARUS LETHARGUS.

LETHARGY.

**MENTAL AND CORPOREAL TORPITUDE, WITH DEEP
. QUIET SLEEP.**

LETHARGY, from the Greek terms γήθη and ἀργὸς, " oblivio pigra," is distinguished from all the preceding species of the present genus by the apparent ease and quietism of the entire system: the limbs retaining that gentle and placid flexion which they are wont to exhibit in natural sleep, and the eyelids being usually closed : by both which signs it is also distinguished from apoplexy.

Lethargy is sometimes produced by congestion or effusion in the brain ; by violent mental commotion, as that of fright or furious anger ; by retrocedent gout, or repelled exanthems ; but more generally by long-continued labour of body, or severe exertion of mind.-

The common causes of sleep, therefore, whether natural or morbid, are in many cases causes of lethargy. The proximate cause, however, of idiopathic lethargy, does not seem to have been sufficiently pointed out ; and on this account it has too frequently, like the preceding species, been confounded with apoplexy, and regarded as a mere modification of it.

We had occasion to take a glance at the general physiology of sleep under the genus EPHIALTES, or nightmare, and observed, that its proximate cause is to be sought for in a torpitude or exhaustion of sensorial power from the ordinary stimulants of the day. Now it is possible that the same effect may be produced by a defective supply of sensorial power as well as by its exhaustion ; and consequently, that the torpitude of sleep may ensue whenever such deficient action or energy exists, even where there is no exposure to its ordinary exciting causes. And this it is, as it appears to me, which constitutes the real difference between

genuine lethargy and sound healthy sleep ; in which sense the former becomes a strictly nervous affection, dependant upon a weak and irregular action of the sensorial organ, accompanied with a diminished production of sensorial power, and this power, so diminished, irregularly distributed over its different departments or ramifications ; being altogether withheld from the external senses and the voluntary organs, while the supply to the involuntary organs is little interfered with, as in the case of common sleep. The faculties of the mind seem also, in most cases, to partake of the torpitude of the external senses ; though, as the whole is a disease of debility, and consequently of irregular action, we can readily account for a few singular cases that have been met with, in which the lethargy has been broken in upon by short returns of sensation, or even of speech, or by an irregular flow of ideas, which the patient is sometimes apt to mistake for sensations. And hence lethargy has been observed under the following varieties :—

a Absolutus.	Without intervals of
Genuine lethargy.	sensation, waking, or
	consciousness.
β Cataphora.	With short remissions
Remissive lethargy.	or intervals of imperfeet waking, sensation, and speech.
γ Vigil.	Perfect lethargy of body,
Imperfect lethargy.	but imperfect lethargy of mind : wandering ideas, and belief of wakefulness during sleep.

The FIRST VARIETY has, in some instances, been considerably protracted. We have examples of its continuance for forty days (*Plott, Natural History of Staffordshire*), and even for seven weeks.—(*Bang. Collect. Soc. Med.*, Havn., ii., 17.) In one instance, it is said to have resulted from insolation, or exposure to the direct rays of the sun-; and at length, with great singularity, to have yielded to a large flow of urine, loaded with pus, that fell to the bottom.—(*Morgagni, de Sed. et Caus. Morb.*, ep. v., 13, 14, Albertino.)

The SECOND VARIETY, or CATAPHORA, is the coma-somnolentum of many writers : and is also a frequent accompaniment of many fevers and other diseases of great debility. It occurs at. times, however, as an idiopathic affection ; and I was some years ago acquainted with a very singular example, that continued for five years. The patient was a young lady of delicate constitution, in her eighteenth year at the time of the attack : her mind had been previously in a state of great anxiety : the remissions recurred irregularly twice or three times a week, and rarely exceeded an hour or two : during these periods, she sighed, ate reluctantly what was offered to her, had occasional egestions, and instantly relapsed into sleep. Her recovery was sudden, for she seemed to awake as from a night's rest, by a more perfect termination of the paroxysm, not followed by a relapse.

A less fortunate case of the same kind is related by Mr. Brewster, and was connected with depressed animal spirits, and probably congestion or plethora. The patient was a female servant about the middle of life. The first paroxysm was preceded by a hemorrhage from the nose, and lasted three days: the next continued six weeks; during which she occasionally swallowed food and had alvine evacuations. She had two subsequent fits, neither of which lasted above a few days. Not long afterward, she hung herself.—(*Edin. Phil. Trans.*, 1817.)

The THIRD VARIETY, or IMPERFECT LETHARGY, is the TYPHOMANIA of the Greek writers; the COMA VIGIL of many later pathologists. It is a frequent sequel upon fevers, or other causes of great nervous debility, in circumstances in which the sensorial power has not recovered its regularity of distribution, or stability of balance: during which the patient uniformly assures his physician and his friends, morning after morning, that he has passed a restless and hurried night, without a moment's sleep, while the nurse has been a witness to his having been asleep the whole night long.

The mode of treatment must depend upon the nature of the cause, as far as we are able to ascertain it. If this have consisted in any suppressed discharge or eruption, we should endeavour to reproduce it by all possible means. If we have reason to suspect compression on the brain, copious bleedings, purgatives, and other reducents, are imperative. And if, as is more commonly the case, it be a strictly nervous affection, and depend on atony and a disturbed production or balance of the sensorial power, the warm nervine irritants, as musk, camphire, valerian, with blisters, sternutatories, and other stimulants, are the means we should have recourse to.

These different processes have been pursued in most ages, but unfortunately they have been pursued indiscriminately: and bleeding, purgatives, and ethers and other diffusible excitants, have been employed on like occasions, or even at the same time. Forestus and Dr. Cheyne, who regarded lethargy as chiefly dependant upon plethora or congestion, seem uniformly to have adhered to a reducent plan; and Celsus, who contemplated it as a nervous affection, equally confines himself to external and internal pungents, and advises pepper, euphorbium, castor, and vinegar, with the fumes of burning galbanum or hartshorn applied to the nostrils: as also shaving the head, fomenting it with a decoction of laurel-leaves or rue, and afterward applying sinapisms or some other rubefacient epithem.

All these are consistent with themselves, how much soever the writers may differ in their view of the proximate cause. Yet, neither line of conduct can be right as a general practice; and hence other practitioners have occasionally intermixed the two, sometimes incongruously; and consequently have done less mischief, as at other times they have done less good.

That genuine lethargy is, not unfrequently, a strictly nervous affection, and even closely connected with an irregular or debilitated state of the mind; and that a reducent plan is not always calculated to afford it radical relief, however it may give a temporary promise, must, I apprehend, be obvious to most practitioners who have paid a due attention to their own circle of cases; but the following example from Dr. Cooke, bearing a close resemblance in its termination to that already quoted from Mr. Brewster, is peculiarly in point, and ought not to be omitted on the present occasion: "A lady about twenty years of age, who had usually enjoyed very good health, was one morning found in a state of profound but quiet sleep, from which she could not be awakened, although the preceding evening she had gone to bed apparently quite well. Various means had been tried with a view of exciting her from this state, but in vain. Under these circumstances, I recommended cupping in the neck; and after she had lost a few ounces of blood in this way, she opened her eyes, perfectly recovered, and remained through the day quite free from all symptoms of disorder. The next morning, and for several successive mornings, she was found in a similar state, from which she was recovered by the same remedy, no stimulating external applications producing any good effect. As she was considerably weakened by repeated depletions, it was determined that, on the next recurrence of the paroxysm, the case should be left to the effects of nature, as long as was consistent with safety. The experiment was tried; and at the end of about thirty hours, she spontaneously awoke, apparently refreshed, and wholly unconscious of her protracted sleep. On the future returns of these paroxysms, which were frequent, the same plan was adopted, and she awoke after intervals of thirty-six, forty-eight, and, on one occasion, sixty-three hours, without seeming to have suffered from want of food or otherwise. In the early part of the disease, various means were employed without the smallest advantage, except that, while under the influence of mercury, which produced a very severe salivation that lasted more than a month, she was free from the complaint. For a considerable length of time, these paroxysms recurred: but at length they gradually left her; and soon afterward she became deranged in mind, in which state I believe she still remains."—(*Treatise on Nervous Diseases*, vol. i., p. 372.)

When, therefore, there are no symptoms leading to a peculiar cause, it will be advisable to bleed by cupping, once or twice, but not oftener; to open the bowels and keep them in a state of slight irritation; to employ blisters or other external stimulants occasionally, and to have recourse to a repeated use of the voltaic trough, sending the line of action from the occiput down the spine, and varying it to the extremities. In the meantime, if the patient can be made to swallow, we should try the effect of musk or camphire, with free doses of the metallic tonics, of which the sulphate of zinc, in doses of a grain three or four times a day, offers the best prospect of success.

SPECIES V.
CARUS APOPLEXIA.
APOPLEXY.

MENTAL AND CORPOREAL TORPITUDE, WITH PUL-
SATION, AND OPPRESSIVE, MOSTLY STERTOR-
OUS, SLEEP.*

THERE is a considerable difference of opinion
among pathologists whether stertor is a necessary and invariable, or only an occasional sign
of apoplexy. Sauvages, Linnéus, Vogel, Sagar,
Forestus (Lib. x., obs. 73), Kirkland (*Comment.*,
p. 16), Young, and by far the greater number
of writers, have arranged it as an essential symptom ; and, hence, the present author was induced to view it in the same light when he published his volume of Nosology. He has since,
however, met with one or two cases of atonic
apoplexy, in which, although the disease proved
fatal, the breathing was at no time noisy or stertorous, though uniformly laborious or oppressive : and he has hence been induced to modify
the specific character in the manner it stands
at the head of the present division ; and thus to
approximate to the opinion of Forestus, Cullen, and Portal, who do not regard stertor as a
necessary apex. Dr. Cullen is generally conceived to have omitted this peculiar mark, in
consequence of his having included asphyxy and
catalepsy, which have no pretensions to stertor,
under the genus APOPLEXIA. But as we shall
have to return to this subject when discussing
the different forms or varieties under which apoplexy shows itself, I shall only further observe
at present, that Dr. Cooke has, with great judgment, steered a middle course in laying down
his own definition, which characterizes apoplexy as " a disease in which the animal functions are suspended, while the vital and natural
functions continue ; respiration being generally
laborious, and frequently attended with stertor."†

Apoplexy is strictly a disease of the nervous
system, dependant upon a suspension of the
sensorial power in almost all its modifications,
sentient, percipient, and motory, with the exception of a certain portion which still continues
to be supplied to the involuntary organs ; the
faculties of the mind participating in the torpitude of the body. In these respects it bears a
very near approach to the preceding species of

CARUS ; it chiefly differs in its being generally
connected with an oppressed state of the vessels of the brain from over-distention or effusion : so generally, indeed, that apoplexy is, by
almost all the writers on the subject, regarded
rather as a disease of the sanguineous than of
the nervous system ; the morbid action of the
latter being supposed to be entirely dependant
on that of the former, and consequently only a
secondary affection.

This view of the subject, however, is by far
too limited : for although, in most cases, the
more prominent symptoms concur with the appearances on dissection in leading us to compression of the brain as the primary cause of
the disease, yet we shall find presently, that it
has sometimes taken place where no such compression seems to have existed, while we have
already had occasion to notice a variety of affections of the head attended with forcible and
severe compression, as inflammation and dropsy
of the brain, that have run their entire course
without any mark of apoplexy whatever : to
which should be added that, while in most other
diseases or lesions accompanied with compression of the brain, and a suspension of sentient
and motory power as a consequence hereof,
such suspension ceases almost the moment the
compression is removed, when the nerves of
feeling and motion, together with the faculties
of the mind, resume their wonted activity, and
evince no tendency to a relapse ; in apoplexy, on
the contrary, the result is always doubtful ; for
a palsy of some part or other is a frequent and
permanent effect, or the mind suffers in some
of its faculties, and a relapse is generally to be
apprehended. So that, though compression of
the brain, and particularly from a morbid state
of the sanguineous and respiratory functions,
may be justly regarded as the ordinary efficient
cause, there seems to be at the same time some
peculiar debility or other diseased condition of
the sensorial system* to which apoplexy is primarily to be referred, and without which it might
not take place ; and which has not been sufficiently adverted to by practitioners. Though
there can be no difficulty in our affirming that,
wherever such a morbid condition exists, compression, from whatever cause, will be sure to
produce the disease.

We may hence see why advancing age should

---

* Another definition is, " Loss of sensation, voluntary motion, and intellect or thought ; respiration, and the action of the heart and general vascular system, being continued."—ED.

† On Nervous Diseases, vol. i., p. 166. Apoplexy is liable to be confounded with syncope and
natural sleep. The following are the marks of
distinction adverted to by Dr. Clutterbuck (see
Cyclop. of Pract. Med., art. APOPLEXY) : in syncope the respiration is suspended, the pulse is not
to be felt at the wrist, the features shrink, and the
surface of the body turns pale and cold. In apoplexy the reverse of all these circumstances takes
place. The distinction between apoplexy and natural sleep can only be made by one being able to
rouse the person from sleep, however profound, by
a certain degree of irritation : this cannot be done,
or but very imperfectly, in apoplexy.—ED.

* Perhaps, instead of these ambiguous expressions, it might be better to say that attacks of apoplexy are mostly preceded by disease of the brain
or its vessels, without which previous disease the
apoplexy would not occur. This remark, however, is liable to exceptions, because we know that
apoplexy may be suddenly induced in the most
healthy subject, if he take an extraordinary quantity of brandy, gin, or other strong spirituous
liquor, into his stomach, in an undiluted state.
Though apoplexy, in the sense of an effusion of
blood in or upon the brain, is not usually occasioned by strangulation, especially where the obstruction of the trachea is complete, it may be produced by it, where the struggle for life is more
considerable, in consequence of the interruption
of respiration being less effectually accomplished.
—ED.

prove a predisposing cause; and account for the statement of Morgagni, who tells us that, of thirty cases of apoplectic patients that fell within the reach of his observation, seventeen were above the age of sixty, and only five below that of forty.* Hippocrates, on a more general estimate, calculated that apoplexies are chiefly (μάλιστα) produced between the fortieth and sixtieth year.—(Aph., sect. vi., 57.) This, indeed, is somewhat earlier than we should expect on the ground of advancing age; but when we take into consideration that it is the precise period in which the mind is most agitated and exhausted with the violent and contending passions of interest, and ambition, and worldly honours, and the blood most frequently determined to the head by this impulse of sudden and irresistible emotions, we shall, perhaps, readily accede to the Hippocratic aphorism as a general rule.

How far apoplexy is occasionally the result of an hereditary influence on the frame, it is not easy to ascertain. Forestus, Portal, and Wepfer, refer to decided instances of such facts within their own knowledge: the first, indeed, relates the history of a father and his three sons, all of whom died in succession of this disease; but as the chronology drops with the second generation, it does not descend quite far enough for the purpose. There is great reason, however, for believing that an hereditary tendency does sometimes show itself; and, as this exists without external or manifest signs, it is probably seated in the sensorial system, and constitutes another of the morbid conditions of this system to which we have referred above, as often giving effect to subordinate causes.

There is no difficulty in conceiving how heat may become a predispodent cause, since nothing tends more effectually to quicken the action of the heart, drive the blood forcibly into the aorta, and, consequently, overload the vessels of the brain. But cold is said to be a predisponent cause as well, and one that operates quite as extensively, while the reason of this has not been at all times very clearly explained. Now, as a hot temperature acts chiefly upon the sanguiferous system, extreme cold acts chiefly upon the sensorial, benumbs the feeling, weakens the muscular fibres, diminishes the sensorial energy, and consequently induces, as we have already seen under one of the varieties of asphyxy, an unconquerable propensity to sleep. And hence, again, in apoplexies produced by severe cold, the primary or predisponent cause is to be sought for in a debilitated state of the nervous system. The Greek physicians are perpetually alluding to this cause as one of great frequency, and the explanation now given does not essentially vary from that offered by Galen.—(De Loc. Aff., lib.

iii., cap. vi.) If, indeed, the cold be exquisitely intense, carus asphyxia is more likely to be produced than carus apoplexia; for we have already observed, under the preceding species, that the very same cause which, operating in a vehement degree, excites the former, operating powerfully, has often a tendency to excite the latter.

The other predisponent causes, so far as they have been traced out, are more obvious to the senses, and, for the most part, more directly referrible to the state of the sanguineous function; as plethora, corpulence, and grossness of habit, a short thick neck, and the free use of wines and heavy fermented liquors. Dr. Cheyne, indeed, believes the last to be so common a cause, as even to produce the disease without any inordinate indulgence whatever: "the daily use," says he, "of wine or spirits will lead a man of a certain age and constitution to apoplexy, as certainly as habitual intoxication."—(Cheyne, p. 146.) This may be true as here limited; but then the limitation must be attended to; in which case we are only told in other words, that wherever such a kind of sensorial debility exists as that which we have already adverted to, the result of age, or habit, or constitution, one man will be as readily led to apoplexy under a moderate use of wine, as another man, destitute of such predisposition, will be under a state of habitual intoxication. With this explanation, however, a moderate use of wine becomes only an accessory, and not a primary cause.

How far there may be any other efficient or exciting causes of apoplexy than compression of some kind or other, it is difficult to determine, though various cases on record should induce us to suppose there are. Hydatids, tumours of almost every consistency, gelatinous, steatomatous, and bony, pus, and indurations of the membranes, have, in various cases, been discovered on dissection, and are generally supposed to operate by compression. But in many instances, these appearances seem to have been too minute for any such effect; and can only fairly be regarded as concomitants or allied powers—as local irritants, stimulating and exhausting the sensorium, and preparing it for attacks of apoplexy against the accession of some superinduced and occasional cause; though, where there exists already a strong predisposition to the disease from hereditary or any other affection, it is not improbable that such local irritants may alone be sufficient to perfect the complaint. And we may hence account for that form of apoplexy which is said to proceed from intestinal worms, or some irritation of the stomach, or from teething; and which, consequently, occurs at an early, instead of at a late period of life, and has been especially denominated apoplexia infantium. Other organs, however, besides the teeth and the stomach, seem not unfrequently to have given occasion to apoplectic attacks from irritation, distention, or organic lesion. Thus, according to M. Portal, superinducing tumours and congestions have been found in the neck, in the breast, or in the

* According to Mr. Hope's paper, read recently before the College of Physicians in London, it would seem that apoplexy is more common and fatal between the ages of forty and fifty, and seventy and eighty, which he thinks may be styled the two apoplectic periods of life. Mr. Hope founds his opinion on the data presented by the records of the St. Mary-le-Bone Infirmary.—D.

abdomen; ossifications in the thoracic and ventral aorta, as well as in the arteries of the upper or lower extremities, in the superior vena cava, and in the right ventricle and valves of the heart, which has also indicated various other changes.—(*Portal, Ch. Résultats de l'Ouverture des Corps*, p. 329.)

Most of these morbid actions and appearances, however, are as common to various other affections of the sensorial system as to apoplexy. We have already noticed them in lethargy, convulsion, epilepsy, various species of cephalæa, and some forms of insanity : and hence, wherever they become causes at all, it is most probable that the disease they immediately produce is regulated by the predisposition of the individual to one, rather than to any other of the above sensorial affections, resulting from family taint, idiosyncrasy, habit, or period of life; and, consequently, that the same exciting or occasional cause which in one person would produce apoplexy, in a second would form epilepsy, in a third convulsion, and in a fourth madness.

It is highly singular that this view of the subject should scarcely ever have been attended to by physicians; and that, while all the writers have pretended to regard apoplexy as a disorder of the nervous system, none of them have suffered such ideas to enter fairly into their pathology, or in any way whatever into their practice ; the nervous organ being supposed by all of them to be in a state of soundness at the time of the attack ; and whatever mischief it suffers to be merely secondary, and consequent upon a morbid state of the bloodvessels, or of some other cause, that as suddenly and effectually interrupts the production and distribution of the sensorial power, as retrocedent gout, mephitic vapours, or narcotic poisons.

Now, all these accidental or effective causes of apoplexy are well known to be causes, also, of the other nervous affections we have just re-

---

* The following reflections on this subject, by Dr. Clutterbuck, appear interesting :—" The opinion that appears to prevail most generally at present, as to the immediate cause of the suspension of functions that constitutes the apoplectic state, is, that the remote causes of the disease, such as extravasated blood, and accumulation of serum, produce a compression of the cerebral substance, thereby interrupting its functions. But, besides that some of the remote causes of apoplexy have no apparent tendency to make any direct pressure on the brain, it must not be overlooked, that the cerebral substance, being in its nature incompressible, cannot, so long as the blood is contained within its vessels, be exposed to greater pressure at one time than another. It must be in some other way, therefore, than by compression of the substance of the brain, that the remote causes act in producing their effect. It cannot be questioned, that pressure on the brain of any kind, if carried to a certain extent, is capable of interrupting the functions of the organ so as to induce apoplexy; but there is good reason to believe that the pressure operates upon the bloodvessels so as to impede mechanically the passage of the blood through them ; in a word, that *interrupted circulation in the brain is the proximate or immediate cause of that temporary suspension of the sensorial functions which constitutes the apoplectic state*."—(See Cyclop. of

ferred to. But if this be the case, how comes it that they should thus vary in their result, and that what in one person and at one period of life should produce apoplexy, should in another person and in another period of life produce lethargy, palsy, convulsions, or epilepsy ? or that some of them should exist without producing any of these diseases, or any other disease whatever ? It is not, perhaps, possible for us to develop the precise condition of the sensorium that leads to any one of these effects rather than to any other; but that there is such a condition, forming a predisponent or remote cause of the specific disease that shows itself, must, I think, be allowed by every one who seriously considers the subject.

Nor is there, in effect, any other means of reconciling the discrepant and opposite opinions that have been held concerning the proximate cause of the disease. This we have stated to be, for the most part, compression, and especially sanguineous compression.* Mr. John Hunter was so strenuously attached to this cause, that he would allow of no other ; M. Rochoux has followed his footsteps (*Dict. de Médecine*, tom. ii., Paris, 1822); and if a man died of apoplexy from atonic gout, and without effusion, the former distinguished it as *a disease similar to apoplexy*. He regarded apoplexy and palsy as one and the same disease, merely differing in degree : and he gives us his sentiments very forcibly in the following words :—" For many years," says he, " I have been particularly attentive to those who have been attacked with a paralytic stroke forming a hemiplegia. I have watched them while alive, that I might have an opportunity to open them while dead : and, in all, I found an injury done to the brain in consequence of the *extravasation of blood*.—I must own, I never saw one of them which had not an extravasation of blood in the brain, except one who died of a gouty affection in the brain,

---

Pract. Med., art. Apoplexy, p. 126.) This intelligent writer then proceeds to show that apoplexy may be brought on by a variety of remote causes, all operating in different ways, but all leading to the same general result—obstructed circulation of the brain. "Whether this be produced by direct external pressure, or by extravasated fluids or tumours within the scull ; whether by arterial excitement, and consequent distention, produced by either alcohol, external heat, or mental emotions ; or whether by any impediment to the return of blood from the brain, by causes influencing the veins; the effect," according to Dr. Clutterbuck's view, "is still the same, and suggests the same general indications of cure ; namely, to restore the circulation of the brain." Some part of this writer's doctrine agrees with the opinion of Dr. Abercrombie, who refers merely to a derangement in the circulation of the brain, without restricting the immediate cause to one principle alone, as Dr. Clutterbuck has done in the foregoing quotation. A correct theory of apoplexy, in relation to its immediate cause, is certainly of the highest importance, as leading to the consideration of what ought to be the principal indication in the treatment of the disease. Thus, Dr. Clutterbuck's views convince him, that the general indication of cure is to restore the circulation of the brain by removing the obstructing cause.—Ed.

with symptoms *similar to apoplexy.*"—(*Treatise on Blood,* &c., p. 213.) ,

In direct hostility to this hypothesis, many other writers of great eminence and experience have contended that compression is no cause whatever, and that an accumulation of blood in the head as a prominent symptom in apoplexy is a doctrine rather than a fact. Of this sentiment is Dr. Abercrombie, who, after examining the question with much ingenuity, brings himself to the following conclusion:—"Upon all these grounds," says he, "I think we must admit that the doctrine of determination to the head is not supported by the principles of pathology, and does not accord with the phenomena of apoplexy."[*] M. Serres, however, a physician of considerable distinction in France, and who followed up this subject for many years by a careful examination of the bodies of persons who died of apoplexy and paralysis, both of the Hôtel Dieu and the Hôpital de la Pitié, has carried his inroad upon the popular doctrine of the day still further; for he has not only in his own opinion completely subverted it, but has endeavoured to establish another doctrine of a very different character upon its ruins.—(*Annuaire Medico-Chirurgicale,* Avril, 1820.) To determine the question, he has gone through a long series of experiments upon the brains of dogs, pigeons, rabbits, and other animals, whose crania were trepanned, their lateral or longitudinal sinuses laid open, and their brains lacerated and excavated in various ways so as to be gorged with effused blood, yet, in none of them did somnolency or any other apoplectic symptom take place. And he hence triumphantly concludes

---

[*] Treatise on Apoplexy, &c., p. 19. If, however, we consult a later publication of this distinguished physician and pathologist, we shall find that, whatever may be his opinion respecting determination of blood to the head as a cause of apoplexy, he himself brings forward examples of apoplexy from pressure on the veins in the neck, and a consequent distention of the vessels of the brain.—(See Pathological and Practical Researches on Diseases of the Brain and the Spinal Cord, p. 204, Edin., 1828.) After adverting to cases from strangulation (cases, however, in which the actual suspension of the functions of the brain might be more justly imputed to the transmission of black or unoxygenated blood to that organ, than to an apoplectic state of it), he notices other examples, "in which persons fall down suddenly in a state of perfect apoplexy, and very speedily recover under appropriate treatment, without retaining any trace of so formidable a malady. The apoplectic attack, as it occurs in such examples as these," he says, "must be supposed to depend upon a cause which acts simply upon the circulating system of the brain, producing there a derangement which takes place speedily, and is often almost as speedily removed. What the precise nature of that derangement may be, is a point of the utmost difficulty to determine," &c. And again, "the apoplectic attack is generally preceded by symptoms indicating some derangement of the circulation in the brain."—(P. 205.) Were the editor bold enough to question the accuracy of some parts of Dr. Abercrombie's valuable treatise, he should be disposed to say that this author comprehends too many different states of disease in

that extravasation of blood does not produce apoplexy, whether lodged between the cranium and the dura mater, or between the dura mater and the brain: whether the blood occupy the great interlobular scissure, and thus lie upon the corpus callosum; whether cavities be made in the fore, the back, or the middle part of the hemispheres, or run from the one into the other ; or, lastly, whether piercing through the corpus callosum, we reach and fill up the ventricles of the brain. "On whatever animal," says he, "we try these experiments, whether on birds, rabbits, or dogs, the result is the same, and hence apoplexy in man ought not to be ascribed to such effusions."

["A person (says Dr. Abercrombie), previously in perfect health, falls down suddenly, deprived of sense and motion, and dies after lying for some time in a state of coma. We find on examination a large coagulum of blood compressing the surface of the brain, or filling its ventricles, and the phenomena of the disease appear to be distinctly accounted for. Another person is cut off with the same symptoms, and we expect to find the same appearances ; but nothing is met with except serous effusion in no great quantity in the ventricles, or only on the surface of the brain. A third is seized in the same manner, and dies after lying for a considerable time in a state of coma, from which nothing can rouse him for an instant ; and, on the most careful examination, we cannot detect in his brain the smallest deviation from the healthy structure."][*]

---

his view of apoplexy. Thus, his 90th case (p. 212) appears to have been only an example of ascites and hydrothorax, where death was preceded by coma and stertor. But if all diseases which exhibit coma and stertor a little before their termination were to be regarded as apoplexies, where would be the limit to this principle of classification? The editor would also say, that apoplexy might be characterized by the suddenness with which the fit takes place, whether preceded by other ailments or not, and that no examples ought to be looked upon as apoplexies in which the coma and loss of sense come on gradually, as they do in the last stage of fevers and other disorders. Apoplectic symptoms, as a critical writer observes, are known to arise from various states of the brain or its parts. It is now, says he, regarded as most expedient to restrict the appellation of apoplexy to that state of the vessels of the brain in which they are either excessively distended with blood, or in which this fluid has escaped, either by exhalation or rupture.—(Edin. Med. Journ., No. xc., p. 83.) Dr. Abercrombie's remarks are particularly interesting, however, as proving that apoplexy should not always be ascribed to fulness of the cerebral vessels, or to extravasation, even though some unknown form of derangement of the circulation in the brain may exist.—Ed.

[*] Pathological and Practical Researches on the Diseases of the Brain and Spinal Cord, p. 202, Edin., 1828. In considering the causes of apoplexy, pathologists must not overlook certain physical conditions of the brain ; as, for instance, its enclosure in an unyielding bony case, whereby it is excluded from the influence of atmospheric pressure. So long as the scull is entire, its cavity is always completely filled by its contents, and there can be no alternate contraction and expan-

How are these discrepancies to be reconciled? by what means are we to account for it, that pressure may be a cause and may not be a cause? and that apoplexy is sometimes found with it and sometimes without it? It is the peculiar state of the sensorium or nervous system at the time that makes all the difference—it is the morbid predisposition or debility, or whatever other deviation from perfect health it may labour under at the moment of the application of the exciting cause, that gives an effect which would not otherwise take place; and something of which in many cases often discovers itself by precursive signs, for a considerable period before the apoplectic incursion. The facts stated by Mr. John Hunter no one can call in question; and we have as little right to question the experiments of M. Serres: the error consists in taking an unsound and a sound state of the brain for like premises, and reasoning from the effects prosion of the cerebral mass, with a vacuity produced by the former between the scull and the membranes of the brain. The contents of the scull, solid as well as fluid, if not absolutely incompressible, at least are so by any force that can be applied to them during life. Yet the bloodvessels within the head will readily yield to pressure, so as to be emptied of their contents; a necessary consequence of which is a stoppage of the circulation in the part so affected. As Dr. Clutterbuck observes (Cyclop. of Pract. Med., art. APOPLEXY), the pressure may be made to take place on any part of the brain, even the most remote from the principal vessels; yet, nevertheless, the pressure, by operating through an incompressible substance, may influence vessels the most distant, so as to impede if not wholly interrupt the cerebral circulation. From these circumstances, the following important conclusions are drawn:—No material variation can take place within a short period in regard to the absolute quantity of blood in the brain. No additional quantity can be admitted into its bloodvessels, because the cavity of the scull is already completely filled by its contents. A plethoric state, or overfulness of the cerebral vessels altogether, though often talked of, can have no real existence; nor, on the other hand, can the quantity of blood within the vessels of the brain be diminished, any more than can wine or other fluid be drawn from a cask without furnishing an equivalent for the portion abstracted from it, by the supply of an equal bulk of air, which, in the case of the brain, can of course find no entrance. No abstraction of blood, therefore, whether it be from the arm or other part of the general system, or from the jugular veins (and still less from the temporal arteries) can have any effect on the bloodvessels of the brain, so as to lessen the absolute quantity of blood contained within them. From the experiments of Dr. Kellie, it was found that in animals bled to death, the brain still contained the usual quantity of blood; and in some cases, the superficial veins were found gorged with blood, and the sinuses full; the rest of the body being at the same time blanched and drained of its blood. In a few instances the brain appeared to contain less blood than usual; but then there was found some serous exudation. When the cranium of the animals subjected to these experiments was perforated before they were bled, the brain was as much emptied of its blood as the rest of the body. In two instances of persons that had been hanged, the cellular membrane of the whole head externally was turgid with blood; but nothing peculiar

duced on one to those that are found to follow on the other. This, in truth, is an error too often committed; and hecatombs of quadrupeds and other animals, in a condition of perfect health, are tortured in a thousand ways for the purpose of determining what they never could determine, though the trials were to be repeated to the end of time; I mean, the effects of certain causes on a diseased state of body in man, from their influence on a sound state of body in brutes.

M. Serres's actual examinations of apoplectic patients after death, however, though conducted also upon a large scale, do not seem to afford much countenance to his hypothesis, nor, in effect, to offer any thing out of the common way. In a considerable number of subjects, there was serous effusion, sanguineous effusion, or both; sometimes in the circumvolutions of the brain, sometimes in the ventricles, sometimes in all these; and not unfrequently the vessels of the meninges appeared distended with was observed in the state of the vessels of the brain itself. When blood is suddenly or rapidly extravasated anywhere within the scull, the space thus occupied can only be furnished by the compression and consequent emptying of the bloodvessels in other parts of the brain; and in the same degree that this happens, it is evident that the circulation of such parts must be interrupted. But in the formation of tumours within the scull, and during the slow accumulation of serum from inflammation or any other cause, the cerebral substance itself may be absorbed to an extent corresponding to the bulk of the tumour, or the quantity of serum deposited. The circulation of the brain may then go on uninterruptedly, and thus the apoplectic symptoms be prevented. But, as Dr. Clutterbuck further explains, although under ordinary circumstances, the absolute quantity of blood contained in the vessels of the brain must remain the same, there may be great differences in regard to its distribution, and the force and velocity with which it is moved. Thus, the arteries of the brain altogether may be unusually distended with blood; but in this case the veins will be in the same degree compressed and emptied, and the circulation of the organ proportionally interrupted, with a corresponding interruption of functions. Again, as the same writer observes, there may be a partial fulness or distention of vessels in one part of the brain only; but this must be at the expense of the rest of the brain, which will be proportionally deprived of the usual supply of blood. In like manner, there may be great diversity with respect to the force and velocity of circulation in the brain; the absolute quantity of blood in the vessels still remaining the same. In this way the functions may be more or less excited, or more or less disturbed. These changes in the state of the cerebral circulation are all independent of the heart. Bloodletting, therefore, however useful in apoplexy, does not become so by diminishing in any degree the absolute quantity of blood in the brain, but by reducing the velocity and impetus of the circulation there, and which it does by influencing the general system. These peculiarities in the condition and circulation of the brain were, as Dr. Clutterbuck notices, long ago demonstrated by the late Dr. Monro, and have been recently confirmed by a variety of experiments instituted by Kellie, Abercrombie, and others, who have drawn from the whole of the investigation the important views and inferences adverted to in the foregoing observations.—ED.

blood, and the membranes themselves thickened. Such appearances seem to furnish something of a stumbling-block to M. Serres's new doctrine, yet he readily gets over the difficulty by satisfying himself that in all these cases the effusion did not produce the apoplexy, but the apoplexy the effusion. In other dissections he found some material alterations in the structure of the brain, but without effusion; and as the class of individuals had evinced palsy rather than apoplexy, he is inclined to think that apoplexy, or that state of the disease in which the stupor is greater and more general, is occasioned by a morbid irritation of the *membranes* of the brain; and palsy, or that state in which the stupor is less, by a morbid change in its *substance*; in consequence of which he proposes to call the first *meningic*, and the second *cerebral* apoplexy. In this conclusion, however, there seems to be a striking mistake; and the very reverse is what we should have expected; for if there be one pathological principle more established than another, it is that stupor and dulness of pain appertain to the parenchymatous irritation or inflammation of an organ, and rousing, restless, and acute pain to its membranous irritation; a principle we have already explained at some length; and whence, indeed, the lancinating pain of pleuritis compared with pneumonitis, and of meningic or brain fever, compared with acute dropsy of the head.—(See vol. i., *Empresma Cephalitis*, Cl. III., Ord. II., Gen. VII., Spe. 1.)

There is far more dependance to be placed upon the painful and unjustifiable series of experiments performed several years since by M. Rolando upon the brains of animals of almost all kinds; and which seem to show, as we have already observed, that animals which possess a perfect brain, derive their sensific power and motific power not jointly from the cerebrum and cerebellum, but separately, the one affording the one power, and the other the other.—(*Saggio sopra la vera Struttura del Cervello*, &c., e sopra le *Funzioni de Sistema Nervosa*, Sassari, 1809.) Stupor and apoplexy were in all these cases produced, not by a morbid irritation of the *membranes* of the brain, as conjectured by M. Serres, but by a morbid irritation of the *substance*, while irritation of the membrane took away neither the sensific nor the motific power.*

The brain, therefore, may be rendered comatose by various causes: but we hold, after all, that the grand exciting cause of apoplexy is compression; and this shows itself in various ways, which are well enumerated by Dr. Cheyne in the following passage:—" I mention first," says he, " the remains of an excited state of the minute arteries of the brain and its membranes, this probably being the most important, as it is the most unvarying appearance; then the extravasation of blood, probably the consequence

of the excited state of the vessels; the turgescence of the venous system; the enlargement of the ventricles, partial or general; and lastly, the serous effusion, which is generally found in various parts of the brain, and which would seem to imply previous absorption of the brain."*

The concluding sentence in this passage appears to indicate that this correct and discriminating pathologist was by no means inattentive to that extraordinary change, which is not unfrequently produced in the structure and tenacity of the brain by various causes of excitement; and exists in a more or less extensive demolition of its substance, so that it is sometimes found to be pulpy or pasty, and at others, the disorganization having proceeded farther, to be as liquescent or diffluent as soup. Morgagni has collected various examples of these and other modes of disintegration; Dr. Baillie has occasionally adverted to them (*Morbid Anatomy*, fascic. x., pl. iii., p. 213, and pl. viii., 227, 228); and Dr. Abercrombie has brought them into a still more prominent notice by an ingenious pathological explanation of their cause.† But in France the subject has been pursued with pe-

---

* Cheyne p. 24. M. Bouilliaud maintains the doctrine, that chronic inflammation of the cerebral vessels, or a diseased state of their coats, has a principal share in the production of apoplexy. (Recherches, &c., in Mém. de la Soc. d'Emul., tom. ix., Paris, 1826.) The connexion between hemorrhage of the brain and disease of the arterial system has been noticed by Morgagni, Lieutaud, Baillie, Hodgson, and others. In one case of apoplexy, recorded by the latter writer, a copious effusion of blood was found beneath the arachnoid coat at the base of the brain, and to have escaped from an aneurismal sac, as large as a horsebean, communicating with the basilar artery, where it divides into the cerebellic and posterior cerebral branches.—(On Diseases of Arteries and Veins, p. 76.) In another instance, detailed by the same surgeon, there was apoplectic hemorrhage from disease of the ramifications on the pia mater (p. 26, case iv.). But a full confirmation of cerebral hemorrhage being frequently connected with disease of the vessels of the brain, may be found in the essay of M. Bouilliaud, who has adduced cases on this point from Lallemand, Serres, De Haen, and other eminent authorities. As a critical writer observes, however, this author can claim no other merit than that of stating a fact " which has been familiarly known to us since the days of Willis, which was converted into a solid and substantial principle by Cullen, and which received the most undeniable confirmation from the researches of Portal and Rochoux in France, and from those of Baillie, Cheyne, and Abercrombie in this country. When," says this same reviewer, " it is remembered how difficult it is to adduce examples of genuine and unequivocal apoplexy from direct impairment of nervous energy, or of what is termed *nervous apoplexy* by Zuliani, Kortum, Kirkland, and Abernethy, it will not be regarded as a proof of too extensive a generalization to maintain, that *apoplexy consists in an affection of the vascular system of the brain only.*"—(See Edin. Med. Journ., No. xc., p. 88.)—Ed.

† Edin. Med. and Surg. Journal, vol. xiv., p. 265. Observations on Chronic Inflammation of the Brain; also, Pathological and Practical Researches on Diseases of the Brain, &c., pp. 81, 86, 129, &c., 8vo., Edin., 1828.

---

* Dr. Stokes, in his lectures on apoplexy, boldly asserts, that the brain must be a very compressible organ; and Dr. Condie, in an able article on the subject, writes as follows: " We should even be inclined to adopt the opinion of Cruveilhier, that the brain is *eminently* compressible."—See Amer. Cycl. of Pract. Med. and Surg., vol. ii.—D.

culiar activity since the publication of the first edition of the present work, and has excited an interest of no ordinary standard. To this change, M. Rochoux has given the name of *ramollissement de cerveau*, or mollities cerebri (*Recherches sur l'Apoplexie*, 8vo., 1814), and its nature and varieties have since been followed up, and systematically arranged with considerable nicety and precision, by M. Rostan (*Recherches sur un Maladie encore peu connué qui a reçu le nom de Ramollissement de Cerveau*, 8vo., 1820) and M. Lallemand (*Recherches Anatomico pathologiques sur l'Encéphale et ses dépendances*, 1821), who have regarded it as an idiopathic affection, and attempted a development of its entire pathology and mode of treatment. Its actual cause is often doubtful; and still more doubtful is it whether it ever exists as a primary disease. That inflammation, consequent on congestion or rupture of the bloodvessels of the brain, is a frequent cause is clear, because the minute and colourless arteries of the part affected are often found striated or infiltrated, as the French call it, with red blood, and a clot of effused blood is traced in the centre. The inflammatory process hereby produced is sometimes violent, and passes rapidly into the suppurative stage, accompanied with severe lancinating pains, and a feeling of constriction round the head, and even delirium; and hence this condition is as common a result of cephalitis as of what we shall presently have occasion to call entonic apoplexy. The soft, pulpy disorganization of the brain is in this case often intermixed with masses of pus, while the general hue of the diseased part is brown or reddish, from a diffusion of the red particles of the blood that have been let loose; and as the extravasated blood becomes more or less decomposed and intermixed with the white or gray matter of the brain, and with effused serum, the colour is found to vary considerably through all the diversities of white, gray, yellow, rosy, amaranthine, deep red, brown, chocolate, and greenish. The gray substance of the brain, however, as less tenacious, is found more generally diffluent and more completely decomposed than the white.

More usually, however, the inflammation is far less violent, or it is even chronic; and the symptoms are those of an obtuse pain in the head, general oppression, occasional vertigo, with indistinctness of memory, and confusion of thought, the pulse evincing but little if any change from a state of health. But as these symptoms are common to various other diseases, their pathognomonic value is small. There are two other signs, however, pointed out by the French monographists as more essentially distinctive, but which the present writer has never had an opportunity of noticing: these are a mouse smell or odour issuing from the body of the patient; and a movement of the lips on one side, accompanied with a rushing or whizzing sound, like what is often exhibited by smokers in the act of smoking tobacco.* For the production of these

last symptoms, however, it is necessary that the disease should be accompanied with hemiplegia, so that one side of the mouth only is capable of motion.

By far the greater number of these symptoms, however, indicate atony rather than eutony of action; and hence, though inflammation is not unfrequently a proximate cause, debility, whether consequent upon inflammation or any other morbid change, is perhaps a more common cause. Hence in our own country this organic mollescence has usually been regarded as a gangrene of the brain, and many of the French pathologists, and especially M. Recamier, incline to interpret it as a result of low atonic or malignant fevers, rather than of phlogtic action. With M. Rostan and M. Lallemand, however, it is ranked as a direct phlogosis, or phlegmasia, not resulting from apoplexy, but necessarily conducting to it and producing it. Yet, as according to their own showing, the leading symptoms are those of turgescence and oppression, with little increase of pulse or other excitement, it should seem to follow that they have in a considerable degree mistaken the cause for the effect, even where inflammation is coexistent.

In reality, though there is no difficulty in accounting for the extravasated blood, or the vascular infiltration, or the depraved colours, which are found in this state of the brain, upon the principle of inflammation, there is a considerable difficulty in explaining upon the same principle the mollification of the diseased area: and it is upon this point that the pathology of the French writers seems chiefly to fail.

The real mode of action, as it appears to the present writer, is the same as that which takes place in mollification of the bones, which we shall explain in a subsequent part of this system; but which, as well as its opposite, fragility of the bones, is always a disease of weakness, local or general. Now we meet with a like deviation from a healthy tenacity of the brain in both these ways; for we find it sometimes too tough, and indeed almost horny (*Morgagni*, passim); as well in the gray as in the white compartments, occasionally, indeed, interspersed with masses of bony matter (see *the accounts of Duverney, Giro, and Moreschi, especially in Gazette de Santé*, Paris, Nov. 11, 1809); and at other times, as in the disease before us, too soft and unresisting; and in both these cases also, if I mistake not, debility will be found the immediate cause, even where inflammation has preceded. The firm and tenacious material which enters so largely into the substance of the brain, and particularly into the white part, is a secretion *sui generis*, and so long as the secernents and absorbents of this organ maintain a healthy action, and precisely counterbalance each other, this material will be duly supplied, and in a healthy state, as it is wanted, and duly removed to make way for a fresh recruit as it becomes worn out. But if the organ from any cause become weakened in its vascular powers, that weakness will extend to one or both the sets of vessels we are now considering, and the result will necessarily be the existence of brainy mat-

---

* These symptoms, justly ascribed to a hemiplegiac state, almost invariably prognosticate a fatal termination of the case.—D.

ter of a depraved and untempered tenacity. In proportion as the compages of the brain becomes looser and less resistible, effusions of serum and red blood, ulceration, gangrene, and a total dissolution of the entire substance, must in many cases follow as a natural result, and in the order here stated. And hence, in cancer of the brain, the substance of the organ is always found in a soft or mollescent state. As a further proof that this peculiar change is for the most part a result of debility, it is admitted by both M. Rostan and M. Lallemand, that it is by far most frequently met with in persons of advanced age; the former, indeed, asserts roundly, that in the whole extent of his practice he has never met with more than one instance, in which he was suspicious of it at or under the age of thirty, and as examination after death was not here allowed him, he does not regard even this case as of any moment.*

It is singular that the congestive fluid, instead

* The softening of textures during life is aseribed by Professor Carswell to three causes.—1. Inflammation; 2. obliteration of arteries; 3. modification of nutrition. It is laid down as a general rule, that every organ or tissue affected with acute inflammation, undergoes at the same time a diminution of consistence. Dr. Carswell represents the process of softening as being accomplished "under the immediate influence of a mechanical agent on the one hand, and a vital agent on the other. Thus, the effused fluids separate mechanically the molecules of the tissue, which the cessation of nutrition had deprived of their vital properties; or, in other words, the cessation of nutrition deprives the molecules of those properties on which their power of aggregation depends, and in this state they are separated and detached by the effused fluids."—(Illustrations of the Elementary Forms of Disease, fasciculus 5.) Softening from obliteration of arteries occurs only in the brain, and at an advanced period of life. "It is," observes Dr. Carswell, "this kind of softening which was first described by M. Rostan, as a disease *sui generis*, as entirely opposite in its nature to inflammation, and which be likened to gangræna senilis. The opinion of this author met with strong opposition from Lallemand of Montpellier, who maintained that softening of the brain is always the consequence of inflammation." But Dr. Carswell considers the latter view as far from the truth as the former is ambiguous and inconclusive; and he thinks that the real nature of this disease, to which the brains of aged persons are so liable, has not hitherto been ascertained. It has been conjectured to originate in ossification of the arteries; yet even M. Rostan, among the great number of cases of softening of the brain detailed in his work, has not given a single instance in which ossification and obliteration of the arteries are mentioned as having been observed on dissection. The coloured engravings contained in Dr. Carswell's publication, illustrative of the softening of various textures, and especially of the brain; are among the finest specimens of the power of the pencil to facilitate the comprehension of the morbid changes to which the several textures of the body are liable. The work in which they are published, entitled "Illustrations of the Elementary Forms of Disease," 4to., Lond., 1833-4, is deserving of every possible encouragement, and should be attentively studied by every medical man desirous of becoming a good pathologist.—Eᴅ.

of proving a material elaborated by the animal frame itself, should sometimes consist of a foreign material recently received into the stomach. Dr. Cooke has given a case strikingly in proof of this, which I shall offer in his own words :—" I am informed by Sir Anthony Carlisle, that a few years ago, a man was brought dead into the Westminster Hospital, who had just drunk a quart of gin for a wager.* The evidences of death being quite conclusive, he was immediately examined, and within the lateral ventricles of the brain was found a considerable quantity of a limpid fluid distinctly impregnated with gin, both to the sense of smell and taste, and even to the test of inflammability. 'The liquid,' says Sir Anthony Carlisle, ' appeared, to the senses of the examining students, as strong as one third gin to two thirds water.' "†

On examining the different sources of a compressed brain, as we have just enumerated them, it will be obvious that they bespeak a very different, and indeed, opposite state of vascular action in different cases; and that, while some of them necessarily imply a vehement and entonic power, others as necessarily imply an infirm and atonic condition. The external symptoms, from the first, speak to the same effect; and hence, from an early period of time,—as early at least as that of La Rivière or Riverius (*Praxis Medica*, 8vo., Lugd., 1670)—apoplexy has been contemplated under two distinct forms or varieties, which have commonly been denominated sanguineous, and pituitous or serous; as though the former proceeded from an overflow of blood highly elaborated by a vigorous and robust constitution, and rushing forward with great impetuosity; and the latter from thin dilute blood, or a leucophlegmatic habit, from the relaxed mouths of whose vessels a serous effusion is perpetually flowing forth. Morgagni has endeavoured to show, but without success, that this distinction was in existence among the Greek writers. It is a distinction, however, that runs not only through his own works, but through those of Boerhaave, Sennert, Mead, Sauvages, and Cullen, and is acknowledged by most practitioners of the present day.

The term pituitous or serous, however, has been objected to as not always expressing the actual state of the brain in atonic apoplexy; since no serum has been found at times in cases where the symptoms of debility have peculiarly led those pathologists to expect it who have employed the distinctive term ; while the cavi-

* Dr. Hosack remarks, in a note to his address delivered before the tempcrance society (Essays, vol. iii., p. 415), "My colleague, Dr. J. W. Francis, Prof. of Obstetrics and Forensic Medicine in the Rutgers Medical College, who has for more than ten years past been engaged as medical witness and adviser in the Criminal Courts of New-York, states to me, that occurrences of this character have repeatedly come before him upon the examination of the bodies of persons who have died from intemperance."—D.

† On Nervous Diseases, vol. i., p. 221. Schrader has a similar case, Observ. Anat. Med., decad. iv., Amsterd., 1674 ; as also Wepffer, Observ. Medico. Pract., p. 7, Scaph., 1722,

ties and interstitial parts of the brain have, on the contrary, been sometimes found as much loaded with blood as in what they denominate sanguineous apoplexy. And hence, Forestus and a few other writers have been disposed to exchange the terms sanguineous and serous, for strong or perfect, and weak or imperfect apoplexy.* How far a modification of this disease, strictly serous, may be said to exist, we shall examine presently ; but that apoplexy is continually showing itself under the two forms of entonic and atonic action, seems to be admitted by all. And as the terms sanguineous and serous do not sufficiently express this change of condition in every instance, the author, in proceeding to treat of these two varieties, will, for the future, distinguish them as follows :—

α	Entonica.	With a hard full pulse, flushed
	Entonic apo-	countenance, and stertorous
	plexy.	breathing.
β	Atonica.	With a feeble pulse, and pale
	Atonic apo-	countenance.
	plexy.	

In ENTONIC APOPLEXY the fit is, for the most part, sudden and without warning; though a dull pain in the head occasionally precedes the attack, accompanied with a sense of weight or heaviness, somnolency and vertigo. The inspirations are deeper than natural ; the face and eyes are red and turgid, and blood bursts from the nostrils. On the incursion of the paroxysm the patient falls to the ground, and lies as in a heavy sleep, from which he cannot be roused. The breathing is strikingly oppressive ; though at first, perhaps, slow and regular, increasing in

* "The distinction which has been proposed," says Dr. Abercrombie, "betwixt sanguineous and serous apoplexy, is not supported by observation. The former is said to be distinguished by flushing of the countenance and strong pulse, and by occurring in persons in the ; ʼ..ur of life ; the latter by paleness of the countenance and weakness of the pulse, and by affecting the aged and infirm; and much importance has been attached to this distinction, upon the ground that the practice which was necessary and proper in one case, would be improper and injurious in the other. I submit, that this distinction is not founded upon observation ; for in point of fact, it will be found, that many of the cases which terminate by serous effusion, exhibit in their early stages all the symptoms which have been assigned to the sanguineous apoplexy ; while many of the cases which are accompanied by paleness of the countenance and feebleness of the pulse, will be found to be purely sanguineous."—(Pathological and Practical Researches on Diseases of the Brain and Spinal Cord, p. 218, 8vo., Edin., 1828.) The divisions of apoplexy, laid down by this interesting writer, are exceedingly judicious. He arranges all cases into three classes :—First, those which are immediately and primarily apoplectic ; secondly, those which begin with an attack of a sudden headache, and pass gradually into apoplexy ; thirdly, those which are distinguished by palsy and loss of speech, without coma.—(P. 208.) However, though the second class of cases are stated to pass gradually into apoplexy, we find, on referring to the details given by Dr. Abercrombie (p. 221), that he only means that the disease is preceded by violent headache, &c., and not that the apoplectic attack itself, when it does come, is not sudden. From the history of such cases he believes, "that they depend upon the immediate rupture of a considerable vessel, without any previous derangement of the circulation, the rupture probably arising from disease of the artery at the part which gives way. At the moment when the rupture occurs, there seems to be a temporary derangement of the functions of the brain, but this is soon recovered from. The circulation then goes on without interruption, until such a quantity of blood has been extravasated as is sufficient to produce coma."—(P. 223.) According to the same authority, the source of the hemorrhage, in this class of cases, is exceedingly various. 1. The most common appears to be the rupture of a vessel of moderate size in the substance of the brain, from which the blood bursts its way by laceration either into the ventricles or to the surface, or in both these directions at once. In general, the hemorrhage cannot be traced to particular vessels, though Dr. Cheyne succeeded in

some instances. A case is described by Serres, in which the rupture took place in the substance of the pons Varolii, and the blood made its way into the occipital fossa. 2. The superficial vessels ; the blood generally communicating betwixt the dura mater and the arachnoid ; but cases are recorded in which it lay beneath the pia mater, and appeared to have been discharged from the retiform plexus of vessels at the base of the brain. 3. From ulceration and rupture of one of the arterial trunks. Dr. Mills has described a case in which the hemorrhage was traced to ulceration of the basilar artery, and a similar affection of the internal carotid is described by Morgagni and Serres. 4. From the vessels of the choroid plexus, as described by De Haen. "This," says Dr. Abercrombie, "may probably be the source of the hemorrhage, when the blood is confined to the ventricle, without any laceration of the substance of the brain." 5. Rupture of one of the sinuses, as in a case described by Dr. Douglas.—(Edin. Med. Ess., vol. vi.) 6. From the rupture of small aneurisms in the basilar artery (Serres), circle of Willis, &c. —(Archiv. Gén. de Méd.) 7. Lastly, Dr. Abercrombie refers to a very uncommon case (Med. Surg. Reg. of New-York), in which the bleeding took place betwixt the dura mater and the bone, from ulceration of a vessel, produced by caries of the inner surface of the left parietal bone. In the most common form of this disease, or that in which the hemorrhage proceeds from a vessel in the substance of the brain, Dr. Abercrombie supposes the rupture to take place from disease of the artery itself, without any relation to that congestive or hemorrhagic condition, making what he terms simple apoplexy. It consists sometimes of ossification of the arteries in various places, and sometimes of that peculiar earthy brittleness, which Scarpa has described as leading to aneurism ; and the canal of the artery will be found in many places to be considerably narrowed or contracted at the hardened parts, and sometimes entirely obliterated. In other cases, numerous branches of the principal arteries of the brain will be found to present a succession of small opaque osseous rings, separated from one another by small portions of the artery in a healthy state. Dr. Abercrombie says that this is a very common appearance in the brains of elderly persons. In some other cases, the inner coat of the artery is much thickened, of a soft pulpy consistence, and very easily separated. —(See Abercrombie's Pathological and Practical Researches on Diseases of the Brain, &c., pp. 239–242.) These observations cannot fail to be highly interesting.—ED.

frequency, weakness, and irregularity, with the progress of the fit, till at length it becomes, in many cases, intermitting and convulsive.

It is in this form of the disease that we chiefly meet with, and are almost sure to find, a snoring or stertorous breathing, which, though not a symptom of apoplexy as a species, may be ranked as a pathognomonic character of the particular form before us. And to the same effect, Dr. Cooke and the most celebrated pathologists who have preceded him. "Boerhaave," says he, "measures the strength of the disease by the degree of stertor; and Portal agrees with him in opinion on this subject; observing, that respiration in apoplexy is greatly impeded, and the motions of the breast are very apparent. We hear a noise of snoring or stertor," he says, "which is great in proportion as the apoplexy is strong. In all the cases of strong apoplexy which I have seen, the respiration in the beginning of the paroxysm was laborious, slow, and stertorous; and in those which proved fatal, this symptom, as far as I can recollect, remained, even when the breathing had become weak and irregular."—(On Nervous Diseases, vol. i., p. 171.) There is also often an accumulation of frothy saliva, or foam, which is occasionally blown away from the lips with considerable force.

The skin is about the ordinary temperature, and covered with a copious perspiration or clammy sweat; the pulse is full and hard, the face flushed, the eyes bloodshot and prominent, and generally closed. The cornea is dull and glassy, and the pupil for the most part dilated. In a few cases, however, there is a tendency to either spastic or convulsive action, spreading sometimes over the limbs, but more generally confined to the muscles of the face; insomuch that, under the first, the teeth are firmly closed, and deglutition is impeded. And where this state exists the pupil is contracted, as in a synizesis, sometimes, indeed, almost to a point. This last feature has been rarely dwelt upon by pathologists, whether of ancient or modern times: but it has not escaped the observant eye of my accurate and learned friend Dr. Cooke:—"In some instances," says he, "I have seen the pupil contracted almost to a point, and a physician of eminence of my acquaintance has likewise observed this appearance of the eyes in apoplexy: yet, although all writers on the subject mention the dilated pupils, I do not find any one, Aretæus among the ancients, and Dr. Cheyne among the moderns, excepted, who has noticed the contracted pupil."—(Ibid., p. 174.)

The paroxysm varies in its duration, from eight to eight-and-forty hours, and sometimes exceeds this period. Dr. Cooke quotes from Forestus the case of a woman, who being seized with an apoplexy, which he calls fortissima, lay in the fit for three days, and afterward recovered. We have already observed, that where it does not prove fatal, it predisposes to a relapse, and often terminates in a lesion of some of the mental faculties, or in a paralysis more or less general: commonly, indeed, in a hemiplegia, which usually takes place on the opposite side of the body from that of the brain

in which the congestion or effusion is found on examination to have taken place. "This," says Dr. Baillie, "would seem to show, that the right side of the body derives its nervous influence from the left side of the brain, and the left side of the body its nervous influence from the right side of the brain. It is rarely, indeed, if ever, that some of the turgid vessels of the brain are not ruptured in this form of the disease, and consequently produce an effusion of blood into some part of the organ of the brain." And, according to the same distinguished writer, the part where the rupture most commonly takes place is its medullary substance near the lateral ventricles, some portion of the extravasated fluid often escaping into these cavities.—(Morbid. Anat., p., 227.)

ATONIC APOPLEXY is the disease of a constitution infirm by nature or enfeebled by age, intemperance, or over-exertion of body or mind. It has more of a purely nervous character, as we have already observed, than the preceding variety, and is more a re... of vascular debility than of vascular surcharge, and consequently where effusion of blood is found, as it often is, in the present form, the vessels have been ruptured, not from habitual distention or vigorous plethora, but from accidental, often indeed slight causes, that have produced a sudden excitement and determination to the head beyond what the vascular. walls are capable of sustaining. Hence, a sudden fit of coughing or vomiting, a sudden fright, or fit of joy, an immoderate fit of laughter (Aretæus de Sign. et Caus. Diut. Morb., lib. i., cap. 7), the jar occasioned by a stumble in walking, or a severe jolt in riding, have brought on the present form of apoplexy, and with so much the more danger as the system possesses less of a remedial or rallying power in itself.

In most of the cases, the effusion detected after death has therefore been as truly sanguineous as in entonic apoplexy; and hence a valid objection to the use of the term sanguineous as descriptive of the entonic form alone. "It is," says M. Portal, "an error to believe that the apoplexy to which old men are so much subject is not sanguineous." Daubenton and Le Roy, members of the Institute, died of this precise kind of the disease at an advanced age; and Zulianus describes a case marked by a pale countenance, and a pulse so weak as scarcely to be felt, which, on examination after death, was found to be an apoplexia verè sanguinea: and another in which, after all the symptoms of what is ordinarily called serous apoplexy had shown themselves, extravasated blood was discovered in the brain, without any effusion of serum, or the smallest moisture in the ventricles.—(See also Burser. de Apoplex., p. 82; Cooke, ut sup.)

It is nevertheless true, that atonic apoplexy is often found with an effusion of serum instead of an effusion of blood, and apparently produced by such serous effusion; and hence, notwithstanding the objections of Dr. Abercrombie, and, in the latter years of his practice, of M. Portal, to serous effusion as a cause at all,* the experi-

* The following conclusions of Dr. Abercrom-

ence and reasoning of Boerhaave, and Hoffmann, and Mead, and Sauvages, and Cullen, must not be abruptly relinquished without far graver proofs than have hitherto been offered : for if it be a question, as Stoll has made it, whether effused serum, when discovered in the brain of those who have died of apoplexy, be a cause of the disease or an effect (*Prælect.*, p. 367),. we may apply the same question to effusion of blood. It is possible, indeed, for effused serum to become occasionally a cause even of entonic apoplexy, or that which, from its symptoms, is ordinarily denominated sanguineous apoplexy ; for it is possible for the exhalants of the brain to participate so largely in the high vascular excitement by which this form of the disease is characterized, as to secrete an undue proportion of effused fluid into any of its cavities, and thus become as direct a cause. of apoplexy as extravasated blood.

. This, however, is not what is generally understood by the term serous apoplexy as distinguished from sanguineous, and, indeed, ought only to be regarded as an effect of sanguineous distention.* Serous apoplexy, properly so called, is strictly the result of a debilitated constitution, and especially of debility existing in the

---

bie, the editor of this work is disposed to adopt as most consonant to facts :— .
1. There is a modification of apoplexy which is fatal, without leaving any morbid appearance that can be discovered in the brain. 2. There is another modification, in which we find serous effusion often in small quantity. 3. The cases which are referrible to these two classes, are not distinguished from each other by any such diversity of symptoms as can be supposed to indicate any essential difference in their nature. 4. Without any apoplectic symptoms, we find serous effusion in the brain in an equal, or in a greater quantity, than in the cases of the second modification. 5. It is therefore probable that, in these cases, the effusion was not the cause of the apoplectic symptoms. 6. It is probable that the cases of the first modification depend upon a cause which is entirely referrible to a derangement of the circulation in the brain distinct from inflammation. 7. It is probable that the cases of the second modification are, at their commencement, of the same nature with those of the first; and that the serous effusion is to be considered as the result of that peculiar derangement of the circulation which constitutes the state of simple apoplexy. In short, Dr. Abercrombie considers the serous modification as simple apoplexy terminating by effusion.—(On Diseases of the Brain, &c., p. 220.) With respect to the impossibility of detecting any morbid appearanecs in some cases of apoplexy, we are not to infer from it that a minute derangement of the structure of the brain, some alteration of its consistence, or some diseased action of its vessels, may not frequently have been concerned in the production of the disease, though overlooked, or not demonstrable, after death.—ED. .

* Here, and in the preceding sentence, the author admits one of Dr. Abercrombie's principal conclusions, somewhat differently expressed, namely, that serous apoplexy is a consequence of some derangement in the cerebral circulation, though what this derangement may be is not defined, further than that it is unaccompanied with any visible morbid appearances in the brain after death.—ED.

excernent vessels of the brain, whether exhalants or absorbents.* I say absorbents, because, although lymphatics have not yet been discovered in this organ, there must be vessels of some kind or other to answer their purpose, and the extremities of the veins have been supposed thus to act ; a supposition which has derived countenance from various experiments of M. Magendie, to which we shall have to advert in the Proem to the sixth class, and which may at least stand as an hypothesis till the proper system of vessels is detected.

Hence, atonic apoplexy rarely makes its attack altogether so incontinently as entonic ; and is commonly preceded by a few warning symptoms. These are often, however, nothing more than the ordinary precursors of other nervous affections, as vertigo, cephalæa, imaginary sounds, a faltering in the speech, a failure in the memory or some other mental faculty, and at length a sense of drowsiness, and a tendency to clonic spasms. On the attack of the paroxysm the patient is as completely prostrated as in the entonic variety, but the symptoms are less violent, though not on this account less alarming, in consequence of the greater debility of the system. The countenance is here pale or sallow instead of being flushed, but at the same time full and bloated ; the pulse is weak and yielding, sometimes, indeed, not easy to be felt ; and the breathing, though always heavy and laborious, not always, as we have already observed, noisy or stertorous. If spasms occur, they are uniformly of the convulsive or clonic kind. The duration of the fit varies, and if the patient recover, he . is more liable to a relapse, and more in danger of hemiplegia or some other form of paralysis, than in the stronger modification of the disease.

From these remarks on the two varieties of apoplexy we may readily see why this complaint, and its ordinary associate or sequel, palsy, should be about equally common to the poor and to the rich : for frequent exposure to cold and wet, severe and long-protracted exercise, and a diet below what is called for, will often be found to produce the same debilitating effects as ease, indolence, luxury, and indulgence at too sumptuous a table. And hence, contrary to what

* Dr. Clutterbuck regards serous apoplexy differently from our author. He conceives that no absolute line of distinction can be drawn between the sanguineous and serous forms of the disease : "they are, in fact, frequently found in combination, or rather to be considered as mere varieties of one and the same affection. Serous accumulations in any of the cavities of the body are in most instances the result of membranous inflammation ; not, in general, of an acute, but rather of a chronic or protracted description. This primary dependance of serous accumulations, or dropsies, as they are called, on inflammation, is not always distinctly seen, on account of the mildness of the inflammatory symptoms at first, and their often having passed away without notice, leaving the accumulation of fluid behind. Still there are but few cases in which the connexion of dropsy with inflammation, as its primary source, may not be traced by accurate inquiry. This applies to the brain as much as to other parts."—See Cyclop. of Pract. Med., art. APOPLEXY, p. 131.—ED.

many would expect, Sir Gilbert Blane has observed from accurate tables, kept with minute attention, and derived from a practice of ten years in St. Thomas's Hospital, and his private consultations, that "there is a considerably greater proportion of apoplexies and palsies among the former than among the latter:" or, in other words, that these disorders bear a larger proportion to other diseases among the lower classes than among those in high life. "Some cases of hemiplegia," says he, "occur in full habits; some in spare and exhausted habits. The former, being most incident to the luxurious and indolent, most frequently occur in private practice, and among the upper ranks of life. The latter occur more among the laborious classes, and among such of the rich as are addicted to exhausting pleasures."—(*Trans. Medico-Chir. Soc.*, vol. iv., p. 124.)*

In forming our prognostic, a special regard must be had to the peculiar character of the disease.' Generally speaking, atonic apoplexy is more dangerous than entonic, for we have here a more barren field to work upon, and nature herself, or the instinctive power of the living frame, has less ability to assist us. As to the rest, in either modification, the degree of danger will be generally measured by the violence of the symptoms. Where, under the first variety, the breathing is not much disturbed, the pupil is relaxed, and there is no appearance of spastic action; and where the perspiration is easy, the skin warm rather than hot, the bowels are readily kept in a due state of evacuation, and more especially where there is any spontaneous hemorrhage, as from the nose or hemorrhoidal vessels, and of sufficient abundance, we may

fairly venture to augur favourably. But where the symptoms are directly opposed to these; where the stertor is deep and very loud (*Dolæus*, p. 144), and particularly where it is accompanied with much foaming at the mouth (*Burser.*, p. 97); where the teeth are firmly clinched, or a spasm has fixed rigidly on the muscles of deglutition, and the pupil, instead of being dilated, is contracted to a point, we have little reason to expect a favourable termination.

The great hazard resulting from this tendency to spastic action, and particularly as evinced in a strongly contracted pupil, is thus forcibly pointed out by Dr. Cooke:—"Among the dangerous signs in apoplexy, many authors mention a dilated state of the pupil of the eye: but the contracted pupil, which I consider to be a still more dangerous appearance, has been scarcely noticed. I am of opinion that this ought to be reckoned among the very worst symptoms of the disease. I never knew a person recover from apoplexy when the pupil was greatly contracted. My opinion on this subject is confirmed by that of Sir Gilbert Blane and Dr. Temple."—(Id., p. 280.)

Dr. Cheyne, in like manner, regards convulsions as a source of great danger: while M. Portal, on the contrary, thinks they sometimes announce a diminution of the morbid cause. The latter reasons from the fact, that when, in living animals, a slight pressure has been made on the exposed brain, convulsions have taken place; while, if the pressure be increased in power, general stupor with stertor and difficult respiration have followed, instead of convulsions; an ingenious conclusion, but not exactly applicable, since in the one case the brain is in a morbid and in the other in a sound state; whence the premises on which the reasoning is founded are not parallel.*

In the treatment of apoplexy, if we be timely consulted during the existence of the precursive signs which have been noticed as occasionally taking place, we shall often find it in our power completely to ward off a paroxysm by bleeding,

---

* "Apoplexy," according to Dr. Condie (Hays' Cyclopedia, vol. ii.), "is of more frequent occurrence in the male than in the female sex: probably from the former being much more addicted than the latter to excesses, both as it regards the body and mind. Of fifty-one apoplectic patients admitted into the General Hospital of Hamburgh during the years 1828 and 1829, fifteen only were females. In Berlin, in 1829, of six hundred and ninety-nine deaths from apoplexy, four hundred and nine took place in males, and two hundred and ninety in females. In Philadelphia, during the three years preceding 1835, the number of deaths from apoplexy was two hundred and nine: of these, one hundred and nineteen occurred in males, and ninety in females. M. Serres, however, found that to the particular form of apoplexy termed by him *meningeal* (that is, apoplexy without paralysis), females are much more liable than males. Out of forty-one cases of this species which fell under his notice, thirty-three were in females, and only eight in males; and the registers of the Salpetrière and Bicêtre make the predominance still greater on the side of the female sex."

The predisposition to a recurrence of apoplexy is much increased after each attack, and popular opinion seems to countenance the belief that the third attack is almost universally fatal. Cases, however, might be adduced, of individuals sustaining ten or more attacks.

Richter (Specielle Therapie) inclines to the opinion that apoplexy sometimes prevails epidemically; and the same belief is entertained by Morgagni, Hoffmann, and others.—D.

* The following passage from Dr. Abercrombie's work, in relation to the prognosis, deserves attention:—"From the facts which have been related, we have reason to believe that there is a modification of apoplexy which is fatal without leaving any morbid appearance, and which probably depends upon a deranged condition in the circulation in the brain. We have also seen grounds for believing that the cases which terminate by effusion are probably at their commencement in this state of simple apoplexy. We have seen farther, that we have no certain mark by which we can ascertain the presence of effusion; and, finally, we have found that even extensive extravasation of blood in the brain may be entirely recovered from by the absorption of the coagulum. These considerations give the strongest encouragement to treat the disease in the most active and persevering manner. They teach us also not to be influenced in our practice by the hypothetical distinction of apoplexy into sanguineous and serous; and, finally, not to be hasty in concluding that the disease has passed into a state in which it is no longer the object of active treatment."—Pathol. and Practical Researches on Dis. of the Brain, p. 288.

purgatives, perfect quiet, and, in the entonic variety, a reducent regimen. Where, however, the pulse and other symptoms give proof of weak vascular action and nervous debility, the depleting plan should be pursued with caution, and it will be better to employ cupping-glasses than venesection, and, in some instances, to limit ourselves to purgatives alone. Yet, whatever be the degree of general debility, if the proofs of compression or distention be clear, as those of drowsiness, vertigo, and a dull pain in the head, it will be as necessary to have recourse to bleeding, either locally or generally, as in entonic apoplexy; for such symptoms will assuredly lead to a fit, unless timely counteracted and subdued.

"In the actual paroxysm of apoplexy," says Dr. Cooke, and I quote his words because it is impossible to exchange them for better, "the patient should, if possible, be immediately carried into a spacious apartment, into which cool air may be freely admitted. He should be placed in a posture which the least favours determination of blood to the head: all ligatures, especially those about the neck, should be speedily removed, and the legs and feet should be placed in warm water, or rubbed with stimulating applications. These means may be employed in all cases of apoplexy" (Burser., p. 288); and are consequently equally applicable to both the forms under which we have contemplated the disease. The collateral means to be had recourse to require discrimination, and it will be most convenient to consider them in relation to the actual form under which the apoplexy presents itself.

In ENTONIC APOPLEXY, copious and repeated bleeding seems, primâ facie, to offer the most rapid and effectual remedy we can have recourse to: yet the opinions of the best practitioners, as well in ancient as in modern times, have been strangely at variance upon this subject. Hippocrates, who regarded apoplexy as chiefly dependant upon a weak and pituitous habit, discountenanced the use of the lancet, as adding to the general debility: and even where it is accompanied with symptoms of strong vascular action, he discountenanced it equally, from an idea that the case was utterly hopeless. The authority of Hippocrates has had too much influence with physicians in all ages, and has extended its baneful effects to recent times, and, in some instances, even to our day. Hence Forestus tells us, that in strong or entonic apoplexy, no courageous plan ought to be attempted, no venesection, no pills: we may, indeed, to please the by-standers, have recourse to the remedia leviora of frictions, and injections, and ligatures round the arms and thighs: "and where," says he, "we have not found these succeed—in rationem sacerdotibus commiserimus."

In our own country, the same timid feeling has been particularly manifested by Dr. Heberden and Dr. Fothergill, but on grounds somewhat different. These excellent pathologists have chiefly regarded apoplexy as a disease of nervous rather than of general debility, and have been fearful of adding to this debility by abstracting blood, and hereby of almost ensuring hemiplegia, or some other form of paralysis. Hence Dr. Heberden speaks with great hesitation concerning the practice, rather than with an absolute and general condemnation of it: he observes, which is true enough, that many persons have been injured by large and repeated bleedings, and then lays down his rule not to bleed either in an attack of apoplexy or palsy, if there would have been just objections to taking away blood before the incursion of either.—(Medical Transactions, i., p. 472.)

Dr. Fothergill, however, expresses himself still more decidedly against bleeding than Dr. Heberden. He suspects that the weakness it occasions checks the natural effort to produce absorption; and that even the hard, and full, and irregular pulse, which seems imperatively to call for a very free use of the lancet, "is often an insufficient guide;" since "it may be that struggle which arises from an exertion of the vires vitæ to restore health." And hence, he adds in another place, "I am of opinion that bleeding in apoplexy is for the most part injurious, and that we should probably render the most effectual aid by endeavouring, in all cases, to procure a plentiful discharge from the bowels: as by these revulsions the head is perhaps much more effectually relieved from plenitude, and that without weakening or interrupting any other effort of nature to relieve herself, than by venesection."*

It is singular that, in drawing such conclusions from the instinctive efforts or remedial power of nature, where a cure has been effected spontaneously, these distinguished writers have not felt more deeply impressed by the salutary effects of spontaneous and copious hemorrhages, as from the nose, the lungs, and the hemorrhoidal vessels, which have never perhaps poured forth blood freely without operating a cure; and that they have not endeavoured to follow these footsteps, as far as they might have done, by substituting an artificial discharge of blood where a natural discharge has not taken place.

Other physicians, however, both in ancient and modern times, have not been equally insensible to this important fact. Galen, though he always hesitated in departing from the practice of Hippocrates, ventured to deviate from him

---

* Works, vol. iii., p. 208. Dr. Clutterbuck seems to lean very much to the doctrines of Heberden and Fothergill; for, in noticing the apoplexy arising from the extravasation of blood in the brain, that form of disease which has attracted the greatest notice, he observes, "this is a case in which bloodletting has been used with little discrimination, and often, there is reason to believe, carried to a hurtful excess. It is evident that the remedy can have no direct effect in removing the extravasated blood; nor can it lessen the quantity of blood altogether within the scull," &c.—(Cyclop. of Pract. Med.) To this some writers would reply, that bleeding is proved by experience to be one of the most powerful means of checking internal hemorrhages, and that in apoplexy it is indicated on this principle, though it may have no direct effect in promoting the absorption of the blood already extravasated.—ED.

upon the point before us. Aretæus, Paulus of Ægina, and Cœlius Aurelianus, carried the remedy of bleeding to a still further extent, and Celsus regarded it as the only means of effecting a cure.—(*De Medecin*, lib. iii., cap. xxvii.)

"The Arabians adopted the practice of the ancients, as far as relates to the employment of bloodletting in the strong apoplexy, and by far the greater number of modern physicians have in this respect followed their example In support of this practice we might adduce the opinion of all who have written on the disease: we might quote from the works of Sydenham, Wepffer, Boerhaave, Van Swieten, Morgagni, Baglivi, Sauvages, Tissot, Mead, Freind, Pitcairn, Hoffmann, Cullen, Portal, Cheyne, and many other eminent modern writers."—(*Cooke*, ut suprà, 292.) As this paragraph is quoted from Dr. Cooke, it is almost superfluous to add his own name to the list of those who strenuously recommend bloodletting.

A question has been made as to the side from which it may be most advantageous to take blood. Aretæus drew it from the sound side, wherever this could be distinguished. Valsalva and Morgagni recommend the same; as does also Cullen, observing that "dissections show that congestions producing apoplexy are always on the side not affected."—(*Pract. of Phys.*, vol. iii., p. 184.) Baglivi recommends bleeding from the diseased side, except where blood is abstracted locally. The question appears to be of no great importance; the grand object in general bleeding is to diminish the quantity and momentum of the circulating fluid, to enable the ruptured vessels to contract with greater facility, and to afford time for an absorption of whatever may have been effused.

In entonic apoplexy, general and local bleeding should go hand in hand; and the quantity drawn should in every instance depend upon the urgency of the symptoms. Dr. Cheyne advises us to begin with abstracting two pounds, and tells us that it will often require a loss of six or eight pounds before the disease will give way.

Dr. Cullen, and many other writers, as Morgagni, Valsalva, and Portal, have recommended that the opening should be made in the temporal artery or the jugular veins. "In all cases of a full habit," says Dr. Cullen, "and where the disease has been preceded by marks of a plethoric state, bloodletting is to be immediately employed, and very largely. In my opinion, it will be most effectual when the blood is taken from the jugular vein; but if that cannot be done, it may be taken from the arm. The opening of the temporal artery, when a large branch can be opened, so as suddenly to pour out a considerable quantity of blood, may also be an effectual remedy; but in execution it is more uncertain, and may be inconvenient. It may in some measure be supplied by cupping and scarifying on the temples or hind-head. This, indeed, should seldom be omitted, and these scarifications are always preferable to the application of leeches."—(Id., vol. iii., p. 182.)

In bleeding from the temporal artery, we may safely let the stream flow as long as it will, for in common it will cease before we have obtained enough, and all tight ligatures about the head, or indeed any other part of the body, should be avoided as much as possible. For the same reason Heister advises that on opening the jugular vein[*] no ligature should be made use of, as the smallest pressure on the part may do harm, by interrupting the circulation of the blood on the external veins of the neck.

M. Dejean of Caen, proposed, not long ago, to the Academy of Sciences, to open the superior longitudinal sinus, after raising the bone which covers it, and asserted that he had employed this mode with great success on strangled dogs.[†] M. Portal and M. Tenon, however, who were appointed commissioners to report on M. Dejean's memoir, agreed that bleeding from the jugular vein is preferable to that from the sinus, as producing the same effect more speedily, and with more facility of restraint when a sufficiency of blood has been taken away.

What seems to be the fair result the author will give in the words of Dr. Cooke. "General opinion, then, as well as reasoning, appears to be very much in favour of free and repeated evacuations of blood, both general and topical, in the strong apoplexy; and I am persuaded that greater advantage may be reasonably expected from this than from any other practice; yet I am very much inclined to think that it may be, and actually sometimes has been, carried too far. I have seen several cases, and heard of many others, in which very large quantities of blood have been drawn without the smallest perceptible advantage, and with an evident and considerable diminution of the strength of the patient."—(Op. cit., p. 311.)[‡]

---

[*] The superior utility of opening this vein is questioned by some of the best practitioners. As Dr. Abercrombie justly observes, "the only jugular vein that can be opened is the external jugular, which has very little communication with the brain, and, consequently, bleeding from it is probably much inferior to bleeding from the temporal artery."—On Dis. of the Brain, p. 289.

[†] The plan of trephining a patient, in order to open the longitudinal sinus for the relief of apoplexy, would be a novelty in operative surgery, equalled only by some of the proceedings of St. John Long.—Ed.

[‡] The opinions of Fothergill and of Heberden on the subject of bloodletting have lost their weight. The abstraction of blood, generally and locally, is now advocated by most clinical observers. On this subject Dr. Condie remarks, "the subtraction of blood is unquestionably one of the most efficacious means we possess for the cure of apoplexy. Employed at a sufficiently early period after the attack, it will frequently very promptly remove the congestion of the cerebral vessels, often prevent extensive extravasation of blood, and preserve the substance of the brain from rupture and disorganization. Even at a later period, it will in many cases greatly ameliorate the symptoms, prevent the extension of the injury which the brain may have already received, promote the absorption of the effused fluids, and the contraction and cicatrization of the apoplectic cavity. Bleeding, it is true, has been objected to in the treatment of apoplexy by a few respectable

The next important means to be pursued is that of exciting the bowels by active purgatives. [This, as Dr. Abercrombie justly remarks, is always to be considered a most important and leading point in the treatment; and, "though, in arresting the progress of the disease, our first reliance is upon large and repeated bleeding, the first decided improvement of the patient is generally under the influence of powerful purging."] The particular purgative is of no importance; whatever will operate most speedily and most effectively is what should be preferred in the first instance:* and hence a combination of calomel and extract of jalap will be found among the best: though a free action may afterward be more conveniently maintained by colocynth or sulphate of magnesia. Dolæus employed calomel so as to excite salivation, from an opinion that all evacuations are useful: and he gives an account of several cures he was hereby enabled to effect, and particularly relates the case of a woman who was in this manner considerably relieved, and died on the cessation of the ptyalism.—(*Dolæus*, p. 149.)

The collateral remedies are of less importance, though some of them may add to the general effect. Emetics are of a very doubtful character in the form of the disease before us, though often highly useful in atonic apoplexy.†

writers; and its use by others is restricted to certain forms of the disease. The objections, however, that have been made to the general employment of bloodletting in the early period of the attack, and its cautious repetition at a more advanced stage, will be found, we apprehend, to be purely hypothetical, and based upon erroneous views of the character of the disease, or to hold good solely against the abuse of the remedy. To say nothing of the concurrent evidence borne in favour of the good effects of bloodletting by the great majority of those medical writers whose opinions on practical subjects are the most deserving of respect, the very symptoms by which the disease is ordinarily accompanied, the morbid state of the brain revealed by dissection, and the fact that spontaneous and copious hemorrhages from the nose, lungs, or hemorrhoidal vessels, have either prevented the occurrence of the attack, when the most unequivocal symptoms of its approach have been present, or completely removed the disease when it has occurred, all press upon the attention of the reflecting practitioner the importance and necessity of bloodletting in the treatment of apoplexy."—(See Hays' American Cyclopedia of Practical Medicine and Surgery, vol. ii., art. Apoplexy.)—D.

* The most efficient purgative is the croton-oil; and, as Dr. Abercrombie observes, if the patient cannot swallow, it may be very conveniently introduced into the stomach, suspended in thick gruel or mucilage, through an elastic gum tube. The operation should be expedited by strong purgative injections.—Op. cit., p. 289.—ED.

† It is much to be regretted that the practice of administering emetics in apoplexy is still pursued by some practitioners. The celebrated and lamented Spurzheim very justly observes, "wherever there is a determination of blood to the head, emetics are contra-indicated; vomiting is admissible only where apoplexy is connected with an overloaded state of the stomach, and then we ought to have recourse merely to tickling the fauces. If

They have been given upon the principle of their producing a sudden prostration of strength and faintness: but this is a result of nausea rather than of vomiting; and we cannot answer that the straining will not renew the extravasation, or even rupture a vessel where no rupture has existed.*

Blisters and sinapisms promise but little in this form of the disease: they tease and irritate to no purpose when applied to the extremities, and are still more injurious when they are made to cover the scalp; for they effectually prevent the use of epithems of cold water, or vinegar, or pounded ice, which afford a rational chance of producing benefit.†

Cordials were in high reputation among the Greek practitioners, from a belief that apoplexy is in almost every case the result of a debilitated and pituitous habit; and the custom has too generally descended to the present day, even where the ground on which it was founded has been relinquished. Stimulants and cordials of all kinds should be sedulously abstained from: and the neutral salts, with small doses of the antimonial powder, or any other cutaneous relaxant, be employed in their stead: cooling dilute drinks should be freely recommended; and if we should hereby be enabled to excite a general moisture on the skin, it may prove of inealculable advantage.

The curative process under our SECOND VARIETY of the disease, or ATONIC APOPLEXY, must vary in many points from the preceding. It is here, if at any time, we should pause before we employ bleeding. Yet, as dissections show us, that even here also compression, and that too from an efflux of blood, is very general, and, either from blood or serum, almost constant,—whatever be the degree of constitutional debility, I can hardly conceive of any case in which we should be justified in withholding the lancet, or

the patient is insensible and cannot swallow, there is danger of suffocating him by introducing any liquid into the mouth. Vomiting always increases the vascular action: the face becomes turgid and suffused; it gives headache, which can be explained only by the congestion of blood in the vessels. Indeed, there is every reason to think that vomiting will bring on apoplexy, and convert a slight attack into a hopeless case rather than cure it."—See Observations on Insanity, by J. G. Spurzheim, London, 1817, p. 49.—D.

* Dr. Abercrombie says, "antimonials may occasionally be useful as an auxiliary, from their known effect in restraining vascular action, provided, in the early stages, they do not occasion vomiting."—(On Dis. of the Brain, p. 288.) In numerous instances, as Dr. Clutterbuck observes, apoplexy is ushered in by vomiting; the disease is then often referred to a disordered state of the stomach as the primary cause; but generally without reason, the disorder of the stomach being mostly secondary, and dependant upon the brain. The mistake is important, as leading to the employment of emetics, the use of which is not unattended with danger.—See Cyclop. of Pract. Med., art. APOPLEXY.—ED.

† Many practitioners will prefer to use warm rather than cold applications in these cases. —D.

the use of cupping-glasses. The argument stands precisely upon the ground of the expediency of bleeding in typhus accompanied with congestion : it is in itself an evil ; but it is only employed as a less evil to fight against a greater. With it we may succeed : without it, in either instance, the case is often hopeless.

Generally speaking, however, local bleeding will here be preferable to that of the lancet ; but cupping should always be preferred to leeches, whose operation is far too slow for the urgency of the occasion. The last, however, are recommended by Burserius, and Forestus quotes an instance in which they succeeded by a formidable application over the entire body.—(*Lib.* x., obs. 76.) Aretæus, after abstracting blood by cupping-glasses, recommends also the use of dry-cupping between the shoulders, and the recommendation is highly ingenious, and worth attending to.—(*De Cur. Morb. Acut.*, i., 4.)

Purgatives, though less violent than in entonic apoplexy, should in like manner be had recourse to : and as we have less danger to apprehend from the use of emetics, they may be given. They have the triple advantage of freeing the stomach from irritating matters, rousing the system generally, and determining from the head to the surface of the body.*

Here also we may use both external and internal stimulants in many cases with considerable success. Of the former, ammonia, camphire, electricity and galvanism, rubefacients and blisters, may be made choice of in succession, and applied alternately to different parts of the body.† Of the latter, we should chiefly confine ourselves to the warmer verticillate plants, as lavender, marjoram, and peppermint, or the warmer siliquose, as horseradish and mustard, or the different forms of ammonia ; yet even of these we are debarred by Dr. Cullen. [In France, nux vomica has been employed ; and in Germany, phosphorus. Dr. Abercrombie (*Pathological and Practical Researches on Diseases of the Brain*, p. 298) is of opinion that all stimulants must be used with considerable caution, and that the patient, during their use, should be kept in a very low state by spare living and occasional evacuations ; and he cannot agree that the diet in paralytic cases ought to be nourishing and restorative.]

In that peculiar kind of apoplexy which is sometimes produced by taking immoderate doses of spirits or some narcotic, and especially opium, in which we meet with an almost instantaneous exhaustion of the nervous power, making a near approach to asphyxy, though with a heavy drowsiness and stertorous breathing, the patient should first have his stomach thoroughly emptied by an emetic of sulphate of copper ; he should be generally stimulated by blisters, and

kept in a state of perpetual motion by walking or other exercise, so as to prevent sleep till the narcotic effect is over. An interesting case of this kind is related by Dr. Marcet.—(*Med.-Chir. Trans.*, vol. i., p. 77.)

After all, it should not be forgotten, that apoplexy is in most, perhaps in all cases, not secondarily alone, but primarily a nervous affection, and dependant upon a predisposition to this disorder in the sensorium itself, if not upon a morbid condition of it : and that hence the patient, though we should recover him from the actual fit, will be subject to a recurrence of it. In this view the interval becomes a period of great importance, and should be as much submitted to a course of remedial treatment as the paroxysm itself.

After entonic apoplexy, the patient should habitually accustom himself to a plain diet, regular exercise, early hours of meals and retirement, and uniform tranquillity of mind : and the state of his bowels should particularly claim his attention. After the atonic variety, the same general plan may be followed with a like good effect, but the diet may be upon a more liberal allowance ; and a course of tonic medicines should form a part of the remedial system. And hence much of the treatment laid down under LIMOSIS Dyspepsia (vol. i.) may be pursued here ; together with the use of the waters of Bath, Buxton, and Leamington.

————

SPECIES VI.

CARUS PARALYSIS.

PALSY.

CORPOREAL TORPITUDE AND MUSCULAR IMMOBILITY MORE OR LESS GENERAL, BUT WITHOUT SOMNOLENCY.

PALSY is a disease which makes a near approach to apoplexy in its general nature and symptoms, and is very frequently a result of it. It is, however, still more strictly, a nervous affection, and less connected with a morbid state of the sanguiferous or the respiratory organs. In examining it more in detail, we shall find that sometimes the motory fibres alone are affected in any considerable degree, while the sentient are only rendered a little more obtuse ; sometimes both kinds are equally torpid, and sometimes several of the faculties of the mind participate in the debility, though they are never so completely lost as in apoplexy.

The Greek writers contemplated the two diseases under the same view, considering them as closely related to each other, or, in other words, as species of the same genus. " The ancients," says Dr. Cooke, who has accurately gone over the entire ground, and taken nothing upon trust, " very generally considered apoplexy and palsy as diseases of the same nature, but different in degree ; apoplexy being a universal palsy, and palsy a partial apoplexy. Aretæus says, apoplexy, paraplegia, paresis, and paralysis, are all of the same kind ; consisting in a loss of sensation, of mind, and of motion. Apoplexy is a palsy of the whole body, of sensation, of mind, and of motion. And on this subject Galen,

————

* After the pathological remarks already delivered on the present disease, it seems that the practice of employing emetics must be attended with some risk of producing a renewal of hemorrhage, or even of occasioning a fresh rupture of the weakened or diseased vessels.—ED.

† Cajeput oil will be found an admirable external application.—D.

Alexander, Trallianus, Ætius, and Paulus Ægineta, agree in opinion with Aretæus. Hippocrates, who in various parts of his works speaks of apoplexy, nowhere, as far as I know, mentions paralysis ; and when he refers to this disease, he employs the term apoplexia. Both Aretæus and Paulus Ægineta represent him as speaking of apoplexy in the leg. Celsus describes palsy and apoplexy by the general terms RESOLUTIO NERVORUM."—(*Treatise on Nervous Diseases*, vol. ii., p. 1.) It is only necessary to add, that paresis and palsy were used sometimes synonymously ; and that, when a distinction was made between them, paresis was regarded as only a very slight or imperfect palsy.

Palsy and apoplexy, however, are something more than the same disease merely varied in degree ; the one, indeed, may lead to and terminate in the other, but they very often exist separately and without any interference ; and notwithstanding their general resemblance, are distinguishable by clear and specific symptoms. But if the Greeks approximated them too closely, the greater part of the nosologists of modern times, as Sauvages, Linnéus, Vogel, Sagar, Cullen, and Young, have placed them too remotely, by regarding each as a distinct genus : the proper nosological arrangement seems to be that of co-species, as they are ranked by Dr. Parr, as well as under the system before us.

The common causes of palsy are usually asserted to be those of palsy : and considering how frequently palsy occurs as a sequel of apoplexy, the assertion has much to support it ; for compression is here also, as well as in apoplexy, a very frequent cause. Yet, as compression does not seem to be the only cause of apoplexy, it is still less so of palsy in all its modifications, and we shall still more frequently have to resolve the disease into some of those causes of general, and especially of nervous debility, which we have already noticed as occasionally giving rise to apoplexy, and which we have more particularly illustrated under the genus CLONUS of the preceding order.

Palsy is often preceded by many of the precursive signs of apoplexy ; and it commonly commences slowly and insidiously ; a single limb, or a part of the body, being at first troubled with an occasional sense of weakness or numbness, which continues for a short time, and then disappears. A single finger is often subject to this token, as is one of the eyes, the tongue, or one side of the face.

The nerves chiefly affected are those subservient to voluntary motion, but the accompanying nerves of feeling in most cases participate in the torpitude, though not in an equal degree, and sometimes not at all. " I never," says Dr. Cooke, " saw a case of palsy in which sensation was entirely lost :" though such cases seem sometimes to have occurred. The action of the involuntary organs, and especially of the heart and lungs, is but little interfered with, though in a few instances something more languid than in a state of ordinary health. And in this respect we perceive a considerable difference between paralysis and apoplexy, in which last the

heart appears to be always oppressed, and the breathing laborious. The faculties of the mind, however, rarely escape without injury, and especially the memory ; insomuch that not only half the vocabulary the patient has been in the habit of using is sometimes forgotten, but the exact meaning of these terms that are remembered ; so that a senseless succession of words is made use of instead of intelligible speech, the patient perpetually misusing one word for another, of which we have given various examples under MORIA *imbecillis*, or MENTAL IMBECILITY. And it is hence not to be wondered at that palsy should occasionally impair all the mental faculties by degrees, and terminate in fatuity or childishness.

We have frequently had occasion to observe, and to prove by examples, that where any one of the external senses is peculiarly obtuse or deficient, the rest are often found in a more than ordinary degree of vigour and acuteness ; " as though the sensorial power were primarily derived from a common source, and the proportions belonging to the organ whose outlet is invalid, were distributed among the other organs." Something of this law seems to operate in many cases of palsy, and is more and more conspicuous in proportion to the extent of the disease : for, in hemiplegia and paraplegia, the half of the body that is unaffected has not unfrequently evinced a morbid increase of feeling. Dr. Heberden attended a paralytic person, whose sense of smell became so exquisite as to furnish perpetual occasions of disgust and uneasiness : and he mentions one case, in which all the senses were exceedingly acute.

It is to this principle we are to resolve it, that where the disease confines itself to the motory nerves of an organ alone, and the sensific are not interfered with, the feeling of the palsied limb itself is sometimes greatly increased, and sometimes exacerbated into a sense of formication, or some other troublesome feeling. " I have seen several instances," says Dr. Cooke, " in which paralytic persons have felt very violent pain in the parts affected, particularly in the shoulder and arm" (Op. cit., p. 5); and the remark, if necessary, might be confirmed from numerous authorities.

Palsy, however, is strictly a disease of nervous debility, and where it shows itself extensively, the whole nervous system is affected by it. The consequence of which is, as we have already shown in treating of entastic, and particularly of clonic spasm, that the sensorial power in all its modifications is communicated irregularly, and its balance perpetually disturbed, so as to operate upon the mind as well as upon the body : whence some parts are too hot and others too cold ; and even the affected limb itself, according to the nature of the affection, and its limitation or extension to different sets of nerves, will be warmer or colder than its natural temperature, and will waste away, or retain its ordinary bulk ; while the passions of the mind will participate in the same morbid irritability, and evince a change from their constitutional tenour. Persons of the mildest and most placid tempers will often discover gusts of peevishness and irascibility : and men of the strongest mental powers have been known to weep like children on the slightest occasions. In a few instances, however, an opposite and far more desirable alteration has been effected. "I had several years ago," says Dr. Cooke, "an opportunity of seeing an illustration of this remark in the case of a much respected friend. The person to whom I allude had always, up to an advanced age, shown an irascible and irritable disposition ; but after an attack of palsy his temper became perfectly placid, and remained so until his death, about two years afterward."— (*On Nervous Diseases*, vol. iii., p. 12.)

It is the general opinion, that paralytic limbs are uniformly colder than in a state of health : and Mr. Henry Earle has ably supported this opinion, upon an extensive scale of examination. —(*Medico-Chirurg. Transact.*, vol. vii.) Dr. Abercrombie, on the contrary, in a correspondence upon this subject with Dr. Cooke, gives it as his opinion, that the paralytic parts do not become colder than natural ; and adds, "that he had long ago observed that they are sometimes warmer than sound limbs, but without being able to account for it." The present author has frequently made the same remark, though he has more commonly found them below the ordinary temperature. The facts, therefore, on both sides, are correctly stated ; and the discrepance is to be resolved into the nature and extent of the sets of nerves that are immediately affected, whether sensific, motific, or both, and into the disturbed and irregular, the hurried or interrupted tenour, with which the nervous influence is distributed.*

The learned Pereboom, who has followed Boerhaave and Heister in attaching himself to the apparently correct doctrine of the Galenic school, that the nerves issuing from the sensorium are of two distinct sorts, one subservient to sensation, and the other to muscular motion, and has so far accorded with the physiology attempted to be established in the commencement of the present volume, has divided palsy, which he describes as a genus, into three species ; a nervous, muscular, and nervo-muscular ; by the first meaning that form of the disease in which there is a deprivation of sense without loss of motion ; by the second, loss of motion while the sensibility remains ; and by the third, loss both of sense and motion.—(*Acad. Nat. Cur. Soc. de Paralysi*, 8vo., Hornæ.) The specific means are here at variance with the physiology ; for, if it be true that muscular motion is as dependant upon the nerves as sensation, then palsy affecting the moving fibres is as much entitled to be called *nervous* as palsy affecting the sentient. Nor are the few cases to be met with of

* According to Dr. Abercrombie, paralytic limbs lose, in some degree, that remarkable power possessed by the living body in a healthy state, of preserving a medium temperature ; and paralytic parts become hotter or colder than sound parts which have been exposed to the same temperature.—Pathological Researches on the Bram, &c., p. 277.

C c 2

privation of feeling, without loss of motion, strictly speaking, to be regarded as palsies. They are rather, as Aretæus has correctly observed, examples of anæsthesia, or morbid want of the sense of feeling, and as such will be found described in the present system under the name of PARAPSIS EXPERS.—(Class IV., Ord. II., Gen. V.)

On this account the present author, in his volume of nosology, thought it better to follow up, though with a considerable degree of simplification, the subdivisions of Sauvages and Cullen, and to distinguish the disease under the three following varieties, founded upon the line or locality of affection :—

a Hemiplegia.	The disease affecting and
Hemiplegic palsy.	confined to one side of the body.
β Paraplegia.	The disease affecting and
Paraplegic palsy.	confined to the lower part of the body on both sides, or any part below the head.
γ Particularis.	The disease affecting and
Local palsy.	confined to particular limbs.

Some nosologists have transferred to this division the local insensibilities and atonies of the external senses, or parts of them, as though they were idiopathic affections. It is rarely, however, or never, as Aretæus has justly remarked, that they are not connected with other symptoms and other derangements of such organs and their respective functions : and hence, they rather belong to the second order of the present class than to paralysis, in the strict sense of the term. They are anæsthesiæ,—νόσοι παραλύτικοι or παρέτικοι, rather than παράλυσεις ; and in the system before us are arranged accordingly.

HEMIPLEGIA, the first of the above varieties of palsy, is far most frequently met with as a sequel of apoplexy, and especially of atonic apoplexy, or that in which the energy of the nervous system is peculiarly diminished and irregular. The usual exciting causes of apoplexy are in consequence of those of palsy, and need not be enumerated in the present place. In a few instances, however, hemiplegia occurs without preceding apoplexy ; and hence distinctly proves that pressure, or at least such a pressure as is demanded to produce somnolency, is not essentially necessary.* Mr. John Hunter, as we have

* Dr. Abercrombie's third class of apoplectic cases is that which he terms paralytic. "The leading phenomenon of this class," he says, "is the paralytic attack without coma, or at least without that complete and permanent coma which occurs in the former classes." He describes the attack as appearing under various forms ; the most common of which is hemiplegia with loss of speech ; but in some cases the speech is not affected ; while in other cases, the loss of speech is at first the only symptom. In some cases again, he observes, one limb only is affected, which is most commonly the arm, though sometimes the leg. Numerous other modifications occur, as palsy of one eyelid, or of the orbicularis muscle ;

already observed, was inclined to think that pressure from effused blood was in every instance the cause both of this disease and of apoplexy; but in allowing, as he has done, that on one occasion at least he was called to a patient who died of a gouty affection of the brain, "*with symptoms similar to apoplexy,*" and without any extravasation whatever, he directly yields the point of compression as a universal cause : for if atonic or retrocedent gout may produce apoplexy or palsy without pressure on the brain, so may many other atonic powers, operating as effectively on the sensorium. One of the most frequent of these powers is a debilitated and paretic state of the liver; and

distortion of the eyes; double vision; twisting of the mouth, &c. Loss of the power of swallowing also occurs occasionally, though more rarely in the cases which do not pass into apoplexy.—(Pathological and Practical Researches on the Diseases of the Brain, &c., p. 245.) The following are the morbid conditions specified by Dr. Abercrombie, as connected with these varieties. 1. Many of the cases have a close analogy to simple apoplexy, and after the patient's death, no particular changes in the brain are found, or only an effusion of serum, often in small quantity. 2. Extravasation of blood of small extent. 3. Softening of the cerebral substance. 4. Inflammation and its consequences.—(P. 247.) 5. Induration of a portion of the brain. 6. Empty cysts, from which the extravasated blood has been absorbed. 7. Extensive disease of the arteries of the brain.—(P. 279.)

An extraordinary case of intermittent hemiplegia of the left side is recorded by Dr. Elliotson in his clinical lectures.—(See Lancet for 1830-1, p. 556.) The paroxysms usually came on at ten o'clock in the morning, every third or fourth day, and, with a single exception, never with a longer interval; but, on one occasion, the complaint left him for sixteen days. He was forty-eight years of age, and had been subject to this affection for two years and a half. The paroxysms lasted from three to four hours. He had been in the East and West Indies, and had had fever both at Bombay and Batavia. Dr. Elliotson believed that this hemiplegia was the effect of malaria, and a form of ague, though not attended with shivering, heat, and sweating. On this principle he gave quinine, at first in doses of five grains every six hours, and the quantity was increased to fifteen. Large doses are often required in quartan ague, and Dr. Elliotson views this as a worse form of disease than quartan, because it occurred every third or fourth day, and the longer the interval between the attacks, the greater the difficulty of cure. The practice was successful, whatever may be the truth of the theory. We must agree with Dr. Elliotson, that, at all events, the case amounts to a proof, that paralysis is not *necessarily* an organic affection; and that hemiplegia does not *necessarily* arise from effusion, or from compression of any kind. If any compression occurred, it could only be during the fit; but Dr. Elliotson inclines to the theory that it was a disorder of function, induced by a particular poison.

Some cases, however, depend upon local affection or injury of the nerves; as the palsy of the deltoid muscle or whole arm, from pressure of the head of the dislocated humerus on the cervical nerves; palsy of one side of the face from an affection of the portio dura, brought on by inflammation of the ear or parotid gland, &c.—Ed.

hence those persons are peculiarly subject to this variety of palsy who have spent the earlier part of their lives in an habitual course of intemperance.* Hoffmann has particularly noticed this cause; and Morgagni describes the case of a man advanced in years, who was attacked with jaundice and hemiplegia simultaneously; the jaundice affecting the hemiplegic side alone, which was the right, and that with so much precision, that the nose was of a deep yellow on the one side, and of its proper colour on the other, which were divided from each other as by a ruled line. Other causes are, exposure to the rays of the sun, drinking cold water and bathing in it when heated, repelled eruptions, and chronic rheumatism.

As apoplexy has its precursive symptoms occasionally, so also has hemiplegia, and particularly when it is connected with a plethoric habit : for, in this case, the veins of the neck and face often appear turgid, there is an obtuse pain in the head, the tongue moves with some difficulty, and particularly on one side, the perception and memory become impaired, and the patient feels a tendency to drivel at one corner of the mouth rather than at the other. The onset, like that of apoplexy, is at last sudden ; and, if the patient be standing, he drops down abruptly on the affected side.

The progress of the disease is uncertain ; and depends very much upon the state of the nervous system at the time of the attack. If there be no chronic debility, nor other morbid condition of the sensorium, the patient will sometimes recover entirely in a week, or even less ; but if this system, or some particular part of it, be in an infirm state, he recovers only imperfectly ; and obtains, perhaps, a thorough or a limited use of the lower limb, while the upper remains immoveable ; or he is compelled to pass through the remainder of a wretched and precarious existence with only one half of his body subservient to his will, the other half being more dead than alive, and withering, perhaps, with a mildew mortification.—(See Cl. III., Ord. IV., Gen. XII., Spe. 2.)

We have stated that in this disease, as indeed in all others accompanied with an atonic disturbance of the nervous energy, there is not only a great irregularity in its supply, but a great and confused disproportion in its distribution to different parts of the body. Dr. Cooke (*On Nervous Diseases*, vol. ii., part i.) and Dr. Abercrombie (*Treatise on Apoplexy and Palsy*) have collected numerous and highly interesting examples, in which the sensific or motific nervous influence was either deficient in some parts, or so accumulated in others, that the most capricious and extraordinary sensations or motions were produced in them.

Sauvages gives a case from Conrad Fabricius of what he calls transverse hemiplegia, in which the disease was confined to the arm on one side, and the foot on the other ; and Ramazzini speaks of a patient whose leg on one side had lost

* Cases of this kind are unfortunately not rare in the United States.—D.

its feeling, but retained its power of motion, while the other leg had lost its power of motion but retained its feeling.* In some instances, indeed, the entire feeling on one side is said to have been lost, and the entire motivity on the other side (*Eph. Nat. Cur.*, passim.) ; and, in a few rare examples, persons during the paroxysms, and even for some time afterward, have felt on the affected side a sensation of pungent heat from cold, and especially polished bodies, and of painful cold from an application of hot bodies.

Where the sensibility is morbidly accumulated in a weak limb, as it often is in hemiplegia, sometimes so much as to give a painful sense of formication, cold not only excites action, but becomes almost as pungent an irritant as an actual cautery ; in the correct language of the poet—

　"Boreæ penetrabile frigus adurat."†

And hence, in climbing lofty mountains, as the Alps and the Andes, the traveller frequently finds his skin more completely blistered from the sharp cold by which he is surrounded, than by an exposure to an equinoctial sun. On the contrary, the morbid halitus or perspiration into which the application of hot bodies often throws a limb, in the same relaxed and debilitated state, produces an unusual sense of coldness in consequence of the evaporation. And we may hence explain the singular case recorded by Dr. Falconer of a gentleman who, after a paralytic attack, felt his shoes very hot when he first put them on, and gradually become cool as they acquired the warmth of his feet ; the reaction and consequent increase of moisture thrown forth from the surface of the feet, producing the difference of sensation.

The case of Professor de Saussure (*Med.-Chir. Trans.*, vol. vii., p. 216) is very singular ; he was gradually attacked with an imperfect hemiplegia, which at first showed its approach by perturbed sensations and vertigo, with a feeling of seasickness, a sight of objects reversed, a difficulty of swallowing liquids, and a total loss of voice, while the powers of the mind remained unimpaired, so that he could watch all his symptoms. Shortly after this the whole of the right side became utterly insensible, the insensible part being divided from the sensible by a geometrical line running down the body in a vertical direction : and in about three months

more, the insensibility of the right side of the head, accompanied with a debility of all the voluntary muscles, was transferred to the left, the right reacquiring its antecedent powers ; but all the right side below the head still continuing to possess its former torpitude. Here, also, there was a very different sense of heat and cold on the opposite sides ; for, while the left was influenced naturally, the right had the falsified sensation just noticed in Dr. Falconer's case, so that in getting into a cold bath or cold bed, the right side had a feeling of heat, while the left side felt cold as it should do. Hot bodies, in like manner, felt cold to the diseased side, apparently from the cause just stated. And that this was the real cause seems manifest from the patient's having often a feeling of a cold dew, or of cold water on the surface, and especially over his face, which induced him to wipe himself as if he had been wet. It is perhaps more singular that, though plunging his right or affected hand into cold water gave him a sense of lukewarmness, plunging it into boiling water gave him a disagreeable sensation, but very different from that of either heat or cold.*

This morbid disturbance and irregular distribution of sensorial power is sometimes productive of the most alarming consequence ; for, in a hemiplegic state of the bowels, some parts are in certain cases so acutely sensible, and others so utterly insensible, that while ordinary purgatives are incapable of exciting evacuations from the torpitude and irresponsibility of the palsied parts, they are sufficient to occasion inflammation, and have actually occasioned it in the parts exacerbated by accumulated sensibility, as certain experiments of M. Magendie have sufficiently established.

It is owing to the same irregular distribution of sensorial power, where every department of the nervous system participates in the diseased state of the sensorium, that we sometimes behold hemiplegia, and particularly imperfect hemiplegia, united with other affections of the same system. The symptoms of hypochondriacism are peculiarly apt to associate with it ; in which case the bravest hero will often lose all his magnanimity, and sit down and weep like a child : and in the celebrated geologist, M. de Saussure, we find a still more complicated instance of hemiplegia, hypochondriacism, and chorea. The disorder crept on by imperceptible degrees, and was accompanied with various anomalies. Both sides were weakened, but the left suffered chiefly ; yet with the aid of a stick he could still drag forward the left leg. By some unknown means he had taken up a morbid notion,

---

* De Morb. Artif., 286. See also Heister, Wahrnehmungen, i., 205. For references to various other facts of this kind, see Abercrombie's Pathol. and Practical Researches on the Diseases of the Brain, p. 275. "A gentleman," says he, "who was under the care of Dr. Hay, of Edinburgh, had two paralytic attacks at the distance of eight months from each other. In the first, there was perfect loss of feeling, with only partial loss of motion ; in the second, there was perfect loss of motion, with only partial loss of feeling," &c. Sir C. Bell's discoveries, and those of C. F. Bellingeri (see Ed. Med. and Surg. Journ., July, 1834), certainly tend to throw light on this curious subject.—ED.

† Virg. Georg., i., 93.

* Dr. Abercrombie remarks, that paralysis generally begins in the extreme parts ; but he has seen one patient who could write distinctly with his arm supported upon a table, after the arm from the shoulder to the elbow was completely paralytic. In a few hours afterward, the hand was also paralytic. He also quotes a case, related by M. Velpeau (Archives Gén., 1825), where the right arm was paralyzed from the shoulder to the middle of the forearm, while the hand was not in the least affected.—See Path. Researches on the Brain, p. 277.—ED.

very common to hypochondriac patients, of the difficulty of passing through a doorway when wide open without being squeezed to death; and hence at the very time in which he could cross his room with a tolerably firm step, the moment he reached the door, which was of capacious breadth and thrown open for his passage, he tottered and precipitated his motions with the jerk of a St. Vitus's dance, as though he were preparing for the most perilous leap : yet as soon as he had accomplished the arduous undertaking, he again became collected, and passed on with comparative ease till he had to encounter another adventure of the same kind, which was sure to try him in the same manner. —(*Medico-Chir. Trans.*, vol. vii., p. 214.) Tulpius gives a somewhat similar case, in which hemiplegia was united with beribery.—(Lib. iv., cap. 5.)

Paraplegia, or the second variety of palsy, has generally been conceived to depend altogether upon a diseased affection of the spine in its bones, ligaments, or interior, most frequently in the region of the loins; in consequence of which the spinal marrow becomes pressed upon or otherwise injured independently of any complaint of the brain. That this is a common cause is unquestionable, and a cause that often operates long without external signs : for the vertebral extension of the dura mater may be thickened, or a serous fluid effused, or blood be extravasated within the vertebral cavity; or a tumour may be formed in some part of it, or the spinal marrow itself may undergo some morbid change. But the best practical observers of the present day concur in opinion that paraplegia, like hemiplegia, is produced still more frequently by causes operating on the brain than confined to the spine. Of this opinion is Dr. Baillie, who ascribes it chiefly to pressure on the brain (*Trans. Med.*, vol. vi., art. ii.), Sir Henry Halford, Sir James Earle, and Mr. Copeland.— (*Treatise upon the Symptoms and Treatment of the Diseased Spine.*) Some kind of affection of the head, indeed, will commonly be discovered from the first, if we accurately attend to all the symptoms; some degree of pain, or giddiness, or sense of weight, or undue drowsiness, or imperfection in the sight. And hence many of the causes of paraplegia are evidently those of hemiplegia, operating probably upon a different part of the brain.

This form of paralysis may take place at any age, but it is more frequent as we advance beyond the middle of life; and Dr. Baillie has observed, that it occurs oftener in men than in women; for which it is by no means difficult to account, considering the greater hurry and activity of life pursued by the former. The disease in many instances makes an insidious approach. There is at first nothing more than a slight numbness in the lower limbs, with an appearance of stiffness or awkwardness in the motion of the muscles : these symptoms increase by degrees; there is great difficulty in walking, and an inability of preserving a balance; the aid of a staff or the arm of an assistant is next demanded : and the urine is found to flow in a

feeble stream, or perhaps involuntarily. The bowels are at first always costive; but as the sphincter loses its power of constriction, the motions at length pass off involuntarily. The disease may continue for years, and the patient at last sink from general exhaustion. It sometimes, but rarely, terminates in a recovery.— (*Practical Essay on the Diseases and Injuries of the Bladder, by Robert Bingham,* 1822.)

When an injured or diseased state of the spine is the origin of paraplegia, the complaint shows itself suddenly, or makes its advances insidiously, according to the nature of the cause : and for a knowledge of this form of the malady we are chiefly indebted to Mr. Pott,[*] who, however, does not think that it properly belongs to the species paralysis, though there seems no sufficient reason why it should not be so arranged, as in truth it has been by most pathologists from the time of Galen, who seems not only to have understood its nature, but to have contemplated it in this view.—(*De Locis Affectis,* lib. iv., cap. vi.) The disease, however, must not be confounded with rhachybia, or distortion of the spine from debility of muscular power, of which we have already treated (Cl. IV., Ord. III., Gen. I., Spe. 3) in the present volume.

It sometimes happens in hemiplegia, that one or more vertebræ have been pushed by sudden force a little out of their proper position; and in this case a considerable degree of numbness, together with less motion in one or both the lower limbs, is almost sure to follow, too often succeeded by a paralysis of the sphincters of the rectum and bladder, and consequently an involuntary discharge of feces and urine : and if the luxation should take place in the dorsal or cervical vertebræ, the organs of digestion may all more or less suffer, the respiration become affected, and the spine itself exhibit a considerable degree of curvature. And the same effects are still more likely to follow, and even to a greater extent and with still more serious mischief, from an idiopathic affection of some part of the spinal chain, arising from inflammation, scrofula, rickets, mollification, or caries; from compression by some effused fluid, or a thickening of its external tunic, or even of the substance of the spine itself; of which, last M. Portal has given a singular example.—(*Anat. Méd.*, p. 117.)

In the last case, the disease for the most part makes its approach slowly, and is often found in weakly and ill-nursed infants. Its precursive symptoms are commonly languor, listlessness, weakness in the knees, and a pale and shrivelled skin. As it advances, there is a difficulty in directing the feet aright when walking, the legs involuntarily cross each other, and the little patient is perpetually stumbling upon level ground, till at length he is incapable of walking at all. In adults, the progress of the disease is more rapid than in childhood.

Like hemiplegia, this variety is sometimes connected with a morbid state of the mental

---

[*] Remarks on that Kind of Palsy of the Lower Limbs which is frequently found to accompany a Curvature of the Spine, 8vo., 1788.

powers, and particularly with hypochondriacism, and this too where the disease proceeds from an organic lesion of the spine. Dr. Cooke has an instructive case in illustration of this in an officer of the army, aged forty-five, who had for many years been exposed to the hardships of a military life, particularly to extremes of heat and cold in various climates. "For two or three years previous to the paralytic attack, he had complained that his state of health was deteriorated, although no precise symptoms of disease could be pointed out either by himself or by his medical friends. His appetite was good, his bowels regular, though inclined to costiveness, and his usual robust appearance was not diminished. He entertained some fanciful notions respecting the state of his health, and from some uneasy sensations about the sacrum, he supposed that he had internal hemorrhoids, though no evidence of their existence could be perceived by his physicians, by whom he was considered as hypochondriacal." After having suffered for two or three years, he gradually lost the power of walking without some support for one of his hands. He went to Bath, and had the hot water pumped upon his loins: soon after which he complained of pain in the lumbar region, which was followed by a collection of fluid behind the great trochanter of the left side, which burst externally, and was discharged daily in considerable quantity. The paraplegia was now complete; the lower extremities being quite useless: the feces and urine, which for a considerable time the patient had with some difficulty retained, came away involuntarily: his strength rapidly wasted; he became much emaciated; and at the end of three months after his return from Bath he died, retaining the use of his senses and his intellectual faculties to almost the last instant of his life. —(*On Nervous Diseases*, vol. ii., part i., p. 43.)

Where the upper part of the spine is affected, the superior limbs are usually divested of mobility or sensibility, or both, while but little disturbance, in a few rare instances, takes place in the inferior. The most singular example of this sort that has occurred to the present writer, is contained in a case related by M. Rullier, of Paris.—(*London Medical and Physical Journal*, July, 1822, p. 80.) The subject was forty-five years of age, and had evinced a slight rachitic tendency from infancy, accompanied, as is often the case, with a considerable precocity of intellectual powers; the dorsal portion of the vertebral column evincing a little distortion, so as to give some degree of elevation to the right shoulder; but which did not proceed further. The patient, from early youth, had indulged himself in every concupiscent indiscretion, and especially in an unbounded and extravagant intercourse with females, which frequently reduced him to a state of exhaustion amounting almost to deliquium. It was not, however, till the age of thirty-four, that he first began to perceive any serious difficulty in the movement of his arms, which was soon connected with some degree of pain and swelling in the distorted part of the vertebral chain. The complaint made a rapid

progress, and the patient in a short time lost the entire use of these limbs, though their sensibility continued to the last, and appeared to grow morbidly acute, as he would not suffer any one to touch them, on account of the pain produced by such contact. He became, indeed, highly irritable in his temper, but could walk a considerable distance, enjoyed company and his usual meals, and still retained an immoderate appetency for venereal pleasures, with the fullest means of indulging it. Hectic fever, however, now attacked him, with phthisis, and he at last fell a sacrifice to such a host of marshalled evils. On a post-obit examination, the chief organs found to be affected were the lungs, and the spinal marrow at the seat of distortion. The last, indeed, presented a very singular appearance. From its origin to the fourth pair of cervical nerves, it was quite natural; but from this point, through an extent of six or seven inches in length, the whole substance of the column was reduced to the most diffluent state of mollification, like what we have already noticed as sometimes found in the brain: while below this length, the cord appeared again to be firm and uninjured; a few flakes of medullary matter were alone found in the morbid fluid which had usurped its place, but altogether disorganized and unconuected. And we here, therefore, behold, to adopt M. Magendie's remarks upon this very marvellous affection, a man enjoying, almost to his last hour, great moral activity, powerful generative faculties, a free movement of his inferior extremities, and a keen sensibility of the superior; who nevertheless, for an uncertain, but probably a very considerable period, had been destitute of one third part of the substance of the spinal marrow; and possessed no kind of communication between the cervical and dorsal portions of this cord,* unless we suppose something of the sort to have been maintained by means of the surrounding membranes; a supposition, however, which is entirely gratuitous, and at most, capable of throwing but little light upon the subject.

LOCAL PALSY is often produced by the general causes of the other varieties, probably operating in a less degree or more partially on the brain. We have already seen that it frequently takes the lead of the general affection, and appears for some days or weeks antecedently, in an imperfect movement of the tongue, or of one eye, or of one side of the mouth, sometimes of one or more of the fingers, or of an entire arm. And if, in this incipient state of the disease, proper evacuants or other means be instantly had recourse to, the paralytic tendency may be subdued, and the complaint limited to these local affections, and in a few days be entirely removed. This variety, however, is often the effect of

* If this were the fact, the case is undoubtedly exceedingly interesting, in a physiological as well as pathological view. However, as a very slight communication between the cervical and dorsal portions of the spinal cord might have existed previously to the dissection, and been inadvertently broken in it, a doubt may be entertained upon this material point.—ED.

other causes tending to destroy the irritability of the nervous system, or particular parts of it ; such as exposure to certain metallic fumes, or other means of absorbing metallic particles, especially those of mercury and lead : and above all, exposure to keen blasts of cold and damp air.* This last is perhaps the most common and effectual cause of local palsy, and is peculiarly operative, where the limb or organ so exposed is in a state of relaxation and perspirable moisture, whether from previous exercise or great heat of the atmosphere. A palsy on one side of the mouth, of the muscles of one eye, of one of the cheeks, of an arm or a leg, is in this manner frequently produced, and becomes at times of very great obstinacy. Occasionally, indeed, the torpitude extends much further than to a single limb, and various organs are involved in its mischief. "A watchman," says Dr. Powell (*Med. Trans.*, vol. v., p. 195), "on quitting his duty after a night of severe cold, was attacked by sudden and violent general pains in his limbs, which soon departed, and left him in a state of universal palsy of the muscles of voluntary motion. He had lost all command over the muscles of his limbs or trunk ; but the joints were unaltered in their external appearance : they were perfectly flexible : and it gave him no pain if you moved them in any direction. The sphincters also of the rectum and bladder had lost their usual powers of retention, and he passed both stools and urine involuntarily and unconsciously. His circulation was not affected in any cognizable degree, and his mind retained its usual powers. His voice was not lost : the hot bath and other remedies were tried in vain ; he died : but on examination, there was no congestion, or effusion, or alteration of structure of any kind discoverable." In this case the motific nerves, or those derived from the anterior trunk of the spinal cord, seem to have been alone affected ; and in those slight palsies, induced by sudden cold or damp applied to one side of the face, and commonly known by the name of *blights*, the nerves that lose their power are branches of the portio dura, the respiratery nerve of Sir Charles Bell, while it is rarely that the twigs of the trigeminus, which commonly accompany them for the purpose of conveying sensation, are united in the mischief.

In the treatment of palsy, it is necessary to distinguish between its attack and its confirmation, and as much as possible to ascertain the nature of its predisponent and exciting cause.

Generally speaking, in hemiplegia, and very frequently in paraplegia, and even in local palsy, the causes of apoplexy are those of the present affection. And as, of these causes, compression

of the brain has appeared to be by far the most frequent in the former disease, so we ought to regard it, and shall generally find it, in the latter. And hence, copious bleeding and purgatives not only recommend themselves to us from the good effects we have already seen them produce in apoplexy, but from the actual and general advantage which has been derived from them in palsy itself. Mr. John Hunter was so fully convinced of the benefit of sanguineous depletion, that he made it his unicum remedium, though he allowed cathartics subordinately. Upon this subject, however, he writes with more force than discrimination. Referring to the stimulant plan pursued by some practitioners, he observes, "This is even carried further than blistering," to which he also objects : "we hardly see a man taken with all the signs of an apoplexy, where a paralysis in some part takes place, or hemiplegia, but he is immediately attacked with cordials, stimulants, electricity, &c. Upon a supposition that it is nervous debility, &c., the poor body is also tortured because it cannot act, the brain not being in a condition to influence the voluntary muscles. We might, with exactly the same propriety, stimulate the fingers, when their muscles are torn to pieces. We ought to bleed at once very largely, especially from the temporal artery, till the patient begins to show signs of recovery, and to continue it till he may begin to become faintish. We should give saline purges freely, to diminish impetus, and promote absorption ; then quietness should be enjoined, and as little exercise of body as possible, and especially to avoid coughing and sneezing. Plain food should be directed, and but little of it."—(*On Blood and Inflammation*, p. 213.)

All this is excellent as a general rule ; but the rule must admit of exceptions. In treating of apoplexy, we have noticed it as dependant on two very different and opposite states of the constitution,—an entonic and an atonic. And the same diversities of constitution are to be found in paralysis. Now, under the entonic state, there can be no question, and there ought to be no exception : and the boldness of the practice should be regulated by the nature of the exciting cause. Where this is over-eating or intoxication, eighteen or twenty ounces of blood may be taken away with advantage, at once ; in a few hours after, twelve or fifteen ounces more ; and the venesection may be repeated a third or even a fourth time, if necessary. Dr. Cross pursued this active plan in the case of a man thirty-five years old, who became hemiplegic from excess of drinking, and at the same time gave calomel to the amount of twenty-five grains to a dose, and in a few days effected a complete cure.—(*Thomson's Annals of Philosophy*, No. xliv., p. 121.) And similar instances of success are to be found in all the writers upon the subject.

Even in atonic apoplexy, it has been observed that venesection is occasionally necessary ; and it may be equally necessary in atonic paralysis ; for here also effusion may take place both of blood and serum : of serum, indeed, more frequently from deficiency than from excess of vigour ; and of blood, from a debilitated state of the vessels,.and their greater facility to be ruptured from slight causes, as a violent fit of coughing or sneezing, of joy or terror. Absorption may not easily take place in this state of constitution ; but emptying the vessels alone will gain space, by stimulating them to contract their diameter.

I cannot better. illustrate this, than by the following case from Dr. Abercrombie :—" An old and very poor woman, aged about seventy, thin, pale, and withered, having gone out to bring water from one of the public wells, on the morning of the 2d of July, 1818, fell down in the street speechless, and completely paralytic on the right side. Nothing was done till about two P. M., when she was found stupid but not comatose, yet completely speechless and para-· lytic : her pulse of good strength, and about ninety-six. She was bled to fifteen ounces. Purgative medicine was ordered, and cold applications to the head : on the 3d she was considerably improved both in speech and motion ; but having become rather worse at night, the bleeding was repeated, and the purgative medicine continued. From this time she improved gradually : at the end of a week .she was able to walk with a little assistance, and speak pretty distinctly ; and by the end of another week, she had entirely recovered her former health."— (*Treatise*, &c., p. 15.) Nothing could be more judicious than this treatment, and the result corresponded with the views of the enlightened practitioner. There can_ be no doubt that, in this case, a vessel had been suddenly ruptured :· the labour in which the patient· was occupied was violent, the.season was that of the summer, and the temperature probably very hot : the stupor and state of the pulse equally indicated compression of the brain.

Thus far, bleeding may be ·allowed, and indeed ought to be imperatively enjoined. But there are some cases in which it is altogether a venture, and others in which it is considered on all hands to be injurious. Even Mr. Hunter himself recoils from the practice where hemipiegia is apparently a result of retrocedent gout ; and if we follow up the spirit of this forbearance, we shall be induced to abstain equally in all instances where there is a like diminution of sensorial power—in all instances of atonic paralysis, let the exciting cause be what it may, where there is no stertor,·no stupor, nor vertigo ; no convulsion, nor other irregular nervous action ; and the pulse, instead of being firm, is feeble and intermittent. For it should never be forgotten that, if many patients have recovered after bleeding, in suspicious circumstances, others have died after it, and probably in consequence of it, while great numbers have derived no benefit whatever. The advice of Dr. Cooke upon this subject is therefore founded on the truest wisdom, and cannot be too extensively committed to memory :—" Each individual case must be viewed in all its circumstances, and by a careful consideration of them our practice should be regulated. Before we prescribe bloodletting in hemiplegia, we must investigate the age,

strength, general constitution, and habits of the patient, and above all, the actual symptoms of the disease. ·In early, or even in somewhat advanced life, if plethora and the various symptoms tending to apoplexy be present, I should not scruple to bleed freely both generally and topically. On the contrary, in great age, debilitated, leuco-phlegmatic habit, dropsical tendency, &c., I should think it right to abstain altogether from this and from every other powerful mode of depletion, unless there be an evident determination to the head, marked by flushing in the countenance, throbbing of the arteries, redness of the eyes."—(*On Nervous Diseases*, vol. ii., part i.; p. 141.)

In·purging, we may proceed with less restraint : for even in debilitated and dropsical habits, stimulating the bowels is almost uniformly beneficial : should there be serous, or·even sanguineous effusion, absorption is hereby powerfully promoted ; and if·there be none, a beneficial revulsion will often be produced, and the stimulus will always be useful. In a very debilitated state of the constitution, however, we should choose the warmer in ·preference to the colder purgatives ; and ·hence jalap, colocynth, or even aloes, in preference to neutral salts : and it will also be serviceable to combine them with some distilled water impregnated with an essential oil, as mint, pennyroyal, juniper, or rosemary.

If we have strong reason to apprehend a sanguineous effusion, emetics ought not.to be employed for a few days ; but if we have no ground of such suspicion, they cannot be had recourse to too soon: In low-or atonic hemiplegia, Stoll first checked the hemiplegia· by emetics, and then carried it off by external and local stimulants, as cantharides, in conjunction with pills of gum ammonia, myrrh, and aloes.*

Such, under different modifications, is the reducent course it seems proper to pursue in the general train of paralytic attacks when they first make their appearance. If this course succeed the patient will soon recover, and, with a view of preventing a relapse, an extension of the reducent or tonic regimen, according to the nature of the case, as we have already noticed in the treatment of apoplexy, is all that we shall have further to prescribe.

But this course may not succeed : the disease may prove obstinate and become confirmed ; and the practitioner be called upon to proceed further.

Having removed, as far as we may be able, all pressure upon the sensorium, and thus given an opportunity of healthful play to its function, our next· business is to reinvigorate its general energy, and extend it to the parts which it has ceased in a greater or less degree to actuate.

Stimulants, external or internal, or both, have been almost uniformly had recourse to for this purpose : but I cannot avoid thinking that the practice has been too indiscriminate, and,. in

* Mat. Med., part ii., p. 92. Few of the best modern practitioners venture to prescribe emetics in any examples of paralysis connected with dis. ease in the head.—Ed.

many cases, far too precipitate. We have observed, that in many cases of hemiplegia, there is not only great local inactivity, but great irregularity of action ; a tumultuous hurry of sensorial power to some parts, with an equal removal of it from others. In all such cases we should proceed gently and palliatively, rather than rapidly and forcibly : and to do nothing is better than to do too much. We should endeavour to allay the nervous commotion, and restore the agitated system to order by internal and external quiet of every kind. The patient should be kept as still as possible in a warm commodious bed and a well-ventilated room. His diet should be plain, with the allowance of a moderate quantity of wine, or wine and water. Camphire, musk, valerian, and other warm sedatives, as ammonia, neutralized with citric acid, are here to be chiefly resorted to, if, indeed, we resort to medicines of any kind ; and to these may be added the less stimulant metallic salts, and especially those of zinc and bismuth. The warm bath may be allowed two or three times a week, and, if the nights be restless, the inquietude may be subdued by hyoscyamus. And, as this form of the disease is often connected with great general debility, and a tendency to hypochondriacism or lowness of spirits, cheerful and exhilarating conversation, and such occasional exercise in a carriage as may be indulged in without fatigue, will form very serviceable auxiliaries. In Pechlin (Lib. iii., obs. 27) is to be found the case of a person called Peyreske, who is said to have been cured of a palsy accompanied with aphonia, by reading some favourite and agreeable authors. This may be an overstatement, or too much stress may be laid on this particular part of the general plan of treatment : but there can be no doubt that, in the form of the disease we are now contemplating, a gentle and insinuating amusement of this kind will not be without its effect.

This tranquillizing and unostentatious plan I have found to answer wonderfully in many cases of that tumultuous and irregular action described in the preceding history. But where the case seems altogether confirmed and chronic, and an entire side, or some other extensive part of the body, shows a fixed loss of sense and voluntary motion, while every other part has resumed its healthy function, we may then, with safety, have recourse to the stimulant practice.

This will consist of external and internal irritants, and Dr. Cullen has given a long and useful table of both. Of the former, the chief are friction by the hand or a flesh-brush ; stimulating liniments prepared of the concentrated acids, or the caustic alkalis inviscated in oil or lard to render them less acrid and corrosive; brine, or a strong solution of sea-salt ; the essential oils of turpentine, or other terebinthinate substances ; and various vegetable acrids, as mustard, garlic, and cantharides, or other blistering insects. The object of all these is the same ; it is that of acting upon the origin of the nervous chain by stimulating it at its extreme end ; and as we have numerous instances of the production of such an effect in a great variety of cases,

particularly in those of trismus and lyssa, or canine madness, the principles of which we have endeavoured to elucidate under these diseases, we have reason to expect a like influence, and of a beneficial instead of a morbid kind, in the applications before us. Generally speaking, however, the irritation produced by the use of many of the siliquose and alliaceous or alkalescent plants, as mustard, horseradish, and garlic, is more uniformly efficacious than that of cantharides ; as the irritation excited is more considerable and of longer duration. Dr. Cullen tells us, that he has reason to believe the use of liquid styrax in the proportion of one part to two of the old black basilicon, a favourite empirical composition, "has been of remarkable service in paralytic cases, and particularly in a debility of the limbs following rickets.*

Many practitioners have, for the same purpose, been in the habit of burning moxa, or cotton alone, on different parts of the affected side. Dupuytren employed the former, and Pascal (*Journ. de Méd.*, tom. lxvi.) the latter ; and both, as they tell us, with great advantage. Baron Larrey speaks in terms of high commendation of the first, and especially in spine-cases, or paraplegia. One of his examples is worth relating. The patient had been a sufferer for three years, and had violent and almost permanent pain in the extremities, tremour, emaciation, and sleeplessness ; the spinous processes of the dorsal vertebræ projected, and were painful on pressure. The moxas were applied in pairs, beginning from the tenth and eleventh dorsal vertebræ. On the first application all pain was removed ; on the second, spontaneous motion was restored ; and, after the use of thirty moxas, the patient walked without support.—(*Recueil de Mémoires de Chirurgie*, &c., 8vo., Paris, 1821.) Others have thought they derived more service from a repeated use of stinging nettles. Some again have employed issues, others setons, others acupuncture, and others the potential or even the actual cautery. This last mode of treatment, however, is best calculated for that form of hemiplegia produced by a diseased spine. Mr. Pott found caustics applied on each side of the spine peculiarly serviceable, and they have been in common employment ever since his recommendation of them.

In the rank of external stimulants, we are to arrange electricity and voltaism. From their well-known and extraordinary power of re-exciting irritability in the muscular fibres of animals that have been for some time dead, it was very reasonable to suppose that either of these stimuli might be employed with very great advantage : and accordingly we meet with them in extensive and popular use from the earliest periods of their having been, if not discovered, at least reduced to scientific management ; and have numerous reports of cases in which the former was tried, and in many instances with advantage,

---

* Mat. Med., vol. ii., part ii., cap. v. The editor has not much faith in the employment of internal stimulants, and believes with Dr. Abercrombie, that the practice is hardly safe unless accompanied by a low regimen.

rather before the middle of the last century.* In several experiments, both have been found highly beneficial; but in various cases also, both have been made use of in vain, and in a few instances, with apparent disadvantage; and those who were at first most sanguine of success, gradually lost their confidence in them.

The fact seems to be, that even at this late period of trial, we are greatly in the dark upon the subject, and have not learned to discriminate the exact modifications of the disease, or the exact modifications of electric power in which alone this active power may be employed with advantage: for that, in both forms, it has been occasionally of very high benefit, is by no means to be disputed: and even at times when communicated by the *gymnotus electricus*, or electric eel itself, of which a singular example is given in the Haerlem Transactions;† the patient having recovered the use of the affected side after a hundred strokes from the fish. Upon the whole, as it is a direct stimulus, it appears better adapted to the atonic than the entonic character of paralysis.

The stimulus of hot water alone is often serviceable in local palsy, especially when it has been produced by cold or damp; and in conjunction with the rubefacients and vesicatories we have just enumerated, or with friction to the part affected by means of the hand or a fleshbrush, and particularly when aided by terebinthinate or other essential oils, will usually succeed in restoring to the affected muscles their wonted power. But where the palsy is more extensive, as in hemiplegia and in many cases of paraplegia, it has been more usual to recommend the stimulus of hot water in conjunction with various active mineral corpuscles held in solution by it: and hence the common resort of paralytic patients in our own country to the waters at Bath, Buxton, and Leamington. Hot baths of this kind are also a direct stimulus; and as such, far more efficacious in paralytics of atonic or dilapidated constitutions, than in those who have suffered from plethoric or entonic fulness, or at least till they have been lowered to the proper standard by a long course of some reducent regimen.

Cold bathing is also a stimulant as well as hot bathing, but a stimulant of a different kind, for it acts indirectly instead of directly. The intention with which it is used, is that of forcibly urging the mouths of the cutaneous vessels into a general entastic or rigid spasm, in order hereby to excite a general reaction, as in the case of the first and second stages of the ague-fit, and thus to draw the torpid muscles into the common range of association. Dr. Cullen seems favourable to this practice under a prudent management. " Cold," says he, " applied to the body for any length of time, is always hurtful to paralytic persons: but if it be not very in-

tense, nor the application long continued, and if at the same time, the body be capable of a brisk reaction, such an application of cold is a powerful stimulant of the whole system, and has often been useful in curing palsy. But if the power of reaction in the body be weak, any application of cold may prove hurtful."—(*Pract. of Phys.*, vol. iv., mclxvi., p. 190.) It is hence only necessary to add, that while the hot mineral baths appear best adapted to cases of atonic paralysis, cold affusion or the cold bath may be employed with most success in accidental palsies of the plethoric and the vigorous.

The ordinary internal stimulants are the mineral waters we have just adverted to, camphire, and other terebinthinate substances, many of the siliquose and alliaceous plants, as mustard, horseradish, garlic, and onions, and a temperate use of wine: the whole of which, however, are proscribed in all cases by many writers of great eminence, and particularly Dr. Cullen and Mr. John Hunter: and which, if allowed at all, should be confined to the atonic form of paralysis, or never be commenced, in any instance of entonic palsy, till the system has been sufficiently reduced for the purpose. And where this has been accomplished, such a class of remedies has often been found of essential service.*

Independently of these, there is a tribe of medicines entitled also to the name of stimulants. I mean several of the acrid poisons, as *arnica montana*, or leopard's bane; *rhus vernix*, varnish sumach; and strychnos, *nux vomica*. All these excite the nervous system to great agitation and spasmodic action; and if the dose be increased, violent convulsions, alternating with tetanus, are sure to ensue: and hence it has been supposed, that they may be rendered effectual in a restoration of motivity to paralytic limbs. The flowers of the arnica, or doronicum, as it was once called, were chiefly employed, though sometimes the leaves were preferred. Dr. Collin was much attached to the former in palsies of all kinds, and affirms that he has found them very generally successful. He gave them in an infusion or decoction, in the proportion of from a drachm to half an ounce, to a pint of the liquid (*Observ. circa Morbos Acutos et Chronicos*, tom. v., p. 108): and, from his recommendation, they were, at one time, very generally adopted, were countenanced by Plenck and Quarin, and experimented upon by Dr. Home.—(*Clinical Experiments, Histories*, &c., Edin., 8vo., 1780.) The last tried them in six cases, but without much success; and they have not been able to maintain their reputation: nor, from the violence and uncertainty of their effects, is it worth while to revive them.

The *rhus vernix*, or varnish sumach, is chiefly indebted for whatever degree of fame it has acquired in paralysis to the recommendation of Dr. Fresnoi. The milky juice of this plant is so acrid as to blister the hands of those who

* Mémoires de l'Academie des Sciences, 1749, p. 40. Jallabert, Expérience sur l'Electricité, Genev., 1749.

† Abhandlungen aus den Schriften der Harlemer und anderer Holländischen Gesellschaften, band i., p. 109.

* Dr. S. Calhoun, of Philadelphia, has proposed the use of the tourniquet for restoring the power of muscles debilitated by long-continued inactivity.—Phil. Journ. of the Med. and Phys. Sc., vol. i., p. 131.—D.

gather its leaves, so that they are obliged to wear gloves. The leaves are employed in decoction and in extract ; and appear not only to act powerfully upon the nervous system, but by urine and perspiration ; and hence the plant has a claim to be considered as an active promoter of absorption as well as a revellent, which may, perhaps, render it serviceable in some cases of paralysis from serious compression of the brain. Of its benefit in some other diseases of a spasmodic or nervous character, and especially in hooping-cough, we have already spoken.

Most of the species of rhus or sumach contain a like pungent acridity in their milky juices, and hence several others of them have occasionally been employed for the same purpose. Dr. Alderson, of Hull, has of late preferred the leaves of the *rhus toxicodendrum*, poison sumach, or poison oak, as it is sometimes, but improperly called : and, in many cases, he has thought it of considerable benefit. He commences with half a grain of the powdered leaves, which he gives three times a day, and gradually increases the dose to four or five grains, till he finds a sense of tingling produced in the paralytic part, accompanied with some degree of subsultus, or a twitching or convulsive motion.*

There are other acrid poisons which have a tendency to produce strong entastic or rigid spasm, most of which possess an intensely bitter principle, and perhaps derive that difference of effect from the tonic power of this very quality. Of these the chief are the strychnos, *nux vomica*, and the *ignatia amara.* Both have hence been employed in paralysis, and the virtues of both seem to be nearly alike ; the former, however, has of late taken the lead upon the recommendation of Dr. Fouquier, of the Hôpital de la Charité at Paris, who has tried it upon a very extensive scale, and apparently with a perfect restoration of health in many cases ; and whose success has been authenticated by similar experiments under the superintendence of MM. Magendie, Husson, Asselin, and other pathologists. He gives it in the form of powder, or alcoholic extract : four grains of the first, and two of the last, are a dose, and may be taken from two to six times a day. He also employs it in injections. In half an hour after administration, the paralyzed muscles have, in various cases, begun to evince contraction : and, what is peculiarly singular, while a spastic contraction is determined to these, the sound parts remain unimplicated in the action. A frequent effect, unquestionably dependant on the bitter principle of the plant, is that of increasing the appetite, and diminishing the number of the alvine evacuations when in excess. Sometimes it produces a temulent effect, and occasions stupor and a sense of intoxication, and, when rashly administered, general tetanus, with all its train

of distressing and frightful symptoms. The most powerful form of this medicine is its alkaline basis, to which the French chymists have lately given the name of strychnine. It has hitherto been chiefly used through the agency of clysters.*

Like all other powerful medicines in their first and indiscriminate use, the nux vomica appears sometimes to have been highly beneficial, sometimes mischievous, and sometimes to have produced violent effects on the nervous system, without an important change of any other kind. Dr. Cooke has collected a variety of cases, in which it has been tried in our own country as well as in France, and this seems to be the general result. The present author has tried it in various instances, but has never been able, from its tendency to temulency, to proceed much more than half as far as some practitioners have gone, who have gradually advanced it from four grains of the powder to twenty-four, three or four times a day. In the case of the late E. Sheffield, Esq., of the Polygon, Somer's Town, mineralogist to the estates of the Duke of Devonshire, and who is well known to have been one of the best practical geologists of his day, the author commenced with two grains alone of the powder given three times daily, as this was a hemiplegia following upon a second fit of atonic apoplexy, with a general debility both of the mental and corporeal powers, the patient being, at the time, rather upwards of sixty years of age. This dose occasioned no manifest effect, and on the third day, August 21, 1819, it was gradually increased to six grains. It now produced a powerful sense of intoxication, but with clonic agitation instead of a tetanic spasm of the paralyzed leg and arm, and great heat down the whole of the affected side. The powder was continued in this proportion for three or four days, but the stupor and vertigo were so considerable and afflictive, that the patient could not be persuaded to proceed with it any longer, and it was in consequence suspended. In the ensuing September 1, he was evidently getting weaker, and recommenced the medicine at his own desire ; the dose was gradually raised from four to six grains three times a day : the same clonic effect was produced, with the same sensation of heat through the whole of the affected side, but without a sense of intoxication. The dose was advanced to eight grains, when the head again became affected, but without any permanent return of muscular power or sensation in the palsied limbs, or any other effect than a few occasional twitches and involuntary movements. Mr. Sheffield could not be persuaded to persevere any further, and the medicine was abandoned. He continued in the same feeble state for about three months, when he fell a sacrifice to a third apoplectic attack, apparently of a much slighter kind.

I have stated that this was a case of atonic affection, and hence there was no opportunity of

---

* Dr. Horsefield, in his inaugural dissertation on the different species of rhus, mentions the efficiency of the toxicodendrum in paralytic affections. " In two instances of hemiplegia," says Dr. Eberle, " I have prescribed the saturated tincture of the rhus with unequivocal benefit."—Practice of Physic, vol. ii.—D.

* Remarques sur la Nux Vomique considerée comme Médicament, par F. M. Coze, &c. ; Journal Universel des Sciences Médicales, Nov., 1819.

giving full play to the power of the nux vomica. But so far as I have seen, I think we may come to the following conclusions : First, that when only small doses can be given without seriously affecting the head, as in cases of great general or nervous debility, the effect is a clonic instead of an entastic or tetanic spasm. Secondly, that, under this effect, it is not calculated to do any permanent good, and often produces mischief. And thirdly, that it is most serviceable in entonic hemiplegia, after the patient has been sufficiently reduced from a state of high energetic health, and especially energetic plethora, to a subdued and temperate state of pulse ; in which state, it may very frequently be employed in doses sufficient to excite strong or entonic spasm.*

Nervous agitation, proportioned to the mode of the disease and the strength of the patient, has often been of peculiar advantage ; and hence, palsy has occasionally been carried off suddenly by a violent fit of mental emotion, as of anger (*Camerar. Memorab.*, cent. v., No. xxx.; *Paulini*, cent. iii., obs. 89 ; *Schenck, Observ.*, lib. i., No. clxxxii.) or fright (*Diemerbroeck, Observ. et Cur. Med.*; *Loeffler, Beyträge sur Wundarzneykunst*, band i.), of both which the examples are very numerous : by a stroke of lightning (*Wilkinson's Case of Mrs. Winder*, 8vo., 1765); and by fevers.—(*Act. Nat. Cur.*, vol. v., obs. 64 ; *Samml. Medicinischen Wahrnehmungen*, band vi., p. 152.) Nor can I do otherwise than think, that one of the most rational and efficacious means of cure in many instances of paralysis, and especially where no great inroad has been made upon the general strength of the constitution, would be a journey into the Hundreds of Essex or some other marshy district, for the purpose of obtaining a sharp attack of a tertian ague, which would most effectually, and I apprehend at the least expense, give us all the advantage of entastic spasm and reaction that we could wish for. In

treating of the tertian intermittent, we observed from Dr. Fordyce, that it has often a tendency to carry off a variety of obstinate and chronic diseases to which the constitution has been long subject, and to restore it to the possession of a better and firmer degree of health.*

In a few cases, hemiplegia is said to have ceased spontaneously by the mere remedial energy of nature ; in one instance, after ten years' standing, and accompanied with loss of voice. —(*Bresl. Samml.*, 1721, pp. 406, 503.) And in a few cases of paraplegia from external injury to the spine, where only one or two vertebræ have in a small degree been displaced from their proper position, the same instinctive or remedial power has alone produced a cure, or greatly alleviated the mischief, by so far thickening the growth of the bones immediately above and below, that the chasm has been filled up, and a line of support restored. The best artificial means of obtaining so salutary an action is by a free and laborious process of friction, vellication, or shampooing, with such intermediate exertion or exercise as the patient may be able to take.†

It is only necessary to add further, that where local palsy‡ has been produced by the fumes or minute divisions of lead or other noxious metals, it is almost always accompanied with symptoms of *colica rhachialgia*, or painter's colic, and is to be remedied by the treatment already laid down under that disease.

---

* Andral thinks that brucea is much better adapted for medicinal purposes than strychnine. —D.

* As the pathology of paralysis shows the very frequent dependance of this disease upon effusion of blood in the head, and certain morbid changes in the brain and spinal marrow, as causes, the editor has less confidence than the author in the scheme here proposed.

† See especially, Shaw on the Nature and Treatment of Distortions to which the Spine and the Bones of the Chest are subject, 8vo., 1823.

‡ In the New-York Med. and Phys. Journal, vol. iii., 430, Dr. Delafield of New-York has published the details of five cases of partial paralysis of the face, which were treated successfully by leeches, cupping, and blistering over the origin of the portio dura, and by the administration of purgatives.—D.

CLASS V.

GENETICA.

DISEASES OF THE SEXUAL FUNCTION.

ORDER I.

    CENOTICA.

        AFFECTING THE FLUIDS.

"   II.

    ORGASTICA.

        AFFECTING THE ORGASM.

"   III.

    CARPOTICA.

        AFFECTING THE IMPREGNATION.

CLASS V.

PHYSIOLOGICAL PROEM.

WE now enter upon the maladies of that important function by which animal life is extended beyond the individual that possesses it, and propagated from generation to generation. To this division of diseases the author has given the classic name of GENETICA, from γείνομαι, "gignor," whence genesis (γένεσις), "origo," "ortus."

In almost every preceding system of nosology, the diseases of this function are scattered through every division of the classification, and are rather to be found by accident, an index, or the aid of the memory, than by any clear methodical clew. Dr. Macbride's classification forms the only exception I am acquainted with; which, however, is rather an attempt at what may be accomplished than the accomplishment itself. His division is into four orders; general and local as proper to men, and general and local as proper to women; thus giving us in the ordinal name little or no leading idea of the nature of the diseases which each subdivision is to include, or any strict one of division between them : for it must be obvious, that many diseases commencing locally very soon become general and affect the entire system, as obstructed menstruation; while others, as abortion or morbid pregnancy, may be both general and local.

Under the present system, therefore, a different arrangement is chosen, and one which will perhaps be found not only more strict to the limits of the respective orders, but more explanatory of the leading features of the various genera or species that are included under them. These orders are three; the first embracing those diseases that affect the sexual fluids; the second those that affect the orgasm; and the third those that affect the impregnation. To the first order is applied the term, CENOTICA (κενώτικα), from κένωσις, "evacuatio," "exinanitio;" to the second, ORGASTICA (ὀργάστικα), from ὀργάζω, "irrito," "incito," and especially libidinose; and to the third, CARPOTICA (καρπότικα), from καρπός, "fructus."

Before we enter upon these divisions, it will perhaps prove advantageous to pursue the plan we have hitherto followed upon commencing the preceding classes; and take a brief survey of the general nature of the function before us, under the following heads :—

I. The Machinery by which it operates.
II. The Process by which it accomplishes its Ultimate End.
III. The Difficulties accompanying this Process, which still remain to be explained.

I. One of the chief characters by which animals and vegetables are distinguished from minerals, is to be found in the mode of their formation or origin. While minerals are produced fortuitously, or by the casual juxtaposition of the different particles that enter into their make, animals and vegetables can only be produced by generation, by a system of organs contrived for this express purpose, and regulated by laws peculiar to themselves.

[In perennial plants (see *Mayo's Outlines of Human Physiology*, p. 462, 2d edit.), the organs of generation are annually shed and reproduced. In animals, the sexual organs are periodically fitted for the function of generation, either by their actual enlargement, or by a determination of blood to them at particular periods. In human beings, the sexual organs are competent to their function during the greater part of life; from the age of puberty to forty-five or fifty, in females; to sixty-five or seventy, or even later, in men.]

Generation is effected in two ways; by the medium of seeds or eggs, and by that of offsets; and it has been supposed that there may be a third way, to which we shall advert hereafter; that of the union of seminal molecules, furnished equally by the male and the female, without the intervention of eggs, which constitutes the leading principle of what has been called the theory of epigenesis.

Many plants are propagable by offsets, and all plants are supposed to be so by eggs or seeds. As we descend in the scale of animal life, we meet in the lowest class, consisting of the worm tribes, with examples of both these modes of propagation also. For, while a production by ova is more commonly adhered to, the hydra or polype is well known to multiply by bulbs or knobs thrown forth from different parts of the body, and the *hirudo viridis*, or green leech, by longitudinal sections, which correspond with the slips or suckers of plants.

In these cases we meet with no distinction of sex; the same individual being capable of continning its own kind by a power of spontaneous generation. In other animals of the worm class, we trace examples of the organs of both sexes united in the same individual, making a near approach to the class of monoicous plants, or those which bear male and female flowers distinct from each other, but on the same stock, as the cucumber; thus constituting proper hermaphrodites, evincing a complexity of sexual structure which is not to be found in any class of animals above that of worms. Some of the intestinal worms are of this description, as the fasciola or fluke, which is at the same time oviparous, the ovaries being placed laterally. The earthworm propagates its kind by a like organization, as does the barnacle, the lamprey, and even the common and conger eel.—(See *Sir Everard Home's paper on some of these animals, Phil. Trans.*, 1823, art. xii.)

The *helix hortensis*, or garden-snail, is hermaphrodite, but incapable of breeding singly. In order to accomplish this it is necessary that one individual should copulate with another, the male organ of each uniting with the female, and the female with the male, when both become impregnated. The manner in which this amour is conducted is singular and highly curious. They make their approach by discharging several small darts at each other, which are of a sharp form and of a horny substance. The quiver is contained within a cavity on the right side of the neck, and the darts are launched with some degree of force, at about the distance of two inches, till the whole are exhausted; and when the war of love is over, its consummation succeeds. The increase is by eggs, which are perfectly round, and about the size of small peas.

There are some animals in which a single impregnation is capable of producing several generations in succession: we have a familiar example of this in the common cock and hen; for a single copulation is here sufficient to give fecundity to as many eggs as will constitute a whole brood. But the same curious fact is still more obvious in various species of insects, and especially in the aphis (puceron, or green-plant louse) through all its divisions, and the *daphnia pulex* of Möller and Latreille (the *monoculus pulex* of Linnæus). In both these a single impregnation will suffice for at least six or seven generations; and in both these, likewise, we have another curious deviation from the common laws of propagation, which is, that in the warmer summer months the young are produced vivaparously, and in the cooler autumnal months, oviparously. It is also very extraordinary that in the aphis, and particularly in the viviparous broods, the offspring are many of them winged, and many of them without wings or distinction of sex; in this respect making an approach to the working-bees, and still more nearly to the working-ants, known till of late by the name of neuters.

For confirmation respecting the generative process which takes place in these two last kinds, we are almost entirely indebted to the nice and persevering labours of the elder and the younger Hüber; who have decidedly proved, that what have hitherto been called neuters, are females with undeveloped female organs, and therefore non-breeders, but whose organs, at least in the case of bees, are capable of development by a more stimulating or richer honey, with which one of them, selected from the rest, is actually treated for this purpose by the general consent of the hive on the accidental loss of a queenbee, or common bearer of the whole, and in order to supply her place. It is these alone that are armed with stings: for the males, or drones, as we commonly call them, are without stings; they are much larger than the non-breeders or workers, of a darker colour, and make a great buz in flying. They are always less numerous in a hive than the workers, and only serve to ensure the impregnation of the few young queens that may be produced in the course of the season, and are regularly massacred by the stings of the workers in the beginning of the autumn. The impregnation of the queen-bee is produced by a process too curious to be passed over. It was conjectured by Swammerdam that this was effected by an aura seminalis thrown forth from the body of the whole of the drones or males collectively. By other naturalists it has been said, but erroneously, to take place from an intermixture of a male milt or sperm with the eggs or spawn of the queen-bee, as in the case of fishes. M. Hüber, however, has sufficiently proved that the queen-bee for this purpose forms an actual coition, and this never in the hive, but during a tour into the air which she takes for this purpose a few days only after her birth, and in the course of which she is sure to meet with some one or other of her numerous seraglio of males. As soon as copulation has been effected she returns to the hive, which is usually in the space of about half an hour, and often bears home with her the full proofs of a connexion in the *ipsa verenda* of the drone; who, thus wounded and deprived of his virility by the violence of her embrace, dies almost immediately afterward. This single impregnation will serve to fecundate all the eggs the queen will lay for two years *at least;* Hüber believes, for the whole of her life; but he has repeated proofs of the former. She begins to lay her eggs, for the bee is unquestionably oviparous, forty-six hours after impregnation, and will commonly lay about three thousand in two months, or at the rate of fifty eggs daily. For the first eleven months she lays none but the eggs of workers; after which she commences a second laying, which consists of drones' eggs alone.

Of the mode of procreation among fishes, in consequence of their living in a different element from our own, we know but little. A few of them, as the squalus, or shark genus, some of the skates, and other cartilaginous fishes, have manifest organs of generation, and unquestionably copulate. The male shark, indeed, is furnished with a peculiar sort of holders for the purpose of maintaining his grasp upon the female amid the utmost violence of the waves, and his penis is cartilaginous or horny. The female produces her young by eggs, which, in several species of this genus, are hatched in her own body, so that the young when cast forth are viviparous.

The blenny produces its young in the same manner; in most species by spawn or eggs hatched externally; but in one or two viviparously, three or four hundred young being thus brought forth at a time. The blenny, however, and by far the greater number of fishes, have no external organ of generation, and appear to have no sexual connexion. The females, in a particular season of the year, seem merely to throw forth their ova, which we call hard roe or spawn, in immense multitudes, in some shallow part of the water in which they reside, where it may be best exposed to the vivific action of the sun's ray; when the male shortly afterward passes over the spawn or hard roe, and discharges upon it his sperm, which we call soft roe or milt. These substances are contained in the respective sexes in two bags that unite near the podex, and at spawning time are very much distended. The spawn and milt thus discharged intermix; and, influenced by the vital warmth of the sun, commence a new action, the result of which is a shoal of young fishes of a definite species.

Yet, though no actual connexion can be traced among the greater number of the class of fishes, something like pairing is often discernible among many of those that have no visible organs of copulation; for if we watch attentively the motions of such as are kept in ponds, we shall find the sexes in great tumult, and apparently struggling together among the grass or rushes at the brink of the water about spawning time; while the male and female salmon, after having ascended a fresh stream to a sufficient height and shallowness for the purpose, are well known to unite in digging a nest or pit in the sand of about eighteen inches in depth, into which the female casts her spawn, and the male immediately afterward ejects his milt; when the nest is covered over with fresh sand by a joint exertion of their tails.

The salmon, the sturgeon, and many other marine fishes, seek out a fresh water stream for this purpose: and their navigations are often of very considerable length before they can satisfy themselves, or obtain a proper gravelly bed. The salmon tribe sometimes make a voyage of several hundred miles, cutting their way against the most rapid currents, leaping over floodgates, or up cataracts of astonishing height; in their endeavour to surmount which they often fail, and tumble back into the water; and, in some places, are in consequence caught in baskets placed in the current for this purpose.

The power of fecundity in fishes surpasses all calculation, and appears almost incredible. It has been said, no doubt in a strain of exaggeration, that a single herring, if suffered to multiply unmolested and undiminished for twenty years, would show a progeny greater in bulk than the globe itself. This species, as also the pilchard, and some others of the genus clupea, as a proof of their great fertility, migrate annually from the arctic regions in shoals of such vast extent, that for miles they are seen to darken the surface of the water.

The mode of procreating among frogs does not much vary from that of fishes. Early in the spring, the male is found upon the back of the female, in close contact with her; but no communication is discoverable, although this contact continues for several days; nor can we trace in the male any external genital organ. After the animals quit each other, the female seeks out some secure and shallow water, in which, like the race of fishes, she deposites her spawn, which consists of small specks held together in a sort of chain or string, by a whitish glutinous liquor that envelops them; and over this the male passes and deposites his sperm, which soon constitutes a part of the glutinous matter itself. The result is a fry of minute tadpoles, whose evolution into the very different form and organization of frogs is one of the most striking curiosities of natural history. In the Surinam toad (*rana pipa*), this process is varied. The female here deposites her eggs or spawn without any attention to order; the male takes up the amorphous mass with his feet, and smears it over her back, driving many of the eggs hereby into a variety of cells that open upon it; and afterward ejecting over them his spermous fluid. These cells are so many nests, in which the eggs are hatched into tadpoles, which are perfected and burst their imprisonment in about three months.

But a volume would not suffice to point out all the singularities exhibited by different animals in the economy of procreation. It is worth while, however, to notice how variously some of the organs of generation are situated in many tribes. In the female libellula, or dragon-fly, the vagina is placed on the upper part of the belly, near the breast. In the male spider, the generative organ is fixed on the extremity of an antenna. In the female *ascaris vermicularis*, or maw-worm, the young are discharged from a minute punctiform aperture a little below the head, which appears, therefore, to constitute the ascarine vagina. In the snail we find this organ placed near the neck, in the immediate vicinity of the spiracle which serves for its lungs. The *tænia solium*, or tapeworm, throws forth its young from the joints.' So some plants bear flowers on the petioles, or edges of the leaves, instead of on the flower-stalk.

In like manner, while the mammæ in the human kind are placed on the chest, and made a graceful and attractive ornament, in all quadrupeds they are placed backward, and concealed by the thighs. In the mare, the teats, which are two, are inguinal ; in the horse, they are singularly placed on the glans penis.

The testes of most animals that possess these organs, and procreate only once a year, are extremely small during the months in which they are not excited. Those of the sparrow, in the winter season, are scarcely larger than a pin's head ; but, in the spring, are of the size of a hazelnut. In man, the testis, before birth, or rather during the early months of pregnancy, is an abdominal viscus : about the seventh month, it descends gradually through the abdominal ring into the scrotum, which it reaches in the eighth month. And if this descent do not take place anterior to birth, it is accomplished with great difficulty, and is rarely completed till the seventh or eighth year. Sometimes, indeed, only one testis descends under these circumstances, and occasionally neither.

There is a set of barbarians at the back of the Cape of Good Hope who appear to be very generally monorchid, or possessed of only a single testis ; and Linnéus, believing this to be a natural and tribual defect, has made them a distinct variety of the human species. Mr. Barrow has noticed the same singularity : but it is doubtful whether, like the want of a beard among the American savages, this destitution is not owing to a barbarous custom of extirpation in early life. It is commonly believed that the productive power of man is greatly impaired, if not totally lost, by a retention of both testes in the abdomen, as in this situation they are seldom completely developed. Mr. Hunter imagines never ; and Zacchias and Riolan concur with him. Mr. Wilson met with one case of this kind, in which the generative power was perfect : and M. Foderé boldly affirms that persons thus incompletely formed are most remarkable for their vigour, thus strangely impeaching the ordinary course of nature.* Yet, in the erinaceus or hedgehog genus, and a few other quadrupeds, they never quit the cavity of the abdomen. In the cock, whose penis is di-

chotomous or two-pronged, they are situated on each side of the backbone.

It has been made a question among physiologists, whether the seminal fluid is secreted by the testes at the moment of the demand, or gradually and imperceptibly in the intervals of copulation, and lodged in the vesiculæ seminales as a reservoir for the generative power to draw upon. The latter is a common opinion. It is, however, opposed, and with very powerful arguments, by Swammerdam and Mr. John Hunter. The secretion found in the vesiculæ seminales is different from that of the testes in the properties of colour and smell ; those of the former being yellow and inodorous, those of the latter whitish, and possessing the odour of the orchis-root, or the down of chestnuts. On the dissection of those who have naturally or accidentally been destitute of one testis, the vesicula of the one side has been found filled with the same fluid, and as largely as that of the other ; and, consequently, the fluid on the vacant side must have been supplied by a secretory action of the vesicula itself. There are no organs of generation that differ so much in their form and comparative size in different animals as these vesicular bags : in the hedgehog they are twice as large as in man, and in many animals they are utterly wanting. They are so in the dog, which continues for a very long time in a state of copulation, and in birds, whose copulation is momentary. They are moreover wanting in most animals whose food is chiefly derived from an animal source, though not in all, as the hedgehog, to which I have just referred, is an example of the contrary.

Mr. Hunter hence concludes that the vesiculæ seminales are not seminal reservoirs, but glands secreting a peculiar mucus, and that the bulb of the urethra is, properly speaking, the receptacle in which the semen is accumulated previously to ejection. Of the actual use of these vesicular bags he confesses himself to be ignorant, yet imagines, that in some way or other, they are subservient to the purposes of generation, though not according to the common conjecture.

In a few rare instances, the uterus and vagina have been found double. Dr. Tiedemann met with two instances of this monstrosity. The organs constituting one of the cases are preserved to this day in the Heidelberg Museum. The individual had been pregnant in one of the sets, and

---

* When one or both of the testes are retained in the abdomen, Mr. Hunter conceives that they are exceedingly imperfect, and incapable of performing their natural function. The editor of this work knows of one example in which this was the case. Mr. Lawrence has seen two cases, in each of which one testis remained in the abdomen, and where the circumstances, ascertained by anatomical examination, corroborated the opinion of Mr. Hunter. In one the body of the gland was not more than half its usual size ; the epididymis, which was very imperfect, ran for about an inch behind the sac of a hernia, which had occurred in the individual, and did not join the body of the testis.

The other case presented exactly the same appearances. A third instance, however, concurring with that noticed by Mr. Wilson, came to the knowledge of Mr. Lawrence. Both of the testes had remained in the abdomen, but were apparently perfect in their structure, and during the patient's life, had executed their functions in a healthy manner.—(Rees's Cyclopædia, art. GENERATION.) It appears, then, that there are exceptions to the conclusion at which Mr. Hunter and some other physiologists arrived on this interesting question ; and that more depends upon the size and structure of the testes being natural, than upon their accidental situation.—ED.

the uterus is here larger than that on the opposite side, which is of the ordinary size. The
woman reached her full time, but died nineteen
days after delivery.*

The ovaria are to the female what the testes
are to the male. They were formerly, indeed,
called female testes, and furnish, on the part of
the female, what is necessary towards the production of a progeny. They are, in fact, two
spheroidal flattened bodies, enclosed between
the folds of the broad ligaments by which the
uterus is suspended. They have no immediate
connexion with the uterus; but near them the
extremity of a tube, which opens on either side
into that organ, hangs with loose fimbriæ in the
cavity of the abdomen, into which it communicates the fimbrial end. This tube is called the
Fallopian, from the name of its discoverer.—
(*Fallop. Observ. Anat.*, 197.) At the age of
puberty the ovaria acquire their full growth, and
continue to weigh about a drachm and a half
each, till menstruation ceases. They contain a
peculiar fluid resembling the white of eggs, once
supposed to be secreted by the glandular structure of various small bodies imbedded in them,
which have been denominated *corpora lutea.*
By some early writers this fluid was contem-

plated as a female semen, forming a counterpart
to the semen of males; but it has since been
held, and the tenet is well supported by anatomical facts, to be a secretion of a different
kind, thrown forth in consequence of the excitement sustained by the separation of one or
more of the minute vesicles which seem to issue
from them as their nucleus or matrix, and which
are themselves regarded by the same school as
the real ovula of subsequent fetuses: to which
subject, however, we shall advert presently.

[Women reach the period of puberty one or
two years before men; and the inhabitants of
warm before those of cold climates. In the
hottest regions of Africa, Asia, and America,
girls arrive at puberty at ten, and even at nine
years of age; in France, not till thirteen, fourteen, or fifteen: while in Sweden, Russia, and
Denmark, this period is not attained till from
two to three years later.* ᵥ

At the time of puberty in the male, the larynx enlarges, the quality of the voice is changed,
the beard grows, the chest and shoulders enlarge, the generative organs are developed,
hair grows upon the pubes, and the secretion of
the seminal fluid begins. In the female, the
breasts and pelvis enlarge, the uterine organs

---

* In August, 1831, Dr. Robert Lee examined
the body of a woman who died eight days after
parturition, from inflammation of the peritoneum and uterus. She had previously borne several living children. The uterus was found to be
divided into two lateral halves, opening into a
common cervix; the os uteri and vagina presenting the appearances usually noticed at that period after delivery. The inner surface of the right
half or cornu, which had contained the fœtus,
was lined by rough irregular flakes of deciduous
membrane, or a layer of fibrin of the blood. One
ovary and one Fallopian tube were connected with
this cornu, and the same was the case with the
unimpregnated one. Both ovaries were enlarged,
but the right was much larger than the left, and
included a distinct corpus luteum. The whole
of the surface of the left cornu was coated with
a delicate membrana decidua, which formed a
shut sac at the cervix, but presented a smooth
circular opening at the uterine orifice of the Fallopian tube, into which its fibres extended, though
to what distance could not be ascertained. Dr.
Lee gives reference to a vast number of what are
termed bilocular, bicorned, bifid, or double uterus,
in all of which, without a single exception, the
uterine appendages consisted of an ovary and one
Fallopian tube annexed to each cornu of the uteri,
and not of two ovaries and two Fallopian tubes, as
the expression double uterus would seem to imply. This kind of malformation has four varieties, which are delineated by Lauth and Cruveilhier:—1st. Where the vagina and the uterus are
separated into two cavities by a septum, without
any thing unusual in the external configuration
of this organ. 2dly. Where the only remarkable
circumstance is the division of the fundus and
body of the uterus into two cornua, as exemplified
in an instance lately published by Mr. Adams.—
(See Med. Gaz. for 1833–4, p. 898.) 3dly. Where
the uterus is bifid, and the cervix and vagina contain a septum. 4thly. Where the vagina forms a
single canal, with a double os uteri. Morand,
Bartholine, Tiedemann, Ollivier, and Dr. Blundell, have related cases of double uterus, in which

impregnation had taken place, and the fœtus had
been retained till the full period; but, according
to Dr. Lee's investigations, none of these authors
have alluded to the presence of a deciduous membrane in the unimpregnated cornu of the uterus.
That such membrane is formed in all similar cases he deems probable, because, in the gravid uterus of the lower animals, the membrane which
surrounds the product of conception invariably
occupies the whole inner surface of both cornua.
At the same time he candidly explains, that in the
examination of the preparation from Dr. Purcell's
remarkable case (see Phil. Trans., vol. lxiv., p.
474), no remains of a membrana decidua were noticed in either the right cornu, which had been
impregnated, or in the left, which had not; though
whether this was owing to accidental decomposition, or intentional removal of such membrane
(as far as the right cornu was concerned), cannot
now be determined.—(See Med. Chir. Trans.,
vol. xvii.) The disposition of the deciduous membrane in the case related by Dr. Lee himself must
have rendered superfœtation impossible, and its
history is adverse to the speculations of M. Cassan on the possibility of superfœtation, where a
double uterus exists. In this case, also, as in ordinary pregnancy, where the inner surface of the
uterus is lined with the deciduous membrane,
Dr. Lee observes, that menstruation must have
been suspended.—See Med. Chir. Trans., vol.
xvii.—ED.

* The age at which the female Indians of North
America reach the period of puberty, has been
generally stated by travellers to be the eighteenth
year: but later observations have proved this assertion to be fallacious. According to Major Long
(Long's Expedition to the Rocky Mountains), the
young squaw has her catamenia in her twelfth or
thirteenth year. Hunter states that menstruation does not occur by two or three years so soon
as among the whites. Both these late travellers,
therefore, fix the period of puberty much earlier
than the European authorities.—(See Clinton's
Letter, in Francis's Denman, 3d edit., New-York,
1829.)—D.

are developed, and a peculiar periodical dis_charge from the uterus commences, which con_tinues, subject to certain suspensions during pregnancy and lactation, as long as the organ is capable of impregnation, or, on the average, about thirty years.]*

It is singular to contemplate the very power_ful influence which the secretion, or even the preparation for secreting the seminal fluid, but still more its ejection, produces over the entire system. On the perfection, and a certain and entonous degree of distention of the natural vessels, ap_parently producing an absorption of the fluid when at rest, the spirits, the vigour, and the general health of man depend. Hence, antece_dently to the full elaboration of the sexual sys_tem, and the secretion of this fluid, the male has scarcely any distinctive character from the female: the face is fair and beardless, the voice shrill, and the courage doubtful. And when_ever, in subsequent life, we find this entonous distention relaxed, we find at the same time languor, debility, and a want of energy both in the corporeal and mental functions. And where the supply is entirely suppressed or cut off by accident, disease, or unnatural mutilation, the whole system is changed, the voice weakened, the beard checked in its growth, and the ster_num expanded: so that the male again sinks down into the female character. These changes occur chiefly where the testicles are extirpated before manhood; but they take place also, though in a less degree, afterward.

In like manner, during the discharge of the seminal fluid in sexual commerce, the most vig_orous frames of the stoutest animals become exhausted by the pleasurable shock: and the feeble frames of many of the insect tribes are incapable of recovering from the exhaustion, and perish immediately afterward; the female alone surviving to give maturity to the eggs hereby fecundated. The same effect occurs after

the same consummation in plants. The stout_est tree, if superfructified, is impaired for bear_ing fruit the next year; while the plants of the feeblest structure die as soon as fructification has taken place. Hence, by preventing fructifi_cation, we are enabled to prolong their duration; for by taking away the styles and stigmas, the filaments and anthers, and especially by pluck_ing off the entire corols of our garden-flowers, we are able of annuals to make biennials, and of biennials, triennials.

In many animals, during the season of their amours, the aroma of the seminal fluid is so strong, and at the same time so extensive in its influence, as to taint the flesh; and hence the flesh of goats at this period is not eatable. Most fishes are extremely emaciated in both sexes at the same time, and from the same cause, and are equally unfit for the table. Stags, in the rutting season, are so exhausted as to be quite lean and feeble, and to retire into the re_cesses of the forest in quest of repose and quiet. They are well known to be totally inadequate to the chase; and hence, for the purpose of maintaining a succession of sporting, they are sometimes castrated, in which state they are called heaviers. If the castration be performed while the horns are shed, these never grow again; and if while the horns are in perfection, they are never shed.*

The male and female raindeer (*cervus taran_dus*) ordinarily cast their horns every year in November. If the male be castrated, the horns will not grow after he is nine years old; and the female, instead of dropping her horns as usual in November, retains them, if gravid, till she fawns, which is about the middle of May. In this case, the usual stimulus necessary for the operation of exfoliation is transferred to another part of the system. And, for the same reason, we often find that a broken bone in a pregnant woman will secrete no callus, and consequently not unite, till after childbirth. In the former case, the roots of the horns are affected by sym_pathy of the general sexual system, of which in_deed they may be said to form a part, and by their superior size are discriminative of the male sex. In the human race, the strong deep voice, char_acteristic of manhood, is rarely acquired if cas_tration be performed in infancy.

There is no animal, perhaps, but shows some sympathetic action of the system at large, or some remote part of it, with the genital organs, when they are in a state of peculiar excitement. The tree-frog (*rana arborea*) has, in the breeding season, a peculiar orbicular pouch attached to its throat; the fore-thumb of the common male toad is at the same season affected with warts; and the females of some of the monkey tribes evince a regular menstruation.

---

* Mayo's Outlines of Human Physiology, p. 463. The menstrual discharge may be stated generally to be "the consequence of a peculiar periodical condition of the bloodvessels of the uterus, fitting it for impregnation, which condi_tion is analogous to that of 'heat' in the inferior animals." In Dr. Hooper's work on the Morbid Anatomy of the Human Uterus, there is an exact representation of the uterus of a woman who was instantaneously killed by an accident during men_struation; and every one must be struck with the resemblance which it bears to the description given by Mr. Cruickshank in the Philosophical Transactions (1797), of the appearances observed by him in rabbits killed during the state of genital excitement, usually called the time of heat. The actual presence of the discharge is the *resolution*, if we may so term it, of the previous condition of the vessels which separate it; for the uterus is fitted for the purposes of impregnation before the menses begin to flow. An instance in proof of this may be given from the Philosophical Trans_actions (1817), of a young woman who bore two children successively without any previous men_struation; which function, in fact, did not show itself externally till after the third pregnancy, which ended in a miscarriage.—Dr. Locock in art. MENSTRUATION, in Cyclop. of Pract. Med.—ED.

* Otto, in his Handbuch der Path. Anatomie, remarks, "I kept a stag for twelve years, which I had castrated when two years old; it put up yearly, when it shed its coat, new long prickers, which were mostly covered with velvet, and were so brittle that the stag never attempted to strike with them; but if angered, used his fore-feet for weapons."—D.

II. The process by which the generative power is able to accomplish its ultimate end, is to the present hour involved in no small degree of mystery ; and has given rise to three distinct and highly ingenious hypotheses, that have a strong claim upon our attention, and which we shall proceed to notice in the order in which they have appeared.

The first and most ancient of these consists in regarding the fœtus in the, womb as the joint production of matter afforded in coition by both sexes, that of the male being secreted by the testes, and that of the female by the.uterus itself, or some collateral organ, as the ovaria, which last, however, is a name of comparatively modern origin, and derived from a supposed office which was not contemplated among the ancients. To this hypothesis has been given the name of EPIGENESIS.

The seed or matter afforded by the female, was regarded by Hippocrates, Aristotle, and Galen, as the menstrual blood or secretion, which they supposed furnished the substance and increment of the fœtus, while the male semen furnished the living principle : Empedocles, Epicurus, and various other physiologists contending, on the contrary, that the father and mother respectively contributed a seminal fluid that equally co-operated in the generation and growth of the fœtus, and stamped it a male or a female, and with features more closely resembling the one or the other, according as the orgasm of either was predominant at the time, or accompanied with a more copious discharge. In the words of Lucretius, who has elegantly compressed the Epicurean doctrine,—

" Et muliebre oritur patrio de semine seclum ;
Maternoque mares exsistunt corpore cretei.
Semper enim partus duplici de.semine constat :
Atque, utri simile est magis id, quodquomque creatur,
Ejus habet plus parte æquâ, quod cernere possis,
Sive virûm suboles, sive est muliebris origo."*

.The distinction of sex, however, was accounted for in a different manner by Hippocrates, who supposed that each of the sexes possesses a strong and a weak seminal fluid ; and very ungallantly asserted that the male fœtus was formed by an intermixture of the robuster fluids of the two sexes, and the female by that of the more imbecile. Lactantius, in quoting the opinion of Aristotle upon this subject, adds, faneifully enough, that the right side of the uterus is the proper chamber of the male fœtus, and the left of the female : a belief which is still prevalent among the vulgar in many parts of Great Britain. But he adds, that if the male, or stronger semen, should by mistake enter the left side of the uterus, a male child may still be conceived ; yet, inasmuch as it occupies the female department, its voice, its face, and its general complexion, will be effeminate. And, on the contrary, if the weaker or female seed should flow into the right side of the uterus, and a female fœtus be begotten, the female will exhibit

* De Rer. Nat., lib. iv., 1220.

many signs of a masculine character, and be inordinately vigorous and muscular.*

The doctrine of epigenesis, under one modification or another, continued to be the leading, if not the only hypothesis of the day, till the beginning of the sixteenth century, when, in consequence of the more accurate examinations and dissections of Sylvius, Vesalius, Fallopius, and De Graaf, the organs which had hitherto been regarded as female testes, and so denominated, were now declared to be repositories of minute ova, and at length named ovaria by Steno in 1667.—(Elem. Myologiæ Specim., p. 117.) We now, therefore, enter upon the second of the three hypotheses above alluded to, which derives the fœtus from rudiments furnished by the mother alone. This hypothesis was originally advanced by Josephus de Aromatariis, as flowing from these anatomical discoveries, but was chiefly brought into notice by Swammerdam and Harvey, who established the doctrine of omne ab ovo. Observing a cluster of about fifteen vesicles in each of the female ovaria, apparently filled with a minute drop of albuminous yellow serum, and perceiving that they appeared to diminish in number in some kind of proportion to the number of parturitions a woman had undergone, it was conceived by these physiologists that such vesicles are inert eggs or ovula, containing miniature embryons of the form to be afterward evolved, one of which, by the pleasurable shock that darts over the whole body, but in an especial degree through this organ, during the act of copulation, is in-

* De Opificio Dei, cap. xii. Mr. Mayo considers it natural to suppose that the sex of the embryo is determined antecedently to impregnation ; but, by what facts he is led to this opinion, is not explained. This part of the subject still continues a complete mystery.† It is a remarkable fact, as Dr. Bostock has observed (Elem. Syst. of Physiology, vol. iii., p. 47), that, although there is no uniform proportion between the number of males and females produced by the same parents, yet that the total number of each sex brought into the world, taking the average of any large community, is nearly the same ; or, more exactly, that we have in all cases a small excess of males. The data that we possess, while they prove that this excess exists in all countries, seem, however, to show that the amount of it differs in different countries. From a very extensive examination made by Hufeland, the numbers in Germany are as 21 to 20.— (Edin. Phil. Journ., vol. v. p. 296.) The census that was taken in England and Wales in 1821, shows the numbers to be nearly 21 and 20.066.‡ But, says Dr. Bostock, to whatever cause we may ascribe the relative proportion, it would appear that the greater number of males who are born is compensated by their greater mortality, whether produced by natural or accidental causes ; for we find, among adults, that the number of females rather exceeds that of males.—Haller, El. Phys., lib. xxviii., p. 1 ; Jameson's Journ., vol. v., p. 200.—ED.

† Sir E. Home thinks that the development of the sex takes place subsequently to impregnation, the ovum being fitted originally to become either male or female.—D.

‡ According to the statistical tables of Dr. Emerson, the proportion in Philadelphia for nine years was as 21 to 19. 43.—D.

stantly thrown into a state of vital activity, detached from the common cluster, and in a short time passes into the uterus through the canal of the Fallopian tube, which spontaneously enlarges for the purpose; where its miniature germe is gradually unfolded and augmented into a sensible fœtus, partaking of the form and figure of the parent stock. The elementary animalcule, it was farther asserted by Harvey, may be occasionally impressed with a resemblance in its features to the father from the electric impulse given in the genial act to every portion of the solids and fluids of the body, and of consequence to the fluid contained in the ovula themselves : but, reasoning from the length of the vagina in cows and many other animals, and an occasional dissection of the human subject soon after coition, he contended that the male semen never did, nor indeed could enter the uterus, and of course could not add any thing to the embryo in its evolution.

Leewenhoeck and Hartsoeker, however, upon a more accurate anatomy of the uterus immediately after copulation, discovered, not only that the projected male semen could enter its cavity, but actually did thus enter, and in some instances which fell within their notice, had clearly ascended into the Fallopian tubes. And now a new doctrine was started, and one altogether opposite to the theory of Harvey. Upon the principle of the former, the father had no immediate connexion with his own child ; he could not bestow upon it a particle of his own matter, and the whole production was the operation of the mother. But, in consequence of this later discovery, it was contended that the entire formation was the work of the father, and that the mother, in her turn, had nothing to do with it : that every particle of the propelled fluid was a true and proper seminium, containing in itself, like the ovulum of the female upon the hypothesis of Harvey, a miniature of all the organs and members of the future fœtus, in due time to be gradually evolved and augmented ; and that the uterus, and possibly the ovulum, into which some one of these male semina or seminia is almost sure of being protruded in the act of generation, offers nothing more than a nest, in which the homunculus or rudimental fœtus is deposited for warmth and nutriment. And, as the former hypothesis appealed to the natural economy of oviparous animals during the period of incubation, that of worms and tadpoles was appealed to by the latter : and a very considerable degree of life and motion was supposed to be discovered and proved by the aid of good magnifying glasses in the simple fluid of the male semen, insomuch that not less than many millions of these homunculi, or unborn manikins, were pointed out as capering in a diameter not greater than than that of the smallest grain of sand, each resembling the tadpole in shape. Delappius, indeed, a celebrated pupil of Leewenhoeck, advanced farther ; for he not only saw these homuncular tadpoles, but pretended to trace one of them bursting through the tunic by which it was swaddled, and exhibiting two arms, two legs, a human head and heart.

Such was the dream of the popular philosophy on the subject of generation indulged in at the period we are now adverting to, and which continued for upwards of a century. It is truly astonishing to reflect on the universality with which this opinion was accredited, and how decisively every anatomist, and indeed every man who pretended to the smallest portion of medical science, was convinced that his children were no more related, in point of generative power, to his own wife, than they were to his neighbour's. It was in vain that Verheyen denied the existence of animalcules in the seminal fluid, and undertook to demonstrate that the motion supposed to be traced there was a mere microscopic delusion : it was in vain to adduce the fact of an equal proportion of paternal and maternal features in almost every family in the world, the undeviating intermixture of features in mules, and other hybrid animals, and the casual transfer of maternal impressions to the unborn progeny, when suddenly frightened in the earlier months of pregnancy. The theory, as it was triumphantly called, of generation ab animalculo maris, was still confidently maintained ; and the mother, it was contended, had nothing to do with the formation of her own offspring, but to give it a warm nest and nourishment.

At length arose the celebrated and indefatigable Buffon, who was not inattentive to the facts before him, nor to the absurdities to which some of them had led. He readily accredited the microscopic motion pointed out by Leewenhoeck in the floating bodies of the male semen, and which Spallanzani has since persuaded himself he has detected, not only in this fluid, but in various others of an animal origin (*Opuscoli de Fisica, Animale, Vegetabile*, &c., vol. ii., 8vo., Milan, 1776), but, instead of admitting them to be animalcules, he regarded them as primordial monads, *molecules organiques*, of a peculiar activity, existing through all nature, and constituting the nutrient elements of living matter : and upon this principle he founded, not indeed a new hypothesis, but a new edition of that of epigenesis, with so much accessory, and in his view of the subject, important matter, as very nearly to entitle it to the character of an original plan. Like the speculations to which it succeeded, it soon acquired a very high degree of popularity.

All organized beings, and hence plants as well as animals, according to the doctrine of M. de Buffon, contain a vast number of these active molecules in every part of their frames, but especially in the generative organs of both sexes, and the seed-vessels of plants, in which they are more numerous than in any other parts. These organic primordia afford nutrition and growth to the animal and vegetable fabrics ; and as soon as these fabrics are matured, and consequently a smaller proportion of such molecules are requisite, their surplus is secreted and strained off for the formation of vegetable and animal seeds. The existence of ovula in the female ovaria, impregnated and detached at the time of conception, is by this hypothesis declared to be a chimera, and their passage into the uterus asserted to be contrary to all observation and fact. The ovaria are once more regarded as female testes, receiving, like those of the male, the surplus of the organic molecules of the body, and secreting them like the latter, for the common purpose of generation. The seminal liquors, thus secerned in the male and female frames, are projected in the act of coition simultaneously into the uterus, and becoming intimately blended there, produce by a kind of fermentation the first filaments of the foetus, which grow and expand like the filaments of plants. To render such combination of seminal fluids productive, however, it was contended that their quantities must be duly proportioned, their powers of action definite, and their solidity, tenacity, or rarefaction, symphonious: and the foetus, it was added, would be either male or female, as the seminal fluid of the man or woman abounded most with organic molecules, and would resemble either the father or the mother, according to the overbalance of the respective elements contributed by each parent.

It is obvious, from this brief view of the subject, that Buffon, in the planning of this hypothesis, did nothing more than avail himself of the anatomical facts of Vesalius, De Graaf, and Harvey, and the supposed discoveries of Leewenhoeck, to revive in a new form the doctrine of the Greek schools, and especially that of Epicurus. The subject, however, was offered to the world with plausible arguments and captivating eloquence, and had soon the good fortune to meet with powerful and enlightened supporters in Maupertuis and Needham, who added some improvements, but of no very great importance, to several of M. de Buffon's tenets; while Haller and Bonet strove hard to revive the hypothesis of female generative power, or that of evolution alone, at first established by Harvey; or rather to erect an edifice, somewhat similar to it, out of the crumbling ruins of the primary building; in doing which they appealed to the phenomena of the vegetable creation with considerable research and some degree of success. But this revived hypothesis, notwithstanding, has never been very generally followed; and is now almost, if not altogether, relinquished, even in Germany.

In like manner, there are several physiologists who have endeavoured to improve the hypothesis of Buffon, of whom it may be sufficient to mention Dr. Darwin and Professor Blumenbach. The alterations, however, are little more than verbal, and consequently of no great importance, and chiefly relate to the subordinate doctrine of organic molecules. For the term organic molecules, Darwin prefers that of vital germes, which he assorts into two kinds, or rather maintains are thus formed by nature, as being secreted or provided by male or female organs, whether animal or vegetable; for in the philosophy of this writer, the two departments tread closely upon each other. In this subdivision of germes, however, the term molecule is still retained, but limited to the female character or department: the vital germes or particles, secreted by the female organs of a bud or flower, or the female organs of an animal,

being by Dr. Darwin denominated *molecules* with formative propensities; while those secreted from the male organs of either department, are called *fibrils* with formative appetences. To the fibrils he assigns a higher degree of organization than to the molecules. Both, however, we are told, have a propensity or an appetence to form or create; as we are told also, that "they reciprocally stimulate and embrace each other, and instantly coalesce; and may thus popularly be compared to the double affinities of chymistry."

In the view of Professor Blumenbach, matter is divided into two kinds, possessing properties essentially different from each other; these are organized and unorganized: unorganized matter is endued with a creative or formative power throughout every particle; and organized matter with a creative or formative effort, a *nisus formativus*, or *bildungstrieb* (*Uber den Bildungstrieb*, 8vo., Göttingen, 1791); as he calls it, a principle, in many respects, similar to that of gravitation, but endowing every separate organ, as soon as it acquires structure, with a vita propria. From the first, he traces the origin of the world in the simple and inorganic state of the mineral kingdom; from the last, the rise of vegetables and animals.

It is only necessary to add further a remark of Mr. John Hunter's, that in plants of all kinds, the seed, properly so called, is produced by the female organization, while the male gives nothing more than the principle of arrangement; and that the same operation and principles take place in many orders of animals.—(*Animal Economy*, p. 55.)

In all these attempts to improve upon the older speculations, there is a great deal that cannot but be regarded as philosophical nugæ. The physiological experiments that have been made, and the anatomical facts that have been discovered, since the days of Harvey, and particularly during the last half century, though they leave the doctrine of generation still surrounded with many difficulties, have sufficiently established the following positions:—

First, that in all ordinary cases, the male semen enters into the uterus at the time of coition; and that in those cases in which it does not or cannot enter immediately, from the extreme length of the vagina, as in some quadrupeds, or from a greater or less degree of imperforation of the vaginal passage, it is conveyed there soon afterward, in consequence of its proximity of situation.

Secondly, that the uterus itself, worked up at this time to the highest pitch of excitement, secretes also some portion of a peculiar fluid, the female semen of the Epicurean philosophers, with which the male semen combines, and which is probably the basis of the membranes soon afterward prepared for the foetus.

Thirdly, that the Fallopian tubes at this period become rigid; their fimbriæ embrace the ovaria; and consequently form a direct channel of communication between the ovaria and the uterus; that what were formerly supposed to be vesicles are real ovula; and that one of them, detached by the momentary shock or excitement, bursts from its nucleus or matrix, enters into one of the open mouths of the fimbriæ of the Fallopian tube, and in consequence, into the tube itself, by which it is conveyed to the uterus; an effect, however, which does not seem to take place during the act of coition, since the ovulum is seldom found, even in the Fallopian tube, till some time afterward : and that, as soon as the ovulum has thus escaped, the. lips of the wound hereby made in the side of the ovary are closed by an external cicatrix, and indented with a small cavity, which forms what is meant by a corpus luteum.

Fourthly, that the cervix of the uterus is from this time closed in its canal towards its upper part, so as to prevent a second fœtation by the introduction of fresh male semen ; while the internal surface of this organ becomes lined with a fine coagulable and plastic lymph, being probably the fluid secreted at the moment of intercourse ; which assumes a thin membranous form, and has been called tunica caduca or decidua, and constitutes the uterine ovum or egg of the fœtus ; this important part of the process seeming to take place about a week after the time of copulation. In the rabbit, Mr. Cruickshank found it as early as the fourth day.

Fifthly, that for the better protection and nutrition of the fœtus, the walls of the uterine ovum are multiplied ; and that hence, while the tunica caduca itself possesses a duplicature, which is called tunica reflexa, there are also two other membranes by which the decidua is lined, denominated chorion and amnion, both which are filled with peculiar fluids ; the fluid of the chorion occupying the space between itself and the amnion, which it surrounds ; and the fluid of the amnion occupying the whole of the interior, which is distended with it like a bladder.*

Sixthly, that the medium of connexion between the fœtus and the mother is the umbilical cord and the placenta,† into which it is distrib-

uted ; the former consisting of an artery from each of the fœtal iliacs, and a vein running to the fœtal liver twisted spirally and surrounded by a common integument ; and the latter consisting of two parts, a uterine or spongy parenchyma, derived from the decidua, and a fœtal parenchyma, consisting of a great multitude of exquisitely beautiful knotty flocculi that cover the chorion, and constitute not only an organ of nutriment, but, as was first ingeniously supposed by Sir Edward Hulse, of oxygenation. In both these organs Sir Everard Home appears, by the assistance of Mr. Bauer's extraordinary microscopical powers, to have detected a few silvery lines, or rather continuous chains of nerves (*Phil. Trans.*, 1825, *Croonian Lecture*), and to have shown the probability of there being an order of vessels in these organs, which were peremptorily denied to exist by Haller. These experiments, however, seem to require confirmation.*

Seventhly, that about the third week, or as soon as the uterine ovum is thus prepared for its reception, we can trace the first vestige of the embryon, oval in its shape, and resembling a minute bean or kidney, swimming in the fluid

---

Albinus represented the placenta to be formed of bloodvessels, cellular tissue, and membranous investments derived from the chorion.—(Annot. Acad.) See a valuable review of Breschet's work, and of Velpeau's Embryologie, in the Edin. Med. and Surg. Journ., No. cxviii., January, 1834.—ED.

* The structure of the human placenta, and its connexion with the uterus, form a subject that has engaged a great deal of attention, and more particularly at the present time, in consequence of the investigations of Dr. Robert Lee, which lead to so different a view from what was promulgated by the two Hunters. In a communication to the Royal Society, Dr. Lee described certain appearances which he observed in the examination of six gravid uteri, and many placentæ expelled in natural labour, which seem to him to warrant the conclusion, that *the human placenta does not consist of two parts, maternal and fœtal ; that no cells exist in its substance; and that there is no communication between the uterus and placenta by large arteries and veins.* The whole of the blood sent to the uterus by the spermatic and hypogastric arteries, except the small portion supplied to its parietes and to the membrana decidua by the inner membrane of the uterus, appears to Dr. Lee to flow into the uterine veins or sinuses, and, after circulating through them, is returned into the general circulation of the mother by the spermatic and hypogastric veins, without entering the substance of the placenta. The deciduous membrane being, according to Dr. Lee, interposed between the umbilical vessels and the uterus, whatever changes take place in the fœtal blood must result from the indirect exposure of this fluid, as it circulates through the placenta, to the maternal blood flowing in the great uterine sinuses.—(See Phil. Trans.) With reference to these points, it merits notice, that M. Velpeau admits that Dr. Lee's statement of the large vessels of the womb not communicating with any corresponding vessels of the placenta, is perfectly well founded ; but he considers Dr. Lee to be erroneous in representing the decidua to be interposed between the womb and the placenta, and, in his own opinion, the chorion adheres directly to the uterine surface, though it is admitted, at the same time, that the uterine sinuses are closed by membranous pulpy matter.—ED.

---

* Dr. William Hunter was the first who gave just views of the decidua, the membrana exterior ovi of Haller, and showed that it consisted, at least at one period of utero-gestation, of two folds. The chorion he described as the third membrane of the ovum from the second to the fifth month, and as the second membrane after the latter period. It was also Dr. Hunter that divided the placenta into the maternal and fœtal portions, which, according to his views, did not communicate with each other. These accounts received implicit belief in the medical schools of England and the continent for nearly half a century.—See Edin. Med. and Surg. Journ., No. cxviii., p. 156.—ED.

† Rouhault, in the Mem. of the Acad. of Sciences for 1714, 1715, and 1716, published descriptions of the placenta, which, he maintained, was produced by a thickening of the chorion, while its spongy tissue was formed solely by an assemblage of capillary veins from the umbilical vessels. He also denied that any anastomoses existed between the vessels of the placenta and those of the womb. In 1734, Dr. Simson, of St. Andrew's. undertook to prove that the placenta was formed from the chorion—a doctrine revived by M. Breschet.—(See his Etudes Anatomiques, &c., de l'Œuf dans l'Espèce Humaine, &c., 4to., Paris, 1832.) In 1754,

of the amnion, and suspended by the umbilical cord, which has now shot forth from the placenta. From this reniform substance the general figure pallulates, the limbs are protruded, and the face takes its rise.

III. The chief difficulties that have been felt, as accompanying these positions, and the general doctrine that flows from them, are the following:—

First, as to the mode by which the male semen is conveyed to the ovulum in the Fallopian tube.

Secondly, the occasional existence of corpora lutea in the ovaria of virgins, or of those who, from misformation, have been incapable of indulging in sexual commerce.

Thirdly, the occasional detection of a full-sized fœtus in the uterus without any placenta,* umbilical cord, or mark of an umbilicus.

The first of these difficulties was originally started, as we have already observed, by Dr. Harvey, who contended that, in the case of cows, whose vagina is very long, as well as in various other cases, the semen cannot possibly reach even the uterus; and that hence there is no reason to suppose it ever reaches it. It was not then known that impregnation commences in the Fallopian tube, and that it must also reach this canal as well; which, by Harvey, would have been received as an objection still more triumphant.

By what means the ejected semen is conveyed into the uterus we do not, indeed, very clearly know, even to the present hour; but that it is so conveyed, and even in animals in which the male organ can by no means come in contact with it, has been proved by incontrovertible facts.† Mr. John Hunter killed a bitch in the act of copulation, and found that the semen was then existing in the cavity of the uterus, in his opinion carried there per saltum. Now, if it reach the uterus, there can be no difficulty in conceiving that it may also reach the Fallopian tubes, which by one end open into the uterus; sucked in, perhaps, as supposed by M. Blumenbach, by the latter organ during the thrilling orgasm of the moment. Leewenhoeck and Hartsocker seem indeed to have removed the difficulty altogether, by having, in some instances, detected the seminal fluid in the Fallopian tubes themselves.‡ And there seems great reason to believe that it has occasionally entered the ovarium, and even produced impregnation in that organ instead of in the uterus, where an obstruction has been offered to the descent of an ovulum into the fimbrial openings of the tube after its detachment: for we cannot otherwise readily account for the formation of fœtuses in the ovarium; facts, however, well known to occur, and of which Mr. Stanley has given a singular instance (*Med. Trans.*, vol. vi., art. xvi.), and Dr. Granville a still more extraordinary example, the fœtus at its examination appearing perfect, and four months old.*

[It appears now to be fully proved, that " *if the canal leading from the orifice of the vagina to the ovaries be interrupted, conception never takes place.* When the interruption results from obliteration of the vagina, the sexual appetite remains unaffected; but when the cause which has produced it is the division of the Fallopian tubes, desire appears to be lost, as well as the capacity of being impregnated." The experiments of Dr. Blundell show that the division of the vagina prevents conception.—(*Med. Chir. Trans.*, vol. x., p. 50.) In several female rabbits, Dr. Haighton divided the Fallopian tubes, and found that the animals invariably lost the sexual appetite. When the Fallopian tube on one side only was divided, the same result generally ensued. In a few cases, however, the animals thus mutilated admitted the male, and became impregnated; but the horn of the uterus, on the side on which the Fallopian tube had been divided, never contained ova.—(See *Phil. Trans.*, vol. lxxxv., p. 108, and *Mayo's Outlines*, p. 471.)]

The second difficulty is also capable of a plausible answer, but not quite so satisfactory as the preceding.

There can be no doubt that the ovarium is directly concerned in the great business of generation, for it is well-known that the operation of spaying or excising the ovaries, corresponds in females to that of castration in males. It takes off not only all power of production, but all desire. And in a recent volume of the Philosophical Transactions, there is the case of a natural defect of this kind in an adult woman, who in like manner had never evinced any inclination for sexual union, and had never men-

---

* A curious case of this kind may be seen in the New-York Med. and Phys. Journal, vol. i., recorded by Dr. Cotton.—D.

† The recent discoveries of Dr. Gartner of Copenhagen, may throw some light on this intricate subject. In some of the mammalia, as the sow and cow, the doctor has been able to trace canals or ducts from the vagina to the ovaries.—D.

‡ In May, 1827, Mr. H. Bond, of Philadelphia, was invited by Dr. S. Tucker to examine the body of a female, between 18 and 20 years of age, who had destroyed herself by taking a large quantity of laudanum. She had passed the whole or the greater part of the night in the arms of a young man, and before break of day destroyed herself by swallowing a strong dose of laudanum. Mr. Bond removed the whole of the genito-urinary organs, and took them home for minute examination.—

Among other circumstances, the following ones were noticed:—"The internal surface of the uterus was lined with a matter having the appearance of semen, and giving out strongly the peculiar odour of that fluid, and the neck of the organ was filled with the same matter. One of the Fallopian tubes (the only one examined) seemed to contain a similar fluid, but the seminal odour was not here well marked. When this matter was removed from the surface of the uterus, the lining membrane appeared extremely vascular, like the conjunctiva in cases of acute ophthalmia, or as if it had been injected with vermilion."—See Lancet for 1833-4, p. 114.—ED

* Phil. Trans., 1820, p. 101. It is contrary to the anatomy of the parts, to fancy that the semen enters the ovary; nor could we explain, by any such doctrine, the occasional formation of parts of the fœtus in the male subject.—ED.

struated; and who on dissection was found, with the deficiency of ovaria, to have the uterus only of the size of an infant's, a very narrow pelvis, and no hair on the pubes.—(*Vol. for the year* 1805, p. 226.)

It seems, also, perfectly clear, that in conception, an ovum does really descend from the ovarium into the uterus within a few days after sexual intercourse has taken place: in proof of which it will be sufficient to quote the following curious historical fact from Sir Everard Home (Id., 1817, p. 252), who appears to have traced its path very accurately:—"A servant maid, twenty-one years of age, died of an epileptic fit seven days after coition, there being circumstances to prove that she could not have seen her lover after the day here adverted to, nor for many days before. The sexual organs were submitted to dissection: the right ovarium had a small torn orifice upon the most prominent part of its external surface, which led to a cavity filled with coagulated blood, and surrounded by a yellowish organized structure: its inner surface was covered with an exudation of coagulable lymph. A minute spherical body, supposed to be an ovum, was concealed in the cavity of the womb among the long fibres of coagulable lymph which covered its inner surface, and especially towards the cervix. This supposed ovum was submitted to the microscopical powers of M. Bauer, who has made various drawings of it, and who detected in it two projecting points, which are considered as the future situations of the heart and brain."

[M. Bauer is stated to have repeatedly verified the preceding observation in animals, and also to have ascertained that the corpora lutea, when the ova are fit for fecundation, burst and expel their contents, and subsequently shrink and disappear. "These interesting observations," says Mr. Mayo (*Outlines of Human Physiology*, p. 466, 2d edit.), "have the advantage of bringing under one theory all the instances of generation with separate organs, by proving that, in the case of mammalia, as in other animals and in plants, an ovum is prepared by the female previously to a fruitful connexion."]

What exact period of time the ovum demands to work its way down the tube into the uterus, has not been very accurately ascertained. That it does not descend at once is admitted on all hands; and there can be no doubt that, in different kinds of animals, a different period is requisite. Mr. Cruickshank, whose experiments were confined to rabbits, ascertained that in this species the ovum demanded for its journey about forty-eight hours. In the case just alluded to seven days had elapsed, and consequently a period perfectly sufficient seems to have been given for the purpose, and there can be little doubt that the minute body observed in the cavity of the uterus, was a genuine impregnated ovum that had completed its travels.

But whence comes it to pass, if the copulative percussion felt through every fibre be the cause of the detachment of ova or ovula from the ovaria, that examples should be found of a like detachment, and consequently of a forma-

tion of corpora lutea, in cases where no copulation has ever taken place? Of the fact itself there is no question.[*] "Upon examining," says Sir Everard Home, "the ovaria of several women who had died virgins, and in whom the hymen was too perfect to admit of the possibility of impregnation, there were not only distinct corpora lutea, but also small cavities round the edge of the ovarium, evidently left by ova that had passed out at some former period, *so that this happens during the state of virginity.*"—(*Phil. Trans.*, 1817, ut suprà.) Professor Blumenbach has met with similar examples.[†] An endeavour has been made to account for the fact, first, by supposing that the females thus circumstanced must have been of a peculiarly amorous disposition, and at particular times morbidly excited by a venereal orgasm originating in their own persons alone, without any intercourse with the male sex. And next, that a high-wrought excitement of this kind may be sufficient to produce such an effect, and to lead to the first and most important step in the generative process. All this is highly ingenious, but we seem at present to want facts to justify us in offering such an explanation. "We cannot doubt," says Sir Everard Home, "that every time a female quadruped is in heat, one or more ova pass from the ovarium to the uterus, whether she receives the male or not."—(*Phil. Trans.*, 1817, ut suprà.) And to the same effect Professor Blumenbach, who first launched this opinion in 1788, before the Royal Society (*Specimen Physiologiæ Comparatæ; Comment. Soc. Reg. Scientiæ Göttengens*, vol. ix., 128) of Gottingen:—"The state of the ovaria," says he, "of women who have died under strong sexual passion, has been found similar to that of rabbits during heat."

---

[*] The fact of birds laying eggs without the co-operation of the male, which eggs, however, are unproductive, is familiarly known.—Ed.

[†] The minute investigations of the latest physiologists seem to have demonstrated clearly that the appearance of corpora lutea is not conclusive that pregnancy has existed. This important principle has been supported by many facts from human and comparative anatomy. To the high names mentioned in the text may be added Blundell, Francis, Granville, Dunglisson, and others. Dr. Francis observes (Notes to Francis's Denman, p. 152), "In my physiological lectures in the University of New-York, as Professor of the Institutes of Medicine, in 1817, I ventured the opinion that the appearance of corpora lutea is not to be deemed decisive of previous pregnancy; I have since found these corpora lutea in two instances where no doubt could exist as to the virginity of the subjects. That undue salacity may induce them, as well as other changes in the ovaria, may be confidently affirmed." Dr. Granville remarks (Graphic Illustrations of Abortion and the Diseases of Menstruation, 4to., London, 1834), "It is inaccurate to state that a woman has been pregnant because a corpus luteum has been found in the ovaria after death, or to calculate the number of children she has borne from the number of corpora lutea so detected. Corpora lutea have been found in the ovaria of very young girls, of unmarried women of the strictest virtue, and in newly-born female infants; and lastly, in steril animals, such as mules."—D.

And in confirmation of this he adds:—"In the body of a young woman, eighteen years of age, who had been brought up in a convent, and had every appearance of being a virgin, Valisneri found five or six vesicles *pushing forward* in one ovarium, and the correspondent Fallopian tube redder and longer than usual, as he had frequently observed in animals during heat. Bonet," he adds, "gives the history of a young lady who died furiously in love with a man of low rank, and whose ovaria were turgid with vesicles of great size." In neither of these cases, however, do we meet with ovula actually detached, and still less with corpora lutea. Add to which, that not only corpora lutea, but detached ovula, and even imperfect fœtation, have at times been found in the ovaries of infants of ten or twelve years of age, who can scarcely be suspected of any such erethism: a very curious instance of which we shall have to quote from Dr. Baillie, under the genus Prœotia.—(Class V., Ord. II., Gen. II., Spe. 2, of the present volume.)

I am aware that the same explanation has been adopted by M. Cuvier; indeed it is difficult to adopt any other; but direct facts in support of it are wanting in him as well as in the authorities just referred to. There is an indirect fact appealed to, however, by the last, which is well worth noticing for its curiosity, whatever degree of bearing it may have upon the present question. After observing that a corpus luteum is not positive evidence of impregnation, he adds, nor does the existence of a decidua in the uterus constitute better evidence of the same, since it has sometimes happened that, at each period of painful menstruation, the excitement of the uterine vessels has produced a perfect decidua, not to be distinguished from that belonging to an ovum. The present author has never met with a case of this kind, but of the fact itself there seems no doubt:* Morgagni has given one striking instance of it in his day (*De Sed. et Caus. Morb. Ep.*), and Mr. Stanley another in our own.—(*Med. Trans.*, vol. vi., art. xvi.) To explain the origin of such a membrane under such circumstances is by no means difficult, as it follows upon the common principle by which other membranous or membrane-like tunics are produced in other hollow organs in a state of peculiar irritation, of which some curious examples have already been offered under DIARRHŒA TUBULARIS.—(Vol. i., p. 137.) The peculiar character of the membrane must necessarily be governed by the character of the organ in which it is formed. Upon the whole, it does not seem to afford much support to the argument in whose favour it is appealed to, and the subject requires further investigation.

* Obstetrical writers have generally noticed the formation of this deciduous membrane. "Sometimes it is small," says Dr. Dewees, "at other times large, and sometimes it resembles the cavity from which it has been expelled; at other times it will be broken into many fragments."—(Diseases of Females, 4th edition, p. 181.) Dr. Granville, in his beautiful "Illustrations of Abortion and the Diseases of Menstruation," has devoted two plates (xi. and xii.) to these formations.—D.

The third difficulty attendant upon the common doctrine of the day, which supposes the fœtus to hold its entire communication with, and to derive its blood, nutriment, and oxygen from the mother by means of the placenta and umbilical cord, is founded upon the occasional instances of fœtuses of large and even full growth being found in the womb, and even brought forth at the proper period, without any placenta, or at least one of any utility, without any umbilical cord, or even a trace of an umbilicus. Admitting the course just glanced at to be the ordinary provision of nature, what is the substitute she employs on these occasions? the means by which the bereft fœtus is supplied with air and nourishment?

The advocates of the doctrine of epigenesis, as new modelled by the hands of Buffon and Darwin, triumphantly appeal to these curious deviations from the established order of nature, as effecting a direct overthrow of the doctrine of evolution by an impregnated ovum; while the supporters of the latter doctrine have too generally cut the question short by a flat denial of such monstrous aberrations.

There is little of the true spirit of philosophy in either conduct. Admitting the existence of such cases, they just as much cripple the one doctrine as the other; for, granting the explanation which is usually offered by the former, the ordinary machinery of a placenta and an umbilical cord becomes immediately a work of supererogation—a bulky and complicated piece of furniture, to which no important use can be assigned, and which the overloaded uterus might be well rid of.

But, on the contrary, to deny the existence of well-established and accumulated facts, merely because we cannot bend them to our own speculation, is still weaker and more reprehensible.* The kangaroo, opossum, and wombat,

* As a great deal of the mystery and obscurity of the process of reproduction in the animal world, and much of the difficulty of explaining several of its phenomena, are naturally connected, as a critical writer justly observes, with the anatomical facts of the new formation at different periods of its progress, it has been always a most essential step in the inquiry to determine the anatomical structure of its different parts. "From this circumstance it has resulted, that all theories of the process of reproduction, framed at periods when anatomy was either little or imperfectly cultivated, and before precision in anatomical inquiry was observed, have been extremely erroneous and fallacious. In the class of warmblooded viviparous animals, or those provided at once with a womb and mammæ, the union of the sexes, if efficient, gives rise to the formation of a new product, which is destined to be attached for a definite time to the inner surface of the womb, in one form of existence or vital action, and thence to be separated in order to become the seat of a different and new species of vital action. The new product thus formed, or ovum, as it is generally denominated, if examined at any given time, is found to consist of certain constituent parts, which may be distinguished into two general divisions; one, which is the germe or rudiment of the future being, and consequently contains more or less completely the representative form or rudiment of all the parts

all breed their young without either placenta or navel-string. The embryons are enclosed in one or more membranes, which are not attached to the coats of the uterus, and are supplied with nourishment, and apparently with air, from a gelatinous matter by which they are surrounded. Hoffmann gives us the case of a fœtus, born in full health and vigour, with the funis sphacelated and divided into two parts.—(*Op. de Pinguedine.*) Vander Wiel gives the history of a living child exhibited without any umbilicus, as a public spectacle (*Observ. Cent. post.*); and, in a foreign collection of literary curiosities, is the case of a hare which was found, on being opened, to contain three leverets, two of them without a placenta or umbilical vessels, and the other with both.—(*Commerc. Liter. Norimberg.*) Ploucquet has collected a list of several other instances in his Initia (*Initia Bibliothecæ, Medico-Pract. et Chirurg.*, tom. iii., p. 554, 4to., Tubing, 1794); but perhaps the most striking example is one which occurred to the present author in December, 1791, an account

---

of that being, and is destined for a comparatively permanent existence; the other certain parts which, either as investments of this rudimental being, or as the medium of its attachment to the inner surface of the womb and its nutrition while there, are limited in the duration of their existence to the period at which the newly-formed being is detached from the body of its mother. If the ovum, or product of generation thus defined, be examined in any of the mammiferous animals, it is found that the former assemblage of parts cannot be recognised with the same distinctness and perfection in the early as in the latter period of utero-gestation; and that there is a period, even after prolific sexual intercourse, in which it cannot be demonstrated in any form. It is different, however, with the second assemblage of parts. The existence of these can be perceived at a very recent period after impregnation; and they are believed on very good evidence, if not to commence, at least to precede the organism of the new body. The great problem in the solution of the principal difficulties of the process of generation is to determine the relation of these two orders of organized parts; to discover how much of the existence and development of the one depends on that of the other; to unfold the mechanism of their formation, and to understand the nature of the process by which they are produced. It is manifest that it is impossible to attain the last of these objects, without a thorough knowledge of the anatomical peculiarities of both assemblages of parts; and if, in any situation, the previous knowledge of the structure of organs be necessary to explain their properties and functions, it is in that of the process of reproduction. There is in this inquiry, however, this peculiar difficulty, that the parts are not at all periods after the process of impregnation exactly the same in appearance and disposition; and it is even uncertain whether they are the same in number. The ovum appears to pass through a succession of stages, in each of which it presents different aspects, and acquires new parts; while some, formerly distinct, disappear, or are blended with others."—(See Edin. Med. and Surg. Jour., No. cxviii., pp. 153, 154.) According to Lobstein, the vesicul umbilicalis, the uses of which are unknown, is restricted to a particular stage of the life of the embryo; and a similar remark applies to the omphalo-mesenteric vessels.—Ed.

of which he gave to the public in 1795.[*] The labour was natural, the child, scarcely less than the ordinary size, was born alive, cried feebly once or twice after birth, and died in about ten minutes. The organization, as well external as internal, was imperfect in many parts. There was no sexual character whatever, neither penis nor pudendum, nor any interior organ of generation: there was no anus nor rectum, no funis, no umbilicus; the minutest investigation could not discover the least trace of any. With the use of a little force, a small shrivelled placenta, or rather the rudiment of a placenta, followed soon after the birth of the child, without a funis or umbilical vessel of any kind, or any other appendage by which it appeared to have been attached to the child. No hemorrhage, nor even discoloration, followed its removal from the uterus. In a quarter of an hour afterward a second living child was protruded into the vagina and delivered with ease, being a perfect boy attached to its proper placenta by a proper funis. The author dissected the first of these shortly after its birth in the presence of two medical friends of distinguished reputation, Dr. Drake of Hadleigh, and Mr. Anderson of Sudbury, both of whom are still able to vouch for the correctness of this statement. On the present occasion, however, it is not necessary to follow up the amorphous appearances any further, as they are already before the public, except to state that the stomach, which was natural, was half filled with a liquid resembling that of the amnios.

This subject has been ably discussed by Professor Monro and Mr. Gibson.[†] The latter, giving full credit to the few histories of the case then before the world, endeavours very ingeniously to account for the nutriment of the fœtus by the liquor amnii, which he conjectures to be the ordinary source of supply, and not the placenta. The chief arguments are, that the embryon is at all times found at an earlier period in the uterus than the placenta itself; which does not appear to be perfected till two or three months after conception; and, consequently, that the embryon must, thus far at least, be supported from some other source than the placenta; and if thus far, why not through the whole term of parturition? That extra-uterine fœtuses have no placenta, and yet obtain the means of growth and evolution from the surrounding parts. That the liquor amnii is analogous in its appearance to the albumen of a hen's egg, which forms the proper nourishment of the young chick; that it is found in the stomach and mouths of viviparous animals when first born; and that it diminishes in its volume in proportion to the growth of the fœtus.[‡]

---

[*] Case of Preternatural Fœtation, with observations: read before the Medical Society of London, Oct. 20, 1794.

[†] Edin. Med. Essays, vol. i., art. xiii.; vol. ii., art. ix., x., xi. See also Dr. Fleming's paper, Phil. Trans., vol. xlix., 1775-6, p. 254.

[‡] The fluid of the vesicula umbilicalis is regarded by M. Velpeau and some other physiologists in a similar light, namely, as a nutritious

To these arguments it was replied by Professor Monro, that we have no satisfactory proof that the liquor amnii is a nutritive fluid at all, and that in the case of amorphous fœtuses, produced without the vestige of a mouth or of any other kind of passage leading to the stomach, it cannot possibly be of any such use : that if the office of the placenta be not that of affording food to the embryo, it becomes those who maintain the contrary to determine what other office can be allotted to it ; and that till this is satisfactorily done, it is more consistent with reason to doubt the few and unsatisfactory cases at that time brought forward, than to perplex ourselves with facts directly contradictory of each other.

For the full scope of the argument, the reader must turn to the Edinburgh Medical E$_{ssays}$ themselves, or, for a close summary, to the present author's observations appended to his own case. It must be admitted that the instances adverted to in the course of the discussion are but few, and most of them stamped with something unsatisfactory. Others, however, might have been advanced even at that time on authorities that would have settled the matter of fact at once, how much soever they might have confounded all explanation. But after the history just given, and the references to other cases by which it may be confirmed, this is not necessary on the present occasion, as it is now well ascertained that the human embryon is always supported for several weeks in the commencement of gestation without a placenta ;* and in various other mammalia, as the mare, ass, camel, and hog, besides those just adverted to, through its entire period. These animals being uniformly destitute of such an organ, the surprise is in some measure removed, which would otherwise be natural on finding a single instance of a like destitution through the whole term of human pregnancy.†

It is singular that the subject of aeration, which forms another difficulty in discussing the question, is not dwelt upon on either side, notwithstanding the ingenious conjecture of Sir Edward Hulse, that the placenta might be an organ of respiration as well as of nutrition, had at this time been before the public for nearly half a century ; and it shows us how slow the best founded theories not unfrequently are in obtaining the meed of public assent, to which they are entitled from the first.

These, however, are only a few of the peculiar difficulties that still accompany the subject of generation, to whatever doctrine we attach ourselves. There are others that are more general, but equally inexplicable. The whole range of extra-uterine fœtuses is of this character ; often formed, and nourished, and developed, without either a placenta or an amnios, and yet sometimes advancing, even in the remote cavity of the ovarium, and perfect in every organ, to the age of at least four months, of which we have already offered an example. A great part of the range of amorphous births defy equally all mental comprehension ; particularly the production of monsters without heads or hearts, some of whom have lived for several days after birth (see *for examples and authorities the author's volume of Nosology*, p. 538) ; others consisting of a head alone, wholly destitute of a trunk, and yet possessing a full development of this organ ; a specimen of which was lately in the possession of Dr. Elfes, of Neuss, on the Rhine (*Hufeland, Journal der Practischen Heilkunde*, Apr., 1816) ; and others again, the whole of whose abdominal and thoracic viscera has been found transposed.‡

Nor less inexplicable is the generative power of transmitting peculiarities of talents, of form,

---

substance—a kind of oil—like the vitelline fluid of the chick ; and he thinks that it contributes to the development of the embryon until the cord and the vessels are formed, and until the ovulum is exactly applied to the inner surface of the womb.—(See his Embryologie, &c., Paris, 1833.) In short, the vesicula umbilicalis seems to him to be analogous to the vitelline sac of the chick, which it resembles in shape, position, its connexion with the intestines, the structure of its parietes, and the quality of its fluid. The theory here adverted to, however, is far from being well established ; and is, perhaps, not better supported than Mr. Gibson's hypothesis respecting the use of the liquor amnii.—ED.

* This statement is at variance, however, with the result of the investigations of M. Velpeau, who describes the development of the placenta as commencing the moment the ovulum enters the uterus, and not, as some writers have represented, three or four months after gestation.—(See his Embryologie, ou Ovologie Humaine, fol., Paris, 1833.) How many unsettled points are there in what may be regarded as the anatomical facts appertaining to this difficult subject !—ED.

† See Phil. Trans., 1822, art. xxix., on the Placenta, by Sir Everard Home, Bart. M. Velpeau infers that the fœtus does not receive from the

womb blood completely elaborated, but a fluid of different chymical properties and general constitution, being more serous, less coagulable, and having much smaller globules.—(Embryologie, &c., Paris, 1833, fol.) However, the editor is disposed to join a critical writer in the belief, that it is physiologically erroneous to imagine it necessary for the fœtus or ovum to receive blood in any shape from the uterus. "What is the use of the complicated but beautiful arrangement of membranes, vessels, and placenta, unless it were that these parts were perfectly competent to derive the materials of blood from the womb, without the intervention of actual vascular canals conveying red, completely-formed blood ? Physiologists, in their inquiry, seem to forget or overlook the fact, that the ovum, after fecundation, is a new being, which has received the principle of life, and that, by virtue of this principle, it is quite capable of attaching itself to any living tissue, and deriving from that tissue the materials of nutriment, as is abundantly evinced in Fallopian and also extra-uterine pregnancies, in which the peritoneum serves as a uterine surface for a time."—See Edin. Med. and Surg. Journ., No. cxviii., p. 174.—ED.

‡ Samson, Phil. Trans., 1674. Smithers, who was executed at the Old Bailey two years ago, for setting fire to a house in Oxford-street, and occasioning the loss of life to some of its inhabitants, furnished an example of such transposition. The preparation is contained in the Museum of the London University.—ED.

or of defects, in a long line of hereditary descent, and occasionally of suspending the peculiarity through a link or two, or an individual or two, with an apparent capriciousness, and then of exhibiting it once more in full vigour.* The vast influence which this recondite but active power possesses, as well over the mind as the body, cannot, at all times, escape the notice of the most inattentive. Not only are wit, beauty, and genius propagable in this manner, but dulness, madness, and deformity of every kind.

[Mr. Mayo supports the opinion, that the physical and moral constitution of the infant have a greater resemblance to those of the father than to those of the mother. The offspring of a black man and a white woman are observed to be darker than that of a black woman by a white. This doctrine, in relation to form, complexion, and moral character, among Europeans at least, has so many exceptions, that its correctness seems doubtful. The following statements, introduced into this gentleman's "Outlines of Physiology," and closely connected with some observations at the commencement of this preliminary physiological discourse, are highly interesting. Some remarkable instances which have recently attracted notice, seem to show that in the higher animals the influence of the male is extended even beyond a single impregnation. A seven eighths Arabian mare, belonging to the Earl of Morton, which had never been bred from before, had a mule by a quagga : subsequently she had three foals by a black Arabian horse. The first two of these are thus described :—They have the character of the Arabian breed as decidedly as can be expected, where fifteen sixteenths of the blood are Arabian; and they are fine specimens of that breed ; but, both in their colour and in the hair of their manes, they have a striking resemblance to the quagga. Their colour is bay, marked more or less like the quagga, in a darker teint. Both are distinguished by the dark line along the ridge of the back, the dark stripes across the forehand, and the dark bars across the back part of the legs. Both their manes are black ; that of the filly is short, stiff, and stands upright : that of the colt is long, but so stiff as to arch upwards, and to hang clear of the sides of the neck ; in which circumstance it resembles that of the hybrid. This is the more remarkable, as the manes of the Arabian breed hang lank, and closer to the neck than those of most others.—(*Phil. Trans.*, 1821, p. 21.) A similar occurrence to the preceding is mentioned by Mr. Giles respecting a litter of pigs, which resembled in colour a former litter by a wild boar. The explanation of these phenomena, preferred by Mr. Mayo, is the supposition that the connexion with the male produces a physical impression, not merely upon the ova which are ripe for impregnation, but upon others, likewise, that are at the time immature. In gallinaceous birds, in turkeys for instance, it is well known that a single coitus will actually impreg-

nate all the ova that are laid during the breeding season. The explanation here quoted he deems more reasonable than any supposed influence of the imagination.—(See *Mayo's Outlines of Human Physiology*, 2d edit., p. 489.)]

Even where accident, or a cause we cannot discern, has produced a preternatural conformation or singularity in a particular organ, it is astonishing to behold how readily it is often copied by the generative power, and how tenaciously it adheres to the future lineage. A preternatural defect in the hand or foot has, in many cases, been so common to the succeeding members of a family, as to lay a foundation in every age and country for the family name, as in that of Varro, Valgius, Flaccus, and Plautus, at Rome. Seleucus had the mark of an anchor on his thigh, and is said to have transmitted it to his posterity ; and supernumerary fingers and toes have descended in a direct line, for many generations, in various countries. Hence, hornless sheep and hornless oxen produce an equally hornless offspring ; and the broad-tailed Asiatic sheep yields a progeny with a tail equally monstrous, often of not less than half a hundred pounds weight. And hence, too, those enormous prominences in the hinder parts of one or two of the nations at the back of the Cape of Good Hope, of which examples have been furnished to us in our own island.

How are we moreover to account for that fearful host of diseases, gout, consumption, scrofula, leprosy, and madness, which, originating perhaps in the first sufferer accidentally, are propagated so deeply and so extensively, that it is difficult to meet with a family whose blood is totally free from all hereditary taint ? By what means this predisposition may be best resisted, it is not easy to determine. But, as there can be no question that intermarriages among the collateral branches of the same family tend more than any thing else to fix, and multiply, and aggravate it, there is reason to believe that unions between total strangers, and perhaps inhabitants of different countries, form the surest antidote. For admitting that such strangers to each other may be tainted on either side with some morbid predisposition peculiar to their respective lineages, each must lose something of its influence by the mixture of a new soil ; and we are not without analogies to render it probable that in their mutual encounter, the one may even destroy the other by a specific power. And hence, nothing can be wiser, on physical as well as on moral grounds, than the restraints which divine and human laws have concurred in laying on marriages between relations ; and though there is something quaint and extravagant, there is something sound at the bottom, in the following remark of the sententious Burton upon this subject :—"And surely," says he, "I think it has been ordered by God's especial providence that, in all ages, there should be, once in six hundred years, a transmigration of nations to amend and purify their blood, as we alter seed upon our land ; and that there should be, as it were, an inundation of those northern Goths and Vandals, and many such like people, which came out of

---

* See Sir E. Home's Paper on Impressions produced on the Fœtus in the Womb.—Phil. Trans., 1825, p. 75.

that continent of Scandia and Sarmatia, as some suppose, and overran, as a deluge, most part of Europe and Africa, to alter, for our good, our complexions, that were much defaced with hereditary infirmities, which by our lust and intemperance we had contracted."—(*Anatomy of Melancholy*, vol. i., part i., sect. ii., p. 89, 8vo.) Boethius informs us of a different and still severer mode of discipline at one time established in Scotland for the same purpose, but which, however successful, would make, I am afraid,

sad havoc in our own day, were it ever to be carried into execution. "If any one," says he, "were visited with the falling sickness, madness, gout, leprosy, or any such dangerous disease, which was likely to be propagated from father to son, he was instantly castrated; if it were a woman, she was debarred all intercourse with men; and if she were found pregnant with such complaint upon her, she and her unborn child were buried alive."—(*De Veterum Scotorum Moribus*, lib. i.)

ORDER I.
CENOTICA.
DISEASES AFFECTING THE FLUIDS.
MORBID DISCHARGES; OR EXCESS, DEFICIENCY, OR IRREGULARITY OF SUCH AS ARE NATURAL.

THIS order, the name of which is derived from Galen, and has been explained already, is designed to include a considerable number of diseases which have hitherto been scattered over every part of a nosological classification, but which are related to each other, as being morbid discharges dependant upon a morbid condition of one or more of the sexual organs. The term employed might have been MEDORRHŒTICA, but that medorrhœa, as a genus, has been already employed by Professor Frank of Paris, in a somewhat different, and, as it appears to the author, peculiarly indistinct sense; as combining, under a single generic name, what seems to be a medley of diseases with no other connexion than locality or contiguity of organs, as mucous piles, fistula in ano, leucorrhœa, clap, gleet, syphilis, phimosis, paraphimosis, and what was formerly called hernia humoralis, by him named epididymitis, the orchitis of the present system. The genera under this order are five, and may be thus expressed:—

I. Paramenia.	Mismenstruation.
II. Leucorrhœa.	Whites.
III. Blennorrhœa.	Gonorrhœa.
IV. Spermorrhœa.	Seminal Flux.
V. Galactia.	Mislactation.

GENUS I.
PARAMENIA.
MISMENSTRUATION.
MORBID EVACUATION OR DEFICIENCY OF THE CATAMENIAL FLUX.

PARAMENIA is a Greek term, derived from παρά, "male," and μὴν, "mensis." The genus is here limited to such diseases as relate to the menstrual flux, or the vessels from which it issues. This fluid is incorrectly regarded as blood by Cullen, Leake, Richerand, and other physiologists; for, in truth, it has hardly any common property with blood, except that of being a liquid of a red colour. It is chiefly distinguished by its not being coagulable; and hence, when coagula are found in it, as in laborious and profuse menstruation, serum or blood is intermixed with it, and extruded either from atonic relaxation or entonic action of the menstrual vessels. "It is," observes Mr. John

Hunter, "neither similar to blood taken from a vein of the same person, nor to that which is extravasated by accident in any other part of the body; but is a species of blood, changed, separated, or thrown off from the common mass by an action of the vessels of the uterus similar to that of secretion; by which action the blood loses the principle of coagulation, and, I suppose, life." Mr. Cruickshank supposes it to be thrown forth from the mouths of the exhaling arteries of the uterus, enlarged periodically for this purpose; and his view of the subject seems to be confirmed by a singular case of prolapse, both of the uterus and vagina, given by Mr. Hill of Dumfries. In this case, the os tincæ appeared like a nipple projecting below the retroverted vagina, which assumed the form of a bag. The patient at times laboured under leucorrhœa; but it was observed that when she menstruated, the discharge flowed entirely from the projecting nipple of the prolapse: while the leucorrhœa proceeded from the surrounding bag alone.—(*Edin. Med. Com.*, vol. iv., p. 91.)[*]

As this distinction has not been sufficiently attended to, either by nosologists or physiologists, many of the diseases occurring in the present arrangement under paramenia have been placed by other writers under a genus named menorrhagia, which, properly speaking, should import hemorrhage (a morbid flow of *blood alone*) from the menstrual vessels. And we have here, therefore, not only a wrong doctrine, but the formation of an improper genus: for menorrhagia or uterine hemorrhage is, correctly speaking, only a species of the genus HÆMORRHAGIA, and will be so found in the present system, in which it occurs in Class III., Order IV. This remark applies directly to Sauvages; and quite as much so to Cullen, who, in his attempt to simplify, has carried the confusion even further than Sauvages. Few diseases, perhaps, of the uterus or uterine passage, can be more distinct from each other than vicarious menstruation, lochial discharge, and sanious ichor; yet

---

[*] The idea that the menstrual fluid is a secretion, is strongly supported by a remark of Sprengel. He says, "arterias equidem certo capillares e villis fundere sanguinem persuadeor, cum a Kaauw Boerhaavii inde temporibus sæpius manifesta visa fuerit ea origo. Quæ arteriæ licet et in hoc viscere continuo in venulas transeant, patuli tameu sunt earum fines in villis massa laxissima cellulosa clausis, e quibus sine laceratione ob impetum majorem, sanguis expeditius effluere potest."—Institut., vol. iii.—D.

all these, with several others equally unallied, are arranged by Sauvages under the genus menorrhagia, though not one of them belongs to it. While Cullen not only copies nearly the whole of these maladies with the names Sauvages has assigned them, but adds to the generic list leucorrhœa or whites, abortion, and the mucous fluid, secreted in the beginning of labour from the glandulæ Nabothi at the orifice of the womb, and hence vulgarly denominated *show* or appearance. Menstruation may be diseased from obstruction, severe pain in its secretion, excess of discharge, transfer to some other organ, or cessation ; thus offering us the five following species, accompanied with distinct symptoms :—

1. Paramenia Ob-　Obstructed Menstruation.
　　structionis.
2. ———— Diffi-　Laborious Menstruation.
　　cilis.
3. ———— Su-　Excessive Menstruation.
　　perflua.
4. ———— Erro-　Vicarious Menstruation.
　　ris.
5. ———— Ces-　Irregular Cessation of the
　　sationis.　　　Menses.

SPECIES I.

PARAMENIA OBSTRUCTIONIS.

OBSTRUCTED MENSTRUATION.*

CATAMENIAL SECRETION OBSTRUCTED IN ITS COURSE ; SENSE OF OPPRESSION ; LANGUOR ; DYSPEPSY.

THIS species, by many writers called menostatio, appears under the two following varieties :—

a Emansio.　The secretion obstructed on its
　Retention of　accession, or first appearance.
　the men-　　The feet and ankles œdematous
　ses.　　　　at night ; the eyes and face in
　　　　　　　the morning.
ß Suppressio.　The secretion obstructed in its
　Suppression　regular periods of recurrence.
　of the men-　Headache, dyspnœa, palpitation
　ses.　　　　of the heart.

In order to explain the FIRST of these VARIE-

---

* The *amenorrhœa* of other medical writers, a term applied to every example of obstructed menstruation except that resulting from pregnancy. Here, however, it is manifest that a variety of affections and many states of the female constitution are disadvantageously confounded together. The non-appearance of the menses in a girl seemingly arrived at puberty, is not at all analogous to the natural cessation of them in a woman that has reached the critical period of life ; and both these forms of amenorrhœa are essentially different from what originates from some chronic inflammation or an organic disease. Again, the latter is not similar in any respect to the stoppage of the menses brought on by impairment of the general health or inertia of the uterus ; while the last mentioned instance is entirely of a different nature from that in which the courses are suddenly suppressed by some accidental cause.—See L. C. Roche, in Dict. de Med. et de Chir. Pratiques, tom. ii., p. 135.—ED.

TIES, or RETENTION OF THE MENSES, by Professor Frank quaintly denominated amenorrhœa (*De Cur. Hom. Morb. Epit.*, tom. vi., lib. vi., part. iii., 8vo., Vienna, 1821) tiruncularum, it is necessary to observe that when the growth of the animal frame is completed or nearly so, the quantity of blood and sensorial power which have hitherto been employed in providing for such growth, constitutes an excess, and must produce plethora by being diffused generally, or congestion by being accumulated locally. Professor Monro contended for the former effect ; Dr. Cullen, with apparently more reason, for the latter. And this last turn it seems to take for the wisest of purposes ; I mean, in order to prepare for a future race, by perfecting that system of organs which is immediately concerned in the process of generation ; and which, during the general growth of the body, has remained dormant and inert, to be developed and perfected alone when every other part of the frame has made a considerable advance towards maturity, and there is, so to speak, more leisure and materials for so important a work. We shall have occasion to touch upon this subject more at large when we come to treat of the genus CHLOROSIS : for the present it will be sufficient to observe, that this accumulation of the nervous energy and sanguineous fluid seems first to show itself among men in the testes, and among women in the ovaria ; and that from the ovaria it spreads to all those organs that are connected with them either by sympathy or unity of intention, chiefly to the uterus and the mammæ ; exciting in the uterus a new action and secretion, which secretion, in order to relieve the organ from the congestion, it is hereby undergoing, is thrown off periodically and by lunar intervals in the form of a blood-like discharge, although, when minutely examined, the discharge, as already stated, is found to consist not of genuine blood, but of a fluid possessing peculiar properties. These properties we have already enlarged upon, and have shown in what they differ from those of proper blood : and it is upon this point that the physiology of Dr. Cullen is strikingly erroneous, for not only in his First Lines, but long afterward in his Materia Medica, he regards the discharge as pure blood, and consequently, the economy of menstruation as a periodical hemorrhage. "I suppose," says he, "that in consequence of the gradual evolution of the system at a certain period of life, the vessels of the uterus are dilated and filled ; and that by this congestion these vessels are stimulated to a stronger action, by which their extremities *are forced open and pour out blood.* According to this idea, it will appear that I suppose the menstrual discharge to be upon the footing of *an active hemorrhagy*, which, by the laws of economy, is disposed to return after a certain interval."*

---

* Mat. Med., vol. ii., p. 587, 4to. In refutation of the notion that menstruation depends on a general plethoric orgasm, Dr. A. T. Thomson, in the second volume of his Elements of Materia Medica, quotes the case of the Hungarian sisters, who were united at the lower part of the back, and lived to the age of twenty-two. The same blood

From the sympathy prevailing between, the uterus and most other organs of the system, we meet not unfrequently with some concomitant affection in various remote parts ; as an appearance of spots on the hands or forehead antecedently to the efflux (*Salmuth*, cent. iii., obs. 18);· or, which is more common, a peculiar sensation or emotion in the breasts.—(*Act. Nat. Cur.*, vol. iii., App., p. 168.)

We cannot explain the reason why this fluid should be thrown off once a month, or by lunar periods, rather than after intervals of any other duration.* But the same remark might have been made, if the periods had been of any other kind ; and will equally apply to the recurrence of intermittent fevers. It is enough that we trace in this action the marks of design and regularity.

The time in which the secretion, and consequently the discharge, commences, varies from many circumstances ; chiefly, however, from those of climate, and of peculiarity of constitution. In warm climates, menstruation appears often as early as at eight or nine years of age ; for here the general growth of the body advances more rapidly than in colder quarters, and the

flowed in the vessels of each, for the abdominal vessels were found after death united at the loins ; yet the uterine function was distinct in each of these individuals, differing in its period, and also in the quantity of the discharge: The menses do not coagulate like blood, nor do they, according to modern statements, contain fibrin ; though this account does not agree with Mr. Brande's observation, that they possess the "properties of a very concentrated solution of blood in diluted serum." M. Lecanu found, that blood drawn from the arm of a woman during the menstrual discharge, contains little more than half of the quantity of globules present in it at other periods.—ED.

* The intervals being exactly those of the course of the moon in the revolution of her orbit, they were supposed to be influenced by this planet ; but were this the case, the menses ought to correspond with one of the phases of the moon's course, which is not the fact. See Dr. A. T. Thomson's Elem. of Materia Med., vol. ii., p. 439. The following are the ages at which, according to the researches of Mr. Roberton, of Manchester, 450 women began to menstruate in this climate :—

In their		In their	
11th year	10	16th year	76
12th year	19	17th year	57
13th year	53	18th year	26
14th year	85	19th year	23
15th year	97	20th year	4

One corollary drawn by Mr. Roberton from this table is, that the natural period of puberty in women of this country, instead of being the fourteenth or fifteenth year, occurs in a much more extended range of ages, and is much more equally distributed throughout that range than authors represent.

In Mr. Roberton's paper, evidence has been collected to prove, in opposition to usual belief, that the age of female puberty in the arctic regions is at least as early as in the temperate zone. In the same document, the reader will also find a statement of various circumstances, which appear to Mr. Roberton to have led travellers to form erroneous conclusions concerning the period of puberty in warm climates.—See Edin. Med. and Surg. Journal for October, 1832, p. 246.

atmosphere is more stimulant. In temperate climates it is usually postponed till the thirteenth or fourteenth year, and in the arctic regions till the nineteenth or twentieth.*

In all climates, however, when the constitution has acquired the age in which it is prepared for the discharge, various causes may accelerate its appearance. Among these we may mention any preternatural degree of heat or fever, or any other stimulus that quickens the circulation. Mauriceau relates a case in which it was brought on suddenly by an attack of a tertian intermittent :· and in like manner, anger, or any other violent emotion of the mind, has been found to produce it as abruptly. The depressing passions, as fear and severe grief, conduce to the same end, though in a different way ; for here there is rather uterine congestion than increased impetus, in consequence of the spastic chill of the small vessels on the surface, which lessens their diameter. Inordinate exercise, or a high temperature of the atmosphere, has in like manner a tendency to hurry on the menstrual tide ; and hence its appearing so early in tropical regions. Dr. Gulbrand, indeed, conceives that even an increase in the elasticity or weight of the atmosphere is sufficient to produce a like effect, and refers to a curious fact in proof of this. In an hospital to which he was one of the physicians, a very considerable number of the female patients were suddenly seized with catamenia : which was the more remarkable, because several of these had, for a considerable time, laboured under a suppression of that discharge, and had been taking emmenagogues to no purpose ; while others had only been free from their regular returns for a few days. On inquiring into the cause, the only one which could be ascertained was a very great augmentation in the weight or pressure of the atmosphere, the mercury in the barometer having attained a height at which it had never been previously observed at Copenhagen, though he does not state the point it had actually reached.—(*De Sanguifluxû Uterino,* 8vo., Hafu.)

* In Lapland, according to Linnæus, women will often menstruate only during the summer months. The difference in the time of life when the menses appear has been mentioned as the reason why women in hot climates are almost universally treated as slaves, and why their influence is so powerful in cold countries, where personal beauty is in less estimation. This is an opinion professed by Hume and Montesquieu (Spirit of the Laws, É. T., b. 16), and is referred to by Dr. Denman :—"In hot climates, women are in the prime of their beauty when they are children in understanding : and when this is matured they are no longer objects of love. In temperate climates, their passions and their minds acquire perfection at, or nearly at the same time : and the united power of their beauty and faculties is supposed to be irresistible."—(Introd. to the Prac. of Midwifery, p. 82.) But, as Dr. Locock well observes, the influence of civilization seems to have been entirely overlooked in this theory; as otherwise the most chivalrous devotion to the fair sex would be found in the savage inhabitants of the countries of perpetual snow.—See Cycl. of Practical Med., art. MENSTRUATION.—ED.

It is possible that other general causes may sometimes operate to a like extent; and hence this disease is said by Stoll, and other writers, to be occasionally epidemic.—(*Rat. Med.*, P. iii., p. 48; *Samml. Med. Wahrnehm.*, b. ix., p. 401.)

Still much depends upon the idiosyncrasy: some girls are of a more rapid growth than others of the same climate; and in some, there is a peculiar sexual precocity, or prematurity of orgasm, that hurries on the discharge before the general growth of the body would lead us to expect it: of which Pecklin gives an example in a girl of seven years of age, who, in the intervals, laboured under a leucorrhœa.* And hence those very early and marvellous stories of pregnancy in girls of not more than nine years old, which, if not well authenticated, and from different and unconnected quarters, might justify a very high degree of skepticism.†

The efflux continues from two to eight or ten days; and the quantity thrown forth varies from four to ten ounces in different individuals: the monthly return running on till the fortieth or fiftieth year, and sometimes, as we shall have occasion to observe hereafter, to a much later period of life.‡

* Lib. i., obs. 24. In the Med. Chir. Trans., Dr. Wall has published the particulars of a child, aged nine years, who had regularly menstruated from the age of nine months, and at two years of age had all the indications of puberty.—ED.

† Haller (Gottl. Eman.), Blumenbach, bibl i., p. 558. Schmid, Act. Helvet., iv., p. 167. Eph. Nat. Cur., dec. iii., an. ii., obs. 172. The following case happened in the practice of Mr. Robert Thorpe, and is recorded by Mr. Roberton of Manchester:—"A girl who worked in a cotton factory became pregnant, as was represented, in her eleventh year. When in labour she was seized with convulsions, but ultimately, without unusual difficulty, was delivered of a full-grown stillborn child. Her recovery was perfectly favourable." Mr. Thorpe and the late Dr. Hardie examined the registers of this girl's birth and christening, and fully satisfied themselves that she had really conceived in her eleventh year, and that at the time of her delivery she was only a few months advanced in her twelfth year. Mr. Thorpe likewise ascertained that she had menstruated before she was pregnant.—See an Inq. into the Natural Hist. of the Menstrual Functions, by John Roberton, Edin. Med. and Surg. Journal for Oct., 1832, p. 231.—ED.

‡ In this climate the function of menstruation lasts, upon the average, for about thirty years of the life of woman, beginning at puberty, and ending somewhere between forty and fifty years of age, *unless interrupted by disease, by pregnancy, or by suckling.*—(See Pract. Comp., by Dr. Gooch, p. if.) It is a popular idea, as Dr. Ramsbotham observes, that some women menstruate *during the whole period of utero-gestation*: even good physiologists and physicians of discernment have adopted the same erroneous opinion. But such a circumstance, he remarks, is perfectly impossible; for, upon impregnation taking place, the uterus becomes lined with a membrane, secreted from its internal surface, which completely closes the orifices of the vessels from which the menses flow. It is certainly true, that some pregnant women are subject to occasional attacks of hemorrhage, both from the uterus and vagina, which may last three or four days. This blood has been taken for the

VOL. II.—E e

It is not always, however, that a retention of the menses to a much later date than sixteen, or even twenty years of age, constitutes disease: for sometimes it never takes place at all, as where the ovaries are absent, or perhaps imperfeet;* or where, instead of precocity in the

menstruous fluid; but it is unlike the menses, inasmuch as it does not return at regular intervals. Although it is impossible for this secretion to continue throughout the whole of pregnancy, the same remark does not hold good with regard to the few early weeks. Dewees is persuaded that women may menstruate till the end of the fourth month, and he supposes that the secretion, in such case, proceeds from the cervix uteri, which before that time is not developed; and Dr. Blundell says he has repeatedly met with cases in which the catamenia flowed for the first two or three months. Dr. Ramsbotham has a patient who always menstruates once after having conceived, though very sparingly.—(See Med. Gaz. for 1833-34, p. 268, Ramsbotham's Lectures.) When women deviate from the natural law, and menstruate during lactation, the milk is observed to be neither sufficiently nutritious nor copious.—(Ib.) During the large proportion of female life allotted for menstruation, there is a great liability to derangements of this process in one form or another; and, as Dr. Locock remarks, the time of the first appearance of the catamenia, and that of their final cessation, are deemed critical periods, when prudence requires the system to be taken great care of. The actual flow of the menstrual discharge itself is also looked upon as a time of great delicacy, and as demanding peculiar attention; so that very few diseases can exist, and very few plans of treatment be recommended, without the presence of the menses in some way influencing the nature of the symptoms or the remedies to be applied. It is in this especially that the character of the female constitution in disease is manifested; for, before puberty, and after the cessation of menstruation, the female differs but little from the male in the character of disease, except in those points which may be considered as accidental, such as organic diseases of the sexual organs.—(See Dr. Locock on the Pathology of Menstruation, in Cyclop. of Pract. Med., part 14.) Dr. Gooch states that menstruation recurs every month with almost mechanical regularity. But though it is unquestionably true, that in a considerable majority of instances, the catamenia recur monthly,—i. e., from the cessation of the secretion at one period, to its reappearance at the next, there elapses an interval of twenty-eight days,—yet "there is a certain proportion of women in whom the interval is not four, but three weeks; another smaller proportion, in whom the interval (apparently in no degree owing to disease) is irregular, being in the same woman at one time three, at another time four, or six, or eight, or even twelve weeks; and in another, but smaller proportion, in whom the catamenia return regularly every fortnight." In all these varieties, the secretion generally continues to flow from about two to six days: in some three or four days longer.—See Roberton's Obs. in Edin. Med. and Surg. Journ., No. cxiii. for Oct., 1832, p. 252.—ED.

* Sometimes the general health and strength continue unimpaired, the growth of the body proceeds rightly, and the circulation is active; but the mammæ are not protuberant; there are no sexual propensities; a slight beard grows on the upper lip; and the general characteristics resemble those of a male. In such a case, the proba-

genital system, there is a constitutional tardiness and want of stimulus ; under which circumstances it appeared for the first time, according to Holdefreund, in one instance, at the age of seventy (*Erzäklungen*, No. iv.) : and in another, that fell under the care of Professor Frank, it never appeared, either in the condition of single or married life, nor had the patient at any time any lochial discharge, though she had produced three healthy children.—(*De Cur. Hom. Morb. Epit.*, tom. vi., lib. vi., part iii., 8vo., Vienna, 1821.) It is only, therefore, when symptoms take place indicating a disordered state of some part or other of the body, and which experience teaches us is apt to arise upon a retention of the menstrual flux, that we can regard such retention as a disease.

These symptoms, as already stated in the definition of the disorder, consist chiefly in a general sense of oppression, languor, and dyspepsy. The languor extends over the whole system, and affects the mind as well as the body : and hence, while the appetite is feeble and capricious, and shows a desire for the most unaccountable and innutrient substances, the mind is capricious and variable, often pleased with trifles, and incapable of fixing on any serious pursuit. The heat of the system is diffused irregularly, and is almost always below the point of health : there is, consequently, great general inactivity, and particularly in the small vessels and extreme parts of the body. The pulse is quick, but low, the breathing attended with labour, the sleep disturbed, the face pale, the feet cold, the nostrils dry, the intestines irregularly confined, and the urine colourless. In some instances there is an occasional discharge of blood, or a blood-like fluid, from a remote organ, as the eyes, the nose, the ears, the nipples, the lungs, the stomach, or even the tips of the fingers, giving examples of the fourth species. There is also, sometimes, an irritable and distressing cough ; and the patient is thought to be on the verge of a decline, or perhaps to be running rapidly through its stages.

A decline, however, does not follow, nor is the disease found fatal, although it should continue, as it has done, not unfrequently, for many years : for if the proper discharge do not take place, the constitution will often in some degree accommodate itself to the morbid circumstances that press upon it, and many of the symptoms will become slighter, or altogether disappear. Most commonly, however, when the patient is supposed to be at the worst, probably from the increased irritation of the system peculiarly directed to the defaulting organs, a little mucous or serous discharge, with a slight show

of colour, is the harbinger of a beneficial change, and is soon succeeded by the proper discharge itself : though it often happens that the efflux is at first not very regular, either as to time or quantity. But this is an evil which generally wears away by degrees.

All the symptoms indicate that retained menstruation is a disease of debility, and there can be little doubt that debility is its primary cause :[*] a want of energy in the secernent vessels of the uterus, that prevents them from fulfilling their office, till the increase of irritability, from the increase of general weakness, at length produces a sufficient degree of stimulus, and thus momentarily supplies the place of strength. The system at large suffers evidently from sympathy.[†]

* There are many cases of retained menstruation, which indicate conclusively that the non-appearance of the menstrual fluid may depend on an entonic state of the system. In such instances, antiphlogistics, and the free use of the lancet, are among the most serviceable emmenagogues.—D.

† Two conditions of body, essentially different, may be connected with the form amenorrhœa, or paramenia, as Dr. Good terms it, now under consideration. In one, puberty is delayed, whether from idiosyncrasy, from want of constitutional energy, or from defective organization : in the other, puberty exists ; the ovaria and the uterus are organically matured ; but their peculiar function is suspended. Dr. Good might have entered further into the consideration of the causes of obstructed menstruation than he has done ; in particular, he might have noticed the frequent difficulty of immediately deciding whether the stoppage of the menses is an original or secondary affection—a cause or an effect—the whole disorder, or merely a symptom. Residence in low, gloomy, damp, marshy places ; food of unwholesome quality, and containing but little nutritious principles in it ; too low a diet ; want of exercise ; labour beyond the strength, and protracted to too late an hour ; are so many circumstances, whose prejudicial influence on female youth will prevent their proper growth, keep them from attaining their strength, and hinder them, though they have exceeded the age of puberty, from possessing the attributes of this enviable stage of life. In women, also, who have already menstruated, similar influences will bring on, first, a diminution of the discharge ; then a retardation of its return by two or three days ; next, still longer intervals ; and at length, complete amenorrhœa. Anæmia, or a deficiency of blood in the system, is another occasional cause of this form of paramenia. Celibacy is likewise generally regarded as giving a tendency to the disorder. Certain it is, that, with many women, sexual intercourse promotes menstruation ; and, as M. Roche observes (Dict. Méd. et de Chir. Pratiques, tom. ii., p. 137), what practitioner has not remarked, that numerous other females, whose courses were always difficult or obstructed before marriage, menstruated copiously and regularly after that change in their condition. But, according to this author, none of the preceding causes of amenorrhœa are so powerful as the existence of any serious chronic disease, whatever may be its nature, whether chronic gastritis, or chronic pneumonia, or pleurisy ; and so frequent does this species of cause seem to him, that he pronounces amenorrhœa in most instances to be a symptom and not a disease. At all events, the observation deserves to be well remembered in practice, by

bilities are, that the ovaries are either absent, or have become so diseased that their functions are entirely lost. A striking instance is related by Mr. Pott, where a precisely similar state was artificially induced by the removal of the ovaries in a young woman ; although, previously to the operation, menstruation, and all the signs of puberty, had regularly existed.—(See Locock, in Cyclop. of Pract. Med., art. MENSTRUATION.)—ED.

Yet menostation may take place from a sup-pression of the menses after they have be-come habitual, as well as from their retention in early life, which constitutes the second va-riety of the disease.

The causes of this form are for the most part those of the preceding, and consist in a torpi-tude of the extreme or secernent vessels of the uterus, produced by anxiety of mind, cold, or suddenly suppressed perspiration ; falls, espe-cially when accompanied with terror, or a gen-eral inertness and flaccidity of the system, and more particularly of the ovaria. Hence the dis-ease may exist equally in a robust and plethoric habit, and in the midst of want and misery. In the last case, however, it is usually a result of weakness alone ; and on this account, it is sometimes found as a sequel of protracted fe-vers.

As this modification of the disease occurs after a habit has been established in the constitution, its symptoms differ in some de-gree from those we have just contemplated. And, as it occurs also both in a state of entony and atony, the symptoms must like-wise differ, according to the state of the con-stitution at the time. If, however, the frame be at the time peculiarly weak and delicate, the signs will not essentially vary from those of the first variety, only that there will be a greater tendency to headache and palpitation of the heart.

If the habit be plethoric, and more particu-larly, if the cause of suppression take place just at the period of menstruation, or during its ef-flux, a feverish heat and aridity of the skin usu-ally make their appearance, the face is flushed, and the eyes red, the head is oppressed, and often aches, with distressing pains down the back, occasionally relieved by a hemorrhage from the nose.

As the principle which should guide us in the mode of treating both these varieties will also extend to the ensuing species, it will be most convenient to defer the consideration of it till that species has passed in review before us. We shall then be able to see how far a common pro-cess may apply, and to contrast the few points in which it will be necessary to institute a dif-ference. All these, indeed, have by many writers, and especially by Dr. Cullen, been included under the term amenorrhœa, which Professor Frank has lately employed in a still wider sense, so as to embrace, not only those three distinct forms of impeded menstruation, but chlorosis as well.—(*De Cur. Hom. Morb. Epit.*, tom. vi., lib. vi., part iii., 8vo., Vienna, 1821.)

---

which means we shall avoid directing all our rem-edies merely to an effect, and leave the cause it-self unremoved. The action of the foregoing causes of amenorrhœa is always gradual; but that of some others is very rapid, provided the period of menstruation is at hand, or the discharge is actual-ly going on. Such is the impression of cold, wheth-er from wet feet, cold bathing, cold drinks, or ex-posure to cold winds, while the individual is in a state of perspiration.—Ed.

E e 2

SPECIES II.
PARAMENIA DIFFICILIS.*
LABORIOUS MENSTRUATION.
CATAMENIA ACCOMPANIED WITH GREAT LOCAL PAIN, AND ESPECIALLY IN THE LOINS ; PART OF THE FLUID COAGULABLE.

In the preceding species, the regular efflux is altogether prevented, as we have already ob-served, by a torpitude of the secerning vessels of the uterus, perhaps of the ovaries also. In the species before us there is no actual suppression, but the quantity thrown forth is for the most part too small, and attended with severe and forcing pains about the hips and region of the loins, that clearly indicate a spasmodic constric-tion of the extreme vessels of the uterus. The secretion is hence extruded with great difficul-ty, and is sometimes perhaps of a morbid char-acter: while, from the force of the action, the mouths of some of the vessels give way, and a small portion of genuine blood becomes in-termixed with the menstrual discharge, forming coagula in the midst of an uncoagulating fluid, and thus drawing a critical line of distinction between the two.

The spastic action, thus commencing in the minute vessels of the uterus, not only spreads externally to the lumbar muscles, but internally to the adjoining organs of the rectum or blad-der, in many instances, indeed, to the kidneys : and hence an obstinate costiveness and suppres-sion of urine are added to the other symptoms, and increase the periodical misery ; the frequent return of which imbitters the life of the patient, and effectually prohibits all hopes of a family ; for, if impregnation should take place in the in-terval, the expulsory force of the pains is sure to detach the embryon from its hold, and to de-stroy the endearing promise which it offers.†
These pains generally recur at the regular pe-riod, but often anticipate it by a day or two, and rarely cease till a week afterward. The dis-ease, moreover, is peculiarly obstinate, and, in some instances, has defied the best exertions of medical science, and has only yielded to time, and the natural cessation of the discharge.

We have frequently had occasion to observe,

---

* The *Dysmenorrhœa* of medical writers in gen-eral.

† Denman and Dewees were of opinion that a female thus affected could not have children ; but the contrary is maintained by Morgagni, Ham-ilton, and Burns. Dr. Ryan has known pain at-tend menstruation for months after marriage, yet conception took place. He mentions two cases: in these no portions of membrane were dischar-ged.—(See Manual of Midwifery, p. 329 ; and Lond. Med. and Surg. Journ., vol. v., 1830.) On this subject Dr. Locock observes, the error has arisen from the facts, that the individuals are par-ticularly liable to abortions at a very early age, which abortions have been supposed to be merely unusually aggravated attacks of the complaint. Nor is the common belief well founded, that preg-nancy is a cure for a previously existing dysme-norrhœa, unless by great care and management the first two or three months are safely passed over. —See Cyclop. of Pract. Med., art. Dysmenor-rhœa.—Ed.

and especially under croup and tubular diarrhœa, that where hollow and mucous organs labour under a certain degree of irritation, a portion of gluten is often thrown forth with the morbid secretion that takes place on the surface, and the result is a formation of a new membrane or membrane-like substance that lines the cavity to a greater or less extent : the nature of this substance being regulated by the nature of the organ in which it takes place. This remark applies particularly to the uterus under the influence of the irritation we are now speaking of ; and consequently, a membrane very much resembling the decidua, or that naturally elaborated by the uterus on impregnation, has been occasionally formed, and discharged in fragments,* during the violence and forcing pain of labori-

* Morgagni, De Sed. et Caus. Morb., ep. xlviii., 12. Denman, Medical Facts and Observations, i., 12. The expulsion of a membranous substance was observed in dysmenorrhœa by Morgagni, who described it as generally consisting of a small bag, containing a fluid, on which account it was usually mistaken at that time for a very early abortion. Afterward the occurrence was more particularly investigated by Dr. Denman, who satisfactorily established the fact, that the membrane was expelled at least as frequently from single as from married women, and that it had the appearance of a triangular cast of the cavity of the uterus, and a resemblance to the membrana decidua. It would seem, according to Dr. Locock, that where a bag containing a fluid was really discovered, it must have been an ovum, at an early period of conception, particularly as such women are very liable to miscarry. Dr. Denman supposed that this membrane, though often not noticed, was expelled in every case of dysmenorrhœa. That he was wrong in this conjecture, as Dr. Locock remarks, is now well known ; for, though occasionally met with, it is by no means common ; and what frequently resembles it at first sight, consists merely of a coagula of blood, with the colouring matter separated from it. From the supposition that the membrane is *always* expelled, and that it consists of coagulable lymph, exuded from the lining of the uterus in consequence of inflammatory action, has arisen, says Dr. Locock, a most mistaken and pernicious treatment, *when universally applied.*—(See Cyclop. of Practical Medicine, art. Dysmenorrhœa.) Dr. Mackintosh considers smallness of the os uteri the most frequent cause of the disease, but he includes also inflammation of the lining membrane of the uterus, or inflammation of the substance of the cervix, and the pressure of tumours, as occasional sources of the complaint. In every museum are specimens of the os uteri being so narrow as to be scarcely capable of admitting a bristle.—(See Ryan's Manual of Midwifery, 3d edit., p. 330.) Dr. Locock believes, that, in the majority of cases, there is not inflammation, but simply irritation of the uterus, the former sometimes taking place, particularly in plethoric and robust constitutions. The women most liable to this complaint seem to him to be those possessing great susceptibility, who are subject to hysterical affections, and who have strong passions and ardent temperaments. Dysmenorrhœa will often occur only at those periods of life when there is great constitutional disturbance, or much mental excitement, as in the early years of menstruation, or shortly after marriage.—See Cyclop. of Pract Med., art. Dysmenorrhœa.—Ed.

ous menstruation. And sometimes the protrusive agony has been so severe as to occasion a displacement or retroversion of the uterus, which has been found forced down, enlarged, with the fundus thrown backward, and the indurated mouth facing the lower edge of the symphysis pubis.—(*Dr. J. Robertson, Edin. Med. and Surg. Journ.*, No. lxxiii.)

Cold, mental emotion, local injury from a fall, and, above all, a peculiar irritability of the uterus itself, are the common causes.

The cure of all the forms of paramenia we have thus far noticed is to be attempted, first, by increasing the tone of the system in general, and next, by exciting the action of the uterine vessels, where they are morbidly torpid, or relaxing them where they are in pain from spasmodic constriction. Both the last, however, are subordinate to the first ; for, if we can once get the system into a state of good general health, the balance of action will be restored, and the organs peculiarly affected will soon fall into the common train of healthful order.

To give strength and activity to the circulation is generally attempted by tonics : to give local action, by stimulants. Both these should be employed conjointly in the two forms of the first species. The astringent tonics, however, are supposed, and apparently with good reason, to be injurious, and in many instances to extend the retardation, or diminish the flow where there is any appearance. Myrrh has long been a favourite medicine ; but its power does not appear to be very considerable in mismenstruation, though it undoubtedly acts as a stimulant in phthisis, and has at times, in highly irritable habits, produced hæmoptysis. The metallic tonics are those on which we can chiefly depend ; and of these, the principal that have been employed are iron and copper.

The first requires less care than the second, and has hence been more frequently recurred to, as the safer. It has been given under a great variety of forms ; but that of the sulphate, or green vitriol, is one of the best and most readily obtained.* It is often tried in union with myrrh ; and where symptoms of dyspepsy exist, and especially acidity in the stomach, the two have been united with carbonate of soda, a combination which makes the celebrated draught, so well known by the name of its inventor, Dr. Griffiths.

Iron is, by some writers, supposed to show an astringent, and by others an aperient power. In different constitutions it may be said to operate both ways. "If, for example," says Dr. Cullen, "a retention of menses depends upon a weakness of the vessels of the uterus, chalybeate medicines, may cure the disease, and thereby appear to be aperient : and on the contrary, in a

* At present, the subcarbonate of iron is frequently preferred, in doses of one or two drachms, thrice a day. The ferrum tartarizatum is also a good preparation. Steel medicines answer well, when the disease is connected with a deficiency of blood in the system, or the state termed anæmia.
—Ed.

menorrhagia, when the disease depends upon a laxity of the extreme vessels of the uterus, iron exhibited, by restoring the tone of these vessels, may show an astringent operation."—(*Mat. Med.*, vol. ii., p. 22, 4to.)

The preparations of copper labour under two disadvantages: they are essentially more astringent than many of the other metals, and at the same time more uncertain in their effect. They are perhaps more soluble in the stomach than any other metallic preparations, wherever there is a sufficient proportion of acid for this purpose: but, as the quantity of acid in this organ is constantly varying, their effect must vary also. Dr. Fordyce advises to avoid cupreous preparations when the intention is to strengthen; but, when we attempt to lessen irritability, he observes that they are extremely useful; and hence their advantage in epilepsy and plethoric hysteria. It is, however, a just remark of Dr. Saunders, that all solutions of metals are sedative and ease pain, or in other words, take off irritability, provided the solution be not too strong. The old tinctura veneris volatilis, consisting of one drachm of filings of copper, infused in twelve drachms of water of ammonia, is one of the simplest and best preparations of this metal, and forms a good substitute for the cuprum ammoniacum, or c. ammoniatum of the Edinburgh and London Pharmacopœias. Boerhaave directs us to begin with three drops as a dose, and gradually to increase it to twenty-four. The chalybeate mineral waters have also been used with considerable success, and the more so as with these are usually conjoined the advantages of travelling, change of air, and a new stimulus given to both the mind and body by novelty of scene, novelty of company, amusing and animating conversation, and exercise of various kinds. With these may also be combined, in the intervals of the menstrual season, and particularly before the discharge has appeared, the use of cold, and especially of sea bathing. An unnecessary apprehension of catching cold by the employment of this powerful tonic has been entertained by many practitioners: with proper care, I have never known it occasion this effect; and it should be only relinquished where no reactive glow succeeds to the chill produced by immersion, and the system is hereby proved to be too debilitated for its use.

The stimulants to be employed under the first species, in conjunction with a tonic plan, are those that operate generally and locally. The general stimulants should consist of those that do not exhaust the excitability or nervous power of the frame, but rather, by the moderation of their effect, and the constancy of their application, support and augment it. Exercise, which we have already recommended, will in this view also be of essential service, as will likewise be uniform warmth; and hence the warmth of a mild climate, and a generous diet, with a temperate use of wine. Hence also the benefit of friction and electricity applied directly to the hypogastric and lumbar regions.*

As the depressing passions produce the disease, the elevating passions have been often known to operate, the best and speediest cure. It has sometimes suddenly yielded to a fit of joy (*Medicin Wochenblatt*, 1782, p. 416), and in one instance, from the violence of the emotion, to a fit of terror.—(*Walther, Thes.*, obs. 37.) We can hence easily see how it may be induced by disappointed love, and removed by a return of hope, and a prospect of approaching happiness. —(*Eph. Nat. Cur.*, dec. i., an. ix., x., obs. 58.)

The stimulants, operating locally in this disease, are known by the name of emmenagogues.* In the old writers the catalogue of these is very numerous. Those most worthy of notice consist of the warmer gums and balsams, as guaiacum, asafœtida, turpentine, and petroleum; castor, and the more irritating cathartics, as aloes, and black hellebore. The last is, in most cases, too stimulant upon the whole range of the intestinal canal, though at one time in high favour as an emmenagogue. Aloes is a particularly valuable medicine. Dr. Adair gave it in combination with cantharides; but in this form it will often be found to produce a troublesome irritation of the rectum or bladder, rather than a salutary stimulus of the uterine vessels.

The *juniperus sabina*, or common savin, is

---

* Alberti Diss. de Vi Electricâ in Amenorrhœ-am, seu Catameniorum obstructionem, Goet., 1764. Birch, Considerations of the Efficacy of Electricity in Female Obstructions, &c., London, 1799.

* Professor A.T. Thomson doubts whether there is any medicinal agent which, when taken into the stomach, exerts a directly stimulant influence on the uterus; though he appears to except savin from this observation, as will be seen in a subsequent note; "but a stimulant effect may be propagated from neighbouring parts to the uterine vessels; hence, some cathartics, which operate chiefly upon the rectum, are found to influence the uterus. When the obstruction of the menses is accompanied with a *florid* complexion, and the colour of the cheeks is the flush of disease, not the glow of health; or when a slight cough, with pain in the chest and difficulty of breathing, accompanies the suppression, bleeding and other antiphlogistic means must be resorted to before taking into consideration the uterine function; and until the general excitement be subdued, the employment of emmenagogues would be injurious. It is questionable whether, in these cases, any of those substances supposed to act directly upon the uterus should be employed. If they can be administered, they will be most likely to prove beneficial when given immediately after the reduction of febrile excitement.

"The employment of emmenagogues is not confined to cases of simple obstruction or suppression. In some females, the pain with which menstruation is accomplished imbitters much of life. This either indicates a peculiar state of the organ itself, or it is the effect of disease, or at least the tendency to it in the organ itself; not, as is sometimes supposed, an increased degree of the irritability of the general system. Some of the substances employed as emmenagogues are supposed directly to lessen uterine irritation, and consequently to facilitate the discharge: they are thus closely allied with sedatives and antispasmodics." —See Dr. A. T. Thomson's Elem. of Materia Med., vol. ii., p. 443.—Ed.

also a valuable medicine, as being both stimulant and slightly aperient, and operating not only locally, but upon the system at large. As the volatile oil, which is the active principle, is dissipated by boiling, the extract is a better preparation. It may be given in powder, extract, or essential oil : of the powder, the dose varies from a scruple to a drachm twice or three times a day : of the extract, from half a scruple to half a drachm ; and of the essential oil, from two to four drops. Dr. Home thought highly of it, and Mr. Hetz has praised it in equal terms.— (*Briefe*, ii., p. 5.) The former declares that, by employing the scruple doses three times a day, he succeeded in three out of five cases.* But the most favourite emmenagogue in his hands was the root of the *rubia tinctorum*, or madder. Of nineteen cases of which he gives an account, fourteen, he tells us, were cured by it. From half a drachm to a drachm was prescribed twice or oftener daily. Dr. Home asserts, that in this quantity it produces scarcely any sensible operation, never quickens the pulse, nor lies heavy on the stomach ; yet that it generally restores the discharge before the twelfth day from the time of its commencement.—(*Clinical Experiments, Histories*, &c., 8vo., 1780.) The present author has never tried it : he has been deterred by the very different and even contradictory accounts of its effects upon the constitution, which have been given by different writers of high authority. While Dr. Home found it thus beneficial in cases of obstructed menstruation, Dr. Parr tells us that it produced a cure in excessive menstruation, but in the former disease effected no change whatever.—(*Med. Dict.*, vol. ii., in verb., p. 524.) From its tinging the urine of a red colour, it has been supposed to be a powerful diuretic ; but even this quality it has been incapable of supporting ; and yet, in the opinion of Dr. Cullen, this seems to be its only pretension to the character of an emmenagogue. —(*Mat. Med.*, vol. ii., p. 553, 4to. edit., comp. with p. 38 of the same.) Given freely to brute animals, Dr. Cullen tells us that it always disorders them very considerably, and appears hurtful to the system. Its direct virtues do not, therefore, seem to have been in any degree ascertained : but let them be what they may, it

has deservedly fallen into disrepute as a remedy for any misaffection of the uterus.

The *athamanta meum*, or spignel, which once rivalled the reputation of madder, seems to have a peculiar influence in stimulating the lower viscera, and especially the uterus and bladder, and is no indifferent sudorific. On this last account, it was at one time highly in favour also in intermittents, and was afterward employed in hysteria and humoral asthma.

It is very probable that in cases of weak action, and especially when combined with a strumous diathesis, the pills or tincture of iodine, as we shall have occasion to notice them when treating of bronchocele, may be attended with beneficial effects. Dr. Coindet regards this medicine, indeed, as one of the most powerful emmenagogues we possess ; and even accounts for its advantages in bronchocele from the sympathy which the uterus and the thyroid gland manifest for each other.—(*Archives Générales de Médecine*, &c., *in Rem.*)

This part of the subject must not be quitted without glancing at a medicine that has lately acquired great popularity in North America as an emmenagogue, and is said to have been employed with unquestionable success. This is spurred rye (*secale cornutum*), or rye vitiated by being invested with the clavis or ergot, a parasitic plant, which we have already had occasion to notice, as producing a powerful effect on the whole system, and especially on the nervous part of it, and the abdominal viscera in general. When taken in such a quantity as to be poisonous, it first excites a sense of tingling or formication, and fiery heat in the extremities, where the action of the system is weakest ; to this succeed cardialgia, and griping pains in the bowels ; and then vertigo, an alternation of clonic and entonic spasms in different parts of the body, and mania or loss of intellect. If the quantity be something smaller than this, it excites that pestilent fever which the French denominate mal des ardens, and in the present work is described under the name of PESTIS *erythematica* (Cl. III., Ord. III., Gen. IV., Spe. 1); while, in a quantity still smaller and long-continued, it seems to spend itself almost entirely on the extremities, as being the weakest part of the body, and to produce that species of GANGRÆNA which is here denominated *ustilaginea*, or MIL. DEW MORTIFICATION.—(Cl. III., Ord. IV., Gen. XII., Spe. 2.)

It is hence a very acrid irritant, and from its peculiar tendency to stimulate the hypogastric viscera, seems often, in minute quantities, to prove a powerful emmenagogue. For this purpose an ounce of spurred rye is boiled down, in a quart of water, to a pint ; half of which is usually taken in the course of the day, both in obstructed and difficult menstruation, and continued for three or four days. The symptoms produced by it are headache, increased heat, and occasioual pain in the hypogastrium, succeeded by a free and easy flow of the menstrual fluid. Advantage has been taken of this effect on another occasion ; for the same medicine has been prescribed in lingering labours, and we are told by

---

* Dr. A. T. Thomson considers savin, or rather the volatile oil of the plant, to be an energetic emmenagogue. From its activity and mode of action, and its proneness to produce uterine hemorrhage, he admits that there is reason for thinking that it is taken into the circulation and carried directly to the organ, on which it exerts a stimulant influence. "This," says the professor, "is not a recent opinion ; for previous to the introduction of the ergot of rye, savin was sometimes employed for the purposes of accelerating parturition and expelling the placenta." As it is apt to excite inflammation of the uterus, he recommends a great deal of caution in its use, and it seems to him only to be adapted to those cases of amenorrhœa which are attended with a pale countenance, and languid circulation. The doses proposed by him are from five to ten grains of it in substance or from two to six minims of the oil, blended with sugar.—See Elem. of Materia Medica, vol. ii., p. 452.—Ed.

Dr. Big_{elow}, with the best success, as good forcing pains are hereby very generally produced speedily.—(*New-Eng. Journ. of Med. and Surg.*, vol. v., No. ii.) In this case Dr. Bigelow, instead of a decoction of spurred rye, prefers giving the crude powder, to the amount of ten grains to a dose. Dr. Chapman, indeed, regards this medicine as chiefly if not solely useful in expediting labour-pains; for, while he asserts that "to the uterus its whole force seems to be exclusively directed, and believes it to be highly beneficial in floodings and other uterine hemorrhages," he tells us, that in repeated trials he has found it of only slender power as an emmenagogue.*

We have hitherto regarded the spur in spurred rye and other grain as a clavus, or species of ustilago. It was formerly, however, conceived to be a disease of the grain itself. M. Decandolle has since described it as a variety of champignon, under the name of sclerotium, from its rendering the grain hard and horny. And M. Virey, in a work reported upon by. M. Desfontaines to the Academy of Sciences of the French Institute, in 1817, has still more lately endeavoured to revive the obsolete opinion, by contending that it is a specific disease of the plant, under which the grain is rendered, not, properly speaking, hard and horny, as is actually the case when infested with the sclerotium, but rather friable, and easily detached.

There is something highly plausible and ingenious in the plan that was at one time tried rather extensively, of compressing the crural arteries by a tourniquet, and thus gorging the organs that lie above and are supplied from collateral branches. By compressing the jugular veins we can easily gorge the head, and endanger extravasation and apoplexy. But it appears upon trial, that the tide thus dammed up in the

* Therapeutics, &c., vol. ii., p. 19, 8vo.; Philadelphia. In inquiring what pretensions the active principle of ergot has to the character of an emmenagogue, Dr. A. T. Thomson observes, that "the chief use to which secale cornutum has hitherto been applied is to produce uterine action, to aid the efforts of parturition when these are insufficient for the expulsion of the child. For this purpose it is administered in doses of from Ʒj. to ʒss, bruised and mixed in f ℥ij of water, at short intervals, until the effect is produced. Ample experience has proved the efficacy of ergot to expel any substance from the uterus, when it is in a state of complete inactivity during the process of parturition. Now, admitting this to be true, these premises are not sufficient to justify the conclusion that it will also aid the menstrual discharge when scanty or suppressed." Dr. Thomson, after examining the theories of its modus operandi, expresses his own belief that it has very slender, if any pretensions to the character of an emmenagogue. "The dose of the secale cornutum," he says, "should not exceed thirty grains. The medicine should be preserved entire in a glass bottle with a ground stopper, and powdered only at the time it is about to be given; and then it may be administered in a glass of wine, which Dr. Balardini has found to be preferable to water. Heat and moisture tend to spoil it. It should always be the growth of the year in which it is prescribed."— See Thomson's Elem. of Mat. Med., vol. ii., p. 470.—Ed.

case before us is thrown back upon too many organs to produce any very sensible effect upon the uterus. Independently of which, the uterus is not, like the brain, exactly enclosed in a bouy box that prohibits a general and equable dilatation of its vessels. In six cases in which Dr. Home made experiment of this remedy, he succeeded but once; and others have been still less successful.—(*Hamilton, Edin. Com.*, vol. ii., art. 31; *Weiz ad Fabric.*, iv., 98.)

Impeded menstruation is sometimes, however, a disease strictly local, and proceeds from the obstruction of the passage by a polypus or other tumour, or an imperforate hymen. In all these cases, the cure must depend upon a removal of the local cause.

Emetics have sometimes been recommended; they rouse the system generally, but have not often been found useful in retention of the menses; though when employed in cases of suppression, and especially at the regular periods of return, or so as to anticipate such return by a few days, they frequently prove a valuable adjunct. If this period be passed by without any salutary effect, and particularly if at the same time the system labour under symptoms of oppression in the head or chest, venesection to the extent of from four to six ounces of blood will be found a very useful palliative, and will have a tendency to keep up that periodical habit of depletion which will probably prove advantageous against the ensuing lunations. Venesection will also be found useful, and often absolutely necessary, where the suspension has suddenly taken place during the flow of the catamenia, from cold, depressing passions, fright, or indeed any other cause.*

In treating the SECOND SPECIES of paramenia, or difficult menstruation, the stimulant part of the process we have thus far recommended must be sedulously abstained from; but the rest may be followed with advantage.† Every thing,

In cases of paramenia obstructionis, Dr. Chapman has derived great benefit from using a decoction of the polygala seneca: Dr. Dewees places great reliance on the volatile tincture of guaiacum. Dr. Hosack has relieved a case of ten years' standing, which had resisted the aloetic and mercurial emmenagogues, by using an injection, per vaginam, of half a drachm of the aqua ammoniæ, and eight ounces of rain water.—(Med. Essays, vol. ii.) This practice has been followed by Dr. Glonninger, and with great benefit.—(New-York Med. and Phys. Journ., vol. iii.) Dr. Lavagna also has succeeded with the same remedy. Dr. London, acting on the suggestions of Hippocrates, who remarked the intimate sympathy between the mammæ and uterus, has cured some cases of amenorrhœa by applying leeches to the mammæ; and Dr. Paterson, of Dublin, has attained the same end by irritating the parts with sinapisms. —(See Boston Med. and Surg. Journal, vol. x., p. 105.)—D.

† Practitioners differ much as to the causes and treatment of paramenia difficilis, a disease which, although not fatal, is extremely difficult to be removed. Dr. Dewees remarks (Diseases of Females), "There appear to be two distinct states of this affection; one where the mammæ sympathize with the uterus by becoming tumid and oftentimes painful, the other where there is no such

indeed, that has a tendency to produce local excitement, and in this respect the conjugal embrace itself, where the patient is married, must be systematically abstained from.* The diet must be plain, and the bowels kept open with neutral salts, or other cooling aperients. And, to allay the strong spasmodic action on which the severe pains in the lumbar and hypogastric regions depend, it will be found highly advantageous, a short time before the expected return of menstruation, to employ relaxants, and especially local relaxants ; and of these, one of the best and pleasantest is the hip-bath, which operates directly on the diseased quarter, and has a tendency to produce the desired effect without weakening the system generally. The ease and comfort of this valuable contrivance are ac-

affection." He thinks the former kind is the more manageable. It may occur in two states of the system ; that of general weakness and debility, or its opposite : in the former case, it is seen in those individuals where the bodily strength has been exhausted by previous disease, or by long-continued labour in an impure atmosphere. In these cases we must attempt to restore the tonic powers of the system ; and the chalybeates, quinine, generous living, moderate exercise in the open air, the tonic mineral water, a change of scene, &c., will be found beneficial. But in the greater number of cases, paramenia difficilis depends on a general entonic state, attended with preternatural fulness of the bloodvessels, and general oppression. In such cases, bloodletting and appropriate cathartics are indispensable ; leeches may be applied to the loins or to the external organs, to be followed by warm fomentations. Campbell recommends the exhibition of an enema of two drachms of asafœtida dissolved in twenty-four ounces of warm water, and the injection of warm water into the vagina until the catamenia have ceased, " to subdue, if possible, that excitement which leads to the effusion of lymph and consequent formation of the membranous and fibrous productions." Osborne, of Dublin, after the means mentioned above, employs small doses of ipecacuanha with opium, belladonna, and the like, to relax the system, and to diminish pain and general distress.
The above remarks apply more particularly to the treatment during the menstrual period. For a radical cure, Dr. Dewees recommends the volatile tincture of guaiacum, to be given with a proper regard to the state of the system: This remedy, observes Dr. Dewees (Diseases of Females, 2d edit., p. 137), has generally been successful, but a perseverance in the use of it for two or three months is sometimes necessary. Dr. Eberle (Practice of Physic, vol. ii., p. 529) recommends the extract of stramonium, given in doses of one eighth of a grain three times daily, commencing about four days before the expected return of the attack. Iodine has lately been used with some success, particularly by Dr. S. A. Cartwright of Mississippi. He remarks (Am. Med. Recorder, vol. xiv.), " Dr. Thompson, of Louisiana, preceded me in resorting to iodine in deranged menstruation. The success which has attended his practice in cases wherein a variety of other remedies had for a long time failed, is a sufficient proof of the beneficial effects of iodine in re-establishing the healthy functions of the uterus, if the proper cases be selected for its exhibition."—D.
* Intercourse should be avoided for about a week before the expected attack.—Dr. Locock, in Cyc. of Pract. Med., art. DYSMENORRHŒA.—ED.

knowledged by almost all who have had recourse to it. Martini and various other writers recommend the cold bath in preference to the hot, and Tissot represents the latter as injurious. But this is to speak without due discrimination. That the cold bath has been found of use in some instances is unquestionable : but only where there has been such a degree of energy in the constitution as to produce a reaction correspondent to the antecedent rigour. The direct effect of the cold bath is to constringe, and consequently, where a spastic contraction exists already, as is mostly the case from local or constitutional debility, to increase the evil. But where the constitution is naturally robust, and but little inroad has hitherto been made upon its strength, the latent energy of the system is capable of resisting the sudden shudder ; an increased action, and consequently an increased and glowing heat, ensue ; the repelled fluids are forced forward ; the blood flows more briskly ; the mouths of the capillary vessels give way in every direction ; the muscular fibres lose their rigidity, and the suppressed secretions, of whatever kind, recommence. And hence it is that cold bathing may sometimes be serviceable in the disease before us, and warm bathing less useful : but these cases are rare, and warm bathing is mostly to be preferred.
Even the hip-bath, however, though it mitigates the pain, occasionally does nothing more : there is the same paucity of discharge, the same intermixture of coagula, and the same tendency to a return of the disease. In such cases it has been common to abstract eight or ten ounces of blood from the loins by cupping, antecedently to the use of the bath ; and this, by diminishing the spastic constriction, has at times diminished in a still greater degree the distressing pain. But I do not think the hip-bath is in general had recourse to early enough. Instead of waiting till the periodical pains return, as is the common practice, I have found it more advantageous to anticipate this period, and to relax the vessels by employing it for two or three nights before the pains are expected. And where in this and every other way it has failed, or the patient, from great delicacy of constitution, has appeared too much exhausted from its use, I have availed myself of the same relaxant power in another way, and, with a like anticipation, have prescribed the use of a broad folded swathe of equal width, as already recommended in peritonitis and hepatitis. The whole should be suffered to remain till the morning, by which time the warmth of the body will he usually found to have evaporated all the moisture, though the skin will still be dewy with perspiration from so powerful a sudorific. I have often found this plan succeed still better than the hip-bath ; and have never known the patient catch cold, or complain of any chilly sensation from it.*

* Where a kind of deciduous membrane has been certainly and habitually expelled, Dr. Locock admits that benefit may be derived from moderate local bloodletting ; but, *as a general practice*, he deems it not requisite; and is of opinion that the extent to which it has been carried in many instances has done serious mischief. From

SPECIES III.
PARAMENIA SUPERFLUA.
SUPERFLUOUS MENSTRUATION.
CATAMENIA EXCESSIVE, AND ACCOMPANIED WITH HEMORRHAGE FROM THE MENSTRUAL VESSELS.

THIS species offers us a disease precisely the reverse of the last, not less in the facility with which the mouths of the vessels give way, than in the quantity of the discharge. It exhibits the two following varieties :—

a Reduplicata.   Excessive from a too fre-
'Reduplicate men-   . quent recurrence.
struation.

β Profusa.   Excessive from too large a
Profuse menstru-   flow at the proper periods.
ation.

the character of the constitutions usually affected, the spasmodic nature of the pain, and the success of a very opposite class of remedies, Dr. Locock concludes that the disease is seldom inflammatory, but arises from a peculiarly irritable condition of the uterine organs. For relieving the pain during the menstrual period he recommends opium, especially combined with ipecacuanha and four or five grains of camphire.—(See also Ramsbotham's Lectures in Med. Gaz. for 1833-4, p. 310.) Immediately before the expected attack, he directs the bowels to be opened by a mild purgative or injection of warm water ; and the patient to put her feet in warm water, or use the warm hip-bath. During the attack, if the pulse be full and frequent, the countenance flushed, and plethora prevail, he approves of cupping on the loins, or the application of leeches to the pudenda or groin. He speaks also favourably of a belladonna plaster applied over the sacrum, and of lotions containing belladonna or opium frequently injected into the vagina. Fomentations to the pubes, loins, and perinæum, are stated to be of great service, and the cautious exhibition of ether, asafœtida, and ammonia, when there is not much feverish excitement, receives the same physician's sanction. With regard to the regulation of the general health during the intervals, as already observed, the patient, if married, is to refrain from sexual intercourse for about a week before the expected attack ; and she may take inwardly some of the preparations of iron. Dr. Locock prefers equal parts of vinum ferri and the spir. ætheris sulph. comp. (ʒss. to ʒj), given two or three times a day ; or the mist. or pil. ferri comp. One useful combination, he says, is the compound extract of colocynth, and the soap and opium pill, in the proportion of two grains of each. But he observes, that on the whole, the natural chalybeate waters answer better than any artificial preparations. Where iron disagrees, zinc is to be tried. With the exception of senega, recommended by Dr. Chapman of Philadelphia, for cases attended with the habitual expulsion of a membrane, vegetable tonics promise little benefit. Cold hip-bathing, and the injection night and morning of cold saturnine lotions into the vagina, are likewise recommended. When dysmenorrhœa and rheumatism have existed in the same patient, guaiacum and colchicum have sometimes cured both disorders.—(See Dr. Locock's Obs. in Cyclop. of Pract. Med., art. Dysmenorrhœa.) Dr. Mackintosh, who adopts the theory of dysmenorrhœa being dependant on constriction of the os uteri, recommends dilating the part with bougies, a practice which, according to Dr. Ramsbotham's report (Med. Gaz., vol. cit., p.

The SECOND VARIETY, or PROFUSE MENSTRUATION, is often technically distinguished by the name of menorrhagia. It is, in effect, the menorrhagia rubra of Cullen, who makes it a distinct affection from metrorrhagia or hemorrhagia uteri, by confining the latter term to a signification of hemorrhage from other vessels of the uterus than those concerned in separating and discharging the catamenial flux.[*]

We have already observed, that we cannot lay down any general rule to determine the exact quantity of fluid that ought to be thrown forth at each lunation, some individuals secreting more and others less ; and the measure varies from four to eight or ten ounces.[†] We can only, therefore, decide that the quantity is immoderate and morbid, when it exceeds what is usually discharged by the individual, or when it is associated with unquestionable symptoms of debility, as paleness of the face, feebleness of the pulse, unwonted fatigue on exercise ; coldness in the extremities, accompanied with an œdematous swelling of the ankles towards the night ; pain in the back in an erect posture ; and various dyspeptic affections.

Either of the varieties may be entonic or atonic, or, in common language, active or passive : but in the first, there is usually a greater degree of local irritability than in the second, so that the secernents are excited, or the extremities of the minute bloodvessels open upon very slight occasions. As the disease may occur under these two different states of body, it may proceed, as Dr. Gulbrand has observed, from an increased impetus in the circulation, a relaxed state of the solids, or an attenuate state of the fluids (*De Sanguine Uterino,* 8vo., Hafn., 1778) : to which he might have added uterine congestion.

Increased impetus usually indicates great robustness of constitution, or an entonic habit, and is not unfrequently connected with uterine ges-

---

310), does not receive the general sanction of the profession.—ED.

* Dr. Mackintosh of Edinburgh, and Mr. Burns of Glasgow, also restrict the name of menorrhagia to cases where, along with the peculiar menstrual secretion, pure blood is expelled ; while other examples, in which the menstrual discharge is merely too copious, are denominated an immoderate flow of the menses.—ED.

† According to Dr. Locock, the quantity lost is, upon an average, about five or six ounces ; " but," says he, " this is merely a general rule : the exceptions are numerous ; and it is only when it becomes an exception to the individual's ordinary habits, that disease should be considered to exist. The effect of climate in these cases is very remarkable ; and what would be considered a very scanty menstruation in the warmer climates of the east, would be deemed menorrhagia in Lapland. A curious blunder was committed in this respect by Dr. Freind, who stated that the quantity of menstrual discharge in this country averaged about twenty ounces—a menorrhagic excess by no means common ; the mistake arising from his having quoted Hippocrates, without reflecting that the δύο κότυλαι Ἀττικαὶ applied only to the females of Greece."— See Cyclop. of Pract. Med., art. MENORRHAGIA. —ED.

tation; and in many cases, the accidental causes are cold, a violent shock or jar, or an accidental blow. . Under this form, the disease commonly yields to venesection, cooling laxatives, and quiet.

Superfluous menstruation from atony, or, in other words, from a relaxed state of the solids, and an attenuate state of the fluids, frequently arises from repeated miscarriages or labours, poverty of diet, and an immoderate indulgence in sexual pleasure. It often próceeds also, and especially in the higher ranks,· from a life of indolent ease and enervating luxury, producing what we have denominated atonic plethora, lax vessels, easily distended by a current of blood superfluous in quantity, but loose and unelaboráte in crasis, and which is reproduced, and perhaps still more abundantly, but at the same time still more loosely, as soon as the excess is attempted to be removed by bleeding.*

Here, therefore, venesection is almost sure to do mischief; we must restrain every luxurious excess as far as it may be in our power, and we may have authority enough to ensure a compliance, which is not always the case; we must employ, at the same time, the milder tonics, with astringents, as kino, catechu, or sulphate of zinc, and carefully guard against costiveness by cool unirritating laxatives. The rhatanyroot appears also, on the authority of Dr. Rath of Nordhausen, to have been peculiarly serviceable in many cases, and particularly in the form of decoction; an ounce being boiled for ten minutes in half a pint of water lightly covered.— (*Hufeland's Journal der practischen Heilkunde*, Jan., 1819.) If the discharge be very considerable, astringent injections of cold water, or, which will commonly be found better, of a solution of alum or zinc, or cold water with a third part of new port wine, should be had recourse to without fail. Early hours are of especial importance, with a due intermixture of moderate exercise, and the use of cold sea-bathing. The Cheltenham waters, as those also of many other chalybeate springs, have often proved serviceable, partly from their own medicinal powers, and partly from the greater purity of air and increase of exercise with which a temporary residence at a watering-place is usually accompanied.†

* In all severe or protracted cases, resisting the usual means of relief, the best practitioners deem it advisable to make an examination of the actual state of the uterus; because symptoms, closely resembling those of menorrhagia, may arise from organic mischief, particularly ulceration, polypus, and inversion of the womb.—Ed.

† On the treatment of paramenia superflua, the able editor of the American edition of Denman's Midwifery makes the following judicious and practical remarks:—

"From the beneficial effects which have occasionally been produced by nausea in the hemorrhage following abortion, it might be inferred that a like advantage might arise from the use of emetics in menorrhagia; and I have, for several years past, adopted this practice in a number of difficult cases with decided relief, where the ordinary means proved unavailing. The principle is not wholly new; as Frank mentions emetics in the list of those

It is a common observation, in moral as well as in physical philosophy, that extremes meet in their effects, or produce like results. There is perhaps no part of natural history in which this is more frequently exemplified than in the sphere of medicine. In the case of apoplexies and palsies, as well as various other diseases, we have had particular occasion to make this remark: and in the genus immediately before us, as well as others closely connected with it, we have another striking instance of its truth. "The proportion of the diseases peculiar to the female sex in the hospital," says Dr. Gilbert Blane, speaking from tables accurately kept by himself for this purpose, "is the same as in private cases; from which it would appear that the unfavourable influence of indolent habits, excessive delicacy, and sensibility of mind and body, in the upper ranks, compensates for the bad effects of hard labour and various privations in the lower orders.*

remedies proper for menorrhagia: yet the paramount relief which is secured in this disease by inducing nausea by small doses of ipecacuanha, repeated within moderate intervals, deserves to be better known. The notion that any peculiar class of remedies possesses a specific action on the uterus, is scarcely any longer recognised as therapeutical; and it is probable that other agents of the materia medica may be found in like manner serviceable, as antimonials, from the well-known consent which exists between the stomach and the uterus, and from the effects which result to the entire vascular system. I have known the discharge disappear after the emetic operation of ipecacuanha; and I have prescribed successfully this article for the same purpose in doses of two, three, or four grains, taken every six hours for several days. The cases on this subject which have lately appeared from the pen of Dr. Osborne of Dublin, give us strong hopes of having acquired the means of better success than heretofore in the treatment of menorrhagia. Dr. Osborne thus states the results of his experience:—'I began the use of ipecacuanha by ordering a scruple to be taken as an emetic at night, and I generally directed an acidulous saline purgative to be administered the following morning. The effect produced exceeded my most sanguine expectations. The discharge either ceased within twenty-four hours, or was so much diminished that no more remedies were necessary to ensure its entire removal. In some few cases it recurred within a short time, but when this did happen, it was only necessary to repeat the emetic once or twice in order to produce a permanent effect. I met with a few individuals in whom the discharge continued with little alteration after the first emetic, but with these I had only to repeat the remedy on the following night; and in one case alone three emetics were taken before the desired effect was produced.'—See Transactions of the Association of King's and Queen's College of Physicians in Ireland, vol. v."—D.

* Paramenia superflua may occur very ten days, be as copious as on ordinary occasions, and yet the patient be apparently in perfect health. Dewees records an interesting case, where a lady had first menstruated at the age of twelve, and continued to do so every ten days until she was forty, except during pregnancy or suckling. Notwithstanding this peculiarity, she was in very good health. Excessive menstruation is to be considered as a disease when it brings on debility, dyspepsy, hysteria,

SPECIES IV.
PARAMENIA ERRORIS.
VICARIOUS MENSTRUATION.

CATAMENIA TRANSFERRED TO AND EXCRETED
AT REMOTE ORGANS.

WE have already noticed the extensive sympathy which the sexual organs maintain with every other part of the system. With the exception of the stomach, which is the grand centre of sympathetic action, there is no organ or set of organs possessed of any thing like so wide an influence. And hence, where, from any particular circumstance, as sudden fright or cold, the mouths of the menstrual vessels become spasmodically contracted at the period of menstruation, and the fluid is not thrown forth, almost every organ seems ready to offer it a vicarious outlet. We have accounts, therefore, of its having been discharged, by substitution, from the eyes, the nostrils, the sockets of the teeth, the ears, the nipples, the stomach, the lungs in the shape of hæmoptysis, the rectum, the bladder, the navel, and the skin generally, as more fully explained in the volume of Nosology, to which the reader may turn at his leisure.

In effect, there is scarcely an organ of the body from which it has not been discharged under different circumstances.* A very singular case is recorded of its being thrown forth from an ulcer in the ankle of a young woman little more than twenty years of age, and which continued to flow at monthly periods, for two or three days at a time, for about five years : after which, some part of the bone having separated in a carious state, the ulcer assuming a more healthy appearance, and the body becoming plumper and stronger, the vicarious outlet was no longer needed, and the menstrual tide returned to its proper channel.†

In all these cases there is a considerable degree of uterine torpitude, and commonly of general debility, while the part forming the temporary outlet is in a state of high irritability or

and the "Protean symptoms of a complication of these affections."—See Ryan's Manual of Midwifery, p. 332, ed. 3.—ED.

* Eph. Nat. Cur., passim. Act. Nat. Cur. Act. Med. Berol. Bertholin. Obs. passim. Cent. passim. Bierling. Thes. Praet. Sennertus, Pract. et Paralip., lib. iv.

† Art. Calder, in Edin. Med. Essays, p. 341. The editor has seen several examples in which the menstrual discharge seemed to be transferred to ulcers. He once visited, with Mr. C. Hutchison, a woman who had an enormous spina bifida, and a sinus in the thigh, from which a bloody discharge took place regularly every month in lieu of ordinary menstruation. Ulcers of the kind now referred to have had the epithet *menstrual* applied to them by Sir Astley Cooper. Baudeloque mentions a woman, aged forty-eight, who had never menstruated, and from the age of fifteen had been attacked every month with vomiting and purging, that used to continue about three or four days. The reader will find some interesting observations on menstruation, and the consequences of its derangement, in Ryan's Manual of Midwifery, ed. 3.—ED.

other diseased action. And hence the remedial process should consist in allaying the remote irritation, strengthening the system generally, and gradually stimulating the uterus to a state of healthy excitement, by the means already recommended.

SPECIES V.
PARAMENIA CESSATIONIS.
IRREGULAR CESSATION OF THE MENSES.

CATAMENIAL FLUX IRREGULAR AT THE TERM OF ITS NATURAL CESSATION ; OCCASIONALLY ACCOMPANIED WITH SYMPTOMS OF DROPSY, GLANDULAR TUMOURS; OR SPURIOUS PREGNANCY.

THE set of organs that are most tardily completed, and soonest exhausted, are those of the sexual system. They arrive latest at perfection, and are the first to become worn out and decrepit. In this early progress to superannuation the secretory vessels of the uterus grow torpid, and, by degrees, the catamenial flux ceases. This cessation, however, has sometimes been protracted to a very late period, and in a few rare instances, the menses have continued nearly, or altogether, through the whole term of life ; we have examples of it, noticed in the volume of Nosology, at seventy-eight and even ninety years of age ; but the usual term is between forty and fifty, except where women marry late in life, in which case, from the postponement of the generative orgasm, they will occasionally breed beyond their fiftieth year.* On approaching the natural term of the

* Childbearing begun at an early age, at sixteen or eighteen for example, rarely goes on through out the whole of what is usually regarded as the natural period for it. The earlier or later termination of childbearing in any country, therefore, as Mr. Roberton observes, will depend upon the average age of marriage which there obtains. In our own country he is led to believe, from facts which he has collected, that the average age of marriage for women is about twenty-one years. Assuming this as correct, he considers the following table as possessing some interest. It is drawn up from the registers of the Manchester lying-in hospital, and shows, on the average of 10,000 instances of pregnancy at all ages, the proportion of women who conceive above the age of forty :—

Of 10,000 pregnant women, 436, or 43 3-5 per 1000, were upwards of 40 years of age.

101, or 10 1-10 per 1000, were in their 41st year.
113, or 11 3-10	42d
70, or 7	43d
58, or 5 4-5	44th
43, or 4 3-10	45th
12, or 1 1-5	46th
13, or 1 3-10	47th
8, or 4-5	48th
6, or 3-5	49th
9, or 9-10	50th
1, or 1-10	52d
1, or 1-10	53d
1, or 1-10	54th

The number of pregnancies, it will be observed, suddenly and greatly diminishes after the age of 45. From the age of 46 to 50, both inclusive, the numbers are nearly equal for each year. Above

cessation of the menses, the sexual organs do not always appear to act in perfect harmony with each other, and perhaps, at times, not even every part of the same organ with every other part. In proof of the first remark, we seem occasionally to meet with a lingering excitement in the ovaria, after all excitement has ceased in the uterus; and we have hence a kind of conceptive stimulation, a physcony of the abdomen, accompanied with peculiar feelings and peculiar cravings, which mimic those of pregnancy, and give the individual room to believe she is really pregnant, and the more so in consequence of the cessation of her lunar discharge, while the uterus takes no part in the process, or merely that of sympathetic irritation, without any change in size or structure.

On the contrary, we may chance to find the uterus itself chiefly if not solely affected with irregular action at this period : evincing sometimes a suppression of menstruation for several months, sometimes a profuse discharge at the proper period, and sometimes a smaller discharge returning every ten or twelve days, often succeeded by leucorrhœa. And not unfrequently the system associates generally in the misaffection, and suffers from oppression, headache, nausea, or universal languor.

All these are cases that require rather to be carefully watched than vigorously practised upon ; and the character of an expectant physician, as the French denominate it, is the whole that is called for. The prime object should be to quiet irregular local irritation, wherever necessary, by gentle laxatives, moderate opiates, or other narcotics, and to prevent any incidental stimulus, mental emotion, or other cause, from interfering with the natural inertness into which the sexual system is progressively sinking. Hence the diet should be nutritive but plain ; the exercise moderate ; and costiveness prevented by lenient, but not cold eccoprotics : aloes, though most usually had recourse to, from its pungency, in earlier life, is one of the worst medicines we can employ at this period, as the sulphate of magnesia, warmed with any pleasant aromatic, is perhaps one of the best.

If the constitution be vigorous and plethoric, and particularly if the head feel oppressed and vertiginous, six or seven ounces of blood may at first be taken from the arm ; but it is a practice we should avoid if possible, from the danger of its being necessarily resorted to again, and at length running into an inconvenient and debilitating habit.*

---

the latter age, the proportion dwindles to one instance of pregnancy in 3333.—(See Roberton on Menstruation, in Edin. Med. and Surg. Journ. for Oct., 1832, p. 254.) Dr. Ryan states that he has known a woman delivered in her sixty-third year. —See his Manual of Midwifery, p. 44, ed. 3.—ED.

* This caution against bloodletting will not be much regarded by American practitioners. The beneficial results of occasional venesection, to secure as it were a vicarious relief, and thus to to guard against that inordinate plethora which so often occurs at the cessation of the catamenia, are well understood, and many formidable symptoms of congestion are relieved by this remedy.—D.

The mammæ, that constantly associate in the changes of the uterus, and constitute a direct part of the sexual system, are at this time, also, not unfrequently in a state of considerable irritation ; and if a cancerous diathesis be lurking in the constitution, such irritation is often found sufficient to excite it into action. And hence, the period before us is that in which cancers of the breast most frequently show themselves.

From the natural paresis into which this important and active system is hereby thrown, a certain surplus of sensorial power seems to be let loose upon the system, which operates in various ways. The ordinary and most favourable mode is that of expending itself upon the adipose membrane generally, in consequence of which a larger portion of animal oil is poured forth, and the body becomes plump and corpulent. The most unfavourable, next to the excitement of a cancerous diathesis into action, is that of irritating some neighbouring organ, as the spleen or liver, and thus working up a distressing parabysma, or visceral turgescence ; or deranging the order of the stomach and laying a foundation for dyspepsy.*

---

* Dr. Marshal Hall, in his Commentaries on the Diseases of Females, recommends particular attention to be paid to the regulation of the bowels, and to diet, air, and exercise, at the cessation of menstruation. When vertigo or drowsiness is an effect of it, he is an advocate for the exhibition of purgatives, and the occasional abstraction of blood by cupping on the nape of the neck, or by the application of leeches. The following passage from Dr. Ryan's Manual of Midwifery is so correctly descriptive of subjects connected with this part of the study of medicine, that the editor deems no apology needed for its insertion :—" When menstruation is about to cease, the period is called ' the change or turn of life,' and many important changes take place in the constitution. The breasts collapse, the fulness of habit disappears, the skin shrivels, and loses its colour and softness, and many diseases appear in the womb and breast which had lain dormant for years. However, when this period has passed, women often enjoy better prospects of health and of long life than the other sex. This period is also designated ' the climacteric, the critical time, the critical age,' and often before its arrival the menstruation is irregular, absent for weeks or months ; the abdomen becomes tumid ; there is loss of appetite in the morning ; and the woman considers herself pregnant, which is never the case. According to the statistical reports of Finlaison, Moret, Chateauneuf, and Lachaise, no more women than men die between the fortieth and fiftieth year ; and Dewees contends that women are not more liable to diseases at this than at any other period of life (meaning, of course, the generality of diseases ; for to cancer we know they are certainly more exposed). The cessation of menstruation, however, is often preceded by gradual decrease or increase of the fluid, nervousness, and all its Protean symptoms ; or more serious diseases appear, so that moderate purgation is often of the greatest advantage. The internal and external orifices of the uterus become obliterated, partially or totally (Dugès) ; or the cervico-uterine orifice (Mayer) ; the uterus and ovaries are atrophied or hypertrophied ; the rugæ of the vagina and mucous membrane of the uterus are relaxed, and pour out a mucous discharge ; the vulva is flaccid and dilated ; there is

GENUS II.
LEUCORRHŒA.
WHITES.

MUCOUS DISCHARGE FROM THE VAGINA, COMMONLY WITHOUT INFECTION ; DISAPPEARING DURING MENSTRUATION.

THE term leucorrhœa, from λευκὸς, "white," and ῥέω, "to flow," is apparently of modern origin, as it is not to be found in either the Greek or Roman writers, and seems first to have been met with in Bonet or Castellus.

This is the *menorrhagia alba* of Dr. Cullen, so denominated because he conceives the evacuation to flow from the same vessels as the catamenia; as also that it is often joined with menorrhagia, or succeeds to it. Its source, however, is yet a point of dispute (*Rat. Med.*, part vii., p. 155): Stoll (*De Notis Virginitatis*, lib. i., prob. 3), Pinæus, and various other distinguished writers, have ascribed it, like Cullen, to the uterus. But as it occurs often in great abundance in pregnant women, in girls of seven, eight, and nine years of age (*Heister, Wahrnehmungen,* b. ii., N. 128 ; *Hoechstetter, Obs. Med.,* dec. iv., cas. i., Schol.), and even in infants, it has been supposed by Wedel (*Diss. de Fluore albo*, Jen., 1743), and most writers of the present day, to flow from the internal surface of the vagina, or at the utmost, from the vagina jointly with the cervix of the uterus. Morgagni is perhaps most correct, who conceives, and appears indeed to have proved by dissections, that in different cases, the morbid secretion issues from both organs ; for he has sometimes found the uterus exhibiting in its internal surface whitish tubercles, tumid vessels, or some other diseased indication, and sometimes the vagina.[*] Frank affirms that he has occasionally, on dissection, traced it issuing from the Fallopian tubes.[†] In the case narrated by Mr. Hill of Dumfries, and noticed under the preceding genus, it was evidently confined to the vagina alone.—(*Edin. Med. Comment.*, iv., p. 91.)

When first secreted it is bland and whitish, but differs in colour and quality under different circumstances, and hence affords the three following species :—

often prolapsus uteri; and the breasts decrease or disappear."—ED.
[*] De Sed. et Caus. Morb., ep. xlviii., art. 12, 14, 16, 17, 18, 19, 27 ; ep. lxii., art. 14. Numerous cases are on record, where, in prolapsus uteri, the leucorrhœal discharge proceeded from the os uteri itself.—(Locock, in Cyclop. of Pract. Med., art. LEUCORRHŒA.) On the other hand, Dr. Jewel believes that the discharge, in ordinary cases, does not issue from the cavity of the uterus.—ED.
[†] De Cur. Hom. Morb. Epit.; tom. v., p. 177, Mannh., 8vo., 1792. The simplest form of leucorrhœa is a mere increase of the natural secretion from the mucous membrane of the vagina. As this membrane is continued to the interior of the uterus and the Fallopian tubes, it is easy to suppose that now and then the lining of these organs may become affected, and the leucorrhœa have a more extensive seat.—Locock, in Cyclop. of Pract. Med., art. LEUCORRHŒA.—ED.

1. Leucorrhœa Communis.	Common Whites.
2. —————— Nabothi.	Labour-show.
3. —————— Senescentium.	Whites of advanced life.

SPECIES I.
LEUCORRHŒA COMMUNIS.
COMMON WHITES.

THE DISCHARGE OF A YELLOWISH-WHITE COLOUR, VERGING TO GREEN.

THIS species is the fluor albus of most writers : the medorrhœa fœminarum insons of Professor Frank. It is found in girls antecedently to menstruation, or on any simple local irritation in the middle of life, and hence also, as just observed, during pregnancy. It is said, in the Berlin Transactions, to be occasionally contagious (*Act. Med. Berol.*, dec. i., vol. v., p. 85) ; and I have met with various cases which seem to justify this remark.[*]

It has occurred as the result of suppressed menstruation :[†] as it is asserted also to have done on a suppressed catarrh (*Act. Erud.*, Lips., 1790, p. 376 ; *Raulin, sur les Fleurs blanches,* p. 329) : and chillness or suppressed perspiration of the feet.—(*Act. Nat. Cur.*, vol. viii., obs. 38.) Local irritations, moreover, are frequent causes. And hence one reason of its being an occasional concomitant of pregnancy ; as also of its being produced by pessaries injudiciously employed, by voluptuous excitements, and uncleanliness. It is said at times to exist as a metastasis, and particularly to appear on a sudden failure of milk during the period of lactation : a failure which may be set down to the list of suppressed discharges.—(*Astruc, de Morb. Mulier.*, lib. i., cap. 10.) Jensen gives a singular case of leucorrhœa that alternated with a pituitous cough.—(*Prod. Act. Hafn.;* p. 160.)

[*] On this point differences of opinion yet prevail. "True leucorrhœa is not infectious ; it produces no disease in a man who cohabits with a female labouring under it."—(Ramsbotham's Lectures, as published in Med. Gaz. for 1833–4, p. 420.) Where the discharge is purulent or of an acrid quality, sexual intercourse, as Dr. Locock observes, will often bring on a train of symptoms in the male very much resembling gonorrhœa. "This, when occurring between husband and wife, has often led to much domestic unhappiness, from the supposition of one party or the other having contracted gonorrhœa from impure connexion. It is important to be able to distinguish between gonorrhœa and common leucorrhœa, to remove or confirm the suspicions ; but it is doubtful whether any very accurate diagnosis can be formed. It has been stated, that in a recent gonorrhœa there is ardor urinæ, which does not accompany leucorrhœa, unless unusually acrid. But how are we to distinguish in a case of this unusually acrid leucorrhœa, or where a gonorrhœa is not recent ? The redness and tumefaction of the labia, nymphæ, &c., only can be seen in a recent gonorrhœa, and they may be seen in severe cases of leucorrhœa, particularly in those following local irritation, or possessing more acute inflammatory action."—See Cyclop. of Pract. Med., art. LEUCORRHŒA.—ED.
[†] It is found also in females who menstruate too copiously.—D

It is most frequently found among the weakly and delicate of crowded cities and humid regions, of a cachectic habit, and who use but little exercise ; especially about the age of puberty, or who, being married, have borne too numerous a family, or been pregnant in too quick a succession. It is also found among the barren, those who cruelly forbear to suckle their own offspring, or who menstruate too sparingly.—(*J. P. Frank, De Cur. Hom. Morb. Epit.*, tom. v., p. 176.)

It is usually accompanied with a sense of languor, and a weakness or pain in the back. And if it become chronic or of long continuance, the countenance looks pale and unhealthy, the stomach is troubled with symptoms of indigestion, the skin is dry and feverish, and the feet œdematous.

The discharge, in its mildest form, is slimy, nearly colourless, or of an opaline hue, and unaccompanied with local irritation. It afterward becomes more opaque and muculent, and is accompanied with a sense of heat, and itching or smarting : in this stage, it is of a yellowish white. But as the disease advances in degree it appears greenish, thinner, more acrid, and highly offensive, and is apt to excoriate the whole surface of the vagina : while there is often a considerable degree of pain in the uterus itself, and even in the loins.

Among novices there is some difficulty in distinguishing the discharge of whites from that of blennorrhœa, which we shall describe presently. But though the appearance of the two fluids is often similar, they may easily be known by their accompanying signs. In blennorrhœa there is local irritation from the first, and this irritation extends through a considerable part of the meatus urinarius, so as to produce a distressing pain in making water ; symptoms which are not found in leucorrhœa.* In the former there is also from the first a swelling of the labia, a more regular though a smaller secretion, and of a more purulent appearance.

When the disease is violent or of long continuance, it leads to great general as well as local debility. It has sometimes been followed by a prolapse of the uterus or vagina (*Boehman, Diss. de Prolapsû et Inversione Uteri.*, *Hal.*, 1745) ; by abortion or miscarriage where there is pregnancy ; and by barrenness where no pregnancy has occurred. When it acts on the system at large, it has given rise to cutaneous eruptions of various kinds (*Klein, Interpres Clinicus*, p. 112), hectic fever (*Hippocr. Aph.*, sect. v.), dropsy, scirrhus, and cancer.—(*Raulin, sur les Fleurs blanches*, tom. i., passim ; *Frank*, ut supr., p. 182.)

The cure is often difficult : but it is of no small importance to be from the first fully acquainted with the nature of its cause and character, for upon this the proper means to be pursued will mainly depend. And hence it will often be necessary to examine the organs themselves.†

---

* Notwithstanding these diagnostic symptoms, distress about the meatus urinarius, and pain in making water, will often be found in leucorrhœa, particularly when of long continuance.—D.

† The following observations by Dr. Locock are

If the cause be uncleanliness, a lodgment of some portion of a late menstrual flux, or any other irritating material in the vagina, nothing more may be necessary than frequent injections of warm water : or, if the vagina itself be much irritated, injections of the diluted solution of the acetate of lead : which last will often, indeed, be found highly serviceable where the discharge proceeds from debility and relaxation, produced by a severe labour or miscarriage, forming no uncommon causes ; as they are also no uncommon effects.

Other astringent injections have often been tried, as green tea, a solution of alum, or sulphate of zinc, a decoction of pomegranate bark, or a solution of catechu. All these are sure to be of service, as tending to wash away the discharge, and keep the parts clean ; and in many cases they will also succeed as astringents ; nor is it always easy to determine which is to be preferred ; for in some cases one answers the purpose best, and in others, another.*

Sir Kenelm Digby recommended a local application of the fume of sulphur (*Medic. Experiment*, p. 65), which may be communicated in various ways ; and so far as this has a tendency to change the nature of the morbid action, by originating a new excitement, it is worthy of attention ; but perhaps the diluted aqua regia bath, of which we have spoken under spasmodic jaundice (*Icter. Spasmodic.*, vol. i.), may prove more advantageous.

The disease, however, is often highly troub-

---

full of judgment and truth :—" Sir Charles M. Clarke," says he, " has classed the diseases of the female genital organs by the nature of the vaginal discharges which are peculiar to them ; and although there are many serious objections to such a mode of classification, yet it proves how important it is to note their several and distinguishing peculiarities. Of the diseases to which females are liable, there is none more common than vaginal discharge of one sort or another ; it attends most of the uterine diseases, and it is extremely common as the result of either local or constitutional disturbance, or of general debility. It is looked upon by the patients themselves as the cause of ill health, or of the symptoms under which they may happen to labour ; whereas, in the majority of instances, the discharge itself can only be considered as a symptom, the effect and result of local or general disorder. By practitioners in general, vaginal discharges have been carelessly attended to ; there has been one common routine of treatment, without investigation ; and it is only when the complaint has been obstinate, that at a later period more minute inquiry has been made, and more rational and scientific plans adopted. So many of the vaginal discharges depend upon uterine disorganization, or some alteration in the position of that organ, that it is advisable in every case, where possible, to make a minute examination per vaginam."—See art. LEUCORRHŒA, in Cyclop. of Pract. Med.—ED.

* Weak solutions of the nitrate of silver are preferred by Dr. Jewel, in the proportion of from one to three grains of the nitrate to each ounce of distilled water. Sometimes he applies the caustic itself to the cervix uteri. At the Lock Hospital, injections, containing ℈ij or ʒss of the nitrate of silver in every ounce of water, have sometimes been employed.—ED.

lesome and obstinate, and hence it has been necessary to employ constitutional as well as local means.

The general remedies that have been had recourse to are almost innumerable. Acids have been taken internally in as concentrated a state as possible, but rarely with much success. The sulphuric acid has been chiefly depended upon: and, in the form of the eau de Rabel, which is that of digesting one part to three of spirit of wine, it was at one period supposed to be almost a specific. The compound, however, has not been able to maintain its reputation, and has long sunk into disuse.

Emetics have been found more useful, as operating by revulsion, and stimulating the system generally, and on this ground a sea voyage, accompanied with seasickness, has often effected a cure. Stimulating the bowels, and particularly in the commencement of the disease, and where the general strength has not been much encroached upon, has, for the same reason, been frequently found useful, as transferring the irritation to a neighbouring organ, and under a more manageable form. And one of the best stimulants for this purpose is sulphate of magnesia. Small doses of calomel have been given daily with the same view, but in general, they have not succeeded. Heister, however, recommended mercury in this disease, even to the extent of salivation (*Wahrnehmungen*, band ii.); yet this is a very doubtful remedy, and even under the best issue, purchases success at a dear rate. A spontaneous salivation has sometimes effected a cure.—(*Eph. Nat. Cur.*, dec. iii., ann. ix., x., obs. 140.) Mr. John Hunter, with a view of changing the nature of the morbid action in its own field, advised mercurial inunctions in the vagina itself.

Other stimulants have been recommended, that operate more generally, and have a peculiar tendency to influence the secretion of mucous membranes, as the terebinthinate preparations, particularly camphire, balsam of copayva, cubebs, and turpentine itself; and there is reason to believe that the second of these has often been useful. It has sometimes been employed in combination with tincture of cantharides: but the latter is in most instances too irritating, whether made use of alone, or with any other medicine.

As the acids have not succeeded, neither have other astringents to any great extent. The argentina, or wild tansy (*potentilla anserina*, Linn.) was at one time in high favour; it was particularly recommended by M. Tournefort, and upon his recommendation very generally adopted. Alum has been supported by a still greater number of advocates for its use; and kino has, perhaps, been employed quite as extensively. Dr. Cullen asserts that he has tried all these alone without success, but that by uniting kino and alum, as in the pulvis stypticus of the Edinburgh College, he obtained not only a most powerful astringent, but one that had occasionally proved serviceable in the present disease. The anserina has justly sunk into oblivion. The rhatany-root is much better entitled to a trial in the form of

a decoction, as already recommended in atonic *paramenia superflua*: though, from its warmth, united with the quality of astringency, it is a still more promising remedy in the leucorrhœa of advanced life.

Upon the whole, the best general treatment we can recommend is a use of the metallic tonics, and especially zinc and iron, in conjunction with a generous but temperate diet, exercise that produces no fatigue, pure air, and change of air, cold bathing, regular and early hours, and especially a course of the mineral waters of Tunbridge or Cheltenham. [In chronic leucorrhœa, the internal and external use of iodine has been tried with benefit (*Gimele ; Omodei, Annali*, &c.); and Dr. Negri and others have tried small doses of the secale cornutum. It is admitted, however, that its efficacy is less prompt than in cases of uterine hemorrhage.— (See *Lond. Med. Gaz.* for 1833–4, p. 369.) When the disorder depends upon suppressed menstruation, M. Guibert finds that upon the menstrual discharge being re-established by bleeding, the leucorrhœa ceases at once.—(*Revue Méd.*, Juillet, 1827.)*

SPECIES II.
LEUCORRHŒA NABOTHI.
LABOUR-SHOW.

THE DISCHARGE SLIMY, AND MOSTLY TINGED WITH BLOOD.

In this species the fluid is secreted by the glandulæ Nabothi, situate on the mouth of the uterus, whence the specific name. It is the *leucorrhœa Nabothi* of Sauvages, and the *hæmorrhagia Nabothi* of Cullen. It is most usually found as the harbinger of labour ; and indicates that the irritation which stimulates the uterus to spasmodic and expulsory contraction, when the full term of pregnancy has been completed, or some accident has hurried forward the process, has now commenced, and that the pains of childbirth may soon be expected. It is probably nothing more than the usual fluid secreted by the glands from which it flows, augmented in quantity in consequence of temporary excitement, and mixed with a small quantity of blood. It is hardly entitled to the name of a hemorrhage, as given by Dr. Cullen, though blood from the uterus often succeeds to it, apparently thrown forth in consequence of the violence of the pains.

In its ordinary occurrence, it is only worthy of notice as a deviation from the common secretions of health, and is rather to be hailed than to become a subject of cure or removal. But there is a state of irritation to which these glands are sometimes subjected that produces the same discharge, and in considerable abun-

---

* When the patient is plethoric, much benefit will sometimes be derived in cases of leucorrhœa from bloodletting. When the pulse is in a proper condition, Dr. Dewees has administered the tincture of cantharides with decided success. This remedy is used until strangury is produced, unless the disease is arrested before. He remarks, "that it rarely withstands a second strangury."
—D

dance, for many weeks or months before labour, and which, for the comfort of the patient, requires a little medical advice and attention.

The irritation may proceed from plethora and distention, or from a weak or relaxed state of the constitution. If from the former, venesection and gentle laxatives will prove the best course we can pursue : if from the latter, a reclined position, easy intestinal evacuations, and such sedatives as may sit most pleasantly on the stomach, and produce least disturbance to the head.

SPECIES III.
LEUCORRHŒA SENESCENTIUM.
WHITES OF ADVANCED LIFE.

THE DISCHARGE THIN, ACRID, FREQUENTLY EXCORIATING AND FETID.

THIS is usually, but not always, connected with a morbid state of the uterus. It commonly shows itself on the cessation of the menses : and is often chronic and obstinate.

The more common diseases of the uterus, with which the discharge is combined, are an incipient cancer, or a polypous fungus. But I have occasionally met with it unconnected with either, and apparently dependant upon a peculiar and chronic irritability of the uterus, or rather, perhaps, of those glands which secrete the fluid that is poured forth during the act of sexual intercourse. A lady, about forty years of age, not long ago applied to me, who had, for more than a twelvemonth, been labouring under a very distressing case of this kind. She had been married from an early period of life, but had never been pregnant. Her general health was good, her temper easy, her imagination peculiarly warm and vivid. She had no local pain, and had ceased to menstruate at the age of about thirty-eight. The discharge, at the time I first saw her, consisted of at least from a quarter to half a pint daily—thick, slimy, brownish, and highly offensive. Every external and internal remedy that could be thought of appeared to be of only temporary avail, and sometimes of no avail whatever, though she certainly derived relief from injections of the *punica granatum*, with a fourth part port wine, which for some time checked the discharge and diminished the fetor. In the meantime, the general strength was preyed upon, the loins became full of pain, the appetite failed, and the sleep was disturbed. Accidental circumstances compelled her, even in this debilitated state, to undertake a voyage to India. During its progress, she suffered severely from seasickness ; but the change hereby produced, or effected by the alteration of climate, proved peculiarly salutary : for she gradually lost the complaint, and recovered her usual health. Hence emetics, change of climate, and the tonic plan already recommended under the first species, seem to be the best course we can pursue in the species before us.*

---

* Sir Charles Clarke has frequently known leucorrhœa, attended by the worst symptoms, subside on the removal of the patient into the country, with very little aid from medicine.—ED.

GENUS III.
BLENNORRHŒA.
GONORRHŒA.

MUCULENT DISCHARGE FROM THE URETHRA OR VAGINA; GENERALLY WITH LOCAL IRRITATION AND DYSURY; NOT DISAPPEARING DURING MENSTRUATION.

BLENNORRHŒA is a Greek compound of modern writers, derived from βλεννά, "mucus," and βέω, "to flow." Sauvages, and after him Cullen, have employed gonorrhœa from γόνος, "semen," and βέω, as a common term for this and SPERMORRHŒA, constituting the ensuing genus, and consisting in an evacuation of semen. Cullen, indeed, has extended the term still further in his First Lines, and hence morbid secretion of mucus, all kinds of venereal contagion and seminal flux, are equally arranged as species of the same generic disease ; and this, too, under a word which imports the last alone : while, to add to the confusion, this very word, in its vulgar sense, is restrained to venereal contagion, which, in its strict meaning, that of seminal flux, it signifies just as much as it does abortion or stone in the bladder. It is high time to make a distinction, and to divide the list of Sauvages into two genera. Blennorrhœa has, indeed, been already employed of late by various writers to denote the first of these genera, and there is no necessity for changing the term.

The genus under Müller (*Müller, Medic. Wochenblatt*, 1784, N. li., *plures species*) is subdivided into numerous species : but the three following include the whole that fairly belong to it :—

1. Blennorrhœa Simplex.	Simple urethral running.
2. —————— Luodes.	Clap.
3. —————— Chronica.	Gleet.

SPECIES I.
BLENNORRHŒA SIMPLEX.
SIMPLE URETHRAL RUNNING.

SIMPLE INCREASED SECRETION FROM THE MUCOUS GLANDS OF THE URETHRA.

THIS definition is given in the words of Dr. Fordyce, and is sufficiently clear and expressive. In effect, the efflux proceeds from mere local irritation, unaccompanied by contagion or virulence of any kind, and is chiefly found in persons in whom the affected organ is in a state of debility ; the occasional causes of irritation being venereal excess, too large an indulgence in spirituous liquors, cold, topical inflammation, too frequent purging, violent exercise on horseback, to which various authors add transferred rheumatic action (*De Plaigne, Journ. de Méd.*, tom. lxxiv. ; *Richter, Chir. Bibl.*, b. iv., p. 508 ; *Pouteau, Œuvres Posthumes*, i.); and occasionally, according to Mr. John Hunter, transferred irritation of the teeth.—(*Natural History of the Teeth.*)

The matter discharged is whitish and mild, producing no excoriation, pain in micturition, or other disquiet. It is the mild gonorrhœa of many writers, the *gonorrhœa pura* of Dr. Cullen, and usually yields without difficulty to rest, emollient injections, and very gentle and cooling purgatives.

SPECIES II.
BLENNORRHŒA LUODES.
CLAP.

MUCULENT DISCHARGE FROM THE URETHRA OR VAGINA, INTERMIXED WITH SPECIFIC VIRUS: BURNING PAIN IN MICTURITION: PRODUCED BY IMPURE COITION: INFECTIOUS.

This is a disorder of far greater mischief and violence than the preceding, and, in contradistinction to it, has been very generally denominated the virulent or malignant gonorrhœa. It is the *gonorrhœa impura* of Cullen.

The disease was for many years supposed to be a local effect of that poison which, when communicated to the system, produces syphilis. It is in truth received in the same manner, and by the same organs—its medium of conveyance being that of cohabitation with an infected person. We are chiefly indebted to Mr. John Hunter for having pointed out the distinction; and there is now scarcely an individual in our own country who has any doubt upon the subject, though there are several who conjecture that it has been derived from the syphilitic venom, changed and softened in its virulence by an introduction into different constitutions. These conjectures are harmless, but they have little ground for support. That it is a disease specifically different from syphilis, is clear from the following facts. Its appearance did not commence till more than a hundred years after that of syphilis;[*] it will continue for months without any syphilitic symptoms, which are rarely, indeed, found connected with it; and where such symptoms have shown themselves, there has been full evidence of a new and different infection, or strong ground for suspicion: the matter of chancre, the pathognomonic symptom of syphilis, when introduced into the urethra, has been found not to produce clap, and the matter of clap inserted under the skin has been proved not to produce syphilis: the common course of mercury, which is the only specific cure for the latter, is a very inconvenient and dilatory way of treating the former; while the local plan, by which the former is conquered with great speed and ease, produces no effect on the latter. It is singular, therefore, that the old and erroneous doctrine of their being one and the same disease should still maintain its ground in France, as it appears to do from M. Sante-Marie's late trea-

tise, as well as various others, on this subject.— (*Méthode pour guérir les Maladies Vénériennes invétérées,* &c., Paris, 1818.)

M. Lagneau, indeed, although he acknowledges that clap or gonorrhœa may have a different origin from syphilis, still endeavours to prove the identity of the former and chancres in the greater number of cases, from the fact that various females have been infected with both complaints by the same man, and various men by the same female.—(*Exposé des Symptomes de la Maladie Vénérienne,* Paris, 1815.) But this will go no further than to show that the individual, communicating both complaints, was infected with both at the same time. What is so common as *porrigo galeata* or scalled-head co-existing with itch; or dysentery with bilious fever, measles, or any other epidemic that may be prevalent together with itself! It is very possible, indeed, that in a few habits or idiosyncrasies, the matter of gonorrhœa may produce chancres or other local sores, or even be followed by constitutional symptoms very closely mimicking those of syphilis: for when treating of this last disease, we shall have to show that such mimicry of symptoms frequently takes place from other impure and local irritants, and with so near a resemblance as to be distinguished with great difficulty from the disease it seems to copy.[*] We have already pointed out the distinctive characters of the malady before us and syphilis; and it is sufficient to observe further, that the anomalous symptoms, if they ever follow genuine clap, occur not in the ordinary course of its march, but as extreme exceptions to its established habits, and are not to be found once in ten thousand examples.[†]

Some of these facts, indeed, were known to physiologists and reasoned from even before the time of Mr. John Hunter; and hence Baglivi contended that virulent gonorrhœa, as it was then called, may be produced by other actimonies than the syphilitic (*De Fibrâ Motice,* &c.), while Zeller, towards the close of the seventeenth century, affirmed that it may originate in either sex without contact (*Diss. de Gonorrhœâ utroque sexú,* Tubing., 1700); and Stoll, in the middle of the eighteenth, that it proceeds from various causes, of which syphilitic contagion is one.—(*Prælect.,* p. 104.) It is due to the merits of Dr. Balfour to observe, that he made the distinction between syphilis and gonorrhœa the

---

[*] As discharges from the urethra have been common from time immemorial, this assertion can hardly be received as correct and certain, inasmuch as it is now impossible to form any judgment respecting the particular nature of those complaints. From what we know of discharges from the urethra, as they appear at the present day, we have every reason to believe that some of those referred to by the ancients, must have been capable of communication from one person to another.—Ed.

[*] The facts recorded in the writings of Mr. Evans and Dr. Hennen, leave no doubt of the fact that sores of various character have arisen on the genitals after connexion with individuals affected only with clap. Whether any of such sores were true Hunterian chancres is another question, of which a different opinion may perhaps be entertained from that of M. Lagneau.—Ed.

[†] Dr. Swediaur enumerates the following species of blennorrhœa: the syphilitic; the herpetic, leprous; scorbutic; the gouty; the rheumatic; the hemorrhoidal; that produced by some substance taken internally or applied externally to the urethra; and blennorrhœa, a stimulo-mechanico.— See his Comprehensive Treatise upon the Symptoms, Consequences, Nature, and Treatment of Venereal or Syphilitic Diseases.—D.

ground of his inaugural dissertation at Edinburgh in 1767, which was nineteen years before the publication of Mr. Hunter's celebrated work.

It is not easy to account for the primary appearance of this or of any other specific poison, but we see daily that most, perhaps all mucous membranes, under a state of some peculiar morbid action, have a tendency to secrete a virulent and even contagious material of some kind or other, the particles of which are in some instances highly volatile, and capable of communicating their specific effect to organs of a like kind, and of propagating their power by assimilation after having been diffused to some distance through the atmosphere, which does not at all times readily dissolve them; though, agreeably to a general law we have formerly pointed out, the more readily, the purer the constitution of the atmosphere.—(Vol. i., corol. 9, p. 344.) We have a manifest proof of this in the muculent discharge of dysentery, in canine catarrh, or the muculent affection in the nostrils of dogs, which is vulgarly called distemper, and in the glanders, possibly also in the farcy, of horses. And although that species of catarrh which we name influenza is probably a miasm, rather dependant on some intemperament of the atmosphere itself in its origin, than on the temperament of the individual who suffers from it; yet this also becomes a contagion in its progress, and is communicable in consequence of such new property, from individual to individual, after a removal into fresh and very remote atmospheres by travelling (see *Catarrhus Epidemicus of this work*, Cl. III., Ord. II., Gen. IX., Spe. 2); while nothing can be more highly contagious than the discharge from the mucous glands of the tunica conjunctiva in purulent ophthalmai, although perhaps a direct contact is necessary for the production of its effect.

In like manner, leucorrhœa, as we have already observed, has sometimes seemed to be contagious; for I have occasionally found a kind of blennorrhœa produced in men, accompanied with a slight pain in the urethra, and some difficulty in making water, upon cohabitation with women who, upon inspection, had no marks whatever of luodic blennorrhœa or clap; and, in some instances, indeed, were wives and matrons of unimpeachable character.

The disease before us, however, has symptoms peculiar to itself, and undoubtedly depends upon a specific virus. The chief of these symptoms are described in the definition. They are generally preceded by a troublesome itching in the glans penis, and a general sense of soreness up the whole course of the urethra; soon after which the discharge appears, on pressing the glans, in the form of a whitish pus oozing from its orifice. In a day or two it increases in quantity, and becomes yellowish; and as the inflammation augments, and the disorder grows more virulent, the yellow is converted into a greenish hue, and the matter loses its purulent appearance, and is thinner and more irritant. The burning or scalding pain that takes place on making water, is usually seated about half an inch within the orifice of the urethra, at which part the passage feels peculiarly straitened, whence the urine flows in a small, interrupted stream: the lips of the urethra are thickened and inflamed, and a general tension is felt up the course of the penis. This last symptom is sometimes extremely violent, and accompanied with involuntary erections; at which time, if the cells of the corpus spongiosum urethræ be united by the adhesive inflammation, and rendered incapable of yielding equally with the corpora cavernosa, the penis is incurvated with intolerable pain. It is to this state of the penis, in which it bears some resemblance to a hard twisted cord, that the French have given the name of CHORDEE. Under these circumstances, we often meet with a troublesome phimosis either of the strangulating or incarcerating kind; in consequence of the increased spread of the inflammation. Sometimes it extends to one or both groins, in which case the glands swell and buboes are often formed: sometimes it reaches to the bladder, the inner surface of which pours forth a cheesy or wheyey fluid, instead of its proper lubicrous secretion, which is blended with the urine; and sometimes the testes participate in the inflammation, become swollen and painful, and excite a considerable degree of fever.

In woman, the chief seat of affection is the vagina; but as this is a less sensible part than the urethra, the pain is seldom so pungent, except when the meatus urinarius and the nymphæ associate and participate in the inflammation.

The disease appears at very different intervals after infection, according to the irritability of the constitution. The usual time is about the fourth or fifth day. But it has shown itself within the first twenty-four hours, and has sometimes continued dormant for a fortnight. Domeier lays down the time from the fourth to the fourteenth day (*Fragmente über die Erkentnis venerischer Krankheiten*, Hanov., 1790); Plenciz fixes it after the tenth.—(*Acta et Observationes Med.*, p. 139.) Sometimes only a very small discharge takes place, while the other symptoms are peculiarly exasperated. To this state of the disease, some practitioners have applied the very absurd name of *gonorrhœa sicca*.

It was at one time imagined that the puriform fluid, which is usually poured forth in considerable abundance, proceeds from an ulcer in the urethra: but it is now well known that it is not necessary for an ulcer or an abscess to exist for the formation of pus, and the dissection of persons who have died while labouring under this disease, has sufficiently shown that the secretion is thrown forth from the internal membrane of the urethra, chiefly at the lacunæ, without the least appearance of ulceration, or even, in most instances, of excoriation.

The cure in the present day is simple; for the venereal clap, like the venereal pox, appears to have lost much of that virulence and severity of character, by passing from one constitution to another, which it evinced on its first detection.[*] Rest, diluent drinks, and an antiphlogis-

---

[*] The statement of clap and the venereal dis-

tic regimen, will often effect a cure alone. But it may be expedited by cooling laxatives and topical applications.

The remedies employed are of two kinds, and of very opposite characters; stimulant and sedative. Both, also, are used generally and locally; with a view of taking off the irritation indirectly, by exciting a new action; or directly, by rendering the parts affected torpid to the existing action, and thus allowing it to die away of its own accord. Many of these medicines, indeed, as well the local as the general, were at one time supposed to be natural antidotes, and to cure by a specific power: an idea, however, which has been long banished from the minds of most practitioners.

The general sedatives that have hitherto been principally employed, are opium, conium, nitre, oily emulsions, and mucilages. The first has often succeeded, but with considerable and very unnecessary inconvenience to the constitution: the others are not much to be depended upon. They may have co-operated with a rigidly reducent diet, but have seldom answered alone.

Employed locally, some of them, and particularly opium, have proved far more beneficial. The best form of this last is that of an injection, rendered somewhat viscid by oil or mucilage.

The stimulant process has, however, been found to answer so much more effectually, that it has almost superseded the use of sedatives.

Formerly this process, also, was employed generally, and it was supposed, and in many cases sufficiently ascertained, that by strongly irritating some other part, the morbid excitement of the urethra would subside, and the organ have time to recover its natural action. And hence the intestines were daily stimulated by cathartics, as neutral salts, mercury, and colocynth, which last was at one time regarded as a specific; or terebinthinates, as camphire, balsam of copayva, and turpentine itself. And sometimes the bladder was treated in the same manner, with diuretics of all kinds, and especially with cantharides.

This plan is still continued in many parts of the east, and particularly in Bengal and Java; where, as we are informed by Mr. Crawfurd, the common remedy, and one to which the disease in those hot regions yields very easily, is that of cubebs, the *piper cubeba* of Linnéus. This pepper, well pounded, is exhibited in a little water, five or six times a day, in the quanti-

tity of a dessert-spoonful, or about three drachms, as well in the ensuing as in the present species, during which time all heating aliments are to be carefully abstained from. The cure, we are told, is entirely completed in two or three days, the ardor urinæ first ceasing, and the discharge again becoming viscid. A slight diarrhœa is sometimes produced, with a flushing in the face, and a sense of heat in the palms of the hands and the soles of the feet. In a few instances, Mr. Crawfurd tells us, inflamed testicles have supervened, an affection which yields easily to the common treatment.—(*Account of the Piper Cubeba*, &c., *Edin. Med. and Surg. Jour.*, No. liii., p. 32.) This plan has of late been extensively made use of at home. Mr. Broughton has given us a result of fifty trials under his own eye; and of these he tells us, that he cured forty-one in less than a month; that five were relieved; one was cured, but relapsed; and three failed. He affirms that it does not disagree with the stomach, is more easily admissible than balsam of copayva, and is not attended with the evils of injections. He employed the medicine two or three times a day; giving, of the powder, from two drachms to half an ounce, and of the wine or tincture from a drachm to half an ounce for the dose.*

There is no necessity, however, for subjecting the constitution to so severe a discipline; for the stimulant process, and particularly that of astringent stimulants, when employed locally, succeeds ordinarily in a few days without any trouble. These consist chiefly of metallic salts in solution, as the muriate and submuriate of mercury, the former in the proportion of three or four grains to eight ounces of water, sulphate of zinc, sulphate of copper, ammoniacal copper, and the acetated solution of lead. The astringent property of most of these, under due management, instead of being found mischievous, gives a check to the morbid secretion, at the same time that it acts as a direct tonic, and rapidly restores the irritated mouths of the exhalants to their healthy and proper action; and this too without the inconvenience of a secondary inflammation. A slight solution of alum alone, indeed, in the proportion of one or two grains to an ounce of water, has, for this purpose, been often employed with sufficient efficacy; though the present author has reason to prefer the sulphate of zinc, which he has usually combined with bole armenic, in the proportion of one scruple of the former and two of the latter to half a pint of water. And he can venture to say, that, through a pretty extensive course of practice for upwards of thirty years, he has never known this composition to fail; and has never perceived it produce any of the inconve-

---

ease having become milder by transmission from one constitution to another, than they were at their origin, is one that can only be received as a suppositiou; for the exact periods of the origin of the venereal disease and of gonorrhœa form a subject involved in considerable obscurity. In the most ancient times, the genitals were also subject to discharges and ulceration; and at the present day, the venereal disease is believed to be either several different specific disorders, or else several forms of one disease, so disguised and modified by the influence of temperament, climate, mode of living, and other causes, as virtually to form cases that seem to have little resemblance to each other, and to require very opposite modes of treatment.—Ed.

* Trans. of the Medico-Chir. Soc., vol. xii., part i., 1822. The cubebs, or Java pepper, as it is termed, still possesses considerable repute for its efficacy in checking gonorrhœas and gleets, and is in common use. It seems to act as a terebinthinate, and like other medicines of this class, if it does good at all, the benefit is perceived as soon as the urine begins to have its odour and other qualities changed by the remedy.—Ed.

niences of stricture or swelled testicle, which were so much, but so groundlessly apprehended, when the stimulating and astringent practice was first introduced.*

The addition of the bole may to some practitioners appear trifling, but it adds to the power of the zinc, probably by giving an increased body to the solution without diminishing its stimulant effect, which would certainly follow by using oil or mucilage in its stead. The sulphate of copper is more irritating than that of zinc, and, in a strong solution, is more likely to produce inflammation; and it is on this account chiefly that the author has confined himself to the latter. It is, in effect, by an analogous practice, that several modifications of purulent ophthalmia, and particularly that of infancy, is most successfully subdued, as we observed when treating of this disease.

It is almost unnecessary to add, that the utmost cleanliness by frequent washing should be maintained from the first appearance of the disease.

Where the complaint, however, is improperly treated with stimulants, and particularly astringent stimulants, or where it has continued too long before application for medical assistance, the whole range of the urethra, or some particular parts of it, are apt to become so irritable as to suffer spasmodic contractions, which commonly pass under the name of strictures, without being so in reality ; and, as we have already observed, this irritation, in some cases, extends to the interior surface of the bladder, and even thickens it. We have often had occasion to remark, that in fibrous structures and canals, the most sensible parts are their extremities ; and this remark is particularly applicable to blennorrhœa, for the portions of the urethra which suffer most from irritation are the interior membrane of the glans and the prostate, particularly the latter, in consequence of its direct connexion with the bladder as well as the urethral canal.

On this account, when a patient once labours under spasmodic constrictions from the disease before us, whatever other parts these may exist in, the introduction of a bougie will be almost sure to prove, that there is also a constriction towards the prostate gland. Generally speaking, it will be found to originate here, and to occur in other parts of the canal from sympathy. But the case will often be reversed, and while the irritation originates in some other part, or in the bladder, it is by sympathy with these that the prostate itself is affected. Mr. Abernethy has pointed out this double source of spasmodic constriction in the prostate, in the clearest manner possible (*Surgical Observations on Diseases of the Urethra*, p. 194, 8vo., 1810) ; and the remarks he has offered upon the propriety of employing or withholding the bougie as an instrument of cure cannot be too deeply imprinted in every student's mind ; the general principle of which is to persevere in its use wherever it appears to blunt the sensibility ; and to pass it as high up the urethra as can be accomplished with this effect, if possible, indeed, through the prostate into the bladder ; but in every instance to desist where a second or third trial of the instrument gives more pain than the first, or to content ourselves with passing it as high as can be done without any such symptoms of increased irritation, and there stopping short ; and only making an occasional trial when we have reason to hope that the morbid sensibility has still further subsided. M. Ducamp thinks, however, that little benefit is to be derived from bougies ; and that suffering them to remain in the urethra is sure to increase the irritation.—(*Traité des Retentions d'Urine par le Rétrécissement de l'Urethre*, &c., Paris, 8vo., 1822.)

SPECIES III.

BLENNORRHŒA CHRONICA.

GLEET.

SLIMY DISCHARGE FROM THE MUCOUS GLANDS OF THE URETHRA, WITHOUT SPECIFIC VENOM OR INFECTION : SLIGHTLY IRRITATING ; CHRONIC.

THIS species is a frequent sequel of a clap that has been ill managed, or has lasted long, and produced an obstinate local debility. But it exists also independently of clap, and is occasioned by strains, excess of venery, and other causes of weakness. The discharge is for the most part a bland and slimy mucus, not accompanied with inflammation, apparently proceeding from a morbid relaxation of the mucous glands of the urethra, and at times, like other discharges from debilitated organs, accompanied with and kept up by irritation, and especially irritation produced by a stricture in the urethra properly so called, or a diseased state of the prostate gland.

In common cases, the disease yields to the local tonics and astringents recommended under the preceding species ; but it is sometimes peculiarly irritable, and bids defiance to all the ingenuity of the medical art. A. Castro gives an instance of its having continued for eighteen years.*

The stimulants ordinarily employed have consisted of copayva, cubebs, or some terebinthinate or resinous balsam in the form of injection ; tincture of ipecacuanha, as recommended by Swediaur ; infusion of cantharides, a favourite remedy with Bartholine ; or a blister applied to the urethra, as advised by Mr. John Hunter and several other writers.

The bougie may here be used, for the most part, more fearlessly than in the preceding species. Its own simple stimulus, if employed regularly once or twice a day, has often proved sufficient : and where this fails, it may be rendered more active by being smeared with turpentine, mercurial ointment, or camphorated liniment ; or armed with nitrate of silver, where

---

* These inconveniences, however, often arise from the use of lead injections, and hence they are now almost universally abandoned.—D.

* De Morb. Mul., p. 68. Here it is to be suspected, that the disease must have depended upon the presence of a stricture in the urethra.—ED.

strictures require it. Even in this species, however, it is a valuable remark of Mr. John Hunter, that before we have recourse to any powerful application, we should well weigh the degree of irritability of the patient's constitution; for we may otherwise run a risk of exciting a violent local inflammation, or of extending the irritation to the testes or the bladder.. Should such an issue unfortunately occur, one of the most salutary injections we can employ is a solution of the extract of hyoscyamus in water. Even in chordees which resisted the influence of opium, Mr. Bell asserts that he has found this medicine advantageous, in the quantity of from one to three grains at a time, and repeated three times a day or oftener. Or we may have recourse to a warm hemlock poultice, applied every night, and made sufficiently large to cover the whole of the perinæum, testes, and penis. I have known this succeed in taking off an habitual irritation, and with it effectually suppressing the discharge, on the third application, in two instances of more than a twelvemonth's standing; and this after stimulants of all kinds, and narcotics of many kinds, and particularly opium, had been tried in succession. The leaves were here employed in a fresh state.

In women, this disease is often mistaken for leucorrhœa; we have pointed out the distinctive character under the last species. Yet the mistake is not of essential consequence, as the same treatment will often effect a cure in both. As the vagina, however, is less irritable than the urethra, gleet in females is a less frequent and troublesome complaint than in males.

GENUS IV.
SPERMORRHŒA.
SEMINAL FLUX.

INVOLUNTARY EMISSION OF SEMINAL FLUID WITH-OUT COPULATION.

The generic name is derived from σπείρω, "sero," "semino;" whence aspermus, "void of seed," gymnospermus, "having the seed naked," a term well known in botany; and hence also numerous other derivatives of the same kind. Gonorrhœa, which is a direct synonyme, would have been retained as the name for this genus, as it is retained by Linnéus, Sagar, and Frank, but from the confused signification in which it has been employed by Sauvages and Cullen; and from its being usually, though most improperly, applied in the present day to blennorrhœa luodes.

The genus offers two varieties, as follow :—

1. Spermorrhœa Enton-　Entonic Seminal Flux.
　ica.

2. ———　Atonica.　Atonic Seminal Flux.

SPECIES I.
SPERMORRHŒA ENTONICA.
ENTONIC SEMINAL FLUX.

INVOLUNTARY EMISSION OF PROPER SEMEN, WITH ERECTION; MOSTLY FROM AN INDULGENCE OF LIBIDINOUS IDEAS.

The usual cause is assigned in the definition,

and it very strikingly points out the influence which the mind bears upon the body, and the necessity of subjecting the passions to the discipline of a chaste and virtuous deportment; since, as there is no passion more debasing than that of gross lust, there is none more mischievous to the general health of the body. It leads the besotted slave straight forward to every other sensuality, and, by becoming at length an established and chronic disease, stupifies the mind, debilitates the body, and is apt to terminate in hectic fever and tabes.

This affection sometimes originates in the body itself; in a local and urgent erethism, produced, as Forestus conjectures (Lib. xxvi., obs. ii.), by a superabundant secretion of seminal fluid in a constitution of entonic health and vigour. And as, in the former case, the body is to be chastised through the mind, in the present the mind is to be chastised through the body : particularly by purgatives and venesection, a low diet and severe exercise. If, however, the patient be single, as is commonly the case, the pleasantest, as well as the most effectual remedy, is to be sought for in marriage.

SPECIES II.
SPERMORRHŒA ATONICA.
ATONIC SEMINAL FLUX.

INVOLUNTARY EMISSION OF A DILUTE AND NEAR-LY PELLUCID SEMINAL FLUID; WITH LIBIDI-NOUS PROPENSITY, BUT WITHOUT ERECTION.

Of this species Sauvages gives us two curious examples : one from Deidier, in which the patient was an exemplary monk, who shrunk with horror at the idea of this involuntary self-pollution, as he regarded it : the other a case in his own practice, in which the patient, a most religious young female, was, as he affirms, driven almost to madness under the same erroneous contemplation of the disease. From his having included a female under this genus, it should seem that Sauvages inclined to the theory of epigenesis, or that which supposes the male and female to contribute equally a seminal fluid in the act of procreation. It is probable that some local irritation is the usual cause. Professor Deidier himself suspected this in the first of the above cases; and referred it rather to a calculus in the bladder, sympathetically affecting the prostate gland, than to any idiopathic disease of the vesiculæ seminales, or the testes. The pious monk found himself most relieved by scourging his legs : a blister applied to the perinæum would probably have relieved him still more effectually. The fluid is a thin degenerate secretion, apparently from the vesiculæ seminales, rather than semen itself. It is sometimes found intermixed with blood; and, in this case, we have a further irritation of a wound or ruptured vessel. The most common cause of this miserable disorder is a previous life of unrestrained concupiscence : and under the debility hereby produced, the morbid discharge is peculiarly apt to flow upon the mere muscular excitement that takes place on evacuating the rec•

tum; and hence follows hard upon a stool.—
(*Art. Med. Berol.*, dec. i., vol. iv., p. 70;
Weichmann De Pollutione, &c., Goet., 1712.)

A cure should be attempted by the daily use
of a bidet of cold seawater, or of early bathing
in the sea, and the internal use of the metallic
tonics. The bowels should be kept lax; but
the warm and irritating purgatives should be
carefully abstained from. Blistering the perinæum, or making a seton in it, has occasionally been found serviceable: as has also a local
use of electricity.*

GENUS V.
GALACTIA.
MISLACTATION.

MORBID FLOW OR DEFICIENCY OF MILK.

THIS includes the greater part of those affections treated of by Dioscorides under the name
of sparganosis, which, however, in his arrangement, embraced, as we observed under PHLEG-
MONE MAMMÆ (Cl. III., Ord. II., Gen. II.,
Spe. 5), many complaints that have little or
no connexion with each other, and particularly
one of the species of BUCNEMIA, or TUMID LEG:
so that it has been necessary to break up the
division, and allot to its different members their
proper positions.

GALACTIA is a Greek term, from γάλα, "lac,"
whence γαλάκτικος, "lacteus." It occurs in
Linnéus and Vogel for the genus now before us,
which by Sauvages and Sagar is written galactirrhœa, literally "milk-flux," in a morbid sense
of the term. The author has preferred GALAC-
TIA as more comprehensive than galactirrhœa,
so as to allow the idea of a depraved or defective, as well as of a superabundant secretion of
milk: all of which are equally entitled to be
comprised under one common head, as excess,
deficiency, or other irregularity of arterial action
in fever. Hitherto, however, from an opposite
fault to that of Dioscorides, these affections have
been separated from each other by many nosologists, and carried to different heads, sometimes
to different orders, and occasionally to different
classes; whence the student has had to hunt
for them through every section of the nosological arrangement. It has already been necessary to make the same remark respecting many
of the species of PARAMENIA; and various other
instances will occur to us in the ensuing orders
of the class we are now explaining.

The flow of milk may become a source of
disease, as being out of season, defective in
quantity, vitiated in quality, transferred to an improper organ, and as discharged from the proper
organ, but in the male sex. These differences
will furnish the present genus with five distinct
species, as follow:—

1. Galactia Præmatura.   Premature Milk-flow.
2. ——— Defectiva.   Deficient Milk-flow.
3. ——— Depravata.   Depraved Milk-flow.
4. ——— Erratica.   Erratic Milk-flow.
5. ——— Virorum.   Milk-flow in Males.

---

* The tincture of cantharides will be found
useful as a local and general stimulant when other
means have failed.—D.

SPECIES I.
GALACTIA PRÆMATURA.
PREMATURE MILK-FLOW.

EFFLUX OF MILK DURING PREGNANCY.

THE mammæ, which maintain the closest
sympathy with the ovaria and uterus, and, in
most animals possessing them, are placed in
their direct vicinity, and which, in truth, are as
much entitled to the character of a sexual organ as any organ of the entire frame, participate
in the development of the generative function
from the first stimulus of puberty. It is then
that the breasts assume a globose plumpness,
and the catamenial flux commences; when
pregnancy takes place, and the uterus enlarges,
the breasts exhibit a correspondent increase of
swell; and when, shortly after childbirth, the
lochial discharge ceases, and the uterus takes
rest, the lacteal discharge is secreted, and
poured forth in immediate succession. The
sympathy continues, however, even after this
rest has commenced, for one of the most effectual means of increasing the flow of milk from
the breasts is a slight excitement of the uterus,
as soon as it has recovered its tone: and hence
the mother of an infant, living with her husband,
and herself in good health, makes a far better
nurse, and even requires a less stimulant regimen, than a stranger, brought from her own
family, and secluded from her husband's visits.
Of this, indeed, many of the rudest and most
barbarous nations, but which are not always inattentive to the voice of nature, have the fullest
conviction; insomuch that the Scythians, according to Herodotus, and the Hottentots in our
own day, irritate the vagina to increase the flow
of milk in their cows and mares.

It sometimes happens, however, that this stimulus of sympathy is carried to excess, even during pregnancy, and that the lactiferous ducts
of the mammæ secrete milk from the ultimate
branches of the arteries sooner than it is wanted.
If the quantity thus separated be small, it is of
no moment; but if it be considerable, some degree of debility is usually produced, with restlessness and pyrexy. And hence Galen observes,
that a premature flow of milk indicates a weakly
child (*Fragm. ex Aphor. Rab. Mois.*, p. 34);
and the collections of medical curiosities contain
various cases, in which it has appeared to be injurious.—(*Act. Nat. Cur.*, vol. iv.) Sauvages
gives an instance, in which a pint and a half
was poured forth daily, as early as the fifth
month. Where the constitution is peculiarly
robust, even this may for some time be borne
with as little mischief as menstruation during
pregnancy: but in ordinary cases, the system
must be weakened by so excessive and unprofitable a discharge. There is another instance
noticed in the volume of Nosology, in which a
pint and a half was poured forth daily at the
fifth month.

The morbid irritation, however, may generally be taken off by venesection, and if this should
not succeed, by a few doses of aperient medicmes.

It has sometimes happened that a like precocity has occurred in young virgins, and that these also have secreted and discharged milk from the proper organ. In many cases this has occurred as a substitute for the catamenial flux, which has been retained or suppressed at the time ;* but more generally it has proceeded from entonic plethora, or a morbid erethism of the sexual organs at the period of puberty (*Hippocr. Aph.*, sect. v., § 39 ; *Vega, Comment. in Hippocr.*, Aph. v., § 39) : and is to be removed by a reducent regimen, bleeding, and purgatives, as just pointed out.

On the other hand, we have occasional instances of a supply of milk in women considerably advanced in life, and who have long ceased to bear children, and even to menstruate. Thus, a woman of sixty-eight is stated by Dr. Stack to have given suck to two of her grandchildren (*Phil. Trans.*, vol. xli., year 1739, 141) ; and another of eighty, in a Swedish journal, is said to have performed the same office.—(See also *Phil. Trans.*, vol. ix., year 1674.) In most of these cases the antiquated nurses have consisted of married women, who had many years before reared families of their own, and whose lactiferous organs were therefore more easily re-excited to the renewed action than if they had never suckled.† The cause has been some peculiar irritation originating in the radicles of the lactiferous ducts, or excited by a transfer of action from the uterus or ovaria, in consequence of a cessation of the menses.

SPECIES II.

GALACTIA DEFECTIVA.

DEFICIENT MILK-FLOW.

INABILITY TO SUCKLE UPON CHILDBIRTH.

THIS is the agalaxis or agalactatio of preceding nosologists, and may proceed from two causes, accompanied with symptoms producing the two following varieties :—

α Atonica.   From want of secretion.
   Atonic inability
   to suckle.

β Organica.   From imperfect nipple or
   Organic inabili-   other organic defect.
   ty to suckle.

To every feeling and considerate mother, inability to suckle is a serious evil ; and, generally speaking, it is an evil of as great a magnitude to the mother herself as to the child ; for a free secretion of milk prevents many present and not a few eventual mischiefs. The health of women during suckling is, in most instances, better than at any period in their lives. Their ap-

petite is excellent, their sleep sound and refreshing, their spirits free, their temper cheerful. But to every conscientious mother there is, superadded to all this, a pleasurable feeling of a still higher and nobler kind ; it is a sense of conscientiously discharging the maternal duty : it is the gratification of beholding the lovely babe, to which she has given birth, saved from the cold caresses of a hireling, to lie in the warm embraces of her own bosom : to grow from the sweet fountain which she furnishes from her own veins, rich, ample, and untainted ; to swell with the tender thrill that shoots through the heart at every little draught which is drawn away from her ; to see the cheeks dimple and the eyes brighten, and the limbs play and the features open ; and to trace in every fresh lineament a softened image of herself, or one dearer to her than herself. This is the luxury that awaits the mother whose unseduced ear still listens to the voice of nature, and estimates the endearments of domestic life at a higher value than the intoxicating charm of fashionable amusements and midnight revels. Though transported with the present, her comforts do not end with the present ; for she has yet to look forward to a term of life in which, when those who have made a sacrifice of maternal duty at the altar of pleasure, are wasting with decline, trembling with palsy, or tormented with the dread of cancer, she will still enjoy the blessing of unbroken health, and sink as on a downy pillow into a tranquil old age.

But though these remarks apply to the greater number of those who, in the career of fashion, abstain from the duty of a mother, they by no means apply to all. There are many excellent mothers who would undergo the severest discipline of pain to accomplish this object ; but after all are not able. There are some, who from the want of a proper nipple, or perhaps the imperfect development of lactiferous ducts, are naturally disqualified for the office ; as there are others whose constitutional debility renders them incapable of secreting their milk in sufficient abundance, or with a sufficient elaboration for healthy food. And in all such cases it is expedient, wherever the means will allow, to seek carefully for the substitute of a foster-mother.

But let not the natural office be abandoned too soon, and particularly where the child is strong and hearty. If the nipple be at fault, much may be done to remedy it. If it be pointed in the breast, it may often be drawn out by exciting a vacuum with the ordinary glass tube invented for the purpose, if dexterously applied ; or, which will often succeed better, by the suction of a woman who is well skilled in the art ; or if these means do not succeed, an artificial nipple may be employed.

And if the breasts be hard and lumpy, and a considerable degree of symptomatic fever supervene, the same kind of suction must be had recourse to twice a day, while the breasts are kept in a constant state of relaxation by gentle friction with warm oil, large cataplasms of bread and water, and a suspensory bandage of flannel

---

* De la Corde, Ergo virgo, menstruis deficientibus, lac in mammis habere potest ? Paris, 1580.

† Dr. Kennedy, of Ashby de la Zouch, has lately recorded a memorable instance of this in the person of Judith Waterford, of that place ; a woman who menstruated during lactation ; who suckled children (many not her own) uninterruptedly through the full course of forty-seven years (three years of which time she was a widow) ; and who, in her eighty-first year, has a moderate but regular secretion of milk.—See Medico-Chirurgical Review for July, 1832.—ED.

passed under the arms and drawn as tight as may be borne without inconvenience.

Even where the milk is not very promising, either in respect to quantity or quality, let not the unhappy mother despair for the first week or two. As her own strength increases, the strength of the milk will often be found to increase also; the milk-vessels will yield with more facility, and the symptomatic pain in the back will subside. Added to which, the matrimonial excitement, to which I have alluded in the preceding species, will in due time be called in to bear its beneficial part ; and the woman who had a hopeless prospect before her, may in due time reap the full harvest of her labours.

SPECIES III.
GALACTIA DEPRAVATA.
DEPRAVED MILK-FLOW.
AFFLUX OF A DILUTE OR VITIATED MILK.

HERE also we have two varieties :—

a Serosa.	Weakened by too large a pro-
Serous milk-	portion of serum.
flow.	
β Contaminata.	Deteriorated by intermixture
Contaminated	with some foreign material.
milk-flow.	

To the FIRST VARIETY we have alluded under the preceding species : for it sometimes happens, that milk, when deficient in quantity, is also of a more dilute quality than it ought to be. But more frequently, as local irritation is a result or concomitant of debility, there is in weakly habits a very large flow of a thin, slightly blue, and almost pellucid milk, containing little sugar, and still less cream. The properties of a sound woman's milk we have already given under CONSUMPTION, and to save an unnecessary repetition, the reader may turn to the passage at his leisure, and compare it with the defective character before us.—(*Marasmus Phthisis*, Cl. III., Ord. IV., Gen. III., Spe. 5.)

In this case, tonics, and a generous diet, afford the best chance of success, and are often employed with full effect.

Under the SECOND VARIETY, the assimilation is imperfect, and the milk has the taste or smell of beer or wine, or some other fluid that has been introduced into the stomach ; proving that the digestive power is weak, and requires correction and invigoration. In other cases, we have examples of black, green, or yellow milk ; probably discoloured by a union with diffused blood.*

---

* Dr. Locock has seen four instances in which it was of a golden yellow colour, and upon standing, a thick layer of bitter cream, as yellow as pure bile, floated on the surface. In neither of these cases was the patient jaundiced ; but a very copious flow of bile being kept up from the intestines by mercurial purgatives, after a few days the yellowness disappeared ; the child till then having been much griped and affected with diarrhœa. In no cases where wet-nurses have been jaundiced, has Dr. Locock seen the milk yellow.—See Cyclop. of Pract. Med., art. LACTATION.—ED.

All violent exertions, whether of body or mind, and hence violent passions, as rage and terror, have a peculiar influence in changing the natural character of milk ; and the depressing passions frequently drive it away entirely.—(*Starch, Archiv. für Geburtshelfer*, b. iii., p. 12., b. ii., p. 3.) It is hence of no small moment that a wet-nurse be of an easy and even temper, and not disposed to mental disturbance.*

SPECIES IV.
GALACTIA ERRATICA.
ERRATIC MILK-FLOW.
MILK TRANSFERRED TO AND DISCHARGED OR ACCUMULATED AT SOME REMOTE ORGANS, OFTEN UNDER A DIFFERENT FORM.

LIKE the menstrual flux, there is scarcely an organ to which the flow of milk has not been transferred under different circumstances, or in different constitutions. And hence the author has adverted in the volume of Nosology to examples of its translation to the fauces, where it has been discharged in the form of ptyalism ; to the general surface of the mammæ, where it has been evacuated in the form of sweat ; to the navel, where it has assumed an ichorous appearance ; to the kidneys, which have thrown it off in an increased flow of urine ; to the eyes, whence it has been discharged as a milky epiphora ; to the veins, which it has overloaded, so as to demand the use of the lancet ; and to the vagina, where it has excited a copious leucorrhœa. It is also said to be frequently translated to the thighs, so as to produce the disease

---

* The qualities of the milk differ considerably during lactation. At first it is thick, yellowish, and has a very large proportion of cream ; several days elapsing before it acquires perfection, in which state it is thin, bluish, and sweet. The quantity of cream varies very much, according to the diet, and the frequency with which the breasts are drawn. " Some milk has decidedly a saline taste, and, at other times, it has been distinctly bitter, so that the child will turn away from the breast in disgust. Its taste and qualities may be easily affected by articles of diet, by passions of the mind, repletion, hot rooms, &c., and the child is more or less disordered by the alteration. Medicines will often affect the milk in a very striking manner ; a purgative given to the nurse will frequently act violently upon the child, without in the least affecting the individual herself. In the same way, alkalis given to the nurse will relieve acidity in the child's stomach ; and mercury, given through a similar medium, will cure syphilitic symptoms in the infant at the breast." Mr. Keate once attended a foreign gentleman, who, in order to promote his biliary secretion, was in the habit of taking asses' milk, medicated by giving the animal a certain quantity of nitrate of mercury. The effect was very marked, and he could bear mercury in no other shape.—(See Dr. Locock's art. LACTATION, in Cyclop. of Pract. Med.) When wet-nurses menstruate, we have the authority of this and other experienced accoucheurs for the observation, that the occurrence has an unfavourable influence on the milk, being likely both to interfere with the duration of the secretion, and to deteriorate its qualities.—See also Dr. Ryan's Manual of Midwifery, p. 667, ed. 3.—ED.

we have already described under the name of BUCNEMIA SPARGANOSIS, but which is clearly unconnected with the state of the milk, or of the breasts.

The causes are chiefly, a sudden exposure of the breasts to cold; cold water drunk improvidently when in a state of perspiration; spirituous potation, and sudden emotion of mind.

The irregular action is best subdued by gentle laxatives, diaphoretics, and perfect quiet in a warm bed. Where ardent spirits have been the cause, the aperients should be more stimulant, and bleeding will often be found necessary.

SPECIES V.
GALACTIA VIRORUM.
MILK-FLOW IN MALES.

MILK SECRETED IN MALES, AND DISCHARGED FROM THE PROPER EMUNCTORY.

A MILKY serum, and sometimes genuine milk, has been found to distil from the nipples of newborn infants of both sexes, and sometimes from boys of a later age.* But various authors, as Schöltz, P. Borelli, and Lauremberg, have given cases of genuine milk discharged in like manner by adult males; occasionally continuing for a long time; and, in some instances, enabling them to perform the office of nurses. In the Commentaries of the St. Petersburgh Academy (tom. iii., p. 278), a flow of milk from the breasts of males is said to be very common in Russia: and Blumenbach has noticed the same peculiarity in the males of various other mammalia.—(*Hannoverich Magazin*, 1787.) Among men, indeed, the discharge appears occasionally to have occurred even in advanced life; for Paullini gives the case of a man who was able to suckle at the age of sixty.—(Cent. ii., obs. 93; *Shacker, Diss. de Lacte Virorum et Virginum.*)

Why man should in every instance possess the same organization as women for secreting and conveying milk, is among the many mysteries of physiology that yet remain to be solved. But as there is little or no sympathy between the mammæ in man and any of the proper organs of generation, as in women, we are at no loss to account for their general sterility and

want of action. Occasionally, however, the lacteal glands in man, or the minute tubes which emerge from them, are more than ordinarily irritable; and throw forth some portion of their proper fluid. And if this irritation be encouraged and supported, there is no reason why such persons may not become wet-nurses as well as females. And hence Dr. Parr inquires, with some degree of quaintness, whether this organization is allotted to both sexes, in order that, "in cases of necessity, men should be able to supply the office of the woman?" Under these circumstances, the discharge, though unquestionably a deviation from the ordinary law of nature, can scarcely be regarded as a disease.

The following, from Captain Franklin's Narrative of his Journey to the Shores of the Polar Sea, is a beautiful exemplification of what Dr. Parr refers to; and I cannot consent to alter the forcible and seamanlike simplicity of the style in which the story is told. "A young Chippewayan had separated from the rest of his band for the purpose of trenching beaver, when his wife, who was his sole companion, and in her first pregnancy, was seized with the pains of labour. She died on the third day after she had given birth to a boy. The husband was inconsolable, and vowed, in his anguish, never to take another woman to wife; but his grief was soon in some degree absorbed in anxiety for the fate of his infant son. To preserve its life he descended to the office of a nurse, so degrading in the eyes of a Chippewayan, as partaking of the duties of a woman. He swaddled it in soft moss, fed it with broth made from the flesh of the deer; and, to still its cries, applied it to his breast, praying earnestly to the Great Master of Life to assist his endeavours. The force of the powerful passion by which he was actuated, produced the same effect in his case as it has done in some others which are recorded: a flow of milk actually took place from his breast. He succeeded in rearing his child, taught him to be a hunter, and, when he attained the age of manhood, chose him a wife from the tribe. The old man kept his vow in never taking a wife for himself, but he delighted in tending his son's children; and when his daughter-in-law used to interfere, saying that it was not the occupation of a man, he was wont to reply, that he had promised to the Great Master of Life, if his child was spared, never to be proud like the other Indians. Our informant (Mr. Wenkel, one of the Association) added, that he had often seen this Indian in his old age, and that his left breast even then retained the unusual size it had acquired in his occupation of nurse."—(P. 157, 4to., Lond., 1823.)

---

* A celebrated anatomist remarks,—"The use of the mammæ in the nourishment of children is known to all the world; but it is not certainly known what the papillæ and areolæ in males can be designed for. Milk has been observed in them in children of both sexes, and this happened to one of my own brothers when he was about two years of age."—Winslow's Anatomy, vol. ii., p. 214.)—ED.

ORDER II.

ORGASTICA.

DISEASES AFFECTING THE ORGASM.

ORGANIC OR CONSTITUTIONAL INFIRMITY, DIS-
ORDERING THE POWER OR THE DESIRE OF
PROCREATING.

The ordinal term ORGASTICA is derived from
ὀργάω, "appeto impatienter; propriè de ani-
mantibus dicitur, quæ turgent libidine." *Scapul.*
Orgasmus is hence used by most writers for salacity in general; though by Linnéus it is employed in a very different sense, being restrained
to *subsultus arteriarum.*

The following are the genera which appertain
to this order :—

  I. Chlorosis.   Green-Sickness.
  II. Prœotia.   Genital Precocity.
  III. Lagnesis.   Lust.
  IV. Agenesia.   Male Sterility.
  V. Aphoria.   Female Sterility.
                    Barrenness.
  VI. Ædoptosis.   Genital Prolapse.

GENUS I.

CHLOROSIS.

GREEN-SICKNESS.

PALE, CHLORID COMPLEXION; LANGUOR; LIST-
LESSNESS; DEPRAVED APPETITE AND DIGES-
TION: THE SEXUAL SECRETIONS DEPRAVED OR
INERT, ESPECIALLY AT THEIR COMMENCE-
MENT.

CHLOROSIS is a derivative from χλόα or χλόη,
"herba virens;" whence, among the Greeks,
χλώρασμα and χλωρίασις, "viror;" "pallor;"
evidently applied to the disease, like our own
term green-sickness, from the pale, lurid, and
greenish cast of the skin.

The causes of this disorder are numerous;
one of the most frequent is menostation, retained or suppressed catamenia; another is excessive menstruation; a third, inability of obtaining the object of desire,—in popular terms,
love-sickness; a fourth is dyspepsy, or any
other source of general debility about the age
of puberty, by which the natural development
of the sexual system and the energy of its secretions are at this time interfered with. Dr.
Parr makes it a question whether love-sickness,
or an ungratified longing for an object of desire,

is ever a cause; but the examples are too numerous to give countenance to any doubts upon
the subject (*Panarol. Jàtrolog, Pentech.*, iii.,
obs. 14; *Ephem. Nat. Cur.*, dec. ii., ann. ix.,
obs. 114); and pining, eager, ungratified desire
for any object whatever, in a particular state of
constitution, whether for an individual or for a
particular circle of society, for home or for
country, is well known in many cases to break
down the general health, and to lay a foundation for chlorosis as well as many other complaints even of a severer kind. We have already noticed it as producing suppressed menstruation; as we have also the opposite state
of disappointment overcome, renewed hope, and
a prospect of connubial happiness, as one of the
best and speediest means of cure.*

Perhaps retained menses and a dyspepsy at the
period of puberty are the most common causes;
and hence chlorosis makes so near an approach
to both these complaints, that some nosologists have merged it altogether in the first, and
others in the second. Dr. Cullen, so far as it
relates to his *opinion*, is an example of the former. Dr. Young, so far as relates to his *arrangement*, of the latter. It is necessary to
attend to this limitation; for, while Dr. Cullen,
in the latter editions of his Synopsis, asserts
"nullam chlorosis speciem veram, præter illam
quæ retentionem menstruorum comitatur, agnos-
cere vellem"—he still continues chlorosis in
all the editions of this work as a distinct genus
from amenorrhœa, or PARAMENIA *obstructionis*,
of which, upon this view of the subject, it should
be only a species or variety. In the same manner, Dr. Young, while he makes chlorosis a
mere species of dyspepsy in his classification,
observes, as though dissatisfied with his arrangement, " I have followed a prevalent opinion, but there are various reasons to think it
is quite as naturally connected with amenorrhœa." Professor Frank has more lately arranged
it as a subdivision or variety of this last complaint.—(*De Cur. Hom. Morb. Epitom.*, tom.
vi., lib. vi., part iii., 8vo., Viennæ, 1821.)

Chlorosis is often, indeed, not only connected
with amenorrhœa, but a consequence of it. Yet
few writers have felt themselves able to adopt
this view of the subject, and to believe it in
every instance a modification of this disease.
Sauvages asserts, that there are daily cases of
chlorosis occurring among children from their

---

* Andral conceives, that certain cases of chlorosis, attended with various functional disorders,
are often entirely the consequence of some defect
in sanguification; a defect whose cause he thinks
must be in the nervous system alone. If this view
be correct, he inquires, what reason is there for
ascribing to irritation and sanguineous congestion
these functional derangements, which are so diversified, comprising epileptic fits, convulsions,
chorea, dyspnœa, palpitations, vomitings, &c.?
On the contrary, he asks, would it not in many
instances be more conformable to truth to impute
these several morbid phenomena to the same cause
which gives rise to them in individuals labouring
under anæmia from not having the benefit of
proper aliment, the influence of the sun, and good
air? What aggravation of the disorder, says he,
would not bleeding here occasion, practised for the

removal of irritation that has no existence! On
the contrary, if you stimulate the nervous system
of many of these chlorotic girls by the physical
and moral emotions of marriage, an improved complexion will soon indicate that hæmatosis or sanguification is going on rightly again, and that in
proportion as the anæmia disappears under the influence of the new condition of the nervous system, so do likewise disappear the difficulty of
breathing, the constant general uneasiness, the
spontaneous lassitude, the indigestion, the pain in
the epigastric region, the pale colour of the urine,
and those numerous and fastidious nervous disorders which really seem as if they were more or less
connected with true organic changes.—See Précis
d'Anatomie Pathologique, par G. Andral, tom. i.,
p. 87.—ED.

cradles; and he has hence, among his chloroses VERÆ, set down one species under the name of *chlorosis infantum*. This, however, is to generalize the term too widely, and to make it include all cases marked by indigestion and a chlorid countenance. Yet I cannot but concur with those authors, who contend that chlorosis is by no means uncommon among females who have *no interruption* of the menstrual flux; though a derangement of some kind or other in quantity, quality, or constituent principles, appears to be always connected with it; and is for the most part the cause or leading symptom. There is even ground for carrying the term, with other authors, still further, and applying it to green-sick boys, as well as green-sick girls, for reasons which will be offered in their proper place.

For the present, it is sufficient to characterize chlorosis as a dysthesis or cachexy, produced by a diseased condition of the sexual functions operating upon the system at large, and hence most common to the age of puberty, in which this function is first called forth by the complete elaboration of organs that have hitherto been inert and undeveloped. "A certain state of the genitals," says Dr. Cullen, and the remark will apply to both sexes equally, "is necessary to give tone and tension to the whole system; and therefore, if the stimulus arising from the genitals be wanting, the whole system may fall into a torpid and flaccid state, and from thence chlorosis may arise."

The genus CHLOROSIS offers the two following species :—

1. Chlorosis Entonica. Entonic Green-sickness.
2. ——— Atonica. Atonic Green-sickness.

SPECIES I.
CHLOROSIS ENTONICA.
ENTONIC GREEN-SICKNESS.

HABIT PLETHORIC; PAIN IN THE HEAD, BACK, OR LOINS; FREQUENT PALPITATIONS AT THE HEART; FLUSHES IN THE FACE; PULSE FULL, TENSE, AND FREQUENT.

CHLOROSIS has been commonly confined to the second or atonic species. But the symptoms and mode of treatment of the disease, as it appears in a vigorous, florid, and full-bosomed country girl, overflowing with health and hilarity, and in a delicate, pale-faced, emaciated town girl, debilitated by an indulgence in a course of luxurious indolence from her infancy, seem to justify and even demand a distinction.

In both cases, there is want of energy of mind, great irregularity in the mental functions, and often a high degree of irritability in the nervous system, clearly proving a very extensive disturbance of the general balance. But they differ in the symptoms enumerated in the definitions, than which no two sets can well be more at variance. They differ also in the remote and proximate causes, and consequently in the mode of treatment.

In the species before us, characterized by a rich and oppilated habit, with a full and tense pulse, and pressive pain in the head or loins, the ordinary causes are catching cold in the feet at the period of the catamenial discharge, by which the constitutional plethora is considerably aggravated, and the plethoric excess itself, even where no cold has been received. For the very reason, that in *dyspermia entonica*, or supererection, as we shall have occasion to observe presently, there is no seminal emission, or as in double-flowering plants there is no efficient development of the sexual distinctions, in the present case there is no sufficient secretion of the genital fluids. And, as we have shown in the Physiological Proem to the present Order, that the maturity of the system in females as well as males depends upon a development of the sexual organization in all its powers, and a certain degree of resorption of its secreted materials, the general frame, how rich soever, and even oppressed with juices of other kinds, must remain incomplete and unripened, and sicken at the time of maturity, for want of this appropriate stimulus. And if such an effect may occur where there is no concomitant source of excitement, we can easily conceive how much more readily it may take place upon catching cold in the feet, or on a sudden and violent mental emotion, or any other cause that may accidentally add to the irritation of the organs immediately affected.

Yet there can be no doubt that the species before us, though the offspring of a redundancy of living power, if neglected, or obstinate and of long continuance, may, and often does, by debilitating the constitution, terminate in the atonic species.

Before such a change, however, takes place, and particularly in the commencement of the disease, we are loudly called upon for general depletion. Copious and not unfrequently repeated venesections will be found necessary: cooling, rather than heating and irritant purgatives, should be interposed; and, where pain about the lumbar region, or any other local irritation, is very troublesome, the hip-bath, or a general warm bath, should be used steadily. And when, by this plan, the sanguiferous entony is subdued, a plain diet, regular exercise, and sober hours, will easily accomplish the rest.

SPECIES II.
CHLOROSIS ATONICA.
ATONIC GREEN-SICKNESS.

HABIT DEBILITATED: GREAT INACTIVITY AND LOVE OF INDULGENCE; DYSPNŒA ON MOVING; LOWER LIMBS COLD AND ŒDEMATOUS, ESPECIALLY AT NIGHT; PULSE QUICK AND FEEBLE.

IN conjunction with the above specific symptoms, there is, in this division of the disease, the same want of energy of mind, and fickleness of temper, and corporeal irritability, which we have already noticed in the preceding, and this too in a much greater degree; abundantly proving a very extensive disturbance of the general balance.

For examples of this species we are to look, not into the quiet and sober retreats of rural life, marked by simple meals, healthful activity, and early hours; but to the gay and glittering routine of town indulgences, and midnight parties, and hot, unventilated atmospheres; the havoc of all which is to be seen in the pale, but bloated countenance, the withering form, emaciated muscles, and departing symmetry of those who are the victims of a life of pleasure; and who, in consequence of their turning night into day, are exhausted, and drowsy, and spiritless, and perhaps confined to their beds all the morning; thus carrying on the inversion of nature, and turning in like manner the day into night.

Under a life of this kind, it is impossible for a growing girl to acquire a healthy maturity; and most happy is it for her that the caprice of fashion, which calls upon her to make this heavy sacrifice of her person for one half the year, drives her, in most cases, into the freshening shades and soberer manners of the country for the other half.

There are other girls, however, who, without these peculiar sources of exhaustion, have so much constitutional debility and relaxation as to be incapable of bearing the double load of growth and sexual development, without manifesting a considerable degree of sickliness in all their functions.

Here, therefore, bleeding and purgatives would only add to the evil; and it behooves us even from the first to employ a strengthening and tonic plan, and to extend it through all the departments of diet, exercise, and medicine: the whole of which, however, may be collected from what has already been observed on the genus PARAMENIA. It is probable, that in many cases of this modification of the disease, the internal use of iodine, either in the form of pills or tincture, amounting to about half a grain to a dose, might be found a very useful stimulant as well as tonic.*

The same kind of debility, which prevents the full development of the sexual organization, and interferes with menstruation in growing girls, prevails not unfrequently in growing boys; and especially when about the age of puberty the growth is rapid, and outruns the general strength of the system. And it is to this state I alluded when observing, a page or two back, that the term chlorosis has occasionally been applied to males as well as to females, at this unsettled period of life. In the volume of Nosology, I have remarked that it is frequently so applied in the east, and especially among Persian writers, who accordingly express one subdivision of the disease by the name

of bimariy hodek بیماری کُرْدَکْ, or *morbus puerorum.* Bonet has followed the oriental extension of the term, and has given instances of its occurring, not only in pubescent, but even adult males; and, in like manner, Sir Gilbert Blane, in his table of diseases under the article chlorosis, observes, that one of his patients affected with this complaint "was a male of seventeen, who had all the characters of this malady, except that which is peculiar to the female sex. He was treated like the others, and recovered under the use of carbonated iron and aloes."—(*Medico-Chir. Trans.*, vol. iv., p. 140.) It is on this account that the definition of chlorosis will be found, in the present work, to vary in some degree from all that have preceded it, so as to render its characters capable of embracing the male as well as the female form of the disease.

GENUS II.
PRŒOTIA.
GENITAL PRECOCITY.

PREMATURE DEVELOPMENT OF SEXUAL ORGANIZATION, OR POWER.

THE generic term PRŒOTIA or PRŒOTES is copied from Theophrastus, and derived from πρωὶ, "præmature." It is, however, peculiarly applied to premature semination.

The genus, as embracing both sexes, comprises the two following species:—

1. Prœotia Masculina.   Male Precocity.
2. ——— Feminina.   Female Precocity.

SPECIES I.
PRŒOTIA MASCULINA.
MALE PRECOCITY.

PREMATURE DEVELOPMENT OF SEXUAL ORGANIZATION IN MALES.

BOTH the mind and body advance, in their ordinary career, by slow and almost imperceptible steps to maturity; faculty after faculty, and function after function, put forth, acquire strength, and become perfected. But occasionally this ordinary course is departed from, and the whole system, as well mental as corporeal, or, which is still more frequent, particular powers or organs, push forward with incredible rapidity. The admirable Crichton, as he is commonly called, and others pre-eminently gifted in the same extensive way, afford instances of the first of these remarks; and those who, in early and even in infant life, have shown a peculiar aptitude for an acquisition of languages, or of music, or numerical arithmetic, give examples of the last kind.

It is not hence much to be wondered at, that a like extraordinary precocity should sometimes exhibit itself in the development of sexual organization and power: and that, from a peculiar degree of local irritation or erethism, the pubes should be found covered with hair, the testes be formed and capable of secreting a seminal fluid

---

* In these cases, the preparations of iron are generally found to be the most successful tonics, and especially the subcarbonate. The treatment may be described in a few words, as consisting of nutritious food, tonics, mild aperients, habitation in a dry, airy situation, chalybeates, sulphate of quinine, and exercise on foot, horseback, &c.— See Ryan's Manual of Midwifery, p. 321, ed. 3.— ED.

and the penis be susceptible of a concupiscent turgescence and erection.

It is not necessary to dwell upon instances of exemplification, which may be traced in great numbers in the writings of physiologists who have been curious upon this subject. Those who are desirous of doing so may turn to the Journal des Sçavans for 1688, and the Philosophical Transactions for 1745. In the former, Boiset gives an instance of this disgusting anticipation in a boy of three years old; in the latter, the subject in the case recorded was two years and eleven months. A simple example at a similar age is well known to have occurred, only a few years since, in a boy who was exhibited by his friends for money to medical practitioners in this metropolis; and may be found, together with various others, minutely described in the first volume of the Medico-Chirurgical Transactions.* Two, of late date, are also detailed in the 11th and 12th vols. of the same work, by Dr. Breschet and Mr. J. F. South.

With respect to moral or even medical treatment, nothing can be worse than this very common practice of a public exposure whenever the case occurs among the poor, who are so strongly tempted to make a profit of it. The orgasm is fed by a repetition of examinations, and the polluting tide that exhausts and debases the body is at length accompanied, even though it should not be so at first, with a polluting pleasure, that in a still greater degree exhausts and debases the mind. An occasional application of leeches to the seat of affection, cooling aperients, a cool, loose, and unirritating lower dress, with the daily use of a bidet of cold water, or iced water, will form the best plan that can be pursued on such occasions; and, by producing a healthful repression, may enable the unhappy infant to grow up with gradual vigour to the possession of a hearty manhood, instead of sinking, as has been sometimes the case, into a premature and tabid old age at the early period of puberty.

---

* In the year 1748, Mr. Dawkes, a surgeon at St. Ives, near Huntingdon, published a small tract, called Prodigium Willinghamense, or an account of a surprising boy, who was buried at Willingham, near Cambridge, upon whom he wrote the following epitaph:—"Stop, traveller, and wondering know, here buried lie the remains of Thomas, son of Thomas and Margaret Hall; who, not one year old, had the signs of manhood; not three, was almost four feet high; endued with uncommon strength, a just proportion of parts, and a stupendous voice; before six he died, as it were, of an advanced age. He was born at this village, October 31, 1741, and in the same departed this life, Sept. 3, 1747."—(See also Phil. Trans., 1744-45.) As Dr. Elliotson has observed, this perfectly authentic case removes all doubts respecting the boy at Salamis, mentioned by Pliny (Hist. Nat., lib. vii., c. 17), as being four feet high, and having reached puberty when only three years old; and respecting the man seen by Craterus, the brother of Antigonus (Phlegon, De Mirab., c. 32), who, in seven years, was an infant, a youth, an adult, a father, an old man, and a corpse.—(Blumenbach's Physiology, 4th edit., note, p. 535.) Premature puberty does not appear to be attended with a proportionally early development of the intellectual faculties.—ED.

SPECIES II.
PRŒOTIA FEMININA.
FEMALE PRECOCITY.

PREMATURE DEVELOPMENT OF SEXUAL ORGANIZATION IN FEMALES.

UNDER the species of obstructed menstruation, we have observed that this secretion, which commonly affords a proof that the sexual organization is developed, and its function completed, takes place at very different periods of life under different circumstances, chiefly those of climate and peculiarity of constitution: and that, though its ordinary epoch is that of thirteen or fourteen, it has sometimes, under the influence of a tropical sun, or a warm and forward temperament, shown itself as early as eight or nine years of age.*

There is hence no difficulty in conceiving that, under the influence of the same kind of local erethism we have noticed in the preceding species, the sexual organization in females may acquire a similar precocity to that in males. And so complete has been the development occasionally, that we have numerous and well-authenticated instances of pregnancy itself occurring at the early age of nine years, on which we shall have to remark more fully in the introductory observations to the third Order of the present Class, when treating of morbid impregnation.

This foremach of nature should be timely checked, for it will otherwise assuredly lead to a very great debility of the system in general, and is usually found to stint the stature, and induce a premature old age. And the means of repression may be the same as those already proposed for male precocity.

The premature development or organization before us does not always seem to be connected with any cupidinous orgasm, or at least, it has occurred under circumstances that render it extremely difficult to entertain any such idea. One of the most singular instances of this kind is a case of extra-uterine fœtation published by Dr. Baillie. It consisted of a suety substance, hair, and the rudiments of four teeth, found in the ovarium of a child of not more than twelve or thirteen years of age, with an infantine uterus, and perfect hymen.—(Phil. Trans., vol. lxxix., p. 71; see also New-York Med. and Physiol. Journ., vol. ii.)

In this case there can be little doubt that an ovulum, by some peculiar irritation, had been excited to the rudimental process of an imperfect conception, and that it had, in consequence, been separated from its niche, and a corpus luteum taken its place. In the Physiological Proem to

---

* Walther, Thes., obs. 40. In some rare cases the menses have appeared in precocious puberty as early as the third or fourth year. Sir Astley Cooper has recorded an instance of this kind (Trans. Med. Chir. Soc., vol. iv.), and others are reported by British practitioners. In one case, the patient was but three years and a half old (Med. Phys. Journ., 1810); and, in another, but two years of age.—(Op. cit., vol. xxviii.) See Ryan's Manual of Midwifery; or, a Compendium of Gynæcology and Paidonosology, 12mo., Lond., 1831, edit. 3, a work replete with useful matter.—ED.

the present Class we have observed, that such changes are occasionally met with in mature virgins, whose organs have afforded ample proof of freedom from sexual commerce; the ordinary mode of accounting for which is by supposing, that although they have never cohabited with the male sex, they have at times felt a very high degree of orgasm or inordinate desire, and that such feeling has been a sufficient excitement to produce such an effect. The author has already expressed himself not satisfied with this explanation ; and the case before us can hardly be resolved into any such cause.*

GENUS III.
L A G N E S I S.
LUST.

INORDINATE DESIRE OF SEXUAL COMMERCE, WITH ORGANIC TURGESCENCE AND ERECTION.

LAGNESIS is a derivative from λάγνης, "libidinosus ;" "præceps in venerem ;" and as a genus, is intended to include the SATYRIASIS and NYMPHOMANIA of Sauvages and later authors ; which chiefly, if not entirely, differ from each other only as appertaining to the male or female sex, and in their symptoms do not, like the preceding genus, offer ground for two distinct species. The proper species belonging to this genus are the following :—

1. Lagnesis Salacitas.   Salacity.
2. ——— Furor.   Lascivious Madness.

SPECIES I.
LAGNESIS SALACITAS.
SALACITY.

THE APPETENCE CAPABLE OF RESTRAINT ; THE EXCITEMENT CHIEFLY CONFINED TO THE SEXUAL SYSTEM.

IN a state of health and civilized society, there are two reasons why mankind are easily capable of restraining within due bounds the animal desire that exists in their frame from the period of puberty till the infirmity of age : the one is of a physical, and the other of a moral kind. The natural orgasm of men differs from

---

* One of the most remarkable instances of Pr. feminina known, is recorded by Dr. D. Rowlett of Kentucky, in the Transylvania Journal of Medicine, October, 1834. The subject of it, when born, was of the usual size, but in a few weeks after birth her hips and breasts began to grow rapidly, and when twelve months old, the menstrual function was established : this appeared regularly until she became pregnant. At the age of ten years and thirteen days she was delivered of a healthy female child, weighing seven pounds and three quarters. The child refused the breast, and was raised by the bottle. Dr. R. remarks: "It is as healthy as is usual for children to be when raised from the bottle ; and at the time of taking these notes it weighed eight and three fourth pounds, and its mother weighed one hundred pounds. She was four feet seven inches high, and had the countenance of a girl not exceeding her in years, but is as intelligent as girls usually are at her age."—D.

that of brutes in being permanent, instead of being periodical, or dependant upon the return of particular seasons : and on this very account, is less violent, more uniform, and kept with comparative facility within proper limits. This is a cause derived from the physical constitution of man. But the power of habit and the early inculcation of a principle of abstinence and chastity in civilized life, form a moral cause of temperance that operates with a still stronger influence than the preceding, and lay down a barrier which, though too often stealthily broken into, yet in the main makes good its post, and serves as a general check upon society.

As man rises in education and moral feeling, he proportionally rises in the power of self-restraint ; and consequently, as he becomes deprived of this wholesome law of discipline, he sinks into self-indulgence and the brutality of savage life. And were it not that the very permanency of the desire, as we have already observed, torpefies and wears out its goad, the savage, destitute of moral discipline, would be at all times as ferocious in his libidinous career as brutes are in the season of returning heat ; when, stung with the periodical ardour, and worked up almost to fury,-the whole frame of the animal is actuated with an unbridled force, his motions are quick and rapid, his eyes glisten, and his nerves seem to circulate fire. Food is neglected ; fences are broken down ; he darts wild through fields and forests, plunges into the deepest rivers, or scales the loftiest rocks and mountains, to meet the object that is ordained by nature to quell the pungent impulse by which he is urged forward (see *Crichton on Mental Derangement,* ii., p. 301):

"Nonne vides ut tota tremor pretentet equorum
Corpora, si tantum notas odor attulit auras ?
Ac neque eos jam fræna virûm, neque verbera sæva,
Non scopuli, rupesque cavæ, atque objecta retardant
Flumina, correptos undâ torquentia montes."*

The power of restraint, however, does not operate alike on all persons, even in the same state of society, and under a common discipline. Period of life, constitution, and habit, produce a considerable difference in this respect, and lay a foundation for the four following varieties of morbid salacity :—

α Pubertatis.   Salacity of youth.
β Senilis.   ——— of age.
γ Entonica.   ——— of full habit.
δ Assueta.   ——— of a debauched life.

The FIRST VARIETY proceeds not so much from organic turgescence as from local irritability : for it is chiefly found in relaxed and delicate frames, weakened by overgrowth, or a life of indolence and indulgence. The action is new, and where, from whatever cause, the irritability is more than ordinary, a degree of excitement is produced which shows itself constitutionally or topically. If in the former way, hysteria, or chorea, or some other nervous affection, is a very frequent effect : if in the latter, a high-wrought and distressing degree of appetence. It is un-

---

* Virg. Georg., lib. iii., 250.

der this state that females are said to be capable of separating ovula from their ovaries, and of forming corpora lutea without actual copulation, in the same manner as the ovaries of quadrupeds that are only capable of breeding in a certain season of the year, exhibit during their heat manifest proofs of excitement, and especially of florid redness, when examined by dissection. I do not think the assertion concerning women is altogether established : but in the case of young men when entering upon, or emerging from pubescence, and of the relaxed and delicate frame just noticed, nothing is more common than involuntary erection and seminal emission during sleep, often connected with a train of amorous ideas excited by the local stimulus, as we have already observed under PARONIRIA SALAX.

It is possible that this affection may occasionally be a result of eutony or plethoric vigour, as well as of atony or delicacy of health : but the last is by far the most common cause.

In the first case we have nothing more to do than to reduce the excess of living power by copious venesections and purgatives, active labour or other exercise, and a low diet. In the second, it will be expedient in a very considerable degree to reverse the plan. We may, indeed, palliate the topical irritation by the use of leeches and cooling laxatives ; but, in conjunction with these, we should employ the unirritant tonics, as the salts of bismuth, zinc, and silver, or the sedative tonics, as the mineral acids, most of the bitters, and the cold bath. By taking off the debility, we take off the irritation ; and by taking off the irritation, we overpower the disease.

The SALACITY OF AGE is a very afflictive malady, and often wears away the hoary form to the last stage of a tabid decline, by the frequency of the orgastic paroxysms, and the drain of seminal emissions without enjoyment. It is usually a result of some accidental cause of irritation in the ovaria, the uterus, the testes, or the prostate gland, and has sometimes followed a stone in the kidneys or bladder ; and is hence best relieved by removing or palliating the local irritation by a warm hip-bath, anodyne injections, or cataplasms of hemlock, or the other umbellate or lurid plants in common use. Where these do not succeed, our only resource is opium and the warmer tonics.

ENTONIC SALACITY, or that of a robust and sanguine temperament, is not always so easily remedied as might at first be supposed. Copious venesections, purgatives, and a reducent diet, and this succeeded by a regular use of neutral salts, and especially of nitre, will often, indeed, be found highly beneficial. But the erethism occasionally becomes chronic, and defies the effects of all medicines whatever, and is excited by the slightest sensible causes, or even by the power of imagination (*Swed. Nov. Nosol. Syst.*, i., p. 231) ; and where there is an excess of irritability in the constitution, and the patient, from a principle of chastity, has sedulously restrained himself from all immoral indulgences, the nervous system, and even the mind itself, have sometimes suffered in a very distressing degree. One or two examples of this we have

already noticed under ECPHRONIA *mania*, or madness. The natural cure is a suitable marriage, wherever this can be accomplished ; but unless the union be of this character, it will often be attempted in vain. Professor Frank of Vienna, in his System of Medical Polity, relates the case of a lady of his acquaintance, of a warm and amorous constitution, who was unfortunately married to a very debilitated and impotent man ; and who, although she often betrayed unawares, by her looks and gestures, the secret fire that consumed her, yet, from a strong moral principle, resisted all criminal gratification. After a long struggle, her health at last gave way : a slow fever seized her, and released her from her sufferings.

The SALACITY OF A DEBAUCHED LIFE, or lechery produced and confirmed by habit, can only be cured by a total change of habit ; which is a discipline that the established debauchee has rarely the courage to attempt. Exercise, change of place and pursuits, cooling laxatives, and a less stimulant diet than he will commonly be found accustomed to, may assist him in the attempt ; but in general, the mind is as corrupt as the body, and the case is hopeless. He perseveres, however, at his peril, for with increasing weakness, he will at length sink into all the miserable train of symptoms characterizing that species of marasmus which is usually expressed by the name of tabes dorsalis.—(Cl. III., Ord. IV., Gen. III., Spe. 4.)

SPECIES II.

LAGNESIS FUROR.

LASCIVIOUS MADNESS.

APPETENCE UNBRIDLED, AND BREAKING THE BOUNDS OF MODEST DEMEANOUR AND CONVERSATION : MORBID AGITATION OF BODY AND MIND.

MOST of the causes of the preceding species are causes of the present, though it shows itself less frequently at the age of puberty. It is in fact very nearly related to the species SALACITAS, though the local irritation is more violent, and the mind participates more generally and in a very different manner. Under the first, the patient has a sufficiency of self-command to conduct himself at all times with decorum, and not to offend the laws and usages of public morals ; and if, as is rarely the case, however, the mind should at length become affected, it is rather by a transfer of the morbid irritation than an extension of it, so that patients thus afflicted very generally lose the venereal erethism, and show no reference to it in the train of their maniacal ideas. In lascivious madness, on the contrary, this last symptom continues in its utmost urgency, all self-command is broken down, the judgment is overpowered, the imagination enkindled and predominant, and the patient is hurried forward by the concupiscent fury like the brute creation in the season of heat, regardless equally of all company and all moral feeling. As it occurs in males, it is the *satyriasis furens* of Cullen ; as it occurs in females, it is the *nymphomania furibunda* of Sauvages.*

The pulse is quick, the breathing short, the patient is sleepless, thirsty, and loathes his food ; the urine is evacuated with difficulty, and there is a continual fever. In women, the disease is often connected with an hysterical temperament, and even commences with a semblance of melancholy (*Delius, Advers.*, fascic. i. ; *Belol, Furor Uterinus, Melancholicus Effectus*, Paris, 1621) ; and I once had an instance of it, from local irritation, shortly after childbirth. The child having suddenly died, and there being no more demand for a flow of milk, the fluid was repelled from the breasts with too little caution, and the uterine region, from the debility it was yet labouring under, became the seat of a transferred irritation. Among females, the disease is strikingly marked by the movements of the body and the salacious appearance of the countenance, and even the language that proceeds from the lips. There is often, indeed, at first, some degree of melancholy, with frequent sighings ; but the eyes roll in wanton glances, the cheeks are flushed, the bosom heaves, and every gesture exhibits the lurking desire, and is enkindled by the distressing flame that burns within.

In some cases, it has unquestionably proceeded from the perpetual friction of an enormous clitoris, making an approach, from its erection, to what Galen calls a female priapism. Büchner, Schurig (*Gynæcolog.*, pp. 2, 17), and Zacutus Lusitanus (*Prax. Admir.*, lib. ii., obs. 91), give numerous examples of this ; and Bartholine has the case of a Venetian woman of pleasure, whose clitoris was rendered bony by frequent use, and consequently became a source of constant irritation.

In hot climates, this kind of enlargement and elongation is by no means uncommon ; and as it becomes a source of uncleanliness as well as of undue excitement, circumcision, or a reduction of the clitoris to its proper size, has been often performed with advantage. The same operation has been proposed for the case before us, and, in some instances, it has succeeded completely. "A young woman," says Richerand, "was so violently affected with this disease as to have recourse to masturbation, which she

repeated so frequently as to reduce herself to the last stage of marasmus. Though sensible of the danger of her situation, she was not possessed of self-command enough to resist the orgastic urgency. Her parents took her to Professor Dubois, who, upon the authority of Levret, proposed an amputation of the clitoris, which was readily assented to. The organ was removed by a single stroke of the bistoury, and all hemorrhage prevented by an application of the cautery. The wound healed easily, and the patient obtained a radical cure of her distressing affection."—(*Nosographie Chirurgicale*, &c.)

Where the cause cannot be easily ascertained, we must employ a general plan of cure. If there be plethora or constitutional fulness, venesection should never be omitted ; and, in most cases, cooling laxatives, a spare diet, with acid fruits and vegetables, cold bathing, local and general, will be found useful. Nitre has often proved beneficial ; and to this may be added conium, aconite, and other narcotics. Camphire is also well worth a trial.

From the infuriate state of the mind in most cases of this malady, Vogel has arranged both satyriasis and nymphomania as species of MANIA. But this is incorrect ; the fury of the mind is merely symptomatic. Parr, on the contrary, has ranked it under LAGNESIS, to which, with great perversion, he applies the term *hallucinatio erotomania*, or love-sickness, more properly a variety of EMPATHEMA *desiderii*, and which, in the present and most other systems, is therefore regarded as a mental malady.

Love-sickness, however, may sometimes be an occasional or exciting cause, and its symptoms may be united with the complaint, and even add to the general effect, of which the History of the Academy of Sciences affords an instance (Ann. 1764, p. 26) ; but in itself it is, as we have already shown, altogether a disease of a different kind ; and where it becomes blended with concupiscent fury, it must be from a concurrence of some of the special causes of the latter, either general or local, which we have just pointed out.

In males, the disease has led to quite as much exhaustion as in females ; Bartholine gives an example of a hundred pollutions daily.

Ages.	Rape on Adults.	Rape on Children.	Total.
Under 21 years,	169	123	292
21 to 30,	105	58	163
30 to 40,	73	59	132
40 to 50,	61	94	155
50 to 60,	32	88	120
60 to 70,	14	166	180
Above 70,	23	318	341
			D.

GENUS IV.
AGENESIA.
MALE STERILITY.

INABILITY TO BEGET OFFSPRING.

THE generic term is a compound from *a*, negative, and γίνομαι, " to beget," and will be found to comprehend the three following species, derived from impotency of power or energy ; an imperfect emission where the power is adequate ; or an incongruity in the copulative influences or fluids upon each other :—

1. Agenesia Impotens.   Male Impotency.
2. ——— Dyspermia.   Seminal Misemission.
3. ——— Incongrua.   Copulative Incongruity.

Among plants we sometimes meet with a like

generative disability, occasionally from imperfectly formed styles or stigmas, stamens, or anthers; sometimes from a suppression of farina, and sometimes from a total destitution of seeds; which last defect is common to *bromelia ananas*; *musca paradisiaca*, or banyan; *artocarpus incisa*, or bread-fruit-tree; and *berberis vulgaris*, or common berberry.

SPECIES I.
AGENESIA IMPOTENS.
MALE IMPOTENCY.
IMPERFECTION OR ABOLITION OF GENERATIVE POWER.

THE species before us is perhaps more generally called by the nosologists anaphrodisia, though this last term has been used in very different senses; sometimes importing a want of desire, sometimes inability, sometimes both; and sometimes only a particular kind of inability; resulting from atony alone. The third species has never hitherto, so far as the author knows, been introduced into any nosological arrangement, although the reader will probably find, as he proceeds, sufficient ground for its admission. And even the first and second, closely as they are connected by nature, have rarely, if ever, been introduced before under the same common division, but been regarded as distinct genera, belonging to distant orders or even classes, and arranged with diseases that have little or no relation to them, of which numerous examples are given in the volume of Nosology.

Impotency in males may proceed from two very distinct causes, showing themselves in different ways, and laying a foundation for the following varieties:—

a Atonica.	Atonic Impotency.
β Organica.	Organic Impotency.

In tl.* FIRST of these, there is a direct imbecility or want of tone; produced chiefly by excess of indulgence, long-continued gleet,* or a paralytic affection of the generative organs. It has also been occasioned by a violent contusion on the loins, a fall on the nates (*Hildan.*, cent. vi., obs. 59), and sabre wounds of the back of the neck. Of the latter, Baron Larrey saw various examples in the campaigns of the French armies.†

Under the two first of these causes, a cure is often effected by time, and local tonics and stimulants, especially cold bathing: and the same process will frequently succeed where the weakness has followed a chronic gleet: in which

---

* This cause is not usually recognised, and, indeed, it is fortunate that impotency is probably never the effect of so common a complaint as an old gleet. Were it otherwise, one half of the male population in London would most certainly be afflicted with impotency in early manhood. Gleets which are attended with and arise from bad strictures in the urethra, are accompanied, it is true, with an impossibility of perfect seminal emission; but here the cause is not the gleet, but the obstruction in the urethra.—ED.

† See Chir. Militaire, &c. Such wounds were observed to bring on atrophy of the testicle.—ED.

VOL. II.—G g

we may also employ the course of remedies already recommended for this complaint.—(*Act. Nat. Cur.*, vol. v., obs. 59.)

Where the impotency results from a paresis or paralysis of the local nerves, or has been brought on by a life of debauchery, the case is nearly hopeless. We have heard much of aphrodisiacs, but there is none on which we can depend in effects of this kind. Wine, which is the ordinary stimulant in the case before us, will rarely succeed even in a single instance; and where it has done so, it has increased the debility afterward. It is, in truth, one of the most common causes of the disease itself.

Cantharides have often been employed, but in the present day they are deservedly distrusted, and flourish rather in proverbs than in practice.* Their effect, as a local stimulant, shows itself rather on the bladder and prostate gland than on the testes, and as a general irritant in increasing the heat and action of the whole system, in which the testes may, perhaps, sometimes have participated. "They are," says Dr. Cullen, "a stimulant and heating substance, and I have had occasion to know them, taken in large quantity as an aphrodisiac, to have excited violent pains in the stomach, and a feverish state over the whole body."—(*Mat. Med.*, vol. ii., p. 563.)

Many of the verticillate plants, as mint and pennyroyal, have been tried in a concentrated state for the same purpose, but with different, and even opposite effects, in the hands of different practitioners. To the present hour they are supposed by many to stimulate the uterus specifically, while they take off the venereal appetence in males. Upon sober and impartial trials, however, they seem to be equally guiltless of both: and may as readily be relinquished for such purposes as the nests of the Java swallow, which are purchased at a high price as a powerful incentive, and form an extensive article of commerce in the east.

The best aphrodisiacs are warm and general tonics, as the stimulant bitters, and the metallic salts, especially the preparations of iron. In China, ginseng has for ages been in high esteem, not only as a general restorative and roborant, but particularly in seminal debilities. Dr. Cullen appears to have thrown it out of practice, by telling us that he knew "a gentleman a little advanced in life, who chewed a quantity of this root every day for several years, but who acknowledged that he never found his venereal faculties in the least improved by it."

Local irritants, in many cases, have undoubtedly been of use, as blisters, caustics, and setons. Electricity is said to have been still more

---

* The remedial powers of the tincture of cantharides certainly deserve to be mentioned in more qualified terms: there are doubtless cases of impotency in which this article can have little or no good effect; but, on the other hand, it has proved serviceable in so many instances, that full confidence is placed in its powers, particularly in the United States, where it has been administered of late years with great freedom.—See Hosack's Appendix to Thomas's Practice of Medicine.—D.

extensively serviceable ; and friction with ammoniated oil, or spirits, or any other rubefacient, is fairly entitled to a trial. Stinging with nettle-leaves (*urtica urens*) was at one time a popular remedy, and flagellation of the loins (*Meibom. de Flagrorum usû in re Venereâ*) or nates (*Riedlin, Linn. Mcd.*, 1696, p. 6), or both, still more so.

In ORGANIC IMPOTENCY, forming our second variety, the chance of success is generally hopeless. This proceeds from a misformation or misorganization of the parts, either natural or accidental : as an amputated, injured, or enormous penis, or a defect or destitution of the testes.[*] Plater introduces brevity or exility of the penis (*Observ.*, lib. i., pp. 249, 250) among the causes, but these evils are generally overcome by habit. An incurvated, retracted, or otherwise distorted form, is also mentioned by many writers ; but such cases seem rather to belong to the ensuing species. An unaccommodating bulk of the organ seems to have been no uncommon cause.— (*Schurig. Gynæcolog.*, p. 226 ; *Wudel, Pathol.*, sect. iii., p. 11.) Schenck gives an instance of this kind, in which the bulk was produced by the monstrosity of a double penis (*Observ.*, lib. iv., N. 2, 8) ; and Albinus relates a case of a divorce obtained against a husband from inability to enter the vagina *ob penem inormem.*—(*Dissert. de Inspectione Corporis, forensis, in causis matrimonialibus fallacibus et dubiis*, Hall., 1740.) A similar litigation with divorce is recorded by Plater.—(*Observ.*, lib. i., p. 250.)

It has been doubted, whether a retention of the testes in the abdomen, or in the path of their descent, will necessarily produce impotency. Swediaur distinctly affirms that impotency is not a consequence, and points out the importance of rightly distinguishing between a real and apparent deficiency, in respect to the one or the other of these two cases.[†]

---

[*] Bad strictures in the urethra, a cause already alluded to in a foregoing page, would rank as a case of organic impotency.—Ed.

[†] Nov. Nosol. Syst., vol. ii., p. 351. This point has been already considered in the present vol., see p. 417. In Sir Astley Cooper's Observations on the Structure and Diseases of the Testes, Lond., 4to., 1830, pp. 52, 53, may be found some interesting facts relating to the subject of this part of Dr. Good's work. From these it appears, that a wasting of one testis at an early period of life does not deprive the individual of the power of procreation. Neither does the removal of one testis always seem to lessen virility. " A gentleman had his testis removed in January, 1821, for an enlargement and great hardness. He recovered in three weeks. His wife, by whom he had already had one child, nursed him during his confinement. In the month of March she proved pregnant, about nine weeks after the performance of the operation." Mr. Headington knew a man who had several children after losing one testicle by an operation. A man, one of whose testicles had been absorbed fourteen years, from wearing a truss for hernia congenita, married, and in due time became a father. It has twice fallen to the lot of Sir Astley Cooper to remove the testicle, where the other had already been lost. In the second case here referred to, the operation was

SPECIES II.
AGENESIA DYSSPERMIA.
SEMINAL MISEMISSION.
IMPERFECT EMISSION OF THE SEMINAL FLUID.

THIS is the dysspermatismus, or, as it is usually but incorrectly spelled, dy-spermatismus, of authors. The termination is varied, not merely on account of greater brevity and simplicity, but in conformity with the parallel Greek compounds, polyspermia, gymnospermia, aspermia, terms well known to every botanist, and the former of which are elegantly introduced into the Linnéan vocabulary.

Imperfection or defect of emission proceeds from numerous causes, accompanied with some change of symptoms as appertaining to each, and laying a foundation for the following varieties :—

α Entonica.	The imperfect emission proceeding from super-erection or priapism.
Entonic misemission.	
β Epileptica.	Rendered imperfect by the incursion of an epileptic spasm produced by sexual excitement during the intercourse.
Epileptic misemission.	
γ Anticipans.	The discharge ejected hastily, prematurely, and without due adjustment.
Anticipating misemission.	
δ Cunctans.	The discharge unduly retarded from hebetude of the genital organs ; and hence not accomplished till the orgasm, on the part of the female, has subsided.
Retarding misemission.	
ε Refluens.	The discharge thrown back into the vesiculæ seminales,[*] or the bladder, before it reaches the extremity of the penis.
Refluent misemission.	

---

performed in Guy's Hospital, in 1801. Four days afterward, the patient informed Sir Astley that he had had, in the preceding night, an emission, which appeared upon his linen. For nearly a twelvemonth, it seems that he had emissions *in coitu*, or the sensation of them. That he then had erections and connexion at long intervals, but without the sensations of emission. After two years, he had erections very rarely and imperfectly, and in time the penis became shrivelled and wasted. It would appear, then, that in this case castration led to a cessation of all seminal emission at the end of a few months. The emission, such as it was, also, could only have been of the fluids secreted by the vesiculæ seminales and prostate gland.—Ed.

[*] The idea, once prevalent, that the vesiculæ seminales were merely reservoirs for the semen, has yielded to the better-founded opinion, that their office is to produce a secretion of their own, which becomes blended with the semen. Mr. Hunter remarked, not only that the fluid contained in the vesiculæ seminales was quite different from semen ; but that, when the testis on one side had been long removed, the same fluid was still found, on dissection, in the corresponding vesicula seminalis. Dr. Good's statement, therefore, respecting the reflux of the semen into the vesiculæ seminales, must be regarded as erroneous.—Ed.

Of the first, or ENTONIC VARIETY, examples are by no means uncommon. Dr. Cockburn gives an instance in a young noble Venetian, who, though married to a fine and healthy young lady, had no seminal emission in the act of union, notwithstanding there was a vigorous erection, while he could discharge very freely in his dreams.—(See a similar case in *Marcel. Donat.*, lib. iv., cap. 18.) As no remedy could be devised at home, the Venetian ambassadors, resident at the different courts of Europe, were requested to consult the niost eminent physicians in their various quarters. The case came in this manner under the notice of Dr. Cockburn, who, hitting accurately upon the cause of the retention, and ascribing it to the violence of the erection, or rather, to the plethora of the penis, whose distention produced a temporary imperforation of the urethra, advised purgative medicines and a slender diet, which soon produced the desired issue.—(*Edin. Med. Essays*, i., p. 270.)

I remember, many years ago, a healthy young couple, who continued without offspring for seven or eight years after marriage, at which period the lady, for the first time, became pregnant, and continued to add to her family every year till she had six or seven children; and in professional conversation with the father, he has clearly made it appear to me that the cause of sterility during the above period was the morbid eutony we are now discussing. Time, that by degrees broke the vigour of the encounter, effected at length a radical cure, and gave him an offspring he had almost despaired of. Mr. J. Hunter recommends opium in this case, as the best allayer of the undue stimulus, and nothing can be more judicious; for M. Bauer has shown, by microscopical drawings, that the corpus spongiosum, as well as the corpora cavernosa, are divided into cells or trellis-work by an infinite number of fine membranous plates, and that the minute arteries which open into them, and fill them with blood in their distended state, are very numerously attended with nerves (*Phil. Trans., communicated by Sir E. Home, Bart.*, 1820, p. 183), the peculiar excitement of which produces the exundation. And hence opium or any other narcotic, by acting as a sedative, and moderating the excitement, must bring down the organ to a desirable scale of tone.

The SECOND VARIETY, or misemission from the incursion of an epileptic fit, it is not difficult to account for. Persons who are predisposed to epilepsy are for the most part of a highly irritable habit; and wherever the predisposition exists, any accidental excitement is sufficient to produce a fresh paroxysm: and hence it is seldom more likely to occur than from the commotion of a sexual embrace. Even death itself has sometimes ensued in consequence of the violence of the venereal paroxysm. Examples of epilepsy from this cause, as collected in the public medical records, are numerous. Among men, one of the most famous instances is that of the celebrated Hunnish chief Attila.—(*Borelli, Amalth. Med. Hist.*, p. 161.)

Morgagni (*De Sed. et Caus. Morb.*, ep. xxvi., art. 13) and Sinbaldus (*Geneanthropia*, p. 794) have given examples among women.

Hence, a life of matrimony had better be relinquished by those who are thus afflicted, as well on their own accounts as on that of their descendants. And where marriage is actually effected, sexual commerce should be sedulously abstained from at the periods in which the disease is accustomed to recur, or during the continuance of those signs by which a paroxysm is usually preceded.

The THIRD and FOURTH VARIETIES, or anticipating and retarding misemission, are put together by Ploucquet under the name of *ejaculatio intempestiva* (*Init. Biblioth.*, tom. iv., p. 61, 4to., Tubing., 1795), and are equally entitled to this character: while the former is, by Schenck, denominated *ejaculatio præmatura*.—(*Observ.*, lib. iv., obs. 46.)

The anticipating or premature variety evinces great nervous irritability in a delicate or relaxed habit; the plethora of the first or entonic variety would produce the best and most effectual cure; but as this is rarely to be accomplished in a constitution of this kind, tonics, a plain but nutritious diet, especially light suppers, and, more especially still, a bidet of cold water before retiring to bed, form the most effectual means of subduing this precession of generative power. In some cases, the afflux has been so quick as to take place even before the vagina has been fairly entered.

The FOURTH or RETARDING VARIETY forms a perfect contrast to the preceding. It imports a sluggishness either of constitution or of local erethism, in consequence of which the seminal flow does not take place till the orgasm of the female has subsided, and fatigue, perhaps disgust, have succeeded to desire. Here, too, general tonics and local stimulants offer the fairest chance of success; and both sting-nettles (*Eph. Nat. Cur.*, dec. ii., ann. v., App., p. 794) and flagellations (*Meibom. and Riedlin.*, loc. citat.), as in some cases of organic impotency, are said to have worked wonders. The variety is generally described under the name of bradyspermatismus.

The REFLUENT VARIETY is chiefly introduced upon the authority of M. Petit (*Mémoires de l'Academie de Chirurgie*, i., p. 434), whose description has been copied by Sauvages. "It consists," he tells us, "in a reflux of the semen into the bladder or vesiculæ seminales, on account of the narrowness of the urethra, in consequence of which there is no semination during the inter-union, and the semen is afterward discharged with the urine."

This narrowness is common to those who have suffered from frequent blennorrhœas, and have hence contracted strictures or indurations in the course of the urethral passage. Deidier adverts to a patient who laboured under a fistula that opened from the vesiculæ seminales into the rectum; in consequence of which, though sound in every other respect, whenever he embraced his wife, scarcely any of the semen escaped from the penis, nearly the whole passing into the intestine, intermixed with a small quantity of urine; and hence his marriage was steril:[*]

In all these cases, the cure of the impotency must depend upon a cure of the local cause of constriction. The *dysspermatismus urethralis, nodosus,* and *mucosus* of Sauvages, and Cullen, who has copied from him, are all resolvable into this variety, as proceeding from like causes, and producing a like effect.

SPECIES III.
AGENESIA INCONGRUA.
COPULATIVE INCONGRUITY.

THE SEMINAL FLUID INACCORDANT, IN ITS CONSTITUENT PRINCIPLES, WITH THE CONSTITUTIONAL DEMAND OF THE RESPECTIVE FEMALE.

ALL the species of this genus are closely connected : yet it is only the first two that have hitherto been noticed by nosologists : nor is there any preceding system, that I am aware of, under which even these two have been introduced into the same subdivision. In almost every instance, indeed, they have been regarded as distinct genera, belonging to distant orders or even classes, and arranged with diseases that have little or no relation to them. Thus, in Sauvages, impotentia, by him called anaphrodisia, occurs in the second order of his sixth class, united with such diseases as "loss of thirst", and "desire of eating;" while dysspermia, or dysspermatismus, is carried forward to the third order of his ninth class. In Cullen, these diseases occur indeed in the same class, a very improper one, that of LOCALES; but under different orders of this class; impotentia being arranged under the second order, with the morbid cravings of the alimentary canal, and some of those of the mind, as nostalgia; and dysspermia being placed under the fifth order, entitled *epischeses*, or SUPPRESSIONS.

The present species is, for the first time, so far as the author knows, introduced into a nosological system; and is derived from personal observation, in full accordance with the scattered remarks of several other writers and practitioners. The principle upon which the species

is founded, belongs strictly to the general doctrine of conception, and has been already explained in the Physiological Proem to the present class. It will hence be sufficient to throw out a few additional hints, for the purpose of bringing the principle more immediately home to the disease before us, and supporting the propriety of its introduction into the general register.

Every one must have noticed occasional instances in which a husband and wife, apparently in sound health and vigour of life, have no increase while together; either of whom, nevertheless, upon the death of the other, has become the parent of a numerous family; and both of whom, in one or two curious instances of divorce, upon a second marriage. In various instances, indeed, the latent cause of sterility, whatever it consists in, seems gradually to diminish, and the pair that was years childless is at length endowed with a progeny. In all this, there seems to be an incongruity, inaccordancy, or want of adaptation, in the constituent principles of the seminal fluid of the male to the sexual organization of the respective female; or upon the hypothesis of the epigenesis, which we have already illustrated, to the seminal fluid of the female. Writers, strictly medical, have not often adverted to this subject, though it is appealed to, and for the most part with approbation, by physiologists of all ages and countries. Sauvages, however, evidently alludes to and admits such a cause in his definition of *disspermatismus serosus,* which is as follows :— "Ejaculatio seminis aquosioris, adeoque ad genesim inepti, quæ species est frequentissimum sterilitatis virilis principium." He illustrates his definition by a case which occurred to Haguenot and Chaptal, who attributed it to the cause in question, and refers for other examples to Etmuller. Cullen expresses himself doubtfully upon this species, "De dysspermatismo seroso Sauvagesii," says he, "mihi non satis constat." Yet his own *gonorrhœa luxorum,* in the present system *spermorrhœa atonica,* and which he explains "humor plerumque pellucidus, sine penis erectione, sed cum libidine, in vigilante, ex urethra fluit," makes so near an approach to it, that the physiologist who admits the one can find little difficulty in admitting the other. The resemblance is indeed close and striking; in the latter disease, the individual labouring under it emits involuntarily, and *without coition,* or even erection, but with a libidinous sensation, a pellucid fluid, apparently of a seminal character, affirmed positively by Sauvages, from whom Cullen derives his species, and to whom he refers, to be an "effluxus seminis;" while, in the former, the same dilute and effete semen, with difficult and imperfect erection, is poured forth *during coition.*

In like manner, Forestus speaks of a proper gonorrhœa, or involuntary emission of the seminal fluid, produced *ex aquositate* (Lib. xxvi., obs. 12), from too watery a condition of the secretion: Timæus, of the same disease occasioned *ex semine acri (Cas.,* p. 188), by a secretion of an acrimonious semen; and Hornung, of hys-

---

[*] Tom. iii., consult. i. That the account here given cannot possibly be correct, is quite obvious ; first, because a communication between the vesicula seminalis and the rectum will not explain the alleged circumstance of nearly the whole of the semen passing into that bowel instead of along the urethra. This is obvious, even if the vesiculæ seminales were reservoirs for the semen, as was once the incorrect supposition ; but now, when it is known that they perform no such office, the insufficiency of the explanation is still more manifest. Secondly, if urine really passed into the rectum, there must have been a fistula between the cavity of the bowel and that of the bladder ; and therefore, in all probability, no such communication between the vesicula seminalis and the rectum ; and the fluid, conjectured to be semen, could have been neither the secretion of the testes, nor that of the vesicula seminalis, but possibly some of the mucus of the inner coat of the bowel itself. The patient's infirmity must have been owing to different causes.—ED.

terics occasioned in married women, who are steril from an "immissio *frigidi* seminis" (*Cista*, p. 487) ; an expression adopted from, or at least employed by Ballonius (Opp. i., p. 120), and supported by Schurig (*Spermatologia*, p. 21) and Ab Heer.—(*Observ. Rar.*, N. 10.)

The explanation, however, now offered, takes a more comprehensive view of the subject, by supposing that the seminal fluid may be secreted, not merely in a state of morbid diluteness, but under various modifications, even in a state of health, of such a condition as to render it inadequate to the purposes of generation in female idiosyncrasies of certain kinds, while it may be perfectly adequate in those of other kinds. In agricultural language, it supposes that the respective seed may not be adapted to the respective soil, however sound in itself. So Parr tells us, on another occasion, that " in some instances, the semen itself seems defective in its essential qualities."—(*Diss.*, *art. Anaphrodisia.*)*

Here, again, the mode of treatment must be regulated by a close attention to the nature of the cause. In most cases, whatever will tend to invigorate the system generally, will best tend to cure the sterility : as a generous diet, exercise, the cold bath, and particularly the use of the bidet or local cold bath. With these may be combined the warm and stimulant resins and balsams, as guaiacum, turpentine, copayva ; and the oxydes of iron, zinc, and silver.

Abstinence by consent for many months has, however, proved a more frequent remedy than any other, and especially where the intercourse has been so incessantly repeated as to break down the staminal strength : and hence the separation produced by a voyage to India, has often proved successful.

GENUS V.
APHORIA.
FEMALE STERILITY. BARRENNESS.
INABILITY TO CONCEIVE OFFSPRING.

APHORIA (ἀφορία), "sterilitas," "infecunditas," from a, negative, and φέρω, "fero," "pario," is a term in common use among the Greek writers. It is singular that the morbid condition it imports has no distinct place in any of our most esteemed nosologists. It may possibly be intended under the anaphrodisia of several of them, though in none of them has the genus any one species that expressly applies to female barrenness.

The proper species belonging to it are the following :—

1. Aphoria Impotens. Barrenness of Impotency.
2. ——— Paramen-　Barrenness of Mismenica.　　struation.
3. ——— Impercita. Barrenness of Irrespondence.
4. ——— Incongrua. Barrenness of Incongruity.

---

* A latent syphilitic taint on the part of the male is an occasional cause of this infirmity. The cure is obvious.—D.

SPECIES I.
APHORIA IMPOTENS.
BARRENNESS OF IMPOTENCY.
IMPERFECTION OR ABOLITION OF CONCEPTIVE POWER.

THIS species runs precisely parallel with the same disease in males, already described under AGENESIA *impotens*, and consequently offers us the two following varieties :—

　α Atonica.　　Atonic Barrenness.
　β Organica.　　Organic Barrenness.

In ATONIC BARRENNESS, there is a direct imbecility or want of tone, rather than a want of desire ; and the ordinary causes are, a life of intemperance of any kind, especially of intemperate indulgence in sexual pleasures, a chronic leucorrhœa, or paralytic affection of the generative organs. It has also been occasioned by violent contusions in the loins or the hypogastric region, and by over-exertion in walking.

The plan of treatment is to be the same as already laid down under atonic sterility or impotency in males ; yet it is seldom that any treatment has afforded success under this variety.

ORGANIC BARRENNESS is produced by some structural hinderance or defect, whether natural or accidental. And this may be of various kinds ; for the vagina may be imperforate, and prohibit not only all intermission of semen, but an entrance of the penis itself. The ovaria may be defective, or even altogether wanting, or not duly developed, or destitute of ovula ; or the fimbriæ may be defective, and incapable of grasping the uterus ; or the Fallopian tube may be obstructed, or impervious, or wanting ; in all which cases barrenness must necessarily ensue. In the case of an impervious vagina, however, unless there be a total occlusion, conception will sometimes follow : for it has occurred where the passage has been so narrow as not to admit the penis ; and occasionally indeed, when, with the same impediment, a rigid and unbroken hymen has offered an additional obstacle, of which the medical records contain abundant examples. Ruysch gives us a singular case of a hymen found unbroken at the time of labour.

These, however, are rare instances ; for the impediment before us is usually a sufficient bar, not only to conception, but to copulation. In such a case, the author was once consulted by a young couple to whom the want of a family was felt as a grievous affliction. The hymen had a small aperture, but was tense and firm, and the ordinary force of an embrace was not sufficient to break it. He explained the nature of the operation to be performed, and added that he had no doubt of a successful issue. The lady was reluctant to submit herself to the hands of a surgeon, and hence, with equal courage and judgment, became her own operator. The impediment was completely removed, and she has since had several children.

In a few instances, however, this will not answer ; for there is a natural narrowness or stricture sometimes found in the vagina which cannot be overcome, at least without a severer operation than most women could be induced to submit to—that I mean of laying it open through the whole length of the contraction. A sponge tent, however, gradually enlarged, or a bougie, has sometimes succeeded. Schurig gives an account of a dissolution of marriage in consequence of an impediment of this kind.—(*Gynæcolog.*, p. 223.)*

SPECIES II.
APHORIA PARAMENICA.
BARRENNESS OF MISMENSTRUATION.

CATAMENIAL DISCHARGE MORBIDLY' RETAINED, SECRETED WITH DIFFICULTY OR IN PROFUSION.

IT is not always necessary to impregnation that a female should menstruate, for we have already observed (see *Paramenia Obstructionis*) that a retention of menses, or rather a want of menstruation, is not always a disease; but only where symptoms occur which indicate a disordered state of some part or other of the body, and which experience teaches us is apt to arise in consequence of such retention. In some cases there is great torpitude or sluggishness in the growth or development, or proper erethism of the ovaries, and menstruation is delayed on this account; and in a few rare instances, we have remarked that it has occurred for the first time after sixty years of age. It may hence easily happen, and we shall presently have occasion to show that it often has done so, that a woman becomes married who has never been subject to this periodical flux; and although it is little to be expected that she should breed till the sexual organs are in a condition to elaborate this secretion, yet if such condition take place after marriage, impregnation may instantly succeed, and prohibit or postpone the efflux which would otherwise take place.—(Class V., Order III., *Carpotica, Introductory remarks*.)

But when there is a manifest retention of the catamenial flux, producing the general symptoms of disorder which we noticed in describing this disease, it is rarely that conception takes place, in consequence of the morbid condition of the organs that form its seat.

For the same reason, it seldom occurs where the periodical flow is accompanied with great and spasmodic pain, is small in quantity, and often deteriorated in quality. And if during any intermediate term conception accidentally commence, the very next paroxysm of distressing pain puts a total end to all hope, by separating the germe from the uterus.

But there must be a healthy degree of tone and energy in the conceptive organs, as well as of ease and quiet, in order that they should prove fruitful; and hence, wherever the menstrual flux is more frequently repeated than in its natural course, or is thrown forth even at its proper time in great profusion, and, as is gener-

ally the case, intermixed with genuine blood, there is as little chance of conception as in difficult menstruation. The organs are too dehilitated for the new process, and not unfrequently there is as little desire as elasticity.

Having thus pointed out the general causes and physiology of barrenness when a result of mismenstruation, it will be obvious that the cure must depend upon a removal of the particular kind of morbid affection that operates at the time, and lays a foundation for the disease, of all which we have already treated under the different species of the genus PARAMENIA, and need not repeat what is there laid down.

SPECIES III.
APHORIA IMPERCITA.
BARRENNESS OF IRRESPONDENCE.

STERILITY PRODUCED BY PERSONAL AVERSION OR WANT OF APPETENCE.

IT is not perhaps altogether impossible that impregnation should take place in the case of a rape, or where there is a great repugnance on the part of the female; for there may be so high a tone of constitutional orgasm as to be beyond the control of the individual who is thus forced, and not to be repressed even by a virtuous recoil and a sense of horror at the time. But this is a possible rather than an actual case, and though the remark may be sufficient to suspend a charge of criminality, the infamy can only be completely wiped away by collateral circumstances.*

In ordinary instances, rude, brutal force is never found to succeed against the consent of the violated person. And for the same reason, wherever there is a personal aversion, a coldness or reserve, instead of an appetence and pleasure, an irresponse in the feelings of the female to those of the male, we have as little reason to hope for a parturient issue. There must be an orgastic shock or percussion sufficient to shoot off an ovulum from its bed, and to urge the fine and irritable fimbriæ of the Fallopian tube to lay hold of the uterus and grasp it tight, by which alone a communication can be opened between this last organ and the ovarium, or the seed cannot reach home to its proper soil and produce a harvest. So observes the first didactic poet of ancient Rome, addressing himself to the Generative Power, in the language not of the voluptuary, but of the physiologist :—

" — par maria, ac monteis, fluviosque rapaceis
Frundiferasque domos avium, camposque virenteis,
Omnibus INCUTIENS blandum per pectora amorem,
Ecficis, et CUPIDE generatim secla propagant."†

---

* A singular case of malformation, occurring in the practice of Dr. Mott, may be seen in the New-York Med. and Phys. Journal, vol. ii., p. 18.—D.

* Dr. Ryan seems to have no hesitation in concluding, from cases to which he refers, that defloration may happen during sleep without the knowledge of the female, or when she is intoxicated, has fainted, or is under the influence of narcotics, and that pregnancy has happened under such circumstances—"facts that demonstrate the absurdity of the English law upon the subject. They also prove that conception may take place after rape."—(See Ryan's Manual of Midwifery, p. 154.)
† De Rer. Nat., i., 17.

" So through the seas, the mountains, and the
    floods,
The verdant meads, and woodlands fill'd with
    song,
SPURK'D BY DESIRE, each palpitating tribe
Hastes, at thy shrine, to plant the future race."

The cause is clear and the effect certain, but
it is a disease immedicable by the healing art,
and can only be attacked by a kind, assiduous,
and winning attention, which, however slighted
at first, will imperceptibly work into the cold
and stony heart as the drops of rain work into
the pavement. It should teach us, however,
the folly of forming family connexions, and endeavouring to keep up a family name, where the
feelings of affection are not engaged on both
sides.

SPECIES IV.
APHORIA INCONGRUA.
BARRENNESS OF INCONGRUITY.
THE CONCEPTIVE POWER INACCORDANT WITH
THE CONSTITUENT PRINCIPLES OF THE SEMI-
NAL FLUID RECEIVED ON THE PART OF THE
MALE.

THIS species runs precisely parallel with the
third under the preceding genus AGENESIA *incongrua*, and the physiological and therapeutic
remarks there offered will equally apply to the
present place.*

GENUS VI.
ÆDOPTOSIS.
GENITAL PROLAPSE.
PROTRUSION OF ONE OR MORE OF THE GENITAL
ORGANS, OR OF EXCRESCENCES ISSUING FROM
THEM INTO THE GENITAL PASSAGE; IMPAIRING
OR OBSTRUCTING ITS COURSE.

ÆDOPTOSIS is a compound term from αἰδοῖον,
" inguen," pl. αἰδοῖα, " pudenda," whence αἰδῶς,
" pudor," and πτῶσις, " lapsus." In like manner,
Sauvages and Sagar use Ædopsophia, applying
the term to the meatus urinarius as well as to
the uterus. Sauvagès, however, expresses the
present disease, but less correctly, by hysteroptosis; for this with strict propriety can denote
only one of the species that fall within its range,
namely, displacement of the uterus.

The genus embraces the five following species:—

1. Ædoptosis Uteri. Falling down of the
                          Womb.
2. ———— Vaginæ. Prolapse of the Vagina.
3. ———— Vesicæ. Prolapse of the Bladder.
4. ———— Compli- Complicated   Genital
          cata.   Prolapse.
5. ———— Polyposa. Genital Excrescence.

* Dr. T. R. Beck has treated, with great perspi-
cuity, the subject of sterility as connected with
juridical medicine.—See his Elements of Med.
Jurisprudence, vol. i. Many interesting remarks
on the same topic may be found in Paris and Fonblanque's Medical Jurisprudence. See likewise
Smith's Forensic Medicine, 3d edition, London;
and Chitty's Medical Jurisprudence, part i., Philadelphia, 1835.—D.

SPECIES I.
ÆDOPTOSIS UTERI.
FALLING DOWN OF THE WOMB:
PROTRUSION OF THE UTERUS INTO THE VAGINA.

THIS may take place in several ways, and
hence offers the following varieties:—

α Simplex.   Simple descent of the Womb.
β Retroversa. Retroverted Womb.
λ Inversa.   Inverted Womb.

In the FIRST VARIETY, or that consisting of a
simple descent of the uterus, the organ retains
its proper posture and figure. Different names
are frequently given to different degrees of this
variety. If the descent be only to the middle
of the vagina, it is called *relaxatio uteri*; if to
the labiæ, *procidentia*; if lower than the labiæ,
prolapsus.* The distinction is of trifling importance; the causes are the same in all, which
are those of debility or violence. The disease
is hence most common to women who have had
numerous families, but is occasionally met with
in virgins after straining, using violent exercise
in dancing or running, or meeting with falls
during menstruation, and hence sometimes in
girls of a very early age. Professor Monro gives
an example of its occurring in an infant of not
more than three years old, preceded by a regular menstruation, or more properly, a discharge
of blood, every three weeks or months, from the
vagina, accompanied with considerable pain in
the belly, loins, and thighs. The case was too
long neglected, as being supposed of little importance; and the uterus, which at first appeared
to be a very small body just peeping out of the
vagina, descended lower and lower, continually
increasing in size, till at length it became as big
as a hand-ball, and entirely blocked up the passage of the pudendum. At this time the returns
of sanguineous discharge had ceased, but a considerable leucorrhœa supervened. The uterus
seems at last to have been strangulated, gangrene ensued, and was soon succeeded by death.
—(*Edin. Med. Essays*, vol. iii., art. xvii., p.
282.)

The disease first shows itself by what is
called a bearing down of the womb, which is a
slight descent produced by a relaxed state of its
ligaments, and its own weight when in an upright position. There is, at this time, an uneasy sensation in the loins, as well as in the inguinal regions, often extending to the labia, and
particularly in walking or standing. There is
also an augmented flow of the natural mucous
secretion in consequence of the local irritation,
which by degrees acquires an irritating quality, excoriates the surrounding parts, and is accompanied with an obstinate leucorrhœa. The
stomach sympathizes with the morbid state of
the womb, the appetite fails, the bowels be-

* Instances are recorded in which the uterus
had been beyond the external parts for two, and
even eighteen years; yet in the latter case, the
woman was not prevented, by the situation of the
womb, from having six children.—See Ashwell,
in London Medical and Surgical Journal, 1830,
vol. iv.—ED.

come irregular and flatulent, and the animal spirits are dejected.

In attempting a cure, we must first restore the prolapsed organ to its proper position, and then retain it there, by a support introduced into the vagina, which should be continued till the ligaments of the womb have recovered their proper tone.* Various pessaries have been invented for this purpose, but that made of the caoutchouc, or elastic gum,† with a ligature to withdraw it at option, appears to be one of the most commodious.‡ Astringent injections, as a solution of alum or sulphate of zinc, of gall, oak bark, or green tea, or even cold water, will generally be found useful ; as will also sponging the body with cold water, or using a hip-bath of seawater. Dr. Clark prefers the vegetable to the mineral injections, having found the latter sometimes too irritating.—(*On the Diseases of Females attended by Discharges*, part i.) New and rough port wine, diluted with an equal quantity of cold water, has proved one of the most valuable injections to which the author has ever had recourse. A sofa or hair mattress should also be used, instead of the relaxing luxury of a down or feather-bed.

Dr. Berchelmann, in a foreign journal, has recommended a far bolder cure, derived from the rash but successful practice of a woman upon herself. This courageous sufferer, having long laboured under a prolapse of the womb, and tried every method in vain, tired out with the continuance of her complaint, cut into the depending substance of the womb with a common kitchen-knife. A considerable hemorrhage ensued ; after which, the vessels collapsing, the organ gradually contracted, and ascended into its proper site ; and she was radically cured of the disease. Having heard of her success, other women in the neighbourhood, afflicted with the same complaint, applied for her assistance, and derived a like cure from the same operation.—(*Acta Philosophico-Medica Soc. Acad.*

---

* It is alleged that it is not an easy matter to occasion a prolapse of the uterus in the dead body, though the broad ligaments have been divided for the purpose: hence, Dr. Dewees conceives that the vagina is the chief support of this organ, which view sufficiently accounts for the tendency to its displacement arising from frequent deliveries, habitual coughs, severe vomitings, and efforts and exertions imprudently made during the menstrual period. Probably the common explanation of the origin of prolapsus uteri from relaxation of those ligaments has little foundation, and whatever elongation they undergo is only an effect.—D.

† Pessaries of this material are most generally used by American practitioners.—D.

‡ In France, the species of pessary generally preferred is that of linen covered with wax, resembling a round or oval disk or plate, with obtuse borders, and open in the centre; or caoutchouc, stuffed with scraped cotton, but of the same mechanic figure. If prolapsus uteri take place soon after delivery, from the woman getting up too early, the immediate application of a pessary would be improper ; the part should be carefully reduced, the patient kept in bed, and mild aperient medicines prescribed. In every case where a pessary is employed, it should be withdrawn and cleaned every third or fourth day.—Ed.

Scient. Princ. Hassiacæ, 4to., Giessæ Cattorum.) It must; however, be useless where the relaxation is seated in the ligaments.*

[When the fundus uteri descends towards the sacrum, or, in other words, between the vagina and rectum, and the os tincæ inclines towards the pubes, the displacement is termed a *retroversion of the womb.* This organ, in fact, is subject to various changes of position, and its axis, with respect to that of the pelvis, may incline backwards, forwards, or to either side. The displacement forwards, which is much less frequent than that backwards, receives the name of *anteversion.* Retroversion is mostly met with in the third or fourth month of pregnancy ; though it sometimes occurs in unimpregnated females, and certain practitioners have even seen it happen oftener in them than in the pregnant.—(*Richter's* Chir. Bibl., b. v., s. 132, b. ix., s. 310; *Stark's Archiv. für die Geburtshulfe,* b. iv., s. 637 ; *Siebold's Journ.,* b. iii., s. 59.) Probably, a retroversion of the womb is never produced all at once, but very gradually, and under the operation of particular circumstances. Thus, at first, the fundus of the organ inclines somewhat lower than usual, and this change by degrees becomes a complete retroversion. As general predisposing causes, may be mentioned a capacious pelvis; deep situation of the viscera ; relaxation of the broad and round ligaments, &c. The occasional causes may be, pregnancy ; immoderate distention of the bladder ; constipation and hard straining at stool ; long continuance in the recumbent posture ; increased weight of the fundus uteri ; and violent efforts.

The symptoms chiefly depend upon the impediments created to the evacuation of the urine and feces, and upon certain morbid changes which occur in the displaced uterus itself. Thus, when a retroversion takes place in pregnancy, the bladder and rectum are suddenly prevented from emptying themselves† ; a sensation of bearing down is experienced, accompanied with tenderness and tension of the abdomen, nausea, and even vomiting, fever, abortion, and sometimes death itself, in consequence of sloughing of the bladder, and effusion of the urine among the viscera. When a finger is introduced into the vagina, the os tincæ is perceived to be behind or above the pubes ; while the fundus uteri is felt making a hard projection at the posterior side of the passage, or that towards the sacrum ; and it presses upon the rectum, within which it may also be felt. The treat-

---

* In what Madame Boivin terms *precipitation*, or *complete prolapsus*, in which the uterus protrudes from the vulva, and hangs between the thighs, covered by the reverted vagina, and containing the bladder and part of the rectum, any rational scheme of relief is entitled to encouragement. With this view is here mentioned Dr. Marshall Hall's method of preventing the return of this extreme protrusion ; it consists in removing a slip of the mucous membrane, which is followed by an arctation of the vagina.—Ed.

† The elevation of the cervix uteri has the effect of compressing the neck of the bladder and the urethra against the os pubis.—Ed.

ment of retroversion consists in emptying the bladder and rectum, and restoring the uterus to its proper position. The first object is to be fulfilled by means of a catheter, the introduction of which will be considerably facilitated, when the portion of the vagina, drawn upward towards the pubes, is pushed downward with the fingers of the left hand. Thus, the orifice and direction of the meatus urinarius, which are sometimes so changed that the passage of the catheter is impracticable, becomes rectified, and the operation succeeds. It has, however, sometimes been found impossible to draw off the urine with a catheter, and absolutely necessary to puncture the bladder.—(*Cheston in Med. Commun.*, vol. ii.) The second indication is to empty the rectum with clysters ; the introduction of which, however, is frequently difficult. After these measures, of which the most efficient is the emptying of the bladder and keeping it in this condition, the uterus often returns spontaneously into its natural position ; and when this does not happen, manual assistance must be given.]

The WOMB is INVERTED when, at the same time that it is displaced or has fallen down, it is turned inside out. This mischievous condition is most commonly produced by unskilfully and violently pulling away the placenta after delivery : and this is only to be remedied by a restoration of the uterus to its proper state before it contracts, without which perpetual barrenness must necessarily ensue, and the patient be subject for life to a difficulty of walking, leucorrhœa, ulceration, and the chance of a scirrhus or cancer.*

SPECIES II.
ÆDOPTOSIS VAGINÆ.
PROLAPSE OF THE VAGINA.
PROTRUSION OF THE UPPER PART OF THE VAGINA INTO THE LOWER.

THIS, like the descent of the uterus, may, according to the degree of the disease, be a relaxation, procidence, prolapse, or complete inversion of the organ. Under all which modifications it has a considerable resemblance to a prolapse of the anus. It appears in the form of a fleshy substance protruding at the back part of the vulva, with an opening in the centre or on one side. At first it is soft, but by continued exposure and irritation, it becomes inflamed, indurated, and ulcerated. The urethra is necessarily turned out of its course ; and if the catheter be required, it should be employed with its point directed backwards and downwards. Its

* The frequent hemorrhage, down-bearing pains, and general weakness, caused by inversion of the uterus, when it does not admit of being rectified, sometimes makes it necessary to remove the part with a double ligature, passed through the neck of the tumour, one part of the silk or twine being tied over the right side of the part, and the other over the left. If severe nervous symptoms follow, opiate injections into the rectum, the warm bath, and bleeding, are the most likely means of appeasing them.—ED.

ordinary causes are those of a prolapse of the womb, and it is to be treated by a like plan of astringent injections and general tonics. Pregnancy commonly performs the best cure ; and where this fails, Dr. Berchelmann, from the success which has accompanied incision in the case of a prolapsed uterus, has recommended scarification, which appears well worthy of trial, though the author has not known it put into practice.*

SPECIES III.
ÆDOPTOSIS VESICÆ.
PROLAPSE OF THE BLADDER.
PROTRUSION OF THE BLADDER INTO THE URINARY PASSAGE.

THIS species is introduced chiefly upon the authority of Sauvages, who gives us two modifications or varieties of it ; one, in which there is a protrusion of the inner membrane, in consequence of its separating from the general substance of the bladder, visible in the meatus urinarius, of the size of a hen's egg, subdiaphonous, and filled with urine ; and the other, in which there is a protrusion of the inner membrane of the neck of the bladder into the same passage. He gives a case of the former variety from Noel, who met with it in a virgin, who was from the first peculiarly troubled with a retention of urine, accompanied with frequent convulsive movements. She soon fell a sacrifice to it, and it was on dissection that the state of the tunic was clearly proved. M. de Sauvages queries whether, on a recurrence of this case, it would be most advisable to make an opening into the protruding sac, or to extirpate it altogether.

The second variety, he tells us, is chiefly found among women who have borne many children, or have been injured by blows or other violence on the lower belly. The protruding cyst, produced by an inversion of the membrane, drops down in the urinary passage to about the length of the little finger, and is sufficiently conspicuous between the labia. Solingen, who met with a case of this kind, returned it by a probe, armed at the upper end with a piece of sponge moistened with an astringent lotion, and afterward endeavoured to retain it in its proper position with a bandage.†

SPECIES IV.
ÆDOPTOSIS COMPLICATA.
COMPLICATED GENITAL PROLAPSE.
PROTRUSION OF DIFFERENT ORGANS COMPLICATED WITH EACH OTHER.

FROM the connexion of the uterus and the vagina with the bladder, a prolapse of either of the

* The operation proposed of late by Dr. Marshall Hall, may be regarded as a revival of this method of treatment.—ED.

† A more common prolapse of the bladder than that noticed by the author, is the cystocele, in which it protrudes through the abdominal ring.—EDITOR.

two former is often complicated with that of the latter, giving us the two following varieties :—

α Utero-vesicalis.   Prolapse of the uterus, drag-
  Utero-vesical   ging the bladder along
  prolapse.   with it.
β Vagino-vesica-   Prolapse of the vagina, drag-
  lis.   ging the bladder along
  Vagino-vesical   with it.
  prolapse.

Under either of these conditions, the bladder being deprived of the expulsory aid of the abdominal muscles, in consequence of its dropping below their action, is incapable of contracting itself sufficiently to evacuate the water it contains : and hence the patient is obliged to squeeze it with her hands or between her thighs.

The causes and mode of treatment have been already described under the two preceding species. The present is the *hysteroptosis composita* of Sauvages.*

SPECIES V.
ÆDOPTOSIS POLYPOSA.
GENITAL EXCRESCENCE.

POLYPOUS OR OTHER CARUNCULAR EXCRESCENCE
IN THE COURSE OF THE GENITAL AVENUE.

This is the *polypus uteri* and *polypus vaginæ* of authors. They issue both from the uterus and the vagina, and hence form two distinct modifications, as follow :—

α Uteri.   Issuing with a slender root
  Polypus of the   mostly from the fundus
  womb.†   of the uterus, and more
                      or less elongating into the
                      vagina.
β Vaginæ.   Issuing from the sides of the
  Polypus of the   vagina, broad and bul-
  vagina.   bous.

The latter excrescences in an incipient state, and particularly when loose and flabby, are sometimes dispersed by stimulant and astringent applications, or a hard compress of sponge or any other elastic material ; and if this cannot be accomplished, they must be destroyed by excision or caustics. It is, rarely that they have a neck narrow enough for the application of a ligature.‡

Polypous excrescences of the womb are, however, a disease of much greater severity ; since the stomach suffers in most cases from sympathy, and consequently the general health, producing all the symptoms we have already noticed under ÆDOPTOSIS *uteri* : which last is not unfrequently a result, if the excrescence be of long continuance and of considerable weight and magnitude.§

---

* For further details on these subjects, see Dr. Clarke's valuable work on the Diseases of Females, and Dr. Dewees's Treatise on the same subject.—D.

† Named by several pathologists of the present day in France, the fibro-cellular tumour of the uterus.—Ed.

‡ In the U. S. Med. and Surg. Journal, vol. i., p. 318, may be seen the details of a case of large sarcomatous tumour in the vagina, occurring in the practice of Dr. N. H. Dering.—D.

§ In particular, the patient suffers great pain in

They are of all sizes and of various degrees of hardness, from that of a soft and yielding sponge to that of firm and substantial leather. Though they commonly grow from the fundus of the uterus, they have sometimes been found to sprout from its sides, and even its cervix, shooting down to different depths of the vagina, and occupying it more or less completely according to their extent. They are generally round in shape and compact in structure, intersected by membranes running in different directions. Sometimes, however, they are oblong, in which case they usually consist of a loose irregular texture with numerous interstitial cavities. Dr. Baillie has given various examples of this diseased production in his tables of Morbid Anatomy.—(See especially fascie. c. ix., plate iv., 1.)

They have been attempted to be removed in different ways, as by caustics, excision, laceration, and ligature. The last, however, is the only method unaccompanied with danger or uncertainty.* Yet even this can rarely be had recourse to without producing the loins, a dragging sensation in the inguinal regions and thighs, and a feeling of weight about the fundament and vagina. Polypi of the womb also frequently bring on hemorrhage, and, after a time, a discharge of mucus, or of a more or less fetid sanies from the vagina. Their pressure on the rectum sometimes interferes with the passage of the feces, and obstinate constipation is the result. Like other organic diseases of the womb, they most frequently form about the critical age, that is to say, between the ages of thirty-eight and fifty. Sometimes the surface of these tumours is smooth, and their substance dense and compact ; in other instances their surface has the irregularity of a fungus, and their consistence is soft. In many cases fibro-cellular tumours of the uterus are not single : so that after the removal of one, another, frequently quite unsuspected, is yet left in the cavity of the uterus, which, continuing to grow and maintain local and general disturbance in the system, with hemorrhage and other kinds of discharges, may ultimately lead to fatal consequences. Sometimes, indeed, uterine polypi, on being drawn down into the vagina with forceps, present a grayish-purple gangrenous appearance, the disorganization being occasionally superficial and of small extent, but sometimes deep and affecting the greater portion of the whole mass. So long as the patient has a reddish or a white mucous discharge, there is no fetor ; the tumour is everywhere uniformly firm ; and, if examined with a speculum, it has the appearance of a white or pink-coloured smooth substance. But when the disease is attended with a sanious discharge, the fetor is intolerably offensive—the stench of gangrene ; and if the parts are examined, the mass has a softness and a fungous look, proportioned to the duration of those symptoms. It is also at this period that the constitution begins to suffer serious impairment ; the skin acquiring a sallow colour, and the patient becoming hectic and emaciated, without either appetite or sleep, and life getting into a state of urgent danger.—Ed.

* Dupuytren has renounced the ligature on account of the difficulties of applying it, and its not including the whole root of the swelling, so that the disease generally recurs, and the patient's grievances partly continue unrelieved. He has observed also, that though the patient may go on well for two or three days, a most offensive discharge then commences, arising from the sloughing of the tumour, and a fatal constitutional de-

course to while the excrescence continues in the womb; and hence the usual method is to defer the operation till from its increase of size and weight it has descended into the vagina, when the removal cannot be attempted too soon. They have sometimes dropped off spontaneously, the peduncle having probably decayed or shrivelled away.*

There is also a variety of excrescence which should not be passed without notice, and which, from its peculiar form and feel, is called the cauliflower excrescence. It arises usually from the surface of the mouth of the uterus, and spreads into the vagina, rarely or never into the cavity of the womb. To the finger it seems to be a portion of placenta, and consists of a mass -of distended bloodvessels surrounded by a membrane, through which oozes profusely the serous part of the blood, and scarcely ever, except when severely handled,'the red globules. The tumour is not tender nor very sensible. The quantity discharged is in proportion to the size of the tumour and the action of the uterine vessels. As the disease advances, the system becomes weakened generally, dyspepsy taking the lead, and dropsy closing the scene.

The cause is seldom ascertainable. While the excrescence is small, it has often been successfully attacked by local bleedings which empty the vessels, by astringent injections, plugging up the vagina, and tightly bracing it with bandages carried round the loins.—(*Obs. on the Dis. of Females*, &c., *by . Ch. Mansfield Clarke,* 8vo., 1821.)

ORDER III.
CARPOTICA.
DISEASES AFFECTING THE IMPREGNATION.

THE ordinal term CARPOTICA is derived from καρπός, "fructus," whence κάρπωσις, "fruitio." In the Physiological Proem to the present class, we have taken a brief survey of the laws and general process of generation, so far as we are acquainted with them. Impregnation constitutes a part, and the most important part, of this wonderful economy; and from the changes that the body undergoes during its action, it can never be surprising that it should often give rise to various diseases. These diseases may be arranged under four genera, including those which occur during the progress of pregnancy; those which occur during the progress of labour; conceptions misplaced; and spurious attempts at conception; the whole of which may be thus expressed:—

I. Paracyesis.	Morbid Pregnancy.
II. Parodynia.	Morbid Labour.
III. Eccyesis.	Extra-uterine Fœtation.
IV. Pseudocyesis.	Spurious Pregnancy.

In the preceding Physiological Proem we have shown that, in order for impregnation to take place, it is necessary the semen of the male should pass from the vagina to the one or other of the ovaries by means of the Fallopian tubes, which lay hold of the uterus by their very fine and sensible fimbriæ, or fringed extremities, with a sort of spastic grasp during the high-wrought shock of the embrace, and thus alone open a pathway for the semen to travel in.

The two ovaries are not merely intended to supply the place of each other, in the event of one being wanting or defective, but, like the testes in men, they seem to increase the extent of the productive power, and enable a female to bear a larger offspring than she would do if she were possessed of one ovary alone. Mr. John Hunter has put this to the test by comparing the number of young produced by a perfect sow, with those of a sow spayed of one ovary, both of the same farrow, and impregnated by a boar of the same farrow also. The spayed sow continued to breed for four years; during which period she had eight farrows, producing a total of seventy-six young. The perfect sow continued to breed for six years; during the first four of which she also had eight farrows, producing a total of eighty-seven young; and during the two ensuing years she had five more farrows,

THE ordinal term CARPOTICA is derived from καρπός, "fructus," whence κάρπωσις, "fruitio." In the Physiological Proem to the present rangement ensues; attended with violent inflammation of the uterus and its appendages, and even of the peritoneum. All these evils Dupuytren refers to the passage of putrid matter into the circulation: and he declares that he has never known them follow the treatment by excision, which is also much less painful than by ligature. The application of the latter is also said to be more liable to bring on uterine phlebitis. According to Dupuytren, the risk of hemorrhage from dividing the pedicle with scissors has been magnified beyond all truth. After two hundred operations of this kind performed by him, there were only two instances of profuse bleeding, which was also readily stopped by plugging up the vagina.—(See Leçons Orales de Clinique Chir., tom. iii., p. 450.) Velpeau has performed the excision of eight uterine polypi, without any trouble from the bleeding. Dupuytren, Lisfranc, Velpeau, and all the best Parisian surgeons, prefer scissors to a bistoury for the division of the pedicle. The tumour is first brought down sufficiently low, partly with hook forceps, and partly by the patient's own efforts; and then the pedicle is cut through. The descent of polypi is facilitated by the moveableness or yielding of the uterus: and in consequence of their fibrous texture, the forceps generally has a sufficient hold upon them for the purpose in view.—ED.

* The spontaneous detachment of uterine polypi by gangrene of the pedicle is so rare, that Baron Dupuytren has seen only one example of it in the whole course of his practice.—(See Leçons Orales de Clinique Chir., tom. iii., p. 438.) When it does happen, the entire pedicle is hardly ever destroyed, so that the element for a reproduction of the tumour remains, keeping up also various inconveniences, which under these circumstances are usually experienced. Dupuytren admits, however, that certain fibrous polypi are detached without any gangrene of their roots; these grow directly beneath the internal membrane of the womb, and scarcely do they begin to protrude beyond the cervix uteri, when, their external covering being very thin, they burst, and after occasioning some bleedings, drop off spontaneously.—ED.

producing a total of seventy-five young, in addition to those of the first four years.—(*Animal Economy*, p. 157.) So that if we may judge from this single experiment, the use of two ovaries, in equal health and activity, enables an animal to breed both more numerously, and for a longer period of time, than the possession of one alone.

Among women, however, the extent of fecundation does not seem to be much interfered with by the defect of a single ovarium, or its means of communication with the uterus, according to a paper of Dr. Granville, read before the Royal Society, April 16, 1813, containing the case of a female, whose uterus was found after death to have had but one set of the lateral appendages, and, consequently, a connexion with but one ovarium, and who, nevertheless, had been the mother of eleven children, several of each sex, with twins on one occasion.

After impregnation has taken place, the membranes produced in the uterus form a complete septum, and consequently a bar to the ascent of any subsequent flow of semen, so as to prohibit the possibility of two or more successive impregnations co-existing in any part of the uterus during the period of a determined gravidity. Children, indeed, have been born within a few weeks, or even months of each other, and hence a colour has been given to the hypothesis, that they may be conceived at different periods of a common parturition; and such births have, in consequence, been distinguished by the name of SUPERFŒTATIONS; but we shall have occasion hereafter, when treating of a plurality of children, to show that it is far more probable, that fœtuses thus born in succession, however they may vary in size or maturity, are real twins, conceived at one and the same time, from the descent of a plurality of ovula into the uterus, instead of a single one, and that the difference of size or maturity depends upon some unknown cause in the dead or puny fœtus, which has killed it or prevented its keeping pace with the other. If, however, a second connexion take place within a few hours of the first, and before the occluding membrane produced on impregnation be formed, a twin may be the result of this additional coition; but the fœtuses will in such case be parallel in their progress to perfection. M. Bouillon has given a curious example of this in a negress, who, at the usual time of pregnancy, was delivered of two male children, full grown, and of like proportions, but the one a negro and the other a mulatto. The mother, after long resistance, confessed that she had had connexion *the same evening* with a white and with a negro.*

---

* Bulletin de la Faculté et de la Société de Médecine, &c., No. iii., 1821. This I presume to be the case originally published by Buffon. In Dr. Ryan's instructive treatise on Midwifery, Dr. Moseley is stated to have related a similar case. Dr. Maton published in the Trans. of the College of Physicians, vol. iv., an example, in which a woman brought forth a healthy infant, and in three calendar months another, apparently at the full time. Desgrange relates a case, in which a wo-

Women are in general capable of breeding as soon as they begin to menstruate, which is the ordinary proof that the organs of conception are fully developed and perfected: and since this discharge, as we have remarked in the Proem just referred to, commences in very early life, and particularly in hot climates, where it has occurred in girls of not more than nine years of age, so we have instances of conception and pregnancy having commenced as early. Baron Haller (Vide *Blumenbach*, bibl. i., p. 558) and Professor Schmidt (*Act. Helvet.*, iv., 162) concur in examples of pregnancy at nine years old: and the medical records confirm these singular histories by numerous instances of a like kind. —(*Eph. Nat. Cur.*, dec. iii., ann. ii., obs. 172.)*

Yet, though menstruation is the ordinary proof that the conceptive powers have acquired a sufficient finish and vigour for their proper function, menstruation itself is not absolutely necessary for impregnation. As there are circumstances that hurry on this secretion before its ordinary term of appearance, there are others that delay it, insomuch that some women pass through a long life without menstruating at all, while others only begin after reaching an adult age, and others again not till the period in which it usually ceases. Now it may happen that a woman whose peculiar habit produces a retardation of menstruation, may marry before this secretion takes place for the first time; and as we have just observed, that she is able to breed as soon as ever she is able to menstruate, the former process may anticipate the latter, and postpone it till the term of pregnancy has been completed. "A young woman," says Sir Everard Home, "was married before she was seventeen, and although she had never menstruated, became pregnant: four months after her delivery she became pregnant a second time;

---

man was delivered of a second healthy child five months and sixteen days after the first; and her husband had had no intercourse with her for sixteen days after her confinement: both children lived. See Ryan's Manual of Midwifery, p. 149, Lond., 1828.—ED.†

* "From a record of the practice of the late Dr. Bland, of London," says Dr. Campbell, "more women conceived between the twenty-sixth and thirtieth year of age, than at an earlier or later period. Of 20,102 women who had children, 85 were from 15 to 20 years of age; 578 from 21 to 25; 699 from 26 to 30; 407 from 31 to 35; 291 from 36 to 40; 36 from 41 to 45; 6 from 46 to 49. In glancing at a record of more than 5000 deliveries in my own practice, I find the most frequent period of conception to be from the 20th to the 26th year; and in this last I can only find 9 deliveries after the age of 42 years."—(Introduction to the Study and Practice of Midwifery, 1833.)—D.

† A case in favour of the theory of superfœtation is stated by Dr. Dewees, in the Medical Museum, vol. i.; and in the practice of Dr. Stearns, a negro woman was delivered of a black child at about the eighth month, and a few hours afterward, of a white fœtus, of about four months.—See also Francis's Denman, p. 663, and Dr. Chapman's paper on the same subject, in the first volume of the Eclectic Repertory.—D.

and, four months after the second delivery, she was a third time pregnant, but miscarried : after this she menstruated for the first time, and continued to do so for several periods, and again became pregnant."—(*Phil. Trans.*, 1817, p. 258.)

There is much difference of opinion as to the period of pregnancy in the human female ; for, while other animals seem to observe great punetuality upon this subject, we meet with so many and such considerable varieties in women, that legislators as well as physicians have not agreed in assigning a common term.* Hippocrates rules it, that we should admit the possibility of a child being born at ten months, but not later,† which is the common term assigned in the book of the Apocrypha entitled Wisdom of Solomon (chap. vii., 2) ; while Haller gives references to women who are said to have gone not only ten, but eleven, twelve, thirteen, and even fourteen months ; most of which, however, are of a suspicious kind. Twelve months, nevertheless, is a term allowed by many physicians, as what may take place under peculiar weaknesses or delicacy of health :‡ and yet it is most probable, that in all these the mother is mistaken as to the proper time of her conception, and imagines herself to have commenced pregnancy for some weeks, or even months, before it actually takes place. In the Gardner peerage cause, tried before a committee for privileges in the House of Lords in 1825-6, nine calendar months were admitted on both sides as constituting the ordinary ultimate range : but a few singular cases were adduced, in which the pregnancy seems to have been protracted at least a month later.§ So that in such anomalies, something, and not a little, must be allowed to moral reputation. The state of menstruation affords no full proof ;

for, as conception may occur without its appearance, so it may continue for many months, or even during the whole term of pregnancy, though most commonly in a smaller quantity than usual. There is a singular case in the Histoire de l'Académie des Sciences, of a living child, born after what is said to have been three years of pregnancy.—(*Hist. de l'Académie des Sciences*, 1753, p. 206.) Few reports of this kind are worth attending to, or entitled to any kind of explanation : but it has sometimes happened, and probably did so in this last case, that a woman conceits herself to be in a state of pregnancy, and has various symptoms that simulate it, for a twelvemonth, or considerably more than a twelvemonth, and particularly towards the cessation of the catamenia, instances of which we shall have occasion to notice under the fourth genus of the present order, entitled PSEUDOCYESIS, or spurious pregnancy ; and if, after such a simulation continued for a year or two, the woman should fall into a state of real pregnancy, she may persuade herself, at the close of the process, that she has been pregnant for the whole of this time.

By the Code Napoleon, the legitimacy of a child born three hundred days after a dissolution of marriage may be questioned. In our own country, the law is to this hour in an unsettled state ; and much nicety of argument has frequently taken place ; of which an example was afforded in the famous question of the Banbury peerage, upon a new-raised distinction of access and generative access. There can be no doubt, however, that a considerable difference in duration may ensue from the state of the mother's health ; for, as the fœtus receives its nourishment from the mother, there is a probability that various deviations from health may retard the maturity of the fœtus. And it is, probably, on this account, that different legislators have assigned different periods of legitimacy ; one of the shortest of which is that determined upon by the faculty of Leipsic, who have been complaisant enough to decide that a child born five months and eight days after the return of the husband, may be considered as legitimate ; and that a fœtus at five months is often a perfect and healthy child :* while the Prussian civil code declares, that an infant born three hundred and two days after the death of the husband shall be considered legitimate.

In the ordinary calculation of our own country, the allowed term does not essentially differ from that in the Code Napoleon : for it extends to nine calendar months, or forty weeks ; but, as there is often much more difficulty in determining the exact day between any two periods of menstruation in which semination has taken effect, it is usual to count the forty weeks from the middle of the interval before it ceases ; or,

* Dr. Merriman, in his able article on Parturition (Med. Chirurg. Trans., Lond., vol. xiii., p. 340), has given a table of the births of 114 mature children, calculated from, but not including, the day when the catamenia were last distinguishable. Of these, 3 were born in the 37th week, 13 in the 38th, 14 in the 39th, 33 in the 40th, 22 in the 41st, 15 in the 42d, 10 in the 43d, and 4 in the 44th.—D.

† According to Dr. Ryan, instances are recorded by Hippocrates, Pliny, Galen, Aristotle, Avicenna, and others, in which pregnancy continued for eleven, twelve, and thirteen months.—Op. cit., p. 168.—Ed.

‡ Büchner, Miscell., 1727, p. 170. Enguin, Jour. de Méd., tom. lxi. Brambilla, Abhandl. der Joseph. Acad. Brand., i., p. 102. Telinont de St. Journ. de Méd., tom. xxvii. Ploucquet, von den Physischen Erfordernissen der Erbfähigkeit der Kinder, p. 69, Treb., 8vo., 1778.

§ Dr. Merriman mentions a case of 309 days. Velpeau states the following :—" A woman in her fourth pregnancy computed that she was four months gone when she came to my amphitheatre. I distinctly felt both the active and passive motions of the fœtus ; appearances of labour took place at the end of the ninth month ; were soon suspended ; did not return for thirty days ; languished a whole week ; so that in fact the delivery did not take place until the three hundred and tenth day."—See an Elementary Treatise on Midwifery, by A. A. L. M. Velpeau, trans. from the French by Ch. D. Meigs, Philadelphia, 1831.—D.

* On the contrary, Dr. Beck is of opinion, that if a mature child be born before the seventh month after connexion, it ought to be considered illegitimate.—(See Ryan's Manual of Midwifery, p. 160.) Dr. Duncan, jun., of Edinburgh, considers the decision in the Gardner peerage case to have been incorrect.—See Edin. Med. Jour., vol. xxvii.—Ed.

in other words, to give a date of forty-two weeks from the last appearance of the menses: and at the expiration of this term, within a few days before or after, the labour may confidently be expected.

In the progress of pregnancy, the size and figure of the uterus, as well as its position, change considerably. In an adult and unimpregnated female, its length is about two inches and a half; its thickness one inch; its breadth at the fundus something less than its length; and at the cervix, about two lines. Before the end of the third month, it has a tendency to dip towards the pelvis, at which period it may be felt to ascend: during the seventh month, it forms a line with the navel: in the eighth month it ascends still higher, reaching midway between this organ and the sternum; and, in the ninth, it almost touches the ensiform cartilage; at the close of which, as though overwhelmed by its own bulk, it begins again to descend, and shortly afterward, from the irritation produced by the weight of the child, or, more probably, from the simple law of instinct, it becomes attacked with a series of spasmodic contractions, extending to the surrounding organs, which constitute the pains of labour, gradually increase in strength, enlarge the mouth of the organ, and protrude the child into the world.

The size of the child at this time varies considerably in different individuals; and seems indeed to exhibit some diversity in different countries. Dr. Hunter, from observations made on some thousands of new-born and perfect children in the British Lying-in Hospital, found that the weight of the smallest was about four pounds, and of the largest eleven pounds two ounces, ordinarily, however, varying from five to eight pounds: whence, as also from his own observations, Dr. Clarke has calculated the average weight at seven pounds five ounces and seven drachms for male children, and six pounds eleven ounces and six drachms for female.— (*Phil. Trans.*, vol. lxxiv.) Dr. Merriman, however, gives one instance, in which the weight reached fourteen pounds; and Sir R. Croft another, in which it reached fifteen pounds.* On the continent, the standard weight seems to be considerably less; for M. Camus reckons it at not more than from five to seven pounds for France, and M. Roederer at from five pounds to

six pounds and a half for Germany. And, consistently with this diminished scale, M. Camus tells us, that out of fifteen hundred and forty-one children examined by himself, the greatest weight was not more than nine pounds, of which there were only sixteen instances; while at the Hospice de la Maternité at Paris, out of twenty thousand perfect births, a few only have reached ten pounds and a half, and none exceeded it.— (*Medical Jurisprudence, by J. Paris, M. D., and J. S. M. Fonblanque, Esq., Barrister at Law*, vol. ii., p. 101.) At this time the standard length of the skeleton, according to M. Beclard, is eighteen inches, that of the spine seven inches and a quarter; the former, at three months from conception, being only six inches, and the latter two inches and two thirds.

If the fœtus be born before the completion of the seventh month, it has but a slender chance of surviving; but there are a few well-authenticated instances of its living when born earlier. Thus Dr. Rodman gives a very satisfactory narration of a child born in 1815, at Paisley, between the fourth and fifth month (*Edin. Med. and Surg. Journ.*, vol. xi.); and Fortunis Liceti, who died at the age of twenty-four, is affirmed by Capuron to have been born at as early a period of pregnancy.*

In natural pregnancy, a strong hearty woman suffers little, considering the great change which many of the most important organs of both the thorax and abdomen are sustaining; and in natural labour, though the returning pains are violent for several hours, there is little or no danger. But numerous unforeseen circumstances may arise from the constitution of the mother, the shape of the pelvis, the figure or position of the child, to produce difficulty, danger, and even death.

In describing the diseases which appertain to the whole of this period, it is not the author's design to do more than to take a general pathological survey, so as to communicate that kind of knowledge upon the subject which every practitioner of the healing art should be acquainted with, even though he may not engage in the obstetric branch of his profession. The minuter and more practical parts, and especially those which relate to the application of instruments, and the mechanical means of assistance, must be sought for in books and lectures ex-

---

* " Dr. Wm. Moore of N. York has had several cases of children born at the natural periods, whose weight was full twelve pounds each. Another practitioner of good authority has furnished me with a similar fact, and I had one under my own observation. Instances also have fallen within the practice of some of my medical brethren, of the child weighing thirteen pounds and upwards. A memorable case of pregnancy occurred in New-York two winters ago, where, from untoward circumstances, the labour was protracted four days, and the life of the mother closely jeoparded in her efforts to expel the child. She was finally relieved by the forceps, and brought forth a dead fœtus, the actual weight of which was sixteen pounds and a half avoirdupois." —See Francis on Med. Jurisprudence, in N. Y. Med. and Phys. Journal, vol. ii.—D.

* In November, 1832, says Dr. Francis, in a note to the editor, " I attended a lady in her accouchement who had advanced but twenty-three weeks in her pregnancy. It was her second labour; the first had been tedious, and she lost her child: during her second gestation, she had suffered a slight attack of the epidemic cholera, which prevailed in New-York that summer, and her health was considerably impaired: over-exercise brought on most unexpectedly the present labour: and within some twenty-five minutes, by one continuous effort, the entire ovum was expelled, the placenta, membranes, and fœtus. They were immediately placed in lukewarm water, and seemingly excited to greater vitality by this means: within a few minutes the child was detached and wrapped up in cotton, and by extreme care survived. As might be supposed, uncommon attention was requisite

pressly appropriated for the purpose, with which it is not his intention to interfere.*

GENUS I.
PARACYESIS.
MORBID PREGNANCY.

THE PROGRESS OF PREGNANCY DISTURBED OR ENDANGERED BY THE SUPERVENTION OF GENERAL OR LOCAL DISORDER.

THE - generic term is derived from παρὰ, "malé," and κύησις, "graviditas." The genus will conveniently embrace the three following species, according as the general system, or organs distinct from those immediately concerned, are disturbed ; as the sexual organs themselves are disturbed ; or as the fruit itself is disturbed and extruded prematurely :—

1. Paracyesis Irritativa.	Constitutional Derangement of Pregnancy.	
2. ——— Uterina.	Local Derangement of Pregnancy.	
3. ——— Abortus.	Miscarriage. Abortion.	

SPECIES I.
PARACYESIS IRRITATIVA.
CONSTITUTIONAL DERANGEMENT OF PREGNANCY.

PREGNANCY EXCITING DISTRESS, OR DISTURBANCE, IN OTHER ORGANS OR FUNCTIONS THAN THOSE PRIMARILY CONCERNED.

THE new condition of the womb operates upon the whole or different parts of the system in various ways. We have frequently had occasion to observe, that there is no organ whatever which exercises a more extensive control over the entire fabric than the uterus, with the exception of the stomach ; and hence many parts are affected by sympathy during its new action, and particularly the brain and the whole of the nervous function. But its change of shape, bulk, and position operates mechanically on other organs, and frequently produces serious mischief by pressure or irritation : these are chiefly the stomach itself, the lungs, the intestinal canal, and the veins of the legs. And hence the evils resulting from these causes may be contemplated under the following varieties :—

α Systatica.	Accompanied with faintings, palpitations, convulsions, or other direct affections of the nervous system.
β Dyspeptica.	Accompanied with indigestion, sickness, and headache.
γ Dyspnoica.	Accompanied with difficult breathing, and occasionally a cough.

---

to its rearing : but it has done as well as most other children, and she is at this time, June, 1835, hearty and well formed."-D.

* The application of instruments, and other details connected with midwifery, are represented in a series of plates, in a work entitled Midwifery Illustrated, by J. P. Maygrier, published by Harper & Brothers, New-York, 1835, 3d edition.—D.

δ Alvina.	Accompanied with derangement of the alvine canal, as costiveness, diarrhœa, or hemorrhoids.
ε Varicosa.	Accompanied with venous dilatation of the lower extremities.

. That the nervous system should often suffer severely, and in various ways, during pregnancy, will not appear singular to those who have attended to the remarks we have already made concerning the close chain of sympathy that prevails between the brain and the sexual organs, from the time of the first development of the latter to their becoming torpid and superannuated on the cessation of the catamenia. But in delicate habits, in which these nervous affections chiefly occur, there is another cause, which is even more powerful than the preceding : and that is, the demand of an additional supply of sensorial power in support of the new process, and, consequently, an additional excitement and exhaustion of the sensorium, persevered in without intermission, and increasing from day to day. This excitement and exhaustion necessarily produce weakness ; and, of course, an irregularity in the distribution of the sensorial energy ; hereby predisposing alike to palpitation of the heart, clonic spasms, and convulsions, according to the law of physiology laid down under the genus CLONUS. Fainting, as has also been previously shown under the genus SYNCOPE, is dependant upon the same deficiency of action, rendered more complete or more protracted in duration.

PALPITATION, in the case before us, is rarely attended with danger, but is often a most distressing symptom. It returns irregularly in the course of the day or night, but particularly after a meal, and very frequently on first lying down in bed. In the capricious state of the nervous system at this time, its return after meals does not seem so much dependant upon the nature of the food as upon the state of the stomach at the moment : it has recurred after a light and plain dinner, and been quiet after a more stimulant dinner ; and then, for a few days, has been most severe after the latter, and least so after the former. For a short time, the digestion has gone on tranquilly under both, and then again excited palpitation, and perhaps in an equal degree under both ; nor has a total abstinence from solid animal food afforded any relief. The pulsatory action is sometimes confined to the heart, sometimes alternates with the cœliac or some other arterial trunk in the abdomen, and sometimes with the temporal arteries. Not long ago, the author was occasionally consulted by a lady, then in her sixth month, who had been most grievously afflicted with this affection from the time of her beginning to breed, and who then continued subject to it till her confinement. None of the antispasmodics afforded much, if any relief ; camphire, in large doses, was found the best palliative ; the narcotics were all tried in vain ; opium maddened the head, and threw out a most distressing lichenous rash. The paroxysms usually continued from two to six or eight hours. Other irritations produced it, as well as those of the stomach, and especially any sudden emotion of the mind.

SYNCOPE or fainting occurs during any period of pregnancy, but chiefly in the stage of the first three months, and especially about the time of quickening. After this period, the general frame acquires a habit of accommodation to the change that has taken place, and is less easily affected. It is ordinarily produced by more than usual exertion, exposure to heat, or any sudden excitement of the mind. It is sometimes of short duration, and the patient does not lose her recollection ; but in other instances, it continues for an hour or upwards. A recumbent position, pungent volatiles, sprinkling the face with cold water, and a free exposure to air, with a moderate use of cordials, offer the speediest means of recovery. The extremities, however, should be kept warm, and the friction of a warm hand be applied to the feet.

One of the worst ailments that ever accompanies the process of gestation is that of CONVULSIONS. They may occur at any period of this process, and their exciting causes are not always manifest. The predisposing causes are, a general weakness or irritability of the nervous system, a constitutional tendency to epilepsy, or any other clonic spasm, and entonic plethora. In all these cases, there is a double danger ; for we have to dread apoplexy from a rupture of bloodvessels in the head ; and abortion or premature labour, from an extension of the spasmodic action to the uterus. No time, therefore, is to be lost, and the remedial process must be as active as it is instant.

Bleeding must be had recourse to immediately, as well in the atonic as in the entonic form of the disease. In the first, indeed, it is of itself an evil, for it will add to the general weakness ; but, as there is already, or by a repetition of the fit will unquestionably be, a considerable determination to the head, and more especially as the vessels in an atonic and relaxed frame yield easily as well to anastomosis as to rupture, it will be a far greater evil to omit it. The quantity of blood, however, that it may be advisable to abstract, must be determined by the concomitant symptoms, so far as they relate to the head. Generally speaking, in weakly habits, the head is only affected secondarily, or by sympathy with the irritation of the uterus, where convulsions make their appearance ; and hence bleeding, in such cases, is to be employed rather as a prophylactic than as an antidote : and it may be sufficient to confine ourselves to the operation of cupping ; at the same time opening the bowels by an adequate repetition of some laxative. After this, opium must be chiefly trusted to, if the spasms still continue : and, on their subsidence, or in their interval, the metallic tonics should be introduced, with the warmer bitters.

Where, however, the constitution is robust, and the convulsions have been preceded, as is often the fact in this case, by a tensive or even heavy pain in the head, vertigo, illusory coruscations before the eyes, or illusory sounds in the ears, the encephalon is itself the immediate seat of the disease, and the bleeding, even in the first instance, should be followed up to fainting, or at least till twenty ounces are drawn away, which it will frequently be necessary to repeat within twenty-four hours afterward ; and, if the practitioner be a skilful operator, it will be better to abstract the blood from the jugular vein, as the good effect will be sooner felt. The hair should be shaved from the head, and ice-water or other frigid lotions* be applied, and very frequently renewed. The bowels must at the same time be purged vigorously, and dilute farinaceous food constitute the whole of the diet. Opium should be abstained from, at least till the general strength is reduced to an atonic state, when, if the paroxysms should still return, it may be had recourse to, in conjunction with antimonial powder, or some other relaxant.

When, in despite of all this treatment, apoplexy has taken place, and is followed by a palsy of a particular organ, or of an entire side, it will often be found that the paralytic affection will continue through the whole course of the pregnancy, and entirely disappear afterward.

SICKNESS, HEARTBURN, and other symptoms of INDIGESTION, are still more common affections than those of the nervous system we have first noticed. These are chiefly troublesome in the commencement of pregnancy, and evidently prove that they proceed, not from any mechanical pressure, either direct or indirect, against the coats of the stomach, but from mere sympathy with the new and irritable state of the uterus : for, as the novelty of this state wears away, and the stomach becomes accustomed to it, the sickness and other dyspeptic symptoms subside gradually, and are rarely troublesome, even when, in the latter months of pregnancy, the uterus has swollen to its utmost extent, from a length of three inches to that of twelve, and has risen nearly as high as the sternum.

The headache which occurs as a dyspeptic symptom, is of a very different kind from that we have just noticed, and is rarely relieved by very copious bleedings ; though the whole of these symptoms are occasionally mitigated by a loss of eight or nine ounces of blood from the arm, or the application of leeches to the epigastric region, as recommended by Dr. Sims and M. Lorentz. Cloths wetted with laudanum, and applied to the pit of the stomach, have also been found serviceable in various cases ; but the most efficacious means consist in the employment of gentle laxatives and a very light diet, to which may be added the use of the aërated alkaline waters, or saline draughts in a state of effervescence.

The fluid discharged from the stomach on these occasions is usually limpid, thin, and watery : but, where there is much straining, a little bile is thrown up at the same time. It is rarely that this kind of vomiting produces any serious evil ; though, when it has become very obstinate, as well as severe, it has sometimes endan-

---

* As we have already stated, tepid applications are preferred by many.—D.

gered a miscarriage. The other symptoms of dyspepsy usually cease with this, and are rather disquieting than sources of any degree of alarm. They may often be palliated by some of the means recommended under LIMOSIS; CARDIALGIA and DYSPEPSIA.

The chief symptoms of DYSPNŒA that become troublesome during pregnancy, are occasional fits of spasmodic anhelation. These are mostly common to those whose respiratory organs are naturally weak, or who are predisposed to hysteria. The paroxysms are of short duration, and usually yield with ease to the warmer sedatives and antispasmodics. A dry and troublesome cough, however, is sometimes combined with this state of the chest, that, if violent, endangers abortion, and has occasionally produced it. Bleeding will here also be advisable as the first step in the curative process. Eight ounces of blood will suffice ; but the depletion must be repeated at distinct intervals if the cough should continue unabated. Gentle laxatives should succeed to the bleeding, and be persevered in as the bowels may require. And to these may be added mucilaginous demulcents, united with such doses of hyoscyamus, conium, or opium, as are found best to agree with the state of the constitution. There is little danger, nevertheless, of this cough terminating in consumption, however troublesome and obstinate it may be in itself, for it is rarely that two superadded actions go forward in the constitution at the same time : and hence, whenever pregnancy takes place in a patient labouring under phthisis, the progress of the latter disease is arrested till the new process has run its course.

DERANGEMENTS OF THE ALVINE CANAL, under some modification or other, accompany most cases of pregnancy, are often very distressing, and by their irritation sometimes hasten on labour-pains before their time.

These affections are of two very opposite kinds. In some instances, the intestines participate in the irritability of the uterus, the peristaltic action is morbidly increased, and there is a troublesome diarrhœa. In others, the larger intestines appear to be rendered torpid, partly by the share of sensorial power which is taken from them in support of the new action, and partly by the pressure of the expanding uterus on their coats. In both cases, piles are a frequent attendant, but particularly in the last.

The diarrhœa varies in different individuals, from a looser flow of proper feces to a muculent secretion, or a dejection of dark-coloured offensive stools, accompanied with a foul tongue and loss of appetite. The first modification requires no remedy, and may be safely left to itself. The second and third import a morbid action of the excretories of the intestines, and are best relieved by small and repeated doses of rhubarb with two grains of ipecacuanha to each (*Burns, Principles of Midwifery,* p. 154), and afterward by infusions of cascarilla, orange-peel, or any other light aromatic bitter.

The costiveness must be carefully guarded against by such aperients as are found upon trial to agree best with the bowels. Where acidity

in the stomach is suspected, magnesia may be employed, and will often prove sufficient: but where this does not exist, the senna electuary, the sulphate of magnesia, or castor-oil, will be found to answer much better. The piles will usually disappear as soon as the bowels are restored to a current state : and, if not, they should be treated according to the plan already laid down under PROCTICA MARISCA.—(Vol. i., p. 195.)

VARICOSE DILATATIONS of the veins of the lower extremities are a frequent, though not often a very troublesome accompaniment of pregnancy. They are chiefly found in women whose occupation obliges them to be much on their feet. Where the affected veins are first perceived to enlarge, the varicose knots may generally be prevented by exchanging the accustomed erect position for a recumbent one, and using the legs but little. Where the varices are actually formed, the legs may be covered with a bandage drawn only with such moderate pressure as to afford gentle support ; for, if carried beyond this, we shall only endanger a worse congestion in some other part not equally guarded against. For the rest, the reader may turn to EXANGIA VARIX, in a preceding part of this work.—(Cl. III., Ord. IV., Gen. XI., Spe. 2.)

Pregnancy may also take place during the existence of abdominal dropsy, or even give rise to it, and the general pressure and enlargement may be so considerable as to threaten suffocation. The ascites will be hereby considerably complicated ; but its mode of treatment will be best considered under the latter disease.—(Infra, Cl. VI., Ord. II., Gen. I., Spe. 5.)*

SPECIES II.
PARACYESIS UTERINA.
LOCAL DERANGEMENT OF PREGNANCY.

PREGNANCY DISTURBED OR ENDANGERED BY SOME DISEASED AFFECTION OF THE UTERUS.

IN the progress of this work, we have seen that, on the commencement and through the course of impregnation, the periodical secretion of the uterus is suspended ; that the organ gradually enlarges from its ordinary size, till in the ninth month it measures ten or twelve inches from top to bottom ; and that, in the course of this enlargement, it changes its position, according to a law that is never departed from in a state of health.

In a state of morbid action, however, or from some accidental injury, the uterus does not always maintain its proper position, nor abstain

* The constitutional derangement of pregnancy is so frequently relieved by venesection, that many American practitioners are in the habit of bleeding at different periods of gestation. The affections of the digestive system, which sometimes annoy the sufferer to a great extent, are often entirely controlled by using prussic acid, given in doses of one drop two or three times a day. Dr. Delafield of New-York, has found this remedy very successful.—D.

from throwing forth not only its ordinary and natural secretions, but other fluids of a morbid character; and hence becomes subject to several varieties of affection, of which it may be sufficient to notice the following:—

a Retroversa.	Retroversion of the uterus.
β Leucorrhoica.	The uterus secreting, or exciting in the vagina, a secretion of leucorrhœa, so as to produce debility.
γ Catamenica.	The catamenia continuing to recur.
δ Hæmorrhagica.	Accompanied with hemorrhage.

A RETROVERSION OF THE UTERUS may be produced in various ways, though it is seldom found except in pregnancy, and between the third and fourth month of this state. This organ, notwithstanding its appendages of broad and round ligaments, is still left pendulous in the hypogastrium: and hence, if the fundus or broad and upper part happen, by a scirrhous induration, or pregnancy, or any other means, to acquire a certain bulk and weight, and if at the same time the cervix, or lower and narrow part, be pushed on one side by any accidental force, as that of the bladder when distended, the broad and upper part will tumble downward, while the narrower part ascends and takes its place. It is this which constitutes a retroverted uterus; but as it occasionally occurs under other stages than that of pregnancy, we have treated of it already under the genus ÆDOPTOSIS UTERI, where we have stated the mode of treatment to be adopted in the case before us.

LEUCORRHŒA is a result of the increased action excited in every part of the uterus, or of the upper part of the vagina, which is inflamed by continuous sympathy. The mucous discharge, denominated leucorrhœa or whites, appears to be secreted from the lower part of the uterus, and the upper part of the latter organ; and hence any excitement operating on the fundus of the womb, may be easily conceived, under a particular condition of the cervix of the uterus and the vagina, or of the system generally, capable of producing this secretion in considerable abundance.

When treating of leucorrhœa as an idiopathic affection, we remarked, that where the discharge is excessive, it produces considerable debility of the system generally, and of the sexual and lumbar regions more particularly; and that when it becomes chronic, it often degenerates into an acrimonious condition, and occasions great disquiet by excoriating the cuticle to a considerable extent.

Both these evils are consequent upon its occurrence in pregnancy, and the first has occasionally threatened abortion. They are to be relieved by the remedial process already pointed out under the genus LEUCORRHŒA.

A continuance of the CATAMENIAL DISCHARGE at the regular periods is also, in many cases of delicate habits, a source of great weakness and discomfort, and sometimes endangers miscarriage or premature labour; in all which instances it ought to be checked by a recumbent position, and particularly a little before the time in which it may be expected, and by the other means already enumerated under PARAMENIA SUPERFLUA. It has sometimes continued, however, in strong and vigorous habits, through the whole period of pregnancy without any serious mischief (Hagedorn, cent. ii., obs. 94); though even here it has usually been found to produce general debility, and many troublesome dyspeptic symptoms.

Hemman* and several other writers give cases of women who have never menstruated except when in a state of pregnancy; such is the degree of irritation which the secretories of the uterus occasionally demand in order to be roused into a due performance of their function. So some persons can only see on a full exposure to a meridian light, and others can only hear when the tympanum is irritated by the noise of a drum or of a carriage, sufficient to deafen all the world around them.

HEMORRHAGE from the uterus is sometimes connected with this irregular return of the periodical discharge; as we have already observed, it is not unfrequently in an unimpregnated state of the organ. In both cases, this is usually a consequence of great general debility, and it is hence the more alarming in any period of parturition, as risking the loss of the uterine fruit. In the delicacy of habit we are now contemplating, bleeding would only add to the debility or predisponent cause; and we must content ourselves with the plan already recommended under atonic hemorrhage of the uterus in a prior class and volume.—(Vol. i., Cl. III., Ord. IV., Gen. II., Spe. 2.) Where the discharge has been induced by external violence or a sudden emotion of the mind, venesection will be the best remedy we can have recourse to, and afterward thirty or five-and-thirty drops of laudanum in a saline draught, with two or three grains of ipecacuanha.

SPECIES III.

PARACYESIS ABORTUS.

MISCARRIAGE. ABORTION.

PREMATURE EXCLUSION OF A DEAD FŒTUS FROM THE UTERUS.

WE have stated, in the introductory remarks to the present order, that the usual term of pregnancy is forty weeks, or nine calendar months. Within this period, however, the fœtus may be morbidly expelled at any time. If the exclusion take place within six weeks after conception, it is usually called MISCARRIAGE; if between six weeks and six months, ABORTION; if during any part of the last three months before the completion of the natural term, PREMATURE LABOUR. Among some writers, however, abortion and miscarriage are used synonymously, and both are made to express an exclusion of the fœtus at any time before the commencement of

---

* Medicinisch-Chirurgische Aufsätze. Berl. 1778. Hopfergärtner, über menschliche Entwickelungen, p. 71, Stutg., 1792.

the seventh month. At seven months the fœtus will often live. It has been born alive, in a few rare instances, at four months (*A. Reyes, Campus Elys., Quest.*, 90, p. 1164); and has as rarely continued alive when born between five and six months.—(*Brouzet, sur l'Education Médicinale des Enfans,* i., p. 37.)

The process of gestation may be checked, however, from its earliest period; for many of the causes of abortion which can operate afterward, may operate throughout the entire term; and hence a miscarriage occurs not unfrequently within three weeks after impregnation, or before the ovum has descended into the uterus. In this case the pains very much resemble those of difficult menstruation; and, with a considerable discharge of clotted or coagulated blood, the tunica decidua passes away alone, having also some resemblance to that imperfect form of it which we have already noticed as being produced in some cases of difficult menstruation, but exhibiting a more completely membranous structure. And here the ovulum escapes unperceived at some subsequent period, and is probably decomposed and incapable of being traced.

In later periods of pregnancy, abortion consists of two parts or stages; the separation of the ovum from the fundus of the womb, and its expulsion from the mouth. Sometimes these take place very nearly simultaneously, but sometimes several days, or even weeks intervene; so that the process of abortion may considerably vary in its duration, and become exceedingly tedious. In several cases I have known the ovum remain undischarged for upwards of six weeks, and in one case, for three months after its separation, and consequently after the death of the fœtus, comparing its size and appearance with the ascertained term of gestation.

Through the whole of this period there is an occasional discharge from the vagina, and often temporary disquietudes, and even contractile pains in the uterus. But both are of a very different kind from those which occur antecedently to the separation of the ovum. The first pains are usually sharp and expulsory, with a free discharge of clotting arterial blood; sometimes indeed in an alarming, though rarely a dangerous profusion; the last are dull and heavy, and the discharge is smaller in quantity, dark, and fetid. We may also judge of the detachment of the ovum, and consequently the death of the fœtus, by the cessation of those sympathetic symptoms which have hitherto connected the stomach and the mammæ with the action of the uterus; as the morning sickness, and the increasing plumpness of the breasts, which not unfrequently are so stimulated as to secrete already a small quantity of milk. On the separation of the ovum from the fundus of the uterus, all these disappear; the stomach may be dyspeptic, but without the usual sickness, and the breasts become more than ordinarily flaccid.

The ovum, when at length discharged, comes away differently in different cases. Sometimes the whole ovum is expelled at once; but more generally it is discharged in detached parts, the

fœtus first escaping with the liquor amnii, or descending with its own proportion of the placenta, the maternal proportion following some hours or even days afterward. And where there are twins, one of the fœtuses, naked or surrounded with its membranes, is usually expelled alone, and the other not till an interval of several hours, or even a day or two; the discharge of blood ceasing, and the patient appearing to be in a state of recovery; so that, in cases of early abortion, it is difficult to determine whether there are twins or not.

The causes of abortion are very numerous; and some of them are rather conjectured than fully ascertained. They may depend upon the ovum itself, upon the uterus itself, or upon the uterus as affected by the nature of the maternal constitution, or accidental lesions.[*]

"The imperfections observable in ova," remarks Dr. Denman, "are of different kinds, and found occasionally in every part; and there is usually a consent between the fœtus and the shell of the ovum, as the placental part and membranes may be called, but not always. For examples have occurred in which the fœtus has died before the termination of the third month, yet the shell, being healthy, has increased to a

---

[*] Abortion, as Dr. Robert Lee observes, is a frequent occurrence in the early months of pregnancy, particularly among women of the lower classes of society, who are exposed to much bodily fatigue and mental anxiety. It is more likely to occur in plethoric, irritable, and nervous subjects; in women who are affected with constitutional diseases, more especially syphilis; in those who have deformity of the bones of the pelvis, or some organic disease of the uterine organs. All the chronic diseases, therefore, to which the uterus and its appendages are liable, may be considered causes of abortion. The production of polypi in the cavity of the uterus, or of fibro-cartilaginous tumours in its walls, and morbid adhesions of the uterus to the surrounding viscera, may all, by impeding the regular enlargement of the gravid uterus, give rise to premature expulsion of its contents. But, according to Dr. R. Lee, by far the most frequent cause of abortion is in the product of conception itself, viz., in a diseased condition of the fœtus or its involucra, by which it is deprived of life, and afterward expelled from the uterus like a foreign body. Sometimes the chorion is thickened, opaque, and extremely irregular, or lobulated on its internal surface. In certain cases, the amnios undergoes similar changes. Blood and serum may also collect between these two membranes; and where abortion takes place after the third month, the placenta has sometimes been found much indurated, and of diminutive size, with calcareous matter deposited in its substance. In other instances the placenta has been unusually large, and its vascular structure converted into a soft fatty substance, or it has contained hydatids. Under these circumstances, the umbilical cord has been remarkably slender, and the fœtus has appeared to perish for want of a proper supply of nourishment, and not from any defect in the supply of its internal parts. Various organic diseases of the brain and other viscera of the fœtus, by extinguishing its life, make it an extraneous body, for the expulsion of which, efforts on the part of the uterus soon commence.—See Cyclop. of Pract. Med., art. ABORTION.—ED

certain size, has remained till the expiration of the ninth month, and then been expelled, according to the genius and constitution of the uterus, though frequently it has been found to have undergone great changes, as, for instance, in many cases of hydatids."—(*Practice of Midwifery*, 5th edit., p. 508, 8vo.)

"It is remarkable," says the same author, "that women who are in the habit of miscarrying go on in a very promising way to a certain time, and then miscarry, not once, but for a number of times, in spite of all the methods that can be contrived and all the medicines that can be given ; so that, besides the force of habit, there is sometimes reason to suspect that the uterus is incapable of distending beyond such size, before it assumes its disposition to act, and that it cannot be quieted till it has excluded the ovum. What I am about to say will not, I hope, be construed as giving a license to irregularity of conduct, which may often be justly assigned as the immediate cause of abortion, or lead to the negligent use of those means that are likely to prevent it. But from the examination of many ova after their expulsion, it has appeared that their longer retention could not have produced any advantage, the fœtus being decayed, or having ceased to grow long before it was expelled. Or the ovum has been in such a state as to become wholly unfit for the purpose it was assigned to answer : so that if we could believe there was a distinct intelligence existing in every part of the body, we should say it was concluded in council that this ovum can never come to perfection, and shall be expelled."—(*Denman*, ubi suprà, p. 508.)

The causes of abortion of a constitutional or accidental kind are more obvious. They may be internal, and depend upon a relaxed or debilitated state of the system generally, and consequently of the uterus as a part of it ; or external, and depend on adventitious circumstances. Violent pressure, as that of tight stays, by preventing the uterus from duly enlarging, is an obvious cause, as is also that of a sudden shock by a fall, or a blow on the abdomen ; violent exertion of every kind is a cause not less obvious, as that of immoderate exercise in dancing, riding, or even walking ; lifting heavy weights ; great straining to evacuate the feces, or too frequent evacuations from a powerful purgative. Violent excitement of the passions, as terror, anxiety, sorrow, or joy. Violent excitement of the external senses by objects of disgust, whether of sight, sound, taste, or even smell ; or whatever else tends to disturb or check the circulation suddenly, and hereby to produce fainting, will often prove a cause of abortion.* And when once this affection has been produced, the organs with difficulty recover their elasticity, and it is extremely apt to recur upon the slightest causes. Plater gives us an account of four-

teen miscarriages in succession (*Observationes*, lib. ii., p. 467) ; Werlhoff, of five within two years (Opp. iii., p. 718) ; and Werloschnig, of not less than eight in a single year.—(*De Curationibus Verno-autumn.*, p. 496.) Wolfius relates the history of a woman who, in the whole course of her life, suffered twenty-two distinct abortions (*Lection. Memor.*, p. 418) ; and Schultz, that of another, who in spite of every remedy miscarried twenty-three times, and uniformly in the third month, probably from an indisposition in the uterus to become distended further, as suggested by Dr. Denman.*

Another and a very frequent cause is plethora, and this whether it be from entony or atony. "The uterus," observes Mr. Burns, "being a large vascular organ, is obedient to the laws of vascular action, while the ovum is more influenced by those regulating new-formed parts : with this difference, however, that new-formed parts or tumours are united firmly to the part from which they grow by all kinds of vessels, and generally by fibrous or cellular substance, while the ovum is connected to the uterus only by very tender and fragile arteries and veins. If, therefore, more blood be sent to the maternal part of the ovum than it can easily receive, and circulate and act under, a rupture of the vessels will take place, and an extravasation and consequent separation be produced ; or even where no rupture is occasioned, the action of the ovum may be so oppressed and disordered as to unfit it for continuing the process of gestation."†

Now in atonic plethora, or that commonly existing in high and fashionable life, among those who use little exercise, live luxuriously, and sleep in soft warm beds, although the action that accompanies the pressure is feeble compared with what occurs in the opposite state, the vessels themselves are feeble also, and their mouths

---

* One of the best accounts of the causes of abortion is contained in Prof. T. R. Beck's Med. Jurisprudence ; art. Infanticide, ed. 1825. An excellent summary of them may be found in Ryan's Manual, p. 193.—Ed.

---

* " I was recently called in attendance on a lady," says Dr. Francis, " who has sustained thirteen abortions in succession during the past nine years : sometimes the gravid womb freed itself of its contents at the completion of the second month : at several other times the duration of gestation was continued to the fifth and sixth months, and in her last pregnancy to the full termination of the eighth month. Vascular irritation or plethora seemed to be the only cause that could be assigned for these accidents. She has never borne a living child."—D.

† Principles of Midwifery, 3d edit., 8vo., p. 191. To use the words of Dr. Robert Lee, the placenta adheres to the uterus by means of the deciduous membrane alone, which is directly applied to the openings of the uterine sinuses. If the impetus of the blood in these be increased by an excited state of the general circulation, or by the irritation of the uterus itself, an unusual afflux of blood to these vessels will take place, and the placenta will be forced from its connexion with the uterus, more or less extensively, by the extravasation of blood from the opening of the uterine sinuses between the placenta and uterus. If this happen to a considerable extent, the process of gestation will be arrested, and, sooner or later, the ovum will be expelled.—See Cyclop. of Pract. Med., art. Abortion.—Ed.

and tunics are exceedingly apt to give way to even a slight impetus ; and hence plethora becomes a frequent cause of abortion in women of a delicate habit and unrestrained indulgence.

Among the robust and the vigorous, however, its mode of operation is still more obvious and direct. An increased flow of blood is here forced urgently into the uterus, which participates irresistibly in the vehemence of the action ; so that if the vessels do not suddenly give way, and hemorrhage instantly occur, the patient feels a tensive weight in the region of the uterus, and shooting pains about the pelvis. "This cause," observes Mr. Burns, "is especially apt to operate in those who are newly married, and who are of a salacious disposition, as the action of the uterus is thus much increased, and the existence of plethora rendered doubly dangerous. In these cases, whenever the menses have become obstructed, all causes tending to increase the circulation must be avoided, and often a temporary separation from the husband is indispensable."—(*Burns*, ut suprà, p. 192.)

The general treatment of abortion consists of two intentions ; that of preventing it when it threatens, and that of safely leading the patient through it when there is little doubt that it has taken place.

The chief symptoms, menacing abortion, are transitory pains in the back, or hypogastric region, or a sudden hemorrhage from the vagina. In all these cases, the first step to be taken is a recumbent position, and when the patient is once placed in this state, we should deliberately examine into the nature of the cause. If there be symptoms of plethora, or oppression, if an accident, or a sudden emotion of the mind, or severe exercise, as of dancing, riding, or even walking, have produced them by disturbing the equilibrium of the circulating system, blood should be immediately taken from the arm, and all irritation removed from the bowels by a gentle laxative or injection.* In plethora, indeed, we may go beyond this, and empty the bowels more freely : yet even here our object should be to reduce without weakening.† In every instance, except where plethora prevails, after abstracting blood, the next best remedy is a full dose of opium, consisting of thirty or forty drops of laudanum, or more if the symptoms be urgent, and repeated every three or four months till the object is obtained.‡ And where the system is

so feeble or emaciated that bleeding is counter-indicated, we must content ourselves with giving sulphuric acid with small doses of digitalis, unless, indeed, there be much tendency to sinking at the stomach, and in this case we must limit our practice to the mineral acids and opium, and gently relieving the bowels.*

By this plan the pains originating from incidental causes are often checked, and the partial separation of the ovum that has commenced is put a stop to. But the remedial process is thus far merely begun ; the patient, for some weeks, must be peculiarly attentive to her diet, which should be light and sparing, and if exercise of any kind be allowed, it should be that of swinging, or of an easy carriage. Cold bathing, and especially cold sea bathing, is of great importance ; and where these cannot conveniently be had, a cold hip or shower-bath may be employed in their stead ; and if there should still be the slightest issue of blood from the vagina, injections of cold water, or of a solution of alum or sulphate of zinc, should be thrown up the passage two or three times a day ; or an icicle, or a snow-ball, be employed as a pessary.

If the habit be peculiarly vigorous and robust, stimulants and softness of bedclothes must be carefully avoided, and the downy couch be exchanged for a hard mattress. But if the constitution be delicate and emaciated, two or three glasses of wine may be allowed daily, and a course of angustura, columbo, or some other bitter tonic, should be entered upon. In either case, however, it is absolutely necessary that sexual connexion should be abstained from for ten days or a fortnight.

It has of late been much the custom to confine women of a very delicate frame, and especially after they have once miscarried, to a recumbent position, from the first symptom of conception through the whole term of gestation. In a few cases this may be a right and advantageous practice ; but in the present day it is employed far too indiscriminately. Among the causes of abortion we have just enumerated, there are many it can never touch, as where the ovum itself is at fault, or there is a natural indisposition in the uterus to expand beyond a certain diameter. In this last case, if we could be sure of it, a tepid hip-bath, employed every evening about the time the abortion is expected, would be a far more likely means of preventing it : for we should act here as in all other affections where our object is to relax and take off

---

* A bad cough is always a dangerous occurrence in pregnancy. Venesection, hyoscyamus, conium, and prussic acid, are the remedies advised by Dr. Ryan.—(Manual, &c., p. 187.) In dyspnœa from the distention of the abdomen interfering with the action of the diaphragm, he recommends antispasmodics.—Ed.

† "Cold applications, and even ice, if it can be procured, should be applied over the pubes."—(See Cyclop. of Pract. Med., art. Abortion.)- Of course the administration of opium should follow, and not precede, the abstraction of blood.—Ed.

‡ Aaskow, Act. Soc. Med. Hafn., tom. i. Even when the case proceeds from plethora, some practitioners have recourse to opium as well as the lancet. Thus Dr. R. Lee gives the following advice :—"A dose of laudanum, or of the liquor opii

sedativus, is to be given, or a starch and laudanum clyster may be administered, to prevent or quiet the uterine contractions. The superacetate of lead is in these cases a valuable remedy. Two grains, combined with a quarter of a grain of opium, may be taken every three hours, until the discharge of blood begins to abate."—Dr. R. Lee, op. et. loc. cit.—Ed.

* In cases of threatened abortion, Dr. Samuel Jackson of Northumberland, Penn., has derived great benefit from applying blisters to the back, or sacrum, and the utility of his practice is confirmed by reports from other practitioners.—See the Am. Journ. of Med. Sc., vol. ii., p. 299.—D.

tension, in which states we uniformly employ warmth and moisture : commonly, indeed, a bread and water poultice. And hence, in the instance before us, one of the best applications we could have recourse to, would be a broad swathe of flannel moistened with warm water and applied round the loins and lower belly every night on going to bed, surrounded externally with a dry swathe of folded linen. This should be worn through the whole night, and continued for a fortnight about the time we have reason to expect a periodical return of abortion from the cause now alluded to.

I was lately requested to join in consultation with an obstetric physician, upon the state of a young married lady of a highly nervous and irritable frame, united with great energy and activity both of mind and body, who had hitherto miscarried about the third month of gestation, by braving all risks, taking walks of many miles at a stretch, or riding on horseback for half the day at a time. She was now once more in the family-way, and had just commenced the discipline of only quitting her bed for the sofa, to which she was carried, and on which she was ordered to repose, with her head quite flat and in a line with her body, and without moving her arms otherwise than to feed herself; and to continue in this motionless state for the ensuing eight months. Without entering into the immediate cause of her former miscarriages, I ventured to express my doubts whether so sudden and extreme a change would not rather, hurry on than prevent abortion. But I recommended that all exertion of body and mind should be moderated, that the diet should be plain, the hours regular, that the position should be generally recumbent, and strictly so for a fortnight, about the time in which abortion might be expected. It was over-ruled, however, to persevere in the plan already adopted from the moment, and every sedentary relief and amusement that could be devised was put in requisition to support the patient's spirits. She went on well for a week : but at the end of this period became irritable, fatigued, and dispirited; and miscarried at about six weeks from conception, instead of advancing to three months, as she had hitherto done.

Even in the case of a delicate and relaxed frame, and of a mind that has no objection to confinement, it is well worth consideration whether the ordinary means of augmenting the general strength and elasticity by such tonics as are found best to agree with the system, and such exercises as may be taken without fatigue, particularly any of those kinds of motion which the Greeks denominated æora, as swinging or sailing, riding in a palanquin, or in a carriage with a sofa-bed or hammock—which, as we observed on a former occasion (*Marasmus Phthisis*, Cl. III., Ord. IV., Gen. III., Spe. 5), instead of exhausting, tranquillize and prove sedative, retard the pulse, produce sleep, and calm the irregularities of every irritable organ—may not be far more likely to serve the patient, than a life of unchanging indolence and undisturbed rest, which cannot fail to add to the general weak-

ness, how much soever the posture it inculcates may favour the quiet of the uterus itself.

We have thus far supposed that there is a mere danger of abortion, and that the symptoms are capable of being suppressed. But if the pains, instead of being local and irregular, should have become regular and contractile before medical assistance is sought for, or should have extended round the body, and been accompanied with strong expulsory efforts, and particularly if in conjunction with those there should have been a considerable degree of hemorrhage, our preventive plan will be in vain : a separation has unquestionably taken place, and to check the descent of the detached ovum would be useless if not mischievous. Even though the pains should have ceased, we can give no encouragement : for such a cessation only affords a stronger proof that the effect is concluded.

If the discharge continue but in small quantity, it is best to let it take its course ; to confine the patient to a bed lightly covered with clothing, and give her five-and-twenty or thirty drops of laudanum. Bleeding is often had recourse to with a view of effecting a revulsion ; it is uncalled for, however, and may do mischief by augmenting the weakness.

But the practitioner often arrives when the discharge is in great abundance, and amounts to a flooding ; and the patient is faint and sinking, and seems ready to expire.

To the inexperienced, these symptoms are truly alarming ; and in a few instances, sudden death appears to have ensued from the exhaustion that accompanies them. But it rarely happens that the patient does not recover in an hour or two from the deliquium ; and even the syncope itself is one of the most effectual means of putting a check to the discharge, by the sudden interruption it gives to all vascular action. Cold, both external and internal, is here of the utmost importance : the bed-curtains should be undrawn, the windows thrown open, and a sheet alone flung over the patient ; while linen wrung out in cold water or ice-water should be applied to the lower parts of the body, and renewed as its temperature becomes warm, withholding the application, however, as soon as the hemorrhage ceases.

Injections should in this case be desisted from ; for the formation of clots of blood around the bleeding vessels should be encouraged as much as possible, instead of being washed away. And for this reason, it is now a common practice to plug the vagina as tight as possible with a sponge or folds of linen, or, what is better, a silk handkerchief, smeared over with oil, that they may be introduced the more easily, and afterward to confine the plug with a T bandage. This plan has been long recommended by Dr. Hamilton, and has been extensively followed with considerable success. Here, also, Dr. Hamilton prescribes large doses of opium as an auxiliary, beginning with five grains, and continuing it in doses of three grains every three hours, till the hemorrhage has entirely ceased. Opium, however, is given with most advantage where the flooding takes place after the expulsion of the ovum; for if this have not occurred, its advantage may be questioned, since it has a direct tendency to interrupt that muscular contraction without which the ovum cannot be expelled. And it should be farther observed, that where opium is had recourse to in such large doses as are above proposed, it must not be dropped suddenly, for the most mischievous consequences would ensue; but must be continued in doses gradually diminishing till it can at length be omitted with prudence.

If the flooding occur after the sixth or seventh month, and the debility be extreme, the hands should be introduced into the uterus as soon as its mouth is sufficiently dilated, and the child turned and brought away. And if, before this time, a considerable degree of irritation be kept up in the womb from the retention of the fœtus or any considerable part of the ovum after its separation, one or two fingers should also be introduced for the purpose of hooking hold of what remains, and bringing it away at once. Such a retention is often exceedingly distressing, and the dead parts continue to drop away in membranous or filmy patches for several weeks, intermixed with a bloody and offensive mucus. And not unfrequently, some danger of a typhus fever is incurred from the corrupt state of the unexpelled mass. In this case, the strength must be supported with a nutritious diet, a liberal allowance of wine, and the use of the warm bitters, with mineral acids. It is also of great importance that the uterus itself be well and frequently washed with stimulant and antiseptic injections, as a solution of alum or sulphate of zinc, a decoction of cinchona or pomegranate bark, a solution of myrrh or benzoin, or, what is better than any of them, negus made with rough port wine. The injection must not be wasted in the vagina, but pass directly into the uterus; and on this account the syringe must be armed with a pipe made for the purpose, and of sufficient length.

The application of cold then, plugging the vagina, opium, and perfect quiet, and where the pulse is full, venesection, are the chief remedies to be employed in abortions, or threatenings of abortions, accompanied with profuse hemorrhage; and where these do not succeed, and especially after the sixth month, immediate delivery should be resorted to. The process, however, of applying cold, should not be continued longer than the hemorrhage demands; for cold itself, when in extreme, is one of the most powerful sources of sensorial exhaustion we are acquainted with. And hence, where the system is constitutionally weak, and particularly where it has been weakened by a recurrence of the same discharge, it may be a question well worth weighing, whether any thing below a moderately cool temperature be allowable even on the first attack? as also whether the application of warm cloths to the stomach and extremities might not be of more advantage? for unless the extremities of the ruptured vessels possess some degree of power, they cannot possibly contract, and the flow of blood must continue. And it is in these cases that benefit has sometimes been found by a still wider departure from the ordinary rules of practice, and the allowance of a little cold negus. So that the utmost degree of judgment is necessary on this occasion, not only how far to carry the established plan, but, on peculiar emergencies, how far to deviate from and even oppose it.

We have said that the hemorrhage which takes place in abortions, however profuse, is rarely accompanied with serious effects. This, however, must be limited to the first time of their taking place: for if they recur frequently in the course of a single gestation, or form a habit of recurrence in subsequent pregnancies, the blood, from such frequent discharges, loses its proper crasis; the strength of the constitution is broken down; and all the functions of the system are performed with considerable languor. The increasing sensorial weakness produces increasing irritability; and hence slighter external impressions occasion severer mischief, and the patient becomes subject to frequent fits of hysteria, and other spasmodic affections. Nor is this all; for the stomach cannot digest its food, the intestines are sluggish, the bile is irregularly secreted, the heart acts feebly; and the whole of this miserable train of symptoms is apt to terminate in dropsy.*

GENUS II.
PARODYNIA.
MORBID LABOUR.

THE PROGRESS OF LABOUR DISTURBED OR ENDANGERED BY IRREGULARITY OF SYMPTOMS, PRESENTATION, OR STRUCTURE.

THE generic term is a Greek compound from παρά, malè, and ὠδίν or ὠδίς-ινος, " dolor parturientis." All the different species of viviparous animals have a term of utero-gestation peculiar to themselves, and to which they adhere with a wonderful precision. Among women we have already said that this term is forty weeks, being nine calendar or ten lunar months. Occasionally, the expulsory process commences within this period, and occasionally extends a little beyond it; but, upon the whole, it is so true to this exact time as clearly to show it to be under the influence of some particular agency, though the nature of such agency has never been satisfactorily pointed out. Sometimes the weight of

* It is observed by Dr. Ryan (Manual, &c., p. 192), that when abortion occurs during the two first months of pregnancy, we can only distinguish it from excessive menstruation by the blood coagulating,—an appearance never witnessed in the menses. Abortion is most common in the first three months, women being then more nervous and irritable than in the subsequent stage of pregnancy. It is also noticed, that consumptive women, who have a great aptitude to conceive, seldom miscarry. It is familiarly known, that such women as marry late in life are particularly liable to the accident. With respect to numerous organic diseases of the uterine organs, and of the embryo and its involucra, acting as causes of abortion, practitioners have no means of preventing or removing them.—Dr. R. Lee, in Cyclop. of Pract. Med., art. ABORTION.—ED.

the child has been supposed to force it downwards at this precise period, and sometimes the uterus has been supposed to contract, from its inability of expanding any farther, and hence from an irritable excitement produced by the pressure of the growing fœtus. By other physiologists it has been ascribed to the increasing activity of the child, and the uneasiness occasioned by its movements. But it is a sufficient answer to all these hypotheses to remark, that a like punctuality is observed, whether the child be small or large, alive or dead ; unless, indeed, the death took place at a premature period of the pregnancy ; for "no fact," says Dr. Denman, "is more incontestably proved, than that a dead child, even though it may have become putrid, is commonly born after a labour as regular and natural in every part of the process as a living one" (*Pract. of Midwifery*, 8vo., 5th edit., p. 255) : and hence we can only resolve it into the ordinary law of instinct or of nature, like that which regulates the term of menstruation, or assert still more intelligibly with Avicenna, that "at the appointed time labour comes on by the command of God."*

In natural labour, which consists in a gradual enlargement of the mouth of the womb and the diameter of the vagina, so as to suffer the child to pass away when urged from above by a repetition of expulsatory contractions of the uterus and all the surrounding muscles,† there is little or no danger, however painful or distressing to the mother. These contractions or labour-pains continue, with a greater or less regularity of interval and recurrence, from two hours to twelve : the process rarely terminating sooner than the former period, or later than the latter ; the ordinary term being about six hours.

But unhappily labours do not always proceed in a natural course ; for sometimes there is a feebleness or irregularity in the muscular action that greatly retards their progress ; or a derangement of some remote organ that sympathizes with the actual state of the uterus, and produces the same effect ; or the mouth of the uterus itself is peculiarly rigid and unyielding ; or the natural presentation of the child's head may be exchanged for some other position ; or the maternal pelvis may be misshapen, and not afford convenient room for the descent of the child ;

---

* This inquiry seems, as Dr. Ramsbotham observes, to promise as much usefulness as the question, why human beings do not grow twenty feet high, or live for five hundred years ?—Ed.
† The action of the uterus is involuntary, which is regarded as "a wise provision of nature, because it is most probable that many women would not have fortitude sufficient to bring on labour voluntarily at the end of the proper term of gestation ; while some might induce action prematurely, either from fear, shame, or other motives. The auxiliary muscles, however, which assist the uterine powers, are, to a certain extent, voluntary ; so that labour may be said to consist of a mixed action, principally involuntary, but partly voluntary ; and it is in the woman's power to aid the contractions of the uterus by the exertion of her own will."—See Dr. Ramsbotham's Lectures, as published in Med. Gaz. for 1833–4.—Ed.

or there may be a plurality of children ; or, even after the birth of the child, the placenta may not follow with its ordinary regularity ; or an alarming hemorrhage may supervene ; each of which conditions becomes a distinct species of disease in the progress of morbid labour, and the whole of which may be arranged as follows :—

1. Parodynia Atonica.   Atonic Labour.
2. ———— Implastica. Unpliant Labour.
3. ———— Sympathet- Complicated Labour-
     ica.
4. ———— Perversa.   Preternatural Presen-
                          tation. Cross-birth.
5. ———— Amorphica. Impracticable Labour.
6. ———— Pluralis.   Multiparous Labour.
7. ———— Secundaria. Sequential Labour.

SPECIES I.

PARODYNIA ATONICA.

ATONIC LABOUR.

LABOUR PROTRACTED BY GENERAL OR LOCAL DE-
BILITY, OR HEBETUDE OF ACTION.

It often happens, in various affections of the system, that a general law is incapable of being carried into effect with promptness and punctuality from weakness or indolence of the organs chiefly concerned in its execution. Thus, when vaccine or variolous fluid is properly inserted under the cuticle, it remains there in many cases for several days beyond its proper period, in a dormant state, from inirritability or indolence in the cutaneous absorbents ; and in the case of smallpox, even where the fluid has been received into the system, whether naturally or by inoculation, and has excited febrile action, this action is, in many instances, very considerably augmented from a like indolence or inirritability of the secernents of the skin, which do not throw off the morbid matter sufficiently on the surface.

A like want of harmonious action very frequently occurs in parturition. The full time has expired—the uterus feels uneasy, and the uneasiness is communicated to the adjoining organs, and there are occasional pains in the back or in the lower belly ; but either from a weakness or hebetude, or both, in the uterus itself, or in the muscles that are to co-operate with it in expelling the child, the pains are not effective, and the labour makes little progress.

It often happens, also, in debilitated habits, that while in some parts of its progress the labour advances kindly and even rapidly, the little strength the patient possesses is worn out, and her pains suddenly cease ; or, what is worse, still continue, but without their expulsory or effective power, and, consequently, do nothing more than tease her, and add to the weakness. This exhaustion will sometimes occur soon after the commencement of the labour, or in its first stage, before the os uteri has dilated, and while the water is slowly accumulating over it ; but in this stage it is more likely to occur, if the membranes should have prematurely given way, and the water have been already evacuated. Yet it occurs also, occasionally, towards the close even of the last stage, and when the head of the child has completely cleared itself of the uterus, and is so broadly resting on the perinæum that a single effective pain or two would be sufficient to send it, without any assistance, into the world.

In the greater number of these cases, to wait with a quiet command of mind, and sooth the patient's desponding spirits by a thousand little insinuating attentions, and a confident assurance that she will do well at last, is the best, if not the only duty to be performed. A stimulant injection, however, of dissolved soap or muriate of soda, will often re-excite the contractions where they flag, or change the nature of the pains where they are ineffective. After this it is often useful to give thirty or five-and-thirty drops of laudanum, and to let the patient remain perfectly quiet. It is not certain in what way the laudanum may act, for it sometimes proves a local stimulant, and sometimes a general sedative; but in either way it will be serviceable, and nearly equally so; for it will either shorten the labour by re-exciting and invigorating the pains, or increase the general strength by producing sleep and quiet.*

In America, it has of late been a common practice to employ spurred rye in cases of this kind, as we have already observed under Paramenia difficilis, for which also it is very generally had recourse to; it being supposed to have a specific power in stimulating the uterus: and the cases adverted to are numerous and authentic, in which it seems to have been serviceable in exciting labour-pains under the present affection.†

If the pulse should be quick and feeble, with languor and a sense of faintness at the stomach, a little mulled wine or some other cordial may be allowed. If the mouth of the womb be lax and dilatable, and the water have accumulated large-ly and protrude upon it as in a bag, advantage is often gained by breaking the membranes and evacuating the fluid, for a new action is hereby given to the uterus, and while it contracts with more force it meets with less resistance, and its mouth is more rapidly expanded. But unless the labour should have advanced to this stage, the membranes should never be interfered with; for their plasticity, and the gradual increase and pressure of their protruding sac against the edges of the os uteri, form the easiest and surest means of enlarging in, while the retention of the fluid in this early stage of parturition lubricates the inner surface of the womb, and tends to keep off heat and irritation.*

For the same reason, if the mouth of the womb be narrow and have hitherto scarcely given way, the application of the finger can be of no advantage. Every attempt to dilate it must be in vain, and only produce irritation, and an increased thickening in its edges: but if it have opened to a diameter of two inches, and be at the same time soft and expansile, advantage should be taken of the pains to dilate it by the introduction of one or two fingers still further, which should only, however, co-operate with the pains, and be employed while they are acting; and, by these conjoint means, the head of the child sometimes passes rapidly and completely out of the uterus.

We have said that it is sometimes apt to lodge in the vagina in consequence of the patient's exhaustion, and an utter cessation of all pains, or of all that are of any avail. The patient should again therefore be suffered to rest, and if faint, be again recruited with some cordial support. Generally speaking, time alone is wanting, and the practitioner must consent to wait; and it will be better for him to retire from his patient, and to wait at a little distance. But if several hours should pass away without any return of expulsory efforts, if there should be frequent or continual pains without any benefit, if the patient's strength should sink, her pulse become weak and frequent, if the mind should show unsteadiness, and there be a tendency to syncope, and if, at the same time, the head be lying clear of the perinæum, the vectis or forceps should be had recourse to, and the woman be delivered by artificial means. This situation forms a general warrant; but for the peculiar circumstances in which such or any other instruments should be employed, the manner of employing them, and the nature of the instruments

---

* Here, instead of laudanum, many practitioners prescribe the acetous solution of opium (Dubl. Pharm.), the liquor opii sedativus, or the acetate or muriate of morphine.—Ed.

† Dr. John Stearns, of New-York, was the first American practitioner who publicly proposed the use of ergot to facilitate lingering labour. In his paper in the New-York Med. and Phys. Journ., vol. i., he has succinctly stated the principles which ought to regulate its employment. He remarks, "The ergot is indicated and may be prescribed, 1st, When, in lingering labours, the child has descended into the pelvis, the parts dilated and relaxed, and the pains having ceased or being too inefficient to advance the labour, there is danger to be apprehended from delay, by exhaustion of strength and vital energy, from hemorrhage, or other alarming symptoms. 2d, When the pains are transferred from the uterus to other parts of the body, or to the whole muscular system, producing general puerperal convulsions. 3d, When, in the early stages of pregnancy, abortion becomes inevitable, accompanied with profuse hemorrhage and feeble uterine contractions. 4th, When the placenta is retained from a deficiency of contraction. 5th, In patients liable to hemorrhage immediately after delivery. 6th, When hemorrhage or lochial discharges are too profuse immediately after delivery, and the uterus continues dilated and relaxed, without any ability to contract.—D.

* The advice, here delivered agrees with that given by the best modern obstetric practitioners. Thus, Dr. Ramsbotham, in his Lectures, strongly recommends the plan of preserving the membranous bag entire as long as possible; or, at least, until it has performed the whole of the office destined for it by nature; namely, the dilatation of the os uteri, the vagina, and in some degree also of the external parts. When the membranes appear externally to the vulva, we may then suppose that they have done all the good that can be expected from them; that their remaining entire may possibly be retarding the labour; and we may in that case venture to rupture them, provided the head present.—See Med. Gaz. for 1833–4, p. 821.—Ed.

themselves, the reader must consult such books as are expressly written upon the subject, and should sedulously attend the lectures and the introductory practice which are so usefully offered to him in this metropolis.*

SPECIES II.

PARODYNIA IMPLASTICA.

UNPLIANT LABOUR.

LABOUR DELAYED OR INJURED FROM IMPLASTICITY OR UNKINDLY DILATATION OF THE SOFT PARTS.

THE tediousness and difficulty of the preceding species of labour proceed chiefly from atony or hebetude of the system generally, or of the local organs particularly. But it often happens, that the parts dilate and the labour proceeds as slowly from an implasticity, or rigid resistance to the expansion and expulsory efforts which should take place, according to the law of nature, at the fulness of time which we are now supposing to be accomplished, and which is sometimes productive of other evils than that of protracted suffering, offering us, indeed, the four following varieties :

a Rigiditatis.	The delay confined to a simple rigidity of the uterus or outer mouth.
β Prolapsa.	Accompanied with prolapse.
γ Hæmorrhagica.	Accompanied with hemorrhage.
δ Lacerans.	Accompanied with laceration of the uterus or perinæum.

RIGIDITY OF THE UTERUS may extend to the entire organ, or be limited to the cervix, or os uteri, as it is called after the cervix has lost its natural form, and partakes of the spherical shape of the fundus. When the former occurs, the practitioner meets with severe pains in the loins, shooting round the lower belly, and producing great contractile efforts of the muscles surrounding the uterus, so as to throw the patient, from the violence of her exertions, into a profuse perspiration, and induce the attendants to believe that the labour is advancing with great speed, while the practitioner himself finds, on examination, that there is no progress whatever ; that the uterus itself does not unite in the expulsory force, the fluid of the amnios does not accumulate over the os uteri, nor the head of the child bear down upon it.

In other cases he finds that the general organ of the uterus does participate in the common action, and force the head of the child downward, but that the mouth of the womb does not dilate or become thinner in consequence hereof ; appearing, on the contrary, in some cases, from a peculiar tenderness and irritation, to grow thicker and tenser, and more intractable.

* See Dr. Dewees's System of Midwifery ; Dr. Meigs's valuable Translation of Velpeau's Midwifery ; Midwifery Illustrated, by J. P. Maygrier, translated from the French by A. Sidney Doane ; Dr. Francis's edition of Denman's Midwifery, &c., &c.

And he not unfrequently finds, even where both the body and mouth of the womb are sufficiently pliable and co-operative with the common intention, and the head of the child has become easily cleared of this organ, that a like rigidity and implasticity exist in the os internum, and that the child, having readily worked its way thus far, is fast locked from this circumstance, and cannot get any further ; and occasionally the rigidity has been found in some part, and particularly the upper part of the vagina, of which Dr. Davis has given a very striking example in a young woman parturient for the first time. The contraction was here a spastic ring, bordering immediately on the orifice of the uterus ; and so inconsiderable that the forefinger could not be made to pass through it.—(*Elements of Operative Midwifery,* &c., 4to., 1825.)

In all cases of this kind, the same means of relaxation should be resorted to as in an irritable or inflammatory tenseness and rigidity of other organs. Blood should be freely abstracted, active purgatives be given by the mouth, and copious emollient injections be administered without much aperient virtue, so that they may for some time remain in the rectum and act as a fomentation. And here also it may be advantageous to apply round the loins and lower belly a broad swathe of flannel wrung out in hot water, and to encircle it with an equally broad band of folded linen, in the manner already recommended in PARAMENIA DIFFICILIS.

In Dr. Davis's case of contracted vagina, after an abstraction of blood to deliquium, which demanded thirty ounces, sixty drops of Battley's sedative solution of opium were also directed to be given, with great judgment as well as with the most desirable success : for in about five hours the child's head had cleared both the orifice of the uterus and the contracted part of the vagina, and was beginning to bear on the os externum ; in about three hours after which, the patient was safely delivered of a living child.

In several cases of rigidity, if no means be adopted to subdue the tension, the protrusive force of the surrounding muscles is sometimes so considerable that, as it cannot expel the child by itself, it goes far to expel the child and the uterus conjointly, the latter being thrust downward into the outward passage, and its mouth projecting out of the vulva, thus constituting a PARTURIENT PROLAPSE.

While the uterus is thus forcibly descending, the attendant should support it, or the head of the child, with two fingers ; if the prolapse be complete, the uterus should be returned into its proper place as quickly as possible ; and if this cannot be done, the child must be turned, and delivery take place as speedily as may be.

In the violence of this struggle, it sometimes happens, moreover, and particularly where the water has escaped, that some of the vessels give way, or the placenta is partly detached, and there is the additional evil of a PROFUSE HEMORRHAGE to contend with.

If this occur in the commencement of labour, venesection should generally be had recourse to, the patient be kept cool and quiet, and take thirty drops of laudanum. If the labour have advanced and is advancing rapidly, and the hemorrhage be not very considerable, we may safely trust to nature to complete the process before any serious mischief ensues. But if the patient be debilitated, or much exhausted, or the labour advance slowly, the woman should be delivered by turning the child, or having recourse to the forceps, according to the progress of the labour, and the position of the child at the time.

But there is a far worse evil than any of these, which results from the implasticity we are now considering: and that is, a rupture or LACERATION, either OF THE VAGINA OF OF THE UTERUS. The causes of laceration are said to be numerous, and it often occurs suddenly and without any known cause: but if we examine into their general nature, we shall find that, except in the case of brutal force or want of skill, they are almost always dependant on a certain degree of implasticity in the lacerated part of the organ, which prevents it from yielding with the uniformity of the other parts, or from a peculiar degree of irritability, that renders it more liable to irregular action or spasm: though there can be no question that, in a very few instances, the laceration has commenced from a cut produced by an occasional sharpness of the edge of the ilium. "Those women," observes Mr. Burns, "are most liable to rupture of the uterus who are very irritable, and subject to cramp; or who have the pelvis contracted, or its brim very sharp, or who have the os uteri very rigid, or any part of the womb indurated. Schulzius relates a case where it was produced by scirrhus of the fundus; and Friedius one where it was owing to a carneo-cartilaginous state of the os uteri."—(*Principles of Midwifery,* 8vo., 3d edit., p. 361.)

Laceration of the fundus of the womb may take place during any part of the labour, when the pains are violent, and the walls of the organ do not act in unison in every part; but the mischief more commonly commences in the cervix, when the head, or the shoulders, or any other part is passing through, and the whole of its circumference does not yield equally.*

Where the accident occurs in the vagina or perinæum, it must necessarily take place after the head has descended from the womb, and is pressing upon the substance of these organs, that, like the lacerating os uteri, does not yield equally in every point.*

In most cases of an implastic rigidity, whether in the body of the uterus itself, or in its cervix, or in the os externum, there is a considerable degree of local irritation, and in many of them a great deal of firm and vigorous action. The parts are not only rigid, but dry, and hot, and tender, and the pulse is generally full, with restlessness and a heated skin. And hence venesection is imperatively called for from an early period of the labour: and there are few cases in which the uterus has not acted afterward with more freedom, and its mouth been rendered laxer, softer, and more compliable. In all such cases, also, an emollient injection several times repeated will advantageously co-operate in taking off the tension, and increasing the expansibility. Here opium should be avoided, but general relaxants, as antimony and ipecacuanha, given in the neutral effervescing draught, may add to the general benefit. The operator must be abstinent till the parts have yielded, and the tension and irritation subsided; for before this, every application of the fingers will only increase the morbid tendency.

The only case in which the use of opium is here to be justified, is where, from the violence of the contractile pains, a considerable and an alarming hemorrhage has ensued, and the state of the os uteri will not allow of the introduction of the hand for the purpose of turning and delivering immediately. In this instance, after venesection and a due administration of emollient and aperient injections, our last dependance must be upon a powerful opiate, for the purpose of allaying the irritation, and taking off the pains.†

And if the force of the expulsory power thrust down the uterus so as to give danger of producing a prolapse, the practitioner must support the organ during the recurrence of the pains, by introducing two fingers into the vagina for this purpose, and the patient must be kept in a recumbent position, without moving from it; and must be instructed to avoid, as much as possible, every expulsory or bearing-down ex-

---

* "This disastrous occurrence is to be dreaded," says Dr. Ryan, "in all cases of transverse labours, unless timely aid be afforded. It is most common in arm presentations, and in deformities of the pelvis. In a word, in all cases where the labour is protracted and violent."—(See Manual, &c., p. 287.) When a woman has already borne children, the os uteri generally dilates very readily in subsequent parturitions; but this is by no means universally the case. Dr. Ramsbotham relates the particulars of a woman whom he attended in her first labour, and the child was born naturally in four or five hours. In her second labour, however, the membranes broke early; the p became exceedingly violent; the head was foaced powerfully against the undilated and rigid os uteri; irregular muscular spasms supervened; and, at the end of about fifty hours from the rupture of the membranes, when the os uteri had not acquired a diameter larger than a shilling, Dr. Ramsbotham, while carefully examining the parts, felt the os

uteri and the cervix give way on the right side, and the head passed at once into the vagina. Bleeding and opium here had failed to bring about the requisite dilatation of the os uteri. The patient died of uterine inflammation on the fourth day after delivery.—See Ramsbotham's Lectures, as published in Med. Gaz. for 1834, p. 161.—ED.

* The following references to cases of ruptured uterus, from falls or blows in the early months of pregnancy, are given by Dr. Ryan, op. cit., p. 441: namely, Phil. Trans., vol. xlv., p. 121; Mém. de l'Acad. des Sciences, 1709; Journ. Méd., 1780; Burns's Midwifery, p. 610; Annals of Med., p. 412; Dublin Med. Trans., 1830, vol. i., New Series, &c.

† In cases of rigidity, where the patients were robust, the celebrated Dr. Hamilton, of Edinburgh, employed venesection; but where they were delicate, the starch and opium clyster.—ED.

ertion while the pain is upon her. If the uterus-have actually protruded into the vagina, a reduction must be instantly attempted: and if this cannot be done, no time should be lost in passing the hand through the cervix, as soon as, without force, it can be sufficiently dilated for this purpose, and delivering the child by turning.

Laceration generally takes place suddenly; though in irritable habits, cramps or other spasmodic affections are often previously complained of in different parts of the body. Mr. Burns has well described the symptoms that succeed:—" When this accident does happen, the woman feels something give way within her, and usually suffers at that time an increase of pain. The presentation disappears more or less speedily, unless the head have fully entered the pelvis; or the uterus contract spasmodically on part of the child, as happened in Bechling's patient. —(Haller, Disput., tom. iii., p. 477.) The pains go off as soon as the child passes through the rent into the abdomen: or, if the presentation be fixed in the pelvis, they become irregular, and gradually decline. The passage of the child into the abdominal cavity is attended with a sensation of strong motion of the belly, and is sometimes productive of convulsions."— (Burns, ut suprà, p. 362.)

It is not necessary to make a distinction between the parts in which the laceration takes place; for, whether it be in the fundus or cervix of the womb, or in the vagina, except where, as just observed, the position is fixed in the pelvis, the part presented instantly disappears, and the child slips imperceptibly through the chasm into the hollow of the abdomen, sometimes with a hemorrhage that threatens life instantly, but sometimes with little or even no hemorrhage whatever.*

This accident will not unfrequently occur towards the close of a labour that promises fair. It is not many years ago when the present author, at that time engaged in this branch of the profession, was requested with all speed to attend, in consultation, upon a lady in Wigmore-street, who was then under the hands of a practitioner of considerable skill and eminence. She had, for about eight hours, been in labour of her first child, herself about thirty-eight years of age, had had natural pains, and been cheered throughout with the prospect of doing well, and even more rapidly than usual, under the circumstances of the case. In fact, the head had completely cleared the os uteri, and was resting on the perinæum, and the obstetric practitioner was flattering himself that, in a quarter of an hour at the farthest, he should be released from his confinement, when he was surprised by a sudden retreat of the child during a pain which he expected would have afforded her great relief, accompanied with an alarming flooding: and it was in this emergency the author of this work was requested to attend. On examination, it was ascertained that a large laceration had

taken place in the uterus, commencing at the cervix, and apparently on the passing of the shoulders; but why any part of it should have torn at this time rather than antecedently, there were no means of determining. It is usual, under these circumstances, to follow up the child with the hand through the rupture into the abdomen, and to endeavour to lay hold of the feet, and withdraw it by turning. The hemorrhage had alarmed the practitioner, and this had not been attempted; and, at the time of the author's arrival, which was about an hour and a half afterward, the attempt was too late, for the pulse was rapidly sinking, the breathing interrupted, and the countenance ghastly; yet the patient had not totally lost her self-possession, and being informed of her situation, begged earnestly to be let alone, and to be suffered to die in quiet.

Where there is little or no hemorrhage, life usually continues much longer, whether the child be extracted or not; mostly about twenty-four hours, though in some cases considerably longer still. Dr. Garthshore attended a patient who lived till the twenty-sixth day, and the Copenhagen Transactions (tom. ii., p. 326) contain the case of a woman who, after being delivered, lingered for three months; and a few marvellous histories are given in the public collections of a natural healing of the uterus, while the child continued as a foreign and extra-fœtal substance in the cavity of the abdomen for many years. Haller has reported a case in which it continued in this state for nine years (Mém. de Paris, 1773); and others relate examples of its remaining for sixteen (Eph. Nat. Cur., dec. i., ann. iii., obs. 12), and even twenty-six years,* or through the entire term of the mother's natural life.†

The only rational hope of saving both the mother and the child, is by following up the latter through the rupture, and delivering it by the feet; but where this cannot be done from the smallness of the dilatation of the os uteri, or from the violent contraction of the uterus between the os uteri and the rent, we have nothing to propose but to leave the event to nature, or

---

* Blood may escape from the vagina, but generally it passes into the cavity of the abdomen, and excites peritonitis.—Ed.

---

* Eph. Nat. Cur., dec. ii., ann. viii., obs. 134. Lieutaud mentions examples in which the fœtus was retained from ten to forty years. When the patient sinks, it is generally from inflammation of the bowels and uterus. In some cases, abscesses follow near the rectum, or in the perinæum, from which the fœtus is discharged piecemeal. Dr. M'Keever's work on Lacerations of the Womb and Vagina, published in 1824, deserves praise, as containing a good deal of information on the subject.—Ed.

† If the woman is saved, the womb decreases, and returns to its former unimpregnated size; the menses return; and she may become pregnant and even bear children before the expulsion of the extra-uterine fœtus.—(Journ. de Méd., tom. v., p. 422; Burns, p. 105.) When the child is retained many years in the abdomen, it becomes enclosed in a cyst. In a case of this kind recorded by Dr. Percival, the fœtus, at the end of twenty-two years, was expelled from the rectum.—(See Ryan's Manual of Midwifery, p. 440.) No doubt some of the instances reported as cases of ruptured uterus, have been in truth extra-uterine conceptions.—Ed.

to extract the child by the Cæsarean operation. We have just seen that, in a few rare instances, the vis medicatrix Naturæ, or instinctive tendency to health, has succeeded in healing the wound, and restoring the patient with the fœtus still inhabiting the belly. But this result is so little to be expected, that an incision into the cavity of the abdomen has not unfrequently been tried, and in some instances unquestionably with success.[*]

SPECIES III.
PARODYNIA SYMPATHETICA.
COMPLICATED LABOUR.

LABOUR RETARDED, OR HARASSED BY SYMPATHETIC DERANGEMENT OF SOME REMOTE ORGAN OR FUNCTION.

We have often had occasion to observe that, with the exception of the stomach, there is no organ that holds such numerous ramifications of sympathy with other organs as the womb; and we hence find the progress of parturition disturbed, and what would otherwise be a natural, converted into a morbid labour, by the interference of various other parts of the body, or the faculties which appertain to them. The whole family of varieties which issue from this source are extremely numerous : but the three following are the chief :—

α Pathematica.　Accompanied with terror or other mental emotion.
β Syncopalis.　Accompanied with fainting.
γ Convulsiva.　Accompanied with convulsions.

In the PATHEMATIC VARIETY, the joint emotions which are usually operative upon the patient's mind, and especially on the first labour, are bashfulness on the presence of her medical attendant, and apprehension for her own safety. There is not a practitioner in the world but must have had numerous instances of a total suspension of pains on his first making his appearance in the chamber. And in some cases, the pains have been completely driven away for four-and-twenty hours, or even a longer term.

There is nothing extraordinary in this, for two powerful morbid actions are seldom found to proceed in the animal frame simultaneously ; and hence pregnancy is well known to arrest phthisis, and the severest pain of a decayed tooth to yield to the dread of having it extracted, while the patient is on his way to the operator's house.

It is hence of great importance, that the bespoken attendant should familiarize himself to his patient before his assistance is required, and endeavour to obtain her entire confidence : and it is better, when he is first ushered into her presence in his professional capacity, that he should say little upon the subject of his visit, direct the conversation to some other topic of general interest, and then withdraw till he is wanted. And if the idea alone of his approach

be peculiarly harassing, it is best for him to be in a remote part of the house in readiness, and not to see his patient till her pains have taken so strong a hold as to be beyond the control of the fancy.

If her apprehensions for herself be very active, and if there be any particular ground for them, it is most reasonable to enter candidly on the question, and to afford her all the consolation that can be administered.

SYNCOPE, in labour, proceeds commonly from a peculiar participation of the stomach in the irritation of the womb, and is hence often connected with a sense of nausea, or with vomiting. Occasionally it occurs also from the exhaustion produced by the violence of the pains : and particularly in relaxed and debilitated habits, in which case the fainting fits sometimes follow up each other in very rapid succession, and require very close attention on the part of the practitioner and the patient's friends.

The usual remedies should here be had recourse to in the first instance ; pungent volatiles should be applied to the nostrils, the patient be in a recumbent position, with the curtains undrawn, and unless the season of the year probibit, with the windows open ; the face, and especially the forehead and temples, should be sprinkled with cold water or ether ; and the usual volatile fetids, aromatics, and terebinthinates, as camphire, should be given by the mouth ; and to these, if necessary, and particularly where the pulse is feeble and fluttering, should be added a glass or two of Madeira, or any other cordial wine, with twenty drops of laudanum.

If this plan should not answer, and especially if the fainting-fits should increase in duration and approximation to each other, the patient must be delivered by the process of turning, as soon as ever the os uteri is sufficiently dilated to let the hand pass without force.

One of the worst and most alarming of the associated symptoms in labour is that of CONVULSIONS, and these are often connected with fainting-fits, and the two alternate with each other. We have already glanced at them generally under SYSPASIA CONVULSIO, but must dwell upon them a little more at large under the present modification.

Convulsions may occur during any period of gestation ; but we are now to consider them as an accompaniment of labour, and as interrupting its progress. Their proximate cause is a peculiar irritation of the nervous system as participating in the irritation of the womb ; and hence it is obvious, that the radical and specific cure is a termination of the labour.

We cannot always trace the link of this peculiar influence of the womb upon the nervous system ; though where there is a predisposition to clonic spasm of any kind, we can readily account for its excitement, and may be under less apprehension, than where it occurs without any such tendency. The occasional causes of fainting are the same as of convulsions : and hence they are apt to follow, and particularly in delicate or debilitated constitutions, on the fatigue and exhaustion of violent and protracted pains,

---

[*] Progrès de la Médecine, 1698, 12mo. Abbandlung der Königl. Schwed. Acad., 1744. Hist. de l'Acad. Royale des Sciences, 1714, p. 29, 1716, p. 32.

great depression of the animal spirits, and profuse hemorrhage. Sometimes, however, they
occur where none of these are present, and
where the patient is of a strong plethoric habit
of body, and especially if it be her first time of
pregnancy ; and are accompanied with, or even
preceded by, a sense of dizziness and oppression
in the head, ringing in the ears, or imperfect
vision; the plethora itself thus forming the occasional cause.

The attendant symptoms are peculiarly violent, sometimes resembling those of hysteria,
sometimes those of epilepsy, but more vehement.
Nothing can restrain the spastic force of a woman when in parturient convulsions, whatever
be her natural weakness. The distortion of the
countenance is more hideous than the most extravagant imagination can conceive ; and the
rapidity with which the eyes open and shut, the
sudden twirlings of the mouth, the foam that collects about the lips, the peculiar hiss that issues
from them, the stertor, the insensibility, and the
jactitating struggle of the limbs, form a picture
of agony that cannot be beheld without horror.

The exciting cause is the irritable state of the
womb ; and whatever be the predisponent or occasional cause, whether a debilitated condition
of the nervous system, or a robust and entonic
fulness of the bloodvessels, it is obvious that
such violence of action cannot take place under
any circumstances without endangering a rupture of the vessels in the head, and consequently
all the mischiefs of apoplexy. It is against this,
indeed, that all practitioners, how much soever
they may disagree upon other points, most cor-
dially endeavour to guard, though it rarely happens that effusion in the brain, and some of its
results, do not take place in spite of all their exertions.

The first step is to open a vein, and bleed copiously from a large orifice till the patient
faints : and if the operator be expert, the best
vein to make choice of is the jugular :* the hair
should be immediately removed from the head,
and lotions of cold water, pounded ice, or the
freezing mixture, produced by dissolving three
or four different sorts of neutral salts in water
at the same time, be applied all over it by wetted napkins, changed for others as soon as they
acquire the least degree of warmth. At the
same time, a purgative injection should be
thrown up the rectum, and five or six grains of
calomel be given by the mouth with a draught
of sulphate of magnesia in infusion of senna.
The paroxysms must, if possible, be put a stop
to, the fatal effects they threaten must be anticipated, and not a moment is to be lost.

This is the general plan ; and it is to be pursued under all circumstances, though its extent,
and particularly in regard to bloodletting, must
be regulated by the strength and energy of the
patient. The local mode of treatment seems to
be somewhat less decided.

* As the only jugular vein that can be opened
is the external, and it does not communicate directly with the sinuses of the brain, modern practitioners do not so frequently bleed in it as their
predecessors were accustomed to do.—Ed.

It may happen that at the attack of the fits,
the os uteri is merely beginning to open, or that
it is of the diameter of a crown-piece, but peculiarly rigid and undilatable. There are practitioners who in this case confine themselves to
the depleting plan, and only wait for the advance
of the labour : but, in the state of the uterus we
are now contemplating, they may have to wait
for some hours before the labour is so far advanced as to render them capable of affording
any manual assistance whatever, while the fits
are perhaps recurring every quarter of an hour,
and threatening fatal mischief to the brain. And
in this case, I cannot but warmly approve of the
bolder, or rather the more judicious advice of
Dr. Bland, who, after a due degree of depletion,
recommends a full dose of opium, for the purpose of allaying the nervous irritation generally,
and particularly that of the uterus, which is the
punctum saliens of the whole. A few hours'
rest may set all to rights, if no vessel have thus
far given way in the head : for when the next
tide of pains returns, it will commence under
very different circumstances, in consequence of
the reducent course of medicine that has been
pursued : and it will rarely be found that the
whole body of the uterus is not rendered more
lax and plastic, and consequently its cervix, and
even the os externum, more yielding and dilatable.

But this is not the common course which the
uterus takes under these circumstances ; for in,
by far the greater number of cases, the whole
of this organ, the cervix as well as the fundus,
is so exhausted in the general contest as to be
more than ordinarily relaxed and flaccid, and dilatable with considerable ease : insomuch that,
if the muscular power of the system were now
concentrated in a common expulsory effort, as
in natural labours, the whole process would terminate in a few minutes. But unfortunately this
muscular exertion, instead of being concentrated, is distracted and erratic, and wanders over
all the muscles and organs of the system, producing general mischief instead of local benefit :
so that whatever pains there may be, they are of
far less use than in a state of harmonious action.
This may be easily ascertained by introducing
the hand on a return of the paroxysm, when the
uterus will be found to contract indeed, but with
a tremulous, undetermined sort of force, perfectly
different from what it does at any other time.

The necessary practice in this case should appear to be obvious and without doubt : the medical attendant seems imperatively called upon
to introduce his hand into the os uteri as soon
as it is sufficiently open for him to do so without
force, to break the membranes if not broken already, lay hold of the child's feet, deliver by
turning, and thus put an end to the convulsions
at once, and consequently to the fatal effects
which seemed to await the mother as well as
the child.

Such was the practice recommended by Mauriceau upwards of a century since : "La convulsion," says he, "fait souvent périr la mère et
l'enfant, si la femme *n'est pas promptement se-
courue par l'accouchement*, qui est le meilleur

remède qu'on puisse apporter à l'une et à l'autre."—(*Traité des Maladies des Femmes grosses*, tom. i., p. 23, 4to., Paris, 1721.) This recommendation was adopted generally, and in our own country successively by Smellie, W. Hunter, and Lowder. And although, in circumstances of so much danger, it was not and could not be always successful, yet it was supposed, and with reason, to be the means of saving the life, as well of the mother as of the child, in very numerous instances in which that of one or of both would otherwise have unquestionably perished. Some forty years after the publication of M. Mauriceau's work, Professor Roederer of Goettingen called this practice in question, and recommended that the patient be left to the natural course of the labour (*Elementa Artis Obstetricæ*, Aph. 679, Goet., 1769, 8vo.) : and we are told by Dr. Denman that in our own country, Dr. Ross, towards the close of last century, "was the first person of late years who had courage to declare his doubt of the propriety of speedy delivery in *all cases* of puerperal convulsions. The observation," continues Dr. Denman (*Practice of Midwifery, ed. by Dr. J. W. Francis*, p. 607, 8vo., 3d edit., 1829), "on which these doubts were founded, was merely practical, and the event of very many cases has since confirmed the justice of his observation, both with respect to mothers and children."

The sweeping extent of this censure seems to show that the practice has often been had recourse to indiscriminately, and without a correct limitation. And the apparent concurrence of Dr. Denman in Dr. Ross's opinion, together with the undecided manner in which he treats of the question in his subsequent pages, has raised up, among the most celebrated obstetric physicians of our own day, various advocates for leaving, in general, to nature, the case of labour accompanied with convulsions, or at least till the natural efforts of the mother are found completely to fail ; and in this last case, as the child's head may be supposed to have cleared the uterus, to have recourse to the perforator or the forceps, according to the nature of the position.

The chief grounds for this proposed delay, as far as I have been able to collect them, are, that the introduction of the hand into the os infernum, in the irritable state of the organ we are now contemplating, is more calculated to renew the convulsions than to put an end to them : that a repetition of them, after due depletion has been employed, is not so dangerous as is generally apprehended, and consequently that immediate delivery is by no means essential to the patient's safety : and lastly, that we are not sure of putting an end to the convulsions, even after delivery is effected ; since it is well known that they have occasionally continued, and sometimes have not commenced, till the process of labour has been long completed.

In reply to this it may be observed, that if a repetition of the convulsive fits be not so dangerous as is commonly apprehended, a practitioner should feel less reluctance in introducing

the hand, even though he were sure of exciting a single fit by so doing : and the more so as this single fit might, perhaps, be the means of terminating the whole, and, consequently, would be a risk bought at a cheap rate. At the same time it should be observed, that general experience does not seem to justify the remark, that a cautious and scientific use of the hand, where the mouth of the womb is sufficiently dilated, becomes a necessary or even a frequent excitement of fresh paroxysms ; and the prediction of such an effect is therefore without sufficient foundation. And if there be a considerable chance, as seems to be admitted, that instrumental assistance will be requisite at last, and that the forceps, or what, in the probability of the child's being still alive, is ten times worse, the perforator, must be called into action, how much more humane is it, as well as scientific, to employ instrumental aid at first, and thus save the pain and the peril of perhaps many hours of suffering—and particularly when the soft, and supple, and plastic instrument of the hand, may supersede the use of the ruder, and rougher, and less manageable tools of art ?

But the most important part of the question is as to the actual degree of danger induced by convulsions : and to determine this, nothing more seems necessary than to put the whole upon the footing of an impending apoplexy. It is possible that no effusion in the brain may have taken place at the time when the depleting plan has been carried into execution ; but if the paroxysms should still recur, surely few men can look at the violence of the struggle which they induce, at the bloated and distended state of the vessels of the face and of the temples, at the force with which the current of blood is determined to the head, at the stertor and comatose state of the patient during the continuance of the fit, without feeling the greatest alarm at every return. And that he does not feel in vain is clear, because in various instances the insensibility continues after the paroxysm is over, accompanies her through the remainder of her labour, and is the harbinger of her death.

Regarding puerperal convulsions, then, as a case of impending apoplexy, produced by an exciting cause which it is often in our power to remove, it should seem to follow as a necessary and incontestable result, that in this, as in every other case in which the same disease is threatened, our first and unwearied attempt should be to remove such cause as far as it may be in our power.

The present author's opinion was once requested upon a case of this very kind ; but it was by the connexions of the patient, who had already fallen a victim to her sufferings. She had been attacked with natural labour-pains, and was attended by a female, who, alarmed by the sudden incursion of a convulsion-fit, sent immediately for male assistance. The practitioner arrived, and a consultation was soon held with several others : the os uteri is admitted to have been at this time open to the size of a crownpiece, soft, lubricous, and dilatable. The depleting and refrigerant plan was, however, confided in alone, and the labour was suffered to take its course. Expulsory pains followed at intervals, but the convulsions followed also, and became more frequent and more aggravated; in about six hours from the time of venesection the patient became permanently insensible; and as the child's head, completely cleared of the uterus, had now descended into the pelvis, it was determined to deliver her by the forceps, which was applied accordingly; and, in about an hour afterward, a dead child was brought into the world, whose appearance sufficiently proved that it had not been long dead.

The source of irritation had now ceased, and with it the convulsions; but the patient continued comatose still; yet even this effect went off in seven hours afterward, and she revived, and gave considerable hopes of recovery. On the second day, however, in consequence of the accession of milk-fever, the convulsions returned, immediately followed with stertor and insensibility, and, on the ensuing day, she died apoplectic.

To reason from a single instance, whether successful or unsuccessful, is often to reason wrong. Yet it is difficult to avoid conjecturing, that if immediate delivery had been taken place as soon as the sanguiferous system had been duly emptied, and when the state of the uterus was so favourable for a trial, two lives might have been spared, both of which were lost under the course pursued.* It is true, the fits returned with the milk-fever, but had the brain been less injured, there would have been far less danger of such return. The cases of Dr. Smellie and of Dr. Perfect concur in justifying such a conjecture: and the following passage of Mr. Burns should be committed to memory by every student and every practitioner. "But this is not all," adverting to the necessity of a free depletion; "for the patient is suffering from a disease connected with the state of the uterus, and the state is got rid of by terminating the labour. Even when convulsions take place very early in labour, the os uteri is generally opened to a certain degree, and the detraction of blood, which has been resorted to on the first attack of the disease, renders the os uteri usually lax and dilatable. In this case, although we have no distinct labour-pains, we must introduce the hand, and slowly dilate it, and deliver the child. I entirely agree with those who are against forcibly opening the os uteri: but I also agree with those who advise the woman to be delivered as

soon as we can possibly do it without violence. There is, I am convinced, no rule of practice more plain or beneficial. Delivery does not, indeed, always save the patient, or even prevent the recurrence of the fits, but it does not thence follow that it ought not to be adopted."—(*Principles of Midwifery*, p. 359, 3d edit, 8vo., 1811.)

SPECIES IV.
PARODYNIA PERVERSA.
CROSS-BIRTH.
LABOUR IMPEDED BY PRETERNATURAL PRESENTATION OF THE FŒTUS OR ITS MEMBRANES.

In the ordinary course of gestation, the fœtus is rolled up into as small a compass as possible, with the breast uppermost and the head dependent, the legs incurvated, and the arms folded: the placenta rises from some part of the fundus uteri, and the umbilical cord hangs at perfect ease in loose folds, or is sometimes turned loosely round the body, thus forming an ellipse, whose longer axis corresponds to the longer axis of the uterus. Why the head rather than the breast, or indeed any other part of the fœtus, should so uniformly constitute the point of presentation, we know not, excepting that it is by far the most commodious point for delivery; and we can hence only resolve it into one of those striking laws of nature, which are ever aiming at accomplishing the best ends by the best means, and afford an unvarying and unequivocal proof of design, united with benevolence and power.*

Here, however, as in every other part of the animal economy, we meet with occasional deviations from the ordinary course of nature, and deviations which are always productive of evil. For it sometimes happens, from incidental causes that are totally concealed from us, that some other part of the child is lowermost, or presents itself instead of the head; or that the placenta rises in an unfavourable part of the womb, or that the navel-string hangs down below the head, and is constantly in danger of being strangled as the child passes through the sharp bones of the pelvis; and hence, we have the following varieties of morbid condition under the present species :—

α Faciei.	Presentation of the face.
β Natium.	———————— of the breech.
γ Pedis.	———————— of one or both feet.

---

* It often happens that the os uteri does not dilate during the most violent convulsions, and consequently delivery cannot be effected. In such cases the French apply the extract of belladonna to dilate the uterine orifice, and when this fails, the woman and infant being in danger, Boelin recommends incisions through the os uteri. In such a case Dr. Ryan joins Dr. Ashwell in preferring the dilatation of the part with the fingers, as affording the mother and infant a much better chance of life. Should the woman die undelivered, the Cæsarean operation ought to be performed shortly after death—in about ten minutes, according to the latter practitioner.—ED.

* M. Viery states, that in those pregnant animals of the multiparient kind which he has dissected, he always found in the horns of the uterus the snouts pointing to the vulva. In a gravid viper which he opened, all the young, eight in number, were placed with their mouths directed towards the external parts. In the egg, the head is always directed to the large end, and that end protrudes first; and the same thing occurs with respect to the ova of fishes. The larvæ of insects pass out with their heads foremost; the chrysalis eats through its silky shell; and the caterpillar through its silky covering. Thus we see that nature is here regulated by one common law.—See Ramsbotham's Lectures, Med. Gaz. for 1834, p. 465.—ED.

δ Brachialis.   Presentation of one or both arms.
ε Transversalis.   ———— of the shoulder.
ζ Funis prolapsi.   Prolapsed navel-string.
η Placentæ.   Presentation of the placenta.

As it is by no means the object of the present work to instruct in the manual or artificial operations of the obstetric art, the author must limit himself to pointing out the different morbid conditions in which such operations will be found necessary. Their nature,-mode of accomplishment, and effective instruments, are only to be learned by works written professedly on the subject, or, which is infinitely better, by an attendance on lectures, and such initiatory practice as the obstetric schools afford. A few general or incidental remarks are all that the author can undertake to add to the above table of morbid presentations.

There is no mode of determining what may be the presentation of a child before the commencement of labour, and, even at that time, it is most prudent for a practitioner to speak with some hesitation on the subject, till the membranes have actually broken, and the position is fully decided. For, though the real presentation is often sufficiently ascertainable through the membranes themselves, and particularly on the natural descent of the head, yet it has occasionally happened that, on the breaking of the membranes, the head has receded, and the shoulder or some other part taken its place ; and there are cases in which the opposite and more fortunate change has occurred, of a recession of a presenting shoulder and a descent of the head in its stead.—(*Joerg, Hist. Part.*, p. 90 ; *Burns*, ut suprà, p. 292.)

There is hence no foundation for those apprehensions which are often entertained by a pregnant woman respecting the misposition of the child, drawn from some peculiar symptom or feeling which she has never been conscious of on former times, as a singularity in the shape of the abdomen, a sense of the child's rising suddenly towards the stomach, or a numb or painful uneasiness in one leg more than in another. These, and hundreds of other anomalous sensations, have occurred in cases where the presentation has at last been found natural, and the labour has proved highly favourable ; while, on the contrary, it is very rarely, when a cross-birth is detected, that it has been particularly apprehended by any precursive tokens whatever. And the minds of the timid may hence be comforted in the midst of all the peculiarities on which they are accustomed to hang with daily alarm.

It will rarely be found necessary to have recourse to any mechanical instrument in any of the varieties we have enumerated above ; and in some of them, as the breech and foot presentations, the expulsory powers of nature generally are sufficient alone, at least till the head descends into the pelvis, at which time it will be found necessary, whenever the arms lie over the head, to introduce a finger or two, and gently draw them down.

Where the face presents, or any other part of the head than the vertex, it was formerly the custom to deliver by turning ; but a skilful practitioner of the present day is commonly able, by a dexterous pressure of one or two fingers against particular parts of the head, and especially if attempted in an early stage of labour, to give the organ a right direction without introducing the hand.

On the presentation, however, of a shoulder, or of one or both arms, it will be expedient to turn as soon as possible ; or in other words, as soon as the mouth of the womb is sufficiently dilated for this purpose. It is singular, that while under the old practice delivery by the feet was often endeavoured in face cases, attempts were made in arm and shoulder cases to bring down the head, and reduce the labour to a natural course. This it seems has been done, and may be done, but with so much fatigue and exhaustion to the patient as to run the risk of incapacitating her for any subsequent efforts, if she do not even fall a sacrifice to a flooding, as in a case related by Dr. Smellie. It is by the successful exertions of Paré and Mauriceau that the better practice of the present day has obtained a triumph over all Europe. Yet in justice to the obstetric practitioners of ancient Greece, it should be observed, that the modern method is little more than a revival of their own, which unaccountably sunk into disfavour : for we are told by Ætius that Philomeles discovered the method, at that time in common use, of turning and delivering children by the feet in all unnatural presentations. Where, however, the child is small or of premature birth, it may sometimes be taken away without changing the presentation : for the obstetric writers abound in examples of delivery effected under such circumstances, by pulling down the arm and drawing the head into the vagina.—(*Gardner, Med. Comment.*, vol. v., 307 ; *Baudelocque*, sect. 1530 ; *Burns*, ut suprà, 303.)

It sometimes happens that the shoulder is so far advanced into the pelvis before the arrival of the practitioner, or from the vehement force of the uterus, that it is impossible to raise or move the child by the utmost power of the operator, and the state of the case seems to leave the woman without any hope of relief. At this very moment, however, and by these very means, the wise and benevolent law of instinct or of nature is interposing to the relief that is despaired of. This wonderful process, though occasionally noticed by earlier writers, and foremost of all perhaps by Schoenheider in the Copenhagen Transactions (*Act. Hafn.*, tom. ii., art. xxiii.), was first fully illustrated and explained by Dr. Denman, who distinguished it by the name of a SPONTANEOUS EVOLUTION. His explanation is best given in his own words :—"As to the manner in which this evolution takes place, I presume that, after the long-continued action of the uterus, the body of the child is brought into such a compacted state as to receive the full force of every returning action. The body in its double state being too large to pass through the pelvis, and the uterus pressing upon its inferior extremities, which are the only parts capable of being moved, the latter are forced gradually lower, making room as they are pressed down for the reception of some other part into the cavity of the uterus which they have evacuated, till, the body turning as it were upon its own axis, the breech of the child is expelled as in an original presentation of that part, and consequently is delivered by nature at the time she least expected it." Dr. J. Hamilton, however, has justly observed, that this evolution can only take place where the action of the uterus can produce no exertion on the presenting part, or where that part is so shaped that it cannot be wedged in the pelvis : and he might have added, where the woman is in full strength, and the uterus is capable of exercising a strong expulsory power. And hence it is a chance that should never be trusted to, or suffered to interfere with the common practice of delivering by the feet, wherever this can be accomplished.*

In all the above cases it is a general rule, and one of great importance, to suffer the water of the amnios to accumulate towards the neck of the womb as largely as possible, and to leave the membranes unbroken as long as may be.

A presentation of the funis is another difficulty often of considerable moment in the progress of labour, for it is obvious that by a check to the pulsation, either actually taking place, or being greatly endangered in every pain by the violent pressure of the head or of any other part against the mouth of the uterus, or afterward against the sides of the pelvis, and consequently against the funis itself, the life of the child is in imminent hazard, and, without the exercise of considerable skill, may inevitably be lost. If it be possible to return the prolapsed part of the funis round the head as it is descending, or to hook it against the hand or some other part so as to keep it clear of pressure, this ought to be done by all means. But if this be impossible, the child must be turned, as soon as turning is practicable from the dilated state of the os internum : or if the head should have reached the pelvis before the accident takes place, the labour must be accelerated by the patient's using her utmost efforts during every pain; and if she be too much exhausted for concentrating her strength, it must be quickened by the use of the forceps. But if the pulsation in the cord have already ceased, and we have hereby a proof that the child is already dead, the labour is to be suffered to take its natural course.

It sometimes happens, however, that after the child is turned, and the head does not follow the body so speedily as could be wished, from the patient being greatly exhausted—and the same frequently occurs in breech cases in consequence

of the protracted length of the labour in this presentation—there is still a considerable danger to the navel-string, from its pressure between the child's head and the pelvis. This should be remedied as much as possible by giving the funis full play between the pains. But it frequently occurs, in spite of the utmost caution, that the pulsation is suspended, and the child is born in a state of asphyxy, and apparently lifeless.

The common practice in this case is to tie the navel-string as quickly as possible, remove the child from the mother to the warmth of the fireplace, and endeavour to stimulate the lungs into action by breathing forcibly into the mouth while the nostrils are closed. Friction with a warm hand, and with the conjoint aid of some pungent volatile, is at the same time applied actively to the chest; and if this do not succeed, the nostrils are attempted to be roused with ammonia, or the fauces with a teaspoonful of brandy and hot water, to excite sneezing or coughing. All this is well; but there is a great, and I am afraid not unfrequently a fatal error, in thus separating the navel-string, and removing the child from the mother. While it continues united, it has two chances of recovery—that of the action of the lungs, and that of the reaction of the umbilical artery. By removing it from the mother we allow it but one chance, and that in my opinion the feeblest. The expansion of the lungs is altogether a new process, and, like other new processes, does not always take place with great promptness, even where the child is in full life and vigour, and the umbilical artery in regular pulsation ; for it is sometimes half a minute, or double this time, before the child begins to cry, which is the first proof of its respiring. But the flow of the blood through the umbilical artery is an established habit, and, like all other habits, has a powerful tendency to recur if we give it time and favour, and must derive an additional tendency from the stimulus of the posterior placental vessels, which are still pulsating and operating with a vis à tergo. Of the various cases of asphyxy on birth which I have witnessed, by far the greater number have proved fatal when treated in the former way, and successful when treated in the latter; and the explanation here given will readily account for the difference.

The PLACENTA itself may also form a preternatural presentation, and add much to the difficulty and the danger of labour. We have said that this rises ordinarily from some part of the fundus of the uterus, though it may originate from its sides, or from some other quarter, for there is no quarter of the womb which may not become its source. Hence it occasionally takes its rise more or less over the mouth of the womb ; and while this part of the womb continues quiescent, it produces no more inconvenience there than anywhere else. But the moment labour commences, or even, in the latter months of parturition, when any cause whatever irritates the mouth of the womb, and in any degree puts it upon the stretch, some of the placental vessels must necessarily become ruptured, and a hemor-

---

* The presentation of the knees has been described by several authors, but this case is exceedingly rare; Madame Boivin has seen four instances of it, Madame Lachapelle none; Campbell also alludes to it in his System of Midwifery. It has been observed by American practitioners, particularly by Francis and Dewees. The general indication in these cases is to deliver by the feet.—D.

rhage ensue. So long as this is small in quantity, and does not frequently return, it will be sufficient to enjoin quiet, a recumbent position, and that the bed be not heated with a profusion of blankets. But if the hemorrhage be considerable, whether before the full time of labour or on its accession, or in any part of it, there is no perfect safety but in delivery, and hereby giving the ruptured vessels an opportunity of closing their mouths. The difficulty is less than a young practitioner might at first expect; for he may be sure from the hemorrhage itself that the os uteri is both dilated and dilatable, since if this did not give way, neither would the vessels which produce the hemorrhage.

Upon the whole, the proportion of unnatural deliveries to natural is but few; and of these it is pleasing also to reflect, that the more they are connected with difficulty or danger, the more rare is their occurrence; insomuch that, comparing the statements of Professor Nægele of Heidelberg (*Uebersicht der Vorfalle in der G. H. Entbindungsanstalt zu Heidelberg,* &c., 1819) with those of several of the most eminent accoucheurs of our own country, as Dr. Bland and Dr. Merriman, we may calculate that a breech case may be expected about once in fifty times, a foot case once in eighty, and the more dangerous presentations of the arm, breast, or funis, scarcely twice in five hundred births.*

SPECIES V.
PARODYNIA AMORPHICA.
IMPRACTICABLE LABOUR.

LABOUR IMPEDED BY MISCONFIGURATION OF THE FŒTUS, OR OF THE MATERNAL PELVIS.

In natural labour, the size of the head is adapted to the diameter of the pelvis it has to pass through: in some children, indeed, the head is rather larger than in others, or has a difference of shape; and we meet with a like difference in the area of the pelvis: and these circumstances may prolong the labour, though the expulsory powers of the mother will ultimately triumph over the resistance.

But it unfortunately happens that the head is sometimes so enlarged by monstrosity of structure, hydrops capitis, or some other disease, or that the maternal pelvis is so deformed in its make, that the child cannot pass through the passage, and delivery becomes altogether impracticable.

There is, however, an intermediate state between the natural size of the pelvis with a head of a natural size applied to it, and that of absolute impracticability from the utter inaccordance of the head to the opening; in which, though the most violent and best-directed pains of the

mother may not be sufficient to produce expulsion, this object may be effected by the assistance of instruments co-operating with the natural efforts.

What space of pelvis is absolutely necessary to enable a living child at its full time to pass through it, has not been very accurately settled by obstetric writers; some maintaining that this cannot take place where the conjugate diameter is less than two inches and a half, though it may till we reach this degree of narrowness; and others that it cannot take effect under three inches. The difference of the size of the head in different children on their birth, and of the thickness of the soft parts within the pelvis in different women, may easily account for this variation in the rule laid down. It is clear, however, from the acknowledgment of both parties, that if the dimension of the pelvis be much under three inches, delivery cannot be accomplished without the loss of the child; and it is also clear that if the head be much enlarged beyond the natural size from any cause whatever, it cannot pass even through the ordinary dimensions; thus giving us the two following sources or varieties of difficult labour from an amorphous cause:—

α A fetû.	The fœtus deformed by a preternatural magnitude of head, or some other morbid protuberance.
β Pelvica.	The pelvis contracted in its diameter by natural deformity, or subsequent disease or injury.

It is by no means easy to determine what is the actual measurement of the hollow of the pelvis in a living woman, and particularly during the time of labour: and hence, how useful soever it may be to be acquainted with what ought to be its precise capacity as taken under other circumstances, the judgment must chiefly determine as to the practicability or impracticability of the passage from a calm attention to the individual case at the time, and particularly where the difficulty proceeds from the form of the child rather than from that of the mother. If, in well weighing the circumstances, the question remain doubtful, the patient should be allowed to proceed with her natural exertions alone, or such only as in addition as the hands may be able to afford, till the strength is considerably exhausted, and the mind participates in the depression of the body. And if, at this time, as will probably be the case, the head has descended so low as to be in contact with the perinæum, and an ear can be felt, it would be imprudent to delay any longer assisting her with the vectis or the forceps.

But the case may not be doubtful, and the passage may be so much contracted as to render all attempts to accomplish delivery by the hands or the ordinary instruments totally ineffectual from the first. In this situation other means must be resorted to, or the mother and the child must both perish, worn out by fatigue, and perhaps rendered gangrenous in the points of contact from irritation and inflammation.

---

* In 71,045 labours occurring in the practice of Madame Lachapelle and others, 70,111 were natural; in 24,214 cases recorded by Madame Boivin and others, the number terminating naturally was 23,795, unnatural cases 256, delivered with forceps 117, with the perforator 31, by symphysiotomy 2, by the Cæsarean section 2, by operations not stated 11.—D.

The means on this occasion are the three following; the practitioner may reduce the head of the child by the crotchet or perforator. He may, in a small degree, enlarge the diameter of the pelvis by dividing the symphysis pubis. Or, he may make a section through the abdomen into the uterus.

The first of these methods is designed to save the mother by a voluntary sacrifice of the child. The two last give a chance to the child, but at an imminent hazard of the mother.

Where the difficulty proceeds from a morbid enlargement of the child's head, the question as to which of these three methods of treatment should be adopted ought not to admit of a moment's delay. The child is, perhaps, dead already, or, if not, it is not likely that it would long survive the deformity it labours under, or live so as to render life a blessing : and the life of a sound woman must not be risked, and still less sacrificed, for the chance of saving an unsound child. The head, therefore, ought to be diminished, and consequently the perforator had recourse to.

But there are instances of a deformity of the pelvis so considerable, that the perforator cannot be employed to any advantage : for how much soever the cranium may have been broken down, there may not be breadth enough to extract the child in any way. And this will always be the case where the range of the pelvis is under an inch and a half from the pubis to the sacrum, or on either side. Dr. Osborn asserts that he once succeeded in removing a child by means of the crotchet, in a case where the widest side of the pelvis was only an inch and three quarters broad, and not more than two inches long (*Osborn's Essays*, p. 203); which is a capacity so narrow as to throw some doubt upon the accuracy of the measurement in the minds of many practitioners (*Burns's Princ. of Midwifery*, p. 351), and certainly so narrow as to form an unparalleled case in the annals of the obstetric art.

In situations, therefore, of this kind, some other plan must be pursued even to save the life of the mother ; and the only plans that can even be thought of are that of dividing the symphysis of the pubes, and that of the Cæsarean section.

Towards the latter months of pregnancy, there seems to be a disposition in the bones of the pelvis to separate at their symphysis, insomuch that some pregnant women are sensible of a motion at the junction of the bones, especially at that of the ossa pubis.—(*Francis's Denman*, p. 98, 484.) This has been known to anatomists for some centuries, and about seventy years ago, for the first time, gave rise to a question, whether advantage might not be taken of this tendency in cases of pelvic contractions, to enlarge the space by dividing the ossa pubis at their symphysis, and thus obtain the same end as is answered by the Cæsarean section, with a considerable diminution of risk. The operation seems first of all to have been proposed by M. Louis of the French Academy of Surgery to Professor Camper of Groningen, who tried it

first on a dead female body, and found it would afford space, and next on a living pig, which, for some days afterward, was incapable either of walking or standing, but in a few weeks perfectly recovered. He was then desirous of trying it upon a young woman condemned to death at Groningen, but did not succeed in his request. Not long afterward, however, it was performed with complete success by M. Sigault of Paris upon the wife of a soldier, who had hitherto borne four children, each of which, from the mother's misformation, was obliged to be extracted piecemeal. The section of the cartilage connecting the ossa pubis, enabled the bones to be separated, according to his account, by a chasm of two inches and a half; and yielded a free passage to the child in four minutes and a half. The wife, with her husband and child, a few weeks afterward, presented themselves to the members of the faculty assembled in their hall. The patient walked steadily, and was found to be perfectly recovered.—(*Med. Comm. Edin.*, vol. v., p. 214.) Mr. Le Roy, who was requested to attend on the occasion, tells us that the same operation was afterward performed by two other practitioners on two other women, and, in both cases, with an equally happy termination. He also observes, that although, in an unimpregnated state, the bones of the pelvis cannot be made to separate upon a division of the symphysis to a space of more than an inch, which would be insufficient for the purposes proposed, the additional softness and flaccidity which take place during pregnancy, as well in the bones and cartilages as in the muscles, is so considerable, that a separation of two inches and a half may be easily effected in labour, and was effected in the above cases, while the same bistoury that divided the soft parts, easily also divided the cartilage.— (*Recherches Historiques et Pratiques sur la Section de la Symphyse du Pubes*, &c., Paris, 8vo., 1778.) In various other parts of the continent, and especially at Mons and in Holland, it has been repeated with complete emancipation both to the child and mother. Dr. J. H. Myers, who witnessed it at Paris, speaks of it in the highest terms of commendation. He says, that the length of the incision does not exceed three inches, and that the whole operation is over in less than five minutes : while, in the Cæsarean operation, the wound is necessarily more than nine inches long, the uterus is divided, and the surrounding viscera are uncovered. "I have seen," says Dr. Myers, "the operation twice performed in this capital with every possible success. The last patient, while I am writing, is in the room, coming to show herself in justice to her operator. It is only eighteen days since the operation was performed, and she is in perfect health, and by no means injured by it."—(*Edin. Med. Comm.*, vol. vii., p. 453.)

The operation however, has been decried, and in some instances has certainly failed ; but there appears to be some doubt whether, in several of these cases at least, if not in all, it was conducted with a sufficient degree of dexterity and skill : for when we are told by one operator that, after the division of the symphysis, he could not effect an opening of much more than a finger's breadth, and by another, that the utmost extent of the hiatus was not more than an inch and a half, and compare these remarks with the following assertion of Dr. Myers upon this very point, it is difficult to come to any other conclusion. " The moment," says he, " the division is made, there is an enlargement of the pelvis, I venture to say, to any extent desired : the last I saw was three inches, accurately measured by an instrument called *pelvimètre*, contrived by M. Trainel." To which we may add, that M. de Lambon performed the operation twice on the same patient ; in the first instance, without injury to the mother : and, in the second, with success to both mother and child.—(*Leake's Practical Observations on the Acute Diseases of Women*, 8vo.)

After these decisive facts in its favour, to which the reader may add others from the volume of Nosology, I cannot but conceive that the prejudice against it, in our own country, has been carried too far. One trial alone has been made among ourselves, and that with an unsuccessful issue. But the chief opposition to it seems to have proceeded from the discountenance of Dr. Denman, added to certain experiments made in relation to it by Dr. William Hunter,* which do not seem to have been conducted under circumstances that can fairly call in question the truth of the preceding statements.

" Immediately," says Dr. Denman, " after the accounts of the operation were brought into this country, wishing, as a matter of duty, to understand the ground of the subject, I had a conference with the late Mr. John Hunter, in which we considered its first principle, its safety ; and after the most serious consideration, it was agreed that, if the utility could be proved, there appeared from the structure of the parts, or from the injury they were likely to sustain by the mere section of the symphysis, no sufficient objection against performing it. Of its real utility it was, however, impossible to decide before many experiments had been made on the DEAD body, to ascertain the degree of enlargement of the capacity of the pelvis, well-formed or distorted, which would be thereby obtained. Such experiments were soon made, and their result published by the late Dr. Hunter ; and these proved on the whole that, in extreme or great degrees of distortion of the pelvis the advantage to be gained was wholly insufficient to allow the head of a child to pass without lessening its bulk ; and, in small degrees of distortion, that the operation was unnecessary, such cases admitting of relief by less desperate methods. They proved, moreover, that irreparable injury would be done by attempts to increase the common advantages gained by the section of the symphysis by straining or tearing asunder the ligaments which

connect the ossa innominata to the sacrum, and to the soft parts contained in the pelvis, particularly to the bladder."—(*Francis's Denman, &c.*, 3d edition, New-York, 1829, p. 486.)

Now it did not require these experiments to prove that this operation, or almost any other, would become mischievous if unskilfully performed ; but surely it was something too much to endeavour to set aside the facts and results known to have taken place in very numerous instances in the *living* body, and to call in question the veracity of those who made them and those who witnessed them, by facts and results made merely on the *dead* body, without one single experiment on the body while alive, and in the peculiar circumstances under which alone it is admitted that the facts and results contended for could possibly take place.

Upon the whole, it is allowed in the passage just quoted, as the concurrent opinion of Dr. Denman himself, Mr. John Hunter, and apparently Dr. William Hunter, and this, too, after " the most serious consideration,"—that " there appears from the structure of the parts, or from the injury they are likely to sustain by the mere section of the symphysis, no sufficient objection against performing the operation." That it will answer in every degree of a contracted pelvis was never asserted by its most sanguine advocates, but only in cases where the constriction was somewhat too considerable to allow of the extraction of the child by the forceps ; and lastly, it is after all admitted by Dr. Denman himself, that where the life of a child is of more than ordinary importance from public or other considerations, and the mother, who is in labour with it, possesses a pelvis so deformed and contracted that it cannot pass through the passage in its present state, " there the section of the symphysis of the ossa pubis might be proposed and performed,—being less horrid to the woman than the Cæsarean operation, and instead of adding to the danger, giving some chance of preserving the life of the child."*

It is perfectly clear, however, that, be the advantages of dividing the symphysis what they may when the pelvis is under certain states of deformity, it is an operation that can never be of any avail where the passage is so narrow that the child cannot be brought away piecemeal even by the use of the perforator. And, in such circumstances, the only alternative is to leave the patient to nature, in the slender and desperate hope, that the pains may gradually wear away as the parts become habituated to the irritation, and the child, as in many cases of extra-uterine fœtation, be thrown out in detached fragments by an abscess ; or to have

---

* See also Osborn's Essay on Laborious Parturition, in which the division of the symphysis pubis is particularly considered, 8vo., Lond., 1783.

* Francis's Denman, ut suprà, 487. On the continent, the section of the symphysis of the pubes was repeated with various success. Thirty-six cases are well authenticated, in which fourteen women died, and half the children were stillborn. It has only been performed once in Great Britain ; Mr. Welchman, the operator, has given the particulars of it in the London Medical Journal for 1790.—See Ramsbotham's Lectures, as published in Med. Gaz. for 1834, p. 404.—ED.

recourse to what has been called the CÆSAREAN OPERATION, and deliver by making a section into the uterus through the abdomen.

The love of offspring, or a sense of duty, has been so prevalent in some women as to induce them to submit to this severe trial in cases where the pelvis has by no means been so straitened as we are now contemplating. And these motives not being confined to any particular age, the operation is of considerable antiquity, and is particularly noticed by the elder Pliny, who tells us, that the elder Scipio Africanus and the first of the Cæsars were brought into the world in this manner, and adds, that the name of Cæsar was hence derived "à cæso matris utero."— (*Hist. Nat.*, lib. vii., cap. ix.) In recent times, one of the earliest cases in which it was submitted to, was that of the wife of a cattle-gelder at · Siegenhausen in Germany, in the beginning of the sixteenth century. The child, it seems, was, from its size, supposed to be incapable of being expelled in the natural way, and the operation was performed by the cattle-gelder himself. Bauhin, in his Appendix to Rousset, who was a warm supporter of the practice, and wrote in favour of it in 1581, tells us that this woman did well, and bore several children afterward in the natural way. There are a few other instances related of its having been executed in a similar way, and with equal success; particularly one performed in Ireland, by an uninstructed midwife, whose instrument was a razor. The case is related by Mr. Duncan Stewart (*Edin. Med. Essays*, vol. v., p. 360), who saw the woman a few days after the operation. She was well in about a month. Among regular practitioners, however, it has been generally opposed on account of its very doubtful result, from the time of Paré and Guillemeau, who warmly resisted its employment. Dr. Hull not long since made a collection of all the cases in which the operation has been performed, both at home and abroad, and calculated them at 231, of which 139, being considerably more than half, had proved successful.—(*Translation of M. Baudelocque's Memoir*, p. 233.) The German collections, indeed, give various examples of its having been repeated several times on the same person: and M. Trestan narrates the extraordinary history of one woman who had submitted to it not fewer than seven times.—(*Journ. de Médecine*, tom. xxxvi., p. 69.) One of the latest examples is, I believe, the case furnished by Dr. Locker, of Zurich, in which the mother and child were both happily preserved.—(*Med. Chir. Trans.*, vol. ix., p. 69.)*

Under this view of the subject, it is singular to observe the general fatality, at least to the mother, with which the Cæsarean section has been followed in our own country. "There are, I think," says Mr. Burns, "histories of twenty cases where this operation has been performed in Britain: out of these only ONE woman has

been saved, but ten children have been preserved."*

At Edinburgh, Mr. Hamilton remarks (*Elements of the Practice of Midwifery*, 8vo.) that it had been performed five times at the date of his publication: and that, in no instance, had the patient had the good fortune to survive it many days. Of the last case he was an eye-witness, and it was only resorted to after every other means had proved ineffectual: the child was saved, but the mother survived only six-and-twenty hours. This ingenious writer enters with great pertinence into the question to what cause so general a failure is to be ascribed. And while he admits that nervous or uterine irritation from the wound, internal hemorrhage, or an extravasation into the cavity of the abdomen, may each have an influence, he is disposed to think, that its ill success is principally to be imputed to the effect which access of air is well known to have on viscera exposed and in a state of irritation. Dr. Monro repeatedly found that, in making even a large aperture by incision into the abdomen of animals, if the wound be quickly closed, the animal readily recovers; but that if the viscera be exposed for only a few minutes to the air, severe pains and fatal convulsions ensue.† And hence Mr. Hamilton recommends that, in performing the Cæsarean operation, the bowels be denuded as little as possible, and the wound be closed with the utmost expedition.

This answer, however, is hardly satisfactory: and I am rather inclined to think, that the comparative want of success at home is owing to the greater reluctance in performing the operation than seems to be manifested in France and Germany; in consequence of which it is rarely determined upon until the woman is too far exhausted, and has an insufficiency of vigour to enable the wounded parts to assume a healing condition. In most of the cases recorded, there does not seem to have been any deficiency of skill; and particularly in that which occurred about five-and-thirty years since, and was attended by Mr. John Hunter and Dr. Ford (*Francis's Denman*, ut suprà, p. 498), and hence the

---

* The Cæsarean operation has been performed but seldom in the United States. The most recent case, which occurred in the practice of Prof. Gibson, of Philadelphia, was successful.—D.

---

* Princip., ut suprà, p. 348. Dr. Ramsbotham, whose lectures have a later date than that of Mr. Burns's work, states, that "out of nearly thirty instances in which this operation has been performed in the British isles, in two only has it proved successful, as far as the preservation of the mother was concerned." The latter physician would restrict this performance to cases of pelvic distortion or tumours. In Britain it is never substituted for craniotomy by choice, but only had recourse to when no other mode of delivery is practicable.—(See Med. Gaz. for 1834, p. 403.) The custom of resorting to it with less delay abroad, is no doubt the reason of its having proved more successful there than in this country, where the woman is usually in a state of extreme danger before the operation is attempted.—ED.

† As the viscera were generally exposed to the air in cases operated upon abroad, which were attended with a considerable proportion of success, such exposure will not account for the greater fatality of the operation in this country.—ED.

unfavourable issue must be resolved into some other cause.

It is happy for the world, and peculiarly so for those who are possessed of a contracted pelvis, and in many cases without knowing it till they are in labour, that a far safer and less painful operation may be had recourse to, where the deformity is known in due time ; I mean that of a PREMATURE DELIVERY. " A great number of instances have occurred," says Dr. Denman, " of women so formed that it was impossible for them to bring forth a living child at the termination of nine months, who have, in my own practice, been blessed with living children by the accidental coming on of labour when they were only seven months advanced in their pregnancy, or several weeks before their due time. But the first account of any artificial method of bringing on premature labour was given to me by Dr. C. Kelly. He informed me, that about the year 1756 there was a consultation of the most eminent men at that time in London to consider of the moral rectitude of, and advantages which might be expected from, this practice ; which met with their general approbation. The first case in which it was deemed necessary and proper, fell under the care of the late Dr. Macauley, and it terminated successfully. The patient was the wife of a linen-draper in the Strand. Dr. Kelly informed me that he himself had practised it ; and among other instances mentioned that he had performed this operation three times upon the same woman, and twice the children had been born living.

" A lady of rank," continues the same writer, " who had been married many years, was soon after her marriage delivered of a living child in the beginning of the eighth month of her pregnancy. She had afterward four children at the full time, all of which were, after very difficult labours, born dead. She applied in her next pregnancy to Dr. Savage, whom I met in consultation. By some accounts she had received, she was prepared for this operation, to which she submitted with great resolution. The membranes were accordingly ruptured, and the waters discharged, early in the eighth month of her pregnancy. On the following day she had a rigour, succeeded by heat and other symptoms of fever, which very much alarmed us for the event. On the third day, however, the pains of labour came on, and she was, after a short time, delivered, to the great comfort and satisfaction of herself and friends, of a small but perfectly healthy child, which is at this time nearly of the same size it would have been had it been born at the full period of utero-gestation ; and it has lived to the state of manhood. In a subsequent pregnancy, the same method was pursued ; but whether the child was of larger size, or the pelvis was become smaller, whether there was any mistake in the reckoning, or whether the child fell into any untoward position, I could not discover, but it was stillborn, though the labour did not continue longer than six hours. Yet, in a third trial, the child was born living and healthy, and she recovered without any unusual incon-

venience or trouble."—(Epist. App. ad Strauss de fœtu, Mussipont., p. 298.)

It is only necessary to add, that at the time in which the labour-pains will come on after thus rupturing the membranes and discharging the waters, is uncertain, and appears to depend much on the irritability of the uterus. It is sometimes delayed, as in the first trial in the case just noticed, for three days, but the labour has sometimes also been found to commence within a few hours.

SPECIES VI.
PARODYNIA PLURALIS.
MULTIPAROUS LABOUR.
LABOUR COMPLICATED BY A PLURALITY OF CHILDREN.

THE fertility of women seems to depend upon various circumstances ; partly, perhaps, the extent or resources of the ovaria, partly constitutional warmth of orgasm, and partly the adaptation of the male semen to the organization of the respective female. Eisenmenger gives us the history of a woman who produced fifty-one children (*Epist. App. ad Strauss de fœtu*, Mussipont., p. 228) ;* and sometimes the fertility seems to pass from generation to generation, in both sexes, though it must be always liable to some variation from the constitution of the family that is married into. I have in my own family, at the time of writing, a young female servant whose mother bore twenty-three children, and brought them up with so much success, that, at the time of the mother's death, she was the youngest of nineteen then living ; and her eldest brother has fourteen children at present, all of whom I believe are in health.

But while some women produce thus rapidly in single succession, there are others that are multiparient, and bring forth occasionally two or even three at a time, more than one ovum being detached by the orgastic shock. Three at a time is not common : I have met with but one instance of it in which the children were all alive and likely to live ; and one instance only occurred to Dr. Denman in the course of upwards of thirty years' practice. Four have occasionally, but very rarely, been brought forth together, and there are a few wonderful stories of five, but which rest on no well-authenticated testimony.†

Twins are mostly produced at a common birth ; but owing to the incidental death of one of them while the other continues alive, there is

---

* A most remarkable instance of fécundity in the human species, is contained in the London Medical Gazette, vol. i., p. 354. The wife of a Russian peasant brought forth fifty-seven children in twenty-one births. They were all living at the same time. In the first four labours, she gave birth to four children at each time ; three in each of the next seven labours ; and she afterward was always delivered of twins. By a second wife, the same man had fifteen children in seven labours. —D.

† In 18,300 cases at the British Lying-in Hospital, no case of triplets occurred. In 20,357 at the Maternité, there were 3 ; and in 59,354 cases, 19. —See Ryan's Manual of Midwifery, p. 290.—Eᴅ,

sometimes a material difference in the time of their expulsion, and consequently, therefore, in their bulk or degree of maturity, giving us the two following varieties :—

α Congruens.	Of equal or nearly equal	
Congruous twin-	growth, and produced at	
ning.	a common birth.	
β Incongruens.	Of unequal growth, and pro-	
Incongruous	duced at different births.	
twinning.		

In CONGRUOUS TWINNING, or ordinary twin-cases, in which there is no great disparity of size between the two, on the birth of the one, it can be pretty easily ascertained that another is still in the womb, by applying the hand to the abdomen : for the limbs, and, if the child be alive, its movements, may generally be felt very distinctly, except, indeed, where an ascites is present, and the practitioner must then have recourse to other tokens.

There are no precise signs by which a woman or her attendant can determine whether she be pregnant of twins or not. Inequalities in the prominence of the abdomen, peculiarities of internal sensation or motion, slowness in the progress of a labour, have been advanced as signs ; but they belong as frequently to the uniparient as to the multiparient, and hence are unentitled to attention.

The claim to priority of birth in a twin case is dependant, not on superiority of strength or any other endowment, but on a closer proximity to the mouth of the uterus alone, and consequently, on a greater convenience of position. Though, when, on the birth of twins, one is found small and emaciated, and the other plump and strong, we have some ground for apprehending that the vigorous child has absorbed the greater part of the nutriment afforded by the mother, as we find not unfrequently in plants shooting from the same spot of earth.

The general rules that govern in morbid labour of individual children, govern equally in morbid labour of twins. The second child is usually delivered with comparatively few pains and little inconvenience, as the parts have been sufficiently dilated by the passage of the first : and, although there is commonly some interval between the termination of the one and the commencement of the other struggle, it is not often that this interval exceeds half an hour or an hour. It has, indeed, in a few instances, extended to whole days ; in one instance to ten (*Hist. de l'Acad. des Sciences*, 1751, p. 107), and in another to seventeen days.—(*De Boset in Verhendelingen van Hurlem*, xii., App. No. 6.) But these are very uncommon cases : and, as mischief may possibly happen to the womb and to the system at large from a long protraction of

uterine irritation, it is now the practice to deliver the second child by art, after having waited four or five hours in vain for a return of expulsory exertions.*

In INCONGRUOUS TWINNING we meet, in different cases, with every possible diversity of perfection of form and term of expulsion, between the co-offspring. Nor is this to be wondered at in either respect. We have already seen that a single fœtus may die during any period of parturition, from a variety of causes ; and hence we may readily conjecture that one of the twins may die at any period, while the other still thrives and remains unaffected. This twin may remain in the womb, and both be expelled together at the full time. But it may happen, also, from the peculiar irritation of the uterus generally, or the peculiar position of the dead fœtus near the cervix, that this organ may be so far stimulated by the death and corrupt state of the fœtal corse and its membranes as to expel it from the body, while the living child receives no injury, continues to thrive, and is maturely delivered at its proper time.

In the latter case, where the dead fœtus has been discharged in the second or third month of pregnancy, the mother, not knowing herself to have been pregnant with twins, has been erroneously conceived, on the arrival of the second birth, to have produced a perfect child within the short term of six or seven months.

In the former case, or that in which the dead fœtus remains quiet in the womb through the remaining term of pregnancy, and both are discharged at a common birth, an opinion equally erroneous was formerly entertained in order to account for the apparent difference of the two in growth and size : for it was supposed that the dead and puny, and apparently premature fœtus, was conceived some months subsequently to the perfect and vigorous child, and hence had not time to reach it in size and perfection : and to this supposed subsequent conception was given the name of SUPERFŒTATION.

We have reason to believe that such a process does occasionally take place in some quadrupeds, whose wombs are so formed as to allow of it : but we have already observed in the preliminary Proem to the present class, as also in the introductory observations to the present order, that in women, from the moment of conception, an efflorescent membrane is formed, which lines the whole cavity of the uterus, and acts as a septum to the ascent of any subsequent tide of male semen ; not to say, further, that the os uteri itself is so plugged up by the secretion of a viscid mucus at the time, as to prevent any communication between this organ and the vagina till the period of pregnancy is completed, And hence the doctrine of superfœtation in wo-

---

* Some practitioners seem not to agree with Dr. Good on this point: the following is the advice delivered by Dr. Ryan. "In all cases, immediately after delivery, the hand is to be placed upon the abdomen to ascertain whether another infant be present ; and if such is the case, the labour should not be provoked for ten or twelve hours, unless some untoward symptoms occur. I have known a woman delivered of one infant on Monday, and the second on the following Thursday, without a bad symptom during the time ; and both infants were born alive. Another case fell under my care, where there was a period of thirty-six hours between the births, and not a pain during the time ; the second infant was born dead. The secale cornutum had its usual good effects in this case."—See Manual of Midwifery, p. 192, ed. 3.

men, excepting under very particular circumstances, has deservedly sunk into general disrepute.—(*Waldschmied, Dissert. de Superfœtatione falsò prætensa,* Hamb., 1727.) For it is possible, however, as we have already observed, for a second fœtation to take place by an additional connexion, within à few hours after the first, and before the formation of the occluding membrane. But in this case the progress of the twins is parallel, and their birth in immediate succession.

The cases of this kind, and formerly ascribed to the exploded cause, are by no means uncommon. Dr. Maton has given a very decided one of a lady delivered at Palermo of a male child, in November, 1807, and again, scarcely three months afterward, in February, 1808, of another male infant, "completely formed."—(*Med. Trans.,* vol. iv., art. xii.) The proportions or powers of the first child are not sufficiently noticed: but we are told that both were born alive; that the elder died when nine days old "without any apparent cause;" and that the younger died also, but after a longer term.

In Henchel we have an account of a minute (*Neue Medicinische und Chirurgische Anmerkungen,* b. ii.) and a mature fœtus born at the same time: and a similar history is given by Mr. Chapman, with the exception of the time, which varied considerably: the dead and minute fœtus, apparently not more than three or four months old, having in this case been born in October, 1816, and the twin, a full-grown child, not till December, just two months afterward.—(*Med. Chir. Trans.,* vol. ix., p. 195.)

In this last instance, however, there can be no doubt that the aborted fœtus had remained quiet in the uterus for some months after its death before it was expelled; which in truth is the only way of reconciling its apparent age and size of not more than three or four months at the time of its expulsion, with the full time or nine months of the mother, completed only two months afterward.

Nor is a quiet and undisturbing continuance in the uterus after the death of the fœtus by any means uncommon, whether the offspring be single or double. We have already given examples of an interval of ten, and even seventeen days, in the case of twins born equally of full size. But where the growth has been discrepant, and the dead fœtus has remained behind unsuspected, it has sometimes been several months before expulsion has taken place. Ruysch gives a case in which it was delayed a twelvemonth after the apparent term of its death, and even then discharged without corruption (*Thesaur. Omnium Max.*): and some of the foreign collections have instances of more than double this time.—(*Neue Samml. Wahrnehmungen,* band iv., p. 241.)

The present author was once engaged in consultation upon the case of a lady in Bedford Row, who had miscarried of a fœtus under three months old, which there was every reason to believe died four months antecedently; as at that time the mother had been attacked with a flooding and rigours, had had various subsequent uterine hemorrhages, and had never been able to quit a recumbent position without producing some return of the bleeding.

SPECIES VII.
PARODYNIA SECUNDARIA.
SEQUENTIAL LABOUR.
DISEASED ACTION OR DISTURBANCE SUCCEEDING DELIVERY.

In ordinary childbirth, the pains of labour may be said to cease with the expulsion of the fœtus: since though sequential, or after-pains, as they are ordinarily called, are not uncommon for a day or two, and are useful in expelling the placenta and its membranes, and a few large coagula of blood that have formed in the uterus, these last are neither violent nor by any means frequent. It sometimes happens, however, that there is almost as much trouble, and as much pain, and as much danger, after the birth of the child as antecedently, so that the labour itself may be fairly said to be protracted into this secondary stage, which offers the following varieties of morbid affection:—

α Retentiva.	Retention of the secundines.
β Dolorosa.	Violent after-pains.
γ Hæmorrhagica.	Violent hemorrhage or flooding.
δ Lochialis.	Inadequate lochial discharge.

In about ten minutes or a quarter of an hour after the birth of the child, the uterus recovers its action, and again exerts itself, though with less force, and consequently slighter pain, to expel what is commonly called the after-birth, consisting of the placenta and its membranes; which, in common cases, are easily separated and thrown off from the sides of the organ. The instinctive or remedial power of nature is just as competent of itself to do this as to expel the child; but as unquestionable benefit is found from assisting in the expulsion in the latter case, a like degree of benefit is also found in the former; and the practitioner, by taking hold of the funis, and gently pulling it during the action of a pain, will in most cases be sure of expediting the passage of the placenta without running the least risk of rudely tearing it from the sides of the uterus, and exciting a hemorrhage.

It will sometimes however be found, that the funis, instead of being fully inserted at its upper extremity into the body of the placenta, originates alone from a few of its vessels, and that from an incautious tug it gives way, and is drawn down by itself, leaving the placenta behind; and consequently putting it entirely out of the practitioner's power to render any collateral assistance.

It also happens, not unfrequently, from the general exhaustion of the system, or the local exhaustion and torpitude of the uterus, that no expulsory pains of any kind follow at the ordinary time, or even for a long period afterward, and consequently, that the placenta is still lying unseparated in the uterus.

On a trial instituted by Dr. W. Hunter and Dr. Sandys, in the Middlesex Hospital, it was found in one case that the placenta, left to the action of the uterus alone, was not rejected till twenty-four hours after delivery; and as no ill consequences followed this experiment, it became soon afterward a practice with many in this metropolis, as it had long before been with still more on the continent, to pay no attention to the placenta, and to leave it to take its course. Great mischief, however, has been in many cases found to ensue from this kind of quietism: for where there is great exhaustion, a sufficiency of natural exertion does not in numerous instances return for three or four days afterward, and sometimes even longer: while the placenta, by remaining in the uterus, keeps up a febrile irritation, and what is infinitely worse, by being in many instances partly, though not wholly detached, and rendered a dead as well as a foreign substance, the detached part putrefies, and produces a fetor through the whole atmosphere of the chamber, sufficient of itself to render the patient sick, and faint, and feverish, if it do not occasion a genuine typhus.

I was lately requested to attend in consultation upon a case of this kind. The patient had had a very difficult labour, and after two or three days of severe suffering, was delivered by the use of the crotchet. She was afterward for a long time in a state of syncope, and the placenta was suffered to remain without any attempt to remove it. She had no expulsory pains for three days; but very great soreness and some degree of laceration in the soft parts, with such a torpitude of the bladder that the water was obliged to be drawn off daily. In about eight-and-forty hours she had a hot dry skin, brown furred tongue, with a quick, small pulse, slight delirium, and occasional shiverings. She was in this state when I was requested to see her. The room, which was small, was insupportable from its stench, notwithstanding all the pains taken to maintain cleanliness, and to cover the fetor by pungent odours. I strenuously advised that the placenta should be instantly removed; but was answered that, as gangrene had already begun, the patient would certainly die, and as certainly sink under the very attempt to bring it away, so that the operator would fall under the charge of having killed her. My reply was, that she would assuredly die if it were not removed, but I was not so certain that she would if it were; that in my judgment, the fetor rather proceeded from the placenta itself than from the ichorous discharge about the vagina, and gave a token of a very extensive separation, though the patient wanted power to expel it from her body. And I could not avoid adding, that if none of the gentlemen present (we made four in all) would venture upon the task, I would take the risk upon myself, though I had long declined the practice, and give the patient this only chance of a recovery. This declaration inspirited the rest; the operation was determined upon: the placenta, as I suspected, was found nearly separated throughout, and half advanced into the vagina, and was removed without difficulty. By the use of the cinchona and the mineral acids, with a nutritive regimen, the patient gradually recovered, and is now in a state of perfect health.

. The modern practice, therefore, of not trusting the placenta to the mere powers of nature when these powers are exhausted or inoperative, is founded upon a principle of the soundest observation. Four or five hours is the utmost time now usually allowed; and if it be retained beyond this period, the operator interferes, brings it away by the funis, if the uterus will hereby become sufficiently stimulated,[*] and if not, or the funis be broken, by cautiously introducing his hand into the uterus, and peeling the placenta gradually from its walls by the action of his fingers.[†]

If the uterus, instead of contracting at its fundus, should contract irregularly and transversely, so as to form what has been called an HOUR-GLASS contraction, the removal of the placenta should take place before this time.

In some irritable habits, on the contrary, the AFTER-PAINS, instead of ceasing gradually, occa-

---

[*] In the Repertorio di Medicina for May, 1826, published at Turin, Dr. Mojon has communicated a new mode of separating the placenta from the uterus. He removes the blood from the umbilical vein, and injects it forcibly with a mixture of vinegar and cold water; if the first injection is not successful, the vein is again emptied, and the same process is repeated. Other practitioners have confirmed the efficacy of this treatment. The committee of the Med. Society at Paris, to whom was referred the memoir of Legras on the subject, close their report by saying, that "the author has proved by facts the safety in all cases of injections into the umbilical vessels after the birth of the child; and also that they are efficient in causing the placenta to separate from the uterus, in arresting hemorrhage from a partial detachment of this body, and finally, in stimulating the uterus when it is inert. It follows also from our views, and from the experiments reported, that the effect of the injections can be regulated by graduating the temperature and quantity of the fluid injected, by rendering it more or less styptic, and by graduating the force with which it is injected. In dangerous hemorrhages the vessels of the placenta should be rapidly distended, and the cold and styptic fluid should thus be sent even to the surface of the uterus."—See the Journ. Gen. de Médecine et de Chirurgie, &c., Avril, 1828.—D.

[†] When the placenta is retained an unusual time, Dr. Ryan recommends friction on the abdomen, grasping the uterus, applying a tight roller, dashing cold water on the abdomen, in order to make the uterus contract, and exhibiting the ergot of rye. If these means fail, and hemorrhage or fainting occur, he advises the separation of the placenta by the assistance of the hand, after which its expulsion will be effected by pressing on the uterus and abdomen so as to make the womb contract. After the birth of the infant, no practitioner should leave his patient previously to the expulsion of the placenta; for, until this has happened, she is never free from danger.—See Ryan's Manual, &c., p. 291. Also, in another part of the same work, we find the following observations: "The cases which cause a necessity for artificial extraction or separation of the placenta, are hemorrhage, convulsions, syncope, inertness of the uterus, spasmodic contraction of the womb, hour-glass contraction, preternatural adhesion, adhesion of the organ to the neck of the uterus, and abortion. Some of these require immediate extraction, as hemorrhage, convulsions, and syncope," &c.—(P. 611.)

sionally continue with little interruption, and with nearly as great violence as those of labour itself ; and this for many hours after the extraction of the placenta.

If such after-pains closely follow the labour, they proceed from a morbid irritation and spasmodic tendency of the uterus alone ; and the best remedy is an anodyne liniment applied to the abdomen, with an active dose of laudanum, which last must be repeated as soon as the first dose has lost its effect, the bowels in the meanwhile being kept regularly open. If such violent pains do not take place till some hours after the evacuation of the placenta, or even the next day, it is highly probable that some large cake of coagulated blood has formed in the uterus, and become a source of irritation. This may often be hooked out by a finger or two introduced for such purpose, and the organ be rendered easy ; if not, an opiate will here be as necessary as in the preceding case.

Hemorrhage, or FLOODING, after delivery, is another evil which the practitioner is not unfrequently called upon to combat. This is sometimes produced by pulling too forcibly at the umbilical cord, and separating the placenta from the walls of the uterus, before its vessels have sufficiently contracted : but the most common cause is an exhausted state of the uterine vessels themselves, and a consequent inability to contract their mouths, so that the blood flows through them without resistance.

The uterus is at this time so stored with blood of its own, that a prodigious rush will often flow from it without producing syncope or any serious evil upon the general system : for it is only till it has lost its own proper supply, and begins to draw upon the corporeal vessels for a recruit, that any alarming impression is perceived. Yet, from the first moment, the attendant should be on his guard, and should have recourse to the means already laid down under flooding occurring in the latter months of pregnancy.* In the present case, however, from the very open state of the mouths of all the uterine vessels that have anastomosed with the placenta, the flooding is here upon some occasions far more profuse and dangerous than at any other period, so that a woman has sometimes been carried off in the course of ten minutes, with a sudden faintness, sinking of the pulse, and wildness of the eyes that is most heartrending.† And, in such a situation, as the living powers are failing apace, and must be supported at all adventures, while cold and astringent applications are still applied to the affected

* Gen. I., Spe. 2, Paracyesis uterina hæmorrhagica ; and compare with Cl. III., Ord. IV., Gen. II., Spe. 2, Hæmorrhagia atonica uteri.

† In cases of this character, the transfusion of blood from the veins of a healthy person into those of the patient, has been recently recommended by Dr. Blundell, and its efficacy is apparently supported by cases occurring in the practice of himself and others. On this operation, Dr. Dewees remarks as follows :—" We do not hesitate to believe these accounts of success, but we very much doubt whether the patient would have died had the remedy been withheld. We believe this prin-

region, we must have recourse to the warmest, the most active, and most diffusible cordials, as Madeira wine or brandy itself in an undiluted state : and if we succeed in rousing the frame from its deadly apathy, we must drop them by degrees, or exchange them for food of a rich and nutritive, but less stimulant description.

When the discharge of blood from the uterus ceases, it is succeeded by a fluid of a different appearance, which is commonly called LOCHIA (λοχια), a term employed by Dioscorides in the sense of secundæ, or the materials evacuated by a lying-in woman after the birth of the child. The nature of this discharge does not seem to have been very fully explained by pathologists. The numerous and expanded bloodvessels of the uterus contract gradually, and particularly in their mouths or outlets ; by which means the fluid they contain, and which is not entirely evacuated by the vagina, is thrown back on the system with so much moderation as to produce no serious evil, and its stimulus is chiefly directed to the breasts. As the mouths of these vessels progressively collapse, the finer part of the blood only, or at least with not more than a small proportion of the red particles, issues from them, and in smaller abundance, and hence the discharge appears less in quantity, and of a more diluted redness. By intermixing with the oxygen of the air, which has a free admission to the sexual organs, this red, as in the case of venous blood, assumes a purple or Modena hue ; and as this hue becomes blended with the yellowish tinge of the serum, it necessarily changes to greenish, which is the colour of the lochial discharge before its cessation.

While this discharge issues in a due proportion to the demand of the idiosyncrasy, for the quantity differs considerably in different women, there is little fever or irritation, and we have no ill consequences to apprehend : but the mouths of these vessels may be irritated by various causes, as catching cold, violent emotions of the mind, the use of too stimulant a diet, or the want of a sympathetic action in the breasts ; and the result, under different circumstances, is of a directly opposite kind. If there be no spasm hereby induced on the mouths of the closing vessels, they will throw off a morbid superabundance of serous fluid, without running perhaps into a hemorrhage, or opening sufficiently to discharge red blood, and the patient will become greatly exhausted and weakened,

cipally on the following grounds :—1st. Because women bear excessive losses of blood without death following. 2d. Because the quantity of blood transmitted to the alien veins does not seem sufficient to prevent death, since but a few ounces have been declared to answer. 3d. Because the additional quantity of blood, though it increases by so much the stock of the patient, does not necessarily or contingently promote the tonic contraction of the uterus, without which all appliances and means to boot will be found unavailing. 4th. Because we have never met with a case where the dormant powers of the uterus could not be roused into successful action if means were timely employed, were of a proper kind, and properly conducted."—D.

have a sense of a prolapse of the uterus, and be peculiarly dispirited in her mind. If, on the contrary, which is more frequently the case, the mouths of the uterine vessels become suddenly and spasmodically closed in consequence of the superinduced irritation, there will be a total and abrupt suppression of the lochia, a sense of great weight and pain will be perceived in the uterus and the whole region of the pubes, a considerable degree of fever will ensue, and the patient will be in danger of a puerperal typhus.

These are the evils which result from a disturbance of the balance of the lochial discharge. In attempting to remedy them, the exciting cause should in the first place be removed as far as this is capable of being accomplished. After which, in the former case, the strength is to be sustained by unirritant tonics, astringents, and a plain nutritive diet : and in the latter, the spasmodic pain, and heat, and other febrile symptoms, are to be subdued by antispasmodics and relaxants, particularly camphire, with small doses of ipécacuanha or antimony. The neutral salts have also in this case proved serviceable, which have the farther advantage of opening and cooling the bowels. It will likewise be found highly useful to foment the abdomen with flannels wrung out of hot water, or, which is far better, to bind a flannel swathe rung out of hot water, in the same manner, round the whole of the abdomen and the back, and to encircle it with a band of folded linen to prevent it from wetting the sheets, and to let it remain on like a cataplasm till it becomes dry by evaporation.

It should not be forgotten, however, that in some women who have healthy labours, there is no lochial discharge whatever ; the bloodvessels of the uterus contracting suddenly and closely as soon as the red blood ceases to flow. I have already pointed out one example of this kind that occurred to Professor Frank, even after a third natural delivery : the patient, moreover, having been from a girl as destitute of menstruation as destitute of lochia ; yet her health was in no respect interfered with.—(*De Cur. Hom. Morb. Epit.*, tom. vi., lib. vi., Pars iii., 8vo., Viennæ, 1824.)

In all the diseases here referred to, cleanliness and purity of air are of the utmost importance : without these, no plan whatever can succeed : and with them, no other plan is often wanted. They are, moreover, of as much moment to the infant as to the mother. It is a striking fact, that in the space of four years, ending in 1784, there died in the Lying-in Hospital of Dublin, at that time a badly ventilated house, 2944 children out of 7650 ; though after the ventilation was improved, the deaths within a like period and from a like number amounted to not more than 279.

GENUS III.

ECCYESIS.

EXTRA-UTERINE FŒTATION.

IMPERFECT FŒTATION IN SOME ORGAN EXTERIOR TO THE UTERUS.

We have shown in the Physiological Proem

to the present class, that the sexual fluid of the male passes, at the time of the embrace or soon afterward, into the uterus, and from the uterus into the Fallopian tube, or even the ovarium, where it impregnates an ovulum, detached from its proper niche by the force of the orgastic percussion. It sometimes happens, however, that the Fallopian tubes, or the openings from the uterus leading into them, are so impacted with fat or some other material, or so straitened in their diameter, that the detached and impregnated ovum is incapable of obtaining a passage into the cavity of the uterus, and is arrested in its course : in which case it must either remain in the tube itself, into which it has thus far proceeded, or drop, at the origin of the fimbriæ, into the hollow of the abdomen. And it has also sometimes occurred, that the ovum or vesicle that has been detached from the ovarium, has been incapable of making its way out of the ovarium itself, and has become impregnated in its original seat, without a possibility of stirring farther.

In all these cases, the progress of impregnation still goes forward, though in an imperfect manner, and with an imperfect development of organs ; and we are hence furnished with the three following distinct species of extra-uterine gestation :—

1. Eccyesis Ovaria.   Ovarian Exfœtation.
2. ———— Tubalis.   Tubal Exfœtation.
3. ———— Abdominalis.   Abdominal Exfœtation.*

It is a very remarkable fact, that the uterus still sympathizes in every one of these species with the imprisoned and impregnated ovum, in whatever part of the body it may happen to be lodged, produces ordinarily the same efflorescent membrane or decidua, which we have already observed it secretes in the commencement of utero-gestation for the reception of the ovum upon its arrival in the uterus, enlarges its capacity, and thickens its walls, as though the fœtus were really present in its interior (see *an exemplification of this in an ovarian exfœtation described by Dr. Granville, Phil. Trans.*, 1820, p. 103) ; exhibits the same symptoms and excites the same caprices of the stomach as those by which utero-gestation is usually distinguished : and at the expiration of the regular period of nine months, and sometimes, as in ordinary pregnancy, even before this, is attacked with spasmodic or expulsory pains, which often continue for some hours, and seldom altogether subside till the organized and extra-uterine substance loses its living power, and becomes the nature of a foreign material to the organs by which it is surrounded. After which, menstruation again returns regularly, as it has hitherto been suspended.

The extra-uterine ovum, in the meanwhile, endowed, in consequence of its impregnation, with a principle of life, continues to grow, whatever be the place of its aberration ; in some instances becomes surrounded with an imperfect kind of placenta, develops the general struc-

* To these species of extra-uterine fœtation may be added a fourth, Eccyesis INTERSTITIALIS, which will be mentioned at the close of the article on E. Abdominalis.—D.

ture of its kind, and exhibits an organized compages of bones, membranes, vessels, viscera, and limbs ; the whole figure being more or less perfect according to circumstances that lie beyond our power of penetration.

After the death of the extra-uterine fœtus, the uterus, and consequently the general frame, frequently become quiet ; and the bulky substance, enveloped in a covering of coagulable lymph, remains for years, or perhaps through the whole of life, with no other inconvenience than that of a heavy weight and tumour in the part in which the dead fœtus is lodged. But in many instances, like any other intrusive or foreign material, it produces great irritation, which is succeeded by the ordinary process of ulcerative inflammation, and an opening is hereby made into the intestines or the vagina, or externally through the integuments of the abdomen, and the indissoluble parts of the fœtus are discharged piecemeal : sometimes the patient sinking during the tedious process, under the exhaustion of a hectic, but, more generally, evincing strength enough to sustain the progressive expulsion, and at length restored to the enjoyment of former health.

SPECIES I.

ECCYESIS OVARIA.

OVARIAN EXFŒTATION.

IMPERFECT FŒTATION OCCURRING IN THE RIGHT OR LEFT OVARIUM.

The physiology and general pathology have been already given so much at large in the paragraphs immediately preceding, that it is only necessary to observe further, that this form of extra-uterine fœtation is very common, as well as distressing. Vater relates a singular case of this kind, producing a kind of general intumescence of the abdomen on the right side, the right ovarium being the seat of the disease, that continued with little variation through a period of three years and a half, with an equal degree of distress and danger to the patient (*Dissert. de Graviditate apparente ex tumore ovarii dextri enormi*, &c.): and other instances are adverted to in the author's volume of Nosology.

It is in this organ more especially, that the rudimental attempts at fœtal organization, the mere sports of nature, are frequently found produced without impregnation, or any contact with the male sex, and sometimes in very young subjects.

One of the most singular cases of this kind is that communicated by Dr. Baillie to the Royal Society in the year 1788.—(*Phil. Trans.*, 1789.) The subject of the case was not more than twelve or thirteen years old, with an infantine uterus and perfect hymen ; and the fœtation consisted of a suety substance, hair, and the rudiments of four teeth.

The same kind of formative ludibria are found, also, in mature life, in women of the most correct lives, and whose chastity has never been impeached. Of this the following is an instance. The subject, an unmarried female, was about

thirty years of age at the time of her death, which took place after a long series of suffering, accompanied with great pain in the region of the bladder, and a considerable swelling of the abdomen. On examining the body, a large tuft of hair, about the size of a hen's egg, was found enclosed in a tumour of the left ovarium, surrounded with a fluid of the thickness of cream. In the bladder was traced a similar tuft of hair, surrounded with a like fluid, which distended and plugged up the organ.—(*Med. Chir. Trans.*, vol. ix., p. 427.)

Such rudiments of organized form have been resolved by the disciples of Buffon into the peculiar activity of his *molecules organiques*, concerning which we have already spoken in the Physiological Proem to the present class, thronging with a more than ordinary proportion in the region or organ in which the preternatural productions have been found to exist : and, by still later physiologists, into a salacious temperament in the individuals who have been the subjects of them, and who are still further said, as we have also remarked in the same Proem, to have a power, when this orgastic erethism is at its utmost heat, as about the period of menstruation, of irritating and even inflaming the ovaria, and occasionally even of detaching one or more ovula, and putting them into a like state of irregular action. And where cases occur in infants, they are ascribed to the same cause operating on a constitution diseased by a morbid precocity.—(See *Præotia feminina*, Ord. I., Gen. II., Spe. 2, of the present class.)

The first of these explanations it is hardly worth while to combat in the present day, and particularly in the present place, after having already illustrated, in the Proem above referred to, the feebleness of its first principles. And, with respect to the second, it is sufficient to observe, that the very same attempts at fœtation are sometimes made and carried quite as far towards completion, in organs that cannot be suspected of any salacious sensation, and even in males as well as in females. Thus, Dr. Huxham gives a case in which the rudiments of an embryo were found in a tumour seated near the anus of a child ;[*] and Mr. Young a still more extraordinary one, yet a case well known, I suppose, to nearly all the medical practitioners of this metropolis from personal inspection, of a large protuberant cyst, containing a nucleus of fœtal rudiments found in the abdomen of a *male* infant about fifteen months old. The child died after a tedious and painful illness. The body was opened, and the cyst examined : " The substance it contained," says Mr. Young, " had unequivocally the shape and characters of a human fœtus :" for a particular description of which the reader must turn to the account itself.—(*Medico-Chir. Trans.*, vol. i., p. 241.)

Upon this subject we can only say, that all such abortive attempts are monstrosities ; and

---

[*] Phil. Trans., vol. xlv., 1748, p. 325.—See also Dr. Edward Phillips's account of a case, in which parts of a fœtus were found in a tumour, situated in the abdomen of a girl two years and a half old. —Med. Chir. Trans., vol. vi., p. 124.—Ed.

that monstrosities are not confined to any particular age, as that of fœtal life, or to any particular organ. They run occasionally through every part of the frame, and every part of life, and appear in the form of cysts, and excrescences, and polypi, and ossifications, and a thousand other morbid deviations from the ordinary march of nature, though they are most frequently found in the first months of impregnation, unquestionably because the excited organs are, at that period, more capable than at any other, of being moulded, by accidental circumstances, into anomalous shapes, and of preserving life under almost every kind of misconstruction and deformity.

In extra-uterine fœtation of whatever kind, or wherever situated, the art of medicine can do but little. If the tumour be free from pain, and the general system not essentially disturbed by it, nothing should be attempted whatever. And if, in a case of irritation and ulcerative inflammation, nature herself seems to point out one particular part for the opening of the abscess rather than another, it will almost always be far better merely to watch her footsteps, and assist her intention, than to attempt a cure or removal of the cyst in any other way ; for we had long ago an opportunity of observing, when treating of INFLAMMATION generally, that, " it is a wise and benevolent law of Providence, and affords an incontrovertible proof of an instinctive remedial power, that inflammation, wherever seated, is always more violent on the side of the inflamed point nearest the surface, and shows a constant tendency to work its way externally rather than internally" (vol. i., p. 427) ; or, in other words, in that direction in which the most salutary end can be obtained with the least essential mischief. And hence, though it may often be found advisable to enlarge an opening made externally by the effort of nature alone, it will generally be injurious to deviate from the spot thus instinctively marked out, and make an opening elsewhere.

The cyst has sometimes lain dormant, or without producing much disturbance, for many years ; and then, from some accidental cause, has become irritated, inflamed, and produced a large abscess : the ovarium, in the progress of the inflammation, forming an adhesion to the integuments of the abdomen, and thus at length breaking externally ; mostly in the course of the linea alba, often near the navel, but sometimes towards the groin. In a few instances, however, the inflammatory action has travelled in some other direction, and sought some other outlet : so that the ovarium has formed an adhesion with the vagina, or the larger intestines, and ultimately opened into them, and the bones and other indissoluble parts of the fœtus have been thrown forth in fragments from the vagina or the anus. Zacutus Lusitanus gives a case, in which the bones of an impregnated ovarium were discharged piecemeal by the anus after the impregnation had continued for twelve years (De Praxi admirandâ, lib. ii., obs. 157) : and Bartholine another of much longer duration, in which an exit was formed in the hypochondrium, after

the fœtus had been imprisoned for not less than eighteen years.

In a few instances, however, the extra-uterine substance has been removed by art without waiting for the formation of an abscess. A successful operation of this kind is related in the Histoire de l'Académie Royale, after a gestation of twenty-seven months, the child being extracted by an incision into the abdomen.—(Hist. de l'Acad. des Sciences, 1714, p. 20 ; 1716, p. 32.) M. Trisen gives a similar example, attended with a like favourable issue (Observ. Chirurg., Leid., 1743, 4to.) : and, in the Edinburgh Medical Commentaries, we have an account of the vagina being laid open for the same purpose.[*]

The fœtus has occasionally been found to acquire a very considerable development and advance towards perfection. Bianchi gives the history of one, that on dissection, after the death of the mother, who carried it fourteen years after its apparent death, weighed eight pounds (Lieutaud, Hist. Anat. Med., i., obs. 1533) ; and Mr. Painter has lately given the case of a lady, who seems to have died in labour of a fœtus of the same kind, that on being taken from the body immediately after death, was found dead, indeed, but complete in its parts, and nearly of the size which is usual at the fifth month of uterine gestation. The Fallopian tubes, apparently too much obstructed at the time of impregnation for a descent of the ovum, were now altogether impervious.—(Lond. Med. Repos., June, 1823.) The uterus itself was not much enlarged, but there was not the ordinary appearance of a deciduous tunic.

SPECIES II.
ECCYESIS TUBALIS.
TUBAL EXFŒTATION.
IMPERFECT FŒTATION OCCURRING IN THE FALLOPIAN TUBE.

DIEMERBROECK has observed, that this is the most common cause under which extra-uterine gestation shows itself (Opera omnia Anatomica, p. 135), and it is at the same time the most dangerous. There is, in truth, less room for distention here than in any of the other cavities in which the exiled ovum may happen to lodge : and hence the overstretched tube has occasionally burst, and the patient has soon fallen a sacrifice to the irritation and fever produced by so large a rent ; while, if this have not taken place from the mischief done to the tube, it has followed nearly as soon from the morbid excitement and inflammation produced in the abdomen in consequence of the sudden entrance of so large a foreign body into its cavity. Dr Middleton, however, has described a singular case of a woman, who carried a fœtus for sixteen years in one of the Fallopian tubes with so little disturbance to the general health of the system,

---

[*] Smith, vol. v., p. 337. Lauverjat extracted an infant by incision through the vagina, and the woman recovered.—See Sabatier, De la Médecine Opératoire, tom. i., p. 136.—ED.

that at this period she became pregnant in the regular way, and appears to have passed through her pregnancy with a favourable issue.—(*Phil. Trans.*, vol. xliii., 1744–5.) The general pathology and mode of treatment run parallel with those of the preceding species.

SPECIES III.
ECCYESIS ABDOMINALIS.
ABDOMINAL EXFŒTATION.
IMPERFECT FŒTATION OCCURRING IN THE CAVITY OF THE ABDOMEN.

An extra-uterine fœtus may be deposited in the cavity of the abdomen by bursting through the walls of the ovarium or Fallopian tube after it has been produced there, or by an accidental drop of the impregnated ovum from the extremity or fringe of the tube in its way to the uterus. In the two former instances, there is danger of great and fatal inflammation; not less from the rent produced in the organ just quitted by the fœtus, than from the irritation which so large a foreign body cannot fail to produce on the organs on which it presses. In the last instance, on the contrary, the substance on its first entrance is so minute, and its growth so gradual, that the contiguous organs suffer little or no irritation, except from some accidental excitement, till at length, indeed, the magnitude of the fœtus may alone be a sufficient cause of morbid action, and lay a foundation for the most serious consequences.

In the introductory remarks to the present genus we observed, that in almost all cases of extra-uterine fœtation, the moment the ovum becomes impregnated, the womb regularly sympathizes in the action, produces a tunica decidua, enlarges, ceases to menstruate, mimics the entire process of utero-gestation, and at the expiration of nine months, is attacked with regular labour-pains. After these have continued for some hours, they gradually cease: and what is still more remarkable, the ex-fœtus, which till this moment is endowed with life, and continues to grow, how imperfect soever its form, dies as though strangled in its imprisonment; and by becoming a dead substance, becomes at the same time a substance obnoxious to the living organs around it, which have hitherto suffered little inconvenience from its proximity; often excites irritation and an abscess, and from such abscess, as we have already observed, is thrown forth piecemeal.

The following history, which is highly curious in itself, forms a striking illustration of the whole of these remarks. It is published by Dr. Bell, of Dublin, from a full knowledge of the entire facts. A young woman, aged twenty-one, after being married fifteen months, had the usual signs of pregnancy, and at the expiration of her reckoning, was attacked with regular labour-pains, which were very violent, for some days, when they gradually left her. But the abdomen still continued to enlarge, while the strength of the patient as gradually failed, and she was reduced to the utmost state of emaciation. Eight

or nine months from the cessation of her labour-pains, she discharged a considerable quantity of fluid from a small aperture at the navel, along with which were perceived some fleshy fibres and pieces of bone. It was proposed to follow up this indication of nature, and make an opening into the abdomen at this very point, large enough to remove the fœtus supposed to be lodged there. This was accomplished by an incision running two inches above and the same length below the navel, when the bones of two full-grown fœtuses were extracted, for little besides bones at that time remained. No hemorrhage ensued, and the patient recovered her health so speedily as to be able to menstruate in about three months. After three months more, she was prevailed upon again to cohabit with her husband, became pregnant, had a natural labour, and bore several children in succession.[*]

In this case it is clear, that the sensations of the uterus, during the development of the twin ex-fœtuses, were those of mere sympathy, as it is also that they ceased to grow, and became dead and irritating substances, after the common term of utero-gestation, or on the cessation of the labour-pains.

This is the usual course; but in some cases the irritation the dead substance excites is less violent, and instead of an ulcerative, an adhesive inflammation is produced, and coagulable lymph is thrown forth, which by the law of nature is gradually transformed into a soft and membranous material, that becomes a sheath or nidus for the dead fœtus, and prevents it from exciting any further irritation. And in this manner an abdominal ex-fœtus has sometimes been borne for a considerable number of years, or even to the end of life, without any serious mischief. In the volume of N*osology* I have referred to various proofs of its having in this way lain quiet for twenty-two, twenty-six, and even forty-six years.

Even in the uterus itself, the whole of this process has in a few rare instances happened, where a morbid cartilaginous membrane has taken the place of the ordinary tissue, or there have been any other means of obstructing the descent of the fœtus, of which the following, cited by M. Fournier, is a striking example. A woman of Soigny, thirty years of age, after four years of marriage and one miscarriage, became pregnant, quickened, and had a flow of milk in her breasts. At nine months, regular symptoms of labour came on; but shortly ceased. In the course of a month she became greatly debilitated, and continued so for a year and a half, during which time her life was often despaired of; after which she recovered strength, but the milk continued in her breasts for thirty years, yet she had never any return of the catamenia. At the age of sixty-one she died of peripneumony, and the body was opened. A tumour, eight pounds in weight, was found attached to the fundus of the

* History of a case in which two fœtuses, that had been carried near twenty-one months, were successfully extracted from the abdomen by incision, &c.

uterus, enclosing a male child, perfectly formed, and of full size for nine months. It did not exhibit any signs of putrefaction, nor exhale any disagreeable smell. It was enveloped in a chorion or amnios, which membranes were ossified, as was also the placenta. The dissection was performed in the presence of two physicians and another surgeon.—(*Dict. des Sciences Médicales,* Art. *Cas Rares.*) Putrefaction, under these circumstances, does not take place; for the imbedded substance is shut out from the chief auxiliary to putrefaction, which is air : but a change of another kind is generally found to prevail, though with some diversity, according to the accidental circumstances that accompany it. And hence the fœtus, on opening the uterus after the death of the mother, or on its own extraction antecedently, has been found sometimes converted into adipocire, or a suety or cétaceous material (*Wagner, Nov. Act. Liter. Maris,* Balth., 1699) making a near approach to it, sometimes into a leathery or cartilaginous structure (*Phil. Trans., various examples,* passim), and sometimes into an osseous or almost stony mass, which has been distinguished by the name of OSTEOPÆDION or LITHOPÆDION.—(*Abhandl. der Josephin. Acad.,* band i. ; *Eyson, Diss. de Fœtû Lapidescente,* Groning., 1661.)

Under these circumstances also, the bulk and weight of the fœtus have considerably varied ; for the fluids having evaporated, it has often been found light and shrivelled ; yet, when loaded with osseous matter, it has been peculiarly heavy. In a structure of somewhat more than ordinary completion, Krohn found the weight amount to four pounds and a half.—(*Fœtûs extra uterum Historia,* Lond., 1791, Gött., Ann. 1791.)

For methodical treatment there is little scope, and this little has been already touched upon under the first species.*

---

* In the Repertoire Gén. d'Anat. et de Physiologie for 1826, Breschet has published six cases of a new species of extra-uterine pregnancy, which may be termed *E. Interstitialis.* Dr. Carswell remarks, " that cases of aberration in the first development and ultimate station of the human embryo like these, were not known to science before these cases were laid before the profession. The facts are singular, yet authentic in all their particulars. It is therefore impossible to deny the existence of another distinct species of pregnancy, *extra muros uteri,* in which the fœtus is lodged among the interstitial elements of that viscus, and has no communication whatever either with the cavity of it on the one side, or the cavity of the abdomen on the other, unless ulceration or laceration take place.

" It is to be remarked, that in all these cases the uterus was found enlarged, its cavity filled with some adventitious production of variable texture, and not always membranaceous, and the Fallopian tube, on the side next to the seat of the embryo of every tumour, invariably impervious. The mother dies from internal hemorrhage, in consequence of laceration of the coats of the cyst containing the embryo. During life, menstruation has ceased in some, and not in other cases of this description."

Figures of two of these cases may be seen in Dr. Carswell's " Graphic Illustrations of Abortion and the Diseases of Menstruation," London, 1834, a work which may be consulted with profit.—D.

GENUS IV.
PSEUDOCYESIS.
SPURIOUS PREGNANCY.

SYMPTOMS OF PREGNANCY WITHOUT IMPREGNATION ; CHIEFLY OCCURRING ON THE CESSATION OF THE CATAMENIA.

In the preceding genus we beheld the uterus excited to action and mimicking the progress of pregnancy, though without any pretensions to it, in consequence of its association with some extra-uterine impregnation. In the present genus there is no proper impregnation anywhere, but a mere irritation derived from the lodgment of some morbid and unorganized substance, which excites a train of feelings, and not unfrequently a change of action, easily recalled from the force of habit. It is on this last account that virgins are rarely, if ever, liable to this affection. Such at least is the general opinion, which appears to be well founded ; " and no case," says Mr. Burns, " that I have met with, contradicts the supposition."

This train of feeling and change of action seem also, at times, excited by a peculiar kind of irritability of the uterus itself, even where there is no substance whatever in its own or any other cavity that can become a stimulus ; and we are hence put into possession of the two fellowing distinct species :—

1. Pseudocyesis Molaris.   Mole.
2. —————— Inanis.   False Conception.

SPECIES I.
PSEUDOCYESIS MOLARIS.
MOLE.

THE UTERUS, IRRITATED BY A COAGULUM OF BLOOD OR OTHER SECRETION LODGED IN ITS CAVITY, OFTEN ASSUMING A FIBROUS APPEARANCE.

A COAGULUM of blood, thrown into the womb by a relaxation of the mouth of the menstrual excernents, or remaining there as a sequel of miscarriage or labour, is perhaps the most common cause of this morbid action and sensation. It was long ago thus explained by Mr. Hewson : " from the blood's being without motion in the cavity of the uterus," and consequently coagulating ; " and hence," continues he, " the origin of those large clots which sometimes come from the cavity, and which, when more condensed by the oozing out of the serum and of the red globules, assume a flesh-like appearance, and have been called moles."—(*Inquiries,* &c, part i., p. 27.) The concretion, indeed, has become sometimes so close and indurated as to resemble the consolidation of a stone ; and hence Mr. Bromfield describes a mole expelled from the uterus, as consisting of a stony mass the size of a child's head.—(*Observ.* ii., p. 156.) And Hancroft has related a similar case.—(*Diss. de Molâ, occasione molæ osseæ in vetulâ inventæ,* Goet., 1746.)

Living blood, however, has a strong tendency at all times, and especially when aided by rest and the warmth of the body, to fabricate vessels and assume a membranous structure. "I have reason to believe," says Mr. J. Hunter, "that the coagulum has the power, under necessary circumstances, to form vessels in and of itself: for although not organic, it is still of a peculiar form, structure, or arrangement. I think I have been able to inject what I suspected to be the beginning of a vascular formation in a coagulum, when it could not derive any vessels from the surrounding parts."* It is probably on this account that we sometimes find the discharged mass or mole evincing something of a fibrous or membranous appearance, and mimicking the structure of an organized substance.

Fragments of a placenta or of its membranes have also sometimes remained unexpelled from the uterus, and have become blended with coagula of blood (*Ruysch, Thesaurus* iii., vi.), and probably of blood aiming as above at a vascular development; and hence the mole has been of a still more complicated character, and has often puzzled practitioners of great judgment and experience.

And occasionally hydatids have found the means of forming a nidus in some one of the sulci of the womb, and by swelling into a considerable vesicular tumour, or various clusters of such tumours, have very considerably added to the enlargement.—(*Eph. Nat. Cur.*, dec. ii., ann. ii., 157, ann. viii., 50, et alibi; *Morgagni de Sed. et Caus. Morb.*, ep, xlviii., 12, &c.) The distinguishing character in this case is the perpetual oozing of a colourless watery fluid from the vagina. The hydatid is usually dispelled by a process resembling labour, which is followed by a profuse and alarming hemorrhage, that, however, seldom proves fatal under proper management.—(*Clarke, Observations on the Diseases of Females*, &c., 8vo., 1821.)

Many writers have described, by the name of moles, the fragments of a fœtus which have long remained in the uterus after its death, and have sometimes been surrounded by an adscititious involucrum, or some part of its placenta or membranes, but so changed by some subsequent chymical or animal operation as to have little resemblance to their original structure.† These

however are rather miscarriages, or remnants of miscarriages, than moles. They manifestly bespeak an impregnation and organic growth in the proper organ, but owing to torpitude or some other diseased condition of the womb, were not expelled at the period of the death of the fœtus. We have already observed in treating of miscarriage, PARACYESIS ABORTUS, and more particularly still under PARACYESIS PLURALIS, that such retention, and almost to an unlimited period, is by no means uncommon, and have illustrated the remark by numerous examples.

Simulating pregnancy, from molar concretions, assumes in many cases so much of the character of genuine impregnation as to be distinguished with considerable difficulty. In general, however, the abdominal swelling increases in the spurious kind far more rapidly than in the real for the first three months, after which it keeps nearly at a stand; the tumour, moreover, is considerably more equable, the breasts are flat, and do not participate in the action, and there is no sense of quickening. There is almost always a retention of the menses.*

If we suspect the disease, the state of the uterus should be examined; and it will often be in the examiner's power to ascertain the fact, and by a skilful introduction of the finger to hook down a part of the mass through the cervix, and hence, by a little dexterity, to remove the whole; but he should be careful not to break the mole into fragments.

Moles, wholly or in fractions, are thrown out by the action of the uterus at different periods— often at three months, more frequently by something like a regular accession of labour-pains at nine; but they occasionally remain much longer: in a case of Riedlin's, for three years (*Lin. Med.*, 1695, p. 297); and in one described by Zuingen

---

*On Blood, &c., p. 92, 4to. edit., 1794. The accuracy of these statements is questioned by some pathologists of the present time.—ED.

† It is supposed "that the embryo may be expelled, and yet the membranes continue to adhere to the uterus, and be completely developed. The membrana decidua is said to acquire a considerable thickness, and the amnion entirely to disappear, while the cavity of the chorion gradually contracting, the mass which remains is only a red fleshy substance, in the centre of which there is sometimes visible a small serous cavity." M. Velpeau and other French pathologists have followed Ruysch in explaining the formation of fleshy moles on this principle; but (according to Dr. R. Lee) though these substances are invariably the product of conception, it is not certain that they are formed by the growth of the membranes, subsequent to the death and expulsion of the embryo. In several cases, no embryo was at any time discharged. —(See Cyclop. of Pract. Med., art. Abortion.) Madame Boivin and Professor Dugès adopt the following arrangement of moles:. 1st. The *false*

germe or ovum; 2d. The *fleshy mole;* and 3d. The *vesicular* or *hydatid mole.* According to this view, all moles are regarded as the vitiated or morbid product of conception, and of course as never formed in any female that has not had sexual intercourse. The first variety—the false germe, occurs in the early days or weeks of conception, in consequence of the formation of a small tumour, or an effusion of blood at the origin of the umbilical vessels, partial detachment of the membranes, and perhaps mere disorder of the circulation by fright, shock, &c.; the embryo dies, and is then dissolved in the water of the amnion, like a flake of gelatin. This blighted ovum seldom remains in the womb beyond two or three months, and cannot then be distinguished from a regular pregnancy at the full time. In general, it is expelled entire and without rupture. Of fleshy moles, two kinds are described—one hollow in the centre, the other solid; both cases referred by these writers to a degeneration of the envelopes of the fœtus. The vesicular mole is ascribed to the same origin. —See Traité Pratique des Maladies de l'Uterus, et de ses Annexes, &c., par Madame Boivin et A. Dugès; of which an instructive analysis is given in the Edinb. Medical and Surgical Journal, Nos. 114-117.—ED.

* The enlargement of the breasts and abdomen comes on more suddenly than in real pregnancy, and in the second month appears more prominent than it would do in the fifth, were such enlargement connected with gestation.—ED.

for not less than seventeen.—(*Theatrum Vitæ Humanæ*, pp. 33, 357.)

SPECIES II.

PSEUDOCYESIS INANIS.

FALSE CONCEPTION.

THE UTERUS VOID OF INTERNAL SUBSTANCE, AND IRRITATED BY SOME UNKNOWN MORBID ACTION.

THERE are two periods during the active power of the womb in which it is peculiarly irritable, and these are at the commencement and at the final termination of the catamenial flux. And hence it sometimes happens at the last period, from some unknown excitement, though generally, perhaps, the increased erethism which, in consequence of such irritation, accompanies the conjugal embrace, that it becomes sensible of feelings and communicates them to the stomach, not unlike what it has formerly sustained in an early stage of impregnation ; and a catenation of actions having thus commenced, every link in the chain that accompanied the whole range of former pregnancies is passed through, and as accurately imitated as if there were a real foundation for them.

This illusory feeling, however, sometimes dies away gradually at the end of three months, but more usually runs on to the end of the ninth, when there is occasionally a feeble attempt at labour-pains, but they come to nothing : and the farce is gradually, and in a few instances suddenly concluded, by a rapid diminution of the abdominal swelling, and a return of the uterus to its proper size.

The most extraordinary case of this kind that has ever occurred to me, is given under the unmeaning name of *nervous pregnancy*, by M. Rusal of Var, in the department of the Charante, in the first number of the *Gazette de Santé* for 1824 ; which is peculiarly characterized by the perpetuity of its annual recurrence for twenty years, or rather through the whole of the patient's life. Mary Gibaud had uniformly enjoyed good health previous to her marriage. This took place when she was about thirty ; shortly after which, menstruation ceased, nausea or sickness was complained of in the morning, the abdomen enlarged, quickening and subsequent motions of the fœtus were supposed to be felt, and at length what were conceived to be labour-pains supervened. These continued while a female midwife was present, for thirty-six hours, but without any enlargement of the os uteri. A surgeon of reputation was applied to, at the moment of whose arrival a considerable uterine hemorrhage took place, accompanied with syncope. The surgeon proceeded instantly to deliver ; but to the astonishment of all present, he found the womb entirely unimpregnated. The hemorrhage took off the pains for two or three hours, at which time they returned again. The surgeon now bled her copiously, and every symptom vanished. At the end of a month, the menstrual excitement not producing any discharge, the same train of feelings were produced in their stead, ran the same round, and terminated in the same way—the same precise order being repeated for twenty times in succession. The patient was from time to time visited by different professors of eminence, and on one occasion was taken to the hospital of Angoulème, where she was tapped, as being supposed to be dropsical ; but no fluid was evacuated. Her breasts through every period were gorged with milk ; and she at length died, in her fifty-first year, of an inflammation of the ear, that spread to the brain.—(See Cl. III., Ord. II., Gen. VII., Spe. 2, *Empresma otitis interna.*)

The ordinary distinctive signs which indicate real from spurious pregnancy under the last species, and which we have already noticed, are equally applicable to the present, and the practitioner should avail himself of them.*

---

* On this subject see Granville's Graphic Illustrations of Abortion, &c.—D.

CLASS VI.
ECCRITICA.
DISEASES OF THE EXCERNENT FUNCTION.

ORDER I.
MESOTICA.
AFFECTING THE PARENCHYMA.

" II.
CATOTICA.
AFFECTING INTERNAL SURFACES.

.. III.
ACROTICA.
AFFECTING THE EXTERNAL SURFACE.

CLASS VI.
PHYSIOLOGICAL PROEM.

THE structure of the solid parts of the body consists of three distinct substances—a filamentous, a parenchymatous, and a cellular or web-like, as it was denominated by Haller, the tissu muqueux of Bordeu (*Recherches sur le Tissu Muqueux ou Organe Cellulaire*, Paris, 1791), and the tela mucosa of Blumenbach.—(*Physiol.*, § 21.) The filamentous is chiefly to be traced in the bony, muscular, and membranous parts: the parenchyma, a term first employed by Erasistratus, and, as we shall show hereafter, in a very different sense from that in which it is used at present, in what are commonly called visceral organs: and the cellular in both. This last, while it serves the purpose of giving support to the vessels and nerves of the fibrous parts, of separating them from each other where necessary, and where necessary of connecting them, is the repository or receptacle of the gelatinous or albuminous material, which constitutes the general substance of the parenchymatous parts, and has peculiar qualities superadded to it, according to the nature of the organ which it imbodies, and the peculiarity of the texture which runs through it: whence the structure of the liver differs from that of the pancreas, the structure of the pancreas from that of the kidneys, and the structure of the lungs, or of the placenta, from all the rest. It is usually supposed to be a condensation of this, that forms the proper membranes which cover the exterior of the viscera, as well as the interior of those that are hollow, and which, as we have already observed (vol. i., *Physiol. Proem*, Cl. I.), are divided into serous, mucous, and fibrous, by Bichat and his followers.

All these parts are perpetually wearing out by their own action, the firm and solid, as well as the most spongy and attenuate. They are

supplied with new materials from the general current of the blood, and have their waste and recrement carried off by a correspondent process.

It is obvious, that for this purpose there must be two distinct sets or systems of vessels; one by which the due recruit is provided, the other by which the refuse or rejected part is removed. —(*Bostock, Elementary System of Physiology*, p. 70, 8vo., 1824.) These vessels are in common language denominated SECRETORIES and ABSORBENTS. They bear the same relation to each other as the arteries and veins: the action, which commences with the former, is carried forward into the latter; and we may further observe, that while the secretories originate from the arteries, the absorbents terminate in the veins. The general function, sustained by these two sets or systems of vessels, is denominated, in the present work, ECCRITICAL or EXCERNENT: the health of this function consists in the balance of power maintained between its respective vessels; and its diseases in the disturbance of such balance. There may be undue secretion with healthy absorption; undue absorption with healthy secretion: or there may be undue or morbid absorption and secretion at the same time.

The refuse matter, however, or that which is no longer fit for use, is not all wasted: nor in reality any of that which falls within the province of the absorbents. Nature is a judicious economist, and divides the eliminated materials into two parts—one consisting of those fluids which, by an intimate union with the newly-formed chyle, and a fresh subaction in the lungs, may once more be adapted for the purposes of general circulation; and the other of those which no elaboration can revive, and whose longer retention in the body would be mischie-

K k 2

vous. It is the province of the absorbent system to take the charge of the whole of the first office; to collect the effete matter from every quarter, and to pour it, by means of innumerable channels that are perpetually uniting, into the thoracic duct, which forwards it progressively to the heart. The really waste and intractable matter, instead of disturbing the action of the absorbents, is at once thrown out of the general system by the mouths of the secernents themselves, as in the case of insensible perspiration; or, where such a perpetual efflux would be inconvenient, is deposited in separate reservoirs, and suffered to accumulate, till the individual has a commodious opportunity of evacuating them, as in the case of the urine and the feces.

Thus far we see into the general economy; but when we come to examine minutely into the nature of either of these sets of vessels, we find that there is much yet to be learned, both as to their structure and the means by which they operate. The subject is of great importance, and may perhaps be best considered under the three following divisions:—

I. The General Nature of the Secernent System.

II. The General Nature of the Absorbent System.

III. The General Effects produced by the Action of these two Systems on each other.

I. It was at one time the common doctrine among physiologists, as well chymical as mechanical, that all the vast variety of animal productions which are traced in the different secretory organs, whether wax, or tears, or milk, or bile, or saliva, were formerly contained in the circulating mass; and that the only office of these organs was to *separate* them respectively from the other materials that enter into the very complex crasis of the blood: whence, indeed, the name of SECERNENTS or SECRETORIES, which mean nothing more than *separating powers*. This action was by the chymists supposed to depend on peculiar attractions, or the play of affinities, which was the explanation advanced by some; or on peculiar ferments, conveyed by the blood to the secernent organ, or pre-existing in it, which was the opinion of others. The mechanical physiologists, on the contrary, ascribed the separation to the peculiar figure or diameter of the secretory vessels, which by their make were only fitted to receive particles of a given form, as prisms where the vessels were triangular, and cubes where they were square. Such was the explanation of Des Cartes: while Boerhaave, not essentially wandering from the same view, supposed the more attenuate secretions to depend upon vessels of a finer bore, and the more viscid upon those of a larger diameter.

Modern chymistry, however, has completely exploded all these and many other hypotheses, founded upon the same common principle, by proving that most of the secerned materials are not formally existent in the blood, and consequently that it is not, strictly speaking, by an act of separation, but of new arrangement or

recomposition, that they are produced out of its elements. [However, notwithstanding it is not always possible to recognise in the blood the elements of every secretion, the quantity of secretion has undoubtedly a relation to the quantity of blood circulating in a part. Thus, when the quantity of milk secreted by the breast is increased after parturition, the arteries of the part are enlarged; and in order to check the growth of a tumour, it is frequently sufficient to tie the main artery leading to it.—(See *Mayo's Outlines of Human Physiology*, p. 116, 2d edit.)]

Not having gained much light from the above researches, physiologists have been led to a critical inquiry into the fabric of the secerning organ, but hitherto without much satisfaction. In its simplest state it seems, as far as it can be traced, to consist of nothing more than single vessels possessing a capillary orifice, as in the Schneiderian membrane.* In a somewhat more compound form we find this orifice opening into a follicle, or minute cavity, of an elliptic shape; and in a still more complicated make, we meet with a glandular apparatus more or less conglomerate, consisting of a congeries of secernent vessels, with or without follicles, and occasionally accompanied with a basin or reservoir for a safe deposite of the secreted or elaborated matter against the time of its being wanted, of which the gall-bladder furnishes us with a well-known example. But, in none of these instances are we able to discover any peculiar device produced by this complication of machinery beyond the mean of affording the means of accumulation: for large as is the organ of the liver, it is in the penicilli, or the pori biliarii alone, that the bile is formed and completely elaborated; the liver is a vast bundle or combination of these, and hence affords an opportunity for a free formation of bile in a collective state, but it has not been ascertained that it affords any thing more. And although in the gall-bladder we find this fluid a little varied after its deposite, and rendered thicker, yellower, and bitterer, the change is nothing more than what must necessarily follow from absorption, or the removal of a part of the finer particles of the bile. The conglomerate glands of the mammæ offer us the same results; for the milk here secreted is as perfect milk in every separate lactiferous tube, as when it flows in an accumulated form from the nipple. And hence follicles themselves may be nothing more than minute reservoirs for the convenient accumulation of such fluids as are deposited in them till they are required for use. Mucus and serum are inspissated by retention, but they rarely undergo any other change. We are obliged, therefore, to conclude with Sir Everard Home, that

* The various substances of which the body consists, or which are thrown out upon its surfaces, or ooze into its cavities, are for the most part separated or secreted from the capillary vessels of the aortic system of arteries. There are probably, as Mr. Mayo has noticed, two exceptions to this statement. The bile appears to be secreted from the capillaries of the vena portæ; and the aqueous vapour from the lungs is perhaps in part supplied from the capillaries of the pulmonary artery.—ED.

"the organs of secretion are principally made up of arteries and veins ; but there is nothing in the different modes in which these vessels ramify that can in any way account for the changes in the blood out of which secretions arise."*

These organs, however, are largely supplied with twigs of small nerves, and it has been an idea long entertained by physiologists, that secretion is chiefly effected through their instrumentality. Sir Everard Home, in his paper inserted in the volume of the Philosophical Transactions just referred to, has observed, "that in fishes which are capable of secreting the electrical fluid, the nerves connected with the electrical organs exceed those that go to all the other parts of the fish in the proportion of twenty to one" (*Phil. Trans.*, 1809, p. 386) : and in confirmation of this view of the subject, it may be remarked, that there are no parts of the body more manifestly affected, and few so much so, as the secretory organs, by mental emotion. The whole surface of the skin is sometimes bedewed with drops of sweat, and even, of blood, by a sudden paroxysm of agony of mind : grief fills the eyes with tears : fear is well known to be a powerful stimulant to the kidneys, and very generally to the alvine canal : anger gives an additional flow, perhaps an additional acrimony, to the bile ; and if urged to violence, renders the saliva poisonous, as we have already observed under the genus LYSSA (vol. ii., p. 292) ; and disappointed hope destroys the digestion, and alters the qualities of the secreted fluids of the stomach. [The saliva, the bile, the urine, and perspiration, are examples of the products of *functional* secretion, as it is sometimes termed, when contrasted with *nutritive* secretion, the object of which is to separate from the blood all the different kinds of matter employed in the growth and incessant renewal of the various textures of the body. Functional secretion is considered to be remarkably under the influence of the nerves. Upon one affection of the mind, the tears flow ; upon a second, the urine ; upon another, the saliva ; yet Mr. Mayo found, upon cutting the nerves of the kidney in a dog, that in half an hour afterward, urine had accumulated in the pelvis of the kidney, and in the ureter, which had been tied.—(*Mayo's Outlines of Human Physiology*, p. 121, 2d edit.) Whether secretion be essentially connected with the influence of the brain and nerves, is a point not yet altogether determined. Many considerations leave no doubt, that the process of secretion in general, and particularly that of functional secretion, is materially affected by the state of the nervous system, especially, as already remarked, by various mental emotions. Whether this fact, which is undisputed, be compatible with other phenomena, proving that se-

cretion may be performed under circumstances wherein the influence of the brain and nerves cannot operate, is another matter for examination. There may not be any thing incompatible in the two positions : the kidney may secrete in an acephalous child, but it may secrete differently, that is to say, more perfectly and freely, in another infant in which the whole nervous system is complete. Mr. Lawrence has briefly summed up the several arguments on each side of this question. Secretion, he observes, is performed by the minute vessels, all the other actions of which are manifestly exempt from the influence of the brain. Capillary circulation ; nutrition, in which the capillaries separate from a common fluid the materials which they convert into all the various animal structures, and thus build up and support the various organs ; the serous and mucous exhalations are all performed in fœtuses without brain or spinal marrow. They go on when the influence of the brain is suspended in apoplexy, compression, and concussion. The two former and cutaneous exhalation are kept up in the limbs of the paralytic, and of animals in which all the nerves have been divided. Nutrition is performed in structures which possess no nerves, as tendon, cartilage, &c. Serum and pus are formed when blisters are applied to paralytic limbs. When the nerves of the eighth pair have been divided, the air-vesicles and tubes of the lungs become loaded with mucous fluid : the same phenomenon takes place in a still greater degree when artificial respiration is carried on in decapitated animals, and has even in this case been set down as the immediate cause of death.—(*Le Gallois, Expériences sur le Principe de la Vie*, &c., p. 240, Paris, 1812.) In the acephalous fœtus, described by Mr. Lawrence, secretion appeared to be independent of the nervous system, as urine was secreted when neither cerebrum nor cerebellum existed.—(*Med. Chir. Trans.*, vol. v., p. 223.)

The foregoing facts clearly prove the possibility of secretion, independently of the brain and nerves : but they are far from proving, that when the brain and nervous system do exist, secretion is beyond their influence. This is a point which the editor deems quite incapable of being established. Even the common action of blushing, the effect of mental emotion, proves that the minute arteries are quickly reached and affected by the nervous influence. The increased determination of blood to the corpora cavernosa, in certain states of the mind, is another proof of the same fact. The profuse perspiration often brought on by fear ; the increased flow of saliva at the sight and smell of food ; the augmented secretion of tears under various affections of the mind ; the copious pale urine, suddenly excreted in hypochondriacal and hysterical persons ; and the decided affection of the biliary secretion in some cases by mental emotion, only admit of explanation by reference to the agency of the nervous system.

Mr. Brodie found that the secretion of the urine does not take place in animals in which, after decapitation, the circulation of the blood was sustained by artificial respiration. This

---

* Phil. Trans., 1809, p. 387. The changes here adverted to are no doubt essentially connected with a peculiarity of organization and vascular arrangement ; but, in addition to these conditions, we are compelled to believe, that the nature, as well as the quantity of the secretion, intimately depends upon the specific action of the secerning or capillary vessels.—ED.

yet prevails.]

Many facts seem to prove, that the secretory organs are very much influenced by the sensorial system ; yet Haller has long ago observed, that the larger branches of the nerves seldom enter into them, and seem purposely to avoid them (*Physiolog.*, tom. ix., passim) : the secernent glands have little sensibility ; and the secretions of plants, which have no nervous system, are as abundant and diversified, and as wonderful in every respect, as those of animals. [In a paralyzed limb, growth, and the common phenomena of reproduction, take place. When the fifth pair of nerves was divided upon the petrous portion of the temporal bone in a rabbit, upon breaking off the crown of an incisor tooth, Mr. Mayo (*Outlines of Human Physiology*, p. 117, 2d edit.) found the part reproduced as rapidly as in an animal in which the nerves were entire. And, as the same writer remarks, the human mola sometimes attains considerable development without either brain or spinal cord. Yet, in the instance of one organ of very delicate fabric, it has been proved, that its nutrition is disturbed upon the division of one of the nerves which supply it. When the fifth pair of nerves is divided close to its origin within a rabbit's scull, the upper portion of the surface of the eye inflames, and the upper segment of the cornea becomes turbid. M. Magendie also found that, if the fifth nerve be destroyed upon the petrous portion of the temporal bone, where it is involved in the ganglion of Gasser, the entire cornea becomes opaque in twenty-four hours, and the opacity daily increases : on the second day, the tunica conjunctiva reddens, and secretes pus ; the iris becomes inflamed and covered with lymph ; and at length the cornea ulcerates, and the humours are discharged.—(*Magendie, Journ. de Physiol.*, tom. iv., pp. 176 and 302.) From what has been stated, it may be concluded, that nutritive secretion is partly independent of the influence of the brain.]

The means, therefore, by which the very extensive and important economy of secretion is effected, seem hitherto, in a very considerable degree, to have eluded all investigation. We behold, nevertheless, the important work proceeding before us, and are in some degree acquainted with its machinery.

The most simple, and at the same time, perhaps, the most copious of the fluids, which are in this manner separated from the blood, is that discharged by very minute secernent vessels, supposed to be terminal or exhalant arteries, which open into all the cavities of the body, and pour forth a fine breathing vapour, or halitus, as it is called, which keeps their surfaces moist, and makes motion easy—an effluvium which must have been noticed by every one who has ever attended the cutting up of a bullock in a slaughter-house. We have formerly had occasion to observe, that arteries terminate in two ways—in minute veins, and in exhalant vessels. The former termination can often be followed up

orifices of the exhalant branches of arteries. Their existence, however, is proved, as Mr. Cruickshank has observed, by their sometimes pouring forth blood instead of vapour, and especially when enlarged in diameter, or acted upon by a more than ordinary vis à tergo. Of this we have an instance in bloody sweat ; as also in the menstrual flux, which, though not blood itself, proceeds, as Dr. Hunter has sufficiently shown, from the mouths of the exhalant arteries of the uterus, periodically altered in their diameter and secernent power.

II. The fluid, thus thrown forth to lubricate internal surfaces, would necessarily accumulate and become inconvenient, if there were not a correspondent set of vessels perpetually at work to carry off the surplus. But such a set of vessels is everywhere distributed over the entire range of the body, as well within as without, to answer this express purpose : and they are hence called ABSORBENTS ; and, from the limpidity of their contained fluid, LYMPHATICS.

Their course has been progressively followed up and developed, from the time of Asellius (*Epistola ad Haller*), who in the year 1622 " reaped the first laurels in this field by his discovery of those vessels on the mesentery, which, from their carrying a milk-white fluid, he denominated LACTEALS" (*Hewson, of the Lymphatic System*, p. 2), and whose researches were confirmed and extended by the valuable labours of Pecquet, Rudbeck, Jollyfe, Bartholine, Glisson, Nuck, and Ruysch, till by the concurrent and finishing demonstrations of Hoffmann and Meckel, and more especially of our own illustrious countrymen, Hewson, the elder Monro, both the Hunters, and Cruickshank, the whole of this curious and elaborate economy was completely explained and illustrated towards the close of the preceding century, and the opposition of Baron Haller was abandoned.*

The vessels of the absorbent system anastomose more frequently than either the veins or the arteries ; for it is a general law of nature, that the smaller the vessels of every kind, the more freely they communicate and unite with each other. We can no more trace their orifices, excepting indeed those of the lacteals, than we can the orifices of the exhalants ; but we can trace their united branches from an early function, and can follow them up singly, or in the confederated form of conglobate glands, till, with the exception of a few that enter the right subclavian vein, they all terminate in the common trunk of the thoracic duct ; which, as

* The claim to the honour of the discovery of the uses of the lymphatics, produced an acrimonious controversy between Drs. Hunter and Monro. Neither of these great anatomists seems to have been aware that the main facts, the cause of this celebrated dispute, had been distinctly mentioned by M. Noguez, in his work L'Anatomie du Corps Humain, ed, 2, 1726.—See an account of the Life, &c., of Wm. Hunter, M. D., by S. F. Simmons, M. D., p. 30.—ED.

we have formerly observed, receives also the tributary stream of the anastomosing lacteals, or the absorbents which drink up the subacted food from the alvine canal, whose orifices are capable of being traced—and pours the whole of this complicated fluid, steadily and slowly, by means of a valve placed for this purpose at its opening, into the subclavian vein of the left side. And as these all perform a common office, are of a like structure, pass through similar glands, and terminate in a common channel, there is strong reason to suppose them to constitute a common system; and hence, as we are capable of tracing up the mouths of the lacteals, we are led to conclude analogically, that the lymphatics have mouths of like kind, and for like purposes, although from their minuteness they have hitherto eluded all detection.

By this contrivance there is a prodigious saving of animalized fluids, which, however they may differ from each other in several properties, are far more easily reducible to genuine blood, than new and unassimilated matter obtained from without.

Yet this is not all; for many of the secretions, whose surplus is thus thrown back upon the system, essentially contribute to its greater vigour and perfection. We have a striking example of this in the absorption of semen, which, as observed on a late occasion (vol. ii., p. 414, *Phys. Proëm*, suprà), gives force and firmness to the voice, and changes the downy hair of the cheeks into a bristly beard; insomuch that those who are castrated in early life, are uniformly deprived of these peculiar features of manhood. The absorption of the surplus matter, secreted by the ovaria at the same age of puberty, produces an equal influence upon the mammary glands, and finishes the character of the female sex, as the preceding absorption completes that of the male. So, absorption of fat from the colon, where, in the opinion of Sir Everard Home, it is formed in great abundance, carries on the growth of the body in youth.*

[Many facts and considerations will apprize the physiological inquirer, that the constituent particles of every texture of the body are always undergoing a change; those which become unfit for longer continuance being withdrawn, and new ones deposited in their place. In this manner, an incessant renovation of the

* Phil. Trans., 1813, p. 157. These opinions respecting the absorption of the semen, of the redundant matter secreted by the ovaries, and fat from the colon, are only to be received as hypotheses. We have no proof that the testis ever produces its particular secretion, except for the purpose of being collected in the bulb of the urethra during the venereal excitement, and of being expelled at the instant when the orgasm takes place. As for the ovaries, we know of no peculiar matter which it is their office to secrete, unless it be the ovula, which nobody supposes to be habitually absorbed. When the testes or ovaries are wanting, or have been removed, the influence upon the constitution is probably rather to be ascribed to the imperfection of an essential part of the genital system, than to the interruption of any supposed absorption of the semen, or of any matter secreted by the ovaries.—Ed.

component matter of the various organs is kept up during life, to which it is unquestionably quite as essential as any of the other great vital functions, though some of these, in consequence of being more obvious to common notice, may have attracted a greater share of attention. In proof of this statement, we need at present merely observe, that while respiration comprehends within itself an example of one modification of absorption without which it would be completely useless, a principal object of the circulation is, that all parts may receive from the blood the new materials expressly intended to replace such as are taken away from them by the organs of absorption; and that, if it were not for the absorbent system, by which the circulation is replenished, the copious deductions from the mass of blood, caused by the various secretions, and the perpetual deposition of new matter in every texture, would speedily bring our existence to a conclusion. Thus, by the reciprocal and harmonious action of the secerning arteries and the absorbents, a change is always taking place in the identity, though not in the nature, of the component matter of every part of the body; and, what is curious, this change is effected, without the part necessarily undergoing any deviation from its ordinary shape, size, and general appearance. However, during the period of growth, the process is so regulated, that the deposition of new particles exceeds the absorption of the old, and the consequence is a gradual enlargement of the body, limbs, and different organs. After this stage of life, whatever increase takes place in the bulk of the body in general, or any of its parts, must originate either from morbid changes of structure, dropsical disease, the formation of tumours, or the accumulation of adipose matter, the absorption of which, in certain constitutions, does not keep pace with its secretion. But although the various parts of the body do not enlarge after the stage of life allotted to growth, many of them lose a considerable portion of their volume in old age, as is exemplified in the muscular system in general, and in the absorbent glands; and even in the infant, while nearly every part is receiving an addition to its size, a few organs, like the thymus gland and the renal capsules, are dwindling away. Now, whenever the body, or any parts of it, receive new particles into their composition, in exchange for the old, as is the case during the whole of life; or whenever the quantity of constituent matter is lessened, and the size of organs consequently reduced; these effects imply the agency of the absorbents, without the co-operation of which the secerning arteries might thicken and increase the volume of parts, but could have no power to produce any of those mutations, in which the removal of some of their component particles is an essential branch of the process. The organs usually believed to effect the species of absorption to which we here refer, are the lymphatic vessels and their glands.

Several cavities in the body are naturally moistened with an exhalation of limpid fluid, and those of the joints are lubricated with synovia; but these and every other secretion, retained for any time within the animal body, are never actually stagnant; for while the arteries are secreting them, the absorbents are actively employed in removing them, so that, in these examples, an uninterrupted renovation is going on, and the quantity of fluid, though continually receiving additions, is prevented by the absorbents from becoming too copious. This function is also commonly ascribed to the lymphatics.

Another form of absorption, entirely distinct from the two preceding ones, yet not less important, is that by which nutritious fluid, the product of digestion, and well known by the name of *chyle*, is taken up from the inner surface of the small intestines, and conveyed into the venous system near the heart. For the performance of this very indispensable function, which, in fact, is *the only one whereby the circulation is known with any degree of certainty to be replenished*, nature has provided a set of vessels, named *lacteals* from their white appearance, which arises from the chyle being seen through their thin and transparent coats. In modern works they are also frequently called *chyliferous vessels* and *nutrient absorbents*. One remarkable peculiarity of the lacteals is, that they generally absorb only chyle, and perhaps never imbibe any other substances; at least, several experiments, undertaken of late years in France, tend to establish this point; though it is one at variance with the result of Mr. Hunter's investigations; a circumstance that will be presently noticed again. But whatever decision may be finally made on this subject, it is acknowledged by all parties, that the lacteals have nothing to do with the removal of the old particles of the body, but only take up those substances which are in contact with the villous coat of the bowels. We have stated that the absorption of chyle by the lacteals is the only process positively known to be instrumental in replenishing the sanguiferous system; an observation justified in the present state of physiological science, by the doubts entertained concerning the origin and uses of the fluid pervading the lymphatics. The common belief is, that the lymphatics absorb all the old and redundant materials of the body, and also various kinds of fluid within its textures and cavities; and that, by some unexplained operation, all these different substances are converted, as soon as they enter into these vessels, into a colourless limpid fluid termed the lymph. The truth is, that nothing has been demonstrably and unequivocally proved about the source of this fluid; and the foregoing hypothesis is absolutely denied by those physiologists who particularly espouse the doctrine of venous absorption. However, although the origin of lymph cannot be said to be known with certainty, its course and destination are perfectly understood; and since the lacteals and lymphatics all terminate in a common trunk, and the chyle and lymph are thus blended together previously to their entrance into the large veins near the heart, there is strong reason for believing that the lymph is concerned in the same function as the chyle. It appears, therefore, that while the

exact use of the lymphatics is a questionable point in physiology, the function of the lacteals, —the conveyance of chyle into the sanguiferous system,—is one that is quite undisputed.]

Lymphatics accompany every part of the general frame so closely, and with so much minuteness of structure, that Mr. Cruickshank has proved them to exist very numerously in the coats of small arteries and veins, and suspects them to be attendants on the vasa vasorum, and equally to enter into their fabric. Wherever they exist they are more richly endowed, as we have just remarked, by very numerous valves, than any other sets of vessels whatever. "A lymphatic valve is a semicircular membrane, or rather of a parabolic shape, attached to the inside of the lymphatic vessels by its circular edge, having its straight edge, corresponding to the diameter, loose or floating in the cavity: in consequence of this contrivance, fluids passing in one direction make the valve lie close to the side of the vessel, and leave the passage free: but attempting to pass in the opposite direction, raise the valve from the side of the vessel, and push its loose edge towards the centre of the cavity. But as this would shut up little more than one half of the cavity, the valves are disposed in pairs exactly opposite to each other, by which means the whole cavity is accurately closed."—(*Cruickshank, Anat. of Absorb. Vessels*, p. 66, 2d edit.)

The distance at which the pairs of valves lie from each other varies exceedingly. The intervals are often equal, and measure an eighth or a sixteenth part of an inch. Yet the interval is, at times, much greater. "I have seen a lymphatic vessel," says Mr. Cruickshank, "run six inches without a single valve appearing in its cavity. Sometimes the trunks are more crowded with valves than the branches, and sometimes I have seen the reverse of this."—(*Loc. citat.*)

In the absorbent system, also, we meet with glands: their form is mostly circular or oval, and somewhat flattened; but we are in the same kind of uncertainty concerning their use, and in some measure concerning their organization, as in respect to those of the secernent system.[*] The vessel that conveys the fluid to one of these glands is called a *vas inferens*, and that which conveys it away a *vas efferens*. The vasa inferentia, or those that enter a gland, are sometimes numerous; they have been detected as amounting to fifteen or twenty: and are sometimes thrice or oftener as many. They are always, however, more numerous than the vasa efferentia, or those which carry on the fluid towards the thoracic duct. The last are consequently, for the most part, of a larger diameter, and sometimes consist of a single vessel alone. It is conceived by many physiologists, that the conglobate mass, which forms the gland, consists of nothing more than convolutions of the vasa inferentia; while others as strenuously contend that they are a congeries of cells, or acini, totally distinct from the absorbent vessels that enter into them. [They are very vascular. Each appears to consist of a soft, fleshy, porous substance, contained in a membranous capsule, the central part being firmer and whiter than the rest. Mercury injected into the vasa inferentia appears to fill a series of cells in an absorbent gland, and then escapes by means of the vasa efferentia. After an injection with wax, the whole substance of the gland seems to consist of convoluted absorbents irregularly dilated, and reciprocally communicating.—(See *Mayo's Outlines of Human Physiology*, p. 213, 2d edit.) The use of the absorbent glands is unknown ; but it would seem that, whatever may be their function, it is most important in young subjects, in whom they are larger and contain a greater proportion of fluid than in more advanced life.]

As in the case of the secernents, we are also unacquainted with the means by which the absorbents act. This, in both instances, is said to be a *vis à tergo*,—a term which gives us little information in either instance, and is peculiarly difficult of comprehension in the latter.* In their most composite state they possess a very low degree of sensibility, and are but little supplied with branches from the larger trunks of nerves.

Abstruse, however, as the process of absorption is to us at present, we have sufficient proofs of the fact. Of six pints of warm water injected into the abdomen of a living dog, not more than four ounces remained at the expiration of six hours. The water accumulated in dropsy of the brain, and deposited in the ventricles, we have every reason to believe, is often absorbed from the cavities ; for the symptoms of the disease have been sometimes marked, and after having made their appearance and been skilfully followed up by remedies, have entirely vanished ; and the water in dropsy of the chest, and even, at times, in ascites, has been as effectually removed.

It has been doubted by some physiologists whether there be any absorbent vessels that open on the surface of the body : yet a multitude of facts seem sufficiently to establish the positive side of this question, though it is not fluids of every kind that can be carried from the skin into the circulating system, and hence their power is by no means universal. Sailors who, when in great thirst, put on shirts wetted with salt water, find considerable relief to this distressing sensation. Dr. Simpson, of St. Andrews', relates the case of a rapid decrease of the water in which the legs of a phrenitic patient were bathed : and De Haen, finding that his dropsical patients filled equally fast, whether they were permitted to drink liquids or not, did not hesitate to assert, that they must absorb from the atmosphere. Spirits, and many volatile irritants, seem to be absorbed more rapidly than water, and there can be no doubt that warmth and friction are two of the means by which the power of absorption is augmented. "A patient of mine," says Mr. Cruickshank, " with a stricture in the œsophagus, received nothing, either solid or liquid, into the stomach for two months : he was exceedingly thirsty, and complained of making no water. I ordered him the warm bath for an hour, morning and evening, for a month : his thirst vanished, and he made water in the same manner as when he used to drink by the mouth, and when the fluid descended readily into the stomach."—(*Anat. of the Absorb. Vessels*, p. 108.) The aliment of nutritive clysters seems in like manner to be often received into the system ; and it is said, though upon more questionable grounds, that cinchona, in decoction, has also been absorbed both from the intestines and the skin.

Narcotic fluids rarely enter to any considerable extent, and never so as to do mischief, respecting which, therefore, the power of the cutaneous absorbents is very limited : and there are few poisonous liquids, with the exception of matter containing the venereal virus, that may not be applied with safety to a sound skin.

[The skin is pointed out by M. Magendie, as an exception to the general law of absorption by veins in all parts of the body. However, if it be deprived of the cuticle, and the bloodvessels of the surface of the cutis be denuded, absorption takes place from it as well as from every other part. After the application of a blister, if the excoriated surface be covered with a substance, the effects of which upon the animal economy are readily recognised, they frequently become very manifest in a few minutes. Arsenic, applied to ulcerated surfaces, has often produced death. In order that the variolous inoculation or vaccination may succeed, every surgeon knows that the virus must be inserted under the cuticle, in contact with the subjacent bloodvessels. But when the cuticle intervenes, unless the substances applied be calculated to attack it chymically, and to irritate the bloodvessels, M. Magendie asserts that no absorption is perceptible. The opinion is quite at variance with the belief, that when the body is immersed in a bath, it absorbs a part of the fluid ; which supposition has led to the occasional employment of nourishing baths of milk, broth, &c.

From a series of very accurate experiments by M. Seguin, it appears that the skin does not ab.

* Dr. S. Cartwright, of Natchez, asserts in his Prize Essay on Absorption, that this power is nothing more nor less than the suction power of the heart extended to the venous radicles, the lymphatics, and the lacteals. All these vessels absorb in consequence of the absorbing or suction power of the heart, into which they ultimately flow. " The veins, lymphatics, and lacteals, all absorb, and their respective fluids receive their motion, not from any hypothetical power resident in the coats of these vessels, whether vital or physical (a power in either case inexplicable and unique in its character), but from the well-known power which results from an inequilibrium or loss of balance in atmospheric pressure. As an effect of this inequilibrium or loss of balance, the heart, the veins, lymphatics, and lacteals, are endowed with a suction power, which enables them to absorb and give motion to the various fluids of every tissue and organ."—See Am. Med. Recorder, vol. xiii., p. 96.—D.

sorb water in which it is immersed. In order to learn whether this was the case with other fluids, he made experiments on persons labouring under venereal complaints. Their feet and legs were kept immersed in baths, composed of sixteen pints of water and three drachms of sublimate, each bath being continued an hour or two, and repeated twice a day. Thirteen patients, subjected to this treatment twenty-eight days, exhibited no signs of absorption. A fourteenth presented manifest indications of it as early as the third bath ; but then he had psoric excoriations on the legs. In two others, similarly circumstanced, the same thing occurred. In general, absorption took place only in subjects whose epidermis was not entirely sound. However, at the temperature of 18° Reaumur, sublimate was sometimes absorbed, but not water. From experiments made with other articles, it was found that the most irritating ones, and those most disposed to combine with the cuticle, were partly absorbed, while others were not so in a perceptible degree. But, according to M. Magendie, what does not happen from simple application, takes place with the assistance of friction. He deems it unquestionable, that mercury, alcohol, opium, camphire, and emetic and purgative medicines, *thus penetrate into the venous system.* They seem to pass through the pores of the cuticle, or the apertures intended for the transmission of hairs, or the insensible perspiration. Besides these experiments, some other very conclusive ones, related by M. Ségalas, leave no doubt that certain poisonous or highly odorous substances, when applied to an internal membranous substance, or to a wound, or rubbed upon the skin, sq as to penetrate the epidermis, *pass directly into the blood, through the coats of the bloodvessels.*]

This double process of secretion and absorption was supposed by the ancients to be performed, not by two distinct sets of vessels expressly formed for the purpose, but by the peculiar construction of the arteries or of the veins, or of both. These are sometimes represented as being porous, and hence, as letting loose contained fluids by transudation, and imbibing extraneous fluids by capillary attraction. There is, in fact, something extremely plausible in this view of the subject, which, in respect to dead animal matter, is allowed to be true, even in our own day. For it is well known that a bladder, filled with blood and suspended in the air, from a cause we shall presently advert to, is readily permeated by oxygen gas, so as to transform the deep Modena hue of the surface of the blood that touches the bladder into a bright scarlet ; and thin fluids, injected into the bloodvessels of a dead body, transude very generally ; insomuch that glue dissolved in water and thrown into the coronary veins, will permeate into the cavity of the pericardium, and, by jellying, even assume its figure. And hence, bile is often found, after death, to pass through the tunics of the gall-bladder, and tinge the transverse arch of the colon, the duodenum, or the pylorus, with a brown, yellow, or green hue, according to its colour at the time.

The doctrine of porosity, or transudation, was hence very generally supported, till the time of Mr. Hewson, by physiologists of the first reputation. Doyle hence speaks, as Mr. Cruickshank has justly observed, of the *porositas animalium,* and wonders that this property should have escaped the attention of Lord Bacon. Even Dr. Hunter and Professor Meckel believed it in respect to certain fluids or certain parts of the body. The experiments of Hewson, J. Hunter, and Cruickshank, have however sufficiently shown that, while vessels, in losing life, lose the property of confining their fluids, they possess this property most accurately so long as the principle of life continues to actuate them.*

There is moreover another method, by which the ancients sometimes accounted for the inhalation and exhalation of fluids, making a much nearer approach to the modern doctrine ; and that is, by the mouths of vessels ; still, however, regarding these vessels as arteries or veins, and particularly the latter. " The soft parts of the body," observes Hippocrates, "attract matter to themselves both from within and from without ; a proof that the whole body exhales and inhales." Upon which passage Galen has the following comment : " For as the veins, by mouths placed in the skin, throw out whatever is redundant of vapour or smoke, so they receive by the same mouths no small quantity from the surrounding air : and this is what Hippocrates means when he says that the whole body exhales and inhales."

This hypothesis of the absorption of veins, without the interference of lymphatics, was revived some years ago by MM. Magendie and Flandrin, of Paris, who made an appeal to experiments which appear highly plausible, and are entitled to a critical examination.

The doctrines hereby attempted to be established are indeed varied in some degree from those of the Greek schools, and are more complex. In few words they may be thus expressed :—that the only general absorbents are the veins—that the lacteals merely absorb the food —that the lymphatics have no absorbent power whatever—and that the villi in the different portions of the intestinal canal are formed in part by venous twigs, which absorb all the fluids in the intestines, with the exception of the chyle, which last is absorbed by the lacteals, and finds its way into the blood through the thoracic duct ; and that these fluids are carried to the heart and lungs directly through the venæ portæ, whose function it is minutely to subdivide and mix with the blood the fluids thus absorbed, which subdivision and intermixture are necessary to prevent their proving detrimental.

M. Magendie further supposes, that the cu-

* Notwithstanding the general accuracy of these observations, the experiments of M. Ségalas prove beyond all doubt, that when certain substances are placed upon the surface of a wound, the excoriated cutis, or an internal membrane in the living body, they find their way directly into the blood through the coats of the bloodvessels.—ED.

tiele has no power of absorption in a sound state, either by veins or lymphatics; but that, if abraded or strongly urged by the pressure of minute substances that enter into its perspirable pores, the subjacent minute veins are thus rendered absorbent.

He supposes the function of the lymphatics to consist in conveying the finer lymph of the blood directly to the heart, as the veins convey the grosser and purple part: and that they rise, as the veins, from terminal arteries.

Proper lymph, in the system of M. Magendie, is that opaline, rose-coloured, sometimes madder-red fluid, which is obtained by puncturing the lymphatics or the thoracic duct, *after a long fast.* It is everywhere similar to itself; and hence differs from the fluid of cavities, which is perpetually varying. He supposes the mistake of confounding the two to proceed from a want of attention to this fact.

One of the chief reasons urged for regarding veins as absorbents is, that membranes which absorb actively have, in his opinion, no demonstrable lymphatics, as the arachnoid. But, according to Bichat, such membranes have no more demonstrable veins than lymphatics; veins are seen to creep on them, but never to enter.

The two principal experiments on which M. Magendie seems to rely in proof that the veins, and not the lymphatics, are absorbents, are the following:—First, M. Delille and himself separated the thigh from the body of a dog, that had been previously rendered insensible by opium. They left the limb attached by nothing but the crural artery and vein. These vessels were isolated by the most cautious dissection to an extent of nearly three inches, and their cellular coat was removed, lest it might conceal some lymphatic vessels. Two grains of the upas tiente were then forcibly thrust into the dog's paw. The effect of this poison was quite as immediate and intense as if the thigh had not been separated from the body: it operated before the fourth minute, and the animal was dead before the tenth. In the second experiment, a small barrel of a quill was introduced into the crural artery, and the vessel fixed upon it by two ligatures. The artery was immediately cut all round between the two ligatures. The same process took place with respect to the crural vein. Yet the poison introduced into the paw produced its effect in the same manner, and as speedily. By compressing the crural vein between the fingers at the moment the action of the poison began to be developed, this action speedily ceased: it reappeared when the vein was left free, and once more ceased on the vein being again compressed.

These experiments are very striking, and, on a cursory view, may be supposed to carry conviction with them; but the confidence of those who have studiously followed the concurrent experiments, and the clear and cautious deductions of our distinguished countrymen, Hewson, both the Hunters, and Cruickshank, supported as they have been by those of Mascagni, and various other able physiologists on the continent,

will not so easily be shaken.[*] Reisseissen has limited his researches to the lungs, but seems to have established the doctrine of a distinct system of absorbents in this organ, by showing that the veins of the lungs do not absorb, and pointing out the occasional cause of error upon this subject.—(*De Fabrica Pulmonum Comm.*, Berolini, 1822.)

We have already observed, that lymphatic absorbents, in the opinion of Mr. Cruickshank, probably in that of all these writers, enter as fully into the tunics of veins and arteries, and even into those of the vasa vasorum, as into any other part of the animal frame: and hence there can be no difficulty in conceiving that the poison, employed in these experiments, might *accompany* the veins by means of their lymphatics. We also observed, that while the lymphatics anastomose or run into each other more frequently than any other set of vessels, their valves, which alone prevent a retrograde course, and direct the contained fluid towards the thoracic duct, are occasionally placed at a considerable distance from each other, in some instances not less than six inches, and that this length of interval occurs in the minute twigs as well as in the trunks. And hence, admitting that, in the veins that were cut or isolated in M. Magendie's experiments, such a vacuity of valves incidentally existed, there is also no difficulty in conceiving by what course the poisons that have already entered into their lymphatics from without should, in consequence of this frequency of anastomosis and destitution of valves, be stimulated to a retrograde course by the violence made use of; and be thrown into the current of the blood from within, by the mouths of those lymphatics that enter into the tunics of the veins; and particularly as the separated vessels were only isolated to a distance of less than three inches, while the lymphatics are occasionally void of valves to double this distance.

In some cases we have reason to believe, that the lymphatics that enter into the tunics of the lacteals, which M. Magendie admits to be a system of absorbents altogether distinct from the veins, are equally destitute of valves in certain parts or directions, and communicate by anastomosis some portion of the chyle and any substance contained in it to the interior of the adjoining veins, and consequently to the blood itself: for the experiments of Sir Everard Home with rhubarb, introduced into the stomach of an animal, after the thoracic duct had been secured by a double ligature, show that this substance, and consequently others as well, is capable of travelling from the stomach into the urinary bladder, notwithstanding this impediment: and there are certain experiments of M. Fohmann (*Anatomische Untersuchungen über den Anastomosis der Lymphatiken mit der Venen,* Heidelberg, 1821), who has paid great attention to the subject, that seem to prove that such anastomosis is not unfrequent. [The researches of Lippi also exhibit a still greater frequency of

* Some observations relating to this statement will be presently introduced.—ED.

communication between the venous and absorbent system. He has demonstrated, that the absorbent vessels in the abdomen communicate freely with the iliac, the spermatic, the renal, the lumbar veins, the vena cava, and with branches of the vena portæ. He has proved, that they communicate as well by opening directly into the great venous trunks, as into the small veins issuing from the conglobate glands, and also by being continuous with the capillary veins. He has also shown, that several absorbent trunks in the belly proceed directly to the pelvis of the kidney, and open into it.—(*Lippi, Illustrazioni Fisiologiche e Patologiche del Sistema Linfatico Chilifero,* Firenze, 1825.) This fact unquestionably tends to corroborate the opinion of Sir Everard Home, that there is a shorter route from the stomach to the bladder, than through the thoracic duct and sanguiferous system. In the singular experiments made with prussiate of potash, by Dr. Wollaston and Dr. Marcet, the blood which was drawn from the arm during the interval of the introduction of this substance into the stomach, and its detection in the urine, did not, on being tested, discover the smallest trace of the prussiate, though it was obvious in the fluid of the urinary bladder. [This is perhaps more explicable by the anatomical facts pointed out by Lippi, than by the conjecture expressed by our author in a former edition, namely, the very diffused state of the prussiate in the entire mass of the blood, and its greater concentration when secreted by the kidneys.]

There is, however, another mode of accounting for the result of M. Magendie's experiments, without abandoning the well-established doctrine of absorption by the lymphatic system. It is a remark which ought never to be lost sight of, that experiments made upon animals in a state either of great pain or of great debility, can give us, by their result, no full proof of the line of conduct pursued by nature in a state of health. In the dead animal body, the valves of the lymphatic vessels very generally lose all elasticity and power of resistance, and transmit fluids in every direction; whence, in all probability, that porosity or transudation which we have already observed as manifest, occasionally, in the stomach and intestines, and in various other organs, on the use of anatomical injections. And hence there can be little doubt, that as an organ makes an approach to the same state of insensibility and irritability, by the severe, if not fatal wounds inflicted on it in the course of such experiments as are here alluded to, the valves of its lymphatic vessels make an approach also to the same state of flaccidity, and allow the fluids, whose course they should resist, to pass in any direction.

The experiments of a like kind, which have, since M. Magendie's communications, been pursued in France by M. Fodere (*Journ. de Physiologie,* Jan., 1823), and in America by Dr. Lawrence and Dr. H. Coates,* are open to the same

* Experiments to determine the Absorbing Power of the Veins and Lymphatics, Philadel. Journ., No. x.

objection. They have been made under circumstances of ebbing vitality or excruciating pain, and a few of them on pieces of animal membrane removed from the parent body. It is admitted candidly, however, by the last two physiologists, that the quill experiment of M. Magendie, in most instances, though not in all, failed in their hands. Even this, however, is in every successful result referred by M. Fohmann to the anastomosing connexion, which he has taken much pains to establish, as existing between various veins and lymphatics, and which we have just adverted to.*.

This altered condition of many parts of the lymphatics in the dead body was sufficiently shown by Mr. Cruickshank, in a course of numerous experiments made at Dr. Hunter's Museum, in the spring of 1773. The organs chiefly injected were the kidney, liver, and lungs of adult human subjects. In one case, he pushed his injection from the artery to the pelvis and ureter without any rupture of the vessels. In another, he injected the pelvis and ureter *from the vein,* which he thought succeeded better than from the artery. In three different kidneys, he injected from the ureter the tubuli uriniferi for a considerable length along the mamillæ; and in one case, a number of the veins on the external surface of the kidneys were evidently filled with the injection. In all these experiments, the colouring matter of the injection was vermilion. In numerous instances, he filled the lymphatics of the lungs and liver with quicksilver; and from the lymphatics of the liver he was able, twice in the adult, and once in the fœtus, to fill the thoracic duct itself.—(*Edin. Med. Com.,* p. 430.)

Dr. Meckel† had already shown the same facts by a similar train of experiments, instituted only a year or two before, and the conclusion he drew from them is in perfect coincidence with the explanation now offered. Dr. Meckel's experiments consisted in injecting mercury with great care, but considerable force, into various lymphatics and minute secreting cavities; and he found that a direct communication took place between such cavities and lymphatics, and the veins in immediate connexion with them: and hence he contended that the lymphatics and the veins are both of them absorbents under particular circumstances; the lymphatics acting ordinarily, and forming the usual channel for carrying off secreted fluids; and the veins acting extraordinarily, and supplying the place of the lymphatics where these are in a state of *morbid torpitude,* or debility, or the cavity is overloaded. He traced this communication particularly in the breasts, in the liver, and in

---

* The ingenious author of the "Study of Medicine" has reasoned in this passage with many strings to his bow. If he adopt Fohmann's explanation, he must evidently give up the conjecture respecting the influence of excruciating pain, and ebbing vitality, in bringing about the results of the experiments in question.—Ed.

† Nova Experimenta et Observationes de finibus venarum et vasorum lymphaticorum in ductus, visceraque excretoria corporis humani, ejusdemque structuræ utilitate, 8vo.

the bladder ; and he thus accounts for the ready passage which bile finds into the blood, when the ductus choledochus is obstructed, as in jaundice; and the urinous fluid, which is often thrown forth from the skin and other organs upon a suppression of the natural secretion.

It follows, therefore, that the experiments of M. Magendie, allowing them to be precisely narrated, are capable of explanation without abruptly overthrowing the established doctrines of preceding physiologists in the same line of pursuit : and we have still ample reason for believing that the economy of absorption is effected by a system of vessels distinct from veins, and, in a state of health, continually holding a balance with the secerning vessels.

[The questions, whether the lymphatics absorb? whether they are the only absorbents of the old particles of the body ? whether the veins are concerned in this or any other branch of the function wholly or in part? and whether the lacteals absorb any other matter but chyle?— all bear so intimately upon many points in pathology and the treatment of disease, that the determination of them in a clear and satisfactory manner is almost, if not quite as desirable, as the settlement of the grand question formerly was about the circulation of the blood.

As having afforded a ground for dissatisfaction with the doctrine that the lymphatics and lacteals were the only absorbents, it may be right to notice the idea entertained by Bichat, Magendie, and some other physiologists, that the capacity of the trunks of the lymphatic system seemed inadequate to the conveyance of the vast quantity of matter that must be absorbed from the various textures and cavities of the body, either in the shape of old particles needing removal in proportion as new ones are deposited, of redundant fluids, of fat, of chyle, &c.—(See Bichat, Anat. Gén., tom. ii., p. 102 ; Magendie, Précis Elém., tom. ii., p. 143.) The opinion tended to raise suspicions of there being some other channels of absorption. As the lymphatics are generally conceived to act upon the matter absorbed at the moment of their imbibing it, and to produce in some inexplicable manner, analogous to the operation of the secerning arteries, certain changes in it, perhaps, much importance cannot be attached to another argument, broached by M. Magendie, namely, that as the lymph is supposed to be taken up by the radicles of the lymphatics from the surfaces of mucous, serous, and synovial membranes, the cellular tissue, the skin, and the parenchyma of every organ, it is presumed to exist in the different cavities of the body. He argues that, though some analogy may seem to exist between the lymph and fluids met with upon serous and other membranes, in the cellular tissue, &c., these fluids readily differ from it, both in their physical and chymical properties. They also differ from each other; so that he conceives that, if this origin of the lymph were to be admitted, various modifications of it would be found ; yet in all parts of the body it appears to be of one description.—(Précis Elém. de Physiol., tom. ii., p. 177.

M. Magendie observes that, before the proofs upon which the common doctrine of absorption by the lymphatics is founded can justly be received as valid, much more requires to be made out than has yet been done. The experiments instituted by Mr. Hunter were designed to prove, first, that the lymphatic vessels are absorbents ; and secondly, that the veins do not absorb. Now, supposing them to be accurate, which M. Magendie endeavours to show is not the case, he argues, that their number is so small, that it is truly astonishing how they should have been deemed sufficient for the subversion of the ancient doctrine. Some strong facts having been already stated in support of the doctrine that the veins absorb, or, at all events, that articles absorbed are partly transmitted into the veins, by anastomoses between these vessels and the lymphatics, we need not enlarge upon this part of the subject. We shall therefore conclude with observing, that any impartial physiologist, who attentively considers the results of the numerous accurate experiments adduced against those of Mr. Hunter, must arrive at the conclusion that the lacteals absorb only chyle, or some of the fluids which happen to be within the alimentary canal when no chyle is present there ; that the mesenteric veins take up other substances; that the small veins in general, and possibly the small arteries, convey a portion of the absorbed matter, by a more direct channel, into the venous system, than that of the thoracic duct ; and that, though the lymphatics are probably absorbents, the source of the lymph in them is yet a questionable point in physiology, and one demanding much more elucidation than it has yet received.* That the experiments of M. Magendie and others have shaken the Hunterian doctrine of absorption, notwithstanding our author's partiality to it, must be candidly acknowledged. The process of absorption, in all its forms, indeed, seems to require more organs than Mr. Hunter has assigned to it, and to be altogether a more complicated function than he has represented it. The greater skill and accuracy, also, with which experimental physiology is now practised, have given the researches of M. Magendie and his colleagues a greater value than those of the immortal physiologist of the preceding century, the glory of his profession and his country. Hence we find, that

---

* M. Magendie observes, nothing affords a more convincing proof of the imperfection of our knowledge of the function of absorption than the ideas of physiologists respecting the lymph. This name is given by some to the serum of the blood ; by others to the fluid in the serous membrane ; by others again, to the serosity of the cellular tissue ; while there are others who consider the fluid which flows from certain scrofulous ulcers as lymph. M. Magendie insists on the propriety of restricting the name of lymph to the liquid contained in the lymphatic vessels and thoracic duct, because, by admitting other significations, a permanence is given to an opinion by no means proved ; viz., that the fluids of the serous membranes and of the cellular tissue, &c. are absorbed by the lymphatic vessels, and transported by them into the venous system.—See Magendie's Elem. Syst. of Physiology, by Milligan, ed. 2, p. 306.—ED.

the opinions of some of the latest writers on physiology are beginning to be materially affected by the facts which have been recently elicited. In proof of this remark, let us merely notice the following passage :—" Of the numerous liquid substances which reach the small intestine, the lacteals appear to absorb chyle only.

"The experiments of Hunter went, indeed, to prove the reverse. When a solution of starch and indigo, or milk and water, was injected by Mr. Hunter into the small intestines of sheep and asses, a bluish or whitish liquid appeared to rise in the lacteals. But there is reason to believe that these observations were not made with sufficient exactness. They have been repeated by M. Flandrin and various physiologists of the present day; and no substance thrown into the bowels, distinguishable by its odour, colour,* or poisonous effects, appeared to enter the lacteals. When Mr. Hunter saw a white fluid rise in the lacteals, after pouring milk into the bowel, we must suppose that some remains of chyle in the small intestine continued to be absorbed; and where the blue liquid was used, the deception probably resulted from the following circumstance. When the lacteals are empty, and are seen against a dusky medium, they appear as blue lines upon the mesentery. I observed this circumstance when repeating the Hunterian experiment upon a rabbit. The lacteals, which, when a solution of starch and indigo was first placed in the cavity of the bowel, were full of chyle, on being examined half an hour afterward, appeared of a clear blue colour; and those present were, for an instant, satisfied that the indigo had been absorbed : but, upon placing a sheet of white paper behind the mesentery, the blue tinge disappeared ; the vessels were seen to be transparent and empty. On removing the white paper, they resumed their blue colour."—(See *Mayo's Outlines of Human Physiology*, p. 223, 2d edit., 8vo., Lond., 1828.) The same writer also believes in the assertion of chyle having been found in the mesenteric veins ; but whether absorbed by these vessels, or poured into them by the lacteals, seems to him not determined. In many places he adverts to the direct termination of lymphatics in the venous system, without the intervention of the thoracic duct. He also considers it proved, that certain poisonous and highly odorous substances, applied to internal membranous surfaces or wounds, or rubbed into the skin, find their way into the blood through the coats of the bloodvessels, as exemplified in the experiments of M. Ségalas. At the same time, he deems it probable that molecular absorption is performed by the lymphatics, as taught by Hunter and others.]

III. In different periods of life, many of the secretions vary considerably in their sensible properties or relative quantity. Thus the bile of the fœtus is sweet, and only acquires a bitter taste after birth. In infancy, perspiration flows more profusely than during manhood : and the testes, which secrete nothing before the age of puberty, at this time acquire activity, and again lose their power in old age.

There are also many of the secernent organs that, in case of necessity, become a substitute for each other. Thus, the perspirable matter of the skin, when suppressed by a sudden chill or any other cause, is often discharged by the kidneys ; the catamenia by the lungs ; and the serum accumulated in dropsies by the intestines.

The secretions are moreover very much affected and increased by any violent commotion of the system generally. In hysteria the flow of urine is greatly augmented, while the absorption of bile seems diminished ; and hence the discharge is nearly colourless. In violent agitation of the mind, the juices of the stomach become more acid than natural ; and sometimes the secernents of the skin, and sometimes those of the larger intestines, are stimulated into increased action ; whence colliquative perspiration, looseness, or both. The heat and commotion of a fever will sometimes produce the same effect, and sometimes a contrary ; the skin being dry, parched, and pricking. And occasionally, the dryness has been so considerable as to produce a sudden separation of the cuticle from the cutis ; of which Mr. Gooch relates a singular instance in a patient, who for several years had once or twice a year an attack of fever, accompanied with a peculiar itching of the skin, and particularly of the hands and wrists, that ended in a total separation of the cuticle from these parts : insomuch that it could easily be turned off from the wrist down to the fingers' ends, so as to form a kind of cuticular glove.—(*Medical and Chirurgical Observations*, 8vo.) The same distinguished writer gives as singular an instance of the effects of solar heat upon the skin of another patient, who had no sooner exposed himself to the direct rays of the sun, than his skin began to be affected with a sense of tickling, became violently hot, as stiff as leather, and as red as vermilion.—(*Op. citat.*) In this case we have an instance of highly excited action in the cutaneous excernents of both kinds, and of the formation of new bloodvessels under the cuticle, followed by a conversion of the cutaneous integument into a coriaceous substance.

There are some parts of the body that waste and become renewed far more rapidly than others ; the fat than the muscles ; the muscles than the bones ; and probably the bones than the skin ; for the die of the madder-root, with which the bones become coloured when this root has for some time formed a part of the daily food of an animal, is carried off far sooner than the coloured lines of charcoal-powder, ashes, soot, and the juices of various plants, when introduced into the substance of the skin by puncturing or tattooing it, a practice common among our sailors, and still more so, and carried to a far greater degree of perfection, among the inhabitants of the South Sea Islands.

* "Chyle never takes the hue of the colouring substances mixed with the food. M. Hallé proved the contrary by direct experiments, which I have lately repeated, and with exactly the same results. Animals which I made eat indigo, saffron, and madder, yielded a chyle whose colour was not at all influenced by those substances."—*Précis Elem. de Physiol.*, tom. ii., par F. Magendie.—Ed.

It has been said, indeed (*Bernouilli, Diss. de Nutritione*, Groning., 1669, 4to.), that the disappearance of madder-colour from the bones, affords no proof that the phosphate of lime, in which it was seated, has itself been carried off at the same time ; because the serum of the blood is found to have a stronger affinity for madder than the phosphate coloured by it ; and hence will gradually attract and remove it, when the animal is no longer fed with the coloured food. The experiment, however, upon which this latter opinion is grounded, has not been hitherto conducted in such a manner as to be directly applicable to the question ; and if it had been, it would afford no proof that a perpetual, though, in that case, a slower change than the madder would exhibit, is not taking place in the bones : nor are we driven to the effects of madder die upon their solid substance as the only foundation for this opinion ; for there is scarcely a bone in the animal system which does not assume a different shape at one period of life compared with its form at another period : a remark that peculiarly applies to the flat bones of the skeleton, and forms the chief cause of that wonderful change which the lower jaw experiences as the individual advances from middle life to old age, and which often gives a different character to the entire face.—(*Gibson, Manchester Memoirs*, vol. i., p. 533.)

It is from this mysterious power of reproduction appertaining to every part of the system, that we are so often able to renew the substance and function of parts that have been wasted by fevers or atrophy, or abruptly destroyed or lopped off by accident.

In the progress of this general economy, every organ and part of the body secretes for itself the nutriment it requires, from the common pabulum of the blood which is conveyed to it, or from secretions which have already been obtained from the blood, and deposited in surrounding cavities, as fat, gelatin, and lymph. And it is probable that the several organs of secretion, like the eye, the ear, and the other distinct organs of sense, are peculiarly affected by peculiar stimulants, and excited to some diversity of sensation.

In Germany, this idea has been pursued so far as, in some hypotheses, and particularly that of M. Hubner (*Comment. de Cœnesthesi*, 1794), to lay a foundation for the doctrine of a sixth sense, to which, as we observed on a former occasion (vol. ii., p. 151, *Physiol. Proem*), has been given the name of *selbstgefühl* or *gemeingefühl*, "self-feeling," or "general feeling." The sensations, however, we are at present alluding to, are not so much general, or those of the whole self, as particular, or limited to the organs in which they originate ; and seem to be a result of different modifications of the nervous influence on which the common sense of touch depends. In most parts of the system these modifications are so inconsiderable as to elude our notice ; but in others we have the fullest proof of such an effect ; for we see the stomach evincing a sense of hunger, the fauces of thirst, the genital organs of venereal orgasm. And in like manner, we find the bladder stimulated by can-

tharides, and the intestinal canal by purgatives ; and we may hence conjecture, that every other part of the system, where any kind of secretion is going forwards, is endowed with a like peculiarity of irritability and sensibility, though not sufficiently keen to attract our attention.

It is hence we meet with that surprising variety of secretions which are furnished, not only by different animals, but even by the same animal in different parts of the body. Hence sugar is secreted by the stomach, and sometimes by the kidneys ; sulphur by the brain ; wax by the ears ; lime by the salivary glands, the secretories of the bones, and, in a state of disease, by the lungs, the kidneys, the arteries, and the exhalants of the skin ; milk by the breasts ; semen by the testes ; the menstrual fluid by the uterus ; urine by the kidneys ; bile by the liver ; muriate of scda by the secernents of almost every organ ; and sweat from every part of the surface.[*]

Hence some animals, as the bee, secrete honey ; others, as the *coccus ilicis*, a large store of wax ; others, as the viper and scorpion, gum, which is the vehicle of their poison ; others thread, as the spider and some species of slug ; and many silk, as the silkworm and the pinna, or nacre, whence Reaumur denominates the pinna the sea- silkworm : it is common to some of the Italian coasts, and its silky beard or byssus is worked at Palermo into very beautiful silk stuffs. There are great numbers of worms, insects, and fishes, that secrete a very pure, and some of them a very strong, phosphorescent light, so as in some regions to enkindle the sea, and in others the sky, into a bright blaze at night. Many animals secrete air ; man himself seems to do so under certain circumstances, but fishes of various kinds more largely, as those furnished with air-bladders, which they fill or exhaust at pleasure, and the sepia, or cuttlefish,

---

[*] No doubt, in the process of glandular secretion, chymical phenomena take place. Several of the secretions are acid, while the blood is alkaline ; and most of them contain proximate principles, which do not exist in the blood, and must be formed in the glands themselves ; but the particular way in which these combinations are effected is unknown. A curious experiment, performed by Wollaston, led him to infer, that a very weak electricity is concerned in the regulation of secretion, and has a marked influence over it. He took a glass tube, two inches long and three quarters of an inch in diameter, and he closed one of its extremities with a bit of bladder. He poured a little water into the tube, with 1-240 part of its weight of muriate of soda ; he wet the bladder on the outside, and placed it on a piece of silver ; he then bent a zinc wire, so that one of its ends touched the silver, and the other entered the tube for about an inch. In the same instant, the external surface of the bladder gave indications of the presence of pure soda ; so that, under the influence of this weak electricity, there was a decomposition of muriate of soda, and the soda, separated from the acid, passed through the bladder. Wollaston thought it not impossible that something analogous might happen in the process of secretion ; but, as M. Magendie justly observes, before this idea can be adopted, more proof of its correctness is required.—ED.

with numerous other seaworms ; and by this power they raise or sink themselves, as they have occasion. The cuttlefish secretes also a natural ink, which it evacuates when pursued by an enemy, and thus converts it into an instrument of defence ; for, by blackening the water all around, it obtains a sufficient concealment, and easily effects its escape. Other animals, and these also chiefly fishes, secrete a very large portion of electric matter, so as to convert their bodies into a powerful battery. The torpedo-ray was well known by the Romans to possess this extraordinary power ; and the *gymnotus electricus* (electric eel) has since been discovered to possess it in a much larger proportion. The genus tetradon, in one species, secretes an electric fluid ; in another, an irritating fluid that stings the hand that touches it ; and in a third, a poisonous matter diffused through the whole of its flesh.

From the same cause we meet with as great and innumerable a variety of secretions among plants, as camphires, gums, balsams, resins : and, as in animals, we often meet with very different secretions in very different parts of the same plant. Thus, the *mimosa nilotica* secerns from its root a fluid as offensive as that of asafœtida ; in the sap of its stem an astringent acid ; its glands give forth gumarabic ; and its flower an odour of a very grateful fragrance : while the MILK-TREE or COW-TREE, the *arbol di lache*, or *palo de vaca*, of South America, overflows with nutritious milk from every part, This is one of the many singular plants noticed by M. Humboldt, in his voyage to the equinoctial regions. It is a native of Venezuela, and belongs to the natural family of the sapotæ ; and its juice, in strict correspondence with its name, is said to possess almost all the properties of cow's milk. M. Humboldt visited the district where it was reported to grow, and found the account true ; but tells us that it is rather more viscous than cow's milk, and has a slight balsamic taste. He drank it plentifully in the evening and early in the morning without any unpleasant effects ; and was told that, when in season, the working people use it with their cassava bread, and always fatten upon it.—(*Annales de Chimie et de Physique*, Juin, 1823, tom. xxiii., p. 19.)

This subject is highly interesting, and might be extended to volumes, but we are already digressing too far. There is no part of the body in which the process of secretion is not going forward ; we trace it, and consequently the fabric which gives rise to it, in the parenchyma, or intermediate substance of organs, in their internal surfaces and outlets, and on the external surface of the entire frame : thus forming three divisions of prominent distinction, both in respect to locality and to the diseases which relate to them. It is on these divisions that the Orders of the present Class are founded.

ORDER I.

MESOTICA.

DISEASES AFFECTING THE PAREN-
CHYMA.

GRAVITY IN THE QUANTITY OR QUALITY OF THE INTERMEDIATE OR CONNECTING SUBSTANCE OF ORGANS ; WITHOUT INFLAMMATION, FEVER, OR OTHER DERANGEMENT OF THE GENERAL HEALTH.

THE classic term ECCRITICA is a derivative from ἐκκρίνω, "secerno," "exhaurio," "to secern or strain off," "to drain or exhaust," and is preferred by the author to any other derivative which κρίνω, its primitive, affords, as equally applicable to the two systems of vessels that enter into the general and important economy illustrated in the preceding Proem. The ordinal term MESOTICA is derived from μέσος, "medius ;" for which PARENCHYMATICA might have been substituted, but that there are two objections to the use of the latter : the first is, that παρὰ is here employed in a different sense from its general signification in the system before us, which is that of "malè," or "perperàm," instead of *per* or *penitus*, its real meaning in parenchyma ; and, consequently, the double signification would trench upon that simplicity and uniformity which it is the direct object of the present nomenclature to maintain. The second objection is, that the term parenchyma (παρίγχυμα) is formed upon a false hypothesis, invented by Erasistratus, who first employed the term, and held that the common mass, or interior substance of a viscus, is produced by concreted blood, strained off through the pores of the bloodvessels which enter into its general structure or membranes.

The order embraces the five following genera :—

I. Polysarcia. Corpulency.
II. Emphyma. Tumour.
III. Parostia. Mis-ossification.
IV. Cyrtosis. Contortion of the Bones.
V. Osthexia. Osthexy.

GENUS I.

POLYSARCIA.

CORPULENCY.

FIRM AND UNWIELDY BULKINESS OF THE BODY OR ITS MEMBERS, FROM AN ENLARGEMENT OF NATURAL PARTS.

POLYSARCIA, from πολύσαρκος, "carnosus," "carne abundans," imports bulkiness from any morbid increase of natural parts, whether fleshy or adipose ; and the present genus is co-extensive with this latitude of interpretation. In medical history, however, we know of no morbid increase of this kind, otherwise than local, except from an accumulation of fat ; and, on this account, Dr. Swediaur has somewhat unnecessarily substituted the name of polypiotes (*Nov. Nosol. Meth. Syst.*, vol. ii., p. 121) for that of polysarcia.

The only organ I know of that evinces any very remarkable increase of natural growth, besides those that secrete animal oil, is the female breast ; for, though we meet with something of the kind occasionally in the scrotum, and especially of négroes, and sometimes in the labia of women in intertropical regions, these* are usually the result of adventitious or foreign matter, tending to suppuration, or some other division of continuity, rather than to a simple but unwieldy enlargement of the natural parenchyma of the organ, not leading to any issue. We may, therefore, contemplate the genus before us under the two following species :—

1. Polysarcia Mammæ.　Pendulous Breasts.
2. ———— Adiposa.　Obesity.

SPECIES I.

POLYSARCIA MAMMÆ.

PENDULOUS BREAST.

BREAST PENDULOUS AND UNWIELDY FROM IN-
CREASE OF ˉNATURAL GROWTH ; WITH OR
WITHOUT PAIN ; HUE PURPLISH.

THIS species is chiefly introduced upon the authority of Sir Astley Cooper, and the description of it I shall give in his own words.

" These glands sometimes grow to an enormous magnitude, about the age of twenty years, so as to hang down upon the abdomen, not from relaxation, but from real increase. I saw a case of this kind in a young woman, aged twenty-three, which began three years prior to my seeing her : tender to the touch, of a dark red colour. She was often costive, but regular in her menstruation." And to this he adds the following case, which was seen by Dr. Babington as well as himself :—"Miss L——, aged seventeen, of a light complexion and delicate constitution, has a remarkable enlargement of her breast. The left is twenty inches from its junction with the chest above to its lower part, and its circumference measures twenty-three inches. The nipple is flattened, the areola excessively expanded. The breast feels as if every lobe of the gland was increased to several times its usual magnitude." The same eminent writer adds, " that the treatment consists in supporting the breasts with a suspensory bandage, in which each of them is to be placed, and which is to be carried over the shoulders." He recommends an occasional use of the hydrargyrum cum cretâ, with rhubarb and subcarbonate of soda.—(*Lectures on the Principles and Practice of Surgery*, vol. ii., p. 218, 8vo., 1825.)†

---

* From the history given of these diseases in the Dictionary of Practical Surgery, the editor believes that p. scroti and p. labii pudendorum, would very properly have constituted here two other species. They have, in fact, no great tendency to suppuration and ulceration ; and even if they had, it might not be a good reason for their exclusion.

† In Hufeland's Journal (part viii., p. 12), a case is described in which the breast hung down to the knees, and measured three feet and three inches in length.—D.

VOL. II.—L l

SPECIES II.

POLYSARCIA ADIPOSA.

OBESITY.

BULKINESS FROM A SUPERABUNDANT ACCUMULA-
TION OF FAT.

THIS species admits of two varieties. For it may be

a Generalis.　　Extending over the body and
General obesity.　limbs.
β Splanchnica.　Confined to the organs or in-
Splanchnic obes-　teguments of the trunk.
ity.

In man and other animals, fat is collected in the follicles of the adipose cellular membrane. When the perspiration becomes profuse in consequence of hard walking or other exercise, a certain portion of animal oil is dissolved in this fluid, which makes the chief, perhaps the only difference, between the matter of perspiration and that of sweat. Fat is hence accumulated by diminished perspiration ; as it is also by the nature of the aliments fed on, and from idiosyncrasy. It is the basis of steatomatous tumours, and contains the sebacic acid, which acts readily on many metals, as lead, copper, and iron. [Many highly important and interesting observations were made on the fat by the celebrated Bichat.—(*Anatomie Gén.*, tom. i., p. 96, &c.) He has pointed out, that while fat is very abundant under the skin, around serous surfaces, and several organs performing extensive motion, there is none of it in the penis, prepuce, scrotum, nor under mucous surfaces, and round arteries, veins, &c. Between the arterial and venous coats, none prevails. Lymphatic glands do not contain it. The brain and spinal marrow are destitute of it. In the interspaces of the nervous fibres, some of it is always found : most frequently it is not very obvious there, but on desiccation, an oily exudation constantly oozes from these fibres, manifestly consisting of fat. Among the muscular fibres it is generally rather plentiful, especially in those of animal life ; for, in those of organic life, very little of it is found. In the bones, where there is none of it, the medullary juice is a substitute for it ; cartilages, fibrous bodies, and fibro-cartilages, are quite free from it. The glandular system sometimes contains it, as is seen in the parotids and round the pelvis of the kidney ; while in other examples, as those of the liver, prostate gland, &c., not the least vestige of it can be traced. The serous and cutaneous systems are never fatty, though they are contiguous to a large quantity of fat. The same is the case with the mucous system : and the fat never has any connexion with the epidermis and hair.

After this cursory view, it appears that the interior of the organic system generally contains very little fat ; and between the different parts of the apparatus themselves there is only a small proportion of it. Thus, between the coats of the stomach, intestines, bladder, &c., between the periosteum and bone, between this and cartilage, between muscle and tendon, there is hardly any adipose matter.

It follows, from this account, that it is chiefly

in the interspaces which the different appara-tuses leave between them, that the fat accumu-lates, and has its cellular reservoirs. Now, when it is examined under this point of view in different regions, it is found, 1. That in the examination of the head, the cranium and face present quite a contrary disposition, the fat being very abundant in the second part, but quite de-ficient in the first, especially in its interior. 2. That the neck contains a very large proportion of it. 3. That in the chest, very little of it is found about the lungs, but a great deal around the heart : that on the outside of this cavity, a considerable mass is found at its upper parts around the breasts. 4. That in the abdomen it abounds, particularly at its posterior part, in the vicinity of the kidney, in the mesentery, and in the omentum. 5. That in the pelvis, its pro-portion is great near the bladder and rectum. 6. That, in the limbs, like the cellular tissue, it is most abundant, as these parts are examined upwards, and about their large articulations.

In the child, the quantity of fat is observed to be proportionally a great deal more consider-able under the skin than anywhere else, espe-cially than in the abdomen, the cellular viscera of which, the omentum in particular, contain at this age none of it. Merely a few flakes of fat are sometimes met with round the kidney, and frequently even they are hardly perceptible. All the rest of the abdominal cavity is destitute of it. The cavity of the thorax scarcely contains more, and always much less in proportion than afterward. Bichat also remarked, that the inter-muscular tissue is almost everywhere without it. One would say, that all the fat is then con-centrated under the skin, at least while the fœtus is healthy.

Towards the adult age, the abdominal fat is proportionally much more considerable than the subcutaneous. An outward plumpness is as unusual about the age of forty, as it is common at that of four or five, the period when, all mus-cular shape being hidden by the superabundance of fat, the body is manifestly rounded.

In old age, nearly all the fat disappears ; and the body wrinkles, grows indurated and lank. In the parts which nature has deprived of fat, the presence of this substance would not have been capable of adapting itself to their func-tions. If the size of the penis had been in-creased by it, this organ would no longer have been adapted to the vagina. The fatty eyelid could not have been opened without difficulty. If it had been introduced into the submucous tissue, it would have lessened the cavity of or-gans lined by mucous surfaces. If it had been diffused in that which surrounds arteries, veins, and excretory vessels, it would equally have ob-structed the calibre of such vessels. Had it been collected in the cerebral cavity, it would have compressed the brain, on account of the resistance of the bony parietes of the scull, &c., which do not yield, like those of the abdomen, when the gastric viscera are loaded with fat. In the thorax, the diaphragm may descend, and besides, the lungs can, without danger, take up less space, when much fat accumulates in the mediastinum. This remark, which is also ap-plicable to the serosity, explains an important phenomenon in diseases ; viz., that a very small quantity of fluid extravasated on the arachnoid coat, is enough to disturb the functions of the brain, while a copious extravasation in the ab-domen or chest, is without actual danger.— (See *Bichat, Anat. Gén.*, tom. i., p. 105.)]

- The grand repository of fat is the cellular texture ; but it is not lodged in the cells of this texture indiscriminately, but in those of a par-ticular kind, and which do not, according to Dr. W. Hunter, communicate with each other, as those which contain air in emphysema or wa-ter in anasarca : in consequence of which, this celebrated physiologist has distinguished the former by the name of adipose, and the latter by that of reticulated, cells.

[That the adipose cells are completely closed, that they do not communicate, as Bichat sup-posed (Ibid., p. 108), and that they differ from those of common cellular membrane in not being pervaded by fluids attempted to be thrown into them, are facts proved, as Professor Béclard (*Bé-clard, Additions à l'Anat. Gén. de Xav. Bichat*, p. 15, 8vo., Paris, 1821) has explained, by va-rious considerations. If we take a portion of adipose membrane, and expose it to a degree of heat sufficient to melt the fat, without injur-ing the structure of the cells, the oily matter will remain in them, and not run out. If a lob-ule of fat be exposed to the rays of the sun, so as to convert the fat into the fluid state, not a particle of it will flow out ; but, if an incision be made into some of the vesicles, the oily li-quid will immediately run out. The same result is obtained when a portion of fat is pressed be-tween the fingers ; the fat does not escape till the vesicles are torn. In the most extensive emphysema, the most considerable anasarca, the effused air, or fluid, never penetrates the adipose vesicles ; the fat continues by itself, quite un-mixed. If this were not the case, would not the fat, when rendered fluid by the ordinary tem-perature of the body during life, constantly gravitate to the lowest situations, and be forced by pressure from one place to another, as hap-pens with respect to the fluid in dropsical per-sons ? In fact, the adipose vessels do not form, like the common cellular substance, a continu-ous whole, but are only contiguous to each oth-er. Another difference is, that the cellular sub-stance exists everywhere, while the adipose membrane is constantly absent from certain parts of the body, even in the fattest individuals. This fact amounts to a proof, that the cellular tissue requires a peculiar organization, without which the fat cannot collect in it. The uses of the cellular and adipose textures are also very dif-ferent. Those of the latter only relate to the fat, which is incessantly secreted into the vesicles, and absorbed from them again ; but the cellular substance forms a common bond of connexion between all the parts, at the same time that it keeps them distinct, facilitates their motions, and maintains the harmony of their functions.]

In many fishes, as the salmon and herring, fat is diffused over the whole body, as though the body were steeped in it. In other genera of fishes, as the ray, it is found in the liver alone. In some few, as the whale, it appears in the form of flakes, and is called blubber, which sometimes amounts to the enormous quantity of three tons in an individual.

[In the dead subject, the fat is almost always solid and congealed; but, in the living, it approaches more to the state of a liquid, at least in certain parts, as about the heart, large vessels, &c. Under the skin, its consistence is always greater. In many experiments, in which Bichat had occasion to open living animals of red warm blood, he never found the fat running, as in the melted state. No doubt, a degree of caloric, equal to our temperature, acting upon the fat out of our bodies, will render it much more fluid than it is in the living subject. While the temperature is also nearly uniform, the degrees of the consistence of the fat vary singularly. There is a striking difference between that of the omentum, which is one of the most fluid in the economy, and that around the kidneys and near the skin, which is much firmer. Many animals of red cold blood have the fat liquid.

In young animals the fat is whitish, and after death exhibits a good deal of consistence. This consistence gives a remarkable firmness and a sort of condensation to the external covering of the human fœtus, while, in the adult, the skin of the dead body, being flaccid and loose, yields to the least impulse communicated to it, in consequence of the state of the subcutaneous fat. In the fœtus, this fat collects in small more or less round globules, giving to the mass of it a granulated appearance. Frequently, there are even very considerable accumulations of it: for example, at this period, there is almost always between the buccinator, the masseter, and the integuments, a sort of ball of fat, making a body quite distinct from the surrounding fat, and which is extracted entire. It contributes very much to the remarkable prominence which the cheeks make at this period of life.

In proportion as we advance in years, the fat grows yellow, and assumes a particular smell and taste. By comparing that of veal with beef, the difference may be readily conceived; and, in the theatres of anatomy, the difference is not less striking between a subject ten years old, and another of sixty.—(Bichat, Anat. Gén., tom. i., p. 182.)]

We are not to conclude with Béclard, however, that fat is only intended for one purpose. It is a bad conductor of heat; and hence, one of its uses is that of keeping the body warm : on which account, those who are encumbered with fat perspire with but a small quantity of exercise, and are almost always too hot. We may hence also see why the warmth of the body is retained by oiling the surface, or wearing oiled skin over it. Fat is supposed, but with little reason, to be of use in lubricating the solids, facilitating their movements, and preventing excessive sensibility. By equally distending the skin, it certainly contributes, where not in excess, to the beauty of the person. In cases of

extreme hunger, or of abstinence from food, fat is reabsorbed, and carried to the bloodvessels; and, from an experiment of Dr. Stark,* it appears to be more capable of supplying the waste of the body than any sort of ordinary food. And hence, there is much probability in the conjecture of Lyonet, that insects, destitute of food, derive their chief nourishment from the fat in which they abound.—(Anat. de la Chenille qui ronge le Bois de Saule, pp. 428, 482, et seq.)

With the exception, however, of the earth of the bones, it is the least animalized of all the substances that enter into the composition of the animal frame. Chymically examined, pure fat contains no azote, which is the peculiar characteristic of animalization; it has also little oxygen, consisting chiefly, indeed, of hydrogen and carbon. "I do not consider," says Mr. John Hunter, "either the fat or the earth of bones, as a part of the animal : they are not animal matter : they have no action within themselves : they have not the principle of life." (On Blood, p. 440.) It is of late formation in the fœtus, scarcely any trace of its existence being discoverable before the fifth month from conception.

The mode of its production is still a matter of controversy. By some it has been supposed to be secreted by peculiar glands, by others merely to transude from exhalant arteries of a peculiar kind. Sir Everard Home has lately started another hypothesis, which is at least highly ingenious, and plausibly supported. He has attempted to prove, that the fat of animals is produced in the larger intestines (especially the colon), out of the recrement of the food and the bile, and afterward conveyed into the system generally by channels yet undiscovered, to contribute towards the common growth of the system, especially in early life.† And some arguments in favour of this opinion may be drawn from the nature of that species of ENTEROLI-THUS, to which in the present system is given the name of scybalum, and from the observations with which it has been illustrated.

Sauvages was desirous of establishing a standard weight of healthy pinguescence; but the attempt is idle, since it varies in almost every individual. The fat of the human frame usually averages about a twentieth part of the whole, but has sometimes amounted to half, or even to four fifths.—(J. P. Frank, de Cur. Morb. Hom. Epit., tom. vi., 8vo., 1821.)

In general obesity, or the variety of adipose

* Hewson, ii., p. 151. The hump of the camel appears to form a sort of reserve, through which, the Arabs say, he is nourished during his long journeys. In a period of plenty, the rapid secretion of fat converts it into a pyramid, equalling a fourth of the animal's entire bulk; but a peregrination through the desert gradually lowers it, so that it becomes scarcely visible. The camel then sinks, and can travel no further till the store is replenished by rest and food.—See Burckhardt's Notes on the Bedouins and Wahabys, 4to., Lond., 1830.—Ed.

† Phil. Trans. for 1813, p. 158, and 1816, p. 301. The subject further pursued in Phil. Trans., 1821, p. 36.

polysarcia immediately before us, the bulk of the body has sometimes been enormous. It has amounted to five hundred, and nearly six hundred pounds, in many instances. Bright, of Maldon, weighed seven hundred and twenty-eight pounds; Lambert, of Leicester, seven hundred and thirty-nine pounds a little before his death, which was in the fortieth year of his age.* The German journals give us examples of men who weighed eight hundred pounds. Yet the Philosophical Transactions furnish perhaps a still more extraordinary example of this disease in a girl, that weighed two hundred and fifty-six pounds, though only four years old.—(N. 185.)†

Where a powerful adipose diathesis prevails, fat is often produced, whatever be the food fed upon. Ale and porter, drunk to excess, are perhaps the most ordinary means; Ackermann gives proofs of the same effect from spirits (*Baldinger*, N. Mag., b. vi., p. 489); and in the Ephemera of Natural Curiosities is the case of an individual, who generated fat faster and in larger quantities upon bread, than upon a meat diet.—(Dec. iii., ann. vii., viii., p. 138.) In every instance, however, indolence and indulgence in sleep seem necessary.

In these cases, the animal oil is sometimes secreted and deposited in the cellular membrane almost as rapidly as water in anasarca; on which account, obesity has by writers been called, and correctly enough, a dropsy of fat. It is, in fact, under particular circumstances, the soonest formed and deposited, and the soonest absorbed, of all the animal secretions.

[Considerable accumulations of fat sometimes appear to take place, as the sudden effect of the influence of the atmosphere. Thus, in the short space of twenty-four hours, a mist will occasionally fatten thrushes, robin-redbreasts, ortolans, &c., in such a degree, that they can hardly get out of the way of the sportsman's gun. This occurrence, which is common in autumn, is not in any case so striking in man.—(*Bichat, Anatomie Gén.*, tom. i., p. 100.)]

For its formation, however, ease of body and mind is indispensable, and perhaps a slight increase of sensorial power beyond the common standard of what has hitherto been the standard of the individual. Hence, those are apt to become fat who suddenly relinquish a habit of hard exercise, either of body or mind, for a life of quiet enjoyment, provided the change be not sufficient to interfere with the general health. And for the same reason, as we have already observed, animals which are castrated, and females that do not breed, or who have just ceased

to breed, grow fat and corpulent with equal ease, the sensorial power intended for the use of the sexual organs, and to be expended at a particular outlet, being hereby thrown back upon the system generally, and transferred to the adipose secernents. And hence, also, the cause of that increase of bulk which most persons experience about the middle of life, when, the muscles having attained their utmost firmness, the stature its full height, and the sexual economy its perfection, there is a less demand for the ordinary supply of sensorial power than has hitherto been made, and the surplus is expended in broadening and rounding the general frame, by filling up the cells of the adipose membrane with animal oil, instead of elongating it.

For all this, however, there must be an ease of body and mind approaching to cheerfulness; on which account plumpness and cheerfulness, or good-humour, are commonly associated in our ideas: for pain and anxiety, that wear away the corporeal substance, generally make their first inroad on the animal oil, and empty the cells of the adipose membrane, before they produce any manifest effect on the muscular fibres, or, as these are collectively termed, the flesh: upon which subject we have already touched in discussing several of the species of the genus MARASMUS.—(Class III., Ord. IV., Gen. III., opening remarks.)

Hence the fat becomes absorbed or carried off, as it is secerned and deposited, more readily than any other animal substance. By sweating, horse-riding, and a spare diet, a Newmarket jockey has not unfrequently reduced himself a stone and a half in a week or ten days (*Code of Health, by Sir John Sinclair*, &c.): and a plump widow has, by weeping, become a skeleton in a month or two.

A moderate increase in the secretion of animal oil rather adds to the facility of motion, and improves the beauty of the person. But if it much exceed this, the play of these different organs upon each other is impeded, the calibre of the bloodvessels is constricted, the pulse oppressed, the breathing laborious, there is an accumulation of blood in the head or heart, a general tendency to palpitation or drowsiness, and a perpetual danger of apoplexy.

[According to Bichat (*Anatomie Gén.*, tom. i., p 98), a considerable embonpoint, far from being a sign of health, almost always denotes weakness of the absorbents intended to take up the fat again, and that, in this respect, it has more analogy with serous infiltrations than is commonly supposed. This assertion is proved by various facts. 1. Every kind of extraordinary embonpoint is attended with a weakness of muscular force, and a state of languor and inertia, in the individual who is the subject of it. 2. In the man, in whom force and vigour predominate, that fatty plumpness which hides the muscular prominences is not seen: the latter are strongly marked. In this respect, the bulk of the body arising from distention by the cellular fat, must be carefully discriminated from that which is produced by the development and fully expressed nutrition of organs. 3. Frequently,

---

* The London butcher, Falstaff, died in his thirty-second year, and his weight was eight hundred pounds. Many histories of preternatural obesity may be seen in a book entitled, " Cursory Remarks on Corpulence, or Obesity, considered as a Disease, &c., by William Wadd, Surgeon," London, 1816, p. 97.—D.

† Dr. M'Naughton, of Albany, has published the particulars of two instructive cases of obesity, arising in two young children of the same family, who at a very early period evinced this tendency to inordinate growth.—D.

the causes which obviously weaken the powers of life, produce a considerable accumulation of fat : such are sloth, rest, copious hemorrhages, the convalescence of certain acute diseases, where the forces 'yet languish while the fat abounds. 4. The fatty state of the muscles is for them a palpable state of debility. 5. Bichat was sometimes convinced, from examining certain emaciated limbs, that the little size which they retain is partly owing to the fat which they contain, and which in proportion is nearly equal to what the healthy limbs contain, while all the other parts are shrunk, the muscles in particular. 6. Castration, which extracts from the vital powers a part of their activity, from nutrition a part of its energy, is very frequently (as already remarked) followed by an excessive degree of obesity. 7. On the other hand, as a certain degree of development in the vital powers is requisite for generation, individuals who are too fat, and in whom that degree is deficient, are generally badly qualified for this function. In women, this fact is remarkable ; and it is not less so in man. In animals, the same thing is observed. In proportion as hens are fattened for our tables, they become less and less suited for laying. Most domestic animals are subject to the same law. One would say that there is a constant and rigorous connexion between the secretion of semen and the exhalation of fat, these two fluids being in the inverse ratio to each other.

From the facts above specified, Bichat infers, that if the moderate deposition of fat indicate strength, its redundance is almost always a sign of weakness, and that, in this respect, there is a kind of connexion between fatty and serous infiltrations. It is to be remarked, however, that leucophlegmasiæ almost always proceed from an organic defect in some viscus or another, particularly the heart, the lungs, the liver, the uterus, and spleen : hence it follows, that they scarcely admit of dispersion, and that death, brought on not by them, but by the organic disease itself, is commonly their termination. On the contrary, such an organic disease rarely accompanies a redundance of fat, which may be consistent with a long life.]

In SPLANCHNIC OBESITY, the encumbered viscera are more or less buried in beds of fat, and usually accompanied with scirrhous affections ; making an approach to some species or other of PARABYSMA, as described in the first Class and second Order of the present system. We have observed, that general obesity may be regarded as a dropsy of animal oil, instead of a dropsy of water. And as the latter disease is sometimes universal, and runs through the whole of the cellular substance, and at others local, and confined to particular cavities, the former also exhibits both these modifications ; and, in the variety before us, is confined to individual organs.*

* Of all the abdominal viscera, the omentum is the most liable to become the seat of a prodigious accumulation of fat. When protruded from the abdomen, and forming the species of hernia termed

It most generally overloads the omentum, and gives that projecting rotundity to the abdomen which is vulgarly distinguished by the name of POT-BELLY, and is well described by Prince Henry, in his address to Falstaff, as " a huge hill of flesh" (*Henry IV.*, part i., act ii.)—" a globe of sinful continents."—(Ibid., part ii., act ii.)*

In attempting a cure of the general disease, the first step is to avoid all the common and more obvious causes as much as possible. Hence, as a life of indolence, and indulgence in eating and drinking, are highly contributory to obesity, the remedial treatment should consist in the use of severe, regular, and habitual exercise, a hard bed, little sleep, and dry and scanty food, derived from vegetables alone, except where, from a singularity of constitution, farinaceous food is found to be a chief source of obesity. And when these are insufficient, we may have recourse to frequent venesection and such medicines as freely evacuate the fluids, whether by the bowels or the skin. And for the same reason, sialagogues, as chewed tobacco (*Borelli*, cent. ii.) and mercury, have occasionally been used with success.—(*Bartholin, Act. Hafn.*, i., obs. 74 ; *Bonet, Sepulchr.*, lib. ii., sect. ii., obs. 36, Appendix.)

Generally speaking, however, the diet and regimen just recommended, with a spare allowance of water, will be sufficient to bring down the highest degree of adipose corpulency. Of this we have a striking example in the history of Mr. Wood, the noted miller of Billericay, in Essex. Born of intemperate parents, he was accustomed to indulge himself in excessive eating, drinking, and indolence, till, in the forty-fourth year of his age, he became unwieldy from his bulk, was almost suffocated, laboured under very ill health from indigestion, and was subject to fits of gout and epilepsy. Fortunately, a friend pointed out to him the Life of Cornaro : and he instantly determined to take Cornaro for his model, and, if necessary, to surpass his abridgments. With great prudence, however, he made his change from a highly superfluous to a very spare diet gradually : first diminishing his ale to a pint a day, and using a much smaller portion of animal food ; till at length, finding the plan work wonders as well in his renewed vigour of mind as of body, he limited himself to a

epiplocele, the displaced portion of it frequently undergoes a similar change, so that the inconvenience of the tumour is seriously aggravated by the size which it attains, and the reduction of the omentum is quite impracticable. In some cases of this kind, however, the mass of fat in the omentum has been so diminished by the effect of frequent purgatives, an abstemious diet approaching to starvation, and long continuance in bed, that the omentum has admitted of being returned into the abdomen.—Ed.

* Dr. Wade has mentioned a case of this kind in the Med. Obs. and Inquiries, vol. iii. Boerhaave relates an instance where the belly of a man grew so large that he was obliged to have it supported by a sash, and had a piece of the table cut out to enable him to reach it with his hands. After death, his omentum weighed thirty pounds.—D.

diet of simple pudding made of sea-biscuit, flour, and skimmed milk, of which he allowed himself a pound and a half about four or five o'clock in the morning for his breakfast, and the same quantity at noon for his dinner. Besides this, he took nothing, either of solids or fluids, for he had at length brought himself to abstain even from water; and found himself easier without it. He went to bed about eight or nine o'clock, rarely slept for more than five or six hours, and hence rose usually at one or two in the morning, and employed himself in laborious exercise of some kind or other till the time of his breakfast. And by this regimen he reduced himself to the condition of a middle-sized man of firm flesh, well-coloured complexion, and sound health.—(*Med. Trans.*, vol. ii., art xvii.) A like plan, or rather something approaching it, the present author once recommended to Mr. Lambert of Leicester, on being consulted concerning the state of his health. But either he had not courage enough to enter upon it, or did not choose to relinquish the profit obtained by making a show of himself in this metropolis. He made his choice, but it was a fatal one, for he fell a sacrifice to it in less than three years afterward.*

When the reduced mode of living thus recommended has been unnecessarily and injudiciously entered upon, and followed up with pertinacity, as in cases where young females are desirous of becoming celebrated for an elegant slenderness of form, it has often been productive of a serious and occasionally of a fatal result. Professor Frank gives a striking example of this in a young lady, who, for the above purpose, had for nearly a twelvemonth greatly diminished her daily food, used severe horse-exercise, and drunk every day a large quantity of vinegar. She at this time was labouring under dyspepsy, hysteria, and a dry cough, with a pungent pain in her side, hectic sweats, and occasionally purulent expectoration: she was pronounced in the last stage of consumption, and her life was entirely despaired of. Frank, however, succeeded in averting this event, by the gradual renewal of a more nutritious diet, and the use of tonics.—(*De Cur. Hom. Morb. Epit.*, tom. vi., lib. vi., 8vo., Viennæ, 1820.)

The local disease is for the most part far less manageable; but it has sometimes yielded to a steady perseverance in the above plan, in connexion with active purgatives, and the application of mercurial ointment to the vicinity of the organ affected; or a free use of calomel in the form of pills.

---

* Professor Graefe relates the following:—A butcher, thirty-seven years of age, weighed three hundred and sixty-three pounds. He was much troubled with difficulty of breathing, and with a sense of suffocation. After trying several modes of treatment and with but slight success, Professor Graefe prescribed twenty drops of the tincture of iodine four times a day. This course was commenced in October, 1825, and in February, 1826, his weight was diminished to one hundred and fifty pounds. The dyspnœa also was completely removed.—D.

GENUS II.

EMPHYMA.

TUMOUR.

GLOMERATION IN THE SUBSTANCE OF ORGANS FROM THE PRODUCTION OF NEW AND ADSCITITIOUS MATTER: SENSATION DULL, GROWTH SLUGGISH.

Phyma, in the present system, is limited to cutaneous tumours or tubers, accompanied with inflammation, as already explained in Class III., Ord. II. Emphyma imports, in contradistinction to phyma, a tumour originating below the integuments, and unaccompanied with inflammation, at least in its commencement; while ecphyma, in Order III. of the present Class, imports, in contradistinction to both, mere superficial extuberauces, confined to the integuments alone. The term *glomeration*, or "heaping into a ball," in the generic definition, is preferred to the more common terms *protuberance* or *extuberance*, because some tumours or emphymata lie so deeply seated below the integuments as to produce no prominence whatever, and are only discoverable by the touch.

The species of this Order, and much of their general character and arrangement, are taken, with a few variations, from Mr. Abernethy's valuable Tract on Tumours.

The subject, indeed, though of a mixed description, is commonly regarded as appertaining rather to the province of surgery than of medicine, from the tendency which most tumours seated on or near the surface have to open externally, or to call for some manual operation. In a general system of the healing art, however, it is necessary to notice them, though it is not the author's intention to dwell upon them at length; but rather to refer the reader, from the few hints he is about to pursue, to Dr. Baron's and Mr. Abernethy's works (*Observations on Tumours*), as the best comments upon them which he can consult:* widely differing, indeed, in their views of the origin of such extraneous growths, but each drawn up with great candour, and appealing to a host of indisputable facts, as we have already had occasion to observe, when treating of hepatic parabysma (Class I., Ord. II., Spe. 1) and tubercular phthisis (Class III., Ord. IV., Gen. III., Spe. 5); to which subjects the reader is referred for an account of the general origin and progress of morbid growths, and other physiological illustrations appertaining to them.

The species embraced by the genus EMPHYMA are the following:—

1. Emphyma Sarcoma.	Sarcomatous Tumour.
2. ———— Encystis.	Encysted Tumour.
	Wen.
3. ———— Exostosis.	Bony Tumour.

---

* In addition to these publications, the editor particularly recommends Dr. Carswell's Illustrations of the Elementary Forms of Disease to be carefully studied. This work presents careful and accurate delineations of the morbid state, and is particularly useful to the pathologist.

SPECIES I.
EMPHYMA SARCOMA.
SARCOMATOUS TUMOUR.
TUMOUR IMMOVEABLE ; FLESHY, AND FIRM TO THE TOUCH.

THE varieties of this species modified in respect to structure and situation, are very numerous. The following, distinguished by the former quality, are chiefly worthy of notice :—

α Carnosum. Fleshy tumour. Vascular throughout: texture simple : when bulky, mapped on the surface with arborescent veins. Found over the body and limbs generally.

β Adiposum. Adipose tumour. Suety throughout: enclosed in a thin capsule of condensed cellular substance : connected by minute vessels. Found chiefly in the fore and back part of the trunk.*

γ Pancreaticum. Pancreatic tumour. Tumour in irregular masses: connected by a loose fibrous substance, like the irregular masses of the pancreas. Found occasionally in the cellular substance, but more usually in convoluted glands : chiefly in the female breast.

δ Cellulosum. Cystose tumour. Derbyshire-neck. Tumour cellulose or cystose : cells oval, currant-sized or grape-sized, containing a serous fluid : sometimes caseous. Found generally, but mostly in the thyroid gland, testis, and ovarium.

ε Scirrhosum. Scirrhous tumour. Hard, rigid, vascular infarction of glandular textures ; indolent, insentient, glabrous ; sometimes shrinking and becoming more indurated. Found in glandular structures, chiefly those of the secernent system.

ζ Mammarium. Mammary tumour. Tumour of the colour, and assuming the texture, of the mammary gland ; dense and whitish ; sometimes softer and brownish : often producing, on extirpation, a malignant ulcer with indurated edges. Found in various parts of the body and limbs.

η Tuberculo-sum. Tuberculous tumour. Formed of firm, round, and clustering tubercles ; pea-sized or bean-sized ; yellowish or brownish red ; wen

ϑ Medullare. Medullary tumour. large, disposed to ulcerate, and produce a painful, malignant, and often fatal sore. Found chiefly in the lymphatic glands of the neck : often simultaneously in other glands and organs. Of a pulpy consistence and brain-like appearance ; whitish ; sometimes reddish-brown ; when large, apt to ulcerate, and produce a sloughing, bleeding, and highly dangerous sore.— Found in different parts : often in the testes ; at times propagating itself along the absorbent vessels to adjoining organs.

All these grow occasionally to an enormous size, particularly the sarcomatous, the adipose, and the medullary.* They are all produced by some increased action or irritation in the part in which they occur, the cause of which it is rarely in our power to ascertain. In general, they commence slowly and imperceptibly, and are seldom accompanied with much pain, whatever be the extent of their growth. They are all more or less organized through the whole of their structure, by which they are particularly distinguished from those of the next species : and it is highly probable that most of the irritating causes which produce any one, produce all the rest, the modification depending on the difference of site, habit, idiosyncrasy, or local misaffection. In their formation, however, there seems to be a greater tendency to inflammation, and especially adhesive inflammation, in the fleshy tumour, or proper sarcoma, than in any of the rest ; and from the more perfect elaboration of its fabric, there is no other form that maintains itself so firmly, or is removed, except by incision, with so much difficulty. The origin of the adipose may, in some degree, be understood from the remark we have offered under the last genus, and particularly under its second variety.†

The scirrhous tumour, when irritated, has a general tendency to run into a cancerous ulcer: for which it is not always easy to account, excepting where there happens to be an hereditary taint in the blood : for neither the tumour, nor its ordinary result, as we observed when treating of carcinus, is by any means confined to a glandular or to any particular structure, though the secernent glands constitute its most common seat. In Mr. Abernethy's treatise, the place of the scirrhous tumour, however, is occupied by

---

* Adipose tumours, as the expression informs us, are composed of fat, but it is finer, more delicate, and of a looser texture, than ordinary fat. They usually lie immediately under the common integuments ; though occasionally they are more deeply seated under the muscles. They are always imbedded in ordinary fat ; so that under the skin of the penis, scrotum, and eyelids, where there is simple cellular membrane, and no fat, they are never met with.—See Chymical Obs. on Fatty Tumours, by Sir Benjamin Brodie, as published in Med. Gaz. for 1834, p. 679.—ED.

* An immense tumour of a sarcomatous character, growing from the outside of the uterus, occurred in a patient under the care of Dr. Mott, and is figured and described in Francis's Denman. The tumour and its excrescences weighed one hundred and two pounds.—D.

† Adipose tumours seem, in some instances, to arise from long-continued pressure, and in others, from slight accident.—See Brodie's Clinical Observations, op. cit.—ED.

another, to which he gives the name of carcinoma, which in the present system is regarded as a modification of the scirrhus, degenerated and ulcerated, mostly by a cancerous diathesis; and in such case appertaining to carcinus, already described in the fourth Order of the third Class; or, where no such diathesis is present, belonging to the same Class and Order, under the genus and species ulcus vitiosum.

The scirrhous tumour is, in fact, the most important of the whole tribe, not only as leading, under peculiar circumstances, and in particular habits, to the most fatal result, but as being more common to every organ than any other variety whatever; and in a few instances, common to almost every organ collectively, or at the same time.*

The other varieties are looser and more spongy, and contain far less of living power: in consequence of which they are more easily disposed to ulcerate, and when in this condition, often spread, and become sordid and malignant from debility alone.

We have said that the tumours of this species will sometimes grow to a vast and preposterous bulk. This is particularly the case with the first variety, or fleshy sarcoma, and more especially when it seats itself in the scrotum, forming the sarcocele, or hernia carnosa, of authors. Negroes are particularly subject to this affection, and in one instance the tumour weighed fifty pounds.—(See Phil. Trans., vol. lxxii., 1783.) Swediaur indeed affirms, that they have occasionally weighed a hundred pounds.—(Nov. Nosol. Meth. System., ii., 529.) The skin of the scrotum is thick, rugose, of a dirty yellow, often covered with exulcerations that emit a fetid ichor. It is said, that among negroes, the disease is more common to the right side of the scrotum than to the left. Stoll, however, has asserted directly the contrary, so far as relates to Europeans, and his remarks are supported by the observations of Pfeffinger and Fredius. He has moreover generalized his assertion by contending that the left ovary of women, as well as the left testicle of men, is more subject to diseases of all kinds than the right.† Baron Larrey describes a sarcoma of the labia among tropical women, of the same nature as the scrotal sarcoma among men.—(Relat. Hist. et Chirurg. de l'Expédition de l'Armée en Egypte, &c., 8vo., Paris, 1803.)

* If the author here refer to scirrhi, strictly so called, or those characterized by a pulpy substance, intersected by radiating or reticulated white bands, he is certainly in error; for this disease cannot be correctly said to be more common to every organ than any other variety of tumour; in persons under a certain age, its occurrence in any organ is rare; and in some organs, its formation has never been observed. On the whole, it is met with in fewer parts than medullary sarcoma, or fungus hæmatodes.—Ed.

† Nov. Act. Physico-Med. Acad. Nat. Cur., tom. iv., Norim. The disease here spoken of is not really one of the testicle itself, but of the scrotum. Modern surgeons would not call it sarcocele, which term they restrict to disease of the testicle itself.—Ed.

The adipose tumour is also frequently of a very large magnitude. Mr. Abernethy gives an instance of one of the thigh that weighed fifteen pounds after extirpation (On Tumours, p. 31, 8vo., 1814), and M. Leske of another, of the weight of nineteen pounds, dissected from the face.—(Auserlesene Abhandlungen, &c., Leipzig, 1774, 8vo.) In the Journal de Médecine is an account of a third, that weighed not less than forty-two pounds.*

M. Leske gives a case, in which what he calls a scirrhous tumour was amputated from the breast, of the enormous weight of sixty-four pounds.—(Op. citat.) [If the epithet scirrhous be here employed to denote the hardened state of parts which is characterized by the peculiar structure that has a tendency to cancerous ulceration, there can be no doubt of a mistake; because it is not the nature of true scirrhus, or of a really cancerous tumour (here particularly excluding from present consideration fungus hæmatodes, or what is sometimes called soft cancer), to acquire a very large size.]

The most unsightly, however, of the whole, is the sarcoma cellulosum, when it fixes on the thyroid gland; in which situation it is often called Botium, Bronchocele, or Goitre; and in our own vernacular language, Derbyshire-neck, from an idea, of considerable antiquity, that the inhabitants of that county are more subject to it than those of other districts: an idea that does not seem to be without foundation; for in a visit which the author lately made to Matlock, he found a much larger number of the poor affected with this disease than he had ever seen before, while the rich escaped; and he found also, that by far the greater part of those who were labouring under it, were not only exposed to all the ordinary evils of poverty, but derived their chief diet from that indigestible and innutritive substance, the Derbyshire oaten cake, which is probably the chief cause of all the glandular and parabysmic enlargements which are so common to that quarter.† We

* Tom. xx., p. 551. The editor remembers an adipose tumour on a man's thigh that weighed nearly fifty pounds. It was removed by Mr. Cline at St. Thomas's Hospital; but in consequence of one part of the swelling having an attachment to the capsular ligament of the hip-joint, the latter was opened, abscesses ensued, and the patient did not recover.—Ed.

† Dr. Francis thinks that the disease is produced by humidity, and explains in this manner its greater prevalence in the vicinity of lakes and rivers. He says it increases with the rainy seasons, and diminishes when the weather becomes cold and dry; and hence argues the reason of its disappearance as the country becomes cleared, a fact observed by him in his western tour. He, however, does not reject the agency of certain waters in aggravating, if not in producing the disease.—(See Cooper's Surg. Dictionary, edited by Dr. D. M. Reese, New-York, 1834, Art. Bronchocele.) Dr. Barton regards bronchocele as having the same origin with remittent and intermittent fevers, and supports his opinion by the consideration, that these two diseases often prevail simultaneously; and farther, persons afflicted with bronchocele are exempt from intermittent fever, although exposed to its exciting cause;

shall see, when treating of cretinism, that a like innutritive diet is one of the most obvious causes of the same appearance as a concomitant in those countries in which cretinism is most frequent. The cells in this protuberance are very numerous, the fluid often viscid, and sometimes gelatinous; so that, when the tumour bursts, as it occasionally does, spontaneously, the contained fluid is apt to drain away very slowly, and has ulcerated with a large sloughy surface, without having half evacuated its contents.

Most of these tumours may be frequently repressed, or resolved, if discovered and attended to in their origin. The fleshy, which always commences with some degree of inflammatory action, should be vigorously attacked with leeches, repeated as often as may be necessary, and afterward with astringents or alterants, as the dilute solution of the acetate of lead for the former purpose, and the mercurial plaster for the latter. An issue or seton in the vicinity will also frequently assist, by producing a transfer of action. If this plan do not succeed, the tumour should be extirpated with the knife without loss of time, or allowing it to acquire any considerable bulk. Baron Larrey affirms, that he has often removed with the knife the largest scrotal sarcomas or adipose swellings, and this with very little pain, and that the wound readily healed.*

The scirrhous tumour is usually indicative of weak, instead of entonic action, in the organ in which it makes its appearance; in consequence of which the lymphatics absorb only the more attenuate part of the secerned fluids, and leave the grosser, which thicken and harden in the parenchyma. There is little irritation at first, but, as the distention and obduration increase, the part becomes stimulated, and as we have already observed, in a scrofulous or cancerous diathesis, is apt to call the latent seminium into action; when the hardened tumour degenerates into a foul ulcer. In an early stage, the disease has yielded to local irritants, which have a tendency to excite an increased action, and of a new kind; and hence the advantage of mercurial applications, or plasters of the gum-resins: and particularly the plaster of ammoniac with quicksilver, which unites the two, and is an admirable preparation. Where, indeed, the irritation is already considerable, the more direct of these stimulants must be abstained from, and the in-

irritants and narcotics may be had recourse to with more advantage, as the preparations of lead, acids of almost every kind, and cataplasms of hemlock, henbane, belladonna, or potato leaves. But here also the best and most effectual relief is to be had in extirpation.

Many of these varieties of tumours, on their first appearance, may be repelled by stimulant applications in conjunction with a steady pressure, wherever this can be applied; for, with the exception of the first, there is little tendency to inflammation in any of them, and, in the greater number, a decided weakness of the living power. They are often, indeed, connected with constitutional debility,* and hence appear simultaneously in different parts of the body. Extirpation, in this case is useless: at least, till the general frame is invigorated by a tonic regimen and course of medicines. And even then, from the peculiar seat or size of the tumour, it will not always be found advisable.

This is particularly true in that variety of the cystous sarcoma which is denominated BRONCHOCELE, GOÎTRE, OR DERBYSHIRE-NECK; and which usually proceeds from an enlargement of the thyroid gland. It is mostly found in females, and, in its commencement, the patient and her friends always turn a deaf ear to the use of the knife, under the hope that it may yield to a course of external and internal medicine; nor is the tumour, indeed, at all times sufficiently defined from the first for any effective use of chirurgical means.† It originates without pain or any discoloration of the skin, and presents a general prominence on the forepart of the neck, that rises so gradually as to be at first almost without an outline. As the prominence increases, it becomes harder and somewhat irregular, commonly with a partial feeling of fluctuation, though, in some instances, the tumour appears to be firm throughout. The skin grows yellowish, and the oppressed veins of the neck become varicose; the respiration is sometimes rendered difficult, and from the same cause the patient is troubled with headaches. The expediency of removing the tumour is at this time highly questionable, and every day increases the difficulty, from the growing diameter of its arteries, and their proximity to the carotids. If, from inattention, or mistaking it for an abscess, it be opened, a hemorrhage often follows, which it is difficult to repress, or which is apt to return from time to time, and has occasionally proved fatal. A soft reddish fungus protrudes through the opening, which yields to the fingers, bleeds

while it is well known that affections of the glands are frequent where intermittents prevail.

Goitre seems to be much more prevalent in some years than in others. According to Dr. Denny, in 1798, one hundred and fifty were affected with this disease at Pittsburg, which contained at that time a population of only one thousand four hundred. In 1806, also, whole families, who had recently settled in the town, were seized with it; and it is stated that at about the same period, the children in one of the common schools were all attacked by it.—See Philadelphia Journ. of the Med. and Phys. Sc., vol. x.—D.

* Relat. Hist. et Chirurg. de l'Expédition de l'Armée en Egypte et en Syrie, 8vo., Paris, 1803. —See the editor's Dictionary of Practical Surgery, 6th edit., art. SCROTUM.

* The doctrine that all new-formed parts or growths, not constituting an original portion of the body, are endued with an inferior degree of vitality to that of parts naturally appertaining to the animal machine, is perfectly correct; but the statement that tumours are connected with constitutional debility, is merely an hypothesis.—ED.

† F. E. Fodéré, Traité du Goitre et du Crétinisme, Paris, 8vo., 1800. No judicious practitioner would ever think of using the knife in the early stage of a bronchocele, especially now that the disease is often treated with considerable success by milder plans.—ED:

when it is touched, and cannot be completely destroyed either by cautery or the knife.* In that form of the tumour, however, which is called the aneurismal, accompanied with a considerable pulsation and enlargement of the superior thyroidal artery, a cure has easily been obtained by an operation; which consists in tying this artery, and thus cutting off the means of supply. Walther, some years ago, pursued this plan with success abroad (*Neue Heilart des Kroffes*, &c., Sulsback, 1817); and Mr. Coates relates a similar case, that has since been attended with a like result in our own country.—(*Trans. of the Medical and Chirurg. Society of London*, vol. x.) Yet even in the more complicated and cellular goître, where the tumour has increased to an enormous extent, and become mapped with innumerable bloodvessels of large diameter, it has in a few instances been attacked and successfully extirpated. One of the boldest operators in this way appears to be M. Hedenus of Dresden, who has lately published a history of not fewer than six cases of this kind, which terminated favourably under his care. In one of these the bronchocele had increased to the size of a skittle-ball, covered the whole of the forepart of the neck, was fourteen inches in circumference at the base, and seven inches in its transverse diameter: it felt firm, tense, and heavy, gave to the hand a sense of pulsation through its whole extent, and considerably affected the breathing, from its pressure on the trachea. The difficulties, however, to be surmounted in the performance of this operation, were chiefly appalling from the vascularity and complexity of the parasitic growth, and the impossibility of taking up many of the bleeding vessels. The operation lasted an hour and a half; and though the patient ultimately recovered, he was several times considered in a state of extreme danger after the part had been removed.†

The internal substance and structure of this tumour differ exceedingly in different cases. It has sometimes been found steatomatous throughout; but more generally, as we have already observed, consists of a fluid varying in viscidity, and in the number of cells or capsules in which it is locked up. It commonly first shows itself in girls who have reached the age of puberty, though it frequently commences at a later period; and is an ordinary symptom of cretinism, as we shall notice when treating of that disease in the course of the present Order. In a few cases, the contained substance is solid, and gives no discharge; and, in some other instances, the morbid growth has evinced a complication of almost every diversity of structure, and especially in those who are constitutionally predisposed to a production of tubers and tubercles. De Haen has given us a striking example

of this in a patient who, after having suffered much from visceral tumours, at length died in a state of dropsy. "In cadavere," says he, "horrendam mole thyroidœam glandulam nactus, publicè dissecui. Mecum auditores mirabantur nullum ferè genus tumorum dari, quin in hac solà thyroidœà inveniretur. Hìc enim steatoma, ibi atheroma, alio in loco purulentus tumor, in alio hydatrius, in alio erat coagulatus sanguis, fluidus ferè in alio, imo hinc glutine locutus plenus erat, alibi calce cum sebo mista, &c. Hæc autem omnia in una eademque thyroidœà glandulà."—(*Rat. Medendi*, pars vii., p. 285.)

Here also we have deficient living power in the organ affected, and very generally in the entire constitution : for it usually appears in girls of relaxed and flaccid fibres, in many cases partly debilitated by growth, and especially where this effect is produced by innutritive food, and partly by a larger flow of catamenia than the general tone of the system can sustain without yielding.

Stimulants and tonics have hence been found generally useful, as have also repeated and long-continued friction with the hand over the area of the tumour, alone or in conjunction with ammoniacal or terebinthinate irritants, chiefly solutions of camphire in spirits. For a reason that does not seem hitherto to have been sufficiently explained, in this kind of tumour, as in those of scrofula, the most successful stimulants are the alkalis : and of these the ammoniacal were formerly believed to be far more so than any of the rest ; and hence the patient was limited altogether to a course of burnt sponge or burnt hartshorn, and at one time to burnt toads. There does not seem, however, to be any particular reason for this predilection, and hence, in a later day, the subcarbonate, or the carbonate of soda, was pretty generally allowed to supply the place of all the other preparations of this kind, as the most convenient form in which the alkali could be given. It was also recommended to be applied externally, in the guise of sea-water, or the bibulous sea-plants, as already described in the treatment of scrofula (Cl. III., Ord. IV., Spe. 1, *Struma vulgaris*): both diseases having many points of resemblance, and especially as being chiefly seated in the glandular parts of the animal frame, and accompanied with great indolence in the lymphatic system.

In the present day, however, every other kind of preparation, as well for the one as the other complaint, has fallen prostrate before the newly-discovered medicine, iodine, so denominated by M. Courtois from its violet hue.* For the purpose before us it has been used both internally and externally. M. Coindet employed

---

* Traité des Maladies Chirurgicales et des Opérations qui leur conviennent, par M. le Baron Boyer, &c., tom. vii., Paris, 1821.
† Gräfe und Walther's Journal du Chirurgie und Augenheilkunde, Berlin, 1822. For an account of which, see Quarterly Journal of Foreign Medicine, No. xix., p. 317.

* This remark is fully confirmed by the experience of American practitioners. In this country bronchocele has been extirpated successfully ; it has been removed by Dr. Coventry's plan, of wearing the muriate of soda over the part affected ; and also by setons and by pressure ; but now we rely principally upon iodine, and many cases might be adduced to prove its efficacy.—See likewise Dr. Gibson's remarks on this subject in the Phil. Journ. of the Med. and Phys. Sc., vol. i.—D.

it in the form of an ointment, which he made by mixing pure iodine or the hydriodate of potash with lard, under an idea that the ill effect it produces, when given injudiciously, may be hereby avoided; and Coster affirms that, by the use of Coindet's ointment, of nearly a hundred individuals affected, more than two thirds were completely cured under his hands.—(*Archives Générales de Médecine*, &c., in re.) M. Brera* thinks it quite as void of mischief, and in most cases more efficacious, employed internally: and uses it in the form of pills or tincture made with pure iodine; or a solution of the hydriodate of potash in distilled water. The dose, in either case, is from a quarter to half a grain three times a day, for an adult.†

When it agrees with the system, the appetite is increased, and the pulse acquires more elasticity and beats stronger; but it has a tendency at the same time to stimulate the salivary glands in the manner of mercury. When it does not agree, it produces a sense of heat and irritation in the fauces, pain in the orbits and balls of the eye, and obscure vision; with tremours or convulsions of the extremities. Dr. Brera, as already observed, has employed it, on account of its absorbent powers, in various cases of parabysma or visceral turgescence, and especially in tubercular formations; and, as is well known, with considerable success: a success which the present author has extensively confirmed by his own practice in all the forms of this remedy. Yet, from the great and general excitement it produces, more judgment is called for in prescribing iodine, whether externally or internally, than is often manifested: and in no case whatever is a bold or daring practice more to be reprobated than in the present. The danger, indeed, is the greater, because the irritation or inflammatory effects are often not visible for a fortnight or three weeks; though, when they have once commenced, they are in many persons very intractable, notwithstanding an utter disuse of the medicine. "I saw two cases, with Dr. Peschier, of Geneva," says Dr. Gairdner, "in which the patients had suffered more than twelve months, and yet their sufferings had undergone little mitigation."—(*Essay on the effects of Iodine on*

the *Human Constitution*, &c., 8vo., London, 1824.) There are some idiosyncrasies, however, that are little affected by its use.

Bronchocele has sometimes been cured spontaneously, an instance of which occurred not long ago to the present author, in a young lady who had, for six or seven years, been successively under the care of all the most skilful physicians and surgeons of this metropolis, and who had nevertheless the mortification of finding the protuberance grow much larger and more unsightly, in spite of frictions, and blisters, and setons, and mercury in every form, and the alkalis, and hemlock, and hyoscyamus, employed jointly or alternately, and in almost every proportion, through the whole of this period. The distended skin at length gave way in various places, and a thin fluid issued from the foramina. This natural discharge was encouraged, and the sac by degrees exhausting itself, the tumour as gradually diminished, and at length completely disappeared.*

SPECIES II.
EMPHYMA ENCYSTIS.
ENCYSTED TUMOUR. WEN.

TUMOUR MOVEABLE; PULPY; OFTEN ELASTIC TO THE TOUCH.

A VERY small change in the power, or mode of action, of a secernent vessel, will often produce a very considerable change in the nature of the fluid which it secretes. Of this we have a clear proof in the thin and acrid lymph poured forth from the mucous membrane of the nostrils in a catarrh, compared with the bland and viscid discharge which lubricates this cavity in a state of health; limpid and mucilaginous at first, but gradually hardening into a horny substance. So the lungs, which, when sound, secrete a mild, when in a morbid condition throw out a tenacious phlegm, a watery or whey-like sanies, or a muculent pus. And we may hence easily account or the great diversity of materials found in the species of tumour before us, which is peculiarly distinguished by being surrounded with a proper cyst, and hence rendered moveable to the touch.

---

* Saggio Clinico sull' Iodio e sulle differenti sui combinazioni e preparazioni, &c., Padua, 1822.
† The tincture is merely a solution of iodine in rectified spirit, in the proportion of two scruples of the former to one ounce of the latter. M. Lugol employs an aqueous solution of iodine, which contains from half a grain to a grain of iodine in a pint of water, in conjunction with twelve grains of muriate of soda. The dose of this preparation is a fluid ounce and a half.—(See Dr. A. T. Thomson's Elem. of Materia Med., vol. i., p. 341.) Lugol uses, however, a great variety of preparations, consisting chiefly of solutions of iodine in distilled water, with a certain proportion of hydriodate of potash. The strength of the solutions differs considerably, and some of them are intended for external use, as lotions, baths, collyria, &c. A particular account of these preparations, and of the cases to which they are adapted, will be found in a work entitled Mém. sur l'Emploi de l'Iode dans les Maladies Scrofuleuses, par J. G. A. Lugol, 8vo., Paris, 1829.—ED.

* Many cases of bronchocele, cured by accidental abscesses and ulceration, are on record. Hence arose the suggestion of employing an issue or seton, as practised with much success by Quadri of Naples. If it were not for the very great efficacy of iodine, the seton would be a valuable mode of treatment. It should be noticed, however, that fatal hemorrhages have sometimes followed it; another reason for preferring the use of iodine. Not long ago the editor was consulted by Mr. Blair, of Great Russell-street, for a bronchocele in a young lady about ten years of age. The internal and external use of iodine was tried, and, in less than two months, the swelling had entirely disappeared. At the Bloomsbury Dispensary he has had several other cases, which have been cured by means of the same remedy. It is not, however, every tumour of the thyroid gland that will yield to this treatment; and he has met with several instances, in which every attempt to disperse the swelling with iodine has failed.—ED.

To follow up the subdivision through the whole of the varieties it offers would be almost endless. The following are chiefly worthy of notice :—

α Steatoma. — Encysted extuberance con-
  Steatome.   taining a fatty or suety
  Adipose wen. substance, apparently se-
                creted from the internal
                surface of the cyst.—
                Found over most parts of
                the body, and varying in
                size, from that of a kid-
                ney-bean to that of a
                pumpkin.

β Atheroma. — Encysted extuberance con-
  Atherome.   taining a mealy or curd-
  Mealy wen.   like substance, sometimes
                intermixed with harder
                corpuscles : apparently se-
                creted as the last. Found
                of different sizes over
                most parts of the body.

γ Melliceris. — Encysted extuberance con-
  Honeyed wen. taining a honey-like fluid.
                Found of different sizes
                over most parts of the
                body.

δ Ganglion. — Encysted extuberance con-
  Ganglion.   taining a colourless fluid ;
                the extuberation fixed
                upon a tendon.

ε Testudo. — Encysted extuberance con-
  Horny wen.   taining a fluid readily hard-
                ening into horn or nail :
                and especially when pro-
                truded externally upon an
                ulceration of the surround-
                ing integuments.

ζ Complicata. — Circumscribed, but incorpo-
  Complicated cyst. rated with the surrounding
                structure ; partly solid,
                partly fluctuating ; skin
                undiscoloured ; tumour
                mostly large, but rarely
                painful, even on pressure,
                or accompanied with con-
                stitutional disturbance.—
                Chiefly seated in the
                breast.

Most of these are supposed by Sir Astley Cooper to be nothing more at first than obstructed and enlarged cutaneous follicles : the sebaceous matter accumulating in the hollow of the follicle, which is lined with cuticle, and expanding it often to a considerable extent by pressure, in consequence of the mouth of the follicle becoming plugged up or entirely closed. When it is plugged up, the obstructed mouth is generally visible by a black dot, which is carbonized sebaceous matter. This being picked off or otherwise removed, a probe may often be easily forced down into the cavity, and the whole of the confined material be squeezed out by pressing the sides of the tumour, even when of some inches in diameter, and this with little pain and no inflammation.* Such Sir Astley

* Surgical Essays, by A. Cooper and B. Trav-

regards as the general history of common encysted tumours seated on the surface. But they will necessarily vary in their structure and contents, from a multiplicity of adventitious circumstances, and perhaps also from idiosyncrasy.

The steatome grows to a larger size than any of the rest. Rhodius gives a case in which it weighed sixty pounds (*Observ. Med.*, cent. iii., Patav., 1657, 8vo.) : and one, weighing twenty-six pounds, was dissected from the scapula.— (*Fabr. Hildan.*, cent. iii., obs. 63.) In its substance, it often makes a near approach to adipocire.*

The ganglion is introduced into the present list from the parity of its nature ; and, in so doing, the author has only followed the example of Mr. Sharp. "The ganglion of the tendon," says he, " is an encysted tumour of the melliceris kind ; but its fluid is generally like the white of an egg. When it is small, it sometimes disperses of itself. Pressure and sudden blows do also remove it ; but, for the most part, it continues, unless it be extirpated."† It is mostly produced by hard labour, or straining a tendon ; and hence is peculiarly common to the wrists of washing-women. In many instances, however, its exciting cause is unknown ; and, in some cases, it appears to depend upon some peculiarity of constitution. It is singular, that it should sometimes disappear during pregnancy, and afterward return. Plater records a case of this kind in the ham, and Bartholine, in the Copenhagen Transactions, another on the wrist.

The horny cyst is described by Vogel, under the name of testudo, here adopted. Mr. Abernethy has glanced at it in his treatise, and Sir Everard Home has more fully described and illustrated it in his cases of horny excrescences on the human body, inserted in the Philosophi-

ers, part ii., 1819. A specimen of encysted tumour, with a bristle in the aperture of the follicle, was lately given by Sir Astley Cooper to the editor, who has placed it in the Museum of the London University.—ED.

* The nineteenth paper in the first volume of the Trans. of the Am. Phil. Society, Philadelphia, 1818, contains the description of a steatomatous tumour successfully extirpated from the back by Dr. Dorsey : the smallest circumference of this tumour was two feet and ten inches, and the largest three feet and nine inches. See likewise the New-York Med. Repository, new series, vol. iii.—D.

† Surgery, chap. xxv., p. 128. Ganglions are swellings containing a viscid, transparent, gelatinous fluid, formed over the fibrous sheaths of tendons, which appear, in some instances, to compose the cyst in which the glairy fluid or gelatinous substance is contained. Such ganglions as are of an oblong shape are produced in this way ; but, according to Dupuytren, the globular ones are on the outside of the fibrous sheaths, with the interior of which, however, they have a communication. When they cannot be dispersed by stimulating applications, pressure, blisters, &c., the surgeon may try to burst them ; and if he cannot succeed in this, he may let out their contents by making a small opening in them with a couching-needle, or the point of a lancet, after which they will admit of being more effectually compressed with a piece of lead, enveloped in linen, and fixed on the part with a bandage.—ED.

cal Transactions : a subject, however, to which we shall have occasion to return when treating of LEPIDOSIS ICTHYIASIS, in the third Order of the present Class.

The COMPLICATED VARIETY is introduced upon the authority of Sir Astley Cooper, and chiefly from his description.—(*Lectures*, vol. ii., pp. 103, 205.) It occurs commonly in the female breast, and apparently, in most instances, is produced by a blow or some other external violence. When first observed, it is not larger, perhaps, than a marble, but it soon becomes larger, till by degrees it reaches the size of a melon, and then suddenly acquires a much ampler ·magnitude. Still, however, the general health of the constitution is but little interfered with; even pressure produces but little pain, though it proves to the finger the existence of numerous cysts, some of them containing others, some a solid material ; but the principal inconvenience is the weight of the breast, by which it is dragged down from the subjacent muscles, and obliged to be supported by a suspensory bandage. In one case, Sir Astley Cooper found that the cyst, or rather the glomeration of cysts, weighed nine pounds ; in another, thirteen. No difficulty was found in the process of healing, as the complaint was altogether local.· The dissected mass appeared for the most part like boiled udder, the interior of which, in some instances, consisted of hydatids ; in some, of numerous lamellæ, like the crystalline lens of the eye ; and in others of serum.

In a few instances, however, apparently from a morbid habit of body, the cyst becomes malignant, and makes an approach towards a scirrhous character. The substance which is effused by the inflammation is more compact, and varies in colour ; in some parts consisting of an adhesive matter, in others being softer, and mixed with the red particles of the blood. A fungous growth sprouts forth soon after, which, when cut through, has the appearance of soft organized matter ; in some parts extremely vascular, in others intermixed with what appears to be coagulated blood, at times with a material resembling putrid brain, or cream tinged by the colouring particles of the blood.

I have stated that the ganglion is sometimes connected with the ·habit or constitution, and the remark may be applied to several of the other varieties. They have hence been found scattered over the whole body (*O'Donnel, Lond. Med. Journ.*, vi., p. 33) ; and, in one instance, appear to have been connate and hereditary.—(*Vogel, Briefen an Haller*, i., Hundest.) In these cases, they will sometimes yield to a general treatment or a change of regimen. Richter gives examples of the ·cure of a steatome, one of the most difficult to be operated upon by internal means, by emetics (*Chir. Bibl.*, band v.) ; and Kaltschmid, by·a diet of great abstinence ;* by which plan, we have already

observed, that adipose corpulence is commonly capable of being removed, and hence not unreasonably advised where there is a tendency to the formation of adipose tumours.

Electricity, and particularly that of the voltaic trough, seems to have been serviceable in dispelling many tumours belonging to this and the last species ; and having omitted it in its proper place, we may here observe, that Dr. Eason of Dublin has given an instance, in which a hard tumour was removed from the breast of a woman who was struck to the floor, and for some time deprived of the use of her limbs, by a stroke of lightning. It was observed to be much softer almost immediately after the accident, and, in a short time, totally disappeared, though it had for a long time resisted the power of every application that could be thought of. —(*Edin. Med. Comment.*, iv., p. 84.)

[With the exception of ganglions, however, which may be cured by rupturing or puncturing the cyst, and ·sometimes by blisters, stimulating liniment, pressure, &c., few encysted tumours admit of being dispersed, but almost always require the employment of the knife. In the operation, the main object is to remove every partiele of the cyst by which the contents of the swelling are secreted ; for, if this be not done, a perfect cure will not be likely to follow. Thus, the editor about four years ago was requested to remove a horn from the surface of the glutæus maximus of an elderly medical practitioner, who had undergone an operation for the same disease many years previously ; but, as a part of the cyst secreting the horny matter had been left, the excrescence returned. The cure is now complete.]

For the rest, the writers on practical surgery must be consulted.

SPECIES III.
EMPHYMA EXOSTOSIS.
BONY TUMOUR.

TUMOUR INELASTIC, OFTEN IMMOVEABLE ; HARD AND BONY TO THE TOUCH.

TUMOURS of this character consist of calculous or hard matter : and are sometimes seated immoveably on a bone, sometimes immoveably on the periosteum, sometimes pendulously in a joint, sometimes either moveably or immoveably in some fleshy part of the body, thus constituting the four following varieties :—

α Ostea.	Immoveable ; protuberant ;
Osteous tumour.	seated on the substance of a bone.
β Periostea.	Immoveable ; protuberant ;
Node.	from a bony enlargement of the periosteum.
γ Pendula.	Bony tumour hanging pendulous into a joint.
Pendulous exostosis.	

----

* Pr. de Steatomate fame curato. Comp. Girard, Lupiologie : ou, Traité des Tumeurs connues sur le Nom des Loupes, Paris, 1775. Sir B. Brodie mentions, in his Clinical Lectures, the power of the liquor potassæ to disperse certain adipose tumours, occurring together in several parts of the body, when taken internally in largish doses for some time.—ED.

δ Exotica.　　　　Bony tumour moveable er im-
Exotic exostosis.　moveable, seated in some
　　　　　　　　　fleshy part of the body.

Lime is one of the substances most easily
secreted in the body of all animals. How far
it may be *formed* in the body, we shall have occasion to notice under the genus OSTHEXIA,
forming the fifth of the present Order. We behold it at an early period of fœtal life, and, in
old age, when every other secretion has diminished or failed altogether, we are perpetually
meeting with examples of a morbid augmentation of this in the coats of the bloodvessels, the
bladder, the brain, and various other organs, afflicting the closing years of life with a variety
of troublesome, and, not unfrequently, highly
painful disorders.

The FIRST VARIETY is found in most of the
bones of the body, but chiefly perhaps in the
bones of the cranium : where they are sometimes excrescent, and composed of bony spicula
resembling crystallizations : sometimes exquisitely hard and glabrous, analogous to ivory (*Baillie, Morb. Anat.*, fascic. x., pl. i., figs. 1, 2), no
doubt from their being composed of phosphate
in a greater measure than carbonate of lime.*

According to their structure, Sir Astley Cooper has subdivided these tumours into cartilaginous and fungous : and according to their seat,
into periosteal, when they commence between
the external surface of the bone and the internal
surface of the periosteum ; and medullary,
when they commence in the medullary membrane and cancellated fabric of the bone.—
(*Surg. Essays, Treatise on Exostosis.*)

This periosteal subdivision includes the SEC-
OND VARIETY of the present species ; which is
chiefly found as a symptom in lues, and is commonly described under the name of *node*. In
some instances, it has occurred as a sequel of
acute rheumatism. And, in both cases, its
treatment must depend upon the nature of the
disease to which it appertains, and must form a
part of the general plan, as we have already observed when discussing these maladies.

The THIRD and FOURTH VARIETIES are chiefly derived from Mr. Abernethy's classification.
The difference of their form and mode of union
with the adjoining parts depends chiefly upon
the difference of their seat. " A woman,"
says Mr. Abernethy, " was admitted into St. Bartholomew's Hospital with a hard tumour on the
ham. It was about four inches in length and
three in breadth. She had also a tumour in
the front of the thigh, a little above the patella,
of lesser size and hardness. The tumour on
the ham, by its pressure on the nerves and vessels, had greatly benumbed the sensibility and

obstructed the circulation of the leg, so that it
was very œdematous. As it appeared impossible to remove this tumour, and as its origin and
connexions were unknown, amputation was resolved on. On examining the amputated limb,
the tumour in the ham could only be divided
with a saw : several slices were taken out of
it by this means, and appeared to consist of coagulable and vascular substance, in the interstices of which a great deal of bony matter was
deposited. The remainder of the tumour was
macerated and dried, and it appeared to be formed of an irregular and compact deposition of the
earth of bone. The tumour on the front of the
thigh was of the same nature with that in the
ham : but containing so little of lime that it
could be cut with a knife. The thigh-bone was
not at all diseased."—(*Surgical Observations,
Classification of Tumours*, p. 102.)

Of the general nature of the exotic variety we
shall have to treat under OSTHEXIA INFARCIENS,
of which perhaps it is only a modification.

These in all instances are cases for surgical
rather than medical treatment, and are seldom
to be cured except by extirpation ; and when this
cannot be done, and the tumour is seated on a
limb, by amputation.

[Dr. Cumin, of Glasgow, defines an exostosis
to be a circumscribed tumour formed on a bone,
and consisting wholly or in part of newly-formed osseous matter. This definition would of
course exclude all cases which commence in the
medullary and cancellous structures. It seems
to him, that the first step in the process by
which an exostosis is produced, is the deposition of cartilage, or of a substance resembling it,
which is afterward followed by the secretion of
bone.

Dr. Cumin divides exostosis into three species :—

1. *Exostosis Cellularis.* The tumour consists of an external crust, within which are numerous bony partitions, together with a quantity
of softer substance, generally of the nature of
mucus, jelly, or cartilage, or atheromatous or
fatty matter. One remarkable variety of this
species is that which contains hydatids.—(See
R. Keate's Case in Med. Chir. Trans., vol. v.)
Another, also pointed out by Dr. Cumin, is exhibited by those swellings on the phalanges of
the fingers and metacarpal bones, which render
the hand deformed and even monstrous. He adverts to the case of an enormous cellular exostosis, described by Kulmus (*Haller, Disput.
Chir.*, tom. v., p. 655), that weighed nearly
five pounds, arose from the clavicle, and consisted partly of bone and partly of cartilage, with
cells containing a pultaceous orange-coloured
substance, resembling marrow. The latter form
of disease is often mentioned by writers under
the name of osteosarcoma, a term rather vaguely
applied.

2. *Exostosis Laminata, vel Petrosa.* The laminated or craggy osseous tumour is represented
by Dr. Cumin as consisting of a mixture of bony
excrescences and cartilage. It has no osseous
shell, and, after maceration, presents the appearance of foliated crystallizations, or craggy

---

* American surgeons have contributed very
much to our stock of knowledge on this subject,
and many brilliant operations have been performed
upon patients affected with this disease. Dr.
Mott's successful excisions of the left clavicle
and of the lower jaw, the removal of the upper maxillary bone by Dr. D. L. Rogers, with similar operations by Stevens, Warren, McLellan, and others, will ever be regarded as happy triumphs of
surgery in the United States.—D.

adherent masses. In some instances of this form of disease, according to the same authority, the new deposition consists, not of osseous substance, but a mere unorganized mass of the earthy salts of bone.

3. *Exostosis Eburnea.* This species, noticed by the greater number of practical writers, is characterized by its excessive hardness and its remarkable whiteness, like that of ivory.— (See *Dr. Cumin's instructive papers in Edin. Med. and Surgical Journ.*, Nos. lxxxii. and lxxxiii.)]

GENUS III.

PAROSTIA.

MIS-OSSIFICATION.

BONES UNTEMPERED IN THEIR SUBSTANCE, AND INCAPABLE OF AFFORDING THEIR PROPER SUPPORT.

PAROSTIA is a compound from παρὰ, "peràm," and ὀστέον, "os, ossis." The genus is new, but sufficiently called for. It includes two species, connected by the common character of an inaccordant secretion of some one of the constituent principles of the bony material, in consequence of which the substance is rendered too brittle, and apt to break on slight concussions or other movements, or too soft, and equally apt to bend. These species are as follow :—

1. Parostia Fragilis. Fragility of the Bones.
2. ———— Flexilis. Flexibility of the Bones.

SPECIES I.

PAROSTIA FRAGILIS.

FRAGILITY OF THE BONES.

SUBSTANCE OF THE BONES BRITTLE, AND APT TO BREAK ON SLIGHT EXERTIONS, WITH LITTLE OR NO PAIN.

BONE, shell, cartilage, and membrane, in their nascent state, are all the same substance, and originate from the coagulable lymph of the blood, which gives forth gelatin, and produces by secretion, though, as already observed, it does not contain, albumen. Membrane is gelatin, with a small proportion of albumen to give it a certain degree of firmness : cartilage is membrane, with a larger proportion of albumen to give it a still greater degree of firmness ; and shell and bone are cartilage, hardened and rendered solid by the insertion of lime into their interior : in the case of shell, the lime being intermixed with a small proportion of phosphoric, and a much larger proportion of carbonic acid ; and in the case of bone, with a small proportion of carbonic and a much larger of phosphoric acid. It is hence obvious, that if the earthy and the animal parts do not bear a proper relation to each other, the bone must be improperly tempered, and unadapted to its office : that if the earthy or calcareous part be deficient, its substance must be soft and yielding ; and that if the animal part be deficient, or the calcareous part in excess, it must lose its cohesive power, become brittle, and apt to break.

It is the second of these morbid states that forms the proximate cause of the species before us, as the first forms the cause of the ensuing species.

PAROSTIA FRAGILIS is the *fragilitas ossium,* or *fragile vitreum,* of authors, and is most frequently found as an attendant upon advanced age. It is also occasionally to be met with as a symptom in lues,[*] struma,[†] porphyra, cancer,[‡] and general intemperance ; and has been known as a sequel of smallpox. When bones are thus affected, they have a tendency to break upon slight and sudden movements. The author was once present at a church in which a lady, nearly seventy years old, in good general health, broke both the thigh-bones in merely kneeling down ; and on being taken hold of to be carried away, had an os humeri also broken, without any violence and with little pain. From the general inirritability of the system, no fever of importance ensued, and, under the influence of a warm bed, and a diluent but somewhat cordial regimen, the bones united in a few weeks. Mr. Gooch relates a similar case of fracture, occasioned by a violent fit of coughing.—(*Observations,* &c., Appendix.)§

---

[*] In the Museum of the University of London is a thigh-bone, which broke as the patient was moving the limb in bed, at a period when he was under the influence of mercury for nodes on the other thigh-bone, which is also in the University Museum.—ED.

[†] In the Museum of the same institution is an os humeri of a scrofulous boy, which was broken by shampooing. This first fracture united ; but a second one happening afterward in another place, a false joint formed. The bone was found to be so brittle after the patient's decease, that when the surgeon was dissecting the limb, a third fracture was produced.—ED.

[‡] Nouveau Journ. de Médecine, tom. i., p. 138. The editor was called, about three years ago, to a gentleman's coachman in Montague Mews, Russell Square, whose thigh broke as he was turning himself in bed. It appeared that he had a cancerous disease of the bladder ; for, after death, a large fungous tumour was found in this organ, situated upon so hard a base, that when felt through the coats of the bladder, it was at first supposed to be a stone. One of the ribs had also undergone a spontaneous fracture ; and both it and the fracture of the femur were surrounded by a mass of scirrhous matter. One section of the femur is in the Museum of the London University, and the other in the editor's possession. The preparations correspond very closely in every respect to the beautiful delineations of cancer of the bones in Dr. Carswell's Illustrations of the Elementary Forms of Disease, fasc. iii. The details of the case are recorded in the Med. Chir. Trans., vol. xvii., p. 51, et seq. See also two cases of fracture of the thigh-bone taking place without any violence, in which a diseased state of the bones appears to have been the predisposing cause of fracture, and concurring with cancer of the breasts, by Thomas Salter, of Poole, Dorset.—Op. cit., vol. xv., p. 186, &c.—ED.

§ In a case under the care of the late Dr. Wright Post, the osseous portion of the thigh-bone was absorbed with great rapidity—the patient, a man between forty-five and fifty years of age, was of a gouty habit, and had been affected with rheuma-

The common cause seems to consist in a general inirritability of the system, and a torpitude of the absorbent powers, which, by carrying off only the finer and more attenuate particles, and suffering the grosser, and particularly the earthy, to accumulate, overcharge the bones with this material.

Hence the best remedy is to be found in a plan of warm tonics, that may supply the system with something of the stimulus it stands in need of, and in a free use of acids, whether mineral or vegetable, that, by their tendency to dissolve calcareous earth, may at least diminish its introduction into the chyliferous vessels in the process of digestion, if they do not reach the assimilating vessels of the bones, and lessen the separation or elaboration at the extremity of the nutritive chain.

Of the mineral acids, the sulphuric will generally be found preferable ; it seldom gripes or nauseates, and almost always promotes the action of the stomach when weak or indolent. It is hence, also, an excellent tonic, and may be persevered in longer than any of the rest. In most cases, the muriatic agrees with the stomach, but not with the bowels, which always become more relaxed during its use than where the other acids are employed. It is on this account, however, peculiarly adapted to cases of habitual constipation. The nitric acid, in a few idiosyncrasies, has proved a very powerful tonic, as well as solvent of animal earth : but, in many cases, it disagrees with the stomach, and produces flatulence, eructation, and other symptoms of indigestion. Where these cannot be employed, we must have recourse to the vegetable acids, and especially the citric or tartaric, the last either in its pure form, or in that of cream of tartar. Lemons and oranges may also be taken copiously, and the carbonic acid, combined with water by means of Nooth's apparatus.[*]

***

tism ; after complaining for about three weeks of pain in the thigh-bone, which however did not prevent him from walking, the pain suddenly became so severe that he was forced to lie down. In the course of the night, the limb was found to be bent at almost a right angle, and so much of the osseous matter was absorbed, that, with the most sedulous application of splints and bandages, the limb could not be kept straight. The limb soon became œdematous, and notwithstanding the liberal use of tonics and other remedies, in about eight months the patient died. On post mortem inspection, the thigh appeared little more than a dense gelatinous mass, and there was scarcely a vestige of the thigh-bone to be found.—See Mott's Medical Magazine, vol. i., p. 153. A much more remarkable case is detailed by Tauvry, in the Mém. de l'Acad. Royale, Paris, 1700 ; viz., that of a girl whose bones were as soft as wax, and bent every time she was moved ; the teeth, however, still retained their original hardness.—D.

* The treatment here advised seems to be suggested by the belief that fragility of the bones is always connected with a state of them in which their earthy part is superabundant. In old age there is always a degree of fragility in the bones, and it is well known, that the proportion of calcareous matter in the bones to the animal and vascular parts of them is then greater than it is in the

SPECIES II.
PAROSTIA FLEXILIS.
FLEXIBILITY OF THE BONES.

SUBSTANCE OF THE BONES SOFT, AND APT TO BEND AND BECOME CROOKED ON SLIGHT EXERTIONS, WITH LITTLE OR NO PAIN.

This is the *mollities ossium* of authors, formerly denominated *spina ventosa*, from its being first noticed on the spine, and accompanied with protuberances which were supposed to proceed from inflation.

Its physiology has been given under the preceding species, with which it is connected in the relation of contrast. As fragility of the bones proceeds from an excess of osseous earth, *flexibility* proceeds from a deficiency of one or more of the elements which constitute it. This deficiency may proceed from two causes, each producing some peculiarity of symptoms, which we shall presently illustrate by examples. For, first, there may be too small a secretion or elaboration of calcareous phosphate to allow a sufficient compactness to the bones : and, secondly, there may be an adequate separation of the calcareous earth, but a deficiency of the phosphoric acid, which, we have already observed, is necessary to give it fixation ; in consequence of which it is often carried back in a loose state into the circulation, and discharged as a recrement by the kidneys or some other emunctory.

The disease is sometimes idiopathic, and occurs sometimes as a symptom of porphyra, diabetes, and some forms of colic. In direct oppositiou to the preceding species, moreover, it is commonly found in the earlier rather than in the later periods of life, and has been observed in infancy.[*] It has occasionally been detected in

***

earlier stages of life. Yet the greasy, oily condition of the bones of an old skeleton, proves that this natural fragility of them is different from that which takes place in younger persons as the result of disease. Other varieties of fragility are attended with a diminution of the quantity of lime, and a corresponding loss of weight in the bones. The fragility of bones from old age is of course incurable ; but with reference to other varieties of the affection, the possibility of curing them will entirely depend on that of curing the original disease. Thus, fragility from cancer may be set down as incurable. It may here be observed, that the latter kind of fragility seems often to depend on the removal of the natural texture of the bones in certain parts of the skeleton, and the deposition of a scirrhous substance in its place.—Ed.

* This observation appears to the editor to be more applicable to rickets than mollities, between which diseases there are several striking differences. In the first place, mollities ossium is an extremely rare disease ; whereas rickets is particularly common. Few instances of mollities have been met with in males, and those females who have been afflicted with it were of, or past, the middle period of life ; whereas rickets is seen principally in children, and perhaps not more in one sex than the other. Another remarkable distinction is, that in rickets the calcareous matter of the bones has been originally deficient ; the bones have never been properly developed from birth ; but before mollities commences they attain their full growth, their texture is perfect, and their

quadrupeds, and of the stoutest kinds, as the ox and the lion. It is sometimes general, and sometimes confined to particular bones.

The cause is commonly obscure : it appears frequently to consist in a morbid state of the digestive organs, but is seated perhaps as often at the other extremity of the great chain of the nutritive powers, in the assimilating or secernent vessels, where it must necessarily elude all detection. In the museum of Professor Prochaska of Vienna, is a preparation of an adult who died of this disease, in which all the vertebræ are glued into one mass, the sacrum being scarcely distinguishable, and the ribs bent inward, and marked by the impression of the arms, which the patient was in the habit of pressing forcibly against his sides. The whole skeleton is extremely light. This last fact is always the case, from the absence of so large a portion of animal earth. An analysis, by Dr. Bostock, of the vertebræ of an adult female who died of the species before us, indicated that the earthy matter was only one eighth part of the weight of the bone, instead of amounting to more than half, which Dr. Bostock estimates to be its proportion in a state of health.—(*Trans. of the Medico-Chirurg. Soc.*, vol. iv., p. 42.)

A singular case of this disease is given by Dr. Hosty of Paris.—(*Phil. Trans.*, vol. xlviii., year 1753.) The patient, a married woman, between thirty and forty years of age, was attacked by it gradually, after several lyings-in, and two falls on the side, which gave her great pain over all her body, but fractured no bone. The first decided symptom was an incurvation of one of the fingers, accompanied with a very considerable discharge of bony or calcareous earth by the urine, which was loaded with it, and gave a copious deposite. The incurvation by degrees extended to all the limbs, so that the feet were at length bent upwards nearly to the head, but without muscular contraction or fracture. The calcareous matter at length ceased to flow towards the bladder, and seems to have been transferred to the salivary glands, from which was discharged a flux of dark discoloured spittle. All the functions of the body were in a state of great disorder ; she had at times a very considerable degree of fever, which was at one period accompanied with headache, delirium, and subsultus tendinum. She died in about a twelvemonth from the commencement of the disease, and all the bones, on being examined,

were found soft and supple, though many of them, as the ribs, were still in some degree friable ; the scalpel, with very little force, ran through the hardest of them. Nothing extraordinary was found in the thoracic or abdominal viscera ; but the right hemisphere of the brain appeared to be one third larger than the left.

In this case the disease evidently commenced in the bones themselves, and seems to have proceeded from a want of phosphoric acid to give compactness to the calcareous earth ; for that there was a sufficiency of this earth, is clear from its being found loose in the fluids, and thrown out as a recrement by the urine and saliva till the whole was removed, and nothing of the bones remained but their cartilaginous or membranous fabric. In a similar case, related by Mr. Thomson, this tendency to the discharge of the absorbed and loose earth of the softened bones at the emunctories of the body was still more considerable. The urine, we are told, for the first two years of the patient's illness, deposited generally a whitish sediment, which, upon evaporation, became like mortar, and, on one or two occasions, he voided a few jagged calculi. After this period the calcareous discharge ceased, the bones having little earth left in their composition, as was sufficiently ascertained on the patient's death, which, however, did not occur till nine years from the commencement of the malady.

[In this case, when the tibia was cut into in the living body, the shell of the bone was of the thickness and solidity of the rind of cheese, and the whole of its interior was occupied by a dusky red or liver-coloured flesh, which was devoid of sensibility. No hemorrhage followed the removal of the osseous covering. The appearances after death were similar to the preceding. The cartilaginous covering of the bones was much thinner than natural ; but their external surface was polished, and, in some parts, elevated into bumps.* In another example, recently described by Mr. Howship, when the periosteum of the thigh-bone was longitudinally divided, the contents proved to be a red, pulpy, or fleshy matter, in some parts much resembling liver ; in one place much softer ; in another, of a grumous consistence, like blood. The whole of the softened femur admitted of a perfect longitudinal division by the knife, through the cylindrical portion, without its meeting with the least trace of ossific matter ; but, towards each extremity, it occasionally encountered a few scattered spiculæ of bone, or a thin external lamina, like a small fragment of paper or egg-shell. The disease seemed to be the effect of a morbid action in the capillary arteries of the medullary membranes. However, although the medullary secretion was everywhere deranged, the matter deposited was by no means uniform

proportion of lime is right, until about the middle period of life, when those peculiar changes in the osseous system begin, which constitute the disease under consideration. In rickets, the bones cannot be suddenly bent in a certain degree without breaking ; but in mollities they are more flexible than a piece of whalebone, the femur having been in some instances on record so soft, that the limb could be bent outwards, so as to bring the outer ankle in contact with the patient's temple. This was exemplified in the case of Madame Supiot, the particulars of whom are published in the Mém. de l'Acad. des Sciences. Mollities ossium, so far as our present information extends, is incurable ; but rickets generally ceases as the child grows up and acquires strength.—Ed.

Vol. II.—M m

---

* Medical Obs. and Inquiries, vol. v., 8vo. The dissection of the subject of this case was made under the direction of Dr. William Hunter, and several of the bones are preserved in the museum which he bequeathed to the University of Glasgow.—See Cumin on Diseases of the Bones, in Ed. Med. Journ., No. lxxxii.—Ed.

in appearance; one mass seemed like coagulated blood; another resembled a portion of gorged liver. At one point, the secreted matter was of a light fibrinous character; at another, it was more like a compact fleshy substance. The periosteum was not materially thickened. The lower parts of the tibia were cut through with ease, but the middle ones resisted the knife. The bones of the pelvis were also so nearly destroyed that they could be cut through with facility, although upon their surface there was a thin osseous shell. The vertebræ, ribs, and sternum, were all so softened as to admit of being easily divided with the knife. The bones of the upper extremities, however, could not be cut through, nor those of the cranium. The viscera, and the cartilages of the joints, were sound.—(*Howship, in Med. Chir. Trans. of Edin.*, vol. ii., p. 152.)]

It is probably to this species we are to refer the singular case translated by Reiske from the Arabic of Ghutzi, of an individual, contemporary with Mahomet, who had no proper bones but those of the cranium, neck, and hands, every other part of the body being pliable as a piece of cloth to the touch of other persons, though the individual could not of his own accord bend a single limb. He was a man, we are told, of the highest dignity, and had acquired celebrity for his wisdom. He was usually carried from place to place in a wicker-basket of palm twigs. —(*Opuscula Medica ex Monumentis Arabum*, 8vo., Hallæ, 1776.)

In some cases there seems to be but little deficiency of phosphoric acid, though there is an evident want of earthy matter; for we meet with no calcareous discharge by any of the emunctories, while the union which takes place between whatever portion of the earth is conveyed to the bones and the phosphoric acid which is secreted at the same time, renders them in some degree friable, though weak, and hence as liable to fracture on slight exertions, as in the preceding species.

A case of this kind was not long ago under the joint care of the author and Mr. Howship. The patient was a lady thirty-five years of age, heretofore in good health: both the thigh-bones had been broken without any violence about a twelvemonth antecedently, and all the other bones showed a strong tendency to softness and compressibility. There was great general debility in all the functions, with a feeble and quickened pulse. By perfect quiet, a recumbent posture on a hard and level couch, and a steady use of a tonic regimen and diet, she was put into a way of recovering. Her general health im-

proved, the extremities of both bones appeared to be united and buried in an irregular mass of callus that clustered around them, and in a few months it was recommended to her to be removed by an easy conveyance to the sea-coast.*

A somewhat similar case, but of greater severity, communicated by Sir John Pringle to the Royal Society, is contained in its forty-eighth volume.—(*Phil. Trans.*, year 1753.) The patient was an unmarried female servant of good character. A parostic diathesis seems from some cause or other to have existed, and to have been brought into action by a tedious and troublesome chlorosis. One of the legs first gave way and snapped as she was walking from the bed to her chair, and soon afterward both the thigh-bones from a little exertion. From this time her general health suffered, her habit became cachectic, and there being an increasing inability to a supply of compact calcareous earth, all the bones became soft and pliable, and bent in every direction without breaking, while those which were broken never united. Her head, however, was throughout scarcely affected, and her mental faculties continued clear to the last. She died in less than nine months from the commencement of the disease, and on examining her body, all the bones were capable of being cut through without turning the edge of the knife.

In one of the two preceding cases, mercury was employed and carried to the extent of producing salivation, yet without any benefit whatever. It is not easy, indeed, to conceive what benefit could be expected from such a plan. The deficiency of one or all the constituents of perfect and healthy earth of bones, is evidently dependant upon local or general debility, though we cannot always discover the cause of this debility, nor the peculiar circumstances connected with it which give rise to this rather than any other effect of diminished energy. And hence the only treatment presenting any hope of success, is that of perfect quiet and a recumbent posture, on a hard mattress or slightly inclined plane, to prevent distortion and fracture, a plain but nutritive and somewhat generous diet, and a course of tonic medicines. In the case of the lady just adverted to, and who was put into a train of recovery, the medicines chiefly employed were various preparations of cinchona and iron, chiefly the pilulæ ferri compositæ, with an allowance of ale instead of wine with her dinner.

Since the first edition of this work, I have learned that this patient, when in the full hope

---

* A further account of this case has been published by my friend Mr. Howship. " The earliest forerunners were debility of vascular action, and especially of the system of voluntary muscles—increasing or diminishing, but always prominent—essentially relieved by tonics, and as essentially aggravated by the excitement of the mercurial influence. One of the most remarkable features in the history, was the relief afforded by sea-air and sea-bathing." In this particular patient, the nervous system was singularly irritable. " The remarkable severity of pain excited in the diseased

member by the action of swallowing, by the slight irritation of a cambric handkerchief touching the face, or even by the mental emotion incident to speaking of her complaint, as well as the sudden excitation of perspiration by drawing the finger over the skin, are circumstances," says Mr. Howship, " that I never had before observed myself, nor met with in the observations of others." Great benefit seems to have resulted from combining tonics and aperients.—See Edin. Med. Chir. Trans., vol. ii., p. 137.—Ed.

of resuming her former health, was suddenly carried off by an attack of pleurisy.*

GENUS IV.
CYRTOSIS.
CONTORTION OF THE BONES.

HEAD BULKY, ESPECIALLY ANTERIORLY: STATURE SHORT AND INCURVATED; FLESH FLABBY, PALE, AND WRINKLED.

THE term CYRTOSIS is derived from the Greek κυρτὸς, "curvus, incurvus, gibbosus," and among the ancients, particularly imported recurvation of the spine, or posterior crookedness, as lordosis, λόρδωσις, imported procurvation of the head and shoulders, or anterior crookedness. It has in recent times more generally been written CYRTONOSOS, literally "morbus incurvus:" but the term νόσος, or morbus, is pleonastic in a system of nosology, and hence CYRTOSIS is preferable.

The genus is intended to include two specific diseases, which have a close connexion in many of their most prominent symptoms, and especially in the sponginess and incurvation of the bones, and in the withered appearance of the flesh, insomuch that the second is by some regarded as only a modification of the first; but which, however, are peculiarly distinguished from each other by the different state of the mental powers. These are:—

1. Cyrtosis Rhachia.	Rickets.†
2. ——— Cretinismus.	Cretinism.

SPECIES I.
CYRTOSIS RHACHIA.
RICKETS.

CHIEFLY AFFECTING THE LIMBS AND BODY:

* From the particulars of her dissection, however, as given by Mr. Howship, and now introduced into the text, it is manifest that the disease had irreparably destroyed the greater part of her skeleton, and that, independently of the pleurisy, she could not have recovered.—ED.

† Some writers would have arranged rickets as a species of mollities ossium. The authority of Dr. Cumin is in support of this view. Thus, the genus softening of bones, he proposes to call *Osteomalakia*, and he divides it into two species: 1. *Osteom. Infantum*, or Rickets; and 2. *Osteom. Adultorum*, or Mollities Ossium.—(See Edin. Med. Journ., No. lxxxii., p. 3.) Cretinism is not necessarily combined with any disease or deformity of the bones resembling that of rickets, but according to late observations is essentially connected with malformation of the head—the cranium being remarkably small, and its bones of extraordinary thickness.—(See Larrey's Mém. de Chir. Milit., tom. i., p. 123.) At the same time, it is a fact that rickets is often conjoined with a state of the scull, in which some parts of it present an extraordinary thickness, while others are as thin as paper, with the tables blended together and incapable of division. Sometimes the parietal bones are seven eighths of an inch in thickness, while in the situation of the fontanelle and sutures, the cranium is surprisingly thin. Hunauld exhibited to the Academy of Sciences a scull in this condition, from the thickened portions of which a mixture of blood and serum could be compressed.—ED.

SPINE CROOKED; RIBS DEPRESSED; ARTICULAR EPIPHYSES ENLARGED AND SPONGY; BELLY TUMID; MENTAL FACULTIES CLEAR, OFTEN PREMATURE.

THERE is some doubt about the origin of both the vernacular names. Cretinism, on its first discovery, was by many writers supposed to be produced by an habitual use of water impregnated with chalk or *creta*, in the low Swiss valleys, where it was earliest traced: and it is commonly supposed that the specific name is derived from this opinion.

The English word *rickets* is usually written, in technical language, rhachitis; a name first given to it by Glisson, and said to be derived from ῥάχις (*rhachis*), the spine, in consequence of the distortion and curvature of this organ, occasioned by its being no longer able to bear the weight of the head and upper extremities. As this malady, however, was first observed in England, and particularly in the western counties, and was *provincially* denominated *rickets*, before it attracted the attention of medical writers, it is more probable that rickets is derived from the Saxon *ricg* or *rick*, "a heap or hump," and particularly as applied to the *back*, which also it denotes in a second sense; so that *ricked* or *ricket* is literally, in its full import, "hump-backed." It is from this root we derive *hay-rick*, "a heap of hay," and not, as Dr. Johnson has given it, from "reek," to smoke. Rhachitis might, however, be a word sufficiently good for the present purpose, were it not for its termination; ITIS, in the medical technology of modern times, implying visceral inflammation, and being limited, by a sort of common consent, to the numerous species of disease arranged in the present method under the genus EMPRESMA, which we have considered already (Vol. i., Cl. III., Ord. II., Gen. VII.); and on this account, in the species before us, rhachitis is exchanged for rhachia.

If this disease were known to the Greeks, we should expect to find it, not indeed under the specific term rhachia, but the generic term cyrtosis; for while neither rhachia nor rhachitis is to be traced among the Greek writers in the sense of diseased action, the latter is common to them in the signification already ascribed to it.

There is much reason for believing, however, that both rickets and cretinism are comparatively of modern date: and it is a singular circumstance, that both these species should have been first noticed, and apparently have made their first appearance, coetaneously. The earliest account we have of rickets is that published by Glisson, as it occurred in England in the middle of the seventeenth century; the first account of cretinism is that of Plater, who met with it about the same time in Carinthia and the Valais. The disease is also common in Navarre, and in many of the valleys of the Pyrenees, particularly that of Luchen; and it has been observed by Sir George Staunton as far off as Chinese Tartary, in a part of the country much resembling Switzerland and Savoy in its Alpine appearance. There are some writers, however, who have endeavoured to trace both species of this genus up to the Greeks and Romans. Thus, Zeviani contends that rickets, if not cretinism, is to be discovered in the Roman names of Vari and Valgi, as also in several passages ridiculing deformity, in Thersites, the supposed Æsop of Greece, as well as in other authors (*Della cura di Bambini, attacati della Rhachitide,* cap. ii., p. 15); but all such remarks are too general; he cannot produce a single passage from the medical writers of antiquity, clearly characterizing the peculiar deformities before us. De Haen has attempted to trace the same disease in the works of Hippocrates, but has failed; and hence it is generally admitted in the present day, and has been so from the time of Glisson himself, supported by the concurrent opinions of Bate, Regemorter, Van Swieten, and Trinka, that both rickets and cretinism are of the recent date we have just assigned to them.

The enlargement of the thyroid gland, called goître or bronchocele, is the most striking feature in the unsightly aspect of a cretin; but this, as Dr. Reeve has observed, is not a constant attendant, nor is there any necessary connexion between goitre and cretinism, notwithstanding the assertions and ingenious reasoning of Fodéré. Cretinism is frequently observed without any affection of the thyroid gland, and this gland, on the contrary, is often very much enlarged, without the slightest degree of that affection of the intellectual faculties by which cretinism is particularly marked.—(*Storr, Alpenreise Vorbereitung,* p. 55.)

In order that the various parts of the body should thrive and enlarge in the infancy of life, it is necessary not only that there be a due supply of nutritious food, but that the entire chain of the nutritive organs, from the digestive to the assimilating powers, should be in a state of sound health, and capable of fulfilling their respective functions. In several of the varieties of atrophy this is not the case. In one or two of them we have reason to believe that the digestive process is imperfect, and that the disease is chiefly seated in the chylific viscera. In others, that proper nutriment, though duly introduced into the blood, is not duly elaborated from it, and converted into the structure of the different parts whose waste it is to supply; and consequently that the disease is chiefly seated in the assimilating powers. And in treating of atrophy, we observed that the one extremity of the nutritive chain so closely harmonizes with the other, that, let the disease commence at which end soever it may, the opposite is affected by sympathy. We also observed, that the different divisions of secernents are not all equally under the influence of a morbid torpitude; since occasionally those that secrete the animal oil cease to act long before any of the rest; whence emaciation occurs, and in many instances continues, for some time, as a solitary symptom: and the individual falls away in plumpness, without being sensible of any other failing.

In rickets, the nutritive organs are disturbed generally through the whole length of the chain; but the chief failure is in a due supply of bony earth, or the phosphoric acid that should combine with it. The evident intention of this kind of supply is to enable the bones to expand and acquire maturity while growing, and to uphold their strength and firmness afterward. And so long as they obtain a sufficient supply, and the waste earth of the bones is proportionably carried off by the absorbents, so long this part of the animal economy continues perfect; but, with the exception of the fat or animal oil, there is, perhaps, no secretion that is so liable to have its proper balance disturbed, whether by excess or deficiency, by a morbid condition of the digestive or of the assimilating powers, as that of bony or calcareous earth.

A deficient formation, then, or elaboration of bony earth, constitutes the proximate cause of both rickets and cretinism.* The remote or exciting causes it is not always in our power to ascertain; yet in numerous, perhaps in most instances, we are capable of tracing them to a want of pure air and a warm and dry atmosphere, nutritious food, regular exercise, cleanliness, and the concomitant evils attendant upon a state of poverty; and hence it is chiefly in the hovels of the poor, the destitute, and the profligate, that both diseases are met with; while the severity of the symptoms is very generally in proportion to the extent or multiplication of these concurrent causes.

But there are other diseases which result from the evils we are now contemplating, as well as rickets or cretinism; such as atrophy, scrofula, scurvy, and typhus fevers: and hence there must be some predisponent cause operating in the present instance, and calling rickets into action rather than any one of the rest. Such cause we do not seem always able to trace; but there is reason to believe that it is sometimes dependant upon an hereditary taint of an diopathic nature, sometimes upon a scrofulous or venereal depravation in the constitution of the father or mother. Such, also, is the opinion of Dr. Cullen. "This disease," says he, "may be justly considered as proceeding from parents: for it often appears in a great number of the same family; and my observation leads me to judge, that it originates more frequently from mothers than from fathers. So far as I can refer the disease of the children to the state of the parents, it has appeared to me

---

* This opinion respecting the cause of cretinism, seems to want a foundation; and with regard to rickets, this disease does not consist merely in a deficiency of the secretion of phosphate of lime; for in addition to the loss of their firmness from that cause, there is a disorganization of their minute texture; and this is so much the fact, that in some aggravated examples on record, the walls of the long cylindrical bones admitted of being entirely removed, so as to expose an internal substance, of homogeneous appearance and cellular texture throughout. The manner in which the side of a long cylindrical bone, bent in consequence of rickets, becomes strengthened and thickened at the lesser curvature of it, to which the line of gravity is now transmitted, is a fact on which Mr. Stanley has made some interesting remarks in a paper inserted in the Med. Chir. Trans.—ED.

most commonly to arise from some weakness, and pretty frequently from a scrofulous habit, in the mother."*—"I must remark, however," continues Dr. Cullen, "that in many cases I have not been able to discern the condition of the parents to which I could refer it."—(*Pract. of Phys.*, vol. iv., book ii., ch. iv., § 1722.)

Rickets seldom appears earlier than the ninth month of infancy, and not often later than the second year,† being preceded, according to Dr. Strack, by a paleness and swelling of the countenance, and a yellow, sulphur hue in that part of the cheeks which should naturally be red. —(*Act. Philosophico-Medico Soc. Acad. Princ. Hassiæ*, &c., 4to., *Giessæ Cathorum.*) In some instances it seems to have originated later ; in every stage, indeed, of a child's growth, till the bones have acquired their full size and firmness (*Thomasin, Journ. de Méd.*, tom. xliii., p. 222): and it is said to have occurred even after this. But, in these late appearances, we are generally capable of tracing the disease to some local injury, which acts as an exciting cause, and, for the most part, unites it with PAROSTIA *flexilis.*

Rhachia, in its ordinary course, commences imperceptibly and advances slowly ; the body becomes gradually emaciated, the flesh flaccid, and the cheeks wan or sallow, with a slight degree of tumefaction. As the flesh diminishes in bulk, the head is found to increase, the sutures gape; and the forehead grows prominent. The spine bends, and is incapable of supporting the weight it has to carry ; the ribs and sternum partake of the distortion ; the former lose their convexity, and the latter projects into a ridge.‡

The same deficiency of bony earth runs through the entire skeleton, and affects not only those parts that are composed chiefly of lime and phosphoric acid, as the flat bones and the middle of the long bones, but the extreme knobs or epiphyses, in which lime is combined as largely with carbonic as with phosphoric acid. And hence the joints are loose and spongy, and in swelling keep pace with the head. In many instances the lime appears to be elaborated, but without its correspondent acids, and consequently without compactness, and to no purpose ; for we can occasionally trace it loose in the urine, in which it forms a calcareous deposite, as though carried off from the blood as a recrement.*

All the assimilating powers participate in the debility in a greater or less degree : the process of dentition is slow and imperfect,† and while the cellular membrane is without animal oil, the muscular fibres are tabid, without energy, and almost inirritable. It does not seem, however, that the sensorial power is much interfered with. Some part, indeed, of what should be sent over the frame at large, appears to be concentrated in the sensorium : so that its equipoise is disturbed, but the general average is not, perhaps, much diminished. And hence the curious and interesting fact, that while the body is generally failing, the mind, in many instances, advances in its faculties, insomuch that a very slight recapitulation of the names of those who have been pre-eminently gifted with mental talents in every age and nation, and have immortalized themselves as poets, philosophers, and even leaders in the field, will put before the eye of persons who have not much attended to this subject, a far greater proportion of the humpbacked and the rickety, than they may hitherto have had any conception of. We had occasion to make a like remark when treating of scrofula, and the same fact occurs almost as strikingly in hec-

---

* Dr. Campbell, in his remarks on rhachia, observes, "I have repeatedly, I think, traced rhachitis to a child having been reared on the milk of a woman who menstruated regularly while nursing." —See his Introduction to the Study and Practice of Midwifery, London, 1833.—D.

† Perhaps it would have been more correct to have assigned a longer space for the common period of the commencement of rickets ; as, for instance, the interval between the eighth month and the third year after birth. The disease may begin, however, in the fœtus : in illustration of which fact there is an excellent preparation in the Museum of the London University. It is questionable whether the bones, after the adult age, ever become affected with rickets for the first time.—Ed.

‡ In individuals who are rickety in a considerable degree, the bones of the lower half of the skeleton are always very diminutive in comparison with those of the upper half ; in other words, they are much less developed : a subject on which some interesting observations were published by Mr. A. Shaw, in the Med. Chir. Trans., vol. xvii., p. 434, et seq. The bones of the upper extremity are not often deformed by rickets, though in the Museum of the London University there is the skeleton of a rickety person, where the pressure of crutches has occasioned remarkable curvatures of the humeri, which are also not rightly developed.—Ed.

* "From some late pathological investigations," says Dr. Francis, "it would seem that there is no deficiency of the phosphate of lime in the constitutions of rickety persons, so far as can be ascertained from the blood. The urine of such persons is often found to be freely saturated with the earthy material, and they frequently suffer from bony deposites in parts where nature never intended such deposites. A most instructive case of this character I saw in consultation with the late Dr. Dyckman, in a patient then about seven years of age. The disorder invaded before the child was two years old. It had long lost the use of its inferior extremities, and in the horizontal position in which it had been for more than three years nourished, its power over the movements of the upper extremities and head was nearly lost. The whole force of the ossific action of the system seemed to be confined to the head ; and this was of great weight, and enlarged to full three times its usual size. Hence the opinion that the bones in rickets only change their shape gradually ; that the arteries of the bones of individuals of a rickety constitution are deficient in the power of separating the phosphate of lime from the blood, so as to deposite it in proper quantity for their support ; and that there is actually no deficiency of this material in the body itself."—See Francis's Denman, 3d edition, p. 125.—D.

† The contrary remark is made by several writers, who adduce the fact in proof of the teeth not being affected by the diseases common to the skeleton, and of their not being vascular. —Ed.

tic fever. The progress of the mind does not necessarily depend upon the general progress of the body : in the ordinary course of things, the one runs parallel with the other ; but, in the great field of pathology, where this course is departed from, we are perpetually called to behold proofs, that these powers are by no means one and indivisible ; and that, even before the hour of death, the spirit gives tokens of an advance towards perfection, while the body in its general crasis is imbecile, or perhaps sinking gradually into ruins.

At the commencement of rickets there is rarely any degree of fever, but, as the disease advances, irritability, as in scrofula, succeeds to inirritability, and a hectic is produced. Or it may happen that the sensorium at last participates in a greater degree with the disease of the rest of the frame, and the mind itself becomes enfeebled, and torpid or fatuous.

In the treatment of rickets, the eye should be directed to the two following intentions : that of strengthening the system generally, and that of facilitating a supply of phosphate of lime to the organs that form the chief seat of disease.

For the former purpose, a pure, dry, and temperate atmosphere, a wholesome diet, regular exercise, of such kind as can be indulged in with least inconvenience, cleanliness, and cold bathing, are of essential importance, and have often worked a cure alone. And it is possibly owing to a more general conviction of the advantage of such a regimen in the present enlightened age, that rickets is a complaint far less common now than it was a century or even half a century ago.

A tonic plan of medicines, however, ought to be interposed, and will effectually co-operate with a tonic regimen. As in infancy we can employ those remedies only which are neither very bulky nor very disgustful, we should, for the purpose immediately before us, make choice of the metallic salts. Mr. Boyle is said to have employed, long ago, with very great success, some kind of ens veneris ; and various preparations of copper have since been made use of, and been highly extolled for their virtues in the present disease, especially by Benevoli and Büchner. Dr. Cullen, however, is persuaded, that the ens veneris of Boyle was a preparation not of copper, but of iron ; in fact, the flores martiales of the old dispensatories ; and there is no doubt that this conjecture is right. From the general irritability of the system, irou, indeed, seems to be more advisable on the present occasion than any other metal ; and its stimulant property is a recommendation.

If the appetite fail, which is not common, and the stomach evince acidity and other dyspeptic symptoms, an occasional emetic will be highly serviceable. The bowels must be kept open with rhubarb or neutral salts ; and if the abdomen be tumid, or there be any other symptoms of an affection of the mesenteric glands, mercury in small doses may be advantageously had recourse to, and combined with the tonic plan.

The means of carrying into execution the second intention, or that of producing a direct supply of osseous matter, is accompanied with more difficulty, nor is it certain that we are in possession of any remedy whatever by which this can be accomplished, though it has often been attempted.

Bone may be regarded as a cancelled fabric of gluten, whose cells are filled up with the earth of lime and a combination of carbonic, and especially phosphoric, acid. In all cases of rhachia there seems to be a deficiency of these acids, but particularly of the phosphoric, and in many cases, a deficiency of the earth as well as of the acids.

Acids, however, of every kind, when in excess, have a tendency to dissolve calcareous earth, instead of concreting it into a solid mass : and hence one of the most effectual means of preventing that tendency to the separation or production of a morbid superabundance of calcareous earth in OSTHEXIA and LITHIA, is a free use of acids as a solvent.

A hint has been taken from this effect, and as the disease before us is of ah opposite kind, and evinces a deficiency of lime, and especially of phosphate of lime, instead of an excess, it has been ingeniously proposed to pursue an opposite practice, and to have recourse to a free use of alkalis and alkalescent earths, especially lime united with phosphoric acid, with a view of obtaining the deficient materials. Baron Haller and De Haen employed for this purpose prepared oyster-shells ; but these consist of lime with carbonic acid, and do not, therefore, offer a proper supply for the basis of bones. M. Bonhomme has of late improved upon this practice, by substituting the phosphate of lime or the powder of bones for its carbonate, and uniting it in equal parts with phosphate of soda : of which compound, the dose is a scruple for an infant given twice a day. And he recommends that the body should also be bathed morning and night with an alkaline solution, consisting of half an ounce of common potass in a pound of spring-water. Abilgaard has carried the alkaline plan still farther, and has employed the fixed alkali internally.—(Collect. Soc. Med. Havn., i., art. i.) And as acidity of the stomach in infants seems to be one cause of the disease, and a principal cause, as conjectured by Cappel[*] and Zeviani,[†] where the digestion is evidently at fault, we may in such circumstances reasonably expect benefit from alkaline preparations or magnesia.

How far any preparation of lime introduced into the stomach may be able to find its way without decomposition through the sanguiferous system to the assimilating vessels, and be secerned in the parts affected, has not been exactly determined. Vauquelin made various experiments upon fowls to decide the question, and M. Bonhomme has since attempted others. To themselves these experiments appeared satis-

---

[*] Versuch einen vollerständigen Abhandlung über die Englische krankheit, &c.

[†] Della cura di Bambini attacati della Rhachitide, cap. ii., p. 80.

factory ; but they are open to some objections which have not been entirely removed. Yet we see every day, in a thousand instances, with what facility substances of almost every kind introduced into the stomach are diffused, with little other change than that of minute division, over every part of the system. Emetics do not act till they reach the circulating system : the colouring matter of the madder-root is conveyed to and tinges the most solid bones : prussiate of potash, turpentine, and various other balsams, enter without change into the bladder. It is hence that rape-seed communicates an intolerable taste to hares that feed upon it ; and that the flesh of sheep feeding upon wormwood acquires the bitter flavour of this plant. So the buckthorn gives a cathartic property to the flesh of thrushes that have swallowed it, and scammony to goats' milk. Partridges that have feasted harmlessly on hellebore often occasion sickness when employed as food ; and when oxen have grazed in a pasture abounding with alliaceous plants, the beef they produce possesses the same taste and smell. And hence phosphate of lime may, in like manner, be conveyed from the stomach to the secernents of the bones, and reach them without chymical decomposition.*

As rhachia is peculiarly distinguished by a great irritability and want of action, rubefacients and other cutaneous stimulants have often been employed, and proved serviceable, as well from the friction that accompanies their use as their own actuating power. These have sometimes been so far heightened as purposely to excite some degree of fever, with a view of carrying off the disease by this means ; as dyspepsy, cephalæa, and chronic rheumatism, have often been carried off by a smart attack of a tertian intermittent. We are told that a practice of this kind prevails very generally in the Western Isles, and is productive of great success. The heating oil of the skate-fish is rubbed, every evening, first upon the wrists and ankles of the patient, which raises a fever of several hours' duration ; and when the inunction upon these parts has lost its effect, it is then applied in like manner to the knees and elbows ; and afterward in like manner to the spine ; so that a certain degree of pyrexy may be daily maintained. And when friction on all these organs is found to fail, as fail it will by degrees, a flannel shirt dipped in the oil is finally had recourse to, and worn on the body, which produces a higher degree of fever than has yet existed ; and continues to be worn, after fresh illinations, till a cure is obtained, which is said to be pretty certain, and usually in a short time.

Many ingenious devices have been executed by surgical instrument-makers for giving support to the limbs that seem mostly to suffer, and for removing the weight of the body from one part to another. In infancy, however, all these are of little avail, and where the disease pervades the entire skeleton, they will always do as much mischief as good, by aiding one part at the expense of another. The best mechanical instruments are a hard incompressible couch, and a level floor, on which the infant may lie at full length, and stretch his limbs as he pleases. The couch, or rather mattress, should be made light and moveable, and especially unyielding, so that he may be carried upon it in the open air for exercise. Moderate warmth is of great service, but a downy bed that gives way to the pressure of the body, and sinks into unequal hollows, cannot fail to increase the incurvation.*

SPECIES II.
CYRTOSIS CRETINISMUS
CRETINISM.

CHIEFLY AFFECTING THE HEAD AND NECK : COUNTENANCE VACANT AND STUPID : MENTAL FACULTIES FEEBLE OR IDIOTIC : SENSIBILITY OBTUSE : MOSTLY WITH ENLARGEMENT OF THE THYROID GLAND.

CRETINISM makes a very close approach to rickets in its general symptoms. It differs principally in the tendency to the peculiar enlargement of the thyroid gland, which in France is denominated goitre, and with us Derbyshire-neck, and in the mental imbecility which accompanies it from the first.

In treating of rhachitis we observed, that while all the functions of the general frame are here in a state of great debility, with the exception of the mental, these last exhibited in many instances a precocity and a vigour rarely found in firm health. On the contrary, in cretinism the organ of the brain seems to follow the fate of the rest of the body, and, in many cases, even to take the lead ; so that the chief imbecility is to be found in this region. For the peculiar symptom of goître, it is not so easy to account. We know so little of the purpose, and even of the fabric, of this gland, as to be incapable of assigning its use in the animal economy ;† and hence it is not much to be

---

* On the Nature and Treatment of the Distortions to which the Spine and Bones of the Chest are subject, &c., by John Shaw, 8vo., 1823.

† For information on this subject, the editor refers the reader to a late publication, entitled, The Anatomy of the Thymus Gland, by Sir Astley Cooper, Bart., 4to., Lond., 1832. The author having ascertained that the thymus secretes all the parts of the blood, and that after birth it does not continue to perform the same office as it does in the fœtus, is led to suggest the following query : —" Is it not probable that the gland is designed to prepare a fluid, well fitted for the fœtal growth and nourishment, from the blood of the mother, before the birth of the fœtus, and consequently before chyle is formed from food ; and that this process continues for a short time after birth, the quantity of fluid secreted from the thymus gradually declining as chylification becomes perfectly established ?" (p. 44.) The anatomical observations, which are quite original, are very curious and instructive.—ED.

---

* The editor has seen several examples of rickets and disunited fractures, where phosphate of lime was freely exhibited to the patients, but without the slightest benefit.

wondered at, that its peculiar tendency to associate, in the present disease, with the morbid condition of the bones and of the intellect, should not hitherto have been ascertained. It does not, however, accompany the other symptoms, though it is, for the most part, an associate.

We have already observed, that cretinism was first distinctly noticed and described by Plater, about the middle of the seventeenth century, as occurring among the poor in Carinthia and the Valais ; and that it was afterward found in a still severer degree in other valleys in Switzerland and the Alps generally ; as it has since been detected in very distant regions where the country exhibits a similarity of features, as among a miserable race called Caggets, inhabiting the hollows of the Pyrenees, whose district and history have been given us by M. Raymond, and as far off as Chinese Tartary, where it is represented as existing by Sir George Staunton.

On the first discovery of cretinism, it was ascribed by some to the use of snow-water, and by others, to the use of water impregnated with calcareous earth : both which opinions are entirely without foundation. The first is sufficiently disproved by observing, that persons born in places contiguous to the glaciers, and who drink no other water than what flows from the melting of ice and snow, are not subject to the disorder ; and that Sir John Pringle and Captain Cook found melted snow or ice-water afford to seamen a peculiarly wholesome beverage : while, on the contrary, the disorder is observed in places where snow is unknown, as at Sumatra. The second is contradicted by the fact, that the common waters of Switzerland, instead of being impregnated with calcareous matter, excel those of most other countries in Europe in purity and flavour. "There is not," observes Dr. Reeve, "a village, nor a valley, but what is enlivened by rivulets, or streams gushing from the rocks. The water usually drunk at La Batia and Martigny is from the river Dranse, which flows from the glacier of St. Bernard, and falls into the Rhone ; it is remarkably free from earthy matter, and well tasted. At Berne, the water is extremely pure ; yet, as Haller remarks, swellings of the throat are not uncommon in both sexes, though cretinism is rare."

As comfortable and genial warmth forms one of the best auxiliaries in attempting the cure of both cretinism and rickets, there can be no doubt that the chill of snow-water, if taken as such, must considerably add to the general debility of the system when labouring under either of these diseases, though there seems no reason for supposing that it would originate either. It is not difficult to explain why water impregnated with calcareous earth should have been regarded as a cause ; for in cretinism, as in rhachia, the calcareous earth designed by nature for building up the bones, is often separated, and floats loose in various fluids of the body, for want of a sufficiency of phosphoric acid to convert it into a phosphate of lime, and give it solidity. And as

it is, in consequence hereof, pretty freely discharged by the urine, it seems to have given rise to the opinion, that such calcareous earth was introduced into the system with the common beverage of the lakes or rivers, and produced the morbid symptoms.

M. de Saussure has assigned a far more probable cause of the disease in referring us to a few other physical features of the Alpine districts, in which it makes its appearance chiefly. The valleys, he tells us, are surrounded by very high mountains, sheltered from currents of fresh air, and exposed to the direct, and, what is worse, the reflected rays of the sun. They are marshy, and the atmosphere is hence humid, close, and oppressive. And when to these chorographical causes we add the domestic ones, which are also well known to prevail very generally among the poor of these regions, such as meager, innutritious food,—concerning which we have already spoken under bronchocele,—indolence, and uncleanliness, with a predisposition to the disease from an hereditary taint of many generations, we can sufficiently account for the prevalence of cretinism in such places, and for the most humiliating characters it is ever found to assume.

The general symptoms of cretinism are those of rhachia ; but the disease shows itself earlier, often at birth, and not unfrequently before this period, apparently commencing with the procreation of the fœtus, and affording the most evident proofs of ancestral contamination.* The child, if not deformed and cachectic at birth, soon becomes so ; the body is stinted in its growth, and the organs in their development ; the abdomen swells, the skin is wrinkled, the muscles are loose and flabby, the throat is covered with a monstrous prominence, the complexion wan, and the countenance vacant and stupid. The cranium bulges out to an enormous size,† and particularly towards the occiput, for it is sometimes depressed on the crown and at the temples ; insomuch that, to a front view, the

---

* The hereditary nature of cretinism is not universally acknowledged : thus, Dr. Bostock mentions cretinism " as one of the most remarkable examples of the influence of external circumstances, both upon the physical and intellectual powers. It consists," he observes, " in a state of mental imbecility, combined with, and probably depending upon, a malformation of the head. It appears to be generated by something peculiar to the atmosphere of the confined valleys, and *does not seem to be hereditary.*"—(Elem. Syst. of Physiology, vol. iii., p. 295.) If, however, this affection depends upon malformation of the scull, one would conclude that the other alleged causes must be abandoned.—ED.

† This statement disagrees with the account given by Larrey of the cases which he saw and particularly examined in the valley of Maurienne. In all these examples, the cranium was remarkably diminutive. The thickness, also, noticed in the bones of the cranium, is repugnant to some of our author's statements respecting the impediment to the secretion of lime in the bones. On the whole, it does not appear that there is any resemblance, or any essential connexion, between rickets and cretinism.—ED.

head in some cases appears even diminutive. The blunted sensibility of these wretched beings renders them indifferent to the action of cold and heat, and even to blows or wounds. " They are generally," observes M. Pinel, " both deaf and dumb. The strongest and most pungent odours scarcely affect them. I know a cretin who devours raw onions and even charcoal with great avidity ; a striking proof of the coarseness and imperfect development of the organ of taste. Their organs of sight and feeling are equally limited in their operation. Of moral affections they seem wholly destitute ; discovering no signs of gratitude for kindness shown to them, nor any attachment to their nearest relations."

The medical treatment, if medicine can ever be of any avail, should be conducted upon the principles and consist of the process laid down under the preceding species.

GENUS V.
OSTHEXIA.
OSTHEXY.

SOFT PARTS MORE OR LESS INDURATED BY A SUPERFLUOUS SECRETION AND DEPOSITE OF OSSIFIC MATTER.

OSTHEXIA is derived from ὀστώδης, " osseous or bony," and ἕξις, " habitus or habit,"—" ossific diathesis or idiosyncrasy." This morbid affection, though repeatedly alluded to and described by miscellaneous writers, has seldom been attended to in nosological arrangements. It does not occur in Dr. Cullen's Classification ; but he alludes to it in his " Catalogue of omitted Diseases," as one of those which he thinks ought not to be omitted.

We have had various occasions for remarking, that, as the calcareous earth, which gives compactness and solidity to the skeleton of the animal frame, becomes waste, and is consequently absorbed and carried off, it is necessary that there should be an equal and regular supply of the same material. This is partly obtained from the lime which enters, in some proportion or other, into almost every kind of nutriment on which we feed : but it seems to be obtained also, and perhaps in a larger proportion, by some chymical elaboration out of the constituent principles of the blood itself : for a healthy animal of any kind appears to supply itself with the requisite quantity of bony earth, whatever be the nature of its food, and though the soil on which it is grown contains no lime whatever, as is the case in several of the Polynesian Islands, and throughout the whole of New South Wales, on the hither side of the Blue Mountains.

In several of the preceding genera we have seen that this material is produced or secreted in deficiency ; on the contrary, in the species appertaining to the present genus, it is produced or secreted in excess ; and deposited, sometimes in single organs for which it is not naturally intended, and sometimes throughout the system at large, occasionally in the parenchyma or general substance of organs, and occasionally

in the membranes or tunics by which they are covered and protected, or in the vessels by which they are furnished with their proper stores.

We see much of this irregularity in old age. The excernent vessels of both sets, absorbents and secretories, partake of the common debility and torpitude of this advanced period. Hence, in all probability, a smaller quantity of lime, as of every other secerned material, is formed at this period, than in the earlier and more vigorous stages of life : but, however small the quantity, it is not carried off with adequate freedom by the debilitated absorbents, and is apt to stagnate, first in the bones themselves, which, as we have already observed, are hereby rendered unduly impacted and brittle, and next in other parts of the system, especially between the muscular and internal coats of the arteries, which are hereby often rendered rigid or even ossific.

This is a natural consequence of the debility of advancing years. But we not unfrequently meet with a like effect in the earlier stages of life, and in persons of the fullest and most vigorous health : in which case, the lime, thus profusely and erratically deposited, is produced and secreted in excess, and consequently by a state of action the very reverse of that we have thus far contemplated.

The mischief, thus originating, lays a foundation, as it appears in the parenchyma, or in the membranes or vessels of organs, for two very distinct trains of symptoms, and may be contemplated under the two following species :—

1. Osthexia Infarciens.　Parenchymatous Osthexy.
2. ———— Implexa.　Vascular Osthexy.

SPECIES I.
OSTHEXIA INFARCIENS.
PARENCHYMATOUS OSTHEXY.

OSSIFIC MATTER DEPOSITED IN NODULES OR AMORPHOUS MASSES, IN THE PARENCHYMA OF ORGANS.

THE most common organs in which calculous concretions are found, are the kidneys and the bladder ; but as in these they form detached and unconnected balls, and are intimately united with local symptoms or a morbid state of these organs, and constitute only one of various kinds of concretions, it will be most convenient to consider them when treating of the particular diseases to which they give rise, or of which they are prominent symptoms.*

The organ in whose interior fabric the present concretions are most usually found, seems to be the pineal gland ; of which almost all the medical and physiological journals, as well domestic as foreign, give numerous examples, as do likewise Diemerbroeck, De Graaf, Schrader, and other monographists. In this gland they

---

* Most of the concretions formed in the kidneys and bladder, do not consist of lime or ossific matter, but of lithic acid ; and even some of those which contain lime are composed, not of the phosphate or carbonate, but of the oxalate of lime. Such is the nature of what are called *mulberry calculi.*—ED

have also been found in other animals than man, chiefly those of the deer kind.

Such deposites are also frequently found in various other parts of the substance of the brain ; in the lungs (*Baillie, Morb. Anat.*, fasc. ii., pl. 6) ; in the substance of the heart, in one instance weighing two ounces (*Burnet, Thesaur. Med. Pract.*, iii., 254) ; in the thymus gland (*Act. Med. Berol.*, tom. i., dec. iii., 28); in the thyroid (*Contuli, de Lapid.*, &c.) ; in the parotid (*Plater, Observ.*, lib. iii., 707), the sublingual, and most other glands ;[*] in the deltoid and most other muscles ;[†] nor is there an organ in which ossification[‡] has not been traced on different occasions. Paullini records one instance of an ossified penis ; in the Ephemera of Natural Curiosities we meet with another (dec. ii., ann. v.) ; and M. Forlenze has lately met with an extensive ossification in the globe of the eye. The sclerotica was natural, but not only the crystalline lens, which is often found in this state, but the iris and the vitreous humour, were completely ossified.[§]

The general pathology we have already given : the symptoms and effects vary to infinity. Most of the above cases seem to have occurred after the meridian of life.

SPECIES II.
OSTHEXIA IMPLEXA.
VASCULAR OSTHEXY.

OSSIFIC MATTER DEPOSITED IN CONCENTRIC LAYERS IN THE TUNICS OF VESSELS OR MEMBRANES, RENDERING THEM RIGID AND UNIMPRESSIBLE.

ALL the vessels and membranes, as well as the more massy or complicated organs of the body, are subject to deposites of phosphate or carbonate of lime, from the causes already

pointed out : some of which are those of weak, and others of entonic action ; the former operating upon the debilitated and the aged, the latter upon the young and vigorous, who labour under a peculiar diathesis or predisposition to the formation of bony earth. The chief modifications appertaining to this species, may be contemplated under the following varieties :—

a Arterialis.   Ossification of the aorta or
  Arterial osthexy. other large arteries.
β·Membranacea.   Ossification of membranous
  Membranous os- or connecting parts.
  thexy.
γ Complicata.   Ossification of different parts
  Complicated os- simultaneously.
  thexy.

Where the DEPOSITE TAKES PLACE IN THE AORTA, it is rarely confined to this artery alone, but spreads to some parts of the heart, and perhaps to the pulmonary, or some other large artery as well. Dr. Baillie gives an instance, in which a considerable portion of the right ventricle and right auricle of the heart was simultaneously affected (*Morb. Anat.*, fasc. v., pl. 2) ; and Morgagni another, in which the ossification extended to the valves, and this too without having produced in the patient either palpitation or dyspnœa.—(*De Sed. et Caus.*, ep. xxiii., 11.) So wonderfully is the instinctive or remedial power of nature capable, in various instances, of accommodating the general system to morbid changes.

We have other examples of the trunk of the aorta being wholly ossified (*Buchner, Miscel.*, 1727, p. 305), and in one case so rigidly, both in its ascending and descending branches, as to compel the sufferer to maintain an erect position.—(*Guattani, de Aneurismate*, &c.)*

---

* Haller, Pr. de induratis corp. hum. partibus, Göett., 1753. Pranser, Diss. de induratione corp. in specie ossium, Leips., 1705.

† In a case occurring in the practice of Dr. David L. Rogers of New-York (Am. Journ. of Med. Sc., vol. xiii., p. 387), the pectoralis major muscle was ossified at its superior part, and extended in the direction of the clavicle to the arm ; the sterno-cleido-mastoideus was ossified from the sternum to its middle portion ; all the muscles going to the scapula were more or less affected. The latissimus dorsi formed a large bony plate from its origin to the angle of the scapula ; and the longissimus dorsi was in a similar condition, extending along the spine like a splint. On examination after death, the ossification was found to be confined to the muscular tissue ; the tendons of the muscles and the vessels were not affected.—D.

‡ Sometimes the author seems to employ the term *ossification* as synonymous with any *calculous* or *earthy formation*, which is by no means correct. In the process of ossification, a peculiar action of the secernent vessels is essentially concerned ; but the production of a calculus in the bladder, salivary ducts, urethra, &c., may arise from a deposite of certain elements, or principles, contained in the urine or saliva.—Ed.

§ Dict. des Sciences Médicales, art. Cas Rares. Many other similar cases are on record, and a very remarkable one is described by Scarpa, in his work on Diseases of the Eye.—Ed.

* A. W. Otto remarks, " that ossification of the arteries appears under various forms ; thus, in rare instances, as little distinct specks of bone in the previously formed plate of cartilage, surrounded by a large vascular circle ; or, more commonly, as a pap-like substance, sometimes white, sometimes yellow, consisting of phosphate of lime and albumen, a milky fluid very similar to fluid lime, which gradually becomes firmer, leather-like, at last bony ; and finally, as earthy or gypsum-like small specks and flakes, not unfrequently exhibiting traces of crystallization. These three kinds of ossification often occur at once in a large artery, for instance the aorta, and then at the same time form more or less numerous isolated or closely approximated irregular bony scales, indeed even actual unbroken bony cylinders, which prevent the approximation of a divided artery, and in the application of a ligature to it, break like a cracked egg-shell. These ossifications have their original seat always between the serous and fibrous coats of the artery, although in their increasing thickness they sometimes destroy, by pressure and irritation, parts of both coats, so that within they are immediately washed by the blood, and project into the cavity of the artery as irregular plates, generally yellow, or as points and processes ; this cavity is often very much narrowed and even filled with them. Ossification of the arteries is but rarely observed in young persons ; very frequently, though by no means as a natural condition, in more advanced age ; perhaps some-

The most troublesome of the membranous ossifications are those of the pleura, of which an example is given by Dr. Baillie in his Morbid Anatomy (fascic. ii., pl. i.) : though the trachea affords at times severe and even fatal examples of this affection (*Kirkring, Specileg. Anat.,* obs. 27), in consequence of the stricture which is hereby occasionally produced. Mr. Chester gives a singular case of the spread of this disease over the thoracic duct, the ileum, and other abdominal viscera.

Yet, in the structure of the arteries, ossification is found more frequently than in any other organ, with the exception of the pineal gland : the cause of which seems to have been regarded as very obscure by Dr. Baillie, and especially when compared with the very few instances in which ossification takes place in the veins.—(*Wardrop's edition of his Works,* vol. i., p. 43.) Yet a probable cause may be pointed out ; and it appears to have been first glanced at by Dr. Hunter, and was afterward followed up with much patient investigation and accuracy of research by Mr. Cruickshank. The former used to send round at his lectures a preparation of the patella, in which he demonstrated that the ossification of that bone began in the arteries running through the centre of the cartilage which, in young subjects, supplies the place of a bony patella. Mr. Cruickshank, on prosecuting the subject, discovered, that all other bones ossify in the same manner, and made preparations in proof of this fact ; distinctly showing that the ossification of bones is not only begun, but carried on and completed, by the ossification of their arteries.

[That cartilages ossify in consequence of the deposition of lime in them by the arteries, is now perfectly established ; but the statement concerning conversion of these arteries themselves into bone, is one that is not at present generally entertained. The internal coat of the arteries, or, to use Bichat's more comprehensive expression, the internal membrane of the whole system of scarlet blood, is noted for its singular tendency in elderly persons to ossify. Bichat calculated, that in every ten subjects past their sixtieth year, the arteries of at least seven have earthy incrustations on them. These ossifications, which never have any thing to do with the proper fibrous or middle coat, always begin upon the external surface of the internal coat, for the incrustation is constantly lined by a thin pellicle, which intervenes between it and the circulating blood, and is obviously the internal coat itself. It is also a remark made by the same physiologist,

what more frequently in men than women ; it is by no means equally common in all parts of the body. Thus we observe it, for instance, in the smaller much more rarely than the larger arteries ; in those of the upper less frequently than in those of the lower extremities ; very rarely in the pulmonary arteries ; the arteries of the walls of the chest and belly, and perhaps those of the alimentary canal and liver, are never ossified : on the contrary, it is common in the aorta, the angle of the carotids, the arteries of the pelvis, brain, thyroid gland, heart, spleen, kidneys," &c., &c.—D.

that these calcareous depositions are not regulated by the laws of common ossification, the cartilaginous state rarely preceding them. The earthy matter is always deposited in detached plates or scales, of greater or lesser breadth ; and the whole artery is seldom converted into one solid tube. Thus, the portions of the internal coat between the scales, were considered by Bichat as so many particular bands ; the arteries thus ossified being composed of numerous pieces, moveable upon each other, and capable in a certain degree of yielding to the impulse of the circulation.

While these earthy plates continue thin, the inside of the artery retains its natural smoothness ; but, when they become thicker, they project into the cavity of the vessel. The thin pellicle covering them, and continuous with the artery, now breaks on a level with their circumference, so that they then adhere merely by their external surface to the proper fibrous coat. Thus, their circumference becomes unequal and rugous ; and if they be numerous, the whole inner surface of the artery is studded with asperities. This course of the disease is frequently exemplified at the origin, and even in other parts of the aorta. The rupture of the inner coat is facilitated by its natural fragility. The ramifications are less frequently the seat of these earthy incrustations than the trunks ; and, as they never occur in the capillary system, Bichat was inclined to think that the common membrane of the system of red blood, in other words, the inner coat of the arteries, does not extend to the capillaries. In the heart is frequently affected, particularly where it forms the aortic and mitral valves. The disease is less common on the inner surface of the left ventricle, auricle, and pulmonary veins, though Bichat had seen instances of it in the latter. This general disposition to ossification is a clear proof that the nature of this membrane is everywhere similar. Bichat imputes the frequent intermission of the pulse in old age to ossification of the lining of the heart : ossifications at the commencement of the aorta also disturb the circulation ; but those of arterial trunks and branches produce no derangement of it.

It is one of Bichat's doctrines, that ossification of the common membrane of the system of red blood is essentially different from those which happen in other parts, inasmuch as it is, as it were, a natural change ; whereas others seem accidental, and are often preceded by inflammation. They are not the result of old age ; but often take place in young persons. He admits that the common membrane of the system of red blood does sometimes ossify in the early stages of life ; but much less frequently than in old age. An ossification of the mitral valves, with which an old man lives very well, and which merely causes an intermission of his pulse, produces the most grievous effects in a younger person,—difficulty of breathing, frequent risk of suffocation, cough, irregular pulse, necessity for constant extension of the trunk, and, in an advanced stage of the case, anasarca, effusion of serum in the chest, spitting of blood,

&c.—(See *Anat. Gén.*, t. i., p. 281.) In the arteries of the abdominal viscera of old subjects, the internal coat is sometimes wrinkled and peculiarly brittle.—(*Soemmering de Corp. Hum. Fabr.*, t. v., p. 58.)

One of the most extensive appearances of this habit acting morbidly on the tunics of vessels, is related by Dr. Heberden (*Med. Trans.*, vol. v., art. xiii.), in the case of a very old man, who at last died suddenly, as well indeed he might, since almost the only viscus that was found, on examination, to be in a healthy state, was the liver. The internal carotid and basilary arteries, with many of their primary branches, were ossified. Through the substance of the lungs, which firmly adhered to their walls, were scattered small calculous tumours. In the heart, the valves of the left auriculo-ventricular opening were partially ossified, those of the aorta completely so, and small depositions of bony matter were found in the tendinous portions of the carneæ columnæ. The coronary artery was ossified through its whole extent. The descending thoracic and abdominal aorta, with all their primary branches, were converted into cylinders of bone, as were the external and internal iliacs. It is not necessary to pursue the description into the morbid appearances of almost every other organ : and I shall only observe farther, that, though the substance of the brain was healthy, the ventricles contained about eight ounces of water. And yet, with all this extent of diseased structure, the patient appeared almost to the last to be of a sound constitution, and free from the usual infirmities of advanced age, with the exception of an habitual deafness ; and he attained upwards of fourscore years of age.

Where this diathesis prevails very decidedly, it sometimes converts, not merely the vessels, but the whole of the tendons and the muscles, into rigid bones, and renders the entire frame as stiff and immoveable as the trunk of a tree. There is a striking illustration of this remark in a case communicated to the Royal Society by Dr. Henry of Enniskillen.—(*Phil. Trans.*, vol. li., year 1759.) The patient was a day-labourer, who had enjoyed good health till the time of his being attacked by this disease. It commenced with a pain and swelling in the right wrist, which gradually assumed a bony hardness, and extended up the course of the muscles as high as the elbow, the whole of which were convert-

ed into a like hardness, and were of double their natural size. The left wrist and arm followed the fate of the right : and the line of ossification next shot down to the extremities of the fingers on both sides, and afterward up to the shoulders, so that the joints were completely anchylosed, and the man was pinioned. At the time of communicating this history, the same ossific mischief had attacked the right ankle, with a like degree of pain, swelling, and bony induration, up the course of the muscles : in which state the man was discharged from the hospital as incurable, after salivation had been tried to no purpose.

Salivation has, indeed, often been tried, probably from its success in removing venereal nodes ; but it does not seem to have been of much avail.

We have pointed out two opposite causes, or rather states of body, in which a tendency to ossification chiefly shows itself. One is that of general debility, and the other of an entonic action in the assimilating organs which are chiefly concerned in the fabrication or separation of lime : and in laying down any plan for relief, it seems necessary to attend to this distinction. Where debility becomes a predisponent of morbid ossification, it is mostly a result or concomitant of old age, a scrofulous diathesis, or atonic gout : and, in all these cases, warmth, a generous diet, and tonic course of medicines, will form the most reasonable curative plan that can be pursued ; and that which will tend most effectually to stimulate the absorbents, and prevent that retardation of bony earth in the lymphatics and vasa vasorum, on which we have already shown the disease to depend in this modification of it.

On the contrary, where it occurs in the middle and vigour of life, and, we have reason to believe, from the existence of too much action in vessels which we cannot very accurately follow up, a reducent plan will be far more likely to prove successful. We should bleed and move the bowels freely, and restrain the patient to a low diet, with a copious allowance of diluent drinks.

And, in both cases, with a view of dissolving, as far as we are able, the calcareous matter that may morbidly exist in the system already, or be on the point of entering into it, we should prescribe a free use of the mineral or vegetable acids, as already recommended under PAROSTIA *fragilis.*

ORDER II.
CATOTICA.
DISEASES AFFECTING INTERNAL SURFACES.

PRAVITY OF THE FLUIDS OR EMUNCTORIES THAT OPEN INTO THE INTERNAL SURFACES OF ORGANS.

CATOTICA is derived from κάτω, "infra," whence κατώτερος and κατώτατος, "inferior," and "infimus." The Order includes four genera, as follow, some of which will be found of extensive range :—

I. Hydrops.   . Dropsy.
II. Emphysema.   Inflation. Wind-Dropsy.
III. Paruria.   Mismicturition.
IV. Lithia.   Urinary Calculus.

GENUS I.
HYDROPS.
DROPSY.

PALE, INDOLENT, AND INELASTIC DISTENTION OF THE BODY OR ITS MEMBERS, FROM ACCUMULATION OF A WATERY FLUID IN NATURAL CAVITIES.

HYDROPS is a Greek term (ὕδρωψ) importing an accumulation of water : and, in nosology, there is no genus of diseases that has been more awkwardly handled. The term hydrops does not occur in Sauvages, Linnéus, or Sagar, and only once in Vógel—in the compound hydrops *scroti*. Linnéus connects anasarca and ascites, its chief species, with tympanites, polysarcia, or corpulence, and graviditas or pregnancy, into one ordinal division, which he names TUMIDOSI, and of which these constitute distinct genera. Sagar arranges all the same under the ordinal division CACHEXIÆ. Vogel pursues the same plan, with the omission of graviditas or pregnancy, which he does not choose to regard as a cachexy. Sauvages employs the term *hydropes*, but only in connexion with *partiales*, in order to restrain it to local dropsies : so that with him, ascites is a hydrops, but anasarca is not a hydrops, and does not even belong to the same order : it is an *intumescentia*, under which, as in the arrangement of Linnéus, it is united with corpulence and pregnancy ; while hydrops *thoracis* is an anhelatio, and occurs in a distinct place and volume.

Dr. Cullen has certainly and very considerably improved upon his predecessors in this range of diseases. After Sauvages, he takes INTUMESCENTIÆ for the name of his order ; but divides it into the four sections of adiposæ, flatuosæ, aquosæ vel hydropes, and solidæ ; while under the third section (the aquosæ vel hydropes) he introduces all the family of dropsies, whether general or local, instead of sending them, with those who preceded him, to different quarters. It would, however, have been a much greater improvement, and have added to the simplicity he aimed at, to have employed hydrops as a generic, instead of hydropes as a tribal or family term. It is to Boerhaave we are indebted for the first use of hydrops as employed in the present method ; and he has been followed by Dr. Macbride and Dr. Young, with a just appreciation of his correctness.

The species of this genus, which extend over the body generally, or almost all the different parts of it, are the following :—

1. Hydrops Cellularis.	Cellular Dropsy.
2. ——— Capitis.	Dropsy of the Head.
3. ——— Spinæ.	——— Spine.
4. ——— Thoracis.	——— Chest.
5. ——— Abdominis.	——— Belly.
6. ——— Ovarii.	——— Ovary
7. ——— Tubalis.	——— Fallopian Tube.
8. ——— Uteri.	——— Womb.
9. ——— Scroti.	——— Scrotum.

Before we enter upon a distinct view of the history and treatment of these several species, it may be convenient to give a glance at the general pathological principles which apply to the whole.

All dropsies proceed from similar causes, which, as they are general or local, produce a general or local disease. The common predisponent cause is debility.* The remote causes are very numerous, and most of them apply to every form under which the disease makes its appearance ; for the accumulation of watery fluid, which constitutes the most prominent symptom of the malady, may be produced by a profuse halitus from the terminal arteries, occasioning too large a supply of that fine lubricating fluid, which, as we have observed in the Physiological Proem to the present class, flows from the surface of all internal organs, and enables them to play with ease and without attrition upon each other ;† it may be produced by a torpid or inactive condition of the correspondent ab-

* This doctrine is rapidly declining. Dr. Armstrong justly observes, that "it is a very important part of modern pathology to ascertain the causes of certain symptoms. When dropsy was supposed to be a disease proceeding necessarily from weakness, almost all cases were fatal. But though experience has fully proved that the theory about weakness being the cause of dropsy is incorrect, it is surprising that such an idea still exists. Dropsy is a mere symptom—the effect of very different conditions."—See Lectures on the Morbid Anatomy, Nature, and Treatment of Acute and Chronic Diseases, p. 841, 8vo., Lond., 1834.—ED.

† For a collection of fluid to take place, so as to constitute dropsy, the cavity in which the secretion occurs must either be completely closed, or, at all events, not permit the effused fluid to escape from the system. The cellular and adipose tissues, and the serous membranes, are therefore the only parts in which the collections of fluid, comprised under the generic term of dropsy, can be formed. Dropsies of mucous membranes are, indeed, sometimes treated of ; but, as Andral explains, no disease of this nature can occur in them, unless their communication with the atmosphere be accidentally interrupted. Thus, the phrase, *dropsy of the stomach*, has been applied to cases in which the pylorus does not readily allow the alimentary matter to pass through it, and this matter being blended with the gastric secretions, a large accumulation of fluid is produced in the stomach. *Dropsy of the uterus* also denotes a case in which, from a contracted state of the os tincæ, an extraordinary quantity of fluid collects

sorbents, occasioning too small a removal of this fluid, when it has answered its purpose and has become waste matter ; or it may be produced by each of these diseased conditions of both sets of vessels operating at the same time ; and it is to this double deviation from healthy action that Dr. Cullen applies the name of an hydropic diathesis.*

If we minutely attend to the histories of those who are suffering from this disease, we shall generally find that they have for some time antecedently been labouring under debility, either general or local ; that they are weakened by protracted fevers, or languishing under the effects of an unkindly lying-in ; that they have unstrung their frames by a long exposure to a cold and moist atmosphere, or have worn themselves out by hard labour ; or, which is still worse, by hard eating and drinking ; or that they are suffering from habitual dyspepsy, or some other malady of the stomach or chylopoëtic organs, especially the liver, which destroys or deranges the digestive process, and hence lays a foundation for atrophy. And for the same reason, innutritious†

or indigestible food is a frequent cause of some species of this disease : as is also great loss of blood from any organ, and especially when such discharge becomes periodical.* Copious and frequently repeated bleeding, for the relief of acute diseases, is also very commonly followed by dropsy.†

Where the digestive organs are in a very morbid state, dropsy may take place as a result of general debility ; but it more commonly occurs from that peculiar sympathy which prevails so strikingly between the two ends of the extensive chain of the nutritive, or, in other words, the digestive and assimilating powers, which we had occasion to explain when treating of marasmus (Cl. III., Ord. IV., Gen. III., opening remarks) : the inertness and relaxation of the excernent vessels being in this case produced by the torpitude of the chylopoëtic viscera ; and the usual forms of dropsy being those of the cellular membrane or of the abdomen. Hence a single indulgence in large draughts of cold drinks, and especially of cold water, when the system is

---

in the womb. Andral has seen one instance, in which, in consequence of an obliteration of the neck of the gall-bladder, this organ was distended, not with bile, but a limpid secretion resembling serum. A small quantity of fluid is always met with in cavities lined by serous membranes, when a body is examined more than thirty hours after death : but this must not be mistaken for a dropsical disease ; it is merely a transudation of the thinner parts of the blood, after life has terminated ; referrible to the commencement of putrefaction, by which the texture both of the blood and the vessels is loosened. Sometimes the fluid that transudes in this way is colourless ; sometimes tinged with blood. According to M. Gendrin, a larger quantity of fluid is generally effused after death in the serous cavities of young subjects than in those of adults, and especially of old persons.—See Gendrin, Hist. Anat. des Inflammations ; Andral, Anat. Pathol., tom. i., p. 316.—ED.

* Although dropsy may be attended with increased exhalation, or diminished absorption, it seemed to Dr. Bateman (and in his opinion the editor coincides), that an investigation of the various causes capable of producing these morbid conditions, proves the exhalant vessels to be most commonly in fault ; and that increased effusion is most frequently the source of dropsy.

† In a part of France which was desolated by famine a few years ago, and where the poor classes could get scarcely any thing but the most common vegetables of the fields to eat, many of these persons became dropsical.—(See Dr. Gaspard's account of the effects of this famine in Magendie's Jour. de Physiologie.) One of the first effects of this wretched diet would certainly be that of lessening the quantity of fibrinous matter in the blood. M. Andral, in his Clinique Médicale, tom. iii., has given an account of several persons who died of dropsy, and in whom no traces of any organic disease could be detected, the only remarkable circumstance being an entire absence of blood both from the large vessels and the capillaries, in lieu of which fluid they contained only a pale reddish serum. The rapid anasarcous and dropsical swellings following the operation of certain poisons, especially those of particular reptiles, are ascribed by Andral to the action of such poisons on the blood, the altered quality of which is evinced by its incapability of coagulating.—ED.

* That cellular and abdominal dropsy are generally associated with debility, can hardly be disputed ; yet, as we see persons linger a long while in the most abject state of weakness, and at length die without exhibiting any signs of dropsy, mere weakness alone, however it may facilitate the occurrence of the disease, cannot be regarded as the essential cause. When disease of the liver, uterus, or lungs, brings on general impairment of the health, and, among other effects, ascites or anasarca, and universal debility and emaciation, we ought rather to look at the disease of the important organ primarily affected as the cause of the dropsy, than to the debility, which is itself only an effect. But that debility sometimes cannot even be suspected as the cause of the effusion must be quite evident, in cases where anasarca is plainly occasioned by pressure, obstructing the circulation in the large venous trunks, independently of any other disease. In examples of diseased liver, the origin of dropsy is mostly referred to obstruction of the circulation in the system of the vena portæ ; a doctrine that furnishes another argument against the essential dependance of dropsy upon debility.

In individuals who become dropsical in the course of chronic diseases, Andral conceives it possible that a state of the blood may exist similar to what happens in persons who have lost too much blood. In fact, in every disease of severity and long duration, this fluid becomes less plentiful and less rich in fibrin. Yet, as is well observed, if this were the only true cause of the dropsy that occurs towards the end of many chronic diseases, why should that disorder so rarely attend pulmonary tubercles, the existence of which must so seriously alter the state of the blood ? And, on the contrary, why should it be so common in cancer of the womb ? Andral affirmed, indeed, that chronic affections of the lungs, even such as are productive of an induration of the greater part of their parenchyma, are seldom, perhaps never, followed by dropsy, unless they happen to be complicated with some disease of the heart, or of some other part, operating as a cause.—Anat. Pathol., tom. i., pp. 330, 332.—ED.

† Andral mentions a case in which large bleedings, practised for the cure of acute peritonitis, left the constitution in such a state, that the mere application of sinapisms to the thighs made them anasarcous.—ED.

generally heated and exhausted, has occasionally proved sufficient to produce dropsy in one of
these forms ; of which we have a striking example in the army of Charles V. during its expedition against Tunis ; the greater part of it, as
we are told by De Haen, having fallen into this
disease, in consequence of the soldiers having
freely quenched their thirst with cold water, in
the midst of great fatigue and perspiration.—
(*Rat. Med.*, part v., 38, 90.)

The sympathetic influence exercised over the
exhalants by a morbid state of the uterus, is not
less manifest : for, in chlorosis, the abdomen becomes tumid, and the lower limbs œdematous ;
and, on the cessation of the catamenia, cellular
and abdominal dropsy are by no means uncommon.*

Such are the general causes of cellular dropsy, as well proximate as predisponent. But there
are a few other causes which it is necessary to
enumerate, as acting occasionally, though the
effects produced by some of them can hardly be
called dropsy in the proper and idiopathic sense
of the term.

In the first place, the absorbents are supposed
by some pathologists, as M. Mezler (*Von der
Wassersucht*) and Dr. Darwin, to be at times
affected with a retrograde action, and hence to
pour forth into various cavities of the body a
considerable mass of fluid, instead of imbibing
and carrying it off. [To this hypothesis, however, the valvular structure of the lymphatics,
not less than the real difference of their contents from the fluid of ordinary dropsy, is a fatal objection.] Next, the exhalants of an organ,
though themselves in a state of health, may
throw forth an undue proportion of fluid in consequence of some stimulus applied to them.
The most common stimulus to which they are
exposed is distention, and that by a retardation
of the blood in the veins, and a consequent accumulation in the arteries. This retardation or
interruption of the flow of venous blood may
arise from diseases of the right ventricle of
the heart or its valves ; from various affections
of the lungs or their surrounding muscles ; from
an upright posture continued without intermission for many days and nights, as is often the
case in monthly nurses ; from a gravid uterus,
whence the œdematous ankles of pregnant women ; from disease of the liver or spleen ; from
obstruction of the veins, aneurisms in the arteries, or steatomatous or other hard tumours in
the vicinity of the larger arterial trunks.

[That simple obstruction to the free passage
of the blood through the veins, and the hinderance thus created to its ready transmission from
the arteries into those vessels, will produce
dropsy, was satisfactorily proved and illustrated
by the experiments of Lower. He applied a
ligature to the ascending vena cava of a dog,
which occasioned its death in a few hours ; and,
upon dissecting the animal, a great collection of
water was found in the abdomen. In other ex-

periments, in which the jugular veins were
tied, all the parts above the ligature became anasarcous, and not filled with extravasated blood,
as had been erroneously anticipated.—(*Tract. de
Corde*, cap. ii.) The obliteration of the principal vein of a limb, and of the collateral branches,
will bring on anasarca ; and so will the pressure of a large tumour, when it is such as interrupts the return of blood through the same vessels. With regard to this part of the subject, it
is worthy of notice, that the extent and situation of the dropsical affection have a strict relation to the point where the venous circulation
is obstructed. Thus, the obliteration of the
femoral or axillary vein, brings on œdema of
the corresponding lower or upper extremity.
The editor has a preparation of obliterated crural vein, taken from a man who died in the
King's Bench Infirmary, with a considerable
œdematous swelling of the corresponding lower
extremity, or rather a tumour somewhat resembling that of phlegmasia dolens. When the
lower vena cava is obliterated, the two lower
limbs become anasarcous ; but no fluid is effused in the peritoneum, or, if any such effusion
happen, it is not till an advanced stage of the
disease, and always consecutively. On the contrary, if the blood cannot circulate freely in the
several portions of the system of the vena portæ, whether in the liver or out of it, the dropsy
commences in the peritoneum. Lastly, if the
venous circulation be obstructed at its very centre, the effect must be felt in every part of the
system, and everywhere there must be a tendency to dropsy. This is what really happens
in organic diseases of the heart.—(See *Andral,
Anat. Pathol.*, tom. i., p. 330.)]

In some cases, inflammation succeeds to distention, and the quantity of fluid poured forth is
still more considerable. It is from this double
source of stimulus, distention and inflammatory
action, that the ventricles of the brain become
filled in meningic cephalitis, and the cavity of
the pericardium occasionally in carditis ; and
hence Dr. Stoker, with a view of exemplifying
and supporting the humoral pathology, has divided dropsies into two kinds, dynamic and ady-
namic ; these evincing too much action, and
those evincing too little (*Pathological Observations*, &c., part i., p. 16, Dubl., 8vo., 1823) :
while other writers have conceived that dropsy
consists, in every instance, of inflammation, or
of an action analogous to it.*

* Joseph Ayre, M. D., Researches into the Nature and Treatment of Dropsy, 8vo., Lond., 1825.
Many facts prove, that one cause of dropsy is inflammation. "A child has inflammation of the
brain, which runs its course in three weeks, and
then the child dies ; and the ventricles of the
brain are found distended with fluid. Another
child has symptoms of hydrocephalus internus,
which goes on more insidiously ; the bones give
way ; and the head becomes tremendously enlarged. It dies, and the body is examined. The
convolutions of the brain are found unfolded, and
there is an immense bag of fluid in the centre ;
this is what is called hydrocephalus chronicus,
and it is most frequently the result of inflammation.
You have examples of the same kind in the spinal

---

* This explanation of the origin of dropsy from
sympathy between the exhalant vessels and other
organs, is quite hypothetical.—Ed.

Thirdly, it is said, that the aqueous fluid of a cavity may be unduly augmented, and consequently dropsy ensue from a rupture of the thoracic duct, or of a large branch of the lacteal vessels. , These, however, are not common causes ; [and, indeed, if an extravasation of the contents of the thoracic duct or lacteals were to happen, the case would have little analogy to dropsy, the fluid of which is neither lymph nor chyle, but always a secretion from the exhalant arteries. Neither is it now generally admitted by modern physicians, that dropsy can originate from any impediment to the flow of the lymph towards the thoracic duct. Such a supposition could only be entertained when that duct itself was obstructed, because the anastomoses of the lymphatics are so numerous that the obliteration of some of them would not hinder the lymph from continuing to circulate. Now, in the few instances recorded of an obliteration of the thoracic duct, dropsy had not invariably taken place ; and when it had, it might rather have depended upon various concomitant lesions. In every case of this kind observed by M. Andral, the course of the lymph in the duct was never completely stopped, but was continued through the medium of collateral branches, which quitted the duct below the obstruction, and joined it again higher up. Theory would also not lead us to suspect obstruction of the thoracic duct to be a cause of dropsy, inasmuch as the functions of the lymphatic system, and the source of the fluid which it contains, are far from being well understood.]—(See *Andral., Anat. Pathol.,* tom. i., p. 331.)

cord from acute or chronic inflammation. Acute or chronic pericarditis occasionally ends by dropsy of the pericardium, or hydrops pericardii. Acute, subacute, or chronic inflammation of the pleura, very often leads to hydrothorax, or dropsy of the chest. A child becomes immensely dropsical from inflammation of the lungs, especially after scarlet fever. On examination of the bodies of phthisical patients, an effusion of fluid in the chest is often found. In acute, subacute, or chronic inflammation of the peritoneum, you find effusion in the belly, which is then called ascites. Upon the same principle hydrocele occurs, or effusion into the tunica vaginalis. Inflammation of the erysipelatous kind produces an effusion into the cellular membrane," &c.—(See Armstrong's Lectures on the Morbid Anatomy, Nature, and Treatment of Acute and Chronic Diseases, p. 841.) Dropsical swellings after scarlet fever, however, sometimes depend upon another cause, specified by Dr. Bright, as will be presently noticed.

It must, indeed, be acknowledged, that dropsy is frequently the effect of inflammation. In proof of this, we may observe with Andral (Anat. Pathol., tom. i.; p. 320), that acute or chronic hydrocephalus is frequently merely a consequence of irritation of the texture of the brain ; that certain examples of ascites are only the sequel of gastro-enteritis ; and that when a mucous membrane or a portion of skin is inflamed, the adjoining cellular tissue often becomes œdematous. The same things are exemplified round an old ulcer, a blister, or even under a sinapism, when the constitution has been enfeebled by chronic disease. Yet it is not to be imagined, that because these cases may be so, every other dropsical affection is preceded either by inflammation or debility.—ED.

Fourthly, rather in opposition to the results of some experiments made by modern physiologists, and already quoted in the Physiological Proem, the skin is said, at times, to be in a condition to absorb moisture too freely from the atmosphere (*Erastus,* disp. iv., p. 206 ; *De Haen, Rat. Med.,* P. iv., p. 125, seq.) ; the stomach is alleged, as in the case of DIPSOSIS *avens,* to demand too large a quantity of liquids to quench its insatiable thirst (*Büchner, Miscell.,* 1730, p. 888 ; *Mondschien,* p. 12) ; and the blood is said to be in a state of preternatural tenuity :[*] and each of these conditions, it is affirmed, has occasionally proved a source of dropsy. The first of these unquestionably occurs at times during dropsy, and all of them may have operated as causes : but preternatural tenuity of blood, adequate to such an effect, is very uncommon, from any cause ; and the remedial power of nature is at no loss for means to carry off a superabundance of fluidity introduced by any means into the system, provided the excernent function itself be not diseased.[†]

* Galen, De Lymph. Caus., lib. iii., cap. viii.; Van Swieten, ad Sect. 1229. A state of general anemia, or extraordinary deficiency of blood in the system, has been noticed by Andral in several individuals who were dropsical at the period of their deaths, and in whom no alteration of the solids could be detected.—Clinique Méd., tom. iii., p. 558.—ED.

† On this part of the subject, our author's sentiments differ from those entertained by some medical writers of considerable eminence, among whom was the late Dr. Bateman. This judicious and respectable physician believed that dropsy might be produced by an immoderate proportion of serous or watery fluids in the bloodvessels, more especially when conjoined with other causes known to be conducive to the disease. "The experiments of Dr. Hales," he observes, "establish the truth of this fact, as fully as those of Lower evince the effect of venous obstruction. Dr. Hales supposed that water, being thinner than the red blood, would pass more readily from the extremity of the arteries into the veins ; and he injected warm water into the arteries of dogs : the event did not answer his expectation ; for the water did not return by the veins, but escaped through the exhalant arteries, through which the red blood could not pass, into the interstices of the cellular membrane, occasioning a dropsical swelling.—(Hæmastat., exp. 21.) When he persisted to inject water through a tube fixed in the carotid artery, although the jugular veins were cut longitudinally, the water did not issue freely by these apertures ; but all the parts of the body began to swell, and a universal dropsy took place."—(Ibid., exp. 14 ; art. DROPSY, Rees's Cyclopædia.) If a copious quantity of blood be taken away from an animal previously to the injection of water into the veins, much more of the latter fluid may be thrown into them before dropsy commences, than when no bleeding has preceded the experiment. On the other hand, if the animal be bled after the dropsy has been induced, the effusion of serous fluid will diminish, and the absorbents resume their wonted activity. The sudden disappearance of an ascites in a person who had an organic disease of the heart, was followed all at once by apoplexy, that proved fatal in a few hours.—(Andral, Anat. Pathol., tom. i., p. 321.) On dissection, no water was found in the peritoneum, nor any traces of extravasated blood in the brain ; but the

[M. Andral inclines to the opinion, that the origin of dropsy sometimes depends upon a diminution of exhalation from the skin and mucous membrane of the lungs, and of the secretion of urine. He is also disposed to believe, that the anasarca which often shows itself in the couvalescence of scarlet fever, is owing to the suppression of cutaneous perspiration during the desquamation of the cuticle.—(*Anat. Pathol.*, tom. i., p. 323.) To Dr. Bright's different explanation of this case, we shall presently refer. If, however, a mere diminution of cutaneous exhalation were an efficient cause of dropsy, it might be supposed that the disease would be much more frequent than it is, and more under the control of atmospheric influence. Why also do we not find it the ordinary consequence of erysipelas, and other affections of the skin, as well as of scarlet fever? M. Andral mentions, in support of his theory, that he has seen a case of dropsy, in which there was only one kidney.—(*Clinique Méd.*, tom. iii.) On the other hand, the editor attended, with Dr. Smith and Mr. Baker, of Staines, a patient, in whom one of the kidneys was completely destroyed, and the capsule converted into a cyst containing three pints of matter. (see *Medical Gazette* for October, 1830); yet no appearances of dropsy presented themselves, the single kidney seeming fully adequate to the function of both. But, notwithstanding this fact, no doubt can be entertained that an interruption of the secretion of urine, carried to a certain degree, may be a cause of dropsy.

Besides the causes of dropsy ordinarily specified by writers, the kidneys are subject to certain alterations, which appear to Dr. Bright, for the following reasons, to be also, in many instances, the primary occasion of increased serous exhalation into the cellular tissue and great cavities. 1. In some cases from an early period, and, in a few, even before the dropsical effusion begins, symptoms of disorder in the kidneys are perceptible, consisting of pain in the

---

several ventricles were enormously distended with a limpid fluid. In this case, Andral concluded that the effusion of water in the ventricles was owing to the redundance of it produced in the circulation by its absorption from the abdomen. Andral refers to other instances, in which anasarca and dropsy of various serous cavities seemed to depend upon no organic disease, as far as dissection could trace it, but upon plethora of the whole system. He gives the particulars of one of these cases, which took place in a young man, about 30, full of strength and life, subject to frequent bleedings from the nose, with eyes habitually turgid, and a universally florid skin, that formed an odd association with the pitting of the subcutaneous cellular membrane. Andral thinks that the dropsy might probably have been removed, and the fatal termination prevented, by copious bleedings. —(Vol. cit.; p. 325.) Dr. Armstrong also enumerates, as one of the causes of dropsy, an excessive quantity either of blood or a watery fluid in the circulation.—(See Lect. on the Morbid Anatomy, Nature, and Treatment of Acute and Chronic Diseases, p. 843.) This form of dropsy, he says, is sometimes connected with inflammation, but sometimes it is not.—Ed.

---

region of those organs, tenderness, or bloody urine, and *in every instance albumen is discharged with the urine*. This last symptom is regarded by Dr. Bright as the pathognomonic sign of the variety of dropsy depending upon renal disease. 2. In some cases of dropsy, no sign whatever of disease of the liver, or of the heart and appendages, can be discovered during life, yet there is albuminous urine, and sometimes other more generally acknowledged signs of derangement of the kidneys. 3. After death, the kidneys are sometimes found to be the only important organs which have undergone morbid changes of structure ; or, at all events, the liver, heart, lungs, and other organs, whose organic changes are known to occasion dropsy by obstructing the passage of the blood, are found in a state of health. 4. In the more numerous cases in which other parts and organs, and particularly the liver, are also diseased, it often happens that the derangement in the structure of the kidneys is much greater than anywhere else, and consequently of much longer standing, so as to show that the diseased state of the liver or other parts is secondary to that of the kidneys, if not produced by it. To these arguments, a critical writer has added another, deduced from the tendency of obstructed secretion of urine to produce dropsy. A few years ago, he attended a case of complete suppression, which lasted about two days : great anasarca was rapidly produced, and as rapidly receded, when, by means of copious bloodletting, purgatives, opium, and warm bathing, the secretion of urine was re-established.

In dropsy from diseased kidney, Dr. Bright found three forms of organic derangement. In the first, or slightest, the kidney is not enlarged, but unnaturally soft, mottled yellow externally, and mottled gray and yellow internally. In a more advanced stage of this variety, portions of the kidney become consolidated, and externally rather tubercular, the projecting parts being paler than the rest of the surface, and incapable of having injection thrown into the arteries. In the *second* species of derangement, the cortical part of the kidney is gradually converted into a granular texture, with a white, opaque, interstitial deposite. In the early stage of this form, the texture of the kidney seems as if it contained fine sand, and is softer than natural. In the advanced stage, the granular structure is obvious externally, and also internally when the kidney is cut open. At the same time, the organ is enlarged. The *third* variety is characterized by external roughness, arising from numerous small projections of a yellow, red, and purplish teint ; and such kidneys have generally a lobulated form and semicartilaginous hardness. Dr. Bright has also seen connected with anasarca a preternatural softness, without any other change, and also a closure of the tubular structure by a white deposite.

Some of the cases of dropsy termed inflammatory, Dr. Bright conceives to depend upon diseased kidney ; as dropsy subsequent to scarlet fever ; anasarca taking place at the approach of mercurial erethism ; and dropsies following exposure to cold and wet in persons debilitated by frequent attacks of syphilis, drunkenness, and other excesses. *In all cases of renal dropsy, the urine is albuminous*; and frequently this is the only sign of the kidneys being diseased. According to Dr. Bostock's experiments, the secretion of albumen seems to be attended with a diminished secretion of urea and of the salts of the urine. It should be recollected, however, that albuminous urine is not necessarily connected with organic disease in the kidney (see *Prout on Diseases of the Urinary Organs*, p. 39); and it is likewise met with in other diseases besides dropsy; but in these, Dr. Bright has always found in the kidneys a change of structure analogous to what he remarked in dropsy. The morbid changes of those organs do not therefore necessarily bring on dropsy, though they may generally do so. *When, in dropsy, the liver or heart, or both, have been found diseased, and not the kidneys, Dr. Bright never observed the urine to be albuminous.*

In the real variety of dropsy, the same author has frequently noticed a strong, well-marked tendency to inflammation, particularly in the serous membranes, requiring vigorous treatment.—(See *Bright's Reports of Medical Cases*, 4to., Lond., 1827.) This will explain his observation respecting what are vaguely called inflammatory dropsies being generally dependant on, or rather associated with, morbid change of the kidney.

In three cases of dropsy where the liver was diseased and the kidneys were sound, Dr. Bright found that the urine was not albuminous; but whether this is a general fact, can only be determined by further investigations.* Accord-

* On this interesting point, the editor avails himself of the sentiments of Dr. Elliotson, who believes that if the kidney be organically affected, have a great congestion of blood in it, or be in an inflammatory state, the urine is generally albuminous. But, on the other hand, he does not think that the circumstance of the urine being albuminous is a proof that the kidney is in this state, at least in a state of organic disease; because he has seen many persons cured of dropsy, and restored to perfect health, who had albuminous urine; and if the kidneys had been originally diseased, it is hardly possible to conceive that a recovery would have ensued: nor could congestion and inflammation of the kidney be suspected, because no symptoms of them existed. He is therefore of opinion, that although it is possible that, in disease of the kidney, and in congestion of that organ, the urine may generally be albuminous, the converse cannot be said; viz., that if the urine be albuminous, we must necessarily conclude that the kidney is in these diseased conditions.—(See Lancet for 1830-31, p. 360.) The editor was consulted in the summer of 1830 for an anasarca in a young man under Mr. Hooper, of the London Road. Several medical practitioners had seen the patient, and very large quantities of water had been occasionally discharged by scarification. The cause of the disease seemed perfectly obscure, as there was no emaciation, no particular debility, the patient complained of no pain in any particular organ, ate well, slept well, and was free from all marks of diseased liver. About three months after the editor had seen him in this state, he died rather suddenly. On dissection, the kidneys were found to be diseased.—ED.

ing to Dr. Crampton, scanty urine, with high red sediments, is seldom wanting in cases connected with diseased liver; and many cases, the details of which he has published, tend to assign much importance to the early appearance of anasarca of the face, as an indication of the disease arising from disease of the heart or pericardium.—(See *Trans. of the Assoc. Physicians, Ireland*, vol. ii., pp. 150, 162, 166, &c.)

From Dr. Bostock's researches it appears probable, that the form of disease in which a yellow or whitish matter is deposited in the natural structure of the liver, consists in the deposition of a principle nearly the same as the cholesterine of bile. It is also suspected that a deposition of the same principle may occur in certain forms of diseased kidney already described. A critical writer mentions, that he lately found it in the fluid of a hydrocele, and also in the fluid of a large osseous cyst, into which one of the kidneys had been converted in a case of dropsy. The inference is, that in certain states of the constitution, the tendency to the production of cholesterine probably forms an important cause of various organic diseases.

In one diseased liver, chymically examined by Dr. Bostock, but in which case no dropsy existed, fatty matter, resembling tallow, was deposited in the meshes of the cellular tissue of that organ. And, in one example of protracted jaundice, accompanying tubercular liver and dropsy, the same distinguished physician found the bile of the gall-bladder to be of an orange-red colour and thin consistence; and that the animal matter in it was almost entirely albumen; none of the usual elements of bile being traced in it.*

From this diversity of causes we may reasonably expect that the dropsical fluid discharged by tapping should exhibit different properties, not only in different organs, but in different cases in the same organ. And hence it is sometimes found nearly as thin as water, incapable of coagulating when exposed to heat, which only renders it turbid; while at other times it flows in a ropy state, and accords, upon exposure to heat, with the natural serum of the blood. A similar discrepance is discoverable in its colour or some other condition: for it has

* See Bright's Reports of Medical Cases, &c., 4to., 1827. After all, the causes of certain dropsies are perfectly obscure. In some cases there is, as Andral justly observes (Anat. Pathol., tom. i., p. 332), no proof of past or existing irritation; of any secretion being suppressed; any alteration of the blood; or any mechanical obstruction of the venous or lymphatic circulation. Such examples he divides into two classes: in one, the dropsy seems to be the primary disorder; in the other, it complicates the latter stages of several chronic affections, though in them the blood undergoes changes which make it resemble that condition of it which induces dropsy in individuals who have lost too much blood. A fancied loss of equilibrium between the action of the absorbents and of the secernent vessels; a presumed alteration in the organic sensibility of the absorbents; or the idea of an irritation affecting the secreting vessels,—he seems to think, are theories destitute of proof and real information.—ED.

sometimes been found black and fetid (*Galeazzi, in Com. Bonon.*, tom. vi.), bloody, sanious, milky (*Willis, Pharmaceutice Rationalis ; Med. Com. of Edin.*, vol. v.), green (*Rücker, Comm. Lib. Nor.*, 1736), yellowish, or peculiarly acrid.— (*Du Verney, Mémoires de Paris,* 1701, p. 193.) [The yellow tinge presented by it when there is jaundice, sometimes depends upon its containing a colouring matter analogous to that of bile. In particular cases, uric acid has also been detected in it.] According to Guattani and Steidele, it has sometimes appeared oily.— (*Guat. de Aneurismatibus ; Steid. Chirurg. Beobacht.*, b. i.) It has been occasionally so alkaline or ammoniacal as to turn sirup of red poppies green (*De Haen, Rat. Med.*, P. xi., p. 214) ; and, according to Dr. M'Lachlan, has sometimes contained so much soda as, by the addition of sulphuric acid, to produce Glauber's salt (*Med. Comm. Edin.*, 9, 2) with little or no trouble.* Dr. Willis has observed a great variety in the proportion of serum discharged by the urine of hydropic patients ; and a variety so perpetually differing as to elude all his attempts, and they were many as well as judicious, to follow up and classify the discrepances.—(*Trans. Medico-Chir. Soc.*, 1812.)†

* Notwithstanding all this diversity, it may be said that the fluid effused either in cavities lined by serous membranes, or in the cellular substance, generally exhibits most of the physical qualities of serum. Like this, it is not spontaneously coagulable ; but it may be coagulated by heat, acids, alcohol, and electricity. Its chymical composition is sometimes exactly similar to that of serum, there being in 1,000 parts, 900 of water, 80 of albumen, and the remainder consisting of salts and an animal matter very like mucus. Sometimes it contains less water and a much larger proportion of albumen than the serum of the blood ; and in other instances, less albumen ; occasionally not more than 20 or 24 parts of it in the 1,000. There may even be a very minute proportion of it, indeed, in the fluid, which then consists almost entirely of water, with some salts in it. In certain cases, a modification of animal matter, the nature of which is not well understood, is blended with the liquid, and lessens its transparency. It sometimes presents itself in the form of flakes ; sometimes in that of minute atoms, which render the whole of the fluid slightly turbid. Andral does not believe that the flakes are necessarily connected with any state of irritation of the serous membrane of the dropsical cavity.—Ed.

† The entonic character of many cases of dropsy, which is so strenuously advocated by the English editor, has long been maintained by many American physicians. Dr. Rush remarks, "that too little action in the arteries should favour dropsical effusions, has long been observed ; but it has been less obvious, that the same effusions are sometimes promoted, and their absorption prevented, by too much action in these vessels. By too much action in the arterial system, I mean a certain morbid excitement in the arteries, accompanied by preternatural force, which is obvious to the sense of touch." "To be convinced of the inflammatory origin of dropsy," says Dr. D. F. Condie, " it is only necessary to examine after death the cavity in which the morbid accumulation is seated. Thus, in hydrothorax and ascites, the pleura and peritoneum will, in very many instances, be found not only highly vascular, but deprived of their nat-

N n 2

COLD AND DIFFUSIVE INTUMESCENCE OF THE SKIN, PITTING BENEATH THE PRESSURE OF THE FINGERS.*

THIS species includes three varieties ; as it is general to the cellular membrane, limited to the limbs, or accompanied with a combination of very peculiar symptoms, and especially severe, and in most cases fatal, dyspnœa :—

a Generalis.	Extending through the cellular membrane of the whole body.†
General dropsy.	

ural transparency and glossy appearance, and covered to a greater or less extent with patches of coagulable lymph. Occasionally, it is true, so great an interval may have elapsed between the existence of the inflammation and the fatal event, as to render it somewhat difficult to recognise the more decided marks of its previous existence : but even in such cases, the thickening of the serous tissue, and the presence of portions of false membrane adhering to the surface of the cavity, or of shreds of coagulable lymph floating in the effused fluid, will indicate with certainty that inflammation must have existed." The same opinion is maintained by Dr. J. C. Cross, of Kentucky, in his Prize Essay on Dropsy, and by other American writers.—D.

* When the serous fluid is effused in considerable quantity, it produces a great deal of swelling, the part or limb undergoing, indeed, an enormous increase of size. In general, the fluid is most copious in depending situations, or those into which it gravitates, and also in parts where the cellular tissue is naturally loose and abundant. The skin, being over the cellular tissue in this state, is always of a paler colour than natural, and on the distention being carried to a certain point, it is thinned, assumes a shining appearance, and not unfrequently bursts, so that a large quantity of the fluid from the neighbouring parts may thus be discharged.—Ed.

† Cases of general dropsy of the cellular tissue are much less common than those of partial extent, especially when the disorder does not depend upon some obstruction of the circulation situated in the heart or large bloodvessels. In numerous examples, only the lower extremities are affected ; and even in others, where the dropsical effusion is universal, it almost constantly begins in the lower limbs. Dr. Bouillaud, by whom these statements are made, is evidently referring to the disease as connected with a general cause ; for certain causes of a local kind may make it take a different course. Instead of *cellular dropsy,* medical writers usually employ the term *anasarca,* which is said to prevail when the quantity of serous fluid in the cellular tissue is copious and more extensively diffused, though, strictly speaking, the cellular membrane of the whole body, or even of the greater portion of it, may not be involved. The serous fluid found in the cavities of the cellular substance, or the serosity, as it is termed by French pathologists, retains its usual properties, both chymical and physical, where the anasarca is free from complication ; but, in particular cases, it is susceptible of changes, as where the disorder is or has been combined with chronic inflammation, or is of long standing. Thus, in one example mentioned by Dr. Bouillaud (Dict. de Méd. et de Chir. Pratiques, tom. i., p.

β Artuum.	Limited to the cellular mem-
Œdema	brane of the limbs, chiefly
	of the feet and ankles;
	and mostly appearing in
	the evening.
γ Dyspnoica.	Œdematous swelling of the
Dyspnetic dropsy.	feet, stiffness and numb-
	ness of the joints; the
	swelling rapidly ascending
	to the belly, with severe
	and mostly fatal dyspnœa.

It is under the first of these varieties that cellular dropsy usually appears as an idiopathic affection. Where the intumescence is confined to the limbs, it is mostly a symptom or result of some other affection, as chlorosis, suppressed catamenia, or any other habitual discharge; a disordered state of the habit produced by a cessation of the catamenial flux : or the weakness incident to protracted fevers, or any other exhausting malady.

The third variety is introduced upon the authority of Mr. W. Hunter, and taken from his Essay, published at Bengal in 1804. The disease appeared with great frequency among the Lascars in the Company's service in 1801. Its attack was sudden, and its progress so rapid, that it frequently destroyed the patient in two days. From the description, it does not seem to have been connected with a scorbutic diathesis; and Mr. Hunter ascribed it to the concurrent

---

321), in which the lower extremities of a woman had long been anasarcous, and as enormously swollen as if they had been affected with elephantiasis, the fluid in the cellular membrane was of a viscid kind, and intimately combined, as it were, with that texture and the skin, into the areolæ of which it had insinuated itself. It appears from a recent analysis of the blood and serum of patients labouring under anasarca, undertaken by Messrs. Brett and Bird, of Guy's Hospital, that the serum is deficient in albumen and its usual salts, while the urine not only has a great deficiency of urea, salts, and animal matter, but is peculiar in containing albumen. They infer from their experiments and observations, that urea, if it ever exist in the circulating fluid, cannot be a cause of the peculiar train of symptoms noticed in patients labouring under anasarca, with coagulable urine.— (See Med. Gaz. for 1832-33, pp. 567-569.) The quantity of serous fluid in the cellular membrane of certain individuals, labouring under anasarca in a great and extensive degree, is supposed to be equal to what is contained in the peritoneum in the largest specimens of ascites. When an incision is made in an anasarcous limb, the depth or thickness of the subcutaneous cellular tissue is found to be vastly increased, sometimes to that of an inch, or an inch and a half, and more. From every point of the wound an abundance of serosity is seen to flow; and if a portion of the cellular tissue be compressed, the fluid issues out of it as from a wet sponge. The cavities of this tissue are increased in size, and while this part is thickened in the manner described, the skin itself is attenuated, pale, dry; and semi-transparent. The muscles of anasarcous individuals are also paler than natural, and, in cases of long standing, are even destitute of their usual red colour.—See Bouillaud, in Dict. de Méd. et de Chir. Pratiques, tom. ii., p. 321.—Ed.

---

causes of breathing an impure atmosphere, suppressed perspiration, want of exercise, and a previous life of intemperance. All or any of these may have been auxiliaries, but the exciting cause does not seem to have been detected. It is a frequent symptom in beribery.

The second and third varieties, however, may be regarded as the opening and concluding stages of cellular dropsy : for, before the disease becomes general, it ordinarily shows itself in the lower limbs, and, in its closing scene, the respiration is peculiarly difficult, and forms one of its most distressing symptoms.

General or local debility is the predisposing cause, ordinarily brought on by hard labour, intemperance, innutritious food, fevers of various kinds, exhausting discharges, or some morbid enlargement of the visceral or thoracic organs, that impedes the circulation of the blood, and produces congestion and distention.

The disease is hence common to all ages, though most frequently found in advanced life : the œdema of the feet and ankles, with which symptom it opens, appears at first only in the evening, and yields to the recumbent position of the night. By degrees it becomes more permanent, and ascends higher, till not only the thighs and hips, but the body at large is affected, the face and eyelids are surcharged and bloated, and the complexion, instead of the ruddy hue of health, is sallow and waxy. A general inactivity pervades all the organs, and consequently all their respective functions. The pulse is slow, often oppressed, and always inelastic : the bowels are costive, the urine for the most part small in quantity, and consequently of a deeper hue than usual : the respiration is troublesome and wheezy, and accompanied with a cough, that brings up a little dilute mucus, which affords no relief to the sense of weight and oppression. The appetite fails, the muscles become weak and flaccid, and the general frame emaciated. Exertion of every kind is a fatigue, and the mind, partaking of the hebetude of the body, engages in study with reluctance, and is overpowered with drowsiness and stupor.

An unquenchable thirst is a common symptom; and when this is the case, the general irritation connected with it sometimes excites a perpetual feverishness, that adds greatly to the general debility. In some parts the skin gives way more readily than in others, and the confined fluid accumulates in bags. At other times the cuticle cracks, or its pores become an outlet for the escape of the fluid, which trickles down in a perpetual ooze. The difficulty of breathing increases partly from the overloaded state of the lungs, and partly from the growing weakness of the muscles of respiration : the pulse becomes feebler and more irregular, slight clonic spasms occasionally ensue, and death puts a termination to the series of suffering. Yet the progress is slow, and the disease sometimes continues for many years.

In attempting a cure of cellular dropsy, and indeed of dropsy in general, for it will be convenient to concentrate the treatment, we should first direct our attention to the nature of its

cause, with a view of palliating or removing it.[*]
We are next to unload the system of the weight
that oppresses it : and lastly, to re-establish the
frame in health and vigour.

Simple œdema, or swelling of the extremities,
is often a symptom or result of some other complaint, as chlorosis, or pregnancy, or some other
cause of distention. In the two last cases, it
may be palliated by bleeding, a recumbent position, and other means adapted to take off the
pressure. In chlorosis, it can only be relieved
by a cure of the primary affection. In like manner, general dropsy may be dependant upon a
habit of intemperance, or a sedentary life, or innutritious food, or an obstinate fit of jaundice :
and, till these are corrected, no medicinal plan for
evacuating the accumulated water can be of any
avail. For, if we could even succeed in carrying it off, it would again collect, so long as the
occasional cause continues to operate.

The occasional cause, however, may no longer exist, as where it has been produced by a
fever or an exanthem, that has at length ceased,
though it has left the constitution an entire
wreck. Or it may exist and be itself incurable,
as where it proceeds from a scirrhous induration
or some other obstruction of one of the larger
viscera of the thorax or abdomen, or is connected with the morbid changes of the kidney very
far advanced, as lately pointed out to the profession by Dr. Bright. In such cases our object
should be to remove with all speed the mischievous effects, and palliate the organic cause, as
far as we are able, according to its peculiar nature, so that it may be less operative hereafter.

A removal of the accumulated fluid from the
cellular membrane generally has been attempted
by internal and external means, as hydragogues
of various kinds, and scarification, or other cutaneous drains.

---

[*] Cellular dropsy, as our author calls it, or anasarca and œdema, are conceived to be produced
in two ways ; in one, secretion that is regularly
going on in the cellular tissue is supposed to be
quickened ; in the other, there is an interruption
or cessation of absorption. One anasarca is sometimes termed *active ;* the other, *passive.* The disease is also divisible into two other forms : one of
which depends upon a cause situated in the parts
where the effusion takes place ; the other upon a
cause that is seated elsewhere.—(See Bouillaud,
in Dict. de Méd., &c., tom. i., p. 322.) The *active*
varieties of anasarca, or those attended with increased secretion, are often thought to be connected with a process, or an increased action, somewhat similar to that of inflammation ; while the
passive forms of the disorder depend upon diminished activity of the lymphatic vessels. But, from
what is stated in the Physiological Proem, it is
questionable whether the lymphatics are the essential organs by which the serosity of the cellular
tissue is absorbed. Many modern pathologists believe, indeed, that a mechanical impediment to the
return of the venous blood is mostly, if not always,
concerned in the production of these *passive* varieties of anasarca. Such impediment has hitherto
been traced only in the large veins and their
branches ; but it may probably exist also in the
minute venous ramifications, the organs by which
the serum of the cellular membrane is not uncommonly suspected to be absorbed.—ED.

The HYDRAGOGUES, or expellents of water,
embrace medicines of all kinds that act powerfully on any of the excretories, though the term
has sometimes been limited to those which operate on the excretories of the intestines alone.
And it becomes us therefore to contemplate
them under the character of purgatives, emetics,
diaphoretics, and diuretics.

The purgatives that have been had recourse
to are of two kinds ; those of general use; and
those that have been supposed to act with some
specific or peculiar virtue in the removal of the
dropsical fluid.

Among the first we may rank calomel, colocynth, gamboge, scammony, jalap, and several
other species of convolvulus, as the greater white
bindweed (convolvulus *Sepium,* Linn.) : the turbeth plant (c. *Turpethum,* Linn.) : and the bras-
sica *marina,* as it is called in the dispensatories
(c. *Soldanella,* Linn.). These may be employed
as drastic purgatives almost indiscriminately,
and their comparative merit will depend upon
their comparative effect ; for one will often be
found to agree best with one constitution and
another with another. We need not here except calomel, unless, indeed, where given for
the purpose of resolving visceral infarctions ;
since, in any other case, it can only be employed
in reference to its influence upon the excretories
generally, and particularly those of the intestinal
canal.

The purgatives that have been supposed to
operate with a specific effect in dropsies are almost innumerable. We must content ourselves
with taking a glance at the following : grana
Tiglia, or bastard ricinus ; elaterium ; elder, and
dwarf elder ; black hellebore ; senega ; and crystals of tartar.

The CROTON *Tiglium,* or bastard ricinus, affording the grana Tiglia of the Pharmacopœias,
is an acrid and powerful drastic in all its parts,
roots, seeds, and expressed oil. The oil is of the
same character as the oil of castor, but a severer
and more acrimonious purge ; insomuch, indeed,
that a single drop, prepared from the dry seeds,
is often a sufficient dose ; while a larger quantity
proves cathartic when rubbed on the navel. In
India, the seeds themselves have long been given
as a hydragogue ; two being sufficient for a robuster constitution, one for a weaklier ; and four
proving sometimes fatal. By far the safest mode
of giving it is in an alcoholic solution, as practised by Dr. Nimmo (*Journ. of Science,* xiii., 62),
since, by such a diffusion, it has less chance of
griping or producing inflammation.[*]

---

[*] According to Professor A. T. Thomson, "the
most common form of giving the oil is that of a pill,
formed by dropping the oil on crumb of bread ; one
or two drops proving a sufficient dose. Or it may
be given with rhubarb, which readily absorbs the
oil, and can be easily formed with a little water
into pills. The purgative property of the rhubarb
is scarcely felt in such small doses. This mode,
however, of administering the oil, has one disadvantage ; namely, it is applied in too concentrated
a state to the portion of the stomach on which it
rests. I have found, that the taste and acrimony
of the medicine are well covered by triturating the
oil with mucilage and sirup of tolu, and diffusing

From the uncertainty and violence of the action of this plant, the ELATERIUM, or inspissated juice of the wild cucumber, is a far preferable medicine for the present purpose. Elaterium itself, however, has been objected to as unduly stimulant : and both Hoffmann and Lister, who, as well as Sydenham, strongly recommend it, observe that its effect in increasing the pulse is perceivable even in the extremities of the fingers. It is on this account that it seems chiefly to have been neglected by Dr. Cullen, who admits that he never tried it by itself, or otherwise than in the proportion of a grain or two in composition with other purgatives. And it is hence, also, that attempts have been made to obtain a milder cathartic from the roots of the plant by infusion in wine or water (*Bouldue, Hist. de l'Acad. Royale des Sciences de Paris*), than from the dried fecula of the juice, which is the part ordinarily employed. Admitting the stimulant power here objected to, it would only become still more serviceable in cold and indolent cases from local or general atony ; but, even in irritable habits, in cellular dropsy, I have found it highly serviceable in a simple and uncombined state, produced, as it ultimately appeared, and especially in one instance, from a thickening of the walls of the heart, in a young lady of only thirteen years of age. It is best-administered in doses of from half a grain or a grain to two grains, repeated every two or three hours for five or six times in succession, according to the extent of its action. Evacuation by the alvine canal is the most effectual of any ; nor can we depend upon any other evacuation, unless this is combined with it.*

The elder-tree and dwarf elder (Sambucus *nigra* and S. *Ebulus*) have been in high estimation as hydragogues by many practitioners. Every part of both the plants has been used ; but the liber or inner bark of the first, and the rob or inspissated juice of the berries of the last, have been chiefly confided in. Dr. Boerhaave asserts, that the expressed juice of the former, given from a drachm to half an ounce at a dose, is the most valuable of all the medicines of this class, where the viscera are sound ; and that it so powerfully dissolves the crasis of the differ-

ent fluids, and excites such abundant discharges, that the patient is ready to faint from sudden inanition. Dr. Sydenham confirms this statement ; asserts that it operates both upwards and downwards, and in no less degree by urine, and adds, that in his hands it has proved successful in a multitude of hydropic cases.—(*Opp.*, pp. 627, 768.) Dr. Brocklesby preferred the interior bark of the dwarf elder (*Œconom. and Med. Observ.*, p. 278), as Sydenham and Boerhaave did that of the black or common elder. Dr. Cullen seems to have been prejudiced against both, though he admits that he never tried them (*Mat. Med.*, vol. i., p. 534) : and it is chiefly, perhaps, from his unfavourable opinion of their virtues, that they seem in our own day to have sunk into an almost total disuse.

The melampodium or black hellebore was at one time a favourite cathartic in dropsies, and has the testimony of high authorities for having very generally proved efficacious and salutary. The ancients found the plant which they employed under this name so severe in its purgative qualities, that they were obliged to use it with great caution ; but we have reason to believe that the black hellebore of the present day is a different production, as it is milder in its effects than the hellebore of Dioscorides, and different in some of its external characters. Its root was the part selected, and the fibres of the roots, or their cortical part, rather than the internal. These were employed either in a watery infusion or extract. Mondschein (*Von der Wassersucht*, &c.) preferred, on all occasions, the latter ; Quarin used either indifferently.—(*Animadversiones*, &c.) Bacher invented a pill which was once in very high reputation, and sold under his own name all over Europe, for the cure of dropsy, in which an extract of this root, obtained, in the first instance, by spirit, formed the chief ingredient ; the others being preparations of myrrh and carduus benedictus. These pills were said to produce a copious evacuation both by stool and urine ; and by this combined effect to carry off the disease. They have, however, had their day, and are gone by, apparently with too little consideration upon the subject ; for the experiments of Daignau and De Horne, and especially the successful trials in the French military hospitals, as related by M. Richard (*Recueil des Observ. de Méd. des Hôpitaux Militaires*, &c., tom. ii., 4to, Paris), to say nothing of Dr. Bacher himself, do not seem to have excited sufficient attention. In our own country, since the days of Dr. Mead, the black hellebore has been limited to the list of emmenagogues, and, even in this view, is rarely employed at present. Whether the plant prove purgative, as has been asserted, when applied to the body externally in the form of fomentations or cataplasms, like the croton, I have never tried.*

---

it through the common almond emulsion."—See Thomson's Elements of Materia Med., vol. ii., p. 345.—ED.

* The active principle of elaterium, constituting one twelfth of its weight, is termed *elatin*, the activity of which as a cathartic is almost incredible ; for "it operates violently when only one minim of an alcoholic tincture, consisting of one grain of elaterium dissolved in ninety-six minims of strong alcohol, is administered : thus, it operates in doses of less than the 96th part of a grain. Elatin has not, however, been employed in its pure state, even in the alcoholic solution, as a cathartic."—(See Thomson's Elements of Materia Medica, vol. ii., p. 350.) The same physician has given elaterium in doses of one sixth of a grain, repeated every four hours ; and he has known it to bring about an evacuation of two gallons of fluid by stool in the course of twenty-four hours. During its operation, it is necessary to keep up the patient's strength with ammonia and camphire, or wine.—ED.

---

* Though this medicine is admitted to produce copious evacuations, both by stool and urine, and to be well fitted to carry off dropsical accumulations, it is now rarely employed, except for the purpose of exciting the uterine organs.—See

The seneka or senega (polygala *Senega*, Linn.) was another medicine much in use about a century ago, and reputed to be of very great importance in dropsy, from its combined action upon the kidneys and intestines, and indeed all the excretories. It reached Europe from America, where it had been immemorially employed by the Senegal Indians, from whom it derives its specific name, as an antidote against the bite of the rattlesnake. The root of the plant is the part chiefly, if not entirely trusted to, and this is given in powder, decoction, or infusion. M. Bouvart found it highly serviceable as a hydragogue, but observes, that notwithstanding this effect, it does not of itself carry off the induration or enlargement of infarcted viscera, and ought to be combined with other means. It was very generally employed by Dr., afterward Sir Francis Milman, in the Middlesex Hospital, and has again found a place in the Materia Medica of the London College. There are unquestionable instances of its efficacy in the removal of dropsy, when it has been carried so far as to operate both by the bowels and the kidneys. It has, however, often failed ; and, as Dr. Cullen observes, is a nauseous medicine, which the stomach does not easily bear in a quantity requisite for success.

A far more agreeable, if not a more effectual medicine in the case of dropsy, is the supertartrate or bitartrate of potass, in vernacular language, the cream or crystals of tartar. In small quantities, and very largely diluted with water or some farinaceous fluid, it quenches the thirst most pleasantly, and at the same time proves powerfully diuretic. But it is as a purgative we are to contemplate it at present : and to give it this effect it must be taken in a much larger quantity, never less than an ounce at a dose, and often considerably above this weight. Thus administered, it proves powerfully cathartic, and excites the action of the absorbents in every part of the system far more effectually than is done by the influence of any entirely neutral salts. "I need hardly say," observes Dr. Cullen, "that upon this operation of exciting the absorbents, is chiefly founded the late frequent use of the crystals of tartar in the cure of dropsy."—(*Materia Medica*, ii., 513, 4to. edit.) Dr. Cullen, in this passage, apparently alludes to the practice of Dr. Home, who was peculiarly friendly to its use ; and in his Clinical Experiments, relates twenty cases in which he tried it, and completed a radical cure in fourteen of them, no relapse occurring, notwithstanding the frequency of such regressions. The practice, however, is of much earlier date than Dr. Cullen seems to imagine ; for Hildanus represents the physicians of his day as at length flying to it as their sheet-anchor, and deriving from it no common benefit.—(Cent. iv., obs. 42.) On the continent it has generally, but very unnecessarily, been united with other and more active materials, as Jalap, gamboge, or some of the neutral salts, chiefly sul-

phate of potass, or common sea-salt. [Supertartrate of potass is preferred by Dr. Bright to more stimulating diuretics *

Another diuretic, deserving particular notice in the consideration of the treatment of dropsy, is the pyrola umbellata, on which Dr. Somerville has published some highly interesting observations. It is a medicine employed by the Indians of North America. Thirty-four pounds avoirdupois of the recent herb produced four pounds of extract, of which five scruples were exhibited by Dr. Somerville in twenty-four hours, either in pills, or dissolved in a little boiling water.—(*Med. Chir. Trans.*, vol. v., p. 340, &c.) The facts stated concerning its efficacy are important ; and it has been tried with success by Dr. Beatty.—(*Trans. of Assoc. Physicians, Ireland*, vol. iv., p. 23.)]

Another powerful source of evacuation that has often been had recourse to for the cure of dropsy, is EMETICS : and, though little in use in the present day, they have weighty testimonies in their favour among earlier physicians. Their mode of action has a resemblance to that of the drastic purgatives ; for, by exciting the stomach to a greater degree of secretion, they excite the system generally ; and, in fact, far more extensively and more powerfully than can be accomplished by mere purgatives, in some degree from the greater labour exerted in the act of vomiting, but chiefly from the closer sympathy which the stomach exercises over every other part of the system than the intestines, or perhaps any other organ can exert. In cases of great debility, however, it must be obvious that such exertion would be too considerable, and would only add to the general weakness ; and it is on this account chiefly that the practice has been of late years very much discontinued in our own country. It is in consequence of this extensive sympathy of the

* Dr. A. T. Thomson's report of the virtues of this medicine is also highly favourable:—"The influence of the bitartrate in dropsical effusions is well authenticated : and indeed every day's experience confirms the confidence in its powers as a diuretic. The emaciation which the continued use of the bitartrate of potassa produces, when taken as a beverage, or in the form of imperial, as it is termed, demonstrates the powerful effect of this salt upon the absorbents ; and it is through the kidneys that the fluid thrown by them into the circulating mass is excreted. I have had," says he, "frequent opportunities of witnessing its beneficial effects in ascites, when this affection is not dependant on hepatic or other visceral obstruction. It is frequently beneficially united with squill, colchicum, and other diuretics, and, when given in a state of solution, with infusion of gentian and other bitter infusions. If the bitartrate have weakened the digestive organs, it may be combined with tartarized iron. In cases which depend on hepatic or other glandular obstructions, its best adjunct is iodine in the form of ointment."—(See Thomson's Elements of Materia Medica, vol. ii., p. 422.) According to this author, the dose for diuretic purposes should never exceed ʒss ; but it should be frequently repeated, until the kidneys are affected, diluting very freely during its employment.—ED.

Thomson's Elements of Materia Medica, vol. ii., p. 341.—ED.

stomach with every part of the system that emetics have often proved peculiarly serviceable in various local dropsies, especially that of the scrotum, when limited to the tunica vaginalis, and that of the ovarium, when discovered in an early stage. And from this cause, in combination with powerful muscular pressure, they have often acted with prompt and peculiar efficacy on ascites, or dropsy of the abdomen: while Withering, Percival, and many of the foreign journals,* abound with cases of the cure of ascites by a spontaneous vomiting.

DIAPHORETICS have also been resorted to as very actively promoting the evacuation of morbid fluids; and many instances are related by Bartholet (*Apud Bonet. Polyalth.*, iv., 47), Quarin (*Animadversiones*, &c.), and others, of the complete success of perspiration when spontaneously excited. Tissot tells us that it was by this means Count Ostermann was cured, a very copious sweat having suddenly burst forth from his feet, which continued for a long time without intermission.

In the Medical Transactions, there is a very interesting case of an equal cure effected by the same means, in a letter from Mr. Mudge to Sir George Baker. The form of the disease was, indeed, an ascites, but it will be more convenient to notice it here, while discussing the treatment of dropsy generally, than to reserve it for the place to which it more immediately belongs. The patient, a female of about forty years old, had laboured under the disease for twenty years: the abdomen was so extremely hard, as well as enlarged, that it was doubtful whether the complaint was not a *parabysma complicatum*, or physcony of various abdominal organs, and tapping was not thought advisable. She was extremely emaciated; had a quick, small pulse, and insatiable thirst, voided little urine, breathed with difficulty, and could not lie down in her bed for fear of suffocation. For an accidental rheumatism in her limbs, she had four doses of Dover's powder prescribed for her, of two scruples in each dose, one dose of which she was to take every night. The first dose relieved the pain in her limbs, but did nothing more. An hour or two after taking the second dose on the ensuing night, she began to void urine in large quantities, which she continued to do through the whole night; and as fast as she discharged the water, her belly softened and sunk; the third dose completed the evacuation. And "thus," observes Mr. Mudge, "was this formidable ascites, which had subsisted nearly twenty years, by a fortunate accident, carried off in eight-and-forty hours." The cure, too, was radical: for the constitution fully recovered itself, and the patient was restored to permanent health.

We may observe from this case, that the viscera are not necessarily injured by being surrounded, or even pressed upon, by a very large accumulation of water, for almost any length of time. It should be noticed, also, in connexion

with this remark, that the patient before us was not much more than in the middle of life, even at the date of her cure; at which period we have more reason to hope for a retention of constitutional health in the midst of a chronic and severe local disease, than at a later age. And there can be no question, that sudorifics will be found more generally successful in establishing a harmony of action between the surface and the kidneys, and produce less relaxation of the system at this than at a more advanced term of life.

But except where there is such a concurrence of favourable points, sudorifics can be but little relied upon in the treatment of dropsy, and are rather of use as auxiliaries than as radical remedies. They are also open to the same objection as emetics: they are apt, as Büchner has well observed, to do mischief by relaxing and debilitating (*Diss. de Diversâ Hydropi Medendi Methodo*, Hal., 1766), and instances are not wanting in which they have very seriously augmented the evil.—(*Piso, de Morb. ex serosa Coll.*, obs. i.)

DIURETICS are a far more valuable class of medicines, and there are few of them that operate by the kidneys alone—the intestines, the lungs, and oftentimes the whole surface of the body, internal as well as external, usually participating in their action.

Of diuretics, the most powerful, if not the most useful, is foxglove. It was in high estimation with Dr. Withering, and Dr. Darwin regards it almost as a specific in dropsies of every kind, though he admits that it does not succeed so certainly in evacuating the fluid from the abdomen as from the thorax and limbs. The preparation usually employed by the latter was a decoction of the fresh green leaves, which, as the plant is a biennial, may be procured at all seasons of the year. Of these he boiled four ounces in two pints of water till only one pint remained, and added two ounces of vinous spirit after the decoction was strained off. Half an ounce of this decoction constituted an ordinary dose, which was given early in the morning, and repeated every hour from three to eight or nine doses, or till sickness or some other disagreeable sensation was induced. In the hands of Sir George Baker, even when used in the form recommended by Dr. Darwin, its success was occasionally very doubtful; while, in some cases, it was highly injurious, without the slightest benefit whatever.—(*Medical Transactions*, vol. iii., art. xvii.) Even where it acts very powerfully as a diuretic, and carries off five or six quarts of water a day, it often excites such incessant nausea, sinking, giddiness, and dimness of sight, and such a retardation and intermission of the pulse, that the increased evacuation by no means compensates for the increased debility. And, by a repetition, it is often found to lose even its diuretic effects.

The powder, made into pills, seems to operate with equal uncertainty. It has sometimes produced a radical cure without any superinduced mischief, but in other cases it has been almost or altogether inert. Sir George Baker

---

* Sammlung Medicinischen Wahrnehmungen, b. viii., p. 220; N. Sammlung, &c., b. viii., p. 114; Schulz. Schwed. Abhandlungen, b. xxi., p. 102.

gives an instance of this inertness, both in the decoction and in pills. In a trial with the former, the dose was six drachms every hour for five successive hours during two days, through the whole of which it had not the least efficacy, not even exciting nausea. In a trial with the latter, three pills, containing a grain of the powder in each, were· given twice a day for several days in succession. They gave no relief whatever, nor produced any other effect than giddiness and dimness of sight.*

It is not wonderful, therefore, that the fortune of foxglove should have been various: that at one time it should have been esteemed a powerful remedy, and at another time been rejected as a plant *totâ substantiâ. venenosa.* Its roots have been tried as well· as· its leaves, and apparently with effects as variable, but less active. It seems to have been first introduced into the London Pharmacopœia in 1721—folia, flores, semen; was discarded in the ensuing edition of 1746, and has since been restored in its folia alone, having encountered a like alternation of favour and proscription in the Edinburgh College. · It is greatly to be wished that some mode or management could be contrived, by which its power of promoting absorption might be exerted, without the usual accompaniment of·its depressive effects. When. recommended so ·strenuously by such characters as Dr. Darwin, and more particularly Dr. Withering, from a large number· of successful cases, it is a medicine which ought not lightly to be rejected from practice, and should rather stimulate our industry to a separation of its medicinal from its mischievous qualities. Upon the whole, the singular fact first noticed by Dr. Withering seems to be sufficiently established, that, in all its forms, it is less injurious to weakly and delicate habits than to those of firmer and tenser fibres.†

The most useful of the. diuretic class of medicines are the siliquose and alliaceous ·tribes; particularly the latter, comprising leeks, onions, garlic, and especially the squill. The .last is always a valuable and important article, and

---

* A tincture of digitalis, prepared by digesting an ounce of the leaves of the herb·in three ounces of alcohol, has been employed in the endemic mode by Dr. Chretien for the last twenty years, and, according to his account, with great·success.— See the Medico-Chirurgical Review, vol. xxvi., p. 208.—D.

† Essay on Digitalis, p. 189. "It is only after ample depletion, or at least such as reduces greatly the pulse, that it affects the capillary system and augments the urinary discharge. It is after tapping and a reduction of arterial action, that decisive advantages are obtained from the employment of foxglove in hydropic affections."—(See Thomson's Elements of Materia Medica, vol. ii., p. 428.) It has been found most beneficial in hydrothorax, and next to that in anasarca. In cases of dropsy following scarlatina, it has been found very useful after purgatives have been freely administered, as well as for the anasarca and ascites occasionally taking place in constitutions broken down by the long use of mercury. The best. adjunct in the latter case is nitric acid, and in·others, bitartrate of potassa, acetate of ammonia, or colchicum.—Op. cit.—Ed.

Sydenham asserts that 'he has cured dropsies by this alone. It has the great advantage of acting generally on the secernent system, and consequently of stimulating the excretories of the alvine canal, as well as those of the kidneys. It sometimes, indeed, proves a powerful purgative ,by itself, but is always an able associate with any of the cathartics just enumerated. It may be given in any form, though its disgusting taste points out that of pills as the ·least incommodious.

When intended to act by the kidneys alone, Dr. Cullen advises that it should be combined with a neutral salt; or, if a mercurial adjunct be preferred, with a solution of corrosive sublimate, which seems to urge its course to the kidneys more quickly· and completely than any other preparation of mercury.—(*Mat. Med.*, vol. ii., part ii., ch. xxi.) It may also be observed, that the dried squill answers better as a diuretic than the fresh; the latter, as being . more acrimonious, usually stimulating the· stomach into an increased excitement, which throws it off by stool or vomiting too. soon· for it to enter into the circulating system.

The *colchicum autumnale,* or meadow saffron, ranks next, perhaps, in point of power as a diuretic, and is much entitled to attention. It is to the enterprising spirit of Dr. Stoerck that we are chiefly·indebted for a knowledge of the virtues of this plant, whose experiments were made principally on his own person. The fresh roots, which is the part he preferred, are highly acrid and stimulating; · a single grain wrapped in crumb of ·bread and taken into the stomach, excites a burning heat and pain·both in· the stomach and bowels, strangury, tenesmus, thirst, and total loss of appetite. And even while cutting the roots,· the acrid vapour that escapes irritates the nostrils and fauces; and the substance held in the fingers or applied to the tip of the tongue, so completely exhausts the sensorial power, that a numbness or torpitude is produced in either organ, and continues ,for a long time afterward.·· According to Stoerck's experiments, this acrimony is best corrected by infusion in vinegar: to which he afterward added twice the quantity.of honey.—(*Libellus de´Radice Colchico Autumnali,* Vindob., 1763, 8vo.) In the form of an acetum, and ·of the strength he proposed, it is given as a preparation in the extant London Pharmacopœia, while most of the other colleges have preferred his oxymel. Stoerck used it under both forms, but perhaps the .best preparation is the wine, as recommended by Sir Everard Home in cases of gout, depurated from all sediment, as already noticed under the latter disease. Stoerck began with a drachm of the oxymel twice·a day, and gradually increased it to an ounce or upwards.

The other diuretics in common use are of less importance, though many of them may be found serviceable auxiliaries, as they may easily enter into the dietetic regimen. These are the sal diureticus or acetate of potash, which very· slightly answers to its name, unless given in, a quantity sufficient to act at the same time as an aperient; nitrous ether; juniper berries, broom leaves, and, which is far better, broom ashes; or either of the fixed alkalis; and the green lettuce, *lactuca virosa*, strongly recommended by Dr. Colin of Vienna, but, as far as it has been tried in this country, greatly beyond its merits.

To this class of remedies we have yet to add dandelion (*leontodon taraxacum*, Linn.) and tobacco. The former of these was at one time supposed to act so powerfully and specifically on the kidneys, as to obtain the name of *lectiminga:* and it is said by some writers to have effected a cure in ascites after every other medicine had failed. It is truly wonderful to see how very little of this virtue it retains in the present day, so as to be scarcely worthy of attention; while, with respect to tobacco, notwithstanding the strenuous recommendation of Dr. Fowler, it is liable to many of the objections already started against foxglove.

The *gratiola officinalis*, or hedge hyssop, was once extensively employed, both in a recent state of its leaves and in their extract, and, like many other simples, it appears to have been injudiciously banished from the Materia Medica. In both forms it is a powerful diuretic, and often a sudorific; and in the quantity of half a drachm of the dry herb, or a drachm of infusion, whether in wine or water, it becomes an active emetic and purgative. It is said to have been peculiarly useful in dropsies consequent upon parabysma, or infarction of the abdominal viscera; and, in such cases, seems still entitled to our attention. As a strong bitter it may, like the *lactuca virosa*, which is also a strong bitter, possess some degree of tonic power, in connexion with its diuretic tendency. The bitter, however, is of a disagreeable and nauseating kind, which it is not easy to correct.*

* In addition to the remedies for dropsy mentioned in the text, the American editor will briefly allude to a few medicines which have been used as hydragogues, and with great success. The different preparations of the root kahinca (chiococca racemosa anguifuga, flore luteo) were introduced to the notice of physicians by Major Langsdorf. This plant grows in South America, and has long been known to the Indians. The French Academy of Medicine intrusted the examination of it to Messrs. Francois, Caventou, and Pelletier, and their memoir, read at the Institute, indicates the kahinca as one of the most powerful means of the Materia Medica to combat dropsy; in fact, it fulfils the same indications as colchicum, squills, nitre, digitalis, &c., and is free from their inconveniences. The best preparation of this medicine is the aqueous extract, which may be given in doses commencing with from twelve to twenty grains, although much larger quantities have been administered without injury: it seems to act more particularly on the large intestines.—See Researches on the Chymical and Medical Properties of the Root of Kahinca, New-York, 1831.

Veratria, also, is a remedy of no little power. According to Dr. Turnbull (An Investigation into the remarkable Medicinal Effects resulting from the external application of Veratria, Washington, 1834), the external application of the ointment of veratria is attended with the happiest effects in diseases attended with aqueous effusion: in these

The EXTERNAL MEANS of evacuating the fluid of cellular dropsy are blisters, setons or issues, punctures, and scarification. The last is least troublesome, and usually most effectual. It is, however, commonly postponed to too late a period, under an idea that sloughing wounds may be produced by the operation, difficult of cure, and tending to gangrene. In blistering, this has often happened; but in scarifying, the fear is unfounded, while any degree of vital energy remains: and it should never be forgotten, that the longer this simple operation is delayed, the more the danger, whatever it may be, is increased. I have never experienced the slightest inconvenience from the practice, and have rarely tried it without some advantage; seldom, indeed, without very great benefit. The wound should be limited to a small crucial incision resembling the letter T on the outside of each knee, as the most dependent organ, a little below the joint. The cut, thus shaped, and very slightly penetrating into the cellular membrane, will not easily close, and consequently the discharge will continue without interruption.*

cases, this remedy acts powerfully as a diuretic. "There appear," says Dr. Turnbull, "to be two states of dropsy in which veratria is useful: one where the pathological condition of the organs on which it depends has been removed, yet where the effused fluid remains, from the inactivity of the absorbents; the other, where the organic change is such that it cannot be radically cured." In cases of the former character, Dr. T. has known the ointment to cure the patient in a week or two, even when the symptoms were extremely serious, and other remedies had failed; and, in instances of the latter kind, much relief has been derived from its use. The ointment is made by combining from fifteen to twenty grains of veratria with an ounce of lard. In order to obtain the full benefit of its application, however, the system of the patient must be properly prepared.

Iodine has lately attracted some attention as a remedy for dropsy. Mr. Hughes has given it in the combination, the hydriodate of potass, with decided benefit; and its value has been tested by some American practitioners.—See the Boston Medical and Surgical Journal, vol. x., pp. 201, 236.

The investigations of Dr. J. H. Griscom and Dr. Knapp, of the remedial virtues of the apocynum cannabinum, or Indian hemp, demand a passing notice. This indigenous plant, which is very common in almost every section of our country, has been proved by many physicians to possess valuable diuretic properties, and in some hopeless cases has saved life. The chymical analysis of Dr. Griscom shows that a decoction, made by boiling two drachms of the root in three pints of water to two, is the best form for use, as its medicinal qualities are imparted to water much more than to alcohol. Three or four wine-glassfuls of this decoction may be given daily.—American Journal of the Medical Sciences, vol. xii.—D.

* Notwithstanding what the author has here stated, all experienced surgeons know that incisions in anasarcous parts are very liable to slough, or to become troublesome, and even dangerous ulcers. Thus, Dr. Armstrong says, "Scarifications for letting out the fluid in anasarca I am very much afraid of. I have frequently seen them become gangrenous, especially below the knee."— (Lectures on the Morbid Anatomy, Nature, and Treatment of Diseases, p. 850.) At all events,

During the progress of hydropic accumulation, there is great dryness of the tongue, and intolerable thirst. And the question has often been agitated, whether, under these circumstances, the patient's strong desire to drink should be gratified. In health, whatever be the quantity of fluid thrown into the blood, it remains there but a short time, and passes off by the kidneys, so that the balance is easily restored ; and hence it is obvious, that one of the most powerful, as well as one of the simplest diuretics in such a state, is a large portion of diluent drink. But dropsy is a state very far removed from that of health ; and, in many cases, a state in which there is a peculiar irritability in the secernents of a particular cavity, or of the cellular membrane generally, which detracts the aqueous fluid of the blood from its other constituents, and pours it forth into the cavity of the morbid organ. And hence it has been very generally concluded, that the greater the quantity of fluid taken into the system, the greater will be the dropsical accumulation ; and, consequently, that a rigid abstinence from drinking is of imperative necessity.

Sir Francis Milman, however, has very satisfactorily shown that, if this discipline be rigidly enforced, a much greater mischief will follow, than by perhaps the utmost latitude of indulgence. For, in the first place, whatever solid food is given, $_u n_{les}$ a due proportion of diluent drink be allowed, it will remain, in an hydropic patient, a hard, dry, and indigested mass in the stomach, and only add a second disease to a first. And next, without diluting fluids, the power of the most active diuretics will remain dormant ; or rather they will irritate and excite pyrexy, instead of taking their proper course to the kidneys. And, once more, as the thirst and general irritation and pyrectic symptoms increase, the surface of the body, harsh, heated, and arid, will imbibe a much larger quantity of fluid from the atmosphere than the patient is asking for his stomach ; for it has been sufficiently proved, that, under the most resolute determination not to drink, a hundred pounds of fluid have in this manner been absorbed by the inhalants of the skin, and introduced into the system in a few days, and the patient has become bulkier to such an extent in spite of his abstinence.

Even in a state of health, or where no dropsy exists, we are, in all probability, perpetually absorbing moisture by the lymphatics of the skin. Professor Home found himself heavier in the morning than he was just before he went to bed in the preceding evening, though he had been perspiring all night, and had received nothing either by the mouth or in any other sensible way. " That the surface of the skin," says Mr. Cruickshank, " absorbs fluids that come in contact with it, I have not the least doubt. A patient of mine, with a stricture in the oesoph-

instead of a crucial incision, very small punctures with the point of a lancet are to be preferred, especially as they answer the purpose of discharging the fluid even better than a single more extensive wound.—Ed.

agus, received nothing either solid or liquid into the stomach for two months ; he was exceedingly thirsty, and complained of making no water. I ordered him the warm bath for an hour, morning and evening, for a month : his thirst vanished, and he made water in the same manner as when he used to drink by the mouth, and when the fluid descended readily into the stomach."—(Anat. of Absorb. Vessels, p. 108, 4to., 1790.)

Under these circumstances, therefore, our first object should be to determine, by measurement, whether the quantity of fluid, discharged by the bladder holds a fair balance with that which is received by the mouth ; and if we find this to be a fact, and so long as it continues to be a fact, we may fearlessly indulge the patient in drinking whatever diluents he may please, and to whatever extent. In some cases, indeed, water alone, when drunk in large abundance, has proved a most powerful diuretic, and has carried off the disease without any other assistance, of which a striking instance occurs in Panarolus (Pentec. ii., obs. 24); and hence Pouteau (Œuvres Posthumes, i.), occasionally advised it in the place of all other aliment whatever ; as does also Sir George Baker (Med. Trans., vol. ii., art. xvii.), who forcibly illustrates the advantage of a free use of diluent drinks, by various cases transmitted to him, in which it operated a radical cure, not only without the assistance of any other remedy, but, in one or two instances, after every medicine that could be thought of had been tried to no purpose.

But the fluid discharged from the kidneys may not be equal, nor indeed bear any proportion, to what is introduced by the mouth ; and we may thus have a manifest proof, that a considerable quantity of the latter is drained off into the morbid cavity. Still we must not entirely interdict the use of ordinary diluents, nor suffer the patient to be tormented with a continued and feverish thirst. If simple diluent drinks will not pass to the kidneys of themselves, it will then be our duty to combine them with some of the saline or acidulous diuretics we have already noticed, which have a peculiar tendency to this organ ; and we shall generally find that, in this state of union, they will accompany the diuretic ingredients, and take the desired course. Of these, one of the most effectual, as well as the most pleasant, is cream of tartar ; and hence this ought to form a part of the ordinary beverage in all extensive dropsies, and especially the cellular and abdominal. Any of the vegetable acids, however, may be employed for the same purpose ; as may also rennet, whey, and buttermilk, and the more acid their taste the better will they answer their end. A decoction of sorrel-leaves makes a pleasant diet-drink for an hydropic patient ; as does likewise an aqueous infusion of sage-leaves with lemon-juice ; both sweetened to the taste. Small stale table-beer, and weak cider, or cider intermixed with water, may in like manner be allowed, with little regard to measure. And it was by the one or other of these, that most of the cures just referred to, as related by Sir George Baker, were effected. In one instance the cider was new, yet it proved equally salutary under the heaviest prognostics. The patient was in his fiftieth year : his legs and thighs had increased to such a magnitude that the cuticle cracked in various places ; he was extremely emaciated,* and so enfeebled as not to be able to quit his bed or return to it without assistance. His thirst was extreme, his desire for new cider inextinguishable, and, his case being regarded as desperate, it was allowed him, mixed with water. He drank it most greedily, seldom in a less quantity than five or six quarts a day ; and, by this indulgence, discharged sixteen or eighteen quarts of urine every twenty-four hours, till the water was totally drained off ; and he obtained a radical cure without any other means whatever. Even ardent spirits, if largely diluted, and joined with a portion of vegetable acid, have been found to stimulate the kidneys : and, in the opinion of Dr. Cullen, may make a part of the ordinary drink.—(*Mat. Med.*, ii., 549.) And it is chiefly owing to the tendency which the neutral salts have to the kidneys, as their proper emunctory, and the sympathy which the secernents of these organs maintain with those of all others, that the cure of dropsy has sometimes been effected by large draughts of seawater alone : though sometimes this has also acted upon the bowels, and produced the same salutary result, by exciting a very copious diarrhœa, of which a striking example is given by Zacutus Lusitanus.—(*Prax. Hist.*, lib. viii., obs. 53.)

It should never be forgotten, however, that dropsy is a disease of debility,* and that the plan of evacuating will rarely of itself effect a cure ; and never, parhaps, except in recent cases, and where little inroad has been made upon the constitution. In all other cases, it should be regarded as a preparatory step alone ; a mere palliative ; and an evil in itself : though an evil of a less kind, to surmount an evil of a greater. And it is for want of due attention to this fact, that the plan of evacuating, and particularly by drastic purgatives, has by many practitioners been carried to a dangerous and even a fatal extreme. Every purgative that does not diminish the general bulk adds to the general disease, by increasing the debility : and if, upon a very few trials, the plan be not found

to answer this salutary purpose, it cannot too soon be desisted from.

The radical cure must, after all, depend upon invigorating the constitution, or restoring the organs particularly affected to a healthy state : for even a total removal of the water affords only a palliative and present relief:

Bitters may sometimes be employed advantageously with diuretics (*Mondschein*, p. 82), or with purgatives.—(*Martius*, obs. 54.)

Bitters, indeed, where the debility does not depend upon visceral obstructions, form one of the most efficacious tonics. They are peculiarly adapted to that general loss of elasticity in the whole system, and that laxity of the exhalants, which constitutes the hydropic diathesis. "It has been alleged," says Dr. Cullen, "that bitters sometimes act as diuretics. And, as the matter of them appears to be often carried to the kidneys, and to change the state of the urine, so it is possible that, in some cases, they may increase the secretion ; but, in many trials, we have never found their operation in this way to be manifest, or at least to be any ways considerable. In one situation, however, it may have appeared to be so. When, in dropsy, bitters moderate that exhalation into the cavities which forms the disease, there must necessarily be a greater proportion of serum carried to the kidneys : and thereby bitters may, without increasing the action of the kidneys, seem to increase the secretion of urine."—(*Mat. Med.*, ii., p. 58.)

To bitters have been added the warmer balsamics and aromatics, and by many physicians the metallic oxydes ; chiefly the different preparations of copper ; though Willis, Boerhaave, Bonet, and Digby, have occasionally preferred those of silver. Iron has generally been abstained from as too heating, though recommended by Grieve (*Med. Com. Edin.*, ix.; ii., 75), Richard (*Journ. de Méd.*, xxix., 140), and Rhumelius.—(*Medic. Spagyr. tripart.*, p. 168.)

When the disease is evidently dependant upon some visceral obstruction, mercury offers a fairer chance of success than any other metal ; and in this case has often been pushed to salivation with the most-salutary result. Du Verney employed it to this extent in an ascitic patient, whom at the same time he tapped ; and, by this double plan, effected a cure ; allowing a regimen of wine and stimulant meals during the process.—(*Mém. de Paris*, 1703, p. 174.) And Rahn assures us that in one case, the disease, though it several times recurred, was in every instance put to flight by a ptyalism excited by mercurial inunction.—(*Medic. Briefwechsel*, b. i., 365.) But where the system is in a state of great general debility, such treatment will only add to the weakness and increase the disease. Small doses of calomel, steadily persisted in, will be here our safest course, with a nutritious and generous diet of flesh-meat two or even three times a day ; shellfish, eggs, spice, and the acrid vegetables, as celery, water-cresses, raw red cabbage, shred fine and eaten as salad.

We have, however, observed, that dropsy occasionally ensues from an undue excitement

---

* The opposition made at the present day to this view of the subject has been already mentioned, and will be noticed again in one of the ensuing notes. Some kinds of dropsy are clearly brought on by interruption of the return of blood from the parts affected.—(See J. Bouillaud, De l'Oblitération des Veines, et de son Influence sur la Formation des Hydropisies partielles, &c., Paris, 1823.) Yet, whoever looks over the remarks of Mr. Hodgson on this subject, published many years ago in his valuable Treatise on the Diseases of the Arteries and Veins, will not, I think, be inclined to set down obstruction of the venous circulation as quite so general a cause of dropsy as M. Bouillaud represents. The latter has attempted, however, in the Dict. de Méd. et de Chir. Pratiques, art. HYDROPISIE, to defend his own view, in opposition to that of Mr. Hodgson. —ED.

of the absorbents or the serous tissues, and is even accompanied with inflammatory action. And, in this case, a free use of the lancet should precede every other remedial method; and will sometimes, as when the stimulus is a retardation of blood in the veins and a consequent accumulation in the arteries, effect a cure of its own accord. It should be, nevertheless, remarked, that dropsies of this form are rather a symptom of some other misaffection, than an original or idiopathic disease.

We have thus far contemplated dropsy as an idiopathic disease, dependant chiefly on constitutional debility :* but there are cases in which it occurs as a transfer of morbid action in some other organ of the system than the cellular

---

* The doctrine of the origin of dropsy from simple debility has been already noticed, and its correctness questioned. Dropsy is undoubtedly very often attended with debility; but this is not its cause. Many dropsies are local, that is to say, restricted to some particular limb or cavity. If they arose from general debility, would they be thus confined to certain situations?—(See Bouillaud, in Dict. de Méd. et de Chir. Pratiques, tom. x., p. 182.) When we find some varieties of dropsy demonstrably proceeding from organic disease of the kidney, liver, heart, or spleen, or from the obstruction or obliteration of the venæ cavæ, vena portæ, or from disease of the heart, surely it is time, at all events, to modify the doctrine relating to the essential dependance of dropsy on debility. Some forms of it, termed active, are unquestionably connected, not with atony of the absorbents, but an increased action of the arteries, leading to an augmentation of secretion and exhalation. These views enable us to perceive the reason why active dropsies, or those accompanied by a process analogous to inflammation, should be treated with much greater success than the passive varieties of the disorder, the result of incurable internal organic diseases. With respect to the prognosis, the following are the sentiments of the late Dr. Armstrong :—"If the cause be inflammation, the prognosis is very often favourable. If it be from some change in the blood, it is favourable, if that change arise from mere disorder. If it arise from organic disease, it is almost invariably unfavourable. It is connected with organic disease most frequently in persons who are advanced in life."— (See Armstrong's Lectures on the Morbid Anatomy, Nature, and Treatment of Diseases, p. 851, 8vo., Lond.; 1834.) In the prognosis, the situation of the dropsy must also be taken into consideration : thus, a dropsy of the pericardium, pleura, or arachnoid membrane, is much more dangerous than one of the tunica vaginalis. An œdema of the lungs or glottis brings on alarming symptoms, and sometimes fatal consequences, though an œdema of one of the limbs may not be attended with any serious inconvenience. Strictly speaking, perhaps, no dropsy is idiopathic, or unconnected with some organic disease of the liver, kidneys, or other viscus, unless we take into the account what may be regarded as a completely local dropsy, the hydrocele, and some other circumscribed effusions. And even when no organic visceral disease can be traced, and the dropsy has followed fever, or some other general disturbance of the health, it is still only an effect, and not an original disease. The same may be said of examples in which it follows inflammation of serous membranes.—ED.

membrane, or whatever other part may be the seat of the hydropic affection ;. and in such cases it is often salutary, and answers the purpose of a counter-irritation, and especially in fevers and inflammatory attacks. "I have," says Dr. Parry, " so often known constitutional maladies suspended, and life evidently lengthened and rendered more comfortable, by the coming on of various dropsical effusions; and, on the contrary, so many persons suffer aggravations of disease or even death, very shortly after the spontaneous disappearance of dropsy, that I cannot avoid considering the effusion as a salutary process rather than as an actual disease."—(Elements of Pathology, &c., vol. ii., 8vo., 1815.)

I have dwelt the longer on this species, because the general observations which it suggests, as well in respect to its causes and history as to its mode of treatment, apply in a very considerable degree to all the rest, concerning which we now shall have little more to do than to enumerate them and point out their distinctive characters.

[In the renal variety of dropsy, described by Dr. Bright, he approves of general and local bloodletting, with the view of checking the progress of the morbid change in the kidney, as well as of combating accidental inflammation in the serous membranes, or a tendency to apoplexy. He has recourse also to mild laxatives and diuretics ; and when he administers squill, he generally combines it with a little opium or hyoscyamus. He is not in favour of employing mercury, which, he says, he has sometimes seen interrupt the good effects of other remedies, often protract the cure, or not at all retard the advance of the disorder to a fatal termination. When tonics are indicated, he has found much benefit arise from combining sulphate of quinine with squill, or from the use of chalybeates, or the uva ursi.—(See Bright's Reports of Med. Cases, &c., 4to., Lond., 1827.)]

SPECIES II.
HYDROPS CAPITIS.
DROPSY OF THE HEAD. WATER IN THE HEAD.

ŒDEMATOUS INTUMESCENCE OF THE HEAD : THE SUTURES OF THE SCULL GAPING.

THIS disease has been strangely confounded by nosologists and practical writers with that inflammation of the brain which apparently commences in its substance or lower part, and, producing effusion into the ventricles, distends them, and thus unites the symptoms of fever and great irritability with those of heaviness, and at length of stupor. The accumulation of fluid is here only an effect, and follows inflammation of the brain as in any other part, and is to be removed by removing the inflammation. It is ordinarily denominated, however, acute or internal hydrocephalus ; but Dr. Cullen has correctly distinguished it from proper hydrocephalus, or dropsy of the head, by placing it in a different part of his classification, and assigning it a different name. In his view it is an apoplexy, and he has hence called it *apoplexia hydrocephalica.* In the present work, it occurs under the name of CEPHALITIS *profunda ;* and in treating of it as a cephalitis, the author has submitted his reasons for not regarding it as an apoplectic affection.*

The disease before us is common to children. A few singular cases are, indeed, recorded of its commencing in adult age (*Hildan.,* cent. iii., obs. 17, 19), and producing an enlargement of the scull by a morbid separation of the sutures ; but these are very rare. That it does, however, occur without such separation and enlargement, and that too occasionally in every period of life, has been proved by a multitude of examinations after death, that have shown the ventricles of the brain distended with fluid, producing a considerable pressure upon the brain. Yet where no such enlargement of the scull takes place, we may sometimes strongly suspect the disease from the symptoms, but cannot during the life of a patient speak with certainty upon the subject.

Dropsy of the head, like that of every other organ, is a disease of debility ; and as we have already observed in the introductory remarks to the present genus, may proceed from a relaxed condition of the secernents of the brain, a torpitude of its absorbents, or from both. The causes of this morbid state we are rarely able to ascertain : yet, in some families, there seems to be a peculiar predisposition to it, since it occurs in many of the children born in succession : and it may sometimes be connected with a scrofulous diathesis.

The immediate seat of the dropsy varies considerably : for sometimes the fluid accumulates between the bones of the cranium and the dura mater ; sometimes between the dura mater or the other membranes and the brain ; and sometimes in the ventricles or convolutions of the organ. With the deficiency of tone, there is also not unfrequently some deficiency of structure or substance : and it is in consequence of this that the fluid, when morbidly secreted or collected in one part, spreads without resistance to another. A deficiency of structure or substance is sometimes found in the brain itself, and sometimes in the cranium. If it occur in the former, a path may be immediately opened for the morbid fluid, accumulated in the ventricles or in any

other interior part, to reach the membranes and distend the scull : and if in the latter, it may even pass beyond the scull, and separate and distend the integuments. I have seen instances of large perforations produced in different parts of the bones by a morbid absorption of the bony earth, as though the trephine had been repeatedly applied, and this too in adult age : and, in some instances, there has been a total absence of the calvaria.—(*Act. Helvet.*, i., 1.) Generally speaking, there is some deficiency of bony earth, as though it were impossible for this secretion to keep pace with the enlargement of the cranium : and hence the bones of the cranium have occasionally been so thin as to be pellucid and transmit the light of a candle, of which Van Swieten gives an instance (*Comment. in Hydrop.*, sect. 1217), from Betbeder (*Histoire de l'Hydro-cephale de Begle,* p. 35) ; or have had their place supplied by a membrane covering the entire range of the sinciput, an example of which will be found in Vesalius.—(*De Corp. Human. fabricâ,* lib. i., cap. 5.)

The dropsical fluid is also said by many writers of high authority to originate in some cases between the integuments and the bone, and to be confined to this quarter ; and hence the disease has been divided into external and internal dropsy of the head. It is possible, indeed, as Van Swieten has justly observed, that since water may be collected in the cellular membrane of the whole body, such an accumulation may take place in the integuments of the head.—(*Comment.*, loc. citat., 1718.) But the pretended cases are so rare, that Van Swieten himself, Petit (*Acadêm. des Sciences, Mem.*, p. 121), and many other writers of high credit, have doubted whether such a form of the disease has ever actually occurred. Yet, should it occasionally take place, there can, I think, be no question that it ought rather to be regarded as a variety of anasarca or cellular dropsy, than hydrocephalus, or dropsy of the head, properly so called. Celsus has been quoted upon the occasion, as confirming the existence of this external modification, and applying to it the name of hydrocephalus : but this is to misunderstand him egregiously. In the passage referred to, he is speaking of internal diseases of the head alone, of cephalæa, and other aches produced by wine or indigestion, by cold or heat, or the rays of the sun, sometimes accompanied with fever, and sometimes without it ; sometimes affecting the whole of its interior, and sometimes only a part :—"modò IN TOTO CAPITE, modò IN PARTE." And then he adds, "præter hæc etiamnum invenitur genus, quod potest longum esse : ubi humor cutem inflat, eaque intumescit, et, prementi digito, cedit : ὑδροκέφαλον Græci appellant."—(*De Medecin.*, lib. iv., cap. ii.) It is manifest, therefore, that the hydrocephalus here noticed, like the other diseases with which it is associated, is an internal affection of the head : and this idea is still farther confirmed by the treatment which he shortly afterward proceeds to prescribe for it.

It is hence highly probable, that the cases which have been called external dropsies of the

---

* From the abundant evidence furnished by the cases and dissections recorded by Dr. Abercrombie, no doubt can be entertained that the disease, commonly called acute hydrocephalus, is originally an inflammatory affection, chiefly seated in the substance of the central parts of the brain ; that it generally terminates in a softening of these parts, or the morbid alteration termed by the French *ramollissement,* combined with serous effusion in the ventricles ; and that it may prove fatal by the softening alone, even of small extent, but with all the symptoms usually considered as characteristic of acute hydrocephalus.—(See Abercrombie's Pathol. and Pract. Researches on Diseases of the Brain, p. 142, &c., 8vo., Edin., 1828.) Many other remarks from this valuable source are introduced into the present work, under the head of cephalitis.—ED.

head, have consisted of internal accumulations spreading to and distending the integuments through channels that were not ascertained, and on this account not supposed to exist.

Were the distinctions of external and internal dropsy of the head necessary to be preserved, it would be far more accurate to limit the former to those modes of the complaint in which the water is confined between the calvaria and the membranes, and the latter to those in which it originates in the cavities of the brain : but as we can rarely, if ever, determine the limits of the collection by the symptoms, it is a distinction which cannot be supported, and would often lead us into error.

The form of the disease, however, which occurs between the calvaria and the dura mater, is by no means common, and hence seldom likely to lead us astray. So little common, indeed, is it, that Dr. Gölis, who probably had more practice in this complaint than any other physician of ancient or modern times, expressly declares, that "he never met with an example of it, and that he knows there are many physicians of extensive practice who have seen as little of it as himself."—(Drs. L. A. Gölis, Abhandlungen über vorzüglicheren Krankheiten, &c., b. i., Wien., 1815.)

Hydrops capitis frequently commences in the fœtus,* and sometimes renders the head so large as to retard the labour, and greatly harass the delivery. Blanchard gives a case, in which four pounds of water were evacuated from the head of a fœtus after its birth. At other times, it does not show itself till some months, or even two or three years, after birth. In most cases the whole head enlarges, attended with a gradual separation of the sutures ; but, in a few cases, the first symptom has been a small, elastic tumour on the upper part of the head, produced by an inequality of the dura mater, and its yielding more readily at the part that presents than in any other quarter. This tumour sometimes grows to a size as large as the

head itself. It is seldom, however, that the walls of the tumour burst ; for the uniform pressure to which they are exposed has a tendency to thicken and harden them. And hence, as the resistance increases, the sutures give way generally, and the tumour frequently disappears and is lost in the general swell.

The brain therefore exhibits, as we have already observed, some misformation or defect, which of itself may constitute a remote cause ; but the proximate cause is a debility of the local secernents, absorbents, or both.* If the debility be confined to these, or the defect in structure do not interfere with the proper development of the mental or corporeal powers of the sensorium, the infant may live and even thrive in every other part, while the water continues to accumulate and the head to become more monstrous, and even insupportable from its own weight : for, provided the pressure applied be very gradual, and unaccompanied with inflammation, the brain, like the stomach and intestines in dropsy of the belly, may be drowned in water for even twenty or thirty years, without serious mischief.—(Coindet, Mémoire sur l'Hydrencephale, &c., Geneva, 1818.) Michaelis relates the case of a patient twenty-nine years old, whose appetite and memory were good, and the pupils of the eyes natural, though the disease had continued from birth.—(Medical Communications, vol. i., art. xxv.) And, in treating of vascular osthexy, I had occasion to notice, from Dr. Heberden, the history of a patient who, with about eight ounces of water in the ventricles of the brain, as appeared on opening him,—and which there was good reason for believing had existed there for many years,—and with scarcely an organ free from disease in his whole body, with the exception of the brain itself, which was found healthy in its substance, was enabled to attain the good old age of upwards of fourscore years with

---

* The disease may begin at a very early period of the embryon ; and M. Otto has seen it in one not further advanced than the sixth week. M. Dugès is not led, however, by this fact to suppose, that the origin of the disease depends upon any retardation in the development of the brain ; for he has ascertained by repeated observation, that the brain of a subject affected with hydrocephalus is perfect with respect to all its parts and configuration, with the exception of those changes which are produced by the distention of the fluid. He has also found, that how thin soever its substance may be, it often weighs, without the fluid, as much as, and even more than, the brain of a healthy individual of the same age as the patient. Chronic hydrocephalus appears to him to be frequently an hereditary complaint, inasmuch as the children of some women are all more or less affected ; and it is an observation made by him, that women who are not very young at the period of their confinement, and who have a redundance of the fluid of the amnios, or a considerable degree of œdema of the lower extremities during pregnancy, are particularly liable to bring forth hydrocephalic children.—See Dict. de Méd. et de Chir. Pratiques, tom. x., p. 131.—Ed.

* No doubt, the pathology of hydrops capitis, or chronic hydrocephalus, is more obscure than that of cephalitis profunda, or acute hydrocephalus ; yet, as Dr. Abercrombie has observed, it is highly probable, that in the disorder under present consideration, the effusion arises from a low degree of inflammatory action in the brain.—(See Pathol. and Pract. Researches on Diseases of the Brain, p. 143.) If this view be adopted, we must not talk of debility, but of an increased action of the secernents. Some distinguished modern pathologists believe that a frequent cause of passive dropsies is an obstruction of the venous circulation ; and Dr. Tonellé has adduced several cases in support of this view, in relation to chronic hydrocephalus. In the fifth volume of the Journ. Hebdomadaire he has inserted the particulars of six instances of obliteration of the venous sinuses of the dura mater, attended with an accumulation of serous fluid under the tunica arachnoides. The fluid which he has likewise found in the ventricles has been constantly the effect of, and in proportion to, such obliteration. Facts of this kind are entitled to the attention of pathologists, though they are not likely to afford an explanation of the causes of hydrocephalus in general. Yet, it is making which some advance to ascertain the circumstances accompany particular examples of the disease. —Ed.

an apparently sound constitution, and free from all the usual infirmities of advancing years, saving the inconvenience of an habitual deafness.

But the torpitude or imbecility of the excernent vessels may extend to the other parts of the brain, and to parts that are immediately connected with the mental faculties ; or the defects of structure that are so often combined with dropsy of the head may extend to the same : and in such cases the hearing, sight, or speech, may be affected : there may be loss of memory, or stupidity, vertigo, epilepsy, or convulsion-fits. The brain has sometimes been found in a spongy or fungous state (*Conrad, Diss. de Hydrocephalo*, Argent., 1778) ; or otherwise disorganized (*Bonet, Sepulchr.*, lib. i., sect. xvi., obs. 9) ; and sometimes tense and slender, with nerves like mucus.—(*Büttner, Beschreibung des innern Wasserkopfs*, &c., Königs., 1773.) The fluid, moreover, may accumulate with rapidity, instead of slowly, as soon as the exciting cause, whatever it may be, is in operation, and the suddenness of the pressure may impede the action of the sanguiferous vessels; and we shall then perceive symptoms of compression ; as a heavy pain in the head, stupor, occasional vomiting, quick pulse, and other febrile concomitants, a perpetual flow of tears from the eyes, or of mucus from the nostrils. And hence dropsy of the head is so frequently a symptom or a sequel of inflammation of the brain, and particularly of parenchymatic inflammation.

In this disease, as in apoplexy, we not unfrequently also meet with that peculiar mollescence of the substance of the brain to which the French pathologists have given the name of ramollissement de cerveau : and which, when treating of apoplexy, we observed, is far more frequently a result of debilitated than of inflammatory or entonic action. Sometimes the entire substance of the organ, as well of the white as of the gray portion, is found in this softened state ; and, in a few instances, a very considerable portion of it is absorbed and carried off, the remaining part being nothing more than a pulpy mass or pouch. "When the cranium," says Dr. Baillie, "is very much enlarged in hydrocephalus, the brain is thinned by absorption into a pulpy bag, and the corpus callosum is burst, so that the water deposited in the ventricles comes in contact with the dura mater at the upper part of the cranium. In this way a hydrocephalus, originally internal, becomes in part external."[*]

Yet even here we have sometimes striking and most singular proofs, that the remedial power of nature is interfering either to obtain a cure, or to render the disease compatible with life, and with the general faculties of the sensorium.

There is an interesting illustration of this remark in a case related by Dr. Donald Monro. A child, at the age of a year and a half, was brought into St. George's Hospital with a head much enlarged from the disease before us. She was feverish, and had a slight stupor. The complaint was peculiarly obstinate, and resisted the use of purges, blisters, issues, bandages, and other remedies. The enlargement proceeded and became chronic, though the fever and stupor gradually diminished, and at length ceased ; yet the head continued to enlarge, and kept an equal proportion with the child's growth : so that, in her eighth year, it measured two feet four inches round, which is nearly a foot more than it ought to have done, and the forehead alone was half the entire length of the face, or four inches out of eight, which is double the proportion it ought to have held,—yet the child was at this time as lively and sensible as most children of her age, and had a strong and peculiarly retentive memory. It was long before she could walk, on account of the vast weight of head she had to carry, and the difficulty of preserving a balance ; but at length she learned to walk also with tolerable ease.—(*Med. Trans.*, vol. ii., p. 359.)

In the following case, the efforts of the remedial power were less successful : but it is peculiarly worthy of notice, as much from the lateness of the age in which the disease commenced, and the sutures were separated, as from the natural struggle there seems to have been to obtain a triumph over it. It is related by Dr. Baillie, in another volume of the same valuable work. The patient was a boy, not less than seven years of age when he first became affected. The pupils, from an early stage, were considerably dilated, and the pulse was somewhat irregular ; he complained of pain towards the back of his head, and was often in a state of stupor. His understanding, however, was clear, and his sight very little impaired almost to the last. He had twice intervals of great promise, for a few weeks, with considerable abatement of all the symptoms, and an appearance of doing well. But in both instances he relapsed, and at the distance of ten months from the commencement, fell under daily attacks of convulsion-fits. It is remarkable that, though his intellect continued unimpaired, the frontal and parietal bones, from the force of the accumulated fluid in every direction, were separated from each other to a distance of from half to three quarters of an inch, notwithstanding that they had been firmly united at their respective sutures before the commencement of the disease. Nearly a pint of water was found in the ventricles.

In many cases, the bones of the scull become peculiarly thin and pellucid, or are altogether deprived of their calcareous earth, and reduced to cartilages. But where the instinctive or remedial power of nature, which is always labouring to restore morbid parts to a state of health, or to enable them in their altered condition to fulfil their proper functions, has succeeded in rendering the diseased brain still capable of exercising

---

[*] Morb. Anat., fascic. x., pl. iii., p. 213. In an embryo, scarcely nine or ten lines in length, M. Dubrueil showed M. Dugès a cranium that was softened, shrivelled up, and perforated at the vertex, without any brain in it. By inflation it immediately became of very large dimensions, with respect to the small size of the being from which it was taken.—See Dict. de Méd. et de Chirurgie Pratiques, tom. x., p. 134.—ED.

some of its faculties, a supply of phosphate of lime is also, in various instances, provided for the bony membrane; which not only reassumes its ordinary firmness, but has sometimes exhibited a density far beyond the usual proportion, and commensurate with the magnitude of the scull, while the cervical vertebræ have been equally strengthened for the purpose of bearing so enormous a load. Hildanus gives a case of this kind in a youth eighteen years old, who had laboured under a dropsy of the head from his third year. The scull was of an immense magnitude (*immensæ magnitudinis*), as well as peculiarly hard and solid. The patient spoke distinctly, but his mind was not equal to his articulation, and he suffered greatly from violent epileptic attacks.—(*Observ. Chirurg.*, cent. iii., obs. xix., p. 199.) "If sculls of this kind," says the Baron Van Swieten, "should be disinhumed in their burial-ground by posterity, there would certainly not be wanting persons who would ascribe them to some gigantic family. If, indeed, the calvaria should be dug up entire, the error may be corrected by observing the size of the upper jaw-bones, which would be found of the ordinary proportion: but if the bones should be separated and single, there could be no appeal to this distinctive mark."*

The disease is always dangerous, from the difficulty of determining its extent, and what degree of cerebral disorganization may accompany it. Where, however, it is limited to a weak condition of the excernents of the brain, it is often remediable, and admits of a radical cure. But where, on the contrary, no favourable impression can be made on the organ, the general frame partakes by degrees of the debility, the vital powers flag, the limbs become emaciated, and death ensues at an uncertain period: or the patient survives, a miserable spectacle to the world and burden to himself; rarely reaching old age, but sometimes enduring life for twenty or even thirty years (*Van Swieten, Comment.*, loc. citat.) before he is released from his sufferings. In a few instances, it is observed by Dr. Coindet, that coma, a dilated pupil, and other symptoms resembling acute hydrocephalus, as it has been called, or profound cephalitis, accompany the disease from its commencement (*Mémoire sur l'Hydrencéphale, &c.*, Geneva, 1818): but I believe the pulse will, in such instances, rarely be found to betray that irritable irregularity in the beat which has been already noticed in the cephalitic disease. On opening the head, twelve or fifteen pints of fluid have often been evacuated: and occasionally not less than twenty-four or twenty-five pints (*Bonet, Sepulchr.*, lib. i., sect. xvi., obs. 1; *Eph. Nat. Cur.*, dec. iii., ann. i., obs. 10), which have the singular property of not jellying even on exposure to heat.—(*Hewson on the Lymph. Syst.*, part ii., p. 193.)

The water has sometimes been found lodged

in a cyst, and, in a few instances, the cerebrum itself has formed a sac for it. Morgagni asserts, that the disease is more common to girls than to boys.—(*De Sed. et Caus. Morb.*, ep. xii., art. 6.)

The cure, as in the preceding species, must be attended by evacuating the water by internal or external means, and by giving tone to the debilitated organs.

Drastic purges can rarely, in this form of the disease, be carried to such an extent as to be of essential service, on account of the early period of life in which it commonly shows itself. For the same reason, diaphoretics have not been generally recommended, or often found serviceable when ventured upon. Diuretics have been more frequently had recourse to, and particularly the digitalis. Dr. Withering was favourable to its use; but it has commonly, as in other forms of dropsy, proved more injurious than beneficial. The best internal medicine is calomel, in small doses, in union with some carminative, for the purpose of keeping up the action of the stomach, a healthy state of which is of great importance. The calomel, however, should be employed rather as a stimulant or tonic, so as to excite the mouths of the torpid vessels to a return of healthy action, than as a purgative, or with a view of producing salivation; except, indeed, where symptoms of inflammation are present, in which case it cannot be given too freely, as already observed under parenchymatic cephalitis.—(Vol. i., p 465.) Where the disease has been unaccompanied with inflammatory symptoms, but nevertheless has been attended with a feverish irritation, and great heaviness, as well as considerable enlargement of the head, the author has found half a grain of calomel, given three times a day, in the manner above proposed, and continued for a month, of essential service: and particularly in a case that occurred to him many years ago, of a little boy who was four years old when the disease first appeared; which, however, had made its attack so insidiously as to escape the observation of the parents till the increased bulk of the head attracted their notice, which was soon afterward succeeded by the symptoms just adverted to. The complaint had increased, the symptoms were more aggravated, and the scull, within six months, had become as large as that of an adult, when the mercurial process was commenced, accompanied with a free fomentation of the head with the solution of the acetate of ammonia, and an occasional use of purgatives. In ten days there was an evident improvement: the child was less languid and feverish, and showed less desire to rest his head perpetually on a chair. The scull no longer augmented; the mental faculties, which had begun to discover hebetude, regained vigour, and the patient, now in his twentieth year, is an undergraduate in one of our universities, exhibiting a development of talents that has already obtained for him various prizes, and gives a promise of considerable success hereafter. The bulk of his head is at this moment very little larger than it was at six years of age: a curious fact

---

* Comment., tom. iv., sect. 1217, p. 123. Monro records the case of a child nine years old, whose cranium was thirty-six inches in circumference. —Ed.

in pathology, though by no means uncommon : since, where the disease forms space enough for a perfect growth of the brain, the calvaria ceases to expand, and the head becomes once more proportioned to the rest of the body.

The external means employed for diminishing the contained fluid, have consisted in local stimulants, as different preparations of ammonia, blisters, and cauteries, and puncturing the integuments.

All local stimulants have a chance of being useful where the disease is seated near the surface, or between the membranes and the cranium, for they tend to excite the absorbents to an increased degree of tone and action, and consequently to a diminution of the general mass. But they do not seem to have much effect when the fluid issues from the convolutions or ventricles of the brain. Blistering the whole of the sinciput has unquestionably been found serviceable, and is perhaps the most effectual external stimulant we can employ.

The water has also been evacuated, in many instances, with full success, by a lancet : and, where the sutures gape very wide, and the integuments are considerably distended, this remedy ought always to be tried. The brain, however, like every other organ, when it has been long accustomed to the stimulus of pressure, cannot suddenly lose such a stimulus without a total loss of energy ; and hence, as it is necessary, in many cases of dropsy of the belly, to stop as soon as we have drawn off a certain portion of water, in order to avoid faintness, it is found equally necessary to evacuate the water from the brain with caution and by separate stages ; for when the whole has been discharged at once, the sensorial exhaustion has been so complete as to produce deliquium and sudden death. Hence six or eight ounces are as much as it may be prudent to let loose at a time in an infant of three or four years of age ; when the orifice should be covered with a piece of adhesive plaster, and an interval of a day or two be allowed. The operation, indeed, is very far from succeeding in every instance: for, in some cases, there is so much internal disease, or even disorganization, that success is not to be obtained by any means. And next, a fresh tide of water will not unfrequently accumulate, and the head become as much distended as before. Still, however, the attempt should be made, and even repeated and repeated again, if a fresh flow of fluid should demand it ; for the disease has occasionally been found to yield to a second or third evacuation, where it has triumphed over the first.

Dr. Vose of Liverpool has published an instructive case of this kind in the second volume of the Medico-Chirurgical Transactions. The patient was seven months old, and the head between two and three times its natural size, when the operation was first performed. On this occasion a couching-needle was made use of, and the orifice was closed when three ounces and five drachms of fluid were evacuated: about an equal quantity was conjectured to dribble from the orifice after the operation : at which

time the infant became extremely faint, and the integuments of the head had shrivelled into the shape of a pendulous bag. He revived, however, with the aid of a little cordial medicine ; and, the water accumulating afresh, a second operation was performed by a bistoury about six weeks after, when eight ounces of fluid were drawn off with little constitutional disturbance ; which was succeeded only nine days later by a third operation, that yielded, by the introduction of a grooved director, twelve ounces, without any interference with the general health whatever. A copious and vicarious discharge of serum from the rectum took place shortly after this third puncture of the integuments, which was succeeded by some degree of deliquium ; but from this also the patient soon recovered ; the head gradually diminished in size, and a complete cure was at length effected.[*]

Formey (Ad Rivierii, Observ. Medic., cent. v.), Pitschel,[†] and several other writers, have recommended compression, with a view of stimulating the torpid mouths of the absorbents to a

----

[*] According to Monro, however, the child was subsequently attacked with symptoms which proved fatal.—(See also Dugès, in Dict. de Méd. et de Chir. Pratiques, tom. x., p. 136.) Mr. Lizars has published a case in the Edin. Med. and Surg. Journ., where he operated about twenty times in the course of three months. The instrument which he commonly employed was a fine trocar, which was introduced to the depth of an inch, at the most lateral part of the anterior fontanelle, so as to avoid the longitudinal sinus. On the discharge of the water, the strabismus and dilatation of the pupil immediately ceased. In some of the later operations, the sutures having become in part closed from the progress of ossification, the head was no longer capable of being adequately compressed, and air rushed in to supply the place of the fluid, but without any ill effects. The same practice has also been adopted in one instance by Dr. Freckleson, of Liverpool ; the lateral ventricles having been punctured four times with safety ; but, in the fifth operation, fourteen ounces of fluid having been suddenly discharged, the child became convulsed, and died on the ninth day. Dr. Conquest has operated on nine children, on four of which he was entirely successful, the individuals having been restored to health. The largest quantity of fluid withdrawn at any one time was twenty ounces and a half ; and the greatest number of operations on one child was five, performed at intervals varying from two to six weeks. The largest total quantity of water removed was fifty-seven ounces, by five successive operations. The trocar was introduced through the coronal suture, below the anterior fontanelle ; and pressure on the head was subsequently made with strips of adhesive plaster. —(See Cyclop. of Pract. Med., art HYDROCEPHALUS, by Dr. Joy, p. 478.) This treatment has likewise been tried by Graefe of Berlin (Journ. für Chirurgie, &c., 1831, b. xv., p. 3), and by Mr. Russell of Edinburgh.—See Edin. Med. and Surg. Journ., July, 1832.—ED.

[†] Anat. and Chir. Anmark, Dresd., 1784. Sir Gilbert Blane was in favour of this practice, aided by the frequent application of leeches.—(See Med. and Physical Journ. for Oct., 1821.) Mr. Barnard made compression with straps of adhesive plaster, and used leeches, with a successful result.—See Med. Repository.—ED.

resumption of their proper action. But no compression can be made on these, whatever they may consist in (for absorbents have not hitherto been detected in the brain), without compressing at the same time parts that are injured by pressure already. Advantage, however, may be taken of the recommendation, after the fluid has been evacuated.*

____

SPECIES III.
HYDROPS SPINÆ.
DROPSY OF THE SPINE.

SOFT FLUCTUATING EXTUBERANCE ON THE SPINE; GAPING VERTEBRÆ.

This is the *spina bifida* of authors, so called from the double channel which is often produced by it through a considerable length of the vertebral column: a natural channel for the spinal marrow, and a morbid channel running in a parallel line, and equally descending from the brain, and filled with the fluid which constitutes the disease.

It is sometimes local ; but, in most instances, is connected with a morbid state of the brain, and directly communicates with it. In this last form, it may be regarded as a compound dropsy of this organ. [As Dr. Abercrombie has noticed, when serous effusion occurs between the dura mater and inner membrane of the cord, the source of it may be attended with ambiguity, on account of the free communication which this space has with the cavity of the cranium, or at least with the cellular texture of the arachnoid coat of the brain. But, as he further explains, when the effusion is contained in the cavity formed betwixt the dura mater and the canal of the vertebræ, there can be no doubt of its connexion with disease of the spinal canal.— (See *Abercrombie's Pathol. and Pract. Researches on Diseases of the Brain*, &c., p. 358, 8vo., Edin., 1828.) In spina bifida, the fluid is always within the dura mater of the cord. On this account, when the disease is combined with hydrocephalus, we see the reason of the communication between the two diseases ; but it is an error to suppose, as our author stated in his last edition, that the dropsical swelling on the spine

is the effect of the water gravitating downwards from the head ; for it is, in fact, the consequence of a malformation of the vertebræ, the ossification of the posterior parts of which is imperfect ; and consequently a protrusion of the dura mater, the cavity of which is filled with fluid, naturally takes place. The dropsical affection of the head does not always accompany the disease of the spine, and is only an accidental complication.]

Dropsy of the spine is mostly congenital, and consequently a disease of fœtal life ; in many instances, however, the tumour does not show itself till some weeks, or even months, after the birth of the child. The degree of danger, as justly observed by Dr. Olivier (*De la Moëlle Epinière, et de ses Maladies*, &c., 8vo., Paris, 1824), must depend upon the structural defect, or other mischief, that exists in the brain or the substance of the spinal marrow. We observed in the last species, that the bones of the cranium are often found imperfect ; and it is hence not to be wondered at, that the bones of the vertebræ should exhibit a like imperfection in the present, and allow a protrusion externally. Fieliz gives a case in which all the spinous processes were deficient, and the dropsy extended through the entire length of the spine.—(In *Richter, Chir. Bibl.*, band ix., p. 185.)

The integuments are here thinner and more disposed to burst than in the head, and hence, if the tumour be left to its natural course, it commonly continues to enlarge till it bursts ;* while, if it be opened, the child, in most cases, dies from exhaustion and deliquium, as in dropsy of the head, provided the water be evacuated entirely : and if it be discharged gradually, an inflammation of the spinal marrow is apt to ensue, which proves as fatal. Hence there is much reason in the advice of Mr. Warner merely to support the tumour, but not to touch it

____

* "Hydrocephalus in its acute form is of frequent occurrence in the United States," says Dr. Hosack, "and this circumstance has led practitioners to look with great circumspectness at the incipient stage of the complaint. The lancet, purgatives of the more drastic sort, and blisters to the more distant parts, are the curative means generally employed." Dr. Rush states, "that the unsuccessful employment of mercury has led him to decline the use of that medicine altogether, except when combined with some active purging articles." The practice of Vose, of Liverpool, of evacuating the water by means of a lancet or trocar, has been successfully employed in this country in several instances. In a recent case, Prof. Mott drew off, on two successive days, about eighteen ounces of fluid, from a child ten months old. The patient, however, died, from a new accumulation of fluid.—D.

O o 2

____

* The rupture of the swelling most frequently, one might say almost always, proves rapidly fatal ; paraplegia, coma, and convulsions usually preceding the death of the patient. It is alleged that, when the tumour bursts during the continuance of the fœtus in the womb, the circumstance is not fatal till a few days after birth, though in general the opening does not heal up. Meckel has given, however, the description of a calf which had, with a hydrocephalocele on the parietal bone, a cicatrix on the loins. But, as the bones were not wrongly formed, the exact nature of the case remains doubtful. M. Dugés has given the particulars of a clearer instance of a rupture of a spina bifida of a human fœtus in utero, and a subsequent cicatrization taking place. The scar in the sacro-lumbar region was large, covering a membranous substance, by which the vertebral canal was not very firmly closed. The child perished six weeks after birth. The cranium contained a great quantity of serosity, though the exact part in which it had accumulated was not noted. There was also some fluid in the vertebral canal, which seemed to be widened at its lower part, where three of the lumbar vertebræ and parts of the sacrum were imperfect. The nerves of the cauda equina adhered to one another, and to the interior of the canal.—See *Dict. de Méd. et de Chir. Pratiques*, tom. x., p. 138.—ED.

otherwise, and, in the meanwhile, to see how far we can give the remedial power of nature an opportunity of exerting itself, by invigorating the frame generally. Something, however, beyond support, may be safely ventured upon ; for a gentle compression, answering the purpose of a truss, and giving the support of artificial vertebræ, may be tried with propriety, and, if found to do no mischief, it should be gradually increased. Sir Astley Cooper has also recommended a much bolder practice ; that of endeavouring to procure an adhesion of the sides of the sac, so as to close the opening from the spine, and to put a radical stop to the disease. There is here, however, much danger from constitutional irritation, yet this eminent and judicious surgeon is well known to have succeeded in one instance.* If the disease extend to the ventricles, it will probably be of little use ; but if it be local, it may ultimately prove successful.

This form of dropsy is mostly fatal ; but there are a few cases on record of a successful termination by the employment of different methods. Thus, Heister, who in his day also recommended compression, gives an example of its having radically yielded to this plan, in union with spirituous liniments (*Wahrnehmungen*, b. ii.) ; and Fantoni (In *Pacchioni Animadvers.*, cit. *Morgagni, De Sed. et Caus.*), and Heilmann (*Prodrom. Act. Hafn.*, p. 136), describe, each of them, an instance of a perfect cure by opening and evacuating the cavity. In all which instances, however, it seems probable, that there was no such communication with the brain, or that the brain or spinal marrow was less affected than they ordinarily appear to be.†

A few singular cases have occurred of young persons protracting a miserable existence under this disease to the age of adolescence.‡ Martini mentions a youth who lived till eleven years old ; and Acrel notices others who survived till seventeen (*Schwed. Abhandl.*, b. x., p. 291, et seq.), but with paralytic sphincters of the anus and bladder : and Cowper speaks of one who attained the age of thirty.

SPECIES IV.

HYDROPS THORACIS.

DROPSY OF THE CHEST.

SENSE OF OPPRESSION IN THE CHEST ; DYSPNŒA

---

* A cure was effected in another example, which was under the care of Mr. F. L. Probart, of Hawarden, North Wales, by repeatedly puncturing the tumour with a fine needle. The particulars are detailed in the Lancet, No. 186.—ED.

† In the Journal Universel for Nov., 1827, two cases of hydrops spinæ are stated to have been cured by puncture. One case was that of a child two months old.—D

‡ Camper saw a case of hydrops spinæ, or spina bifida, where cicatrization followed the rupture of the tumour in a patient 20 years of age, who was living eight years after this event. The editor once visited, with Mr. Copland Hutchison, a young woman at least 18 or 20 years old, with an enormous spina bifida over the lumbar region and sacrum.—ED.

ON EXERCISE, OR DECUMBITURE ; LIVID COUNTENANCE ; URINE RED AND SPARE ; PULSE IRREGULAR ; ŒDEMATOUS EXTREMITIES ; PALPITATION, AND STARTINGS DURING SLEEP.

THIS is the hydrothorax of authors ; and the secreted fluid, in direct opposition to that of hydrocephalus, commonly, perhaps always, jellies upon exposure to heat.

Sauvages, who has made this disease a genus, gives a considerable number of species under it, derived from the particular part or cavity of the thorax which is occupied, or the peculiar nature of the effusion ; as hydrops mediastini, pleuræ, pericardii, hydatidosus ; to which he might have added pulmonalis, as the water is, perhaps, sometimes effused into the cellular texture of the lungs. But these can never, with any degree of certainty, be distinguished from each other till after death. The distinction of Avenbrugger, into dropsy of one side and dropsy of both sides of the chest, is of little practical importance. "It is," observes M. Corvisart, in his comment on the *Inventum novum*, "a mere difference of quantity ;" and would, in his opinion, be better expressed by the terms partial and complete.

[However, if the statements of Laennec be correct, the foregoing distinction is not altogether so useless ; for, according to the latter excellent pathologist, *idiopathic hydrothorax commonly exists only on one side.* Its anatomical characters, he says, are simply an accumulation of serum in the cavity of the pleura ; this membrane being quite healthy in other respects ; and the lung being compressed towards the mediastinum, flaccid, and destitute of air.* He has seen this form of the disease unaccompanied by any other dropsical affection, or any organic lesion to which it could be ascribed. In one case of this kind, the right pleura contained twelve pounds of a colourless, limpid serum.†]

The complaint at its origin excites little or no observation, and it continues its course imperceptibly ; there is at length found to be some difficulty of breathing, particularly on exertion or motion of any kind, or when the body is in a recumbent position, usually accompanied with a dry and troublesome cough, and an œdema of the ankles towards the evening. Then follow, in quick succession, the symptoms enumerated in the definition, several of which I have drawn directly from my friend Sir L. Maclean's very accurate arrangement of them.—(*Inquiry into the Nature, Causes, and Cure of Hydrothorax,* 8vo., 1810.) The difficulty of breathing be-

---

* The lung of the same side as the effused fluid is pushed towards the spine and the upper part of the chest, while the diaphragm, the liver, and the spleen, according to the side that happens to be the seat of dropsy, are propelled downwards. When the fluid is in the left sac of the pleura. it is sometimes exceedingly copious, displacing the heart from the left to the right side of the thorax.—EN.

† See Laennec on Diseases of the Chest, p. 485, 2d edit., transl. by Forbes. The pleura is of a paler colour than natural, but in other respects sound.

comes at length peculiarly distressing, and the patient can obtain no rest but in an erect posture ; while, even in this condition, he often starts suddenly in his sleep, calls vehemently for the windows to be opened, and feels in danger of suffocation.[*] His eyes stare about in great anxiety, the livid hue of his cheeks is intermixed with a deadly paleness, his pulse is weak and irregular, and as soon as the constrictive spasm of the chest is over, he relapses into a state of drowsiness and insensibility. The disease is often connected with some organic derangement of the heart ; and M. Corvisart conceives, that several of the above symptoms only belong to it when such a connexion exists, and the dropsy is merely symptomatic. He objects even to the signs of starting in sleep, anxiety of the præcordia, inability to lie down, and irregular pulse :—which he affirms indicate alone an organic disease of the heart or large vessels.[†] If the effusion be confined to one side, the side thus surcharged becomes more rounded, and the intercostal spaces augment in size as the water accumulates ; while the œdema of the extremities is confined to the same side.

[According to Laennec, percussion yields a dead, dull, flat sound, and the stethoscope indicates the absence of respiration everywhere except at the roots of the lungs. The peculiar sound which he terms œgophonism, and is explained in the section on phthisis in the first volume of this work, he also found to prevail in cases of hydrops pectoris.]

The disease, contrary to the preceding species, is mostly to be found in advanced life, and its duration chiefly depends upon the strength and habit of the patient at the time of its incursion. It is hence, in some cases, of long continuance, while in others, the patient is suddenly cut off during one of the violent spasms which at length attack him, as well awake as in the midst of sleep. [Hydrops thoracis is considered by many to be a very common disease, and a frequent cause of death. When truly idiopathic, however, and existing in a degree sufficient of itself to produce death, Laennec regarded it as one of the rarest diseases,[‡] and he did not

rate its fatality higher than one in two thousand deaths. He had often known hypertrophy of the heart, aneurism of the aorta, irregular consumption, and even scirrhus of the stomach or liver, mistaken for this affection, when there was no co-existing effusion in the pleura, or at least none except what took place immediately before death. The common notion of the frequency of hydrops thoracis is ascribed by Laennec in a great measure to sero-purulent effusions being generally confounded with it. Symptomatic hydrothorax, however, he admits, is as frequent as the idiopathic is rare (see *Laennec on Diseases of the Chest*, &c., p. 484–488, 2d edit., *trans. by Forbes*) ; though, as Dr. Darwall has explained, this symptom only occurs in a very early stage, while there is but a small quantity of fluid effused. Afterward, the only information derived from the stethoscope is a want of respiration everywhere excepting at the root of the lungs.—(*Dr. Darwall, in Cyclop. of Pract. Med.*, art. HYDROTHORAX.)]

The causes are those of dropsy in general,[*] upon which we have already enlarged, acting more immediately upon the organs of the chest, and inducing some organic affection of the heart, lungs, or larger arteries. We also sometimes find, upon dissection, that the disease has been produced, or considerably augmented, by a number of hydatids (*tænia hydatis*, Linn.), some of which appear to be floating loosely in the effused fluid, and others to adhere to particular parts of the internal surface of the pleura, constituting the *hydrothorax hydatidosus* of Sauvages. [In the rare examples of idiopathic hydrops thoracis, the cause is obscure, though probably dependant upon some change in the action of the exhalant vessels of the pleura. One remark made by Laennec (op. cit., p. 486) on this point deserves notice, as it coincides with the opinions of all the best writers in this country on dropsical diseases ; namely, that whatever may be the difference between a case of hydrothorax ic, we are by no means inclined to coincide with his views. If idiopathic hydrothorax mean any thing, it means a disease in which effusion of serum is the only affection, and in which there is neither inflammation of the pleuræ, nor serious disease of any other organ. Such an affection we have never seen, nor have we found upon record any satisfactory example of it."—See Cyclop. of Practical Med., art. HYDROTHORAX.—ED.

.[*] When the collection of fluid is only within one cavity of the pleura, the patient ordinarily lies on the diseased side of the chest, in order that the sound side may expand the more freely for the performance of respiration. It is when the fluid occupies both sides of the chest that the patients usually sit up in their beds, with great anxiety in their countenances, and all the respiratory muscles in energetic action.—ED.

[†] The editor has no doubt that Corvisart's observations are perfectly well founded ; and that some of the symptoms enumerated by our author convey no information on the nature of the case. Dr. Maclean's work is, as Dr. Forbes candidly states, entitled to notice, as illustrating the power of digitalis in this disease ; but it abounds in grievous errors in pathology and diagnosis.—ED.

[‡] On this part of the subject the opinion of Dr. Darwall deserves attention :—" Although," says he, " so celebrated an author as Laennec has divided hydrothorax into idiopathic and symptomat-

[*] The French pathologists divide hydrothorax into two kinds ; one termed *active*, and consisting in an augmented secretion from the pleura ; the other called *passive*, and proceeding from a diminution in the absorbent power of the extremities of the veins, or from some impediment to the circulation of the blood in the venous trunks to which the smaller veins tend. The latter case, like other dropsies, may depend upon some obstruction of the stream of blood at the very centre of the circulation, namely, in the heart itself. Affections of the lungs and of the heart are those in which hydrothorax presents itself as a complication, and, as Dr. Darwall justly observes (Cyclop. of Pract. Med., art. HYDROTHORAX), it is by its interfering with the functions of those organs, that suspicion of the presence of effusion is often first excited.—ED.

and an acute pleurisy, or between a case of ascites from general debility or organic disease of the heart or liver, and the same disease from an attack of peritonitis, or, in short, whatever may be the difference in general between a dropsy and an inflammation, there can be no doubt that these affections, so opposite in their extreme degrees, are nevertheless often very nearly allied in their slighter shades. We frequently find in the serum of ascites or hydrothorax filaments of albumen, almost as solid as a false membrane. Symptomatic hydrothorax, according to Laennec, may accompany almost every disease, acute or chronic, general or local. Its presence almost always denotes their approaching and fatal termination, and often precedes it only a few moments. It is perhaps not more frequent in cases of ascites and general anasarca than in other diseases. It is most commonly met with in persons dead of acute fever, disease of the heart, or tubercles, or cancer. Its symptoms, which resemble those of the idiopathic disease, Laennec says, do not in general make their appearance but a few days, or even hours, before death.—(Op. cit., transl. by Forbes, 2d edit., p. 488.)]

The only decisive symptom in this disease is the fluctuation of water in the chest, whenever it can be ascertained ; for several of the other signs are often wanting, or, in a separate state, are to be found in other complaints of the chest. as well as in dropsy, more particularly in asthma and empyema. And, hence, in determining the presence of this disorder, we are to look for them conjointly, and not to depend upon any one when alone. Even when associated, we are sometimes in obscurity : and the difficulty of indicating the disease by any set of symptoms has been sufficiently pointed out by De Haen (Rat. Med., P. v., p. 97) ; while Lentin (In Blumenbach Biblioth., iii.), Stoerck (Ann. Med., ii., p. 266), and Rufus (Ad River. Observ. Med.), have given instances of its existence without any symptoms whatever ; and Morgagni with few or none.—(De Sed. et Caus. Morb., ep. xvi., art. 2, 4, 6, 8, 11.) Bonet observes that dyspnœa (Ep. cit., art. 28, 30) is not an indication common to all cases,* and Morgagni, that startings during sleep, or on waking, do not always accompany the disease, and may certainly exist without it. Hoffmann and Baglivi have given, as an additional symptom, intumescence and torpitude of the left hand and arm ; but even this affection, or the more ordinary one of laborious respiration, has existed without water in the chest. De Rueff relates a singular case in a man who was attacked with most of the symptoms jointly,

* Sepulchr., lib. ii., sect. i., obs. 72, 84. On the contrary, Laennec affirms, that the chief and almost the only symptom of this disease is the impeded respiration. This observation is probably correct ; for, though Bonet makes exceptions, there is much ground for believing that he refers to cases in which the effusion occurred only a little while before death, and where, of course, during the course of the disease which actually destroyed the patient, no particular difficulty of breathing might have been noticed.—Ed.

at the age of about sixty, and was supposed to be in the last stage of this disease. He recovered by an ordinary course of medicine, and died at the age of eighty, with his chest perfectly sound to the last.*

The general principles to be attended to in the mode of treatment, are the same as have already been laid down under HYDROPS cellularis. Dr. Ferriar employed elaterium equally in both affections, and, in the present disease, with a degree of success that chiefly brought it once more into popular use.† The squill is here a more valuable medicine than in most other species ; as, independently of its diuretic virtue, it affords great relief to the dry and teasing cough, and in some degree, perhaps, to the pressure of the fluid itself, by exciting the excretories of the lungs to an increased discharge of mucus. Digitalis, as in other species of the same genus, is a doubtful remedy ; its diuretic effects are considerable ; but, however cautiously administered, it too often sinks the pulse, and diminishes the vital energy generally ; and is particularly distressing, from its producing nausea and endangering deliquium ; results which ought more especially to be guarded against in dropsy of the chest, as it is, in most cases, not merely a disease of debility, but of enfeebled age. Sir L. Maclean is a firm friend to its use in almost every case : but even he is obliged to admit, that the state of the pulse, the stomach, the bowels, and the sensorial function, should be attentively observed by every one who prescribes it. And, under the following provision, which he immediately lays down, there can be no difficulty in consenting to employ it. "If these be carefully watched, and the medicine withdrawn as soon as any of them are materially af-

* Nov. Act. Acad. Nat. Cur., tom. iv., 4to., Norimb. According to Dr. Darwall, the earliest symptom of effusion is an œdematous state of the eyelids, occurring chiefly in the morning ; and often only remembered when the feet and ankles have been observed to swell in the evening. Then, in cases depending on disease of the heart, the external œdema increases, the dyspnœa and the difficulty of lying down become more distressing, the œdema of the face augments, and the lips become livid, and at times almost black. The termination is observed, in many cases, to be very sudden, and in fat individuals sometimes a very slight effort is sufficient to break the thread of life. When hydrothorax succeeds to bronchitis and pneumonia, the palpitation and other cardiac symptoms are said, by Dr. Darwall, to be generally absent, and increased dyspnœa is the only circumstance manifested. Previously to this, however, the face and feet swell, as in the former example. The patient then requires the head and shoulders to be raised, and is at length unable to lie down at all. The termination is seldom so sudden as when the heart is diseased, nor is the countenance so livid and purple.—See Cyclop. of Pract. Med., art. HYDROTHORAX.—Ed.

† In cases of hydrops thoracis there is no remedy more efficient than elaterium, which has been given in this form of dropsy with more advantage than in any other. It may be administered in doses of one sixth or one quarter of a grain, to be repeated two or three times a day, according to the state of the patient.—D.

fected, I hesitate not to affirm, that no serious inconvenience will ever ensue from it, and that it may be administered with as much safety as any of the more active medicines in daily use."[*] Laennec considered diuretics and purgatives the chief means of relief.

Blisters are, in many cases, of considerable avail; they act more directly, and therefore more rapidly and effectually, than in most other modes of dropsy, and should be among the first remedies we have recourse to.

The strong symptoms of congestion under which the heart seems, in some instances to labour, have occasionally induced practitioners to try the effect of venesection : and there are cases in which it has unquestionably been found serviceable : as that more especially related by Dr Home, in which he employed it seven times in the course of eighteen days, and hereby produced a cure.[†] I am induced to think, however, that, in this example, the dropsy was an effect of the obstruction under which the heart laboured, rather than that the obstruction was an effect of the dropsy. And, in all cases of this kind, no practice can be more prudent. But, when the dropsy is primary and idiopathic, all such obstructions will be more safely and even more effectually relieved by a quick and drastic purge, than by venesection.[‡]

Opium is a medicine that seems peculiarly adapted to many of the symptoms ; but by itself it succeeds very rarely, heating the skin, and exciting stupor rather than refreshing sleep. When mixed, however, with the squill-pill, or with small doses of ipecacuanha, and, if the bowels be confined, with two or three grains of calomel, it often succeeds in charming the spasmodic struggle of the night, and obtaining for the patient a few hours of pleasant oblivion.

Besides blisters as external revellents, setons and caustics have sometimes been made use of, and especially in the arms or legs. Baglivi preferred the cautery, and applied it to the latter (*Opp.*, p. 103) ; Zacutus Lusitanus to both, and employed it in connexion with diuretics and tonics.—(*Prax. Admir.*, lib. i., obs. 112.)

Tapping is another external means of evacuating the water. The practice is of ancient date, and is described by most of the Greek writers. To avoid the effect of a dangerous deliquium from a sudden removal of the pressure, Hippocrates allowed, in many instances, thirteen days before the fluid was entirely drawn off. And to prevent the inconvenience resulting from a collapse of the integuments and the necessity of a fresh opening, or the retention of a cannula in the orifice through the whole of this period, he advised that a small perforation should be made in one of the ribs, and that the trocar should enter through this foramen.—(Περὶ Ἔθνος Παθῶν, lib. liii., p. 544.)

There are two very powerful objections, however, to the use of the trocar. The first is common to most dropsies, and consists in its offering, in most instances, nothing more than a palliative. The second is peculiar to the present species, and consists in the uncertainty of drawing off any water whatever, from the obscurity or complicated nature of the complaint, upon which we have touched already. If the fluid be lodged in the pericardium, the duplicature of the mediastinum, or the cellular texture of the lungs, it is obvious that the operation must be to no purpose. And yet, with the rare exception of a palpable fluctuation in the chest, we have no set of symptoms that will certainly discriminate these different forms of the disease. It must be also equally in vain if the fluid be confined in a cyst, as has occasionally proved a fact, unless the operator should have the good fortune to pierce the cyst by accident. And in a few instances again, the fluid, which has at all times a striking tendency to become inspissated, has been found so viscid as not to flow : of which Saviard has given us a striking example.—(*Recueil d'Obs. Chirurgicales,* &c., Paris, 1784.)

A considerable pause is necessary, therefore, before tapping is decided upon : nor ought it ever to be employed till the ordinary internal means have been tried to no purpose. But when these have been tried and without avail ; and more especially when we have reason to ascribe the disease to local debility or some local obstruction rather than to a general decline of the constitution ; and more especially still when we have the satisfaction of ascertaining a fluctuation, or of noticing, as has sometimes occurred, that the ribs bulge out on

---

[*] Inquiry into the Nature, &c. of Hydrothorax, p. 171. Dr. Forbes has offered one valuable practical observation on the employment of diuretics :—"The undoubted fact," says he, "of a serous effusion being an almost uniform attendant on the inflammation of serous membranes, ought to make us slow to trust to mere diuretics, and other similar remedies, in cases wherein we have strong reason for suspecting dropsical effusion in the chest."—(See Laennec on the Chest, note in p. 487, 2d edition.) Dr. Darwall admits, that the relief afforded by elaterium and croton-oil is more speedy than that obtained by diuretics ; but he says, they cannot be employed in a debilitated state of the system.—Cyclop. of Pract. Med., art. HYDROTHORAX.—ED.

[†] Clinical Experiments, p. 346. It appears to Dr. Darwall, that two circumstances may occur in hydrothorax, rendering bloodletting necessary ; 1st, Pleurisy, acute or subacute ; and, 2d, Congestion in the lungs. The latter is peculiarly liable to happen when hydrothorax is connected with valvular disease of the heart. In the former case he deems local bleeding, especially cupping, always the best.—See Cyclop. of Pract. Med., art. HYDROTHORAX.—ED.

[‡] A note made on this part of the subject by Dr. Forbes merits attention. "Dropsy of the chest," he says, "frequently accompanies organic disease of the heart ; but still more frequently is the latter disease, when unattended by any effusion into the pleura, mistaken for the former. In cases of this kind, the stethoscope is of great use in directing the treatment ; as the means so successful in relieving the dropsical affection, are at best useless in the lesions of the heart."—(See Laennec on Dis. of the Chest, p. 489, 2d edit.) Andral states, that a diminution in the capacity of the right ventricle, without any other alteration of the heart, frequently accompanies dropsy.—Anat. Pathol., t. ii., p. 292.—ED.

the affected side, the operation may be ventured upon.

In a case in which all the precautionary steps just mentioned had preceded, and where a fluctuation was clear, Dr. Archer of Dublin drew off eleven pints* at once by tapping, and the patient found instant relief, and was tolerably well for at least three years afterward.†

On the continent the operation of tapping is far more frequently tried than in our own country; and the German Miscellanies are full of cases of a successful event. In the volume of Nosology I have given an account of many of these; in several of which the water evacuated appears to have been very considerable. Thus, in one instance, a hundred and fifty pounds were discharged at a single time; in others, between four and five hundred pounds by different tappings within the year: and in a single example, nearly seven thousand pints, in eighty operations, during a period of twenty-five years, through which the patient laboured under this complaint; having hereby prolonged a miserable existence, which doubtless would have terminated without it much earlier, but which, perhaps, was hardly worth prolonging at such an expense. In the Berlin Medical Transactions, there is a case of a cure effected by an accidental wound made into the thorax, by which the whole of the water escaped at once.—(*Act. Med. Berol.*, vol. x., dec. i., p. 44.)

In a few rare instances we have reason to believe that the disease ceased spontaneously, judging from the trifling remedies that were employed.‡

SPECIES V.
HYDROPS ABDOMINIS.
DROPSY OF THE BELLY.

TENSE, HEAVY, AND EQUABLE INTUMESCENCE OF THE WHOLE BELLY; DISTINCTLY FLUCTUATING TO THE HAND UPON A SLIGHT STROKE BEING GIVEN TO THE OPPOSITE SIDE.

THIS is the ascites of nosologists. It is some-

---

* M. Itard estimates the largest quantity of fluid ordinarily met with in hydrothorax at twelve or fourteen pints; but Portal cites an instance in which sixteen were contained in the chest; and Dr. Darwall saw one case, arising from an aneurism of the arteria innominata, where the quantity was fourteen or fifteen pints.—ED.

† Transact. of the King and Queen's College, Dublin, vol. ii., p. 1. Dr. Darwall considers this case to have been one of empyema, as having been preceded by pleurisy.—(See Cyclop. of Pract. Med., art. HYDROTHORAX.) Empyema being usually confined to one side of the chest, and the opposite lung comparatively empty, there is a greater prospect of benefit from discharging the fluid. On the other hand, as in hydrothorax both sides of the chest are affected, though perhaps not in an equal degree, and, as when the disease is so far advanced as to demand an operation, the cellular tissue of the lungs themselves is probably likewise the seat of effusion, the usefulness of the practice seems to Dr. Darwall very problematical.—ED.

‡ Hydrothorax being generally, perhaps always, merely a consequence of some other disease, it is

---

times a result of general debility, operating chiefly on the exhalants that open on the internal surface of the peritoneum;* sometimes occasioned by local debility or some other disease of one or more of the abdominal organs, considerably infarcted and enlarged, and sometimes a metastasis or secondary disease produced by repelled gout, exanthems, or other cutaneous eruptions: examples of all which are to be found in Morgagni (*De Sed. et Caus. Morb.*, ep. xxxviii., art. 49), and offer the three following varieties, which may not unfrequently be applied to the preceding species;—

α Atonica. Preceded by general debility Atonic dropsy of of the constitution. the belly.

β Parabysmica. Preceded by or accompanied Parabysmic drop- with oppilation or indura- sy of the belly. ted enlargement of one or more of the abdominal viscera.

γ Metastatica. From repelled gout, exan- Metastatic dropsy thems, or other cutaneous of the belly. eruptions.

In the FIRST VARIETY, the fluid is found in the cavity of the abdomen. It is produced by any of the causes of general debility operating on an hydropic diathesis; and is frequently a result of scurvy or various fevers.

In the SECOND VARIETY, the organ most commonly affected is the liver, which is occasionally loaded with hydatids, and has sometimes weighed twelve pounds.† The gall-bladder is often proportionally enlarged and turgid, and has occasionally been found with an obliterated meatus, full of a coffee-like fluid, and together with its contents has weighed upwards of ten pounds.‡

---

only by removing the latter that a permanent cure of the dropsy can be accomplished; and, as Dr. Darwall observes, the goodness of our practice will depend very much upon the accuracy of our diagnosis relative to the original cause of the effusion. —ED.

* That there is strong reason for suspecting many dropsical effusions to depend upon increased exhalation, and not diminished absorption, has been already noticed. We have also adverted to the modern theory, now generally received, that dropsy is frequently connected with inflammation of serous membranes, and consequently that the effused serum is often the product, rather of an increased action of the vessels than of their relaxation and debility.—ED.

† Dr. Elliotson observes, that when ascites is not the result of acute or decided inflammation, there are marks of structural change; and the dropsy is by some ascribed to disease of the liver, so frequently is that organ affected. "Where, however, the peritoneum is diseased, you will find that portion covering the liver very thick, quite white, and opaque; and I do not believe that ascites arises from disease of the liver, but from a structural change in the peritoneum itself." The peritoneum is described not only as becoming thick, but assuming a satin whiteness.—(See Lectures delivered at the London University, as reported in Med. Gaz. for 1832–33, p. 452.) However, Dr. Elliotson adds, that he has seldom opened a case of ascites in which the liver was not diseased in some part or another.—ED.

‡ The morbid changes in the kidneys, described

The accumulation has also sometimes been discovered in the omentum (*De Haen, Rát. Med.,* Pr. iv., p. 95 ; *Senberlich, P. de Hydrope Omenti Saccato,* Fr. 1752); or sides of the intestines.' —(*Frank, in Commentation,* Goetting., vii., 74.) In this second variety the disease is often denominated an encysted dropsy ; a term, however, which will quite as well apply to dropsies of the ovaria, the Fallopian tube, and even the uterus and scrotum, as to that of the liver.

In the THIRD VARIETY, the fluid is commonly deposited in the cavity of the abdomen ; and is far more easily removed than in either of the others ; often yielding, indeed, to a few drastic purges alone ; except where, as sometimes happens in metastatic dropsy from repelled gout, the constitution has been broken down by a long succession of previous paroxysms.

Under the veil of dropsy, pregnancy has often been purposely disguised ; and sometimes, on the contrary, where pregnancy has been ardently wished for, and has actually taken place, it has been mistaken for a case of ascites ; while, in a few instances, both have coexisted. Mauriceau, indeed, mentions a case of pregnancy recurring a second time along with dropsy (*Traité des Maladies des Femmes Grosses,* ii., pp. 59–204) : and in an hydropic diathesis, there is a general tendency to the latter whenever the former makes its appearance. If dropsy occur at a period of life when the catamenia are on the point of naturally taking their leave, and where the patient has been married for many years without ever having been impregnated, it is not always easy, from the collateral signs, to distinguish between the two. A lady, under these circumstances, was a few years ago attended for several months by three or four of the most celebrated physicians of this metropolis, one of whom was a practitioner in midwifery, and concurred with the rest in affirming that her disease was an encysted dropsy of the abdomen. She was in consequence put under a very active series of different evacuants ; a fresh plan being had recourse to as soon as the preceding had failed ; and was successively purged, blistered, salivated, treated with powerful diuretics, and the warm bath, but equally to no purpose : for the swelling still increased, and became firmer ; the face and general form were emaciated, the breathing was laborious, the discharge of urine small, and the appetite intractable ; till at length these threatening symptoms were followed by a succession of sudden and excruciating pains, that by the domestics, who were not prepared for their appearance, were supposed to be the forerunners of a speedy dissolution, but which fortunately terminated before the arrival of a single medical attendant, in giving birth to an in-

fant that, like its mother, had wonderfully withstood the whole of the preceding medical warfare without injury.

In all common cases, the best means we can take to guard against deception are to inquire into the state of the menses, of the mammæ, and of the swelling itself. If the menses continue regular, if the mammæ appear flat or shrivelled, with a contracted and light-coloured areola, and if the intumescence fluctuate, there can be no doubt of its being a case of dropsy : but if, on the contrary, the mammæ appear plump and globular, with a broad and deep-coloured areola ; if we can learn, which, in cases where pregnancy is wished to be concealed, we often cannot do, that the catamenia have for some time been obstructed ; and if the swelling appear uniformly hard and solid, and more especially if it be seated chiefly just above the symphysis of the pubes, or, provided it be higher, if it be round and circumscribed,—though we may occasionally err, there can be little or no doubt, in most instances, of the existence of pregnancy. The most difficult of all cases is that in which dropsy and pregnancy take place simultaneously. It is a most distressing combination for the patient, and is usually treated with palliatives alone till the time of childbirth. Chambon advises, that in urgent cases the legs and feet should be scarified.—(*Maladies des Femmes,* tom. i., p. 28.) But sometimes there is danger of instantaneous suffocation from the rapidity with which the dropsy advances, and the disproportionate dilatation of the peritoneum, the abdominal muscles, and the integuments. Scarpa has noticed such cases, and recommends immediate tapping, and that the trocar be introduced between the edge of the rectus muscle in the left hypochondrium and the margin of the false ribs ; in which situation it will run the least risk of injuring the uterus.—(*Sulla Gravidanza susseguita de Ascite,* &c., Freviso, 1817.) The reaction, however, which takes place in the abdominal muscles and organs thus suddenly set at liberty, is apt to bring on labour-pains, and consequently to produce a miscarriage ; and on this account the present author would recommend that the fluid should be drawn off at intervals, and not wholly at a single sitting.

The ordinary causes of dropsy of the abdomen are those of cellular dropsy, of which we have treated at considerable length already, and to which the reader may therefore refer himself : the only difference being, as in dropsy of the chest, that the excrements of these cavities are, from particular circumstances, more open at the time to the influence of whatever may happen to be the cause, than the excrements of the cellular membrane, or of any other part of the system. From the extent, however, of the abdominal region, and the connexion of its cavity with so many large and important viscera, and especially with the liver, we can be at no loss in accounting for a more frequent appearance of dropsy under this species than under any other.

The general symptoms, moreover, are those of cellular dropsy. The appetite flags, there is the same aversion to motion and sluggishness

---

by Dr. Bright as leading to dropsy, as well as the deposition of cholesterine in the diseased livers of dropsical persons, have been already particularly brought before the reader's notice in the section on cellular dropsy. The frequency of a diminution in the capacity of the right ventricle of the heart in dropsical persons, without any other change of this organ, is another interesting fact to which Andral has invited attention, as already mentioned.—ED.

when engaged in it, the same intolerable thirst, dryness of the skin, and diminution of all the natural discharges. The peculiar symptoms, as distinct from cellular dropsy, are the gradual swelling of the belly, and, as a consequence of this, a dry, irritable cough, and difficulty of respiration.*

It is often difficult to determine whether the water be seated in the cavity of the abdomen or in a distinct cyst. But, generally speaking, if we have previously had reason to suspect a diseased condition of one of the ovaries, or if the swelling be _local_ or unequal, and the constitution do not seem to enter readily into the morbid action, we may suspect the dropsy to be of the encysted form. While, on the contrary, if the animal frame evince general weakness, if the limbs be œdematous, the appetite fail, and the secretions be concurrently small and restricted, there is good reason for believing that the fluid is effused in the cavity of the peritoneum.

The treatment of ascites, as to its general principles and plan, must be the same as that already laid down for anasarca or cellular dropsy :† but here, instead of evacuating the water by scarification, we can often advantageously draw it off at once by tapping. Where, indeed, the dropsy is of the encysted kind, our efforts will sometimes prove in vain ; for we may either miss the proper viscus, or the fluid, lodged in the separate vesicles of a vast aggregation of hydatids, amounting sometimes to seven, eight, or nine thousand at a time (*Commerc. Nor.*, 1731, p. 271), cannot be set free. But, where it lies in the peritoneal sac alone, or on the outside of this sac alone, we can often afford very

great relief by this simple process, and sometimes an effectual cure. It ought, therefore, by no means to be delayed, as it often is, till the debility, from being local, has become general ; nor can the operation be too soon performed after a fluctuation is distinctly felt, and the swelling from its bulk has become troublesome to the breathing, and interferes with the night's rest. Nor should we be deterred if the first evacuation do not fully succeed. On the contrary, if the general strength seem to augment for some time after the operation, the appetite to improve, and the usual symptoms of the disease to diminish, we may take courage from our first success, and augur still more favourably from a second, or even a third attempt, if it should be necessary. Various cases have fallen to the lot of the author, in which a radical cure has been completed in this manner : nor are instances wanting in which the patient has only recovered after the twelfth time of operating. Hautesierk gives an instance of cure after sixty tappings within two years and a half, in conjunction with a steady use of aperients and tonics (*Recueil*, ii.) ; and Martin, in the Swedish Transactions, relates another instance of an infant of four years old restored after a second use of the trocar, in conjunction with a like course of medicines. The support of a broad belt or bandage should always be had recourse to afterward, which should be drawn as tight as the patient can bear it with comfort, for the pressure will tend to prevent a reaccumulation. In a few instances, indeed, it has proved stimulant enough to excite the absorbents into rapid action, and carry off

---

* As in most other dropsies, there is generally very little urine ; and so long as there is not disease of the heart, or pleuritis, or bronchitis, many patients breathe with an enormous collection of fluid in the abdomen, much better than might be expected. The swelling begins below, and gradually ascends, till the whole abdomen is distended with the fluid.—ED.

† In every case, the cause of the disease must be considered before a judicious practice can be determined upon ; in particular, the practitioner should consider whether the cause be inflammation, plethora, obstruction to the return of blood, or some change in the blood itself, or whether the dropsy be encysted. " If dropsy be connected with inflammation, the urine is scanty and high-coloured, and on boiling it, or adding to it nitric acid, it very often, but not always, deposites albumen."— (See Armstrong's Lect. on the Morbid Anatomy, Nature, and Treatment of Acute and Chronic Diseases, p. 848.) If, with this state of urine, the pulse should be hard and frequent, the tongue furred, and the skin hot towards night, Dr. Armstrong recommends bleeding, purging, and a regulated diet, assisted by digitalis, squill, calomel, or colchicum. If obstruction to the return of blood be the cause of ascites, he prescribes alteratives every second night, and daily purging by calomel, elaterium, or turpentine, with alkalis, and a regulated diet. Where the bronchial mucous membrane is affected, he is in favour of purging, diaphoretics, and a regulated temperature. If the heart be obstructed, he praises alteratives, purging, and moderate bloodletting, with a bland diet, and rest. If ascites depend upon plethora, the means of relief recommended by this physician are bleeding, pur-

ging, a low diet, and the warm bath. If ascites be conjoined with some change in the blood, proceeding from disorder of the digestive organs, he prescribes gentle laxatives daily, and mild alteratives every other night, with fresh air, a bland diet, and venesection or leeches, if requisite.

All medical practitioners now agree, that the kind of treatment called for by ascites must depend very much upon the settlement of the question, whether inflammation is present or not ? If it be present, the cure of it will generally remove the dropsy ; but when no inflammation exists, elaterium, cream of tartar, or other hydragogue purgatives, may be autiously tried. Dr. Elliotson begins with one fourth of a grain of elaterium every other day ; and if the patient bear this medicine well, the dose is gradually increased to a grain or a grain and a half, though occasionally to five grams. While elaterium is thus prescribed every other day, the patient should be supported with wine, "so that while you drain him well, you make him some sort of amends for it." When there is organic disease, Dr. Elliotson prescribes mercury or iodine. "If," says he, "you choose to treat the disease with diuretics, which is frequently a good practice, squills, digitalis, and mercury, answer exceedingly well. This is not so certain a practice as treating the case by hydragogues, which are also diuretics ; but if you adopt it, you will frequently find that the kidneys will not act, and yet, if you tap the patient, they will act directly."—(See Lectures delivered at the London University, as published in Med. Gaz. for 1832–33, p. 453.) These valuable observations agree precisely with what every man of experience must have remarked.—ED.

the water without the operation of tapping.—(*Hasson, Annuaire Medico-Chirurgical.*)

Internal evacuants, therefore, as far as the strength will allow, and tonic restoratives generally, should be called to our aid through the entire process of cure, as already recommended under HYDROPS *cellularis*. The thirst, which is often unconquerable, and the most distressing of all the symptoms, may be allayed, as we have already pointed out, by a free use of subacid drinks, the desire for which is by no means to be repressed, as the absorbents of the skin are always stimulated by the irritation of an ungratified desire to imbibe far more fluid from the atmosphere than any indulgence in drinking can amount to. As ordinary food, the alliaceous plants, which give an agreeable excitement to the stomach, and at the same time quicken the action of the kidneys, will be found highly useful: and asparagus, which in an inferior degree answers the last of these purposes, may make a pleasant change in its season.

It must be confessed that tapping is often employed without radical success ; for the disease, under all its modifications, is too often incurable. Yet, even in the worst of cases, it has its advantage as a palliative ; and it is no small consolation to be able to procure temporary ease and comfort in the long progress of a chronic, but fatal disease.

In some instances, the quantity of fluid evacuated by the operation of tapping has been enormous. It has often amounted to eight gallons at a time, and Dr. Stoerck gives an instance of twelve gallons and a half.—(*Ann. Med.*, i., p. 149.) Guattani relates a case, in which thirty pints of an oily fluid were discharged by a single paracentesis. This disease was produced by an aneurismal affection.—(*De Aneurismatibus.*) The operation has frequently been repeated forty or fifty times upon the same patient; and sometimes much oftener. In one case it was practised ninety-eight times within three years.—(*Edin. Med Communications*, vol. iv., p. 378.) And another case is recorded, in which the operation was repeated a hundred and forty-three times.—(*N. Samml. Med. Wahrnehmungen*, b. iii., p. 94.) Dr. Scott, of Harwich, performed the operation twenty-four times in only fifteen months, and drew off a hundred and sixteen gallons in the whole.—(*Edin. Med. Comment.*, vol. vi., p. 441.)

Occasionally, both abdominal and cellular dropsy have been carried off by a spontaneous flow of water from some organ or other. In the latter species, most frequently by a natural fontanel in some one of the extremities, as the hand, foot, or scrotum.—(*Riedlin, Linn. Med.*, 1696, p. 258 ; *Schenck*, lib. iii., sect. ii., obs. 136, ex *Hollerio*, obs. 140, 141.) In the former, by a spontaneous rupture of the protuberant umbilicus, of which the instances are very numerous :* and hence many operators, taking a hint from this spontaneous mode of cure, have

preferred making an incision into the umbilicus with a lancet to the use of the trocar. Paullini relates a singular mode of operation, and which, though it completely succeeded, is not likely to be had recourse to very often. The patient, not submitting to the use of the trocar, had the good fortune to be gored in the belly by a bull; the opening proved effectual, and he recovered.—(Cent. ii., obs. 10.) [Of late, a new proposal has been made, and even put in practice, to tap the abdomen through the fundus of the bladder, and then to maintain the communication between the cavity of the peritoneum and that of the bladder. In the case, however, related by Dr. Andrew Buchanan (see *Glasgow Medical Journ.*, vol. i., p. 195), the latter object was not effected, so that no opportunity was afforded of estimating the good or bad consequences of it. The risk of an extravasation of urine in the abdomen, however, and the dangerous irritation likely to attend any attempt to keep up a fistulous communication of the kind referred to, are considerations adverse to the success of the plan.]

There are also a few instances of a subsidence of the accumulation upon a spontaneous efflux of some other kind ; especially of blood, and chiefly from the hemorrhoidal vessels.—(*Saviard, Observ. Chir.*, p. 150.) Where, indeed, as has sometimes happened, abdominal or cellular dropsy, or both, have been produced from inflammatory oppilation, on suddenly catching cold, free venesection has proved the most effectual, and sometimes the only means of carrying it off, which in a few instances it has, with a general freedom of action to the kidneys, as well as to other organs, almost instantaneously.*

SPECIES VI. ˉ ˍ

HYDROPS OVARII.

DROPSY OF THE OVARY.

HEAVY INTUMESCENCE OF THE ILIAC REGION ON ONE OR BOTH SIDES ; GRADUALLY SPREADING OVER THE BELLY ; WITH OBSCURE FLUCTUATION.

THERE is the same difficulty in distinguishing this disease from pregnancy as in dropsy of the belly: and, consequently, the same mistakes have occasionally been made. There is also quite as much difficulty in distinguishing it from the parabysmic variety of abdominal dropsy, especially when the liver is the organ enlarged and filled with hydatids. Yet, in this last case, the confusion is of less consequence, as the general mode of treatment will not essentially vary. Pregnancy, when it first alters the shape, produces an enlargement immediately over the pubes, which progressively ascends, and when it reaches the umbilicus, assumes an indefinite boundary. In the atonic or common variety of

---

* Desportes, Hist. de Malad. de St. Domingue, ii., 122. Schenck, lib. iii., sect. ii., obs. 147. Forestus, lib. xix., obs. 33.

* Edin. Med. and Surg. Journ., No. lxxi., Dr. Graham. The rest of the treatment of *hydrops ab. dominis* will be found under the head of *hydrops cellularis*. It is always an advisable plan, when the water is diminishing, to have the abdomen well bandaged.—ED.

abdominal dropsy, the swelling of the belly is general and undefined from the first. And in dropsy of the ovary or ovaries, it commences laterally, on one or both sides, according as one or both ovaries are affected. And it is hence of the utmost importance to attend to the patient's own statement of the origin of the disease and the progressive increase of the swelling. It is generally moveable when the patient is laid on her back; and as the orifice of the uterus moves also with the motion of the tumour, by passing the finger up the vagina, we may thus obtain another distinctive symptom. When there are several cysts in the ovary, we may perceive irregularities in the external tumour.*

This disease is sometimes found in pregnant women; but far more commonly in the unimpregnated and the barren. It is also met with in the young, and those who regularly menstruate, as well as in those whose term of menstruation has just ceased. The accumulation of fluid is often very considerable.† Morand drew off four hundred and twenty-seven pints within ten months (*Mém. de l'Acad. de Chir.*, ii.; 448); and Martineau four hundred and ninety-five within a year; and, from the same patient, six thousand six hundred and thirty-one pints, by eighty punctures, within twenty-five years.‡

There is a tombstone near Dartford in Kent,

* Encysted dropsy of the ovary may usually be discriminated from ascites by the following circumstances:—The tumour commences on one side of the abdomen, its surface is unequal, and its fluctuation, if felt at all, is very unequal. The health is at first but little impaired, and the thirst, scanty urine, and other symptoms which characterize general dropsy, are wanting. The catamenia are usually extremely irregular, or altogether suppressed. According to Dr. Seymour, when both ovaria are diseased, the menses are always absent. —(See Illustrations of some of the principal Diseases of the Ovaria, 8vo., Lond.; 1830; and Dr. R. Lee, in Cyclop. of Pract. Med., art. Ovaria.) Ovarian cysts are often combined with considerable enlargement of the ovary itself, which becomes converted into a whitish, hard, cartilaginous mass, resembling a fibrous tumour of the uterus. Portions of such tumours of the ovary sometimes have calcareous matter deposited in them, while, in other instances, instead of being converted into solid earthy matter, they undergo a softening process, by which their fibrous structure is completely destroyed, and large irregular cavities formed, containing a dark-coloured gelatinous fluid. Dr. Seymour has described these ovarian tumours under the term of scirrhus of the ovaria, though, as Dr. R. Lee justly observes, they are not of a malignant nature, and have no tendency to degenerate into cancer.—Op. et loco cit.—Ed.

† Haller remarks (Disp. Med., vol. iv., p. 449), "Monstrosum hoc ovarium e sede sua exemtum et cum utero recisum statira ponderatum 100 libras cum dimidia œquaverat."—D.

‡ Phil. Trans., 1784, p. 471. The cyst is preserved in the Hunterian Collection. Dr. Elliotson saw one instance in which 84 pints were drawn off by a single tapping; and Mr. Chevalier another, in which 636 pints were discharged.—(See Med. Gaz. for 1832-33, p. 454; and Med. Chir. Trans.) The fluid of ovarial dropsies is found to be exceedingly greasy, and to contain a substance analogous to adipocire. Dr. Bostock terms it albumino-

erected to the memory of Ann, daughter of John Mumford, Esq., of Sutton Place, which proceeds to tell us, that "her death was occasioned by a dropsy, for which, in the space of three years and ten months, she was tapped one hundred and fifty-five times. She died the 14th of May, 1778, in the twenty-third year of her age, an example of patience, fortitude, and resignation." The species of dropsy is not indeed stated, but Sir Astley Cooper, who has also referred to this monument (*Lectures*, vol. ii., p. 374, 8vo., 1825), regards it, and with much probability, as an ovarian case.

The disease commences, and indeed often continues for years, without much affection of the general health; yet it is insidious, and the constitution at length suffers and falls a prey to it; the exceptions, indeed, are rare.* Yet Dr. Baillie knew of one instance in which the disease disappeared spontaneously, after it had existed for nearly thirty years, and the patient remained in good health permanently.†

serous matter, and says that it differs from cholesterine.—(See Med. Chir. Trans., vol. xv.) The fluid often looks like coffee, pea soup, or melted jelly.* The thicker and darker the fluid, and the more it abounds in flakes of greasy matter, the worse is the prognosis, in relation to the prospect of a cure, or even of long relief from an operation, because those circumstances manifest that the interior of the cyst has been at times the seat of inflammation, which is then apt to follow paracentesis, and to prove fatal.—Ed.

* The injurious effects on the system proceed from the pressure and irritation of the cysts on the abdominal and pelvic viscera. A portion of the cyst may descend between the bladder and rectum, and thus interrupt the evacuation of the urine and feces. The symptoms of a stricture of the rectum may be thus excited. The editor has attended several cases of ovarial dropsy, in which he has been obliged to draw off the urine with a catheter. In a lady who was under the care of Dr. R. Lee, the pressure of an ovarian or uterine tumour upon the neck of the bladder, rendered the use of the same instrument indispensable.—(See Cyclop. of Pract. Med., art. Ovaria; also Dr. Park and Dr. Merriman's papers in the Med. Chir. Trans., vols. iii. and x.) Interruption to the return of blood from the lower limbs and pelvic viscera, and inflammation and suppuration of the cyst, are other sources of annoyance and danger sometimes occurring.—Ed.

† Lectures and Observations on Medicine, 1825, unpublished. Dr. Mead records one example in which eighteen pints of fluid were discharged from

* On examining a fatal case occurring in the practice of Prof. Mott, and recorded by Dr. Francis, the following appearances presented themselves. "Upon laying open the abdominal parietes, several pints of fluid were found in the peritoneal cavity. The abdomen was filled with an immense congeries of tumours, of different sizes, from that of a pea or small marble to those of a capacity to contain several quarts; they were of various shapes, and were occupied with fluids of different degrees of consistence and colour. In some the fluid was quite thin and pale; in others, altogether gelatinous and inodorous; and in others again, the contained mass was composed of substances resembling pieces of fleshy matter, and fetid."—N. York Med. and Phys. Journ., vol. ii.—D.

Internal medicines have been rarely found efficacious, and, when tried, must consist of those already noticed in the treatment of cellular dropsy.* Tapping affords the same ease as in abdominal dropsy, and the operation is to be performed in the same manner.' I had lately a lady under my care for six or seven years, who required the operation to be performed at first every six months, afterward every three months, and at length every month or six weeks. She rose from it extremely refreshed, and in good spirits; and often on the same evening joined a party of friends, and was sometimes present at a musical entertainment. In about six years, however, her health completely gave way, and she sunk under the disease.

So little, however, is the general health interfered with for the first year or two, that the patient occasionally becomes pregnant while the accumulation continues to increase, and often produces a living offspring.† Sir L. Maclean has given an interesting case of this kind, in which there was not only an extensive dropsy, but an abscess of the ovary, and a discharge of pus as well as of water on tapping, which was performed five times during a single pregnancy. The patient passed easily through her labour, but died within five months afterward upon a bursting of the abscess into the peritoneal sac. On examining the body, two pints of "a thick, brown, well-digested pus were found to have escaped into the cavity of the abdomen, and three pints more in the ovarian sac. The opening was large enough to admit of three fingers, and the external surface of both the large and small intestines was found inflamed, and verging in some places on gangrene."—(*Inquiry into the Nature,* &c., *of Hydrothorax,* appx., p. 1, 8vo., 1810.)

The fluid is in this species, also, sometimes lodged in a cyst, occasionally in many cysts,‡

---

the navel, in consequence of a rupture of the sac; and the particulars of another case are given by Dr. Blundell, in which a lady, afflicted with ovarian dropsy, fell from her carriage and received a violent blow on the abdomen, followed by a considerable evacuation of urine; she recovered, married, and dying ultimately of retroversion of the uterus, was carefully examined, when it was ascertained that the ovarial cyst had been ruptured by the former accident, and its contents had been effused in the cavity of the peritoneum, whence it had been absorbed.—Ed.

* Mercury and iodine are the medicines principally tried, and this sometimes both externally and internally, though even with less success than in ascites; for it would appear that either the inner surface of an ovarial cyst is not so actively absorbent as the peritoneum, or is less readily influenced than that membrane by medicines to quicken the action of those vessels by which alone the accumulated fluid might be removed.—Ed.

† A case of this kind occurred in the practice of Dr. Francis and Dr. Mott. The patient had suffered from hydrops ovarii for seven years; she became pregnant, although the tumour was so large as to cause difficulty of breathing and much spasmodic suffering. At the end of the eighth month of pregnancy, she was delivered of a living and healthy child.—D.

‡ In Dr. Seymour's work on the ovaria, it is

---

or perhaps hydatids, and there is great difficulty in ascertaining its exact situation, and consequently in puncturing it, and especially in evacuating the water when there is more than one cyst. A distinguished and skilful friend of the author's not long since made an attempt on a lady who had been affected with the disease for some years; yet unfortunately not a drop of serum issued, but instead of it a pint of blood. The swelling of the abdomen has since increased to an enormous size; internal medicines have proved of little avail, and she has not consented to another trial of the trocar. It was probably from an equal want of success, that Tozzetti long since declared the operation to be of no avail (*Osservazioni,* &c.); and that Morgagni denounced it not only as useless, but mischievous.* Le Dran endeavoured to effect a permanent cure afterward by incision and suppuration, as in the radical cure for scrotal dropsy. Other practitioners have used injections of port wine; and others again have forced a tent into the wound made with the trocar. These have sometimes succeeded; but a dangerous inflammation is too apt to follow, and occasionally death itself.—(*Francis's Denman,* ch. iii., sect. xii.) Dr. Percival relates a cure produced by vomiting, in which a salutary transfer of action seems to have taken place.—(Ep. ii., p. 156.) [Mr. Abernethy, after paracentesis, prevented another accumulation of fluid in the sac by repeatedly blistering the integuments; but the plan has rarely answered.]

Extirpation of the diseased ovarium was rather proposed than practised by the surgeons of the preceding century.' De Haen regarded the operation as doubtful (*Rat. Med.,* p. iv., c. iii., sect. iii.), and Morgagni asserted it to be impossible.—(*De Sed. et Caus. Morb.,* ep. xxxviii.,

---

stated, that "the first form of this disease, and the simplest, is from an enlargement or alteration of the corpora Graafiana." This opinion is corroborated by the authority of Cruveilhier. The case of two or more cysts is attributed to the enlargement of two or more vesicles.—(See Illustrations of some of the principal Diseases of the Ovaria, pp. 44, 45, 8vo., Lond., 1830.) As cysts with a fibrous covering are formed in parts where this explanation of their origin is out of the question, the subject appears far from being well determined.—Ed.

* De Sed. et Caus. Morb., ep. xxxviii., art. 68, 69. Professor Delpech gives many reasons in support of the same view.—(Chirurgie Clinique de Montpellier, 4to., 1823–28, 2 tomes.) So long as an ovarial dropsy does not occasion very urgent symptoms, the editor always recommends the patient not to be in a hurry to undergo paracentesis. Dr. Elliotson also remarks, that the best practice, in cases of encysted dropsy of the ovary, is to support the patient's strength, to put off tapping as long as possible, and give no medicine whatever, except it be iodine.—(Lectures delivered at the London University, as reported in Med. Gaz. for 1832–33, p. 455.) One consideration offered by this able physician against resorting to the operation early is, that there may be many cysts at first, which afterward unite into each other, so that the fluid now admits of being effectually discharged, which was evidently not the case in an earlier stage.—Ed.

art. 69, 70.) L'Aumonier, however, chief surgeon of the Rouen hospital, successfully extracted the organ upwards of fifty years ago ; and a few other practitioners have operated with a like favourable issue since, and especially in several parts of America. Thus Dr. Smith of Yale College, Connecticut, has completely succeeded in removing the organ, notwithstanding the operation was impeded by numerous adhesions (*American Med. Rev.*, 1822) ; while Dr. M'Dowell of Kentucky* has not only, in several cases, extirpated, with a full restoration to health, a dropsical or otherwise diseased ovarium, but laid open the peritoneum to a great extent, for extirpating other tumours in the abdomen.—(*Lizars, in Edin. Med. Journ.*, No. lxxxi., p. 250, and No. lxxxiv.) It must be admitted, however, that the operation is a very hazardous one, and, in spite of Dr. M'Dowell's success, often useless, even when it does not prove fatal. Mr. Lizars of Edinburgh, with as much skill and judgment as have perhaps ever been evinced, succeeded but once in three distinct cases ; and even in this he did not venture to extract the other ovary, though evidently in a morbid state. In his second case, the patient died in about eight-and-forty hours after the operation. In the third, the tumour was so adherent to other organs, and especially so thickly inosculated with the omentum, that excision was impracticable. The patient recovered from the section, but with an entire retention of the disease.†

SPECIES VII.
HYDROPS TUBALIS.
DROPSY OF THE FALLOPIAN TUBE.

HEAVY, ELONGATED INTUMESCENCE OF THE ILIAC REGION, SPREADING TRANSVERSELY ; WITH OBSCURE FLUCTUATION.

THIS species is not common. Dr. Baillie, however, among others, has particularly noticed and described it in his morbid anatomy, in a case referred to in the volume of Nosology. Its mode of treatment is that of dropsy of the ovarium. Tapping may be attempted ; but, as the water lies frequently in hydatid vesicles or distinct sacs, success is doubtful.

The quantity of fluid is for the most part larger than in the ovarium. Munick mentions a case in which the distended tube contained a hundred and ten pints of fluid (*Apud Manget*) ; Harder in one in which the fluid measured a hundred and forty pints (*Apiar.*, obs. 87, 88) ; and

* Dr. M'Dowell has recorded five cases in which this operation was successful. The ovarium has been extirpated also by Dr. D. L. Rogers of New-York. The patient recovered, but died with dysentery eighteen months after the operation. Dr. Alban G. Smith has likewise performed the same operation, and with highly beneficial results.—D.

† Observations on Extraction of Diseased Ovaria, illustrated by Plates, fol., Edin., 1825. For an ingenious account of the structure and formation of ovarial cysts, the reader should consult Dr. Hodgkin's paper in the Med. Chir. Trans., vol. xv. —ED.

Cyprani another, that afforded a hundred and fifty pints at a single tapping.—(*Epistola historiam exhibens fœtûs humani ex tuba excisi*, Leid., 1700.) Weiss describes a case of complicated dropsy, distending both the ovarium and the Fallopian tube.—(*Abhandl. einer ungewöhnlichen Krankheit*, &c., Rastadt, 1785.)

The causes and progress, as well as general mode of treatment, are those of dropsy of the ovary. Its chief distinctive symptom is the elongated line which the swelling assumes, and the direction it takes towards the iliac region on the one side or on the other.

SPECIES VIII.
HYDROPS UTERI.
DROPSY OF THE WOMB.

HEAVY, CIRCUMSCRIBED PROTUBERANCE IN THE HYPOGASTRIUM, WITH OBSCURE FLUCTUATION ; PROGRESSIVELY ENLARGING, WITHOUT ISCHURY OR PREGNANCY ; MOUTH OF THE WOMB THIN, AND YIELDING TO THE TOUCH.

SAUVAGES makes not less than seven species of this disease, which he calls hydrometra, and which with him occurs as a genus. The distinctions, however, are of too little account to call for such a subdivision ; and one or two of the species have been by many writers regarded as doubtful, particularly the hydrometra gravidarum, or dropsy of the womb during pregnancy.—(*Clarke, Observations on the Diseases of Females*, &c., 8vo., 1821.) Dr. Cullen conceives it to be altogether unfounded, and hence makes the symptom of *citra graviditatem* a pathognomonic character of the complaint. But to this subject we shall have to return presently.

The disease is rarely, however, to be met with in the cavity of the uterus, and when this is the case, the orifice is perfectly closed. It is much more frequently to be found in a particular cyst, or the walls of a hydatid, or a cluster of hydatids, or between the tunics of the organ.* It is for the most part the result of a scirrhous or some other morbid change in the organ. A membranous or cellular dropsy is the variety most commonly assumed, in which the uterus

* Dr. Denman thought that hydrops uteri might be regarded as only a large hydatid ; for, according to his experience, whenever water was discharged in a case of this kind, a membranous bag was afterward expelled, although after some interval ; and this bag, when inflated, assumed the form of the distended uterus, of which it appeared to be a tunic.

Clarke (Dis. of Females) asserts that sometimes, from the discharge of hydatids, flooding takes place, more alarming than that which ensues from the separation of the placenta, because the latter occupies but a limited space ; whereas, hydatids may spring from any part of the internal cavity of the uterus. In a late formidable case of hydatids of this organ, the discharge was preceded by excessive flooding ; a diseased mass then followed, much resembling that figured by Clarke in his Diseases of Females ; the morbid preparation is in the possession of Dr. J. W. Borrowe.—D.

is sometimes distended to an enormous size, and the abdomen seems to be labouring under an anasarca.

The water, when in the cavity of the uterus, may often be evacuated by a cannula introduced into the mouth of the organ ; and if this should be prevented by a scirrhus, cicatrix, or tubercle lying over its mouth, a rupture of the sac in which the fluid is lodged may sometimes be produced by a violent shock of electricity passed through the hypogastric region, hard exercise, or emetics.

A sudden fall has often had the same effect. Tozzetti relates a case of cellular dropsy of the womb, which extended down the thigh and leg on one side, and disappeared by a spontaneous discharge of the water from the cuticle of the leg affected.—(Osservazioni Mediche, Firens., 1752.)

The uterus has also been said to be sometimes affected with dropsy, in consequence of a conveyance of the water, accumulated in the cavity of the abdomen in dropsy of the belly, into the uterine cavity, by means of the fringy termination of the Fallopian tubes. Of this cause, however, there does not appear to be any satisfactory proof. "Yet I must confess," says Dr. Denman, " I have seen some cases of water collected, and repeatedly discharged from the uterus, in the state of childbed, which I was unable to explain on any other principle." —(Francis's Denman, ch. iii., sect. ix.) Possibly, in this last case, a better explanation might have been sought for in an irritable state of the vessels that throw forth the liquor amnii during pregnancy itself, and which, under this kind of stimulus, may have secreted it to excess.

This, in effect, is the commonly supposed cause of a dropsy of the uterus while in a state of pregnancy ; which, however denied by some writers, appears to be very sufficiently established, and to be even capable of removal by the operation of paracentesis. Langio (lib. i., epist. xxix.) and Lamper (Dissert. de Hydrope) recommend this mode of treatment, and Scarpa gives an instance of its curative effect. " In October, 1808," says he, " my colleague Nessi successfully punctured the dropsical uterus of a countrywoman, aged thirty-five years, who in the fifth month of her pregnancy was threatened with suffocation. The perforation was made in the linea alba, between the pubes and the umbilicus. The woman gave birth to two children, who died soon after. The patient rose on the fourteenth day from that of the operation, but was seized with menorrhagia, which, however, was productive of no ultimate evil." This result is to be expected ; for we have already observed, that even tapping in ascites during pregnancy is apt to lead to a like issue. Scarpa himself was also consulted in a case of dropsy of the abdomen, in conjunction with a probable dropsy of the womb. On performing the operation for the former, as we have already described it, from twenty-five to thirty pounds of fluid were evacuated, and the patient immediately felt great relief. But, on the ensuing night, labour-pains were induced, and two fœtuses of

six months old were expelled, which died in a few seconds ; antecedently to the birth of which, upon a rupture of the membranes, not less than fifteen pounds of liquor amnii, as calculated by the attendants, were thrown forth as by a flood. The patient had a rapid recovery, and, in a few years, became twice pregnant, and was delivered with facility.—(Sulla Gravidanza sussiguita de Ascite, Trevisis, 1818.)

The internal treatment of this species of dropsy is that of the preceding.

———

SPECIES IX.
HYDROPS SCROTI.
DROPSY OF THE SCROTUM.

SOFT, TRANSPARENT, PYRIFORM INTUMESCENCE OF THE SCROTUM ; PROGRESSIVELY ENLARGING, WITHOUT PAIN.

THIS is the hydrocele of Heister and other writers ; and offers the two following varieties :

a Vaginalis.　The fluid contained in the
Vaginal dropsy of　tunica vaginalis or sur-
the scrotum.　rounding sheath of the
　testis.
β Cellularis.　The fluid contained in the
Cellular dropsy of　cellular membrane of the
the scrotum.　scrotum.

The ordinary causes of the FIRST VARIETY are not known with any degree of certainty. In the majority of cases, it seems to be unconnected with any particular state of the health or constitution. It has, however, been known to follow concussion of the scrotum, though, in almost all cases, no such cause can be suspected. Van der Harr asserts, that it occurs more frequently on the left than on the right side.— (Waarneeminge.) Delattre describes a congenital example of it.*

The SECOND VARIETY takes easily the pressure of the finger, and is mostly an accompaniment of general cellular dropsy, or a prelude to it. If it be an idiopathic affection, it may be removed by scarification.

The vaginal dropsy of the scrotum is the proper disease, and is elastic to the touch. It sometimes takes place with great rapidity, but in general very slowly. In some cases the tunic is extremely distended, and the whole scrotum rendered transparent, so that a candle may be seen through its contents.

On the Malabar coast, Kœmpfer asserts that the disease is endemic :† and the scrotum has been sometimes found to weigh sixty pounds.— (Mémoires de Paris, 1711, p. 30.) And Mr. D. Johnson of the Bengal establishment tells us,

———

* Journ. de Méd., tom. xxxii. By a congenital hydrocele is now usually signified that form of the disease in which the communication between the cavities of the peritoneum and tunica vaginalis is unclosed, and fluid collects within the latter.—ED.

† Amœnitat. Exotic. Here probably Kœmpfer must be referring to the sarcomatous enlargement of the scrotum so frequent in hot climates, and not to hydrocele, the weight of which is much less than that of a solid tumour.—ED.

that the native surgeons cure it sometimes by a cataplasm of tobacco-leaves, and sometimes by one of pounded indigo-leaves, and crude sal ammoniac. He adds, that they perform occasionally the operation for a radical cure by incision.—(*Miscellaneous Observations on certain indigenous Customs, Diseases, &c., in India.*)

In recent cases, emetics have appeared peculiarly serviceable ; and astringents and stimulants may be tried in the form of cataplasms or fomentations ; as vinegar, with or without a solution of muriate of ammonia, or neutralized with subcarbonate of ammonia.* When there is much pain, leeches should be previously applied. If this do not succeed, the sac must be opened, and the fluid be evacuated by a lancet† or the trocar. But the water soon reaccumulates, and the same palliative must usually be had recourse to three or four times a year. Van Swieten mentions the case of a dignified ecclesiastic, who was obliged to have the operation performed every three months for twenty years in succession.—(*Comment.* ad § 252.) And I had lately a patient who submitted to it as often, for many years of the latter part of his life, though he did not live so long as Van Swieten's patient.

The only radical cure we are acquainted with is that of obliterating the cavity, by exciting an inflammation in the vaginal and albugineous tunics. By this method the two tunics are made to adhere together, and, the cavity being destroyed, there can be no subsequent accumulation. Thus, inflammation may be excited by an incision, a seton, a caustic, the introduction of an irritating fluid by means of a syringe, as brandy, diluted spirits of wine, diluted port wine, or a solution of corrosive sublimate. The cure by injection is that to which modern surgeons have generally given the preference, as being the mildest and most effectual. Within the last few years, however, a more simple method has been proposed ; though experience has not yet decided so fully in its favour as in that of the treatment by injection.

Mr. Kinder Wood, after evacuating the fluid, draws forward with a small hook " that portion of the tunica vaginalis presenting at the external opening, and cuts it away with a pair of scissors, immediately closing the external opening with adhesive plaster ; by which means a moderate inflammation of the membrane will be ensured, and I am led to hope," says the ingenious writer, " that the success will be frequent."—(*Trans. of the Medico-Chir. Soc.*, vol. ix., p. 49.) In effect, Mr. Wood gives various instances of complete success. The piece snipped off is very small, and little inconvenience is suffered. The inflammation under this mode

of operating is so inconsiderable as to be confined to the tunica vaginalis alone, and consequently the cavity between the two tunics is not obliterated, as is obvious by the testis being still able to roll to a considerable extent within the scrotum. This plan, therefore, is best adapted for dropsies of recent standing, and where the sac is not much thickened and indurated. In old and obdurate cases, it will mostly be found necessary to carry the inflammation so far as to obliterate the cavity.*

Mr. Wood does not seem to be aware, that Mr. John Douglas employed a similar remedy as a radical cure in the dropsy of the scrotum, and recommended it in his Treatise on Hydrocele, published in this metropolis in 1755. Celsus appears also to have glanced at the same practice.—(*De Medecin.*, lib. vii., cap. 21.)

In a case on which the author was consulted some few years ago, the patient, a gentleman far advanced in life, and who had been regularly tapped about once in three months for five or six years antecedently, found a considerable hemorrhage ensue shortly after the last operation, but which yielded on immersing the scrotum into water chilled to the freezing point. The hemorrhage, however, returned within two days, and the scrotum was again as much distended, though manifestly with blood, as before the trocar had been applied. It was clear, either that in this HÆMATOCELE, as it has been sometimes called, a pretty large artery had been accidentally wounded, or that the internal parts were in a very morbid condition. To ascertain the real fact, and put a stop to the discharge, the scrotal and vaginal tunics were immediately laid open from the top to the bottom, and a pretty strong pressure made between the testicle and the sides of the latter tunic with folds of lint, which effectually restrained the hemorrhage. On examining the organ more closely on the ensuing day, a foul and spongy ulcer was detected on the tunica albuginea, from which the hemorrhage had proceeded : by a course of warm digestive dressing, however, both the wound and the ulcer healed, and a radical cure of the dropsy was completely accomplished.—(See, for a case somewhat similar, *Edin. Med. Ess.*, art. xiv., by *Mr. Jamieson*)

A variety of this disease has occasionally been found in an accumulation of fluid in the tunica vaginalis of the spermatic cord, owing to a defective adherence of the peritoneal covering of this organ through its entire length, and hence the possibility of a collection of fluids in the unattached parts. A cure, as in scrotal hydrocele, is obtained either by injection or incision.†

The clitoris has sometimes been found af-

---

* Stimulating applications do not very often succeed on adult subjects, though sometimes they do so on children. Dupuytren informs us, that he has often dispersed hydroceles by blistering the scrotum.—ED.

† The lancet is a bad instrument for the purpose, because it is more apt than the trocar to occasion hemorrhage within the tunica vaginalis. —ED.

* Recent observations prove, that a radical cure is often brought about on another principle, namely, by some change in the action of the vessels which secrete the redundant fluid.—ED.

† Tyrrell's edit. of Sir A. Cooper's Lect., vol. ii., p. 111. The best practice is to lay open the tumour, and then fill the cavity with lint. The excision of the anterior part of the cyst is unnecessary.—ED.

fected with the second or cellular variety, and acquired a considerable size. The earliest writer who seems to have noticed this sort of dropsy is Aëtius (tetrab. iv., serm. ii., c. 22; serm. iv., c. 100); and it has since been described or adverted to by Van. Swieten (*Comment.* ad § 1227), Saviard (*Nouveau Recueil*, &c.), Manoury (*Journ. de Méd.*, 1790), and various others, under the name of *hydrocele muliebris* or *fœminina.*

GENUS II.
EMPHYSEMA.
INFLATION. WIND-DROPSY.

ELASTIC AND SONOROUS DISTENTION OF THE BODY OR ITS MEMBERS, FROM AIR ACCUMULATED IN NATURAL CAVITIES IN WHICH IT IS NOT COMMONLY PRESENT.

THE term EMPHYSEMA is derived from ἐμ– or ἐν– and φυσάω, "inflo," "flatu distendo." It has often been made a question by what means the air is obtained in various cavities, in which it is found in great abundance ; for we cannot always trace its introduction from without, nor ascribe it to a putrefactive process. Fantoni found air seated between the tunics of the gallbladder, and Hildanus in the muscles. "In one instance," observes Mr. J. Hunter, "I have discovered air in an abscess, which could not have been received from the external air ; nor could it have arisen from putrefaction."—(*Animal Economy*, p. 207.) The case is singular, and well entitled to attention, but too long to be copied. From this and various other circumstances, Mr. Hunter conceived the opinion, that air is often secreted by animal organs, or separated from the juices conveyed to them : and he appeals, in confirmation of this opinion, to the experiments of Dr. Ingenhouz upon vegetables. I have not had an opportunity of reading these experiments, but that such a sort of secretion exists in plants must be obvious to every one who carefully examines the inflated legume of the different species of bladder-senna (colutea), and the capsules of several other shrubs quite as common in our gardens, and which can only become inflated by a separation or secretion of air from the surrounding vessels. Yet an appeal to a variety of curious facts in the economy of numerous animals will perhaps answer the purpose much better, as leading us more directly to the point. The *sepia officinalis*, or cuttlefish, and the *argonauta nautilus,* the ordinary parasitic inhabitant of which—for we do not know the animal that rears the shell —has a very near resemblance to the cuttlefish, and, as suspected by Rafinesque, and since determined by Cranch, is a species of ocythoë (*Phil. Trans.*, 1817, p. 293), introduce air at option into the numerous cells of the backbone, and thus render themselves specifically lighter whenever they wish to ascend from the depths of the sea to the surface ; and, in like manner, exhaust the backbone of its air, and thus render themselves specifically heavier, whenever they wish to descend. All fishes, possessing a sound or air-bladder, are equally capable of sup-

plying this organ with air, first for the purpose of balancing themselves, and next apparently for that of raising themselves towards the surface. In all these cases, the air thus introduced and accumulated appears to be a direct secretion : at least, we cannot otherwise account for its presence, as we can easily do in the bones of birds, whose cells are filled with air ; for we can here trace an immediate communication with the air-cells of the lungs ; and Dr. Baillie was induced to regard as a secretion the air accumulated in one or more emphysematous affections that occurred in his practice.[*]

"There is no difficulty," says he, "in conceiving the possibility of this action taking place. It is just as easy to conceive air secreted from the blood by the action of the vessels, as the secretion of the bile, milk, or any other secreted fluid." The case he chiefly depended upon is of a very singular character, from the extent of the disease. The patient was a girl about ten years of age, placed under his care in St. George's Hospital. The pulse was felt with difficulty, from the elevation of the skin, and the crackling of air under the fingers. There was the same elevation and crackling in the back, breast, belly, and thighs ; and it was obvious that there was some accumulation of water in the cellular membrane of the legs and face. The cause was unascertainable, but there had been no local injury. The patient died the next day ; and on examining the body, independently of the free influx of air already observed over the cellular membrane of the surface, the stomach was found distended almost as far as it could stretch, the intestinal canal was moderately filled with it, and various other vacuities gave proofs of its existence. About a gallon of water was found in the cavity of the abdomen.

Mr. Bauer has lately shown, that a gas is constantly shooting forth in small bubbles from the roots of plants into the slimy papulæ by which they are surrounded ; and that it is by this means that the slimy matter becomes elongated, is rendered vascular, and converted into hair or down. Mr. Brande has also shown that gas, meaning hereby carbonic acid gas, exists in a considerable quantity in the blood while circulating in the arteries and veins, and is very largely poured forth from blood placed, while warm, under the receiver of an airpump, so as to give an appearance of effervescence. He calculates that two cubic inches are extricated from every ounce of blood thus experimented upon, the venous and arterial blood containing an equal proportion. And Sir Everard Home has hence ingeniously conjectured, that it is by the escape of bubbles of this gas through the serum, in cases of coagulated blood, that new vessels are formed, as also that granulations are produced in pus ; from which it appears that the same gas escapes with equal freedom.

---

[*] Trans. of a Soc. for the improvement of Med. and Chir. Knowledge. Dr. Davy has offered facts confirming the same opinion, in his Observations on Air found in the Pleura in a Case of Pneumato-thorax, &c.—Phil. Trans., 1823, p. 496.

These results of Mr. Brande are in perfect accordance with the well-known experiments of Dr. Hales and Baron Haller upon the same subject, which of late years appear to have been too much neglected, if not discredited. The former asserts that, in distilling blood, a thirty-third· part of the whole proved to be air : and the latter confirms the assertion : ." utlque," says he, " ferè trigesima tertia pars totius sanguinis verus est aër." The inquiry has smee been followed up by Dr. Davy, who has not only confirmed many of the same results, but given an accurate analysis of the air thus, in various cases, accumulated.—(*Observations on Air found in the Pleura*, &c., *Phil. Trans.*, 1823.) From all which we may reasonably conjecture, that the body of air found in certain cases of emphysema is produced, like other fluids found in the different cavities of the animal frame, by a process of secretion. The species are the three following :—

1. Emphysema Cellulare. Cellular Inflation.
2. ———Abdom- inis. Tympany.
3. ———Uteri. Inflation of the Womb.

There are probably many others ; but these are the only ones which have been hitherto distinctly pointed-out.

SPECIES I.
EMPHYSEMA CELLULARE.
CELLULAR INFLATION.

TENSE, GLABROUS, DIFFUSIVE INTUMESCENCE OF THE SKIN, CRACKLING BENEATH THE PRESSURE OF THE FINGER.

This is the pneumatosis of Sauvages and Cullen, and consists in a distention of the cellular membrane by air instead of by water, as in *hydrops cellularis* or anasarca. The distention is sometimes limited to particular parts of the body, and sometimes extends over the entire frame.

From the remarks we have just offered on the probable separation or secretion of air from the blood, this disease may originate from various causes, and exhibit itself under various modifications ;* but the two following are the only extensive forms under which it has hitherto been traced :—

a A vulnere thora- cis. From a wound in the chest, with sense of suffocation.
Traumatic emphysema.

* One variety, not noticed by our author, is that occasionally following the rupture of the air-cells of the lungs in a violent fit of coughing. The pathology of this case was first explained by M. Louis, in the Mém. de l'Acad. de Chirugie, where he details instances of it from the excessive coughing attending the lodgment of extraneous substances in the trachea. Another example of what is sometimes called idiopathic emphysema, brought on by cough subsequent to pneumonia in an infant, is recorded by Dr. A. S. Ireland.—See Trans. of Assoc. Physicians, vol. iii., p. 112, Duhl., 1820.—ED.

β A veneno. From fish-poison or other
Impoisoned emphysema. venom ; with extensive signs of gangrene and putrescence.

For the FIRST OF THESE VARIETIES, there is no great difficulty in accounting. If a wound penetrate the chest so as to enter any part of the lungs, and divide some of the larger branches of the bronchiæ or the air-cells, the inspired air, instead of being confined to its proper channels, will rush immediately into the chest, and fill up its whole cavity ; as it will also frequently into the cellular membrane of the lungs, and the parietes of the chest, whence it will find a passage into the cellular membrane of the entire body, and produce a universal inflation.

This last effect is highly troublesome and distressing : but the first is productive of the utmost alarm. The lungs, compressed on every side by the extravasated air, are incapable of expansion ; and there is consequently an instantaneous danger of suffocation. The patient labours for breath with all his might, and labours to but little purpose ; his cheeks are livid, his senses soon become stupified, the heart palpitates violently, the pulse is rapid but small ; and, without speedy relief, death must inevitably ensue. The distress is moreover sometimes aggravated by the excitement of a cough, in the fits of which, if any considerable bloodvessel have been burst, blood is expectorated along with the rejected mucus. [The thoracic parietes are manifestly distended, the ribs are more or less separated, and the diaphragm projects into the cavity of the abdomen. When the disease exists on the left side of the chest, that muscle is propelled considerably downwards ; and, when it is on the right side, the liver is pushed below the margin of the ribs.— (See *Laennec on Dis. of the Chest*, p. 492, 2d edit. by Forbes.)] It is this form of emphysema which constitutes the pneumo-thorax of Itard and Laennec, or the pneumato-thorax, as it is more correctly called, of Dr. John Davy, who has described two cases in which the communication seems to have been produced by a suppurated tubercle that formed an opening from some branch of the bronchiæ into the sac of the pleura.*

[According to Laennec, the certain diagnosis of this affection is afforded by the comparison of the results of percussion and mediate auscultation. Whenever we find one side of the chest sounding more distinctly than the other, and, at the same time, perceive the respiration very well in the least sonorous side, and not at all in the other, we may be assured that there exists pneumo-thorax on the latter.]

Mr. Kelly, in the Edinburgh Medical Commentarles, has given a very singular case of this affection from a like cause, in which the inflation extended widely over the body. The patient, almost fifty-seven years of age, had long laboured under a chronic cough and difficulty of

* Phil. Trans., 1823, ut supra. Laennec's experience taught him to believe this to be the most common of all the forms of pneumo-thorax.

breathing. The emphysema began to appear 'on the second day, after a most violent fit of coughing, laborious respiration, and pain in the side. It soon covered the whole right side to the scrotum, which was also much inflated, producing a crackling sound upon pressure; and, gradually widening its course, by the fourth day it extended over the whole body. - It was at first conceived that air bad entered from without into the cellular membrane by means of some wound in the side; but no such injury or any other channel of communication could be discovered. The symptoms, however, were so pressing, that it was at length determined, under the advice of Dr. Munro, to afford an escape for the air, by an opening into the cavity of the chest. The pleura was in consequence tapped; when, upon withdrawing the perforator, such a blast of wind issued through the cannula as to blow out a lighted candle three or four times successively.[*] The patient immediately became easy and free from oppression, and his pulse fell from above a hundred strokes in a minute to ninety. Punctures were at the same time made into the cellular membrane in different parts of the body, and from these also the imprisoned air puffed out upon pressure, but not otherwise. The patient recovered gradually, and in about three weeks ate and slept as well as he had done at any time for thirty years before. For nearly a twelvemonth he continued to enjoy a good state of health: but, about the close of this period, he was again attacked with a cough, a pain in the chest, and a difficulty of breathing; a hectic fever followed, and he died in about six weeks. On opening the thorax, Mr. Kelly tells us, that he found the lungs "in a very putrid diseased state, with some tubercles on the external surface of the right lobe; there was extensive adhesion to the pleura, particularly at the place where the pain had been felt most keenly before the perforation; and, on making an incision into the right lobe, an abscess was discovered, which contained about four ounces of fetid purulent matter."—(*Edin. Med. Comment.*, vol. ii., p. 427.) We are hence, I think, led to conjecture, that the emphysema was in this case produced by the bursting of a former abscess in the right lobe of the lungs, accompanied with a rupture of one or more of the bronchial vessels, in consequence of which the same effect followed as if a wound had been inflicted from without.

[The manner of making an opening into the chest must be learned by reference to the writers on surgery; and to the same sources of information the reader should turn for an account of the treatment of emphysema from wounded lungs.]

The inflation which follows so suddenly and so extensively in the SECOND VARIETY, or upon the introduction of fish-poison, or that of several species of the mushroom or numerous other edible venoms into the stomach, it is not so easy to account for. In most of the cases, there is so violent and general a disturbance of every function, as to produce extreme and instantaneous debility : all the precursors of putrescence are present, and speedy dissolution is threatened. Every part of the body is swollen and inflated, particularly the stomach and intestines, the vapour of which, when examined after death, is found to consist of a fetid and putrid gas; a blackish and greenish froth is discharged from the mouth; clonic or tetanic spasms play wildly over all the muscles; the chest labours with suffocation; the brain is stupified; and broad livid or gangrenous spots spread over the body; and on dissection are found still more freely, and of larger diameter, on the surface of most of the thoracic and visceral organs. The most effectual remedies against all such inflations are the most powerful antiseptics : as acids, alcohol, and the aromatics.

We never cease to find a free extrication of air whenever the body or any part of it is running rapidly into a state of putrefaction : and hence another cause of cellular emphysema, and a cause that is perpetually occurring to us in gangrene.

SPECIES II.
EMPHYSEMA ABDOMINIS
TYMPANY.

TENSE, LIGHT, AND EQUABLE INTUMESCENCE OF THE BELLY; DISTINCTLY RESONANT TO A STROKE OF THE HAND.

THIS disease is the tympanites of authors, so called from the drum-like sound which is given on striking the belly with the hand.

Tympanites, however, is by most writers applied principally to an enormous collection or evolution of air in some part or other of the alvine canal, constituting the *tympanites intestinalis* of Sauvages: and it is to this disease alone that Dr. Cullen confines his attention, when treating of the subject in his First Lines. This flatulent distention he ascribes to an atony of the muscular fibres of the intestines, accompanied with a spasmodic constriction in parts of the canal, by which means the passage of the air is in some places interrupted. In this view of the case, however, tympany, instead of being entitled to the rank of a distinct genus, is nothing more than a symptom or sequel of some other enteric affection, as dyspepsy, colic, worms, or hysteria : and hence the remedies applicable to these are what Dr. Cullen recommends for tympanites, namely, avoiding flatulent food, laxatives, and tonics.

Mr. John Hunter seems to have conceived that a tympany of the stomach or intestines may exist as an idiopathic complaint. " I am inclined," says he, " to believe, that the stomach has a power of forming air and letting it loose from the blood by a kind of secretion. We cannot, however, bring any absolute proof of this taking place in the stomach, as it may in all cases be referred to a defect in digestion :

---

* In a case recently reported in Dr. Johnson's Med. Chir. Review, the same thing happened when Mr. Guthrie made an opening into the chest. In this instance, the operation gave temporary relief; but the patient survived only a short time.
—ED.

P p 2

but we have instances of its being found in other cavities, where no secondary cause can be assigned."—(*On the Animal Economy*, p. 206, 4to., 1792.) He alludes chiefly to an extrication of air in the uterus, which we shall have occasion to notice in our next species.

In concurrence with these remarks, it may also be observed, that some persons are said to have a power of producing ventricular distentions voluntarily, which it is difficult to account for, except by a voluntary power of secreting air for this purpose, or forcing it down the œsophagus, which will be still less readily allowed. Morgagni (*De Sed. et Caus. Morb.*, ep. xxxviii.; art. 23 ; *Collect. Soc. Med. Hafn.*, ii., p. 73) and other writers have hence treated of this form of the disease, as well as of that in which the flatus is lodged in the peritoneal sac : while others have contended that this is the only form, and that a peritoneal tympany has no real existence.*

If an idiopathic tympany of the stomach should ever be decidedly ascertained, its cure must be attempted by the remedies for flatus of any other kind : but at present, the only disease we can fairly contemplate as entitled to the name of tympanites, or *emphysema abdominis*, notwithstanding the incredulity of some practitioners, is that in which the resonant swelling of the belly is produced by air collected in the sac of the peritoneum. It is undoubtedly a rare disease, though we must contend, in the language of Dr. Cullen, that "from several dissections, it is unquestionable that such a disease has sometimes truly occurred:" nor can we suppose such accurate and cautious pathologists as Heister (*Wahrnehmungen*, i., art. 15), Lieutaud (*Hist. Anat.*, v., p. 432), and Bell (*On Ulcers and Tumours*, vol. ii.), who have respectively given examples of it, to have been successively deceived upon the subject. Admitting it to be produced by secretion, its occasional causes are still very obscure. It has been said to follow jaundice and morbid affections of the abdominal viscera ; debility produced by fever ; hysteria ; violent passions or other emotions of the mind : and probably all these may have operated in different cases.

The ordinary natural cure seems to consist in an escape of the air from the umbilicus by an outlet produced by an abscess or ulceration of this protuberant organ, or a sudden and fortunate rupture of its integuments. Morgagni and several later writers (*Guisard, Pratique de Chir.*, tom. i., p. 134) give us well-authenticated cases of an occurrence of the first of these, and Stoerck of both.—(*Ann. Med.*, ii., pp. 190, 193, 194.) We are thus led by nature herself to try the effects of tapping, or making an artificial

opening into the cavity of the abdomen, in the case of wind-dropsy as well as in that of water-dropsy : and here, from the protruded state of the umbilicus, the lancet may conveniently be introduced at this point. The belly should, at the time of the operation, be well swathed with a broad girth, which may be tightened at option, and should be kept as tight as the patient can bear it, as well for the purpose of general support, as for that of expelling the air within, and preventing the entrance of air from without.

Van Swieten dissuaded his pupils from this operation (*Ad Sect.*, 1251) ; and Cembalusier (*Pneumatopathol.*, p. 503 ; *Dusseau, Journ. de Méd.*, 1779), and a few others, have since asserted that it does not answer. But in most of these cases we have reason to believe that the seat of the disease was mistaken, and that the flatulence existed in the intestinal canal rather than in the peritoneal sac.

Antecedently, however, to the operation of the paracentesis, we may try the effect of sending shocks of the electric aura through the abdomen. Cold fomentations, moreover, or even pounded ice, may be applied externally, and gelid drinks be swallowed copiously at the same time. This plan is said to have answered occasionally.—(*Theden, N. Bemerkungen und Erfahrungen*, ii., p. 251.) And it is obvious that a tonic regimen, with free exercise, and particularly equitation, and, where it can be had recourse to, sea-bathing, should be entered upon as soon as the tympany is dispersed.

There is a singular case of flatulent distention inserted in the Edinburgh Medical Essays, by Professor Monro, which is called a tympany, but does not seem to have been exterior to the intestinal canal ; and hence, if a tympany at all, must have been produced by a secretion of air into the stomach or bowels, as conjectured by Mr. J. Hunter. The patient was a young woman, aged twenty-two. The inflation continued for at least three months, the belly being sometimes so extremely distended as to endanger its bursting, and sometimes considerably detumefied, at which last period a variety of unequal and protuberant balls were felt all over the abdomen, and seemed to indicate so many intestinal constrictions. The patient's appetite continued good; she was very costive, and menstruated only at intervals of several months. She was at length attacked with borborygmi, and a day or two afterward had such explosions of wind ἄνω καὶ κάτω, that none of the other patients would remain in the same room, and hardly on the same floor with her. From this time she recovered gradually.—(*Edin. Med. Essays*, vol. i., art. xxxi.)

SPECIES III.

EMPHYSEMA UTERI.

INFLATION OF THE WOMB.

LIGHT, TENSE, CIRCUMSCRIBED PROTUBERANCE IN THE HYPOGASTRIUM ; OBSCURELY SONOROUS ; WIND OCCASIONALLY DISCHARGED THROUGH THE MOUTH OF THE UTERUS.

THIS is the physometra of Sauvages and later

---

* Littre, Mém. de l'Acad. des Sciences, 1713, p. 235. Dr. Elliotson believes that tympanites, in the sense of a great collection of air in the peritoneum, usually takes place from an aperture existing in the intestines, so that the air escapes.—(See Lectures delivered at the London University, as reported in the Med. Gaz. for 1832–33, p. 456.) Whether this opinion has ever been verified by *post mortem* examinations, is not stated.—ED.

nosologists. Like the last species, it is by no means a frequent complaint, and not easy to be accounted for, except upon the principle of a secretion of air ; and hence the existence of this species, as well as of the last, has been denied by several writers who do not happen to have met with examples of it. The description given of it is somewhat obscure in most of the pathologists ; but there seems, upon the whole, sufficient reason for admitting it into the list of morbid affections. "It has been said," observes Dr. Denman, " that wind may be collected and retained in the cavity of the uterus till it is distended in such a manner as to resemble pregnancy, and to produce its usual symptoms ; and that by a sudden eruption of the wind, the tumefaction of the abdomen has been removed, and the patient immediately reduced to her proper size. Of this complaint I have never seen an example : but many cases have occurred to me of temporary explosions of wind from the uterus, which there was no power of restraining."—(*Francis's Denman*, chap. iii., sect. x.)

The uterus is one of those organs referred to under our last species, as supposed by Mr. John Hunter to have a power of secreting or separating air from the blood : and as he has examined the subject with critical accuracy in direct reference to the present complaint, his remarks are particularly entitled to our attention. " I have been informed," says he, " of persons who have had air in the uterus or vagina, without having been sensible of it but by its escaping from them without their being able to prevent it : and who, from this circumstance, have been kept in constant alarm lest it should make a noise in its passage, having no power to retard it as when it is contained in the rectum. The fact being so extraordinary made me somewhat incredulous ; but rendered me more inquisitive, in the hope of being enabled to ascertain and account for it : and those of whom I have been led to inquire, have always made the natural distincti between air passing from the vagina and by the anus : that from the anus they feel and can retain, but that in the vagina they cannot ; nor are they aware of it till it passes. A woman, whom I attended with Sir John Pringle, informed us of this fact, but mentioned it only as a disagreeable thing. I was anxious to determine if there were any communication between the vagina and rectum, and was allowed to examine, but discovered nothing uncommon in the structure of these parts. She died some time after ; and being permitted to open the body, I found no disease either in the vagina or the uterus. Since that time I have had opportunities of inquiring of a number of women concerning this circumstance, and by three or four have been informed of the same fact, with all the circumstances above-mentioned."—(*Animal Economy*, p. 406, 4to., 1792.)

The only difficulty in the case is the means by which air can thus become accumulated in the cavity of the uterus ; for, admitting this fact, of which there can no longer, I should think, be any doubt, we can easily conceive a disten-

tion to the utmost power of the organ in consequence of an obstruction of the mouth of the womb from spasm, a coagulum of blood, or any other viscid material. And hence, in all the cases of this disease which have descended to us, we find such a closure described as existing whenever the organ has been examined. Thus, in the instance related by Eisenmenger (*Collect. Historia fœtus Mussi-pontani*, &c.), we are told that the uterus was completely impervious ; and a like account is given of a similar instance recorded in the Ephemera of Natural Curiosities. Palfin (*Description des parties de la femme qui servent à la génération*, Leid., 1708) gives a case, in which the obstruction proceeded from a hydatid cyst that had fixed at the mouth of the uterus, and Fernelius (*Patholog.*, lib. iv., cap. xv.) another, in which the obstruction, and consequently the inflation, returned periodically. Dr. Denman intimates that this affection is sometimes accompanied with spasmodic pains, resembling those of labour ; and the same remark will apply to dropsy of the womb, which so much resembles it. The fact is, that the uterus, when once enlarged by whatever means, and stimulated, has a natural tendency to run into a series of expulsory exertions in order to free itself from its burden, and to excite all the surrounding muscles into the same train of action ; and hence natural labour, false conception, uterine dropsy, and inflation, produce the same effect, though perhaps in different degrees.

As an occasional discharge of wind from the vagina affords temporary ease, we should take a hint from this effect ; and endeavour first to evacuate the confined air entirely, by a cannula introduced into the os tincæ ; and secondly, to invigorate the weakened organ by the use of some tonic injection, as a solution of catechu, alum, sulphate of zinc, or diluted port wine.

GENUS III.

PARURIA.

MISMICTURITION.

MORBID SECRETION OR DISCHARGE OF URINE.

THE term PARURIA is a Greek derivation from παρά, "perperam," and οὐρέω, "mingo." The genus is intended to include the ischuria, dysuria, pyuria, enuresis, diabetes, and several other divisions and subdivisions of authors, which, like the different species of the preceding genus, lie scattered, in most of the nosologies, through widely different parts of the general arrangement. Thus, in Cullen, diabetes occurs in the second class of his system ; enuresis in the fourth order of his fourth class ; and ischuria and dysuria in the fifth order of the same class: All these, however, form a natural group ; and several of them have characters scarcely diversified enough for distinct species, instead of forming distinct genera. DYSURIA might have been employed instead of PARURIA, as a generic term for the whole ; but as it has been usually limited to the third species in the present arrangement, it has been thought better to propose a new term, than to run the risk of confusion by retaining the old term in a new sense.

The species that justly belong to the present genus appear to be the following :—

1. Paruria Inops. -   Destitution of Urine.
2. ——— Retentionis. Stoppage of Urine.
3. ——— Stillatitia. Strangury.
4. ——— Mellita. . Scacharine Urine.
5. ——— Incontinens. Incontinence of Urine.
6. ——— Incocta. Unassimilated Urine.
7. ——— Erratica. ' Erratic Urine.

From this group of family diseases we may perceive that the urine is sometimes deranged in its quantity, sometimes in its quality, and sometimes in its outlet : and that, in its quality, it is deranged in two ways ; by being made a medium for foreign materials, and by being imperfectly elaborated. The most important principle which it seems to carry off from the constitution, is the urea, or that of the uric acid : and it has been ingeniously remarked by M. Berard, in his Analysis of Animal Substances, " that as this is the most azotized of all the animal principles, the secretion of urine appears to have for its object a separation of the excess of azote from the blood, as respiration separates from it the excess of carbon."

SPECIES I.
PARURIA INOPS.
DESTITUTION OF URINE.

URINE NOT SECRETED BY THE KIDNEYS : NO DE-
SIRE TO MAKE WATER, NOR SENSE OF FULNESS
IN ANY PART OF THE URINARY TRACK.

A DEFICIENT secretion of urine is often a result of renal inflammation, in which case, however, there is necessarily a considerable degree of pain and tenderness in the lumbar region. It sometimes proceeds from transferred gout, of which Mr. Howship relates a striking instance in a case that occurred to Mr. Heaviside. In this case, also, there is usually great pain in the loins, a symptom which was very prominent in the exemplification now alluded to. The gout disappeared from the foot suddenly on walking home at night in the cold. The patient, a general officer, made little water through the night, less the ensuing day, and none the day after. The catheter was then passed, and the bladder was found empty.* But the present species occurs occasionally as an idiopathic affection, sometimes followed rapidly by great danger to the general fabric, sometimes assuming a chronic form, and running on for a considerable period of time without danger, and sometimes existing as a constitutional affection coeval with the birth of the individual.—(See Spe. 7 of the present genus, *P. erratica.*)

Dr. Parr relates a case that occurred in his

own practice, in which no urine was apparently secreted for six weeks (*Dict. in verb. Ischuria*); and Haller gives a similar case that lasted twenty-two weeks.—(*Bibl. Med.*, Pr. ii., p. 200.) In the Philosophical Transactions (vol. xxviii., year 1783) we meet with various instances of a similar deficiency ; among the most singular of which is the case of a youth of seventeen years of age, described by Dr. Richardson, who had never made water from his birth, nor had felt the least uneasiness on this account, being healthy, vigorous, and active.

Let it not be supposed, however, that the constituent principles of so important a recrement as the urine remain in the system, and load the blood, without danger. The outlet at which these are separated and discharged is not always manifest, and hence they sometimes appear not to be separated and discharged at all ; though, if the state of the patient be critically examined into by an accurate pathologist, the vicarious channel will generally be detected, and most of the cases that must at present range under the species before us would be transferred to that of *paruria erratica.*

The two most common emunctories that supply the place of the kidneys are the skin and the bowels. In Dr. Parr's case, he states that there was no vicarious evacuation, except a profuse sweat for a day or two, and he adds, that there was no suspicion of imposture, as the patient was in an hospital and constantly watched. But we have no account of the state of the bowels. In Dr. Richardson's case of a natural destitution of urine, the patient is admitted to have laboured under an habitual diarrhœa, though with little uneasiness, and the discharge of the urinary elements is very correctly ascribed to the intestinal flux.*

---

* Dr. Salmon A. Arnold, of Providence, R. I., has recorded the case of a young woman (see New-England Journal of Medicine and Surgery, Boston, 1825) who laboured under a retention of urine for two years, and through the integuments of whose lumbar region a fluid resembling urine oozed in abundance, whenever the catheter was not introduced at the usual periods. In September, 1822, seventy-two hours once elapsed without the instrument having been used : in the course of this delay, a liquid, completely like urine, is stated to have been discharged from the right ear ; first by drops, and then in a larger quantity at a time. The discharge continued on the following days, amounting to about eight ounces in each twenty-four hours, and always preceded by painful sensations in the eye and ear. Whenever the discharge happened to be interrupted or diminished, a general anxiety used to come on, with severe headache, and then delirium. Occasionally violent spasms, like those of opisthotonos, were produced by the same cause, followed by syncope and complete insensibility. Deafness and loss of sight afterward occurred in the right ear and eye. These symptoms continued till the end of 1824, the discharge issuing alternately from both ears and the left eye, which became considerably inflamed. In March, 1823, the patient began to vomit up a fluid precisely similar to urine. In April, the right breast became swollen, tense, and painful, and shortly afterward some drops of fluid were discharged from the nipple. In twenty-four

---

* Practical Treatise on the Symptoms, Causes, &c. of some of the most important Complaints that affect the Secretion and Excretion of the Urine, part i., ch. i., sect. ii. The suppression of the secretion of urine in Asiatic cholera is one of the usual effects of that extraordinary disease.—EDITOR.

The effects that result from a retention of the urinary elements in the system are, a loss of energy and a growing torpitude in every function, proving that the sensorium is directly debilitated, and rendered incapable of producing the nervous influence. It is hence to be expected that the brain should evince torpitude in a greater degree than any other organ, and become oppressed and comatose, as though in a state of apoplexy.* Nor is it difficult to account for these effects, since they naturally follow from the blood being surcharged with that excess of azote which, as we have just observed, it appears

---

hours these phenomena ceased, but reappeared a week afterward, and now the liquid voided was of a lemon colour, and was proved by analysis to contain urea. In May, 1823, after some pain and tension about the hypogastric region, a fluid, exactly like what had been evacuated from the preceding organs, began to ooze from the navel. A similar evacuation next commenced from the nostrils. The fluid from all these quarters was analyzed, and found to contain urea. It contained, likewise, the alkaline sulphates, muriates, and phosphates. During the foregoing occurrences, a small but varying quantity of urine continued to be voided from the bladder; and occasionally the urinary fluid discharged at different points was preceded by an oozing of blood. When care was taken to pass the catheter very often, the discharges were lessened, but not entirely stopped. In the autumn of 1824, notwithstanding the evacuation of urinary fluid from the right ear, breast, and navel still continued, though in a diminished quantity, the patient was not severely ill, and could get up and walk about. At that time a good deal of urine was passed in the regular way; and the evacuation of a similar liquid from the eye, stomach, and nostrils, had for some time ceased.†

From the various facts here recited, M. Andral infers, that the blood contains, in variable proportions, the elements of all the secretions; that, under ordinary circumstances, these elements are separated from the circulation only by those organs whose special structure is adapted to bring about such separation; but that, under particular states, these elements may be separated from the circulation by other channels than those regularly intended for the purpose; not, indeed, in the condition of perfect secretions, but in a more simple form, containing the elements of those secretions.—See Andral, Anat. Pathol., tom. i., p. 357.—ED.

* We have known of a case of this kind, from a sudden suppression of urine in a patient affected with diabetes.—D.

† This case is minutely detailed in the Am. Journ. of Med. Sc., vol. i. The following table, extracted from that paper, shows the quantities of urine discharged from various parts of the body during a period of ten days.

1824.	Bladder.	Right Ear.	Breast.	Navel.	Nose.	Left Eye.
July 20	16	15	12	18	2	2
21	10	32	36	17	1	1½
22	16	30	16	10		
23	14	35	20	36	3	3
24	10	32	8	16	14	13
25	12	30	16	30	16	6
26	20	46	16	38	16	8
27	16	52	16	48	17	6
28	12	40	17	37	16	8
29	16	47	15	20	16	8
30	10	54	16	44	16	5

—D.

---

to be the office of the urine to carry off.* The destructive power of azotic gas to animal life is known to every one, as is also its further power of increasing the coagulability of the blood.

I do not know, however, that the great and pressing danger of having the constituent principles of the urine thrown back into the blood had been distinctly pointed out by any physician, when Sir Henry Halford communicated some valuable observations on the subject. "A very corpulent, robust farmer, of about fifty-five years of age, was seized with a rigour, which induced him to send for his apothecary. He had not made water, it appeared, for twenty-four hours: but there was no pain, no sense of weight in the loins, no distention in any part of the abdomen; and therefore no alarm was taken till the following morning, when it was thought proper to ascertain whether there was any water in the bladder, by the introduction of the catheter; and none was found. I was then called, and another inquiry was made some few hours afterward, by one of the most eminent surgeons in London, whether the bladder contained any urine or not, when it appeared clearly that there was none. The patient sat up in bed and conversed as usual, complaining of some nausea, but of nothing material, in his own view; and I remember that his friends expressed their surprise that so much importance should be attached to so little apparent illness. The patient's pulse was somewhat slower than usual, and sometimes he was heavy and oppressed. I ventured to state, that if we should not succeed in making the kidneys act, the patient would soon become comatose, and would probably die the following night; for this was the course of the malady in every other instance which I had seen. It happened so; he died in thirty hours after this, in a state of stupefaction."—(Med. Trans., vol. vi., p. 310.)

To this short history Sir Henry has added the following remarks, which are of too much importance to be omitted. "All the patients who have fallen under my care, were fat, corpulent men, between fifty and sixty years of age; and, in three of them, there was observed a strong urinous smell in the perspiration twenty-four hours before death;" evidently proving that, in these cases, the instinctive or remedial power of nature, aided by the constitutional vigour of the respective patients, was endeavouring to convert the exhalants of the skin into a substitute for the palsied kidneys, but was not able completely to succeed. This view of the danger that results generally from having the elementary principles of the urine thrown back into the blood, thus strikingly pointed out by Sir Henry Halford, has since been confirmed by Dr. Baillie's opinion, as contained in his posthumous volume. "There is," says he, "a great difference in the

* On this subject, the experiments of M. Ch. Chossat are highly interesting.—See Mém. sur l'Analyse des Fonctions 'Urinaires; Journ. de Physiol. Expér., par F. Magendie, tom. v., p. 65, et seq. Whether the blood of persons afflicted with paruria inops be really surcharged with azote, is a point that must not be regarded as certain, until determined by chymical researches.—ED.

hazard of a patient's situation, whether the kidneys separate a little urine or none at all. In the first case be generally recovers, and in the second very rarely. It is curious that life should terminate so soon when the functions of the kidneys have become totally suspended. A person who receives no nourishment whatever into the stomach, or by any other means, will live longer."—(*Lect. and Obs. on Medicine, by the late Matthew Baillie, M. D.*, 1825, unpub.)

In attempting a cure of *paruria inops*, we ought, in the first instance, whatever be its cause, to take a hint from the light of nature which is thus thrown upon us : and, as the excretories of the skin and of the kidneys are so perpetually assisting each other in almost every way, excite the former by active diaphoretics to take upon themselves for a time the office of the latter, and carry off the urea that should be discharged by the kidneys.

We should next endeavour to restore the kidneys to their natural action by gentle stimulants or diuretics, as the alliaceous and siliquose plants, especially horseradish and mustard, the aromatic resins and balsams, especially those of turpentine, copayva, and the essential oil of juniper. Digitalis is of little avail, and in idiopathic diseases of the kidneys, does not often exhibit a diuretic effect. If given at all, it should be in conjunction with tincture of cantharides, or the spirit of nitric ether.

Stimulants may, at the same time, be applied externally, as the hot bath, or strokes of the electric or voltaic fluid passed through the loins ; to which may succeed rubefacients and blisters.

In the meanwhile, the alvine canal should be gently excited by neutral salts ; and juniper tea, broom tea, or imperial, may alternately form the common drink. The juice of the birch-tree (*betula alba*) will often, however, prove a better diuretic than any of these. It is easily obtained by wounding the trunk, and, when fresh, is a sweetish and limpid fluid, in its concrete state affording a brownish manna. It has the advantage of being slightly aperient, as well as powerfully diuretic. [However, if the case were connected with gravel and inflammation in the kidneys, the diuretic treatment should be abandoned for the antiphlogistic.]

SPECIES II.
PARURIA RETENTIONIS.
STOPPAGE OF URINE.

URINE TOTALLY OBSTRUCTED IN ITS FLOW ; WITH A SENSE OF WEIGHT OR UNEASINESS IN SOME PART OF THE URINARY TRACK.

This is the ischuria of many writers, and though, like the preceding species, it is equally without a flow of urine, it differs widely from it in other circumstances. In *paruria inops*, the excretories of the kidneys are inactive, and consequently no urine is produced. In the species now before us, the secernents possess an adequate power, but the secretion is obstructed in its passage. And, as it may be obstructed in different organs, and in numerous ways in each organ, we have the following varieties :—

α Renalis.	Pain and sense of weight in
Renal stoppage	the region of the kidneys,
of urine.	without any swelling in
	the hypogastrium.
β Ureterica	With pain or sense of weight
Ureteric stop-	in the region of the ure-
page of urine.	ters.
γ Vesicalis.	With protuberance in the
Vesical stoppage	hypogastrium ; frequent
of urine.	desire to make water ;
	and pain at the neck of
	the bladder.
δ Urethralis.	With protuberance in the hy-
Urethral stop-	pogastrium ; frequent de-
page of urine.	sire to make water ; and
	a sense of obstruction in
	the urethra, resisting the
	introduction of a catheter.

OBSTRUCTION OF URINE may take place IN THE KIDNEYS from a variety of causes, as spasm, calculous concretions, inflammation, or abscess ; and the tumour or swelling, which occurs in any of these states, may be so considerable as to prevent the fluid from flowing into the pelvis of the kidneys as it becomes secreted by the tubules, or out of the pelvis when it has collected there. [This is the renal ischuria of Sauvages, and is characterized by the following circumstances : —It supervenes upon some previous affection of the kidneys, and is accompanied by pain, or an uneasy sense of weight in the loins. There is no tumour in the hypogastrium, such as a distended bladder would occasion, nor any desire to make water. The most frequent cause of the disease is inflammation, or calculi of the kidneys or ureters. The symptoms at first are sometimes not very urgent. Thus, in an example recorded by Dr. Teeling, its peculiarity was the quantity of gravelly matter in one kidney, with the complete stoppage of the ureter on one side, and the evidently inflamed condition of the other kidney, and that neither of these occurrences should have been marked by any local urgent pain or sickness of the stomach, and scarcely any fever. The patient had been subject to calculous and gouty symptoms.—(See *Dr. Teeling's case of Sup. of Urine, Trans. of Assoc. Physicians*, vol. iv., p. 169, 8vo., Dublin, 1824.)]

The kidneys lie so deep, that their intumescence is often imperceptible to the eye, or even to the touch. At times, however, they become wonderfully augmented as the process of inflammation proceeds. Cabrolius gives us the history of a purulent kidney that weighed fourteen pounds.—(*Cabrol. Observ.*, p. 28.) And where the enlargement is accompanied with but little inflammation, proceeds gradually, and does not enter into a suppurative state, the organ not unfrequently becomes much more enormous, and has sometimes been found to weigh from thirty-five to forty pounds.—(*Commerc. Liter. Nor.*, 1731, p. 32 ; 1737, p. 326.)

In this condition there is no difficulty in conceiving a total obstruction to the flow of the urine, even when elaborated in sufficient abundance. But the kidney, on the contrary, sometimes wastes away instead of enlarging, and this so much as to become a shrivelled sac, and not exceed a drachm in weight; and as the sinus of the kidney contracts with its body, the organ at its extreme point is sometimes found imperforate; and hence how small soever may be the quantity of fluid which, in this morbid condition, may be separated from the blood, none whatever can pass into the ureter; and if both the kidneys concur in the same emaciation, this also must form as effectual a cause of the disease before us as any other,

When the STOPPAGE OF URINE exists in the URETERS, the causes may be as numerous and nearly of the same kind as when the kidneys are at fault: for here also we occasionally meet with calculous concretions, inflammation, and spasm: to which we may add grumous blood, viscid mucus, and a closed orifice in consequence of ulceration.

VESICAL RETENTION OF URINE is produced by inflammation, pressure upon the neck of the bladder, irritation, or paresis. Pressure upon the neck of the bladder may be occasioned by distention of the rectum from scybala, or other enterolithic concretions, inflammation, abscesses, or piles; or by distention of the vagina from inflammation, or a lodgment of the menstrual flux in consequence of an inperforate hymen. Irritation may be excited by a calculus, or too long a voluntary retention of urine, as often happens on our being so closely impacted in large assemblies or public courts, or so powerfully arrested by the interest or eloquence of a subject discussed in such places, that we cannot consent to retire so soon as we ought: whence the sphincter of the bladder, from being voluntarily, becomes at length spasmodically constricted, and the urine cannot escape.

Atony or paralysis of the bladder, by which its propulsive power is destroyed, is a frequent cause; whence, as Saviard has observed, it is often met with in paraplegia (*Observ. Chirurgiques*): and, as Morand remarks, in injuries to the spine.—(*Vermischte Schriften*, b. ii.) And hence, I have occasionally found it an attendant upon severe and long-protracted attacks of lumbar rheumatism (see also *Snowden, in the Lond. Med. Journ.*), as most practitioners have probably done of injuries to the kidneys, ureters, urethra, prostate gland, or penis. I have witnessed it in infancy from the irritation of teething, where dentition has been attended with difficulty.

In URETHRAL RETENTION OF URINE, the causes do not essentially vary from those already noticed; such as inflammation, the lodgment of a calculus, viscid mucus, and grumous blood. To which are to be added, the ligature of a strangulating phimosis; irritation from a blennorrhœa or clap; strictures; the absorption of cantharides from blistered surfaces.*

---

* In this last example, the secretion of urine is always much diminished, though the patient is tormented with a constant desire to attempt micturition. The case, as Dr. Davy remarks, is attended with a phlogosis of the pelvis of the kidney, or of the lining of the bladder, ureters, or some part of the urethra, and even with an effusion of blood under the epithelium.—Edin. Med. Journ., No. xcvii., p. 315.—ED.

There is always danger from a retention of urine when it has continued so long as to distend and prove painful to the bladder; and the danger is of two kinds: first, that of an inflammation of the distressed organ; and next, that of resorption, and a refluence of the urea and other constituent parts of the urine, as noticed under the preceding species.

The retention, however, has occasionally continued for a considerable period without mischief. It has lasted from a week to a fortnight. —(*Eph. Nat. Cur.*, passim; *Cornar. Obs.*, N. 21.) Marcellus Donatus gives a case of six months' standing (lib. iv., cap. 27, 28); and Paullini another of habitual retention.—(Cent. ii., obs. 26.) But, in all these, an observant practitioner will perceive the two following accompaniments: firstly, a constitutional or superinduced hebetude of the muscular coat of the bladder, so as to indispose it to inflammation; and, secondly, a resorption of the urinary fluid, and its evacuation by some vicarious channel, as already remarked under *paruria inops*. We have there stated, that the two most commonly substituted outlets are the excretories of the bowels and of the skin. Dr. Perceval gives an instance of the latter, in which the perspirable matter was so much supersaturated with the ammoniacal salt of the refluent urine as to crystallize on the surface of the body, and this to such an extent that the skin was covered all over with a white saline powder.—(*Edin. Med. Com.*, vol. v., 437.) Sometimes it has been thrown out from the stomach intermixed with blood, in the form of a hæmatemesis (*Act. Nat. Cur.*, iii., obs. 6); and sometimes from the nostrils, with the same intermixture, in the form of an epistaxis.—(Idem., dec. ii., an. iv., obs. 63.) And where the absorbents of the bladder have been too torpid for action, it has regurgitated through the ureters into the pelvis of the kidneys, and been resumed by the absorbents of these organs, instead of by those of the former.—(*Petit, Traité*, &c., *Œuvres Posthumes*, tom. iii., p. 2; see also Spe. 7 of the present Genus, P. erratica.)

The quantity retained, and afterward discharged, or found in the bladder on dissection, has often been very considerable. It has occasionally amounted to eight or nine pints; and there is a case given by M. Vildé, in the Journ. de Médecine, in which it equalled sixteen pints.

In all the varieties thus pointed out, the mode of management must be regulated by the cause, as far as we are able to ascertain it.

If we have reason to believe the suppression to be strictly renal, from the symptoms just adverted to, and particularly from ascertaining that there is no water in the bladder or ureters, whether it proceed from inflammation or stone, we shall do right, in most cases, to employ relaxants and mild aperients; and, where the pain is violent, venesection, succeeded by anodynes. But it sometimes happens, that the obstruction is produced by a parabysmic enlargement or coacervation of the substance of the kidney, without inflammation. If this should occur in both kidneys at the same time, which is rarely the case, we have little chance of success by any plan that can be laid down. If it be confined to one, the sound kidney will-often become a substitute for the diseased, and perform double duty; and we may here attempt a resolution of the enlargement, by minute doses of mercury continued for some weeks, unless salivation should ensue, and render it necessary to intermit our practice. A mercurial plaster, with ammoniacum, should also be worn constantly over the region of the affected organ.

The same plan must be pursued, if we have reason to suspect the obstruction is confined to the ureters. The passage of a calculus is the chief cause of this variety of retained urine; and, independently of the sense of pain and weight in the region of the ureters, which an impacted calculus produces, we have commonly, also, a feeling of numbness in either leg, and a retraction of one of the testicles in men, symptoms with which all men of experience are familiarly acquainted. Opium and relaxants are here the chief, if not the only means we can rationally employ. The suppression is seldom total: for the opposite ureter is rarely so much affected by sympathy as to be spasmodically contracted, and equally to oppose the flow of the urine.

The most common variety of this disease is that of vesical retention, or a retention of water in the bladder. This is usually produced by inflammation or spasm, by which the sphincter of the bladder becomes contracted and rigidly closed. Inflammation is to be relieved by the ordinary means; and, in addition to these, by anodyne clysters and fomentations, a warm bath, warm liniments, especially of camphire or essential oil of turpentine, and blisters to the perinæum. Spasm is excited by various causes: a stone in the bladder will do it; the irritation of gonorrhœa, or inattention to the call of nature, will bring it on. Spasm is for the most part to be treated, and will in most cases be subdued, by the method just proposed for inflammation; to which we may add camphire and opium by the mouth, and bladders of warm water applied to the pubes and perinæum, or, which is better, the warm bath itself. Camphire has the double advantage of being a sedative as well as an active diuretic; but, combined with opium, we obtain a much more powerful medicine than either affords when employed singly. If the retention proceed from Spanish flies, camphire alone will often answer; though in this case it is far better to combine with it mucilaginous diluents, as gumarabic dissolved in barley-water.* Several of the terebinthinate oils have also been employed with great advantage: as the oil of juniper, which is, in fact, nothing more than an essential oil very carefully distilled from

the fresh cones of the trees which yield the common turpentine; and the balsamum hungaricum, which is an exudation from the tops of the pinus silvestris, and proves sudorific as well as diuretic. Another remedy of early origin, and which has preserved its reputation to our own day, is the dandelion, the *leontodon taraxacum* of Linnæus. It was at one time regarded as a panacea, and prescribed for almost every disease by which the system is invaded, as gout, jaundice, hypochondrias, dropsy, consumption, parabysmas of every species, as well as gravel and other diseases of the bladder; and was equally employed in its roots, stalks, and leaves. It is now chiefly used as a deobstruent; but it possesses unquestionably diuretic powers, and hence, indeed, its vulgar name of piss-a-bed.

If the joint use of these means should fail, the water is usually evacuated by the introduction of a bougie or catheter, though the irritation is sometimes increased by the use of these instruments; and the spasm (stricture), or the thickening at the prostate or about the neck of the bladder, is often so considerable as to prevent an introduction of even the smallest of them.

If, however, no catheter can be passed, all other usual means fail, and the distress be alarming, nothing remains but to puncture the bladder. The circumstances, however, demanding this operation, and the considerations by which the mode of doing it should be determined, must be learned by reference to surgical writers.

The urethral retention, as already pointed out, arises also from inflammation, which is to be treated in the ordinary way; or from a calculus or a stricture, both which are best removed by the application of a bougie. In the last case, the bougie, if it pass without much pain, should be continued daily, and progressively enlarged in its size. It has often been employed with a tip of lunar or alkaline caustic, and, in many instances, with perfect success; but very great caution is requisite in the use of a caustic bougie; and, even in the hands of the most skilful, it has sometimes proved highly mischievous. When a simple bougie is employed, Ferrand (*Blegny Zod.*, ann. 1681) advises that, if the water do not flow immediately, it should be reintroduced and left in the urethra; and I have myself advised such a retention of the bougie-catheter through an entire night with considerable advantage; for the water, which would not flow at first, has gradually trickled, and given some relief to the over-distended bladder, which has hereby progressively recovered its tone and propulsive power; so that the water before morning has been propelled in a stream. But this is a plan only to be pursued where the organ has too little, instead of too much irritability, and, consequently, where there is no danger of inflammation.

---

* Instead of these medicines, or the spirit of nitric ether usually prescribed, Dr. Davy finds the best mode of relief to be the introduction of the catheter, not with the view of drawing off the urine, but simply for the purpose of letting the instrument remain a few seconds in the neck of the bladder.—(Edin. Med. Journ., No. xcvii., p. 315.) One would not be inclined to repose much confidence in this practice, especially when it is considered that the urethra is in a state of phlogosis.—Ed.

SPÉCIES III.

PARURIA STILLATITIA.

STRANGURY.

PAINFUL AND STILLATITIOUS EMISSION OF URINE.

This is the dysuria of Sauvages and later writers. In the preceding species, there is an entire stoppage of the urine ; in the present it flows, but with pain and by drops. Several of the causes are those of *paruria retentionis ;* but others are peculiar to the species itself; and, as they are accompanied with some diversity in the symptoms, they lay a foundation for the following varieties :—

. α Spasmodica.	Spasmodic Strangury.
β Ardens.	Scalding Strangury.
γ Callosa.	Callous Strangury.
δ Mucosa.	Mucous Strangury.
ε Helminthica.	Vermiculous Strangury.
ζ Polyposa.	Polypose Strangury.

The FIRST VARIETY is characterized by a spasmodic constriction of the sphincter, or some other part of the urinary canal, catenating with spasmodic action in some adjoining part. The spasmodic actions, of which this variety is a concomitant, are chiefly those of hysteria, colic, and spasm in the kidneys. It is hence a secondary affection, and the cure must depend on curing the diseases which have occasioned it. Opium and the digitalis will often afford speedy relief, when given in combination.

In the SECOND VARIETY there is also a spasmodic constriction, but of a different kind, and making it more of a primary affection; whence Sauvages and others have distinguished it by the name of *dysuria primaria.* It is excited by an external or internal use of various stimulants, as acrid foods, or cantharides taken internally ; and is accompanied with a sense of scalding as the urine is discharged.

This is also a frequent result of blisters ; and to avoid it in this case, the patient should be always advised to drink freely of warm diluents in a mucilaginous form. Gumarabic, marshmallows root, the jelly of the orchis or salep, infusion of quince-seed, linseed, or decoction of oatmeal or barley, may be employed with equal benefit.*

Camphire has also been employed with great advantage, and acts on the double principle of being a diuretic and a sedative. It is often found to act in the same manner when applied externally, and even when intermixed with the blister-plaster itself, as though in some constitutions it possesses a specific influence over the bladder ; upon which subject Dr. Perceval has penned the following note in his Commentary to the volume of Nosology :—" In three instances, blisters sprinkled with camphire were repeatedly applied without strangury, and as uniformly, when the camphire was omitted, with the concurrence of that symptom. I will not say that in all constitutions camphire will obviate strangury ; nor in all constitutions will cantharides without camphire produce it."†

* One of the most valuable articles in the materia medica for these affections, is an infusion of the buchu leaves; this remedy has been used by many with singular benefit.—D.

† Dr. Davy's mode of relieving strangury from the absorption of cantharides has already been mentioned under Spe. 2. It is probable, that mixing camphire with the blistering-plaster only operates on the principle of dilution.—ED.

It will commonly be found useful, and sometimes absolutely necessary, in this variety, from whatever cause produced, to employ neutral aperients : and, with them, the means just recommended in cases of cantharides will rarely fail to succeed in most other cases. If not, the practitioner should have recourse to a decisive dose of opium.

Strangury is also occasioned by a CALLOUS THICKENING of the membrane of the urethra, producing a permanent stricture. Some interesting examples of this may be seen in Dr. Baillie's Plates of Morbid Anatomy.—(Fascic. iii., pl. iv., v.)

The most common situation of a stricture is just behind the bulb of the urethra, though it may take place in any other part. M. Ducamp has invented an ingenious instrument for determining the exact point, consisting of a sound graduated into inches, half inches, and lines, which at once determines the distance of the obstruction from the orifice of the urethra. In five cases out of six, however, he found the obstruction seated not higher up than from four and a half to five and a half inches, and he is inclined to think that this is rather higher than occurs in general (*Traité des Rétentions d' Urine,* &c., Paris, 8vo., 1822), which is contrary to the ordinary calculation in our own country. A stricture of this kind " consists," says Dr. Baillie, " of an approximation, for a short extent, of the sides of the canal to each other. Sometimes there is a mere line of approximation, and not uncommonly the sides of the urethra approach to each other for some considerable length, as, for instance, nearly an inch. The surface of the urethra at the stricture is often sound, but not unfrequently it is more or less thickened." It is this thickening which produces the variety of strangury before us ; and Mr. Bauer has satisfactorily explained these effects by a series of microscopical plates, which show us that spasmodic strictures in the urethra are produced, not from a contraction of any supposed circular fibres in the inner tunic, but by a contraction of a greater or less portion of the fibres of the exterior and surrounding fibres of the muscular coat, which may take place through the entire ring, or only on one side.—(*Phil. Trans.,* 1820, p. 186.) The sides of the urethra are sometimes approximated so nearly by its tumefaction that the stricture will only allow a bristle to pass through it : and hence ulcers are occasionally formed in the prostate gland, and fistulæ in the perinæum ; and the diameter of the urethra between the stricture and the bladder is enlarged by the accumulation and pressure of the urine in that situation ; of all which Dr. Baillie has also given examples.

The pain in micturition is sometimes peculiarly distressing ; the limbs tremble, the face becomes flushed, and the feces issue at the same time, so that the patient is obliged to pass his water in the same position in which he goes to stool. M. Ducamp gives the case of a merchant labouring under this complaint, in whom the violent straining produced a large inguinal hernia : and refers to others who were afflicted with stricture of the rectum from the same cause.*

When the prostate or urethra is thus highly irritable, palliation only can be resorted to; but where the thickening is recent, and there is little irritation, a skilful use of a bougie will sometimes afford temporary relief; after which, by gradually employing those of a larger diameter, the stricture will often give way and the canal widen, so as to allow the water to flow with considerable comfort. M. Ducamp objects to the use of bougies, from the mischief they produce when unskilfully applied.—(*Traité des Réten-tions d'Urine*, &c., ut suprà.) But the objection is too indiscriminate : and the plan is, after all, less adventurous than any application of caustic, although in the more cautious, but more complicated way, proposed by himself.

In the variety which we have called MUCOUS STRANGURY, the urine is intermixed with a secretion of acrimonious mucus, of a whitish or greenish hue, which is frequently a sequel of gout, lues, or blennorrhœa. It is often, however, produced by cold, and in this last case forms the *catarrhus vesicæ* of various authors : so denominated from its being conceived that the bladder and urethra are affected in the same manner as the nostrils in a coryza. The constriction therefore depends upon an excoriated or irritable state of the urethra or neck of the bladder, and, at times, of the mucous membrane of the bladder itself.—(*Tacheron, Recherches Anatomico-Pathologiques sur la Médecine Pratique*, in loco.) And hence the warm bath, or sitting in a bidet of warm water, is often of considerable service. Warm and diluent injections have also frequently been found, as well as diluent and demulcent drinks, of great advantage.† A very severe case of this kind occurred not long since to the author, in a lady of the middle of life, who had about three months before suffered much from a laborious labour, in which a dead child was brought into the world by the use of the single blade. The bladder, irritated in the course of the labour, was long affected with irregular action, but at length appeared to have recovered its tone. A sudden exposure to cold brought back the irritability, the mucous discharge was considerable, and the micturition so constant and painful, that, for two nights in succession, the patient evacuated the bladder, or strove to evacuate it, nearly forty times each night. The plan above recommended was diligently pursued, and at night the body swathed with flannel wrung out in hot water, with an outer swathe of a towel. Forty drops of laudanum were given at bedtime, and repeated doses of

tincture of hyoscyamus in the day. On the third day the disease subsided, and vanished in the evening. If this variety continue long, it is apt to produce an obstinate and very narrow stricture, of which ulceration and fistulæ in perinæo are frequent results.*

Strangury is sometimes accompanied with a DISCHARGE OF WORMS of a peculiar kind, and proceeds from the irritation they excite. Of this we have various instances in the Ephemerides of Natural Curiosities (dec. i., ann. ix., x., obs. 113 ; dec. ii., ann. i., obs. 104 ; ann. vi., obs. 31 ; dec. iii., ann. i., obs. 82 ; ann. ii., obs. 203), in some of which the worms were found in the bladder after death, and in others discharged by the urethra during life : and a like fact is alluded to by Dr. Frank, though he does not seem to have witnessed it himself.—(*De Cur. Hom. Morb. Epit.*, tom. v., p. 79.) They are described as of different forms in different cases, sometimes resembling the larves of insects ; sometimes distinctly cucurbitinous, of the fasciola, fluke, or gourd kind. Dr. Barry of Dublin has given the case of a solitary worm discharged by the urethra of a man aged fifty, "above an inch in length, of the thickness of the smallest sort of eel, and not unlike it in shape, ending in a sharp-pointed tail." It was dead, but did not seem to have been dead long. The patient had for several years been in the habit of discharging urine mixed with blood, but unaccompanied with pain either in the bladder or urethra. During the whole of this time he had been feverish ; and gradually lost his appetite, much his strength decay, and had become tabid and hectic : from all of which he speedily recovered as soon as this cause of irritation was removed.—(*Edin. Med. Ess.*, vol. v., part ii., art. lxxii., p. 289.) M. Demet has lately given a similar case, but of a more complicated kind. The patient was a man of fifty years of age, who had through a great part of his life been subject to anomalous pains in the lumbar region and abdomen, and, in adolescence, to a frequent nasal hemorrhage. One day, at the period now spoken of, after passing much blood by the urethra, he voided by the same channel a round worm *fourteen inches in length, of the size of a goose-quill :* after which he found himself greatly relieved, and the hæmaturia ceased. In the course of three months, he voided by the same passage fifty worms, apparently of the same species, but of different sizes. He had notice of their forthcoming by a sense of heat in the urinary canal, and a slight febrile excitement, which went off as soon as the worms were ejected. They were uniformly dead when discharged.—(*Dict. des Sciences, Medicales*, art. CAS RARES.)

We have also an example of a like vermicule, highly gregarious, and of considerable length, in an interesting paper inserted by Mr. Lawrence in

---

* Traité des Rétentions d'Urine, &c., Paris, 8vo., 1822. In Sir Astley Cooper's work on Hernia is the account of a patient with strictures, who had several hernial protrusions brought on by the efforts of the abdominal muscles to empty the bladder. In fact, the frequency of hernia, as a consequence of old and bad strictures in the urethra, is well known to all experienced surgeons.—ED.

† In all cases of mucous strangury, the sanative powers of the uva ursi deserve to be remembered.—D.

* It is scarcely necessary to remind practical men, that the catarrh of the bladder, as it is here called, does not produce the stricture, but is generally the effect of it, or of disease of the prostate gland, or of some irritation in the neighbourhood of the bladder.—ED

the second volume of the Medico-Chirurgical Transactions. The patient was a female, aged twenty-four, and had long laboured under a severe irritation of the bladder, which was ascribed to a calculus. She at length discharged three or four worms of a nondescript kind, and continued to discharge more, especially when their removal was aided by injections into the bladder, or the catheter had remained in the urethra for the night. The evacuation of these animals continued for at least a twelvemonth. Twenty-two were once passed at a time ; and the whole number could not be less than from eight hundred to a thousand. A smaller kind was also occasionally evacuated. The larger were usually from four to six inches in length ; one of them measured eight. For the most part, they were discharged dead.

The subject is obscure, but it may be observed, that the ova of various species of worms, and even worms themselves, are occasionally found in many animal fluids, and have been especially detected in the bloodvessels, where they have been hatched into grubs or vermi-

cules, for the most part of an undecided character ; though some, observed in the mesenteric arteries of asses, have been referred to the genus strongylus.—(Hodgson on the Diseases of Arteries.) And in like manner, Dr. Frank assures us, that he has found ascarides both in the bladder and kidneys of dogs, particularly in polypous concretions in these organs.—(De Cur. Hom. Morb. Epit., tom. v., p. 76.) Dr. Barry supposes his isolated worm to have travelled in the form of an ovum as far as to the extremity of an exhaling artery opening into the bladder ; to have found, in this place, a proper nidus and nourishment for the purpose of being hatched into a larve or grub, and of growing to the size it had assumed when thrown out of the urethra ; and, in consequence of this progressive growth, and the proportional dilatation of the vessel in which it was lodged, he accounts for the discharge of blood without pain. If a worm reach the bladder alive and full of eggs, we have no difficulty in accounting for a succession of progenies.[*]

---

* The editor, through the kindness of his friend Mr. Docker, late of Canterbury, has been furnished with the particulars of a young woman, upwards of twenty years of age, who has been under the care of Mr. Law, of Penrith, in Cumberland, since October, 1830, and has discharged several thousand portions of tænia from the meatus urinarius. In a letter, dated Penrith, Aug. 29, 1833, Mr. Law states, that " she first felt a sensation like that of a rupture of the bladder, when in the act of stooping to cut a corn, in August, 1829. From that time she had discharges of bloody urine occasionally, with the sensation of something moving in the bladder, more particularly so after each evacuation, and had concluded that this was a worm. However, no mention was made of this to any one, although her health was impaired, until I was called to attend her for an attack of laryngitis, in October, 1830. Blisters being used, brought on retention of urine, with cystitis, which rendered the use of the catheter necessary. After this had been conquered, she mentioned her feelings and apprehensions to me, which for some time I treated as imaginary, till at length, from the greatly disturbed state of the mucous membrane of the bladder, evidenced by deposition, in large quantities, of a white sediment in the urine, I was led to try the exhibition of spirit. terebinth., both by the mouth and injection. Great irritation ensued, but a small portion (about eight joints) of tænia was discharged, per urethram, alive. This led me to the determination to try the effect of opiate solutions, frequently injected into the bladder, which, by keeping the worm constantly under its influence, might destroy it. This persevered in for three days answered the purpose ; all motion of the worm ceased ; and, by an expansion of the urethra, its discharge was effected in large quantities, but in so decayed and broken a state that its parts could not be numbered ; but I am certain that these could not have been less than 2000 joints. With these there was much hemorrhage, also membranes and other substances. From this date, January, 1831, to the beginning of April of the same year, there were no indications of more tænia ; yet the urine was generally tinged with blood, and deposited the white sediment in less quantities than formerly. During this period an anodyne injection had been used almost

daily, as the irritation of the bladder was considerable. At this time she again felt the motion of tænia, and I again resorted to frequent opiate injections, but without success for some days, and then determined upon the administration of spirit. terebinth. by the mouth, a teaspoonful of which was taken on the morning of the 18th of April, and which passed by the bladder in an hour and a half, bringing off some portions of the worm in a recent state, with a net-like membrane. From this date to September 20th, there were passed from the bladder, per urethram, 1239 joints of different sizes, from one third to the eighth of an inch in width, and which were all preserved, with portions of net-like membrane, and fungi, either like the liver or the muscles of a fowl, and sometimes of a fleshy fibrous substance, having the appearance of the muscular coat of the bladder, with a shaggy surface on one side, resembling the villous coat of the intestines. These were brought away almost daily, while the urine diminished in quantity, rarely exceeding four ounces in twenty-four hours. A pause ensued from the last date to November 16th, of the same year ; during which time neither worm nor substances passed off, but the fluid discharged was bloody, and always highly offensive. On this day the spirit. terebinth. was again administered, and brought off in an hour two small pieces of net-like cellular tissue, with nine joints of middle-sized worm interwoven with it. From this time to January 18th, 1832, there were 773 joints preserved of different sizes, and these were generally accompanied with membrane and fungi of different kinds. From this date to March 27th, there were no portions of tænia passed ; but on that day the spirit. terebinth. was again taken, and before May 1st, 853 joints passed, making a total of 2865 now in my possession, besides a very small and apparently perfect worm of twenty-nine joints. During the period mentioned there have been at different times profuse hemorrhages from the intestines, surmised to arise from the ascending colon, which have reduced my patient to a very weak state. She is now (August 23d) in tolerable health, but again bringing away from the use of the spirit. terebinth., more tænia. On the 21st instant there came off four joints of a small worm, with two small fungi.

" Among the singular and unaccountable phenomena accompanying this affection, is the rapidity with which spirit. terebinth. now passes from the stomach to the bladder. It is invariably felt in the bladder in less than twenty seconds from being taken; and its evacuation, per urethram, rarely exceeds two minutes: on one occasion it passed in one minute and a quarter; and from the recent appearance of the worm and fungi, seems to separate them in passing.

"Mr. Docker is in possession of some specimens of the worm, fungi, and membranes."

In a later communication to Mr. Docker, the following additional particulars of this remarkable case are given:—.

"*Tuesday Evening, April 15th,* 1834.

"My dear Cousin,

"I am very sorry that I have hitherto been unable to send you the specimens of tænia, &c. as you requested, and now do so in a great hurry, in order to avail myself of a gentleman's visit to London, who has kindly offered to take a box for me. My engagements during the absence of my young man at Edinburgh were so many, that I could not find time to make a selection of my tænia, &c. for Mr. Cooper until his return, and now send you a few specimens of the different sizes, with those of the fungi, muscular substances, as I call them, and the net-like membranes. I also enclose a copy or two of my memoranda regarding the effects of the spirit. terebinth., and also the results for a few days (which may be taken as a fair sample of the whole). You will see by the former the rapid passage of the spirit. terebinth. from the stomach to the bladder, and the increase of that rapidity by degrees to its present point, about eight seconds, and its evacuation in less than a minute, when the orifice is not obstructed by much substance. This is an interesting phenomenon, and worthy of the particular attention of the anatomist and physiologist. As you have been an eye-witness, with many other medical men, it is a fact which can admit of no doubt. The second phenomenon is also remarkable and interesting : the small secretion of fluid by the kidneys. This is always increased by the spirit. terebinth. on the day following its exhibition. The cups which are used by the patient hold four ounces and a half each. I do not know whether you have sufficient data from which to make out the case ; but if Mr. Cooper wishes for a view of the whole case, I shall be happy to try to make it out for him. The nidus of the worms is still undestroyed, and I am now about to try some of the preparations of iron held in solution. The general health (if it may be so called) of my patient is better than heretofore ; and I am yet using occasionally the spirit. terebinth., although it seems to distress her much. Perhaps you will be kind enough to see Mr. Cooper, and forward the box to him, with my memoranda.

"Believe me, dear cousin, affectionately yours,
"Thos. Law."

Copy of Memoranda made from March 24 to June, 1833, in the Case of Jane Stephenson.

Date.	Spiritus Terebinthinæ administered.	Time of evacuation from bladder.	Tænia and other substances evacuated.
March 24.	ℨ jss. 1 p. m.	28 minutes	66 joints in one piece, 1 piece of fatty cellular membrane, and 5 small livery pieces.
25.	ℨ jss. 11 a. m.	20 minutes	46 joints of tænia unconnected, but in a fresh state.
			82 joints of tænia, different sizes ; 1 large piece of net-like membrane.
26.	ℨ j. ¼ past 10 a. m.	15 minutes	Size.
27.	ℨ j. 11 a. m.	28 minutes	122 joints, different sizes, and 2 net-like membranes.
28.	None.	Fluid bloody, 7 oz.	None.
29.	ℨ j. 12 noon	24 minutes	162 joints ; a few small livery substances.
30.	ℨ j. 10 a. m.	15 minutes	160 joints, different sizes.
April 1.	ℨ jss. 10 a. m.	12 minutes	34 joints, nearly of same size.
4.	ℨ jss. a. m.	11 minutes	165 joints, different sizes.
10.	ℨ jss. a. m.	11 minutes	46 joints, 1 membrane.
11.	ℨ jss. a. m.	10 minutes	86 joints, 2 membranes.
12.	ℨ jss. a. m.	11 minutes	28 joints, 1 membrane.
14.	ℨ jss. a. m.	Not noted	48 joints, 1 membrane in a decayed state.
15.	None administered, as the tæniæ were now in a decayed state		60 joints, 1 membrane.
16.	None		35 joints, 1 membrane.
17.	None		25 joints.
18.	None		6 joints, ¼ inch wide ; 27 joints, middle-sized.
24.	ℨ jss. 10 a. m.	Not noted	35 joints.
26.	ℨ ij. 10 a. m.	3 minutes	3 joints, large ; 20 joints, middle-sized.
27.	ℨ ij.	3½ minutes	2 joints, large ; 6 joints, middle-sized.
May 4.	ℨ ij. 10 a. m.	In half a minute felt in bladder,* came off in 2¾ minutes	No tænia ; fungus, weighing, ℨ ij.

* This was the first day on which the rapid passage to the bladder was noticed.

Strangury is also sometimes produced in consequence of the orifice of the bladder, or canal of the urethra; or both, being obstructed by the formation of a ᴘᴏʟʏᴘᴏᴜs ᴇxᴄʀᴇsᴄᴇɴᴄᴇ.* Dr. Baillie's Morbid Anatomy furnishes sev-eral examples of this variety ; which, in most cases, is only to be radically cured by an extirpation of the substance which produces the obstruction (fascie.- ix., plate iii.), wherever it can be laid hold of. When small, however, and

Date.	Spiritus Terebin- thinæ administered.	Time of evacuation from bladder.	Tænia and other substances evacu- ated.
	As there was no appearance of tæniæ or fungi, and the patient felt weak, the spirit. terebinth. was suspended till June 25, when it was again tried.		
June 25.	ʒ ij. 10 a. m.	Felt in bladder in 20 seconds, eva- cuated in less than 2 minutes.	No tænia, but a piece of fungus, with a piece of substance like fasciculi of muscular fibres.
27.	ʒ ij. 10 a. m.	Felt in bladder in 15 seconds, and evacuated in 2 minutes.	

Memoranda from January 29, 1834.

Date.	Spiritus Tere- binthinæ admin- istered.	Time when felt in blad- der.	Time of evacua- tion.	Results.
Jan. 29.	ʒ iij. 10 a. m.	14 seconds	40 seconds	69 joints of tænia, many livery fungi, and muscular fasciculi.
Feb. 1.	ʒ iij.	15 seconds	1 min. 10 sec.	38 joints connected and 5 separa- ted, both fresh ; livery fungi, and muscular fasciculi.
2. 3. 4.	None.			
5.	ʒ iij.	10 seconds	52 seconds	18 joints, fungi, and fasciculi.
7.	ʒ ij.	20 seconds	1¼ minutes	70 joints, fungi, fasciculi, and net.
11.	ʒ iij.	10 seconds	2 minutes	100 joints, 3 sizes, livery fungi, and muscular substances.
15.	ʒ ij.	9 seconds	45 seconds	1 thick reticulated membrane, with muscular substances.
19.	ʒ iij.	8 seconds	2¼ minutes	102 joints, fungi, and musc. sub.
22.	ʒ iij.	8 seconds	1 min. 40 sec.	92 joints, muscular substances.
24.	ʒ ij.	10 seconds	54 seconds	Muscular substances, but no joints.
25.	ʒ iij.	9 seconds	1 min. 20 sec.	65 joints, musc. sub., and fungi.
27.	ʒ iij.	Not noted	- - - -	7 joints, fungi, livery and musc. sub.
March 3.	ʒ iij.	8 seconds	1 min. 8 sec.	19 joints, many muscular sub.
8.	ʒ iij.	10 seconds	1 min. 10 sec.	28 joints, ditto.
14.	ʒ iij.	9 seconds	1 min. 5 sec.	16 joints, ditto.

Day and hour.	Quantity of urine. 1st evacuation.	Remarks.	1st injection.	Remarks.	Cups taken in 24 h.	2d injection, which remains.
Nov. 8, from 5 to 7 p. m.	ʒ iij. 2 dr.	Nearly col- ourless	Aq. tepid. ʒ ij.	Returned in quantity ʒ iij. ʒ vij.	3	Aq. ʒ x. Tr. opii ʒ ij.
Nov. 9.	ʒ ij. ʒ vj.	Brown and resinous	Aq. tepid. ʒ ij.	ʒ vij. pale	4½	Same.
10·	ʒ iijss.	Tinged with blood	Same	ʒ iij. ʒ vi.	3	Same.
11.	ʒ iijss.	- - - -	Same	ʒ iijss.	3	Same.
12.	ʒ ijss.	Red	Same	ʒ iijss.	3	Same.
13.	ʒ iij. ʒ vj.	Red	Same	ʒ iijss.	3	Same.

The editor returns his best thanks to Mr. Law for the foregoing particulars, which would have been more complete had they comprised a state-ment of the condition of the alvine evacuations. Professors Elliotson and Carswell, who have ex-amined some of the specimens of tænia kindly forwarded to Mr. Cooper, conclude with him, that in this singular case, some communication exists between the bladder and the bowels. If the patient were to die, an examination of her body would be desirable. In one of the last numbers of the London Med. and Surg. Journ., is a case where a lumbricus was voided from the bladder ; but no other instance, excepting that under Mr. Law, is known of tæniæ being expelled from that organ.—Eᴅ.

* Tumours sometimes form in the bladder and obstruct the flow of urine into the urethra ; but with respect to the formation of polypi and ca-runcles in the urethra, it is now well known, that what the old surgeons used to regard in this light, was usually only common strictures. The ex-crescences spoken of by Dr. Perceval, as situated near the neck of the bladder, were probably what Sir Everard Home has described as the effect of some conditions of the prostate gland.—Eᴅ.

in the form of caruncles, these excrescences have sometimes separated spontaneously, and been thrown out by the urethra, with very great relief to the sufferer, and have been followed by a perfect cure.—(*Fabric. Hildan.,*-cent. iv., obs. 53 ; *Art. Nat. Cur.,* vol. i., obs. 13.)*

Upon this variety, my venerable friend Dr. Perceval has added the following note in his manuscript Commentary on the Nosology, from which the present work has been so often enriched :—" It might not be amiss to insist on a case which sometimes deceives young practitioners,—ischuria cum stranguria. A copious draining of urine took place for several days in a patient with a swelled belly. Death supervening, the bladder was found distended to an enormous bulk, and the parietes of the abdomen wasted. Two excrescences near the neck of the bladder internally had almost closed its outlet, and interfered with the action of the sphincter.". Where the irritation is considerable, these excrescences sometimes ulcerate, and form fungous sores, with great distress and gnawing pains, that shoot into the hips and posterior muscles of the thighs, though the exact mischief cannot be ascertained till after death ; of which Mr. Bingham has given an example.—(*On the Diseases and Injuries of the Bladder,* &c., 8vo., Lond., 1822.)

SPECIES IV.
PARURIA MELLITA.
SACCHARINE URINE.

URINE DISCHARGED FREELY, FOR THE MOST PART PROFUSELY ; OF A VIOLET SMELL AND SWEET TASTE ; WITH GREAT THIRST, AND GENERAL DEBILITY.

THIS is the diabetes, diabetes Anglicus, or diabetes mellitus of authors ; from διαβήτης, importing " a siphon," or rather from διαβαίνω, " transco." Diabetes, among the Greek and Roman, and indeed among modern physicians till the time of Willis, imported simply a flux of urine, either crude or aqueous—for no distinction was made between the two—and both were named indifferently diabetes, dipsacus from the accompanying thirst, urinary diarrhœa, urinal dropsy, and hyderus (ὕδερος), or water-flux. — (*Galen, de Crisibus,* lib. i., cap. xii.) The writers among the ancients who seem chiefly to have noticed it, are Galen, Aretæus, and Trallian. The form of diabetes to which we are now directing our attention, Galen describes as having a resemblance to lientery, from the rapidity with which the solids and fluids of the body seem to be converted into a crude and liquid mass, and hurried forward to the kidneys ; and to canine appetite, from the voracity and thirst which are its peculiar symptoms. He supposes a high degree of appetence or irritation to exist in the substance of the kidneys, in consequence of

which it attracts the matter of urine with great vehemence from the vena cava ; and an equal degree of atony and relaxation to exist in its orifices or pores, so that the same matter flows off unchanged as soon as it reaches them.—(*De Loc. Affect.,* lib. vi., cap. iii., *compared with De Crisibus,* lib. i., cap. xii.)

This general view of the subject was adopted, with a few additions, by Aretæus, and, without any, by Trallian ; and seems to have descended, with little variation, as we have just observed, till the time of Willis, who first called the attention of practitioners to the curious and important fact, that the urine of diabetic patients seems in many cases to contain a saccharine principle. In his time, however, these cases were not duly distinguished, and hence, in Sauvages, who was well acquainted with Willis's discovery, diabetes signifies equally an immoderate flux of urine from hysteria, gout, fever, spirituous potation, as well as urine combined with saccharine matter : though the only relation which the last has to the rest is that of its being *usually* secreted in a preternatural quantity : but, as even this last quality, though mostly, is not always the case, it should be distinguished by some other name than that of diabetes, and form a distinct division : or, if the name of diabetes be applied to it, it should be given to it exclusively. Dr. Young, who retains the name in the latter sense, and employs it as that of a genus, justly allows but one species to the genus, the *diabetes mellitus* of Cullen, and describes the *diabetes insipidus** under the genus and species of *hyperuresis aquosus.* The distinction indeed is so clear, and has been so generally admitted for nearly the last half century, that it is wonderful Professor Frank, with all his fondness for generalization, should have turned to the erroneous view of the early writers, and again confounded genuine diabetes with hyderus or water-flux, the enuresis of most writers. There is great doubt whether this last ever exists as an idiopathic affection. Cullen himself, indeed, candidly expresses the uncertainty of his mind upon the subject :—" Almost all the cases of diabetes of late times," he observes, " exhibit saccharine urine, ita ut dubium sit, an alia diabetes idiopathicæ et permanentis species revera detur." If such be found, it will probably be nothing more than a variety of the next species in the present arrangement, PARURIA INCONTINENS : while the honeyed diabetes, or saccharine urine, ought to be studied as a distinct affection.†

---

* In diabetes insipidus, the urine is almost exclusively composed of water and a small proportion of animal matter.—See Andral, Anat. Pathol., tom. ii., p. 657.—ED.

: † M. Renauldin (Dict. des Sciences Méd.), Dr. Prout, and the generality of modern writers on diabetes, agree in the propriety of confining this term to the disease in which the urine contains sugar, the paruria mellita of our author. Dr. J. L. Bardsley does not assent, however, to this view of the subject ; and he maintains that there are several instances on record of patients dying under all the symptoms of diabetes, yet without the slightest indication of sugar in the urine. Here, he argues,

---

* The late Prof. E. D. Smith, of S. Carolina, cured a female affected with this variety of paruria by mechanical compression ; a small piece of cane was worn in the urethra, and in a fortnight the patient recovered.—Phil. Journ., vol. i., p. 148.—D.

The pathology of this disease is still involved in a considerable degree of obscurity : for, though anatomy has pointed out a few morbid changes that exist more or less extensively in the urinary or digestive organs, and chymistry has sufficiently explained to us the morbid character of the discharge, they have thrown less light upon its origin than could be wished for, and have hitherto led to no satisfactory opinion upon the subject. Even the seat of the disorder is, to the present hour, a point of controversy.

Saccharine or honeyed paruria is rarely, though sometimes,* found in early life, but is often a sequel to a life of intemperance, on which account it is occasionally connected with a morbid state of the liver. It makes its approach insidiously, and often arises to a considerable degree, and exists for some weeks, without being particularly attended to. If the urinary symptoms take the lead, it is without the patient's noticing them, for the first morbid change he is sensible of is in the stomach. At this time, to adopt the description of Dr. Latham, " it is attended, for the most part, with a very voracious appetite, and with an insatiable thirst ; with a dry, harsh skin,† and clammy, not parched, but sometimes reddish tongue ; and with a frequent excretion of very white saliva, not inspissated, yet scarcely fluid. As the disease proceeds, it is accompanied often with a hay-like scent or odour issuing from the body, with a similar sort of halitus exhaling from the lungs, and with a state of mind dubious and forgetful : the patient being dissatisfied, fretful, and distrusting, ever anxious indeed for relief, but wavering and unsteady in the means advised for the purpose of procuring it."—(*Facts and Opinions concerning Diabetes*, &c., p. 1.)

In the meantime, the kidneys discharge a fluid usually very limpid, though sometimes

slightly tinged with green, like a diluted mixture of honey and water, and possessing a saccharine taste, more or less powerful. The quantity, in a few rare instances, has been found not much increased beyond the ordinary flow, but, for the most part, the secretion is greatly augmented, and not unfrequently amounts to forty, or upwards of forty pints, in the course of a day and night.*

The pulse varies in different individuals, but for the most part is quicker than in health ; and, not unfrequently, there is a sense of weight or even acute pain in the loins, occasionally spreading to the hypochondria, a symptom which Aretæus notices as one of the earliest that appears ; the uneasiness extending still lower, till, as the same writer remarks, a sympathetic smarting is felt at the extremity of the penis whenever the patient makes water.

The flesh wastes rapidly ; and as the emaciation advances, " cramps," says Dr. Latham, " or spasms of the extremities, sometimes supervene, the pulse is more quick and feeble, and the saliva more glutinous. And when the strength is almost exhausted, in a still more advanced stage of the disease, the lower extremities often become œdematous, and the skin cold and damp : the diabetic discharge is then frequently much diminished, and is sometimes even found to become more urinous for a few hours before death closes the distressing scene."

A pulmonic affection occasionally accompanies or precedes the attack ; Dr. Bardsley, indeed, affirms that he does not recollect a case that was entirely free from this symptom. And it is probably on this account, as also from the feverish state of the pulse, which by some writers has been supposed to partake of a hectic character, that by MM. Nicholas and Gueudeville the disease has been denominated *phthisurie sucrée.—(Recherches et Expériences Médicales et Chimiques sur la Diabète sucrée*, 8vo., Paris, 1803.) The state of the bowels is extremely variable, though there is commonly a troublesome costiveness ; sometimes, indeed, so much so, that the feces are peculiarly hardened and scybalous. In a few instances, the disease seems to be connected with family predisposition. Mr. Storer has noticed a case of this kind in his communication with Dr. Rollo ; and M. Isenflamm has given the history of seven children of the same parents who fell victims to it in succession.†

---

that it would not be fair to assume its presence in a latent state ; for, says he, it may be latent in the most incidental case of hysterical enuresis, and then how could the name of diabetes be refused to this fortuitous symptom ?—(Cyclop. of Pract. Med., art. DIABETES.) Certain cases, in which an excess of urea in the urine is a characteristic symptom, have been, according to Dr. Prout, mistaken for what writers term diabetes insipidus.— See an Inquiry into the Nature and Treatment of Diabetes, Calculus, &c., London, 1825, 2d edit.—ED.

* Latham's Facts and Opinions, p. 176. Dr. Bardsley has witnessed two instances of the disease in children under six years of age ; and a very clear example, connected with the process of dentition, is related by Morton. Dr. Watt also met with one case in a boy only three years old.—ED.

† It is observed by Dr. Marsh, 1st, That, in many of the cases whose histories are recorded, the earliest disturbance in the general health could be distinctly traced to some cause acting upon the skin, and producing derangement of its functions. 2dly, Every case of diabetes mellitus is accompanied with a peculiarly morbid condition of the skin. 3dly, None of the remedies employed produced the slightest benefit until the skin began to relax, and a sweat to appear on the surface.—See Dublin Hospital Reports, vol. iv., p. 432.—ED.

* Frank, De Cur. Hom. Morb. Epit., tom. v., p. 44. This author relates the particulars of a case in which fifty-two pounds were discharged in twenty-four hours ; and instances are by no means uncommon of from twenty-five to thirty-five pints having been voided every day for weeks and months together.—(See Dr. Copland's Dict. of Pract. Med., art. DIABETES, p. 507.) Fonseca saw an instance, in which the incredible quantity of two hundred pints of urine were discharged in twenty-four hours.—ED.

† Versuch einiger practischer Anmerkungen über die Eingeweide, &c., Erlang., 1784. The same thing is noticed by Dr. Prout, who knew a mother, an uncle, a brother, and a sister, all affected with the disease ; and it is singular that an

Professor Frank, who, during a practice of twenty years in Germany, met with but three cases of this complaint, though afterward with seven in the course of eight years in Italy, adds to the preceding symptoms, that the skin is scaly as well as arid.—(*De Cur. Hom. Morb. Epit.*, tom. v., p. 39, Mannh., 8vo., 1792.)

The real nature of the fluid evacuated has been very sufficiently determined, both in our own country and on the continent, by chymists of the first authority, who have concurrently ascertained, that while it is destitute of its proper animal salts, it is loaded with the new ingredient of saccharine matter. [Dr. Prout suspects that the urine is albuminous before it becomes saccharine; and, as Dr. Marsh* observes, the determination of this fact would be of importance, with a view of enabling the practitioner to prevent the full development of the disease.]

Dr. Dobson, from a pound of urine, collected an ounce of saccharine substance: and Mr. Cruickshank, from thirty-six ounces troy, obtained in like manner, by evaporation, not less than three ounces and a quarter: which, from the quantity discharged by the patient, would have amounted to not less than twenty-nine ounces every twenty-four hours. A patient, however, under Dr. Frank, but who was in the last stage of the disease, evacuated his urine in a much higher degree of concentration; while the general amount was not more than in a state of health; for from two pints the saccharine matter obtained weighed not less than six ounces.†

Chevreul has shown that, by concentrating this morbid urine, and setting it aside, we may obtain a deposite of sugar in a crystallized state.‡

excess of urea seemed in some cases of this kind to constitute the first step towards the presence of saccharine matter; and, as an able critic remarks, when we couple with this the fact, related p. 82 of Dr. Prout's work, of the effect of opium in changing the urine from six or eight pints, sp. gr. 1.038, containing a large proportion of white sugar, and very little urea, to two pints, sp. gr. 1.174, with an excess of urea, and apparently no sugar, we must agree with Dr. Prout, that this alternation of a principle containing nearly half its weight of azote, with another containing no azote at all, is perhaps one of the most singular facts in physiology.—See Edin. Med. Journ., No. lxxxvii., p. 382.—ED.

* See Dublin Hospital Reports, vol. iii., p. 461. Dr. Elliotson states, that he never had a patient labouring under diabetes, in whom the feeling of sexual power and desire had not ceased entirely, or become very much impaired.—(Lectures at the Lond. Univ., as reported in Med. Gaz. for 1832-3, p. 727.) Very often there is redness and soreness of the end of the urethra. Dr. Elliotson has even seen phymosis, which may arise from the irritating quality of the fluid.—ED.

† De Cur. Hom. Morb. Epit., tom. v., p. 47. One patient, under Dr. Elliotson, made but three pints of urine in a day, a quantity less than what he drank; while Dr. Heberden mentions a case in which the urine amounted to double the quantity of drink.—See Med. Lectures delivered at Lond. Univ., as reported in Med. Gaz., 1832-3, p. 728. —ED.

‡ The saccharine matter of diabetic urine has

The absence of animal salts has been ascertained not less satisfactorily. MM. Nicholas and Gueudeville showed, by a series of experiments in 1802, that the saccharine urine contains no urea,* and no uric nor benzoic acid; that the phosphoric salts exist in a very small proportion; and that, in consequence of its sugar, it will enter into the vinous and acetous fermentation, and yield an alcohol of a disagreeable odour.—(*Recherches et Expériences*, ut suprà citat.) The same results have since been obtained by MM. Dupuytren and Thénard, by experiments still more satisfactory. They also found an albuminous substance in the urine, which is always discharged in a sensible form when the disease begins to take a favourable change, and is the constant harbinger of a return of the proper animal salts; for, after having appeared for a little while, it gradually diminishes and yields its place to the urea and uric acid. Dr. Henry appears also to have arrived at many of the same conclusions, though by a somewhat different process.†

Dissection has also been had recourse to for collateral information on this complicated malady: but its researches have been less successful than those of the chymists. The only organ in which any morbid structure has been clearly ascertained, is the kidneys.‡ Mr. Cruickshank

hitherto been generally deemed to be similar to that of the grape; but of late, M. Chevallier has found that it is analogous to that of the sugar-cane.— See Dict. de Méd. et de Chir. Pratiques, tom. vi., p. 249.—ED.

* It has been supposed, says Dr. Elliotson, that the sugar is dependant upon the deficiency of urea; and urea and sugar are known to contain the same q t of hydrogen exactly; but the quantity of carbon and oxygen in sugar is twice that in urea. It has therefore been supposed, that there is only a morbid change in the composition of the urine—that instead of urea you have sugar. However, it is contended by Dr. Elliotson that this is not accurate, because he has seen a large quantity of sugar in the urine where there was a considerable quantity of urea: still he admits, that in proportion as the one is deficient, the other is frequently abundant.—(Med. Lectures at the Lond. Univ., &c., op. cit.) Recent investigations made by M. Barruel, senior, tend to, prove, indeed, that there is a certain quantity of urea in diabetic urine; while in some instances not a particle of uric acid could be detected, so that the chymical character of diabetic urine is considered by some experimenters as consisting rather in the absence of this acid than of urea.—See Dict. de Med. et de Chir. Pratiques, tom. vi., pp. 249, 250.—ED.

† Med. Chir. Transact., vol. x. See also Note sur le Diabètes sucré, by MM. Vauquelin and Ségalas, in Magendie's Jour., tom. iv., p. 355, where the correctness of the results obtained from the analysis of diabetic urine by the above-mentioned French chymists, is illustrated by further examinations.—ED.

‡ The disorder often extends to the bladder, which is contracted, and thicker than in the normal state: the ureters also are sometimes dilated. The gastro-intestinal mucous membrane presents traces of inflammation almost constantly.—See Roche and Sanson's Nouv. El. de Path. Medico. Chirurgicale, tome seconde.—D.

affirms generally, that " the arteries of the kidneys are, on these occasions, preternaturally enlarged, particularly those of the cryptæ, or minute glands which secrete the urine."— (*On the Lacteals and Lymphatics*, p. 69.) And this state of inflammation or morbid activity is confirmed by Dr. Baillie in his " Account of a Case of Diabetes, with an Examination of the Appearances after Death,"[*] in which he tells us that " the veins upon the surface were much fuller of blood than usual, putting on an arborescent appearance. When the substance of both kidneys was cut into, it was observed to be everywhere much more crowded with bloodvessels than in a natural state, so as in some parts to approach to the appearance of inflammation. Both kidneys had the same degree of firmness to the touch as when healthy : but, I think, were hardly so firm as kidneys usually are, the vessels of which are so much filled with blood. It is difficult to speak very accurately about nice differences in degrees of sensation, unless they can be brought into immediate comparison. A very small quantity of a whitish fluid, a good deal resembling pus, was squeezed out from one or two infundibula in both kidneys, but there was no appearance of ulceration in either."[†]

These premises, taken conjointly or separately, according to the light in which they may be viewed by different persons, open an abundant field for speculation concerning the nature of the malady : and hence an infinity of hypotheses have been offered, of which the following are the chief :

I. The disease is dependant upon a morbid

action of the stomach, or some of the chylifacient viscera, which necessarily, therefore, constitute its seat.

II. The disease is dependant upon a dyscrasy or intemperament of the blood, produced by a morbid action of the assimilating powers.

III. The disease is dependant upon a retrograde motion of the lacteals, and is consequently seated in the lacteal vessels.

IV. The disease is dependant upon a morbid condition of the kidneys, and seated in these organs.[*]

I. The first of these hypotheses, though not the most ancient, has been by far the most commonly received, and is, perhaps, the most prevalent in the present day. It is derived from observing the increased action which exists in the stomach, and probably also in the collatitious viscera, in conjunction with the untempered fluid which is discharged by the kidneys, whose morbid crasis is referred to these organs. But even here there has been much difficulty in determining which of the digestive viscera is principally in fault. Dr. Mead having remarked that the disease is frequently to be traced among those who have lived intemperately, and particularly who have indulged in an excess of spirits and other fermented liquors, ascribed it to the liver, and the idea was very generally received in his day. Dr. Rollo has since, and certainly with more plausibility, fixed the seat of the disease in the stomach, and confined it to this organ : conceiving it to consist " in an increased action and secretion, with a vitiation of the gastric fluid, and probably too active a state of the lacteal absorbents ; while the kidneys and other parts of the system, as the head and skin, are only affected secondarily."

According to this hypothesis, the blood is formed imperfectly from the first ; and the morbid change of animal salts for sugar is the work of the stomach or its auxiliary organs, which are immediately influenced by it. It is a strong if not a fatal objection to this view of the subject, that the blood, before it reaches the kidneys, is found, upon the most accurate experiments to which it has hitherto been submitted, " to contain the salts of the blood, but no trace whatever of sugar." The experiments I allude to are those of Dr. Wollaston and Dr. Marcet.—(*Phil. Trans.*, vol. cit., 1811, p. 96.) Prior experiments had indeed been made under the superintendence of Dr. Rollo, which induced those engaged in them to conjecture that some small portion of sugar might exist in the blood ; but these trials led to no definite conclusion, and did not satisfy the experimenters themselves. The results of Wollaston have since been confirmed by other experiments of Nicholas, Sorg, Thénard, Bostock, and MM. Vauquelin and Ségalas.[†]

II. The second hypothesis, or that which regards the disease as dependant upon a dyscrasy or intemperament of the blood, produced by a morbid action of the assimilating powers, is of parallel date with the preceding, and has had the successive support of many of the ablest and most distinguished pathologists, from its origin to our own day. It was first started by Dr. Willis, and immediately followed his discovery of the saccharine property of diabetic urine. "Diabetes," he says, "is rather an immediate affection of the blood than of the kidneys, and thence derives its origin; for the mass of the blood becomes, so to speak, melted down, and is too copiously dissolved into a state of serosity: which is sufficiently manifest from the prodigious increase of the quantity of urine, which cannot arise from any other cause than from this solution and waste of blood." He admits, however, that the orifices are at this time peculiarly relaxed and patulous, in consequence of which the untempered fluid passes off with a greater ease and rapidity.

This hypothesis of Willis was readily embraced by his distinguished contemporary Sydenham, who fortified himself in the same by observing, that those who have long laboured under an intermittent, and have been unskilfully treated, and, especially old persons, sometimes fall into a diabetes, from a crude or debilitated condition of the blood. And hence he tells us, in his letter to Dr. Brady, that "the curative indication must be completely directed towards invigorating and strengthening the blood, as well as restraining the preternatural flux of urine."

Thus advanced and advocated by two of the brightest luminaries that have ever enlightened the medical world, it cannot be a matter of surprise, that this opinion should have been extensively adopted. In truth, it was espoused on the continent as well as at home, and, in 1784, gave birth to M. Place's able dissertation (*Diss. de verâ Diabetis causâ in defectû assimilationis quærenda*, Goett., 1784); and continued to be the prevailing opinion till the appearance of Dr. Rollo's work, to which we have just adverted; and even since the appearance of this work, it has been still warmly and ably maintained by Dr. Latham, who, while he pays all the homage to Dr. Rollo's labours and abilities to which they are entitled, and scrupulously adopts the general principles of his practice, opposes his doctrine of a morbid condition of the stomach (*Facts and Observations*, &c., p. 230), which, as well as the kidneys (Id., p. 110), he believes to be perfectly sound in its action. "I must take leave," says Dr. Latham, "to differ in opinion most materially from Dr. Rollo,

who seems to consider this most enormous appetite as such an evil in diabetes, as to endeavour, by every possible means, to repress it, having founded his theory principally upon the idea, that on this action of the stomach depends the evolution of sugar, with the whole train of consequent symptoms: whereas, I consider the appetite, however great it may be, and which I would never check by medicines, as a natural sensation, calling into its full exercise that organ, through which the constant waste of the body must be directly supplied, and without which the patient must soon inevitably perish: and I look upon the more moderate appetite, which takes place usually in a few days after a strict conformity to animal diet, as the surest sign of convalescence, inasmuch as I hold it in proof, that the blood being thereby rendered firmer in its crasis, there is less disposition in it to be decomposed, and consequently (as is the fact), that there must soon be a diminished discharge of nutritious matter from the kidneys."

An opinion promulgated and maintained in succession by authorities so high, and names so dear to the HEALING ART, ought not to be lightly called in question: but it is as difficult to reconcile the present notion as the preceding with the existence of the ordinary salts and the nonexistence of sugar in the blood of diabetic patients. Dr. Latham, however, has argued the point with great and elaborate ingenuity, and has endeavoured to show, by a train of reasoning which is worthy of attention, that the sugar, in respect to its elements, may exist in the blood, though the substance itself be not discoverable in it, being "so weakly and loosely oxygenated as to be again readily evolved by the secretory action of the kidneys; not from any fault in the kidneys themselves, but from the regular and natural exercise of their function, in separating from the imperfect blood such matters as are not properly combined with it."—(Op. cit., p. 97.)

III. A bold and plausible effort was made, between forty and fifty years ago, to get rid of the stumbling-block of the absence of sugar from the blood, by showing, that provided it were once formed by the digestive organs, there is no necessity for its travelling in this direction. This hypothesis was brought forward by that very acute and ingenious physiologist, Mr. Charles Darwin, in an essay presented to the Æsculapian Society of Edinburgh in 1778. In this essay he endeavoured to account for the disease of saccharine urine by a retrograde motion of the lymphatics of the kidneys. Having endeavoured to establish the general principle of a retrograde lymphatic action, he proceeds to remark, that all the branches of the lymphatic system have a certain sympathy with each other, insomuch that when one branch is stimulated into any unusual motion, some other branch has its motions either increased, or decreased, or inverted at the same time: thus, when a man drinks a moderate quantity of vinous spirit, the whole system acts with more energy by concert with the stomach and intestines, as is seen from the glow on the skin, and the in-

tom. iv., p. 355. Vauquelin found no sugar in the blood of a person whose urine actually contained one seventh part of sugar; he could detect no urea in the blood of the same individual, though he gave him a large quantity by the mouth for several days. He also states, that an opposite occurrence was here manifested to what is seen in scurvy; namely, the blood did not putrefy so soon as that of a healthy subject.—ED.

crease of strength and activity; but when, says he, a greater quantity of this inebriating material is drunk, at the same time that the lacteals are quickened in their power of absorbing it, the urinary branches of the absorbents, which are connected with the lacteals by many anastomoses, have their motions inverted, and a large quantity of pale, unanimalized urine is hereby discharged. Where, continues Mr. Darwin, this ingurgitation of too much vinous spirit occurs often, the urinary branches of absorbents at length gain a habit of inverting their motions whenever the lacteals are much stimulated: and the whole or a greater part of the chyle is thus carried to the bladder without entering the circulation, and the body becomes emaciated: while the urine is necessarily sweet and of the colour of whey. And on this account Mr. Darwin proposed to denominate the species before us a *chyliferous diabetes.*

This hypothesis, for, ingenious as it is, it has never been entitled to a higher character, became at one time also very popular, and was supported by the talents of the celebrated author of Zoonomia, the father of its ingenious inventor. A few singular facts, which have occurred since the decease of both these writers, seem at first sight to give it a little colourable support: such as the rapid passage of certain substances from the stomach to the bladder, apparently, according to the experiments of Dr. Wollaston and Dr. Marcet, without their taking the course of the circulation; and M. Magendie's experiments upon the lymphatic system, and the doctrine he has founded upon them. How much soever this speculation may have been caught up hastily by men of warm imagination, or those who are fond of novelty, the soberer physiologists have never been made converts to it. "In the diabetes," says Mr. Cruickshank, "it has been supposed, that the chyle flows retrograde from the thoracic duct into the lymphatics of the kidney, from them into the cryptæ, so into the tubuli uriniferi, thence into the infundibula, pelvis, ureter, and so into the bladder. This opinion is mere supposition, depending on no experiments. And, besides that all such opinions should be rejected, why should the chyle flow retrograde into the lymphatics of the kidney and not into the lacteals themselves? And why are not the feces fraught with a similar fluid as well as the urine? The arteries of the kidneys are on these occasions preternaturally enlarged, particularly those of the cryptæ, or minute glands which secrete the urine. And it is infinitely more probable, that the fluid of the diabetes arises from some remarkable change in the vessels usually secreting the urine, than from any imaginary retrograde motion of the chyle through the lymphatics of the kidneys."—(*On the Lacteals and Lymphatics*, p. 69.) Neither will this hypothesis account for the sweetness of urine in diabetes; for Dr. Baillie has sufficiently shown, that chyle itself has very little sweetness belonging to it at any time, and is totally incapable of supplying the large quantity of saccharine matter which diabetic urine evinces. Even Dr.

Wollaston prefers a state of doubt, concerning the course pursued by the above-mentioned substances, to an adoption of this conjecture, notwithstanding the ready solution it offers to his experiments. "With respect," says he, "to Dr. Darwin's conception of a retrograde action of the absorbents, it is so strongly opposed by the known structure of that system of vessels, that I believe few persons will admit it to be in any degree probable."—(*Phil. Trans.*, ut suprà, 1811, p. 105.)

Professor Frank seems to have been equally struck with the plausibility of the hypothesis, and the objections to which it is open. And hence, without abandoning it, he endeavours to mould it into a less objectionable form. He gives up the doctrine of a retrograde motion, but still conjectures that the disease is seated in the lymphatic system generally, with which the urinary combines in excitement; and consists in a stimulation of both these systems by some specific virus, formed within, or introduced from without, and operating with a reverse effect to the virus of lyssa, or canine madness; so that, while the latter engenders a hydrophobia or dread of liquids, this excites an inextinguishable desire of drinking; and he particularly alludes, in illustration, to the virus of the DIPSAS, or serpent of the ancients, which was proverbial for producing this effect; and hence, as we have already observed, gave rise to one of the names by which this disease was distinguished in earlier ages. He supposes that, from the irritability thus induced in the lymphatic system, every other part of the general frame is exhausted of its nutrition and healthy power; and that the fluids thus morbidly carried off are hurried forward, and especially that of the chyle, and of the cutaneous exhalants, to the kidneys, which concur in the same diseased action, and constitute the flow of urine, and especially of saccharine urine, by which the disease is peculiarly characterized.—(*De Curand. Hom. Morb. Epit.*, tom. v., p. 54, Mannh., 8vo., 1782.) But this is rather to make an exchange of difficulties than to free the explanation from such impediments; and, in truth, to render the machinery still more complicated than under Mr. Charles Darwin's hands. Upon this view of the subject, the kidneys play merely an under part, and are only secondarily affected; yet, admitting the real seat of the disease to be the lymphatics, why the urinary secernents should thus make common cause with them in the general strife in which they are engaged, rather than those of the intestines, the skin, or any other organ, we are not informed. Nor have we any lamp to explain to us the nature of the specific poison here adverted to; or the path by which the chyle must travel to the kidneys, without passing through the general current of the blood.

IV. We come now to the fourth hypothesis to which the disease before us has given rise, and which places it primarily and idiopathically in the kidneys. These form, indeed, the most ostensible seat, and hence, as we have already seen, they were the first suspected, and were supposed by the Greek writers to be in a state of great relaxation and debility, and hence also of great irritability. To this irritability was ascribed their morbid activity, and the accumulation of blood with which they were overloaded; while their weakened and relaxed condition allowed the serous or more liquid parts of the blood to pass off through the patulous mouths of the excretories without restraint or change, and, consequently, in a crude and inelaborated form, like the food in a lientery.

Such was the explanation of Galen: and of all the hypotheses before us, there is no one that seems to be so fully confirmed, as well by the symptoms of the disease during its progress, as by the appearances it offers upon dissection. The anatomists have hence generally adopted this opinion, which is to be found in Bonet (*Sepulchr.*; lib. iii., sect. xxvi., obs. 1), Ruysch (*Observ. Anat. Chir.*, N. 13), and Cruickshank (*On the Lacteals and Lymphatics*, p. 69); and in proof that it has of late been gaining additional ground among physicians and medical practitioners in general, as well on the continent as in our own country, it may be sufficient to refer to the writings of Richter, the works of MM. Nicholas and Gueudeville, and MM. Dupuytren and Thénard, already quoted, and the communications of Mr. Watt, Dr. Henry, and, still more lately, of Dr. Satterley; several of whom, however, conceive the stomach, or some other chylifactive organ, to be affected at the same time secondarily or sympathetically.*

By far the greater number of these writers regard the irritation of the kidneys as connected with inflammation, though several of them ascribe it to a spasm. The latter seem to reason from the pain found occasionally in the region of the loins, and the limpidity and enormous quantity of the fluid that is discharged, which in their opinion is analogous to that evacuated in hysteria or hypochondria; such was the opinion of Camerarius upwards of a century ago (*Diss. de Diabete Hypochondriacorum Periodico*, Tub., 1696), and it is that of Richter and Gueudeville in our own day: "La phthisurie," says the last, for under this name he describes saccharine urine, "est une consomption entretenue par une deviation SPASMODIQUE et continuelle des sucs nutritifs non animalisés, sur l'organe urinaire."—(*Recherches et Expériences Médicales*, &c., 8vo., Paris, 1803.)

* Hypertrophy of the kidneys in diabetic cases is the alteration which dissections prove to be a more common change in them than any other, as authenticated by Andral and Dezeimeris; yet it would be venturing too far to set down this state of the kidneys as essentially concerned in the production of diabetes, because certain cases are recorded in which the kidneys do not appear to have been affected with hypertrophy One such example is related by M. Demours.—(Journ. Universel des Sciences Méd., tom. xiv., p. 121, 1819.) And, as Dr. Bouillaud remarks, even if hypertrophy of the kidneys would account for the increased secretion of urine, it could not explain how the modifications in the chymical composition and in the quality of this fluid were produced.—See Dict. de Méd. et de Chir. Prat., tom. vi., p. 253.—Ed.

There seems, after all, but little to support this doctrine, and yet it was adopted by Cullen, and that so completely as to induce him to arrange diabetes in his Class Neuroses, and Order Spasmi, immediately before hysteria and hydrophobia. His reason for doing so is contained in the following passage in his First Lines:— "As hardly any secretion can be increased without an increased action of the vessels concerned in it, and as *some* instances of this disease are *attended* with affections manifestly spasmodic, I have had no doubt of arranging the diabetes under the order of Spasmi."—(*Pract. of Phys.*, Aph. 1504.) A more unsatisfactory reason has perhaps never been offered, nor does the author himself seem satisfied with it, for we find him shortly afterward, not, indeed, like M. Gueudeville, uniting it with another cause to give it potency, but abandoning it for this auxiliary cause, which seems to be adopted exclusively; for he adds, within a few aphorisms, "I think it probable that, *in most cases*, the proximate cause is some fault in the assimilatory powers, or those employed in converting alimentary matter into the proper animal fluids."—(Id., Aph. 1512.)

But, admitting the kidneys to be in a morbid and highly irritable state, which is the oldest and apparently the best-supported doctrine upon the subject, and that this state is connected with an inflammatory action of a peculiar kind, what necessity is there for supposing an idiopathic affection of any other part, whether the stomach or the nerves, the chylifacient or the assimilating powers? And why may not every other derangement, that marks the progress of the disease, be regarded as consequent upon the renal mischief? I ask the question with all the deference due to the distinguished authorities that have passed in review before us, the value of whose writings, and the extent of whose talents, no man is more sensible of than myself; but I ask it also, after having studiously attended to the nature of these derangements, both in theory and in all the practice which has fallen to my own lot, and with a strong disposition to believe that the whole can be traced and resolved into this single and original source, and consequently that diabetes is a far less complicated disease than has hitherto been imagined.

That an inordinate excitement of the kidneys is capable of augmenting the urinary secretion, whatever be the cause of such excitement, is obvious to every one who has attended to the stimulant effects of spirits drunk to excess, hysteria, and several other irregular actions of the nervous system, and the whole tribe of diuretics. From a morbid irritation of the kidneys alone, we may, I think, satisfactorily account for the largest quantity of water that is ever discharged in the disease before us, and see with what peculiar force it was denominated by the Greeks HYDERUS (ὕδερος), or water-flux, as also HYDROPS *matellæ*, or URINAL DROPSY.

This analogy will be still more obvious from our following up the common forms of dropsy to their ordinary consequences, and comparing them with the consequences of diabetes. As the watery parts of the blood in cellular or abdominal dropsy are drawn off with great rapidity and profusion to a single organ, every other organ becomes necessarily desiccated and exhausted ; the skin is harsh and dry, the muscles lean and rigid, the bloodvessels collapsed, the bowels costive, and the adipose cells emptied of their oil. Every part of the system is faint, and languishes for a supply ; and hence that intolerable thirst which oppresses the fauces and stomach, and urges them by an increased action to satisfy the general demand. This is a necessary effect of so profuse a depletion, be the cause what it may ; and we have reason, therefore, to augur, à priori, that such an effect must follow in this form of the Greek HYDERUS, or water-flux. That it *does* follow we have already seen ; and we are hence led almost insensibly to adopt, in its fullest latitude, the correct doctrine of Dr. Latham, that " the increased appetite in this last disease, however great it may be, is a natural sensation, calling into its full exercise that organ, through which the constant waste of the body must be directly supplied, and without which the patient must soon inevitably perish."—(*Pract. Treatise,* &c., i., p. 417.)

From a morbid excitement, then, a weak and irritable inflammation, if I may be allowed the expression, of the kidneys alone, we are able to account, not only for all the local symptoms of an enormous flux of water, lumbar or hypochondriac pains, and occasionally fulness, and the post-obit appearances of distended or " preternaturally enlarged arteries," as observed by Mr. Cruickshank ; " bloodvessels more crowded than in a natural state, so as in some parts to approach to the appearance of inflammation," as observed by Dr. Baillie ; " ossified arteries," as observed by Mr. Gooch ; and "a glutinous infarction of the parenchyma of the kidneys," as observed in other cases by Plenciz (*Acta et Observationes Med.,* p. 153); but also for all the constitutional symptoms of a dry, harsh, and heated skin,[*]

general emaciation and sense of exhaustion, depression of animal spirits, great thirst, and voracious appetite. In dropsy, indeed, the appetite is not uniformly voracious, nor is it always so in diabetes : but that inanition of almost every kind has a tendency to produce this symptom, where the tone of the stomach is not interfered with, or has re-established itself, is manifest from its occurring so commonly after severe fatigue, long fasting, protracted fevers, or any other exhausting state of body. And hence the very existence of the symptom in diabetes is a direct proof, that the action of the stomach, instead of being morbid, is perfectly sound, though inordinately excited.[*]

But, it may perhaps be said, the grand question still remains untouched. How are we to account for that crude, fused, or dissolved state of the blood, which appears so conspicuously in diabetes, and which reduces it from an animalized to a vegetable crasis ? Now, upon this point, let us fairly put to ourselves this previous question :—Does such a state of the blood appear at all ? and is it in fact reduced or changed in any respect from its animalized character antecedently to its arrival at the morbid organ of the kidneys ? So far as we have been able to obtain information from chymical experiments, the blood of a diabetic patient continues in full possession of its animalized qualities, and evinces no approach towards those of vegetable fluids : and, so far as we can judge from its being drawn from the arm during life, instead of evincing a thin, dissolved, and colourless state, it discovers that very condition which we should anticipate as a natural consequence of a very copious abstraction of its serous or more liquid principles. For we are told, without a dissentient voice, by those who have drawn blood freely and repeatedly during the disease, that it has the

---

neys, is mostly only one of the consequences of gastritis.—ED.

[*] Relating to the question concerning the connexion of diabetes with the digestive organs, some curious experiments are related by Dr. Krimer, of Halle.—(See Horn's Archivs, 1819.) In some animals, he artificially produced diabetes by injecting into their stomachs diabetic urine. He also observed the effects of certain kinds of food on the urine of animals. In his opinion the experiments prove, that particular kinds of grain, viz., rye, ergoted rye, oats, and rice, diminish the activity of the nervous system, and especially of the par vagum, whereby the urine is rendered very dense. Its usual constituents, uric acid and urea, disappear, and their place is supplied by albumen and the colouring matter of the blood. The difference of effect of cane sugar and diabetic sugar, when injected into the stomach or the venous system, is also worthy of notice. Dr. Krimer infers, that the secretion of the urine partly depends upon the par vagum, and that a diminished action of this nerve produces an increased quantity of solid matter in the urine ; and though not of sugar, at least of albumen, mucus, and red particles of the blood. He thinks it possible that diabetes may depend upon a similar state of the par vagum. After all, however, this is ascribing the disease only to a peculiar action of the secernent vessels of the kidney ; a fact of which there can be no doubt, in whatever way excited.—ED.

---

[*] As already remarked, however, it is observed by Dr. Marsh, that in many of the cases whose histories are recorded, the earliest disturbance in the general health could distinctly be traced to some cause acting upon the skin, and producing derangement of its functions.—(See Dublin Hospital Reports, vol. iii., p. 432.) So Dr. Marsh's view of the pathology of diabetes, somewhat modified, had an advocate in the late Dr. Armstrong, who observes, "the kidneys have naturally been examined after death, and in some instances they have been found inflamed : but in others, little or nothing morbid has been discovered ; and from the peculiar state of the skin, stools, urine, &c., it is probable, that the affection of the kidneys is the ultimate result of disorder of the skin, of the mucous membranes of the stomach and intestines, and of the liver."—(See Armstrong on the Morbid Anatomy, Nature, and Treatment of Diseases, p. 837.) Perhaps, of the pathology of diabetes, it is best at present to acknowledge our ignorance. This remark is applicable to several other theories which might be specified, as, for instance, to that of M. Dezeimeris (Mém. de la Soc. d'Emulation, tom. ix.), who, mistaking a mere coincidence for a true cause, maintains that diabetes, or, what seems to him the same thing, irritation of the kid-

general appearance of treacle ; is thicker than natural from the drain of its finer parts, and darker from a closer approximation of its red corpuscles, little capable of coagulability from its loss of coagulable lymph, and hence not separating by rest into a proper serum and crassamentum. And we are told farther, that wherever venesection has been serviceable, and the renal flux has diminished, the blood instantly assumes a greater disposition to coagulate, and loses the darkness of its hue.*

The chief reason, after all, for supposing that this change from an animalized to a vegetable, or rather from an uric to an oxalic character, takes place in the blood itself, is from the difficulty of conceiving how it can take place in the kidneys : the difficulty of explaining how an organ, whose common function is to secern alkalis, and an acid strictly animal, should be brought to secern an acid directly vegetable. But, in the first place, is the difficulty one which is diminished by transferring this wonderful change of action to the assimilating powers, or to the stomach, or to any other organ ? For let us lay the fault where we will, we are still involved in the dilemma of supposing, that an animal structure, whose healthy function consists in the formation of ammonia, has its action so perverted by the disease before us as to produce sugar in its stead. And hence, by enlisting the assimilating powers into service upon the present occasion, we only gain two levers instead of one. We place the globe upon the elephant instead of upon the tortoise, but we have still to inquire what it is that supports the latter ?

There are, however, if I mistake not, various pathological and physiological facts perpetually occurring before our eyes, which, if properly applied, may at least reconcile us to this supposed anomaly, if they do not explain its nature : a very few of which I will briefly advert to.

We see a tendency in most animal organs to produce sugar under particular circumstances, whatever be the character of their ordinary secretion ; and this both in cases of health, where we have no ground for supposing an imperfectly animalized fluid, and in cases of disease, where such a change may perhaps be contended for and supported : and we see this also, and equally, under an animal and under a vegetable diet ; in some instances, indeed, most so where the former predominates. No one, if he did not know the fact, would predict that the breast of a healthy woman, which forms no sugar at any other time, would become a saccharine fountain immediately after childbirth ; and still less so that an animal diet, or a mixed diet of animal and vegetable food, would produce a larger abundance than a vegetable diet alone : and least of all, that woman's milk produced by animal food would yield more sugar in a given quantity than ass's, goat's, sheep's, or cow's ; and less caseous matter than any of these quad-

rupeds (*Expérimens des MM. Stipriaan, Livis-cius, et D. Bondt, in Mém. de la Soc. de Méd. à Paris*, 1788), though this last is the only matter of a strictly animalized quality which milk of any kind contains.

This, however, is a natural process. Yet, under the action of a morbid influence, sugar is often produced in other organs, while what should be sugar in the mammæ is changed to some other substance. Under the genus Ptyalismus we have observed, that the saliva is sometimes so impregnated with a saccharine principle as to acquire the name of P. *mellitus :* it is indeed by some authors represented as having the sweetness of honey. Pus, under various circumstances, evinces a sweetish taste, and hence the occasional sweetness of the sputum in consumptive patients. So in fevers of various kinds, as we have already had several occasions to observe, and particularly in hectic fever, the sweat throws forth a vapour strongly impregnated with acetous acid.

It is unnecessary to pursue these illustrations any further. Candidly reflected upon, they cannot fail, I think, to diminish in a considerable degree the repugnance which the mind at first feels in admitting a secretion of sugar by an organ, whose common function is so inaccordant with such a production : and consequently they co-operate in leading us to the conclusion, which it has been the design of these remarks to arrive at, that *paruria mellita*, or diabetes, is a disease seated in the kidneys alone, and dependant upon a peculiar irritability or inflammation of the renal organ.†

With regard to the predisposing or occasional causes of this disease, however, we are still involved in considerable darkness ; with the exception, that whatever debilitates the system seems at times to become a predisponent, and only requires some peculiar local excitement to give birth to the disease, without which it is in vain to expect that it should take place. Hence it occurs to us, in some instances, as a consequence of old age : in others, of a consti-

---

* Vol. i., p. 64. In diabetes, or paruria mellita, MM. Vauquelin and Ségalas, who carefully analyzed the saliva, as already observed, found no saccharine matter in it.—See Magendie's Journ., tom. iv.—Ed.

† On the pathology of diabetes, Dr. Elliotson delivers the following opinions :—" As to the real nature of the disease, some declare it is situated in the kidney, others that it is situated in the stomach. Now, many of the symptoms are as easily explained on one supposition as on the other. Many of them are referrible altogether to the discharge of fluid. The thirst and the dryness of the skin are evidently referrible to the loss of fluid. So again, the costiveness, the emaciation, the hunger, the debility, the sensation of sinking at the stomach, are all referrible to the mere loss of so much substance as must be lost in the production of sugar. But the absence of sugar in the blood, and the very frequent absence of dyspepsy, or any thing connected with the stomach, except the hunger (which the excessive loss will explain), make it appear to me most probable that the disease is situated in the kidney."—See Med. Lectures delivered at the Lond. Univ., as reported in Med. Gaz., 1832-33, p. 730.—Ed.

---

* MM. Vauquelin and Ségalas have recently analyzed the blood and saliva of diabetic patients, without finding the least particle of sugar in them. —See Magendie's Journ. de Physiologie Expér., tom. iv., p. 355.—Ed.

tution broken down by intemperance, or other illicit gratifications ; in others, again, of a diseased liver, diseased lungs,* or atonic gout, and particularly of chronic carbuncles, or ill-conditioned sores approaching to their nature, and showing, like themselves, a considerable degree of constitutional debility.†

I am greatly obliged to Dr. Latham for calling my attention to this last fact while drawing up the present history of the disease, and for referring me, in support of his own opinion upon this subject, to the following passage in Cheselden : " There is sometimes a large kind of bile or carbuncle in this membrane, which first makes a large slough and a number of small holes through the skin, which in time mortifies and casts off ; but the longer the slough is suffered to remain, the more it discharges, and the more advantage to the patient : at the latter end of which case the matter has a bloody tincture and a bilious smell, exactly like what comes from ulcers in the liver ; and both these cases are attended with SWEET URINE as in DIABETES." —(*Anatomy*, 8vo., p. 139.)

In concurrence with this remark of Cheselden, Dr. Latham informs me in a letter as follows : " I have a patient at this moment, whose diabetes was first observed after a long confinement from carbuncle : he is upwards of seventy, and is moreover afflicted with a mucous discharge from the internal coats of the bladder." Not dissimilar to which is the following case, which is well worthy of notice, and occurs among the earliest, in Dr. Latham's treatise on this disease. " About the year 1789, there was a most remarkable case of diabetes in St. Bartholomew's Hospital, under the immediate care of the late greatly to be lamented Dr. David Pitcairn. The patient's history of himself was this : that a rat had bitten him between the finger and thumb, that his arm had swelled violently, and that biles and abscesses had formed, not only in that arm, but in other parts of the body : that his health from that time had decayed, and emaciation followed. His urine had then the true diabetic character, both in quantity and qual-

---

* See Case in Latham's Tracts, &c., p. 142, as also the remarks already quoted from Dr. Bardsley. The majority of patients whom Dr. Elliotson has attended for diabetes have died of phthisis, which is a very common termination of the complaint.— See Lectures delivered at London Univ., as reported in Med. Gaz. for 1832-33, p. 728.—ED.

† According to Roche and Sanson, diabetes is generally attributed to excessive indulgence in warm, watery, acidulated, fermented drinks, as tea, cider, beer, &c. ; to the abuse of alcoholic liquors, and of diuretic drugs ; to the action of cantharides ; in short, to whatever increases the action of the kidneys. Among its causes, also, are injuries of the lumbar region, the presence of calculi in the kidneys, the sudden suppression of a cutaneous affection and of a profuse perspiration, all which causes directly or indirectly irritate the urinary apparatus. " The disease is more common," say they, " in males than in females, and is most frequent in cold and moist countries."—See their very valuable work, entitled, Nouveaux Elemens de Pathologie Medico-Chirurgicale, troisième edition, Paris, 1833.—D.

ity : the saccharine part was in very great proportion, constantly oozing through the common earthen pot over the glazing, and affording an infinity of pure saccharine crystals, adhering like boar-frost to the outside of the utensil, and which were collected by myself and by every medical pupil daily, in great abundance."—(*Facts and Opinions*, p. 134.)

How far the grand agent in this change of renal action, admitting the disease to be seated in the kidneys, is to be ascribed to a change in the quality or intensity of the nervous power transmitted to it, or, as the chymists call it, in the state of the animal electricity of the organ, to which power Dr. Wollaston has referred the production and distinction of all the secretions, I am not prepared to say : but the subject ought not to be concluded without noticing this conjecture, which at the same time imports, on the part of those who hold it, an admission of the general principles of the disease which I have endeavoured to support. " Since," says Dr. Wollaston, " we have become acquainted with the surprising chymical effects of the lowest states of electricity, I have been inclined to hope that we might from that source derive some explanation of such phenomena. But, though I have referred secretion in general to the agency of the electric power with which the nerves appear to be endued, and am thereby *reconciled to the secretion of acid urine from blood that is known to be alkaline,* which before that time seemed highly paradoxical, and although the transfer of the prussiate of potash, of sugar, or of other substances, may equally be effected by the same power as acting cause, still the channel through which they are conveyed remains to be discovered by direct experiment."—(*Philosoph. Trans.*, 1811, p. 105.)

While such is the diversity of opinions which have been held concerning the pathology of honeyed paruria, it cannot be a matter of much surprise, that the proposed plans of treatment should also exhibit a very great discrepance.

On a first glance, indeed, and without keeping the grounds of these distinct opinions in view, nothing can be more discordant or chaotic than the remedial processes proposed by different individuals. Tonics, cardiacs, astringents, and the fullest indulgence of the voracious appetite in meals of animal food, with a total prohibition of vegetable nutriment, on the one side ; and emetics, diaphoretics, and venesections to deliquium, and again and again repeated, on the other : while opium in large doses takes a middle stand, as though equally offering a truce to the patient and the practitioner.

It is easy, however, to redeem the therapeusia of the present day from the charge of inconsistency and confusion, to which at first sight it may possibly lie open. Different views of the disease have led to different intentions : but so long as these intentions have been clearly adhered to, how much soever they may vary in their respective courses, they are free from the imputation of absurdity. These intentions have been chiefly the following :—

.I. To invigorate the debilitated **organs,**

whether local or general, and to give firmness and coagulability to the blood.

This was the object of all the Greek physicians, and it regulated the practice to a very late period in the history of the disease. "The vital intention," says Dr. Willis, "is performed by an incrassating and moderately cooling diet ; by refreshing cordials, and by proper and seasonable hypnotics." Hence agglutinants of all kinds were called into use, as tragacanth, gum-arabic, and the albumen of eggs ; and these were united with astringents, as rhubarb, cinnamon, and lime-water, with or without an anodyne draught at evening, as might be thought prudent. Sydenham carried the tonic and cardiac part of this plan considerably further than Willis : for while the latter chiefly limited his patients to milk or a farinaceous diet, the former allowed them an animal diet with a vinous beverage. "Let the patient," says he, "eat food of easy digestion, such as veal, mutton, and the like, and abstain from all sorts of fruit and garden-stuff, and at all his meals drink Spanish wine."

This plan continued in force, with little variation, except as to the proportionate allowance of animal and vegetable food, till within the last thirty years ; the chief tonic medicines being the warm gums or resins, astringents, and bitters. Alum and alum whey appear to have been in particular estimation with most practitioners. They were especially recommended by Dr. Dover and Dr. Brocklesby in our own country, and by Dr. Herz (Sell, Neue Beiträge, i., 124) on the continent. Dr. Brisbane and Dr. Oostendyk (Samml. auserl. Abhandl. für Pract. aerzte, b. i., 179), on the contrary, assert, that in their hands they were of no use whatever. Sir Clifton Wintringham applied alum dissolved in vinegar, as a lotion, to the loins. The other astringents that have been chiefly had recourse to are lime-water, as noticed already, chalybeate waters, kino and catechu in tincture, powder, and decoction ; none of which, however, seem to have been eminently serviceable ; while cantharides as a local astringent has been exposed to a very extensive range of experiment, both at home and abroad. Dr. Morgan gave it in the tincture, Dr. Herz in the form of powder, and both esteemed it salutary. Dr. Brisbane tried it in the first of these ways, giving from twenty to thirty drops twice a day : but appears to have been as dissatisfied with cantharides as with alum, and declares that all astringents are hurtful, as Amatus Lusitanus (cent. v., cur. 33) asserted long before that they are of no use.

The practice of Professor Frank seems to have been as feeble as his hypothesis. Though he notices the above remedies, together with various others, he seems to place more dependance upon a blister applied to the os sacrum, or the internal use of asafœtida, valerian, and myrrh, than upon any other course of medicine whatever : telling us, towards the close of his chapter, that a pupil of his employed the vesicating plaster as above with a happier success than any other plan, and hereby succeeded in restoring two diabetic patients to former health :

while, for himself, in true diabetes mellitus, after alum, tincture of cantharides, Dover's powder with camphire, decoction of bark with simarouba, and myrrh with sulphate of iron (sal martis), had completely failed, he obtained a manifest decrease of urine by asafœtida, with valerian and a watery infusion of myrrh : and at length, by the aid of cuprum ammoniacale, given twice a day in doses of from half a grain to a grain, acquired for his patient a restoration to perfect health, which he confirmed by a generous diet.

II. A second intention of pathologists in the present disease has been that of adding to the deficient animal salts, and resisting the secretion of sugar, by confining the patient to a course of diet and medicines calculated to yield the former and to counteract the latter.*

This intention may have been indirectly acted upon by some part of the process we have just noticed, and particularly by the dietetic plan of Sydenham : but it is to Dr. Rollo that the medical world is immediately indebted for its full illustration, and the means of carrying it directly into effect, which consists in enforcing upon the patient an entire abstinence from every species of vegetable matter, and consequently limiting him to a diet of animal food alone : some form of hepatized ammonia being employed as an auxiliary in the meantime. Narcotics, as under the preceding intention, are also occasionally prescribed by Dr. Rollo : and, in accordance with his doctrine, that the stomach is the chief seat of morbid action, and that the thirst and voracity are indications of such action, the aid of an emetic is occasionally called in to allay the high-wrought excitement.

From this last part of Dr. Rollo's curative method, Dr. Latham appears to dissent upon the ground, and in the present author's opinion a correct ground, that the increased action of the stomach proceeds from a sound instead of from a morbid appetence : but to the injunction of an exclusive use of animal food, and a total abstinence from fermented and fermentable liquors, he accedes, with a full conviction of its importance, and without permitting the smallest deviation.† And as Dr. Rollo, with a view of com-

* As the sugar of diabetic urine is, as the French express themselves, not azotized, it was conceived that its formation might be prevented by restricting the patient to a diet of substances abounding in azote, as animal food in general, and greasy articles. Nicholas and Gueudeville, and afterward MM. Dupuytren and Thénard, attested the usefulness of this practice, which, as the text explains, was first proposed by Dr. Rollo.—ED.

† As a remedy for saccharine urine, however, Dr. Prout has little reliance on a diet exclusively animal. According to his experience, it lessens the quantity and deepens the colour of the urine, and thus disguises the saccharine matter ; but, as far as he has been able to ascertain, it does not diminish the specific gravity of the secretion. Other writers, however, besides Rollo, assert that the disease has been suspended or materially benefited by an animal diet.—(See Edin. Med. Journ., No. lxxxvii., p. 337 ; Magendie's Journal, tom. iv., p. 361, &c.) An exclusively animal diet, Dr. Marsh admits, may alter the sensible proper-

pleting the intention of supplying the readiest means for a recruit of the deficient animal salts, prescribed hepatized ammonia as an auxiliary, Dr. Latham, for the same purpose, prescribes phosphoric acid, having observed in various cases of the disease an evident deficiency in the supply of phosphate of lime.

[On the chymical principle of introducing into the system the substances observed to be deficient in diabetic urine, M. Rochoux proposed the trial of urea itself as a remedy for diabetes. For several days it was given to a patient, whose urine was most carefully analyzed during the continuance of the plan, in order to ascertain whether any of the urea taken into the stomach found its way into the urine. None, however, could be detected; but the quantity of urine secreted was increased.* It seems, then, as if the plan of communicating to the urine its natural qualities, by exhibiting phosphoric acid, hepatized ammonia, and urea, on chymical principles, offers no prospect of any essential benefit.]

III. Some of the indications of the disease, however, have given rise to a much bolder intention. We have already seen that, from a few of its symptoms, and the appearances discoverable on dissection, there is reason to apprehend an irritable and inflammatory state of the kidneys: and it has hence been attempted to cut short the complaint, and, so to speak, to strangle this condition at its birth, by copious and repeated bleedings. Le Fevre appears to have adopted and acted upon this principle almost as early as the beginning of the preceding century (Opera, p. 134, Verunt., 1737, 4to.); but he does not seem to have obtained any considerable number of converts to his opinion; and it is to Dr. Watt, of Glasgow, that we are principally indebted for whatever advantages may have resulted from this mode of practice in our own day; and particularly for trusting to it mainly or exclusively, and carrying it to a very formidable extent. The plan pursued by Dr. Watt has since been pursued by Dr. Satterley, and the success obtained by the former has apparently been more than equalled by the latter, in the course of various trials.—(See Med. Trans., vol. v., art. i.)

[With regard to venesection, it is to be regretted that similar success has not been obtained by other practitioners. Dr. Prout says that no advantage is derived from bleeding, except in the acute stage of diabetes; and even in that, a critical writer assures us that his experience does not confirm the expectations raised by the reports of Dr. Watt.† Whether

venesection, however, is particularly dangerous in diabetic habits, on account of the tendency of a wound in them to produce diffuse inflammation, may be questioned. It deserves notice, at the same time, that Dr. Prout inclines to this belief, and that two cases of diffuse inflammation from this cause, in diabetic subjects, are reported by Dr. Duncan, jun.]*

In Dr. Satterley's case, there was the local symptom of great pain in the loins, which in the first is described as having been "first severe, but at times excessively acute." Here also the testicles were occasionally retracted; and in one of two female cases there was a distressing itching in the pudendum: so that there is reason to conclude that these instances were accompanied with a more than ordinary degree of irritability or inflammation.† "This," says Dr. Satterley, "is the extent of my experience respecting bleeding in diabetes: an experience that fully warrants my asserting the safety, and I think the efficacy, of the practice, in some species of this complaint."

IV. It has, however, been thought possible by other practitioners, to subdue the irritation, whether local or general, and which is often strikingly conspicuous, by powerful narcotics repeated in quick succession; and thus to obtain a cure without that increase of debility which, in many cases, must necessarily ensue upon an active plan of depletion—and this has constituted a fourth intention.

Anodynes, though of no great potency, were occasionally administered by Willis and Sydenham: and their benefit was expressly insisted upon by Buckwald.—(Dissert. de Diabetis Curatione, &c.) The ordinary form has been that of Dover's powder, thus aiming at a diaphoretic as well as a sedative effect: and, in this form, it has sometimes been found successful, particularly in a case published by Dr. M'Cormick (Edin. Med. Comment., vol. ix., art. ii., p. 56), and more lately by Dr. Marsh of Dublin (Dublin Hospital Reports, vol. iii., 8vo., 1822); but I am not aware that narcotics alone have been relied upon, or their effects completely ascertained, before the late experiments of Dr. P. Warren, an interesting statement of which he has communicated in the same work that contains Dr. Satterley's practice in venesection.— (Vide suprà.) These experiments embrace the

the vapour or tepid bath, and the pulv. ipecac, comp., aided by purgatives, leeches to the epigastrium, &c.—(Dublin Hospital Reports, vol. iii.) Dr. Barry combines an animal diet with the vapour bath, and occasional topical bleeding, and has recorded an example of the success of such treatment.—See Lancet, No. ccxxxviii., p. 926.—Ed.

* Dr. V. Mott remarks (Am. Med. and Phil. Reg., vol. i., p. 349) that he was an eyewitness of the beneficial effects of bleeding in paruria mellita, in the Royal Infirmary at Edinburgh, in the practice of that very eminent physician, James Hamilton.—D.

† Dr. Ayre, whose pathological opinions lead him to refer diabetes to a local disease of the kidneys, puts great faith in the efficacy of cupping on the loins, a practice, also, of which Dr. Baillie has spoken favourably, as we shall presently find.—Ed.

ties of the urine, and materially diminish its quantity, but he says that it will effect little towards the removal of the disease.—(See Dubl. Hospital Reports, vol. iii., p. 431.)—Ed.

* MM. Vauquelin and Ségalas, in Magendie's Journ. de Physiol., tom. iv., pp. 356-358, Paris, 1825.

† Edin. Med. Journ., No. lxxxvii., p. 337. When the disease is recent, and the strength not too far exhausted. Dr. Marsh approves of bleeding; but his principal reliance is on diaphoretics, especially

pr g g of two cases that occurred under Dr. Warren's care in St. George's Hospital. In the first he directed his attention, like Dr. M'Cormick, to opium, in conjunction with some relaxant; and hence made choice of the compound powder of ipecacuanha. So far as the present cases go, however, they prove very satisfactorily, that whatever benefit is derivable from the use of this valuable medicine, depends far more upon its sedative than its sudorific power.* Dr. Warren, indeed, seems rather to have found the latter a clog upon his exertions, as he could not carry the opium far enough to produce a permanent effect, on account of the nausea or vomiting occasioned by the ipecacuanha, from which symptoms no benefit whatever appeared to be derived. In his first case, therefore, he soon trusted to opium alone, and persevered in the same practice through the second.†

These patients also were in the prime or middle of life; the one aged twenty-two, the other thirty-eight; and both had been declining for some months antecedently to their applying to St. George's Hospital for relief. The first seems to have been worn down by the fatigue of journeying, and was considerably disordered, before the attack of diabetes, in his stomach and bowels. When received into the hospital, however, with this last complaint upon him, he had considerable pain in his back and loins. Of the origin of the second case, no account is given. To ascertain whether an animal diet would succeed by itself, or whether it be of any collateral advantage, the patients were sometimes restricted to animal food alone, to opium alone, and to opium with a mixed diet of animal and vegetable food. It appears to me, from the tables, that the animal régimen was of advantage, but certainly not alone capable of effecting a cure; for, in every instance, the quantity of urine increased and became sweeter, whatever the diet employed, as soon as the opium was diminished. Dr. Warren, however, is inclined to think, that it was of no avail whatever; and consequently, the second patient had no restriction upon his food, whether animal or vegetable. The quantity of opium given was considerable. When Dover's powder was employed, it was gradually increased from a scruple to a drachm twice a

day. And when opium was employed alone, or with kino, with which it was for a short time mixed, but without any perceptible advantage, it was augmented from four grains to six grains and a half twice a day in one patient, and to five grains four times a day in the other. It is singular, that the opium seldom produced constipation. Few other medicines were employed.*

The sum of the whole appears to be, that *paruria mellita* attacks persons of very different ages, constitutions, and habits, and hence, in different cases, demands a different mode of treatment: and that the morbid action is seated in the kidneys; with the irritable, and often inflammatory state of which, all parts of the system more or less sympathize. It appears that, under a diet of animal food strictly adhered to, the tendency to an excessive secretion, and particularly to a secretion of saccharine matter, is much less than under any other kind of regimen, though, from idiosyncrasy or some other cause, this rule occasionally admits of exceptions.† It appears also that the irritation is in some instances capable of being allayed, and at length completely subdued, by a perseverance in copious doses of opium, and in others by a free use of the lancet, leading more rapidly to a like effect. As the irritability of the affected organ is connected with debility and relaxation, tonics are frequently found serviceable, and particularly the astringents: those mostly so that are conveyed to the kidneys with the least degree of decomposition. And hence the advantage that has been so often found to result from a use of lime-water, alum whey, and many of the mineral springs. The mineral acids are, on this account, a medicine of very great importance, and in some instances have been found to effect a cure alone; of which Mr. Earnest has given a striking proof in a professional journal of reputation.—(*Medical Journ.*, vol. xiii.) Their sedative virtue is nearly equal to their tonic, and they surpass every other remedy in their power of quenching the distressing symptom of intolerable thirst. Cinchona and various other bitters have been tried, but have rarely proved successful. Some benefit has occasionally been derived from irritants applied to the loins, and especially from caustics; but these have also failed. The colchicum autumnale, since its revival, has been had recourse to by several practitioners; and, in some cases, apparently with far more success than opium.

How advantageous soever the plan of san-

---

* On the contrary, Dr. Marsh, from the consideration of various facts, arrives at the conclusion, that interruption of the cutaneous functions has a great share in the production of the disease, and that opium acts beneficially by its sudorific qualities.—ED.

† Opium increases the lithic acid urea, and lessens the sugar. Dr. Elliotson, once finding a man dying of diabetes, gave him opium so freely, that it induced stupor and some degree of delirium; and, in the course of sixty hours, the quantity of urine was reduced from eight pints to two in the twenty four hours; and from being very heavy, it lost the greater part of its morbid specific gravity, and absolutely the whole of the sugar; indeed, urea was produced in excess—the urine contained more urea than it ought to do in health.—See Lectures delivered at Lond. Univ., as reported in Med. Gaz., 1832-3, p. 731.—ED.

* Med. Trans., vol. iv., art. xvi., p. 188. Dr. Sharkey has published two cases, in which a cure was effected by the exhibition of phosphate of soda. He was induced to try this medicine, on account of its effect in diminishing the quantity of urine.—(See Trans. of Assoc. Phys. Ireland, vol. iv., p. 379.) The dose given at first was an ounce, and it was afterward diminished to a drachm thrice a day. The rigorous animal diet recommended by Rollo was found unnecessary.—ED.

† We have seen, however, that Dr. Prout's investigations led him to believe that an animal diet does not lessen the saccharine secretion, but only conceals the sugar, by rendering the colour of the urine deeper, and its consistence thicker.—ED.

guineous depletion may be found occasionally, it is clear that it cannot be had recourse to generally ; for the present disease is, for the most part, though by no means always, a result of advanced years and of a debilitated constitution. Under such circumstances, indeed, it has uniformly occurred to the present writer, in the few instances he has been called upon to superintend it, in which, while the thirst was intense, the appetite by no means kept pace with it, and was sometimes found to fail completely.' When, on the contrary, the constitution does not seem seriously affected, and the soundness, and, indeed, vigour, of the stomach and collatitious viscera, are sufficiently proved, by the perpetual desire of food to supply the waste that is taking place, a free use of the lancet may probably be allowed, as offering what may be called a royal road to the object of our wishes : but the practice should, I think, be limited to this state of the animal frame ; since, while this favourable condition of the digestive organs remains, whatever be the prostration of strength induced by the lancet, it will soon be recovered from.

. By what means an animal diet effects the beneficial change ascribed by some writers to its use, has never, that I know of, been distinctly pointed out : but there is a fact of a very singular kind that has lately been discovered in animal chymistry, which is, I think, capable of throwing a considerable light upon the subject. In healthy urine, the predominant principle is that of uric acid ; in diabetic, that of saccharine or oxalic. The uric acid, indeed, exists so largely in sound urine as to be always in excess, as we shall have occasion to observe under LITHIA, or URINARY CALCULUS. It is not only a strictly animal acid, but, till of late years, was supposed to exist in no other urine than that of man ; though it has since been found, but in smaller proportion, in the urine of various other animals. Whatever, then, has a tendency to reverse the nature of the acid secretion in the disease before us, to produce uric instead of oxalic acid, and in this respect to restore to the urine its natural principle, must go far towards a cure of the disease, as well by taking off from the kidneys a source of irritation, and hereby diminishing the quantity of the secretion, as by contributing to the soundness of the urine itself: Now the physiological fact I refer to is, that animal food has a direct tendency to induce this effect; for Dr. Wollaston has satisfactorily ascertained, that a greater quantity of uric acid is produced in the dung of birds in proportion as they feed on animal food : and he has hence ingeniously suggested, that where there is an opposite tendency in the system to that we are now contemplating, a tendency to the secretion of an excess of uric acid, as in the formation of uric calculi and gouty concretions, this evil may possibly be obviated by a vegetable diet.*

---

* The observations of several American practitioners, to be found in the different periodical journals, while they add to existing facts as to the nature of paruria mellita, have contributed but little to our knowledge of its treatment.

Since the above was written, and the second edition of this work published, Dr. Baillie's posthumous volume has put us into possession of his mode of treating saccharine urine.' It may appear to many feeble, as much of his practice may do ; but long experience, which had made him sage, had made him also cautious and skeptical of medical means. His chief dependance was upon laudanum combined with some bitter, as infusion of rhubarb or columbo. The quantity of laudanum he proposes daily is fifty drops, and the dose of the bitter to be repeated three or four times within the same period. Bleeding, both local and general, is often, he thinks, useful, as " the bloodvessels of the kidneys in this disease are generally more or less distended with blood. The diet should be temperate, and consist CHIEFLY of animal food ; and the best kind of drink is, upon the whole, Bristol water."—(Lectures, &c., 1825, unpublished.) He thus seems rather to wait for the disease to assume a favourable turn, than to lead it to such.*

In an able paper, entitled Thoughts on Diabetes, Dr. Chapman, of Philadelphia, strongly recommends the use of the carbonate of iron, while he admits also that benefit may be derived from general and local bloodletting, and a close adherence to an animal diet.—(Phil. Journal of Med. and Phys. Sc., vol. xiv.) Dr. Samuel Jackson, of Northumberland, has successfully treated a case of it. " We directed the patient," says he,' " to take Dover's powder every evening as freely as his stomach would bear it, and at the same time to put his feet for several hours into a tub of hot water, under the bed-clothes, while he lay extended on his back and well covered." By these means, and by the use of a tonic mixture of bark, ginger, and iron-rust, and at the same time an animal diet, the patient soon improved. In two months, the urine was reduced from five and six gallons in the twenty-four hours to about two quarts, and his skin was rendered natural to the touch, as also healthy in its functions; in fact, the cure appeared to be complete.—(Am. Journ. of Med. Sc., vol. iii.)

Prof. Hall, of the University of Maryland, has lately published a case of this disease successfully treated by the internal use of the tincture of cantharides ; and Hufeland, in his journal for February, 1834, states an instance which was cured by the employment of kreosote, given to the extent of eight drops a day.

Dr. Francis informs me, that in a formidable case of diabetes occurring in his practice, where the patient, a male, 27 years old, discharged from eight to ten quarts of urine daily, the disorder was much mitigated by the internal use of iodine. In five days after commencing with this remedy, the quantity of urine was reduced to two quarts; at this time the patient complained of great debility; and the kreosote was employed ; while, however, the tonic powers of the system were benefited, the discharge of urine increased; the kreosote was now suspended, the iodine was resumed, and with immediate benefit to the patient. —D.

* If the patient's strength would bear it, Dr. Elliotson would recommend venesection, and a confinement as much as possible to animal diet, opium and the phosphate of iron being also prescribed. He considers it likewise advisable to make the patient wear plenty of clothes, so as to keep the skin warm. Warm clothing, and exercise till sweating is produced, have been advised;

SPECIES V.

PARURIA INCONTINENS.

INCONTINENCE OF URINE.

**FREQUENT OR PERPETUAL DISCHARGE OF URINE,
WITH DIFFICULTY OF RETAINING IT.**

T_{HIS} is the enuresis of most of the nosologists, and admits of four varieties from diversity of cause and mode of treatment, with often a slight diversity in the symptoms.

a. Acris.   From a peculiar acrimony in
Acrimonious in-   the fluid secreted.
' continence of
. urine.

β Irritata. ·   From a peculiar irritation in
Irritative inconti-   some part of the urinary
nence of urine.   channel.

γ Atonica.   From atony of the sphincter
Atonic inconti-   of the bladder.
nence of urine.

δ Aquosa.   · From superabundant secre-
Flux of aqueous ·   tion : the fluid limpid and
urine. ·   dilute. .

In the FIRST VARIETY, proceeding from a peculiar acrimony of the secreted fluid, the cause and effect are mostly temporary ; as too large a portion of spirits combined with certain essential oils, as that of the juniper-berry. Diluents and cooling laxatives offer the best cure.

In the SECOND VARIETY, the irritation usually proceeds from sand or gravel, or some foreign substance, as hairs, accidentally introduced into the urethra. We have some accounts, however, of a discharge of hairs in such quantities that it is not possible to ascribe the affection to an accidental cause ; and we should rather, perhaps, resolve them into a preternatural growth of hair in the bladder itself ; an idea the more tenable, as we shall have to observe, in due time, that calculi of the bladder have occasionally been discharged, or found after death, surmounted with down. In this case the disease may be regarded as a species of trichosis, under which name it is described by Goelicke (*Dissert. de Trichosi,* Frankf., 1724), as it is under that of trichiasis by Scultetus.—(*Trichiasis admiranda, seu Morbus Pilaris,* &c., Noric., 1658.) But, at present, we are in want of decisive information upon the subject. If the last view be correct, filling the bladder with injections of lime-water, or any other depilatory liquid, of as much acrimony as the bladder will bear without injuring its inter-

yet he has known persons perspire profusely in the disease, without any good being done.— (See Med. Lectures, delivered at the Lond. Univ., as reported in Med. Gaz. 1832-3, p. 731.) The difficulty of curing paruria mellita may be understood from the following facts : " Within the last six or seven years," says Dr. Prout, " nearly twenty cases of diabetes have fallen under my observation ; and, among these, I have never, but in *one* instance, and in that *for a very short time only,* seen the urine of a diabetic patient rendered quite natural." Of twenty-nine diabetic patients under Dr. Bardsley, sixteen eventually died, eight recovered, and the fate of the other five was unknown.—See Cyclop. of Pract. Med., art. DIABETES.—ED.

nal and mucous surface, will be the best mode of cure.*

Frequently, however, the irritation is that of simple debility : and hence, tonics and stimulants, as the terebinthinates, or even the tincture of cantharides, may be employed internally with success, while externally we prescribe blisters to the perinæum, or the cold water of a bidet. Pressure is also of great service in many instances. In the sixth volume of the Medico-Chirurgical Transactions, Mr. Hyslop gives a case of nine years' standing, in which a cure was effected in three days by binding a bougie tightly to the urethra, through its course, by means of adhesive plaster. And Mr. Burns gives another case, in the same volume, in which great benefit was derived from a similar plan : which is also in many instances equally adapted to the next variety.

In INCONTINENCE OF URINE FROM AN ATONY of the sphincter of the bladder, the same means may be had recourse to, though with less hope of success.†

---

* In acute cystitis, the contact of the urine with the bladder is often productive of so much agony, that the latter organ will not retain the smallest quantity of it, and it dribbles away as fast as it descends from the kidneys.—ED.

† The subject of incontinence of urine is rather more diversified than our author makes it, whose case, referred to acrimonious urine as a cause, is rather of a doubtful nature, and not, perhaps, recognised in practice. The fibres of the detrusor and those of the sphincter are naturally antagonists to one another : thus, in the healthy state of the parts, the action of the sphincter at most periods predominates over that of the muscular fibres of the parietes of the bladder, so as to confine the urine in that receptacle, in which it accumulates, and produces distention. Now, when this is carried to a certain degree, an inclination to discharge the urine is felt ; the will relaxes the sphincter, the abdominal muscles are put in action, the bladder itself contracts, and the urine is expelled. The natural order of things, however, here described, is liable to be deranged by various causes. 1st. In consequence of certain acute diseases, complicated with diminution of the nervous influence, stupor, or coma, or of violent concussion of the brain, apoplexy, extreme intoxication, or injuries of the medulla spinalis, it is common to find patients voiding their urine by drops, incessantly and unconsciously. In almost all such cases, the urine first collects in the bladder, and does not begin to dribble away through the urethra until the bladder has been distended to a certain point, beyond which it will not yield further. Here, the stronger the contractile power of the sphincter is, the more tardy is this evacuation, *par regorgement,* as it is termed by French practitioners. On the contrary, when the sphincter is considerably weakened or paralyzed, the bladder expels the urine almost as soon as it receives it, and undergoes but little or no distention. 2d. Old men, especially those addicted to excesses, are very subject to incontinence of urine, usually preceded by retention. The bladder, at first weakened, gradually becomes more and more paralytic, emptying itself in the commencement of the infirmity very slowly, next retaining continually increasing quantities of urine, and at length continually discharging the overflowings by drops. 3d. In persons afflicted with strictures in the urethra,

Stoll recommends the use of acetum armoracium, which, from combining a stimulant with a tonic and astringent power, may possibly be found serviceable, and is certainly worthy of trial.—(*Prælect.,* p. 287.) Small shocks of electricity passed from the pubes to the perinæum seem also to have succeeded in a few cases. But the best radical cure seems to be obtained by cantharides applied in the form of vesicatories, or taken in that of tincture, so as even to produce a strangury where this can be accomplished ; which is in fact nothing more than stimulating the muscles that have lost their tone into a new and even excessive action : for such an action, when once effected, can often be moderated and made regular. Mr. Bingham has given one or two instructive cases of a result (*Practical Essay on the Diseases and Injuries of the Bladder,* &c., 1822) of this kind.*

an incontinence of urine *par régorgement* sometimes takes place ; in general, as surgeons well know, in these cases, the urine accumulates in the bladder, its evacuation being difficult, incomplete, and accompanied by a good deal of effort. The neck of the bladder, however, may become weakened, distended, and perfectly inert. The prostatic and membranous portions of the urethra may undergo similar changes ; and M. Bégin has several times found, in the dead subject, those parts of the canal situated behind the urethra, so dilated as to represent a kind of second bladder. Under these circumstances, the stricture then becomes the only obstacle to the escape of the urine, which may continually dribble away.—(See art. Incontinence, in Dict. des Sciences Méd., tom. x.) Some examples of incontinence of urine are brought on by various mechanical causes, as the division of the neck of the bladder in lithotomy ; the forcible extraction of calculi ; a fungous tumour arising from a diseased prostate gland ; the pressure of the head of the fœtus on the bladder in the latter months of pregnancy ; or fistulous communications between the bladder and rectum, or between the bladder and the vagina. In addition to the numerous varieties of incontinence of urine already specified, another particularly common one remains to be mentioned ; namely, the case seen in children, whose bladders, not being very capacious, yet extremely irritable, contract during sleep, and the urine wets the bed. In the daytime, however, the influence of the will suffices to prevent the urine from being discharged, and consequently the infirmity is only nocturnal and incomplete.—Ed.

* M. Ribes has known the nux vomica, or strychnine, cure the incontinence of urine which occurs in persons afflicted with incomplete paraplegia ; but M. Bégin has tried it without success. —(See Dict. de Méd. et de Chir. Pratiques, tom. x., p. 387.) In old men, incontinence of urine is often combined with a full state of the bladder, which has lost its power of contraction. Here the regular use of the catheter, which is to be allowed to remain in the urethra, is of important service ; for, without it, no other means will avail. Some practitioners also inject into the bladder lotions containing the chloride of soda, or composed of sulphurous or chalybeate waters, in a diluted or concentrated form. They apply cloths wetted with ice-cold water to the hypogastrium and perinæum, or put the patient in the cold bath. Others prefer large blisters over the sacrum, pubes, or perinæum ; or have recourse to strong spirituous liniments. With these remedies

As the perpetual dribbling of the urine in this, and even the preceding variety, is always troublesome, and often produces excoriation, the patient will find it very convenient to be provided with a light urinary receptacle. This, for males, may consist of a small bag of oiled silk, worn as a glove for the penis, with a small piece of sponge placed in it as an absorbent. The simplest contrivance for females is a larger piece of soft sponge loosely attached to the pudendum.

The fourth variety, or flux of aqueous urine, is often a nervous affection, as in hysteria or hypochondrias ; but it more generally proceeds from a relaxation of the mouths of the cryptæ or tubuli uriniferi, which, in consequence, suffer a much larger quantity of fluid, and with too little elaboration, to pass through them than they should do.*

In treating of *paruria mellita*, we observed that, antecedently to the discovery of the singular secretion of sugar in the genuine form of this disease, the term diabetes, by which it was commonly expressed, imported an extraordinary or profuse flow of urine, whether watery or saccharine : whence the term was made to embrace at least two affections of the kidneys of very different kinds ; as a simple relaxation of the mouths of the urinary tubules from debility, and vehement excitement and a morbid change of action ; the former expressed by *diabetes insipidus*, and the latter by *d. mellitus*. The variety we are now contemplating constitutes the first of these ; as the second runs parallel with the preceding species. It is the *urina aquosa* (*De Crisibus*, lib. i., cap. xii.) of Galen, which was also by himself, as well as the Greek writers in general, blended with the *urina mellita*, from their not having been acquainted with the difference of their constituent principles, and of the state of the kidneys in the one case and in the other ; and hence both were equally described by them under the names of hyderus, or water-flux, and hydrops matellæ, or urinal dropsy ; and, as Professor Frank has even in the present day followed or rather revived the Greek import of diabetes, his enuresis embraces the preceding varieties, but omits the present ; as included under the former.—(*De Cur. Hom. Morb. Epit.*, tom. v. p. 68.)

As this variety, like the preceding, is dependant on a debilitated state of the organ, it should be attacked with the same remedies, and particularly with astringent tonics and stimu-

may be united the internal administration of quinine, chalybeates in the form of medicine, or mineral waters, and, as our author recommends, the tincture of cantharides in prudently regulated doses.—Ed.

* The doctrine of augmented secretion from relaxation of the secernent organs is too mechanical a theory to carry with it much probability. Increased secretion always implies, in the view mostly adopted by the best modern pathologists, an increased action of the secerning vessels. Without this, however open and relaxed the excretory tubes of a gland might be, it is manifest that no augmented secretion would take place.— Ed.

lants, both local and general. Blisters, applied to the loins, will be found often useful, as may also tincture of cantharides, in doses of from twenty drops to half a drachm or even a drachm The warm and resinous balsams will moreover frequently afford aid, as turpentine and balsam of copayva, or the essential oil of juniper.

The quantity discharged under this variety of the disease, has occasionally been enormous,* amounting to from thirty to forty pints a day, and sometimes more, for one, two, or even three months, without intermission ; many examples of which are offered in the volume of Nosology. Fonseca mentions a case of two hundred pints evacuated daily, but, for what term of time, is uncertain.†

SPECIES VI.
PARURIA INCOCTA.
UNASSIMILATED URINE.

URINE IMPREGNATED WITH FLUIDS TAKEN IN-
TO THE STOMACH, AND EXCRETED WITHOUT
CHANGE.

THE Greek pathologists evidently allude to this morbid state of the urinary organs in comparing some varieties of their diabetes, or urinary diarrhœa, to a lientery, or *lævitas intestinorum*, under which last the food is described by them as evacuated in a crude and undigested state, with very little alteration from the condition in which it was introduced into the stomach.

The experiments of Sir Everard Home, and those of Dr. Wollaston and Dr. Marcet, all contained in the Philosophical Transactions for the year 1811, show that rhubarb and prussiate of potash may pass from the stomach into the bladder without undergoing any decomposition ; and, in these cases, apparently without taking the course of the bloodvessels. By what other path it is possible for them to have travelled, is to this moment a subject of mere conjecture ; upon which, however, the author has offered a few hints in the Physiological Proem to the

* In a case occurring in the practice of Prof. Chapman, of Philadelphia, no less than ninety-eight pints of urine were voided in twelve hours.— (Phil. Jour. of the Med. and Phys. Sc., vol. xiv., p. 324.) Morgagni mentions, that "within ninety-four days, a maiden at Venice expelled three thousand six hundred and seventy-four pints of urine : and another at Bologna, in the space of ninety-seven days, discharged four thousand one hundred and seventy-one pints. Both of them drank little or nothing, and, like persons labouring under hydrophobia, they were extremely thirsty, yet abhorred the sight of liquids."—(See Cook's Morgagni, vol. ii., p. 346.)—D.

† De Naturæ Artisque Miraculis, p. 538. The treatment of incontinence of urine must always be regulated by a consideration of its cause. Mostly it is only the effect of some other injury or disease, and then the cure depends upon the removal of the latter. The nocturnal form of the complaint, so common in children, requires that they should be waked, and desired to make water, once or twice in the course of the night. They should also be kept from drinking tea or other diluent fluids in the evening.—ED.

present class. Oil of almonds has frequently reached the bladder with an equal destitution of change, and has been discharged in the form of oil by the urethra (*Bachotoni, Comment. Bonon.*, tom. ii., part i.) ; and oil of turpentine and juniper pass off in the same manner. Actuarius mentions a discharge of urine of a blue colour from a boy, who had taken a bitter pill designed for another patient, but does not state the materials. Urine, containing a sediment resembling Prussian blue, was discharged copiously by a patient in a low fever, about three days before his death :* it afterward became greenish, and possessed a strong ammoniacal smell. Another case is related by the same author of a discharge of blue urine from a woman of sixty, without mischief. We do not know, however, that either of these two last cases was connected with any thing introduced into the stomach, and the blue or dark-coloured matter consisted probably of extravasated venous blood, intermixed with the yellow or other tinge of the urine ; and perhaps we are to ascribe to a like cause a case related by Dr. Marcet, in which the urine was black, or rather became so, soon after being discharged, in a boy seventeen years old, and apparently healthy, and who had laboured under this affection from his birth. It was, however, accompanied with this peculiarity, that although in this state it was almost imputrescible, whenever occasionally the preternatural colour was lost, it became putrid very rapidly. Dr. Prout, who analyzed it, thought he discerned some new substance in combination *with ammonia*.—(*Trans. of Medico-Chir. Soc.*, vol. xii., part i., 1822.) This has been supposed to be a peculiar acid ; and it has been suggested that it should be distinguished by the epithet MELANIC.

There is also a secretion of reddish turbid urine, depositing an abundance of a lateritious or pink-coloured sediment : this is a peculiar sign of inflammatory fever, which rarely, if ever, occurs without it ; though the lighter pink deposites take place occasionally also when no fever is present. The colouring material has been named by M. Prout ROSACIC ACID ; and appears, from experiments and remarks of Dr. Prout, to consist essentially of lithate of ammonia or of soda, teinted by purpurate of ammonia : the purpurate itself being a combination of nitric and lithic acid, both secreted conjointly by the kidneys.†

Swediaur, under his genus dysuresia, enumerates urines of various other kinds.—(*Nov. Nosol. Meth. Syst.*, ii., 61.) And occasionally such morbid changes are to be found during

* M. Jules Cloquet, in 1823, communicated to the Acad. R. de Méd. at Paris, the case of a child thirteen years of age, who, for three days, while labouring under enteritis, voided urine of a perfectly blue colour. Another member of the Academy also states, that he had noticed a similar occurrence in a man afflicted with acute rheumatism.—Archiv. Gén. de Méd., Juin, 1823.—ED.

† Inquiry into the Nature and Treatment of Diabetes. Calculus, &c. By William Prout, M. D., 2d edit., pp. 16, 17, 125 ; 1825.

paroxysms of hysteria, though more commonly the urine is then destitute of its natural colour. —(*Practical Essay on the Diseases and Injuries of the Bladder*, &c., 1822.)

Copious diluents, mucilaginous or farinaceous, will at all times afford the best means of deterging the kidneys of any such untempered materials as those we are now contemplating; and if the colour should appear to proceed from a rupture of bloodvessels in the same organs, the affection will become a variety of hæmaturia, and should be treated accordingly.—(See p. 11 of the present volume.)

[Dr. Prout, in his valuable publication, first considers diseases in which an albuminous principle in the urine is a characteristic symptom. Here it occurs very rarely in the serous, and much more frequently in the chylous form, or in an intermediate state. An extraordinary case of chylous urine fell under the care of Dr. Elliotson. The urine was chylous at every period; but what was voided in the evening had such a resemblance to chyle, that Dr. Prout doubts whether he should have discovered the difference if it had been presented to him as a specimen of chyle. It consisted of a solid coagulum of a white colour, and having the shape of the vessel, like blancmange. Dr. Prout has seen the ordinary forms of this disease mostly in persons beyond the middle age, of an irritable scrofulous habit, and impaired digestive powers, and who have been free livers. In such habits, and perhaps in others, under certain circumstances, he conceives that this condition of the urine may be excited by a long course of mercury, stimulating diuretics, violent passions of the mind, or exposure to cold. Frequently, however, the particular cause cannot be traced.

Slight degrees of this affection may exist for years without becoming worse, or producing any serious effects on the constitution. Even in the extraordinary case under Dr. Elliotson, the constitutional symptoms were by no means severe, and it did not interfere with the generative powers.

The treatment, Dr. Prout says, must depend upon the disease with which it is complicated. Considered as a symptom, however, it may be useful in teaching us to avoid stimulant diuretics, especially alkaline ones. According to this intelligent physician, sedatives and tonics may be occasionally beneficial.*]

SPECIES VII.
PARURIA ERRATICA.
ERRATIC URINE.

URINE DISCHARGED AT SOME FOREIGN OUTLET.

UNDER the preceding species, we have seen that certain substances, introduced into the stomach, will find their way unchanged to the kidneys. The present species presents to us a singularity of a different and almost opposite

---

* See Prout's Inquiry into the Nature, &c., of Diabetes, Calculus, &c., 2d ed., 8vo., Lond., 1825. The second chapter of this work treats of diseases in which an excess of urea is a characteristile.

Vol. II.—R r

---

kind, by showing us that the urine itself, in a certain condition of the organ that secretes it, or of the system generally, may travel from the kidneys to other regions in a form equally unchanged.* We know nothing of the means by which all this is accomplished; but we can sometimes avail ourselves of the fact itself, by employing a variety of medicines, which, in consequence of their being able, in this manner, to arrive at a definite organ without being decomposed in the general current of the blood, are supposed to have a specific influence upon such quarter, and have often been denominated specifics for such an effect; as cantharides in respect to the bladder, demulcents in respect to the lungs, and cinchona in respect to the irritable fibre.

This disease has often been described under the name of uroplania, which is nothing more than a Greek compound for " erratic urine," as it is here denominated; but it has seldom been introduced into nosological arrangements. The cases, however, are so numerous and distinct, in writers of good authority, that it ought not to be rejected. In most instances, it is not a vicarious discharge; or, in other words, a secretion of a different kind, compensating for a destitution of urine, but a discharge of a urinous fluid, apparently absorbed after its secretion by the kidneys, and conveyed to the outlet from which it issues by a path or under a protection that has hitherto never been explained. We sometimes meet with it while there is a free secretion of urine by the kidneys, and a free passage by the bladder and urethra, in which case alone it can be called a disease. On other occasions we find it, as already observed under PARURIA *inops*, performing a remedial part, and travelling in the new direction to carry off recrementory matter that cannot be discharged at its proper outlet, nor retained in the blood without mischief.†

---

* See Spe. 2, δ of the present genus, urethral stoppage of urine.

† A remarkable instance of vicarious discharge of urine occurred in the practice of Dr. Isaac Senter, and is recorded in the first volume of the Transactions of the Phil. College of Physicians. The patient was a girl sixteen years old, who, after suffering for a year from some pulmonary affection, difficulty of breathing, vomiting of blood, &c., became affected with a suppression of urine, which continued for four days; and during this time she was unable to void a drop. The sixth day she vomited water which, she said, tasted in every respect like urine; and, as the vomiting continued, the swelling and soreness at the lower part of the belly was relieved. " I saved," says Dr. Senter, " the water that she brought up this way, and compared it with what I drew off from the bladder, and found it the same in every respect." After a little time the urine was mixed with gravel. The vomiting of urine and gravel continued at times for three years, during which period it passed at times from the finus and navel. On examining this female after death, the bladder was found healthy and free from gravel. Another case, similar to this in many respects, is recorded by Dr. C. Ticknor in the American Journ. of Med. Sciences, vol. xiv.—D.

It has, in different persons, been evacuated by the rectum, salivary glands, the skin at the navel, and by a fistulous opening in the perinæum, and has sometimes been found, on post-obit examinations, filling the ventricles of the brain. Mr. Howship relates a singular case, in which the secretion was discharged alternately, and in an almost incredible deluge each time, from the kidneys and the bowels, with long intervals of suppression, occasionally extending to six weeks or two months ; an examination by the catheter proving that no water existed in the bladder during these periods. At one of these irregular tides, twenty-two quarts were passed by the bladder in occasional spasmodic gushes within three days : and at another two gallons of urine were passed daily by the rectum for four days in succession. The patient was a lady twenty-four years old at the commencement of the disease, which, at the time of writing, had continued, with little variation, for nearly four years, apparently without much serious inroad on her constitution.* It does not seem to have been accurately ascertained, whether the discharge from the bowels was genuine urine or a substituted fluid.

The volume of Nosology gives a reference to cases and authorities, illustrating each of these forms of discharge : and additional ones are probably to be met with in other writings.

GENUS IV.

LITHIA.

URINARY CALCULUS.

MORBID SECRETION OR ACCUMULATION OF CALCULOUS MATTER IN THE URINARY CAVITIES.

LITHIA is a Greek term from λίθος, whence λιθιάω, "calculo laboro." It has often been written lithiasis, which is here exchanged for lithia, since iasis, in the present arrangement, is limited, as a termination, to words indicating diseases affecting the skin or cuticle.

The name of lithus or lithiasis, as used by Aretæus and Aurelianus, and that of calculus or sabulum, as employed by Celsus and Pliny, sufficiently evince the elementary principles of which the Greeks and Romans conceived urinary calculi to consist. The mistake is not to be wondered at when we reflect, that it was only between thirty and forty years ago that these principles were detected with any degree of accuracy ; and that we are indebted to the minute and elaborate experiments of Fourcroy and Vauquelin for an analysis that, till their

time, though successively pursued by Hales, Boyle, Boerhaave, and Slare, had been left in a very unsatisfactory state ; and which even since this period has required the further corrections of Wollaston, Marcet, Cruickshank, Berzelius, Brande, Prout, and various other animal chymists, to produce all the success we could desire. So general was the belief that the calculi of the bladder were formed in the same manner and consisted of the same materials as the stones of the mineral kingdom, that Dr. Shirley published a learned book as late as 1671, which is now become extremely scarce, entitled, "Of the causes of stones in the greater world, in order to find out the causes and cure of the stones in man."

The urinary secretion in a state of health is one of the most compound fluids of the animal system ; and consists of various acids and alkalis, the former, however, bearing a preponderancy, with a certain proportion of calcareous earth, and other materials which it is not necessary to dwell upon at present. The acid first discovered in it was the phosphoric, which was traced by Brandt and Kunckel, whence the experiments of Boyle, from which he obtained phosphorus. The important discovery of uric acid was reserved for Scheele, who detected it in 1776 : as he did also benzoic acid, chiefly confined to the urine of children, but alleged by Dr. Prout not to form part of healthy urine. Prout has since proved that it contains also carbonic acid, and a peculiar resin like that of bile ; and other acids, in smaller proportion, have more lately been ascertained by Thénard and Berzelius.* Hence the calcareous earth that is separated by the kidneys, as we have had occasion to observe that it is also by most other organs of the body in a state of health or of disease, is productive of numerous compounds, as carbonate of lime, phosphate of lime, oxalate of lime ; together with compounds still more complicated by an intermixture of the lime with the urinary alkalis. But as, in a state of health, the urine is always found to contain calcareous earth under some form or other, in a morbid state it is also found to contain magnesian earth, more or less united with the other materials, both acid and alkaline. In many cases, moreover, the natural acids or the natural alkalis are secreted in excess, in others in deficiency. And from all these circumstances it is easy to conceive, that a very great variety of concretions, or calculi, may at times take place either in the kidneys or in the bladder. How far these varieties extend, has, perhaps,

---

* Practical Treatise, &c., on Complaints that affect the Secretion of Urine, 8vo., 1823. One of the most extraordinary cases on record is that of Mary Burton, aged 27 years, who laboured under a retention of urine, and who, whenever the introduction of the catheter was deferred beyond the regular period, used to discharge from the ears, breasts, nostrils, and one of her eyes, a fluid exactly similar to urine. The particulars, which are given by Dr. Salmon A. Arnold, in the New-England Journal of Medicine and Surgery for October, 1825, have been stated in a previous note to the subject of paruria retentionis.—ED.

* The researches of Dr. Prout tend to prove, that *healthy urine* contains water, urea, lithic acid, lactic acid, and its accompanying animal matters ; sulphuric acid, phosphoric acid, muriatic acid, fluoric acid ?, potash, soda, ammonia, lime, magnesia, silex ?, and mucus of the bladder. *Diseased urine,* according to the same authority, contains albumen, fibrin, red particles, nitric acid, erythric acid, purpuric acid, melanic acid ?, oxalic acid, benzoic acid, carbonic acid, xanthic oxyde, cystic oxyde, Prussian blue, sugar, and bile.—See Prout's Inq. into the Nature, &c., of Diabetes, Calculus, &c., 2d edit., 8vo., Lond., 1825.—ED.

not fully been determined to the present day; but ,the number which has been detected and analyzed is now very considerable, and has been increasing ever since Dr. Wollaston's valuable essay on this subject, which appeared in the Philosophical Transactions for the year 1797, and laid a foundation for the arrangement. Among those which have been subsequently ascertained, a few, and especially the cystic oxyde, have been discovered by himself; and the whole are thus enumerated by Dr. Marcet in a still later production of highly distinguished merit :*—1. *Lithic calculus*, composed chiefly of lithic or uric acid. 2. *Earth-bone calculus*, consisting chiefly of phosphate of lime. 3. *Ammoniaco-magnesian phosphate* or *calculus*, in which this triple salt obviously prevails. 4. *Fusible calculus*, consisting of a mixture of the two former. 5. *Mulberry calculus*, or oxalate of lime. 6. *Cystic calculus*, consisting of the substance called by Dr. Wollaston cystic oxyde. 7. *Alternating calculus*, or a concretion composed of two or more different species arranged in alternate layers. 8. *Compound calculus*, the ingredients of which are so intimately mixed as not to be separable without chymical analysis. 9. *Calculus* from the *prostate gland*, of a peculiar kind, and consisting, according to Dr. Wollaston, " of phosphate of lime not distinctly stratified, and tinged by the secretion of the prostate gland." The two not hitherto described are, 10. *Xanthic oxyde*, making an approach to the cystic calculus, but giving, which that does not, a bright lemon residuum on evaporating its nitric solution. And, 11. *Fibrinous calculus*, so called from its possessing properties exactly similar to those of the fibrin of the blood, and no doubt formed by a deposite from this fluid.†

Of these, a few only are commonly found in the bladder, though most of those which are found in the kidneys are found also in the bladder, and in reality constitute the common nuclei of the calculous concretions of this last organ ; the augmentation, resulting from other constituent principles of the urine, gradually separating and incrusting them as they lie in the bladder in an undisturbed state.

The symptoms, moreover, of renal and vesical calculi differ as widely as their component parts, and hence point out the necessity of subdividing the genus into the two following species :—

1. Lithia Renalis.　Renal Calculus.
2. ——— Vesicalis.　Vesical Calculus.

* Essay on the Chymical History and Medical Treatment of Calculous Disorders.

† The solid concretions, or urinary calculi, though presenting numerous varieties, are generally composed, as Dr. Prout has ably explained, of four elementary substances only :—lithic acid and its compounds, oxalate of lime, cystic oxyde, and the earthy phosphates. From a table drawn up by this author from the contents of several museums, in which were 823 calculi, the comparative frequency of each species was as follows :— lithic acid, 294; mulberry, 113 ; phosphates, 3; alternating calculi, 186 ; mixed compound, 25.— EDITOR.

SPECIES I.
LITHIA RENALIS.
RENAL CALCULUS.

PAIN IN THE LOINS, SHOOTING DOWN TOWARDS THE TESTES OR THIGHS ; INCREASED BY EXERCISE ; URINE OFTEN DEPOSITING A SABULOUS SEDIMENT.

THE calculous matter of the kidneys sometimes passes off in minute and imperceptible grains with the urine, which are only noticed by their concreting or crystallizing about the sides of the vessel that receives it ; and sometimes collects and forms very troublesome spherules or nodules in the substance or pelvis of the kidneys : thus offering the two following varieties :—

α Arenosa.　　　Pain slight, and unfrequent :
Urinary sand.　free discharge of sabulous
　　　　　　　granules.

β Calculosa.　　Pain mostly severe and con-
Urinary gravel.　stant ; sabulous discharge
　　　　　　　small, and occurring but
　　　　　　　seldom ; calculus varying
　　　　　　　in size, often large, and
　　　　　　　obstructing the pelvis or
　　　　　　　ureter of the kidney.

Urinary sand, or the sabulous matter deposited on the sides or bottom of a receiving vessel, is of two kinds, WHITE and RED:* and it is of great importance to distinguish the one from the other, as they proceed from very different causes, and require a different, and, indeed, opposite mode of treatment. Mr. Brande has published an excellent treatise upon this subject in his Quarterly Journal ; and, in the remarks about to be offered upon this species, I shall avail myself in no small degree of the benefit of his labours, in connexion with those of Dr. Marcet; to which I have already referred.

The urine, in a healthy state, is always an

* Dr. Prout, whose important writings on this subject our author has not availed himself of, divides the deposites which occasionally take place in the urine into three kinds : the amorphous ; the crystallized, or gravel ; and the solid concretions, or calculi. The amorphous sediments indicate an excess of lithic acid, and consist essentially of lithic acid, combined with a base, generally ammonia. They are of a yellow, red, or pink colour. The yellow are the sediments of health ; the red denote feverish or inflammatory action, especially when on the decline ; while the pink generally indicate fever of an irritable nature, as hectic, and occur in the urine of dropsical individuals, and of those labouring under chronic visceral affections, particularly of the liver. According to Dr. Prout's researches, the colour of these deposites depends upon two substances : the first, an ingredient of healthy urine, which forms the yellow deposites ; and the other, purpuric acid, upon which the pink sediment depends ; while the red, or lateritious, is a mixture of both. The crystallized deposites are also of three kinds : viz., of lithic acid, by far the most frequent, and always red ; the triple phosphate of magnesia and ammonia, always white ; and the oxalate of lime, extremely rare, of a blackish-green colour.—See Prout's Inquiry into the Nature, &c. of Diabetes, Calculus, &c., Lond, 1825, 2d edit.—ED.

acid secretion, and it is the excess of its acid that holds the earthy salts in solution. If, from any cause, it be deprived of this excess, or, in other words, the secretion of its acid be morbidly diminished, the earthy parts are no longer held in solution, and a tendency to form a WHITE SAND or CALCAREOUS DEPOSITE immediately commences. And that this is the real source of its production is manifest, from the simple experiment of mixing a little alkali with recently voided urine ; for the alkali has no sooner exercised its affinity for the acid than the urine throws down a white powder. And hence a like deposite will not unfrequently take place upon using magnesia too freely.

A knowledge of the cause of this modification of urinary sand puts us at once into an easy mode of curing it ; a mode, however, which was first pointed out to the world by Dr. Wollaston. It consists in introducing into the system some other acid as a substitute for that which is wanting to the kidneys. All the acids seem to answer this purpose ; but as the sulphuric usually sits more easily on the stomach than any other of the mineral acids, it is entitled to a preference ; and the more so on account of its superior tonic powers, and consequently its better adaptation to the chylifactive organs, a debility which is no unfrequent cause of the complaint. The vegetable acids, nevertheless, may be interposed with the sulphuric, or, where the stomach is very delicate, entirely supersede their use. Of these the citric is the pleasantest, and can be persevered in for the longest period of time, especially in the case of children. The tartaric, however, and especially in the form of cream of tartar, has the advantage of gently operating upon the bowels, which is always a beneficial effect. Carbonic acid, whether taken in the form of effervescing saline draughts, or simply dissolved in water by means of Nooth's apparatus, will also be found a useful and pleasant auxiliary. The general diet should be of the same description, and be as largely as possible intermixed with salads, acids, fruits, and especially oranges. Malt liquor should be abstained from ; and, if the habit of the patient require that he should continue the use of wine, champaign or claret should be preferred to madeira or port.

It is possible, however, that this modification may be the result of too large a secretion of calcareous earth, instead of too small, a secretion of acid ; yet, the effect being the same, the same mode of treatment will be advisable.

But the acid may be in excess, instead of in deficiency, or, which is nearly the same thing, the natural secretion of calcareous earth may itself be deficient, while the acid retains its usual measure : and, in this case, the acid itself has a tendency to form a deposite by crystallizing into minute and red spiculæ—and hence the modification of RED SAND, that is so frequently found coating the sides and bottom of chamber utensils.*

This, like the preceding, is sometimes voided in a concrete or crystallized state, or the urine may be voided clear, and the deposite not take place till some hours afterward. The last is ordinarily the result of some temporary cause, and is of no importance, as it disappears with the cause that produces it. The first is of more serious consideration, as it indicates a lithic diathesis, that may lead to a formation of large and mischievous calculi, and is a pretty certain harbinger of the variety we shall have to notice under the name of gravel.

As acids form the best preventive and cure in the preceding case, alkalis present an equal, or nearly equal remedy in the present, with the exception that the tendency to produce urinary red sand is more likely to run into a habit, and is hence less easily extirpated, than that to produce white.

It has, in fact, been long known, that concrete uric acid is soluble in the caustic fixed alkalis ; and these were, in consequence hereof, the earliest forms of alkali adverted to for this deposite. But it has since been ascertained, that the alkaline carbonates and subcarbonates are equally effectual. And, as the latter are far less apt to disagree with the stomach than the former, they have very generally taken their place. Of the alkalis and alkaline carbonates, soda has commonly been found to answer the purpose best. It is, indeed, chiefly effectual in its pure state, but it is most convenient to use it in a milder form ; and of all the forms it offers, that of soda-water is the pleasantest, and may be persevered in for the longest period of time. Nevertheless, there are some constitutions in which potash and its carbonate prove more effectual than soda ; a remark for which we are indebted to Sir Gilbert Blane, who, on this account, has occasionally given it the preference, and for the sake of rendering it more palatable, has sometimes partly saturated it with lemon-juice or citric acid ; and when there has been severe or protracted pain, producing considerable irritation, has united it with opium.—(*Trans. of a Society for improving Med. and Chir. Knowledge*, vol. iii., p. 358.) A drachm of the carbonate of either of the fixed alkalis will form a moderate dose for an adult, and may be repeated two or three times a day, taken during the effervescence produced by the addition of half an ounce of lemon-juice to the menstruum, which may consist of two ounces of water sweetened with honey.

Ammonia and its subcarbonate have been had recourse to, and with great advantage, where symptoms of indigestion have been brought on by the fixed alkalis ; and particularly in cases in which red gravel is connected with gout, and the two diseases show a disposition to alternate.

Magnesia is also of considerable use, as has

---

* Dr. P_{rout}'s explanation of this part of the subject is different : according to his views, the precipitation of lithic acid depends upon the presence in the urine of a free acid, commonly the muriatic, sometimes the phosphoric or sulphuric, and occasionally other acids, which act by decomposing saline compounds, and setting a destructible acid free, which is the immediate cause of the deposition of lithic acid and gravel.—ED.

been lately shown by Mr. Brande —(*Phil. Trans.*, year 1810, p. 136; 1813, p. 213.) Taken in free and frequent doses, it has often succeeded in checking the tendency to a formation of sand and gravel, and has kept many individuals free from this complaint for very long periods of time, who have been constitutionally predisposed to it. Nevertheless it is not calculated to supersede the use of the alkalis, but may be employed as a convenient adjunct, or supply their place for a time when the patient has become tired of using them.

There is some doubt as to the manner in which the acids employed to correct a secretion of white sand, and the alkalis that of red, fulfil their object; whether indirectly, by a peculiar action on the chylifacient organs, so as to render the fresh supply of nutriment more easily disposed to yield an acid in the one case, and less easily in the other; or directly, by passing unchanged along the current of the blood, and arriving at the kidneys in their proper forms. There is a difficulty attending both these views; but as uric acid, though soluble in the caustic alkalis, is found not to be soluble in their carbonates and subcarbonates, the benefit of alkaline medicines does not seem referrible to their solvent powers. And hence it is, on the whole, more probable that both acids and alkalis produce an indirect influence on the kidneys, as we have already had occasion to observe that animal food does in saccharine urine, by a peculiar influence on the chylifacient viscera, or the nutritive materials during their subaction.

There is also another class of medicines which have long stood the test, and been proved to possess a truly remedial power in all urinary concretions of the kind before us—I mean astringents. So considerable is their efficacy, that De Heucher ascribes to them an expulsory power, in his treatise entitled " Calculus per astringentia pellendus." Their real mode of action has probably been pointed out by Dr. Cullen in a passage in which he has anticipated much of the reasoning of the present day concerning the benefit of alkalis, and has hereby given an additional proof of the strength of his judgment. Speaking of the leaves of the uva ursi, he says, that this medicine, " not only from the experiments of the late De Haen, but also from my own, I have found to be often powerful in relieving the symptoms of calculus. This plant is manifestly a powerful astringent; and in what manner this and other astringents are useful in the cases mentioned, may be difficult to explain: but I shall offer a conjecture upon the subject. Their powerful attraction of acid we have mentioned above; and that thereby they may be useful in calculous cases is rendered probable by this, that the medicines which of late have been found the most powerful in relieving the symptoms of calculus, are a variety of alkalis which are known to do this without their acting at all in dissolving the stone."—(*Mat. Med.*, part ii., chap. i., p. 13.) Their virtue as a stomachic tonic ought also to be taken into consideration, as well as their absorbent power.

The SECOND VARIETY of the lithic concretion we are now contemplating, and which, from its tendency to form larger masses, is usually denominated GRAVEL, is of far greater importance than the preceding, from the actual pain that is suffered in most cases, and the danger there always exists of the conversion of such nodules into calculi of the bladder. One of the largest and most extraordinary instances of this kind is to be found in the museum of the London College of Surgeons, belonging to Mr. Hunter's collection, by whom it was taken from the body of Mrs. ——, a niece of Sir Richard Steele, of the weight of seven ounces and a half. She was never known to have had a nephritic symptom till just before her death, when she was suddenly attacked with a violent pain, which produced a fever that destroyed her.

Of the eleven classes of urinary calculi enumerated by Dr. Marcet, there are rarely more than three that are found passing through the natural passages of the kidneys, though others are traced occasionally as imbedded in the pelvis or substance of the kidneys. These three are the uric, oxalic, and cystic; and of these, the two last are very rare productions in comparison with the first. " Out of fifty-eight cases of kidney calculi," says Mr. Brande, " fifty-one were uric, six oxalic, and one cystic." The phosphates seem never to form calculi in the kidneys, for which it is difficult to assign a reason.

The uric calculi, as voided immediately from the kidneys, are of a yellowish or reddish-brown colour, somewhat hard, and soluble in caustic potash. They exhale the smell of burnt horn before the blowpipe, and, when heated with nitric acid, produce the peculiar red compound which Dr. Prout has called rosacic acid. The oxalic calculi vary considerably in appearance. They are generally of a grayish-brown colour, and made up of numerous small cohering spherules, and have sometimes a polished surface, and resemble hemp-seeds. They are easily recognised by their insolubility in dilute muriatic acid, and by swelling up under the blowpipe, and burning into a white ash consisting of pure lime. The cystic calculi have a yellowish colour and a crystallized appearance; they are soluble in dilute muriatic acid, and in diluted solution of potash. Dr. Wollaston has remarked that, when heated in the flame of a spirit-lamp or by the blowpipe, they exhale a peculiar fetid smell, by which they may readily be characterized.—(*Brande, Journal*, &c., vol. viii., p. 67.)

The usual symptoms by which this variety is marked, are those of pressure and irritation: as a fixed pain in the region of the affected kidney, with a numbness of the thigh on the same side, the pain alternating with a sense of weight. The pain is sometimes very acute, and accompanied with nausea and deliquium, proving that the calculus has entered the ureter, and is working its way down into the bladder; after which the pain ceases till it reaches the urethra, or, by remaining in the bladder, it becomes incrusted with other materials, and forms a vesical calculus. During the whole of the passage from the kidneys, the urine is usually high-coloured, and deposites a reddish or reddish-brown sediment, occasionally not unlike the grounds of coffee, and evidently giving proof of the laceration of bloodvessels by the angular points of the calculus. It is a very singular fact, and has been properly noticed by Dr. Heberden, that during the most violent pain at any time endured from this cause, there is rarely any acceleration of the pulse : in the same manner as the torture sustamed by the passage of a gall-stone through the gall-ducts produces as little effect upon it. If, however, the flow of the urine be obstructed by the calculus, as sometimes happens, the ordinary constitutional symptoms take place which characterize that affection, as a general sense of uneasiness, heat, thirst, a quickened pulse, and other pyretic concomitants : sickness at the stomach, costiveness, sleepless nights, and at length coma, intermitting pulse, convulsions, and death : and all this even while the pain, or weight in the loins, is not peculiarly distressing. We have often had occasion to observe, that when a morbid change takes place in an organ very gradually, it may proceed to almost any extent without any acute suffering on the part of the patient, and sometimes without any suffering- whatever. The same fact not unfrequently occurs in the disease before us, of which a remarkable instance is related by Dr. Marcet, in a patient who died of a dropsy in the chest, without having made any complaint of the state of his urinary organs, though one of his kidneys was found, on dissection, to be distended by a large collection of calculi.

Sometimes a stone in the kidney, when very large, may be felt through the loins. " Mr. Cline informed me," observes Sir Astley Cooper, " that a patient consulted him who had this disease, in whom he could distinctly feel the stone by pressing firmly on the loins. The patient's general health would not, at that time, bear an operation, otherwise Mr. Cline would have removed the stone by incision."—(*Lectures*, &c., vol. ii., p. 222, 8vo., 1825.)

The proximate cause of the formation of uric calculi we have already shown to be an excess of uric acid : that of the oxalic and cystic is not quite so obvious—a point, however, of less importance, from the unfrequency of their occurrence. The predisposing and occasional causes of all of them are too often involved in obscurity. In many persons, there is an hereditary tendency to this complaint ; general indolence, or a sedentary life, becomes a predisponent in others ; too large an indulgence in fermented liquors, and the luxuries of the table generally, form a predisponent in a third class ; but the chief cause of this kind we are acquainted with, is a want of constitutional vigour, and especially in the digestive organs. The periods of life in which this disease occurs most frequently, are from infancy to the age of puberty, and in declining years ; while it is rarely found during the busy and restless term of mature virility.

It is for the same reason that the disease of gravel is so frequently connected with gout, which has a peculiar tendency to debilitate the digestive organs. " The calculous cachexy of the urinary system," says Dr. Swediaur, " often resembles the podagric cachexy, to which, indeed, it bears a strong analogy. Both are hereditary, occasionally endemic. As gout is for the most part observed in regions abounding in wines, lithia is chiefly traced where malt liquors are the ordinary beverage ; and hence, in Europe we are not without examples of it, even in infancy. Almost all cases of gout, occurring after the middle of life, are combined with calculous urine ; while the last proves at times a metastasis of the first."—(*Nov. Nosol. Meth. Syst.*, vol. ii., 259.)

The process of treatment must, for the most part, be derived from these causes. As a preventive of that modification of calculus which is by far the most frequent, we have already advised the use of alkalis and alkaline carbonates. When the digestive organs are weak, the diet should be light but generous ; warm and bitter tonics will always be found serviceable ; the bowels should never be suffered to become costive, and should occasionally be stimulated by brisk, purgatives, which tend equally to remove acidities from the stomach, and to stimulate the kidneys to a more healthy action. Indolence and a sedentary life must give way to exercise, and especially equitation, which is by far the best kind of exercise for the present purpose ; and whatever will tend to promote an increased determination towards the surface, and a frequent glow on the skin, will prove a valuable auxiliary : for the skin itself becomes, in this affection, an outlet for the discharge of a redundance of acid, as may be observed by the simple experiment of tying a piece of paper stained with litmus about the neck ; which, in even a state of common health, will often be changed to a red colour, by the acid thrown off in the ordinary course of perspiration.

Of the mischievous effects of a luxurious diet, and the advantage of abstinence, M. Magendie has given a very striking example in the case of a merchant of one of the Hanseatic towns, who was habitually afflicted with the complaint before us. " In the year 1814, this gentleman," he tells us, " was possessed of a considerable fortune, lived in an appropriate style, and kept a very good table, of which he himself made no very sparing use. He was at this time troubled with the gravel. Some political measure unexpectedly took place, which caused him the loss of his whole fortune, and obliged him to take refuge in England, where he passed nearly a year in a state bordering upon extreme distress, which obliged him to submit to numberless privations ; but his gravel disappeared. By degrees, he succeeded in re-establishing his affairs ; he resumed his old habits, and the gravel very shortly began to return. A second reverse occasioned him once more the loss of all he had acquired. He went to France almost without the means of subsistence, when, his diet being in proportion to his exhausted resources, the gravel a second time vanished. Again his industry restored him to comfortable circumstances ; again he indulged in the pleasures of the table, and had to pay the tax of his old complaint."—(*Recherches Physiologiques et Médicales sur les*

Causes, les Symptoms, et le Traitement de la Gravelle, 8vo., Paris, 1818.)

It may at first sight appear a singular fact, but the remarks just offered will tend to explain it, that mariners are rarely subject to stone or gravel. Upon this subject Mr. Hutchinson has published a valuable article (*Trans. of the Medico-Chirurg. Society,* vol. ix.), from which it appears that out of ninety-six thousand six hundred and ninety-seven patients, admitted in the course of sixteen years into the three grand coast hospitals of Plymouth, Haslar, and Deal, not more than eight had laboured under either species of lithia. Whence it is inferred, that the occupation, diet, activity, and regimen, of a maritime life, are the best preservatives against all such affections : such as an animal aliment largely combined with the alkaline stimulus of muriate of soda ; a farinaceous, for the most part, instead of any other vegetable diet ; great exercise, and that free exhalation from the skin at night, which is so well known to take place among sailors in the royal navy, in consequence of their being compelled to sleep closely together.[*] And, as the disease appears to be equally uncommon in tropical climates, we have here an easy explanation of the cause of its infrequency. In our own country it appears, from the tables of the Norwich hospital, to be more frequent in Norfolk than in any other county of the same population.

It only remains to be observed, that during the paroxysm of pain produced by the passage of a calculus through the ureter, our chief object should be to allay the irritation and mitigate the distress. The warm bath is here a valuable remedy ; friction on the loins, with rubefacient irritants combined with narcotics, often affords relief : but the present author has found most benefit from a flannel swathe wrung out in hot water and folded about the loins ; being suffered to remain there for hours wrapped round, to confine the moisture, with an outer swathe of calico or linen. If these do not answer, opium, and in free doses, must be had recourse to

---

SPECIES II.

LITHIA VESICALIS.

STONE IN THE BLADDER.

FREQUENT DESIRE OF MAKING WATER, WITH A DIFFICULTY OF DISCHARGE ; PENIS RIGID,

---

[*] Here several other circumstances should be taken into the account, as explaining, perhaps more certainly, the rarity of calculi in the royal navy. First, the small number of children in it. Secondly, boys with any complaints about the urinary organs, would naturally not be sent to sea. Thirdly, the custom of discharging from the service all men above a certain age. Similar considerations will probably explain the rarity of stone cases in the army. According to the investigations of Dr. Prout, between puberty and the age of forty, there is less tendency to lithic acid deposite than at any other period of life. About forty, lithic acid is apt to be discharged ; and about sixty, the urine sometimes becomes neutral, and the earthy phosphates are deposited.—ED.

WITH ACUTE PAIN AT THE GLANS : SONOROUS RESISTANCE TO THE SOUND WHEN SEARCHING THE BLADDER.

THE substances, vulgarly called stones in the bladder, are for the most part of a very composite structure. They originate from a nucleus, which may consist of any morbid or foreign material, that can accidentally obtain an entrance and a lodgment in the bladder ; the body of the calculus being formed out of such constituent parts of the urine as are most easily detached and attracted : which gradually incrust around it, and concrete into a mass, for the most part far too large to pass through the urethra.

The most common of these nuclei is a kidney calculus itself, and consequently a crystallized spherule or nodule of uric acid ; and when the acid is habitually in excess, the coating of the vesicular calculus may consist of this alone or chiefly : but, from the great variety of materials, as earths, alkalis, and other acids, besides uric, and sometimes blood and mucus, which enter into the composition of the urine at this time, it is not often that a calculus of the bladder is a crystallization of uric acid alone.

In the introductory remarks upon the present genus, we observed that the different kinds of calculi discovered in the human bladder had been treated of by Dr. Wollaston, as far as they were then known, in a very masterly essay upon this subject, published in the Philosophical Transactions for the year 1797 : he has since enumerated them as follows :—

1. Uric acid calculus.

2. Fusible, triple, or ammoniaco-magnesian phosphate.

3. Bone-earth calculus, or phosphate of lime.

4. Mulberry calculus, or oxalate of lime.

5. Cystic oxyde.

The cystic oxyde is not contained in the article above referred to, as not having been discovered at the time : but it has since been detected by the same excellent chymist, and named as above.

We have also observed that various other calculous masses have still more lately been ascertained by the analyses of other experimenters, and that the whole number, as arranged by Dr. Marcet, amounts, in the present day, to eleven or twelve. Their names we have already given : nor is it worth while, in a work devoted to practical medicine, to notice them any further, as they are rarely to be met with in comparison to the five arranged above, and, when met with, will not call for any essential difference in the mode of treatment.

In effect, they have been found equally different in composition, form, size, and colour ; from the weight of half a drachm to that of several pounds ; purple, jasper-hued, red, brown, crystalline, cineritious, versicoloured : in one or two instances covered with down (*Blegny, Zodiac.,* ann. iv., Febr., obs. 4), apparently produced from the surface of the bladder, from which, as we have already had to observe, hairs are occasionally discharged with the urine.—(Gen. III., Spe. 5, part. in cont.) They have also been

found solid, perforated, hollow, compact, crumbling, glabrous, rough, and spinous (*Bartholin,
Act. Hafn.*, tom. ii., obs. 85), and, in a few instances, combined with iron.—(*Act. Erudit.*,
Leips., 1627, p. 332; *Dotæus, Ep. ad Wald-
schmidt*, p. 253.)

They seem sometimes to form very rapidly ;
and when the patient has already discharged
one or two, and the urethra has in consequence
become more than ordinarily dilated, they occasionally pass off in great numbers in a short
space of time. We have hence, in different
professional journals and transactions, accounts
of a hundred and twenty voided in the course
of three days (*Eph. Nat. Cur.*, dec. iii., ann. v.,
vi., p. 99) ; two thousand in the course of two
years (*Gründlicher Bericht, von Blatterstein*),
and three hundred of a pretty large size within
the same term.—(*Hildan. Fabric.*, cent. i., obs.
89.) The largest discharged in this manner,
which has ever occurred to me in reading,
weighed five ounces. Dr. Huxham describes
one instance of such a fact (*Huxh.*, vol. iii., p.
42) ; and another is given in a distinguished
foreign miscellany.—(*Sammlung. Med. Wahrnehmungen*, b. viii., p. 258.) By females they
have often been discharged of the weight of two
ounces and a half ; and my excellent friend, Dr.
Yelloly, mentions a calculus of nearly three
ounces and a half (*Trans. of the Medico-Chir.
Society*, vol. vi.): in one case we are told of a
stone, thus evacuated, that weighed twelve
ounces.—(*Eph. Nat. Cur.*, dec. ii., ann. v., obs.
71.)

But, when extracted by art, they have been
found considerably larger, and occasionally of
enormous size on dissection, when the patient
has died without a removal of the calculus.
"The largest stone," observes Sir Astley Cooper,
"which I have successfully extracted, weighed
near six ounces. At the Norfolk and Norwich
Hospital there is one of eight ounces. Mr.
Mayo, of Winchester, removed one, in fractured
portions, of fifteen ounces. I have one in my
possession which I extracted, but not successfully, weighing sixteen ounces.* We have a
morsel of a stone, given to the collection by Mr.
Foster, which, I understand, was twenty-nine
ounces in weight. One in Trinity College Library, at Cambridge, weighs thirty-two ounces
and seven drachms. But the largest stone
which has ever been found in the human body, is
that given to the College of Surgeons by Sir
James Earle : this weighed forty-four ounces."
—(*Lectures*, &c., vol. ii., p. 232, 8vo., 1825.)
When their size is small there is often a numerous aggregation. The same distinguished surgeon tells us that he once extracted nine at a
time ; once thirty-seven ; and once not fewer
than a hundred and forty-two ; some of which
were as large as marbles.

The general character of the URIC CALCULUS
has been given already. Its texture, when

---

* Dr. Valentine Mott recently extracted from a
man a calculus measuring nearly twelve inches in
circumference, and weighing upwards of seventeen ounces avoirdupois. The patient, however,
died the fifth day after the operation.—D.

formed in the bladder, is commonly laminated ;
and when cut into halves, a distinct nucleus of
uric acid is almost always perceptible. Its exterior is generally smoother than that of other
calculi, except the calculus of bone-earth, or
phosphate of lime.—(*Brande's Journal*, vol. viii.,
p. 207.)

The appearance of the second, or FUSIBLE
CALCULUS, is generally white, and often resembles chalk in its texture. Strongly heated before the blowpipe, this substance evolves ammonia, and readily fuses ; whence the name assigned to it. It often breaks into layers, and
exhibits a glittering appearance when broken.

The third division, consisting of the BONE-
EARTH CALCULUS, or phosphate of lime, unmixed
with any other substance, has a pale-brown
smooth surface ; and when sawn through, is
found of a laminated texture, and easily separates into concentric crusts. This calculus is
peculiarly difficult of fusion.

The fourth division, embracing the MULBERRY
CALCULUS, or oxalate of lime, is of a rough and
tuberculated exterior, and of a deep reddish-
brown or mulberry colour, probably produced by
a mixture of blood that has escaped from some
lacerated vessel, whence the name assigned to
it. The nucleus is generally oxalic, and of renal origin ; but it is sometimes uric. It is also
frequently enveloped by the fusible calculus.

The fifth, or CYSTIC CALCULUS, has a crystalline appearance, but of a peculiar greasy lustre,
and is somewhat tough when cut. Its colour is
a pale fawn, bordering upon straw-yellow. It is
very rare.

Such are the calculi which are principally
found in the bladder ; and we may readily conceive with what facility they are formed there,
when an accidental tendency is given to their
formation by a lodgment of any thing that may
serve as a nucleus, by noticing the deposites
of phosphates of lime and other materials that
are perpetually incrusting every substance over
which a current of urine is frequently passing ;
as the public drains in our streets, which are
daily exhibiting them in regular crystals.

The ordinary causes of renal calculi are necessarily those of vesical calculi, but any local injury or infirmity which prevents the urine from
passing off freely from the bladder, accelerates
their formation and enlargement, not only by the
confinement it causes, but by the decomposition
which rest soon produces, in which case it becomes ammoniacal, and a larger portion of the
phosphates will be precipitated. And hence,
an obstruction in the urethra of any kind, but
particularly a diseased prostate, becomes a frequent auxiliary, and sometimes even a primary
cause, of the formation of a stone, without any
mischief in the kidneys, or any disordered secretion of urine.—(*Ibid.*, p. 210.) "The bladder," says Sir Everard Home, "never being
completely emptied, the dregs of urine, if I may
be allowed the expression, being never evacuated, a calculus, formed on a nucleus of the ammoniaco-magnesian phosphate and mucus, is
produced, when it would not have been produced
under other circumstances. This species of

stone, or a stone upon such a nucleus, can only be produced where the bladder is unable to empty itself. It may, therefore, be arranged among the consequences of the enlargement of the middle lobe of the prostate gland."—(*On the Diseases of the Prostate Gland*, vol. i., p. 40.)

It does not appear, from the experiments or observations of Dr. Marcet, that a difference in the waters of different places is much, if at all, concerned in the production of calculous disorders: nor have we any satisfactory evidence of their being more prevalent in cider countries than in others, notwithstanding the general opinion that they are so. But we are yet in want of sufficient data upon this subject to speak with much decision.

As the disease of stone in the bladder is very generally a sequel of calculi in the kidneys, the symptoms indicative of the preceding species form, in most instances, the first symptoms of the present. Yet occasionally, from causes we have just pointed out, the concretion commences in the bladder, and the symptoms of an affected kidney are not experienced. One of the first signs of a stone in the bladder is an uneasy sensation at the point of the urethra, occurring in conjunction with a discharge of urine that deposites red or white sand, or after having occasionally voided small calculi or fragments of a larger. This pain is sympathetic, and proceeds from the irritation of the prostate or the neck of the bladder, agreeably to a law of nature we have often found it necessary to recur to, which ordains that the extremities of nerves which enter into the fabric of an organ, and particularly of mucous canals, should possess a keener reciprocity of feeling than any intermediate part, and consequently participate with more acuteness in any diseased action. This uneasy sensation at the point of the urethra is at first only perceived on using any violent or jolting exercise; or in a frequent desire to make water, which is often voided by drops or in small quantities; or, if in a stream, the current stops suddenly, while the patient is still conscious that the bladder is not fully emptied, and has still an inclination to evacuate more, but without a power of doing so. As the stone increases in size, there is also a dull pain about the neck of the bladder, the rectum partakes of the irritation, and produces a troublesome tenesmus, or frequent desire to go to stool. When the pain is trifling, the urine is often limpid; as the saline or earthy materials, from their confinement in the bladder, arrange themselves around the growing calculus, and enlarge it by a new coating; but when the irritation is considerable, there is often a mucous sediment in the water, and sometimes a discoloration from blood. The region of uneasiness extends its boundary,* the stomach participates in the dis-

quiet, sleepless nights ensue, with pyrexy, anxiety, and dejection of spirits: all which symptoms are increased by exercise of every kind, and particularly by equitation. Several of these signs may indicate a primary disease of the prostate or neck of the bladder; but the occasional discharge of calculous fragments, or deposite of urine loaded with uric acid, or phosphate of lime, is sufficiently pathognomonic. It is usual, however, in all such cases, to examine the bladder with a sound, which commonly puts the question beyond all dispute: though, if the calculus be lodged in a peculiar sac, or the fasciculi of the bladder, or lurk behind some morbid enlargement of the prostate gland, the sound may not detect it, and the experimenter may deceive himself and the patient in respect to the nature of the disease.

The treatment of this malady offers two indications, a palliative and a radical.

The palliative may be applied to relieve the actual symptoms, and to prevent a further enlargement of the calculus.

The symptoms vary greatly in different cases: partly, indeed, from the size of the calculus itself, but quite as much from the constitutional irritability of the bladder, and the particular quarter of it in which it is seated. In a few persons, the bladder has possessed so little morbid excitement, that stones of considerable magnitude have been found in this organ after death, without having produced any very serious inconvenience during life. If the calculus be immediately seated on the neck of the bladder, it is, however, almost impossible for the most impassive not to suffer severely at times. But the stone has sometimes found a fortunate lodgment between the muscular fascicles of the bladder, where it has become imbedded as in a pouch, and a train of morbid symptoms, which have antecedently shown themselves, have gradually disappeared in proportion as this change has been effected.

Mr. Nourse showed to the Royal Society the bladder of a man, in which not less than six sacs or bags were in this manner produced by a protrusion of the internal coat of the bladder through the muscular, and which contained altogether nine stones.—(*Mem.*, 462, sect. 3.) The stones are sometimes fixed so firmly, that it is impossible to separate them by the forceps in performing the operation of lithotomy, without tearing the bladder or cutting one side of the sac: which last method, M. Garangeot informs us he once tried with success. In several other cases, however, that he has described, the vessels of the bladder had spread luxuriantly over the stone, and apparently grown into it; and the extraction was followed by a mortal hemorrhage.—(*Mém. de l'Acad. de Chir.*, tom. i.) Generally speaking, calculi, when seated in pouches of this kind, continue without much disturbance for years, and sometimes for the whole of a man's natural life, of which Dr. Marcet has given various striking examples in his treatise.

Art cannot scoop out such convenient receptacles, but it may do something to allay the

---

* "In severe cases of stone," says Prout, "I have often witnessed a painful or uneasy sensation experienced by patients at the bottom of the foot, sometimes amounting to pain, at other times to a sensation of numbness or itching. This circumstance has been noticed by other surgeons." —See Colhoun's Prout, p. 202.—D.

irritability of the bladder when severely excited, and in this manner palliate the distressing pain that is often endured. This may frequently be accomplished by the warm bath ; by rubefacients impregnated with opium applied to the region of the pubes, and in the course of the perinæum ; by cooling aperients, and a steady use of sedatives, particularly of conium, and the carbonate of soda, which last seems to have a peculiar influence in diminishing the irritability of the organ. If these do not answer, we must have recourse to opium, which will often succecd best, and with least inconvenience to the constitution, if introduced into the anus in the form of a suppository.*

Our next intention should be to prevent, as far as possible, an augmentation of the calculus already existing in the bladder.

In order to accomplish this, it will be necessary to inform ourselves of its chymical constituents ; for otherwise, any method we may propose will probably do harm. From the remarks already made, it is obvious that the chief constituent principles of the calculi in the bladder, like those in the kidneys, are uric acid and bone-earth, or phosphate of lime. If the former predominate, the urine will often throw down a precipitate or incrustation of red sand ; if the latter, of white sand : and, in the former case, as there is an excess of uric acid, our remedial force must be derived from the alkalis and alkaline preparations to which we have already adverted under the preceding species : in the latter case, as there is in all probability a deficiency of acid, we must have recourse to an opposite mode of treatment, and employ the mineral and vegetable acids, with a diet chiefly composed of vegetables, as recommended above under renal calculus.

But the calculus may consist of both ; for it may exhibit, and often does, a nucleus of crystallized uric acid with laminæ of phosphate of lime, magnesia, or some other substance ; or by carrying either of the above processes to an extreme, we may convert one morbid action into another. For if, by the use of alkalis, we diminish too much the secretion of uric acid, we may let loose the calcareous earth, which, in a healthy proportion, it always holds in solution, and hereby increase the vesical calculus by supplying it with this material ; while, on the contrary, by an undue use of acids, when these are required to a certain extent, we may obtain a secretion of uric acid in a morbid excess, and augment the stone in the bladder by a crystallization of an opposite kind. Hence a very considerable degree of skill and caution is requisite in the mode of treatment, and the character of the urine should be watched perpetually.

* The celebrated Franklin had taken large quantities of blackberry jam for the pain of stone, and found benefit from it ; but discovered at length that the medicinal part of the jam resided wholly in the sugar. From half a pint of sirup, prepared by boiling down sugar in water, taken just before he went to bed, he declared that he found the same relief that he did from a dose of opium.—D.

Nor, when the calculus is of a still more composite kind, can either of these plans be attended with all the success they seem to ensure, so that the augmentation will sometimes be found to pr   e in spite of the best directed efforts.

From the success that has attended the use of the *colchicum autumnale* in many cases of gout, and the tendency there is in many cases of this disease to form calculi in the joints, Mr. Brande has ingeniously thrown out the idea of trying the virtue of the colchicum in the disease before us, and hints that he has received from one quarter a very flattering account of its success, though not sufficiently precise for publication. If the reasoning pursued in examining the powers and effects of the colchicum in that part of the present work which is allotted to the history of gout be correct, we can have little hope of any permanent advantage from its use in respect to the lithic concretions before us.

There is something perhaps more plausible in the remedial regimen proposed by M. Magendie, who, on reflecting that azote is an essential constituent of urea and uric acid, advises that the patient be confined to food that possesses no sensible portion of azote, as sugar (*Recherches Physiol. et Méd.*, &c., ut suprà), gum, olive-oil, butter, and a vegetable diet generally : thus treating it with a dietetic course directly the reverse of what is now generally proposed for *paruria mellita*, or diabetes.*

From the whole that has been advanced, not only under the present genus, but also under much of the preceding, it is obvious that the soundness of the urine keeps pace, in a considerable degree, with the soundness of the stomach and its auxiliary organs, and is dependant upon them : and hence, in calculus concretions of every kind, it is of the utmost importance that the chylifacient viscera, and the whole course of the intestinal canal, should be kept in as healthy a state as possible.

Astringents and bitters offer to us the best remedies for this purpose. From the supposed absorbent power of the former, Dr. Cullen, as we have already seen, ascribes to them much of the peculiar benefit resulting from the use of alkalis and magnesia, independently of their decided virtue as a tonic : nor ought we, while upon this subject, to overlook the advantage which, in calculi of uric acid at least, the same distinguished writer asserts that he derived from the use of soap, which he ascribes entirely to its correcting acidity in the stomach (*Mat.*

* In the lithic acid diathesis, Dr. Prout recommends alkaline remedies, or neutral salts, containing a vegetable acid, assisted with alteratives and purgatives. In the oxalate of lime diathesis, he has seen benefit follow the attempt to change it into the lithic acid diathesis by exhibiting muriatic acid. In the phosphatic diathesis, he has recourse to the free use of opium ; and when the distressing symptoms are relieved, he prescribes the mineral acids, cinchona, uva ursi, and different preparations of iron and other tonics, joined with opium. Alkalis, and salts of vegetable acids, and mercury, he recommends to be avoided ; and he deems animal diet preferable to acescent food. —ED.

Med., part ii., chap. x., p. 402); thus acting the same-part as magnesia, and in many cases with greater potency.

If such be the difficulty of preventing a calculus already formed in the bladder from enlarging, we may readily see how hopeless must be every attempt at dissolving the matter that has already become crystallized or concreted. Calculi of uric acid will dissolve in caustic alkalis, but in no alkalis of less power ; nor can those of the phosphates be acted upon by acids of any kind, except in a state far too concentrated for medical use. "These considerations," says Mr. Brande, "independently of more urgent reasons, show the futility of attempting the solution of a stone of the bladder by the injection of acid and alkaline solutions. In respect to the alkalis, if sufficiently strong to act upon the uric crust of the calculus, they would certainly injure the coats of the bladder ; they would also become inactive by combination with the acids of the urine, and they would form a dangerous precipitate from the same cause. The acids, even when very largely diluted, and qualified with opium, always excite great irritation. They cannot, therefore, be applied strong enough to dissolve any appreciable portion of the stone, and the uric nucleus always remains as an ultimate obstacle to success."—(*Journal*, vol. viii., p. 215.) The greatest impediment of all, however, consists in the difficulty of ascertaining the nature of the surface of the stone that is to be acted upon, and the diversity of substances of which its various laminæ very frequently consist ; insomuch, that had we glasses that could give us an insight into the bladder, and unfold to us the nature of the first layer, and could we even remove this superficial crust by a solvent of one kind, we should be perpetually meeting with other crusts that would require other lithontriptics ; while the very means we employ to dissolve them, by decomposing the principles of the urine, would build up fresh layers more rapidly than we could hope to destroy those already concreted.

In truth, if we examine the most famous lithontriptics that have had their day, we shall find, that by far the greater number of them were calculated to deceive either their own inventors or the public, by a palliative rather than a solvent power. Some of them were oleaginous or mucilaginous ; others, that contained a considerable portion of alkali, contained also some narcotic preparation ; while a third sort seem to have acted by a diluent power alone, in consequence of being taken into the stomach or injected into the bladder in a very large quantity ; and by these means all had a tendency to appease the irritation. Even Mrs. Stephens's rude and operose preparations, which exercised so much of the analytical skill of Dr. Hales, and Dr. Hartley, and Dr. Lobb, and Dr. Jurin, and many other celebrated characters of their day, were combined with opium when the patient was in pain, and with aperients when he was costive ; and through their entire use, with an abstinence from port wines and other fermented liquors, salt meats, and heating condiments, and with rest

and a reclined position instead of exercise : and with these auxiliaries, there is no great difficulty in supposing she might often succeed in allaying a painful fit of stone or irritation of the bladder, whatever may be the talismanic virtue of her egg-shells, and pounded snails, and best Alicant soap, and cresses, and burdock, and parsley, and fennel, and hips, and haws, and the twenty or thirty other materials that held a seat in the general council.—(See *a full account of them in Edin. Med. Essays*, vol. v., part ii., art. lxix.)

How far filling the bladder with sedative or demulcent injections may succeed in diminishing irritation and alleviating pain, has not perhaps been sufficiently tried ; but from the supposed success of many of the old lithontriptics employed in this way, and whose virtue can be ascribed to no other cause, it is a practice worth adventuring upon in the present age of physiological experiments. When, however, there is much disease of the prostate or bulb of the urethra, the attempt should be desisted from ; but whenever the sound can enter without much pain, we need not be afraid of increasing the irritation. This operation is of very ancient date, and of equally extensive range, as appears from a brief account, published in a professional journal of considerable merit, of the manner in which it is performed in the present era, and has been from time immemorial, in the dominions of Muscat, beyond the mountains of Sohair, in Arabia. The instrument employed is a catheter of gold made long enough to pass directly into the bladder, so as to avoid injuring any part of the urethra with such solvent as might be had recourse to. The usual form, it appears,—and I notice it for the purpose of confirming the remark I have made upon the nature of such lithontriptics as have been most in vogue in every age,—consists of a weak ley of alkali or alkaline ashes, united with a certain proportion of mutton suet and opium.—(*Edin. Med. Comm.*, vol. iii., p. 334.) And when we are gravely told that this preparation never fails to *dissolve* the stone, we are at no loss to settle the account upon this subject, and can trace the real cause of whatever degree of ease that may have been derived from such an injection, and can allow that even the alkali itself, if not in too concentrated a state, may have been of occasional advantage. MM. Prevost and Dumas have since tried an application of the galvanic fluid for the same purpose, but it does not appear, with a success that is likely to render such an attempt popular.

When, however, all these means of relief fail, and the general health is worn out by a long succession of pain and anxiety, nothing remains but the operation of extraction. The shortness and expansibility of the urethra in women, which allows, as we have already seen, a passage for calculi of a considerable calibre to pass naturally, has suggested an idea of the possibility of introducing a stone-forceps into the female bladder, so as to supply the place of lithotomy. The first hint of this kind that has occurred to me is to be found in the Gallicinium Medicopracticum of Gockel, published at Ulm in 1700. It was afterward taken up, perhaps originally started, by Mr. Bromfield, who ingeniously advised, that the urethra should, for this purpose, be dilated by forcing water through the gut of a fowl introduced into the urethra as an expansile cannula. Mr. Thomas has since, by the use of a sponge tent gradually enlarged for the purpose, succeeded in introducing his finger into the bladder, and bringing away an ivory earpick, which had been incautiously used as a catheter, and had slipped into the cavity of this organ (*Trans. of the Medico-Chir. Society*, vol. i., p. 124) : and Sir Astley Cooper has still more lately devised an instrument, that by a gradually enlarging pressure, by means of its opening blades, will accomplish the same object in a single night, or even a few hours, and has rendered an extraction of calculi from the female bladder a comparatively simple and easy operation, attended indeed with little inconvenience.

M. Civiale has taken advantage of this wonderful power of dilatation in the urethra, and has endeavoured to avail himself of it in males as well as in females ; not, indeed, with a view of bringing away a calculus of any considerable size through the male urethra in an *entire* state, but by grinding, or, as we should now perhaps call it, *macadamizing*, the stone into granules so fine as to pass without difficulty. The instrument is highly ingenious, whatever becomes of its general success, and this plan has justly obtained a panegyric from MM. Chaussier and Percy, appointed as a committee to examine into its pretensions by the Royal Academy of Sciences. It consists of a *straight* and hollow cylinder, of a diameter as large as the urethra can be made to admit; through this tube, when it has entered the bladder, is introduced another instrument made of steel, and consisting of three elastic and curved claws, capable of seizing and fixing the stone when projected. It consists also, besides such pincers, of a stillet of the same metal, at the extremity of which is a circular saw, which can be worked upon the stone, and abrade it till it is entirely comminuted, without injuring the bladder. It has already been tried on the dead, and in a few instances on the living body : but its general success is still doubtful. " Yet," observe the committee, " notwithstanding its inefficacy in some cases, and the difficulty of its application in others, it cannot fail to form an epoch in the annals of the healing art, nor to be regarded as one of its most ingenious and precious resources." Some such machine seems to have been suggested by one or two individuals antecedently, but Dr. Civiale is unquestionably the first who has produced and made trial of it.

This, however, is a method that can never be applied to males,* nor even successfully to

* Were this a treatise on surgery, the editor would here not only have corrected this part of the author's text, but have paid a tribute of praise to the several individuals by whom lithotrity and lithotripsy have been brought to their present state of efficiency ; and this more especially in relation to male subjects, to which Dr Good pronounces them unadapted, though it is for them alone they are principally of value ; the female urethra being so

females, except when the calculus is comparatively of small dimensions, or the meatus is so far dilated by the passage of former calculi as to render it unnecessary.* In all other cases, lithotomy offers the only means of removing the indissoluble stone from the bladder ; and for the various modes in which this is performed, the reader must consult the writers on practical surgery.

Calculi, thus extracted, have been found of all weights and bulks. A stone from a quarter of an ounce to half an ounce may perhaps be regarded as the ordinary average : but they have sometimes grown to a much larger size; and have still been safely extracted. The largest for which lithotomy seems at any time to have been undertaken in this country, weighed forty-four ounces,

short and dilatable, that calculi may generally be removed without any necessity for lithotomy. The dexterity of Baron Heurteloup, and the great ingenuity and power of his instruments in these operations, the editor has witnessed on several occasions ; and an opportunity of making a similar observation was kindly afforded, at the editor's request, by the Baron, last winter, to the whole of the surgical class of the London University, when he gave a full account of the instruments, and demonstrated their use on a patient brought into the theatre for the purpose. By these remarks the editor would not have it supposed, however, that he means to ascribe all the merit of bringing these operations to their modern state of improvement to any one individual ; and, in addition to the names of Civiale and Heurteloup, those of Le Roi d'Etiolle, Costello, and others, are entitled to be mentioned with commendation.—Ed.

* The operation of lithotrity has been performed successfully in the United States by Dr. Alban G. Smith of Cincinnati, Dr. Randolph of Philadelphia, and Dr. Depeyre of New-York. M. Blandin, the celebrated surgeon at the hospital Beaujon, in Paris, has ably discussed the relative merits of lithotomy and lithotrity. The following are his conclusions : 1. Hemorrhage is much more frequent and more alarming after lithotomy than after lithotrity. 2. The rectum, peritoneum, and other important organs, may be wounded in lithotomy. These accidents have been known to occur in lithotrity ; but not certainly with the present improved instruments. 3. Urinary infiltration is not uncommon after lithotomy ; rare, very rare, after lithotrity. 4. Phlebitis occurs much more frequently after lithotomy than after lithotrity ; indeed, only one instance after the latter operation is recorded. The same remark applies to peritonitis, urinary fistulæ, &c. On the other hand, it may be urged in favour of lithotomy, 1. The pain and nervous accidents are, on the whole, more severe, more prolonged, and of more frequent occurrence, after lithotrity than after lithotomy. 2. Cystitis is a sequence of lithotrity more frequently than of lithotomy. 3. The inflammation of the prostate gland, terminating in abscesses and producing retention of urine and other serious accidents, is," of greater importance" after lithotrity than after lithotomy. 4. In lithotrity, the extremity of an instrument may be broken off and left behind in the bladder. 5. The chance of reproduction of the calculus is greater after lithotrity than after lithotomy, although the conclusions of Civiale are directly opposite. (See Parallele entre la Taille et la Lithotritie, by P. F. Blandin, Paris, 1834, reviewed in the Medico-Chirurgical Review, vol. xxvi.)—D.

and was sixteen inches in length. The operation was attempted by Mr. Cline (*On Sir David Ogilvie*), but the stone could not be brought away, and the patient died in a few days.—(*Phil. Trans.*, year 1809. *By Sir James Earle presented to the College of Surgeons.*) In a foreign journal of high reputation, we have an account of a calculus found in the bladder after death, that weighed four pounds and a half, or seventy-two ounces, and seems to have filled nearly the whole of its cavity.—(*Bresl. Sammlung*, band ii., 1724, 434, 11.)

ORDER III.

ACROTICA.

DISEASES AFFECTING THE EXTERNAL SURFACE.

PRAVITY OF THE FLUIDS OR EMUNCTORIES THAT OPEN ON THE EXTERNAL SURFACE ; WITHOUT FEVER, OR OTHER INTERNAL AFFECTION, AS A NECESSARY ACCOMPANIMENT.

ACROTICA is a Greek term, from ἄκρος, "summus," whence ἀκρότης, ητος, "summitas," "cacumen." The excretories of the skin form a most important outlet of the system, and although the fluid they secrete is, in a state of health, less complicated than that of the kidneys, under a variety of circumstances it becomes more so. It is to this quarter that all the deleterious or poisonous matter, produced by eruptive fevers, is directed by the remedial power of nature, as that in which it can be thrown off with least evil to the constitution.* By the close sympathy which the surface of the body holds with the stomach, the heart, the lungs, and the kidneys, its excretories are almost perpetually varying in their action, and still more so from their direct exposure to the changeable state of the atmosphere : in consequence of which they are one moment chilled, torpid, and collapsed, and perhaps the next violently excited and irritated ; now dry and contracted ; now relaxed, and streaming with moisture ; now secreting their natural fluid alone ; and now charged with extraneous matter of various kinds.

But the mouths of the cutaneous exhalants are in their own nature peculiarly delicate and tender ; and hence the necessity of their being covered by the epithelium of a fine cuticle, which defends them in a considerable degree from the rudeness of external impressions or irritants with which the air is impregnated.† This defence, however, they frequently lose ; often from external violence, and often also, from the acrimony or roughness of the materials that are

thus transmitted to them, and which excoriate as effectually as friction, a keen frosty northeast wind, or the direct rays of a tropical sun. And at times the absorbents of the skin are torpid or weak in their action ; and the finer parts only of the fluids that are secerned are imbibed and carried off, while the grosser parts remain and accumulate in the cutaneous follicles. And hence a great variety of superficial eruptions, papulous, pustulous, and ichorous, squammose, or furfuraceous. And not unfrequently there is a constitutional irritability of the skin, which not only renders it peculiarly liable to be excited by slight causes in every part, but to sympathize in the morbid action through its whole extent, in whatever part it may commence : and hence the spread of eruptions to a greater or less extent, sometimes, indeed, over the entire surface. A knowledge of this fact is of great importance, for we can often avail ourselves of it in the treatment of constitutional or organic affections of considerable severity or danger ; and by exciting a temporary irritation on the skin, mitigate or entirely subdue the original malady. All the benefits derived from the eruptions produced by the tartar-emetic ointment,* blisters, sinapisms, and the entire host of counter-irritants, as applied to the surface, are dependant upon this extensive and important principle in pathology.

From these sources of affection, a variety of complaints must necessarily take their rise, none of them perhaps fatal to life, but many of them peculiarly troublesome and obstinate. They may be arranged under the following genera :—

I. Ephidrosis.	Morbid Sweat.
II. Exanthesis.	Cutaneous Blush.
III. Exormia.	Papulous Skin.
IV. Lepidosis.	Scale Skin.
V. Ecphlysis.	Blains.
VI. Ecpyesis.	Scall. Tetter.
VII. Malis.	Cutaneous Vermination.
VIII. Ecphyma.	Cutaneous Excrescence.
IX. Trichosis.	Morbid Hair.
X. Epichrosis.	Macular Skin.

Most of these genera contain numerous species, many of which, though by no means all, form a part of Dr. Willan's arrangement, and have been described by himself or my late excellent friend Dr. Bateman, of whose labours I shall avail myself, as far as they may answer the present purpose. By Professor Frank they have been marshalled under the term IMPETI-

---

* Whether any deleterious matter is actually thrown off in this manner, is a doctrine that will probably not be satisfactory to many good pathologists. It is the particular character of certain diseases to produce, among other effects, increased perspiration, spots, efflorescences, and various kinds of eruptions, as they are commonly termed ; yet there is no proof that these affections constitute so many modes for the passage of deleterious matter out of the system. To the editor, this language appears only allowable in a figurative sense. —ED.

† Lectures on the general Structure of the Human Body, and on the Anatomy and Functions of the Skin, &c. By Thomas Chevalier, F. R. S., &c., lect. vi., vii., London, 1823.

* Letter to C. H. Parry, M. D., F. R. S., on the Influence of Artificial Eruptions in certain Diseases, &c. By Edward Jenner, Esq., M. D., 4to., Lond., 1822.

GINES, employed, but with a latitude never assigned it before, as the name of a class, divided into the two orders of MACULOSÆ and DEPASCENTES.

GENUS I.
EPHIDROSIS.
MORBID SWEAT.
PRETERNATURAL SECRETION OF CUTANEOUS PERSPIRATION.

EPHIDROSIS (ἐφίδρωσις) is a Greek term for "sudor." The matter of sweat and that of insensible perspiration are nearly the same; the former consisting of the latter with a small intermixture of animal oil. It is affirmed by some writers, that there are persons who never perspire. This demands ample proof; for experience teaches us, that all warm-blooded animals either perspire by the skin, or have some vicarious evacuation that supplies its place, as in the place of the dog kind, in which an increased discharge of saliva seems to answer the purpose; though, in violent agony, I have known a Newfoundland dog thrown into a sweat that has drenched the whole of his thick and wavy hair. In cold-blooded animals we sometimes find partial secretions, as in the lizards, the exudation from some of which, particularly the lacerta geitja of the Cape of Good Hope, is highly acrid: and, as it touches the hands and feet of men, occasionally produces dangerous gangrenes. Generally speaking, however, cold-blooded animals secrete but a small quantity of fluid from the surface, and consequently suffer but little exhaustion or diminution of weight, and can live long without nourishment: and it is hence probable that, among mankind, those who throw off but a small quantity of halitus, may exist upon a very spare supply of food; which may afford a solution to many of the wonderful stories of fasting persons, most of whom seem to have passed sedentary and inactive lives, recorded in the scientific journals of different countries, a subject we have already discussed (vol. i., Cl., I., Ord. I., Limosis expers, p. 82): for the matter of insensible perspiration is calculated, upon an average, as being daily equal in weight to half the food introduced into the stomach in the course of the day. Thus, if a man of good health and middle age, weighing about 146lbs. avoirdupois, eat and drink at the rate of fifty-six ounces in twenty-four hours, he will commonly be found to lose about twenty-eight ounces within the same period by insensible perspiration: sixteen ounces during the two thirds of this period allotted to wakefulness, and twelve ounces during the remaining third allotted to sleep.

It sometimes happens that this evacuation is secreted in excess, and becomes sensible, so as to render the whole, or various parts of the body, and especially the palms of the hands, covered with moisture, without any misaffection of the system. It is to this species that the term ephidrosis has been usually applied and limited by nosologists. Sauvages, however, has employed it in a wider signification, so as to include various other species, and perhaps correctly; though Cullen inclines to regard all but the first as merely symptomatic of some other complaint.

The following appear to be those which are chiefly entitled to a specific rank :—

1. Ephidrosis	Profusa.	Profuse Sweat.
2. ————	Cruenta.	Bloody Sweat.
3. ————	Partialis.	Partial Sweat.
4. ————	Discolor.	Coloured Sweat.
5. ————	Olens.	Scented Sweat.
6. ————	Arenosa.	Sandy Sweat.

SPECIES I.
EPHIDROSIS PROFUSA.
PROFUSE SWEAT.
CUTANEOUS PERSPIRATION SECRETED PROFUSELY.

THIS is commonly a result of relaxed fibres: the mouths of the cutaneous exhalants being too loose and patulous,* and the perspirable fluid flowing forth copiously and rapidly upon very slight exertions, sometimes without any exertion at all; as we have already seen the urine flows in paruria aquosa, and the serum in various species of dropsy. It is the hyperhydrosis of Swediaur.

There is here, generally speaking, less solution of animal oil than in perspiration produced by exercise or hard labour (Büchner, Diss. de Sudore Colliquativo, Hal., 1757): but from the drain that is perpetually taking place, no animal oil accumulates, and the frame is usually slender. Corpulent persons also perspire much, but this is altogether from a different cause, being that of the weight they have to carry, and the labour with which breathing and every other function are performed, in consequence of the general oppression of the system. Here also an extenuation of the frame would soon follow, but that, from the peculiar diathesis which so readily predisposes to the formation of fat, the supply is always equal to, and for the most part continues to exceed, the waste, unless a more than ordinary course of exertion be engaged in.

In persons of relaxed fibres, but whose general health is sound, I have frequently perceived that there is no particular liability to catch cold, notwithstanding this tendency to perspiration; and have very often seen it suddenly checked

---

* This hypothesis of increased secretion being dependant on too relaxed a state of the secement or excretory vessels, is rather a favourite one with our author, as appears from various passages in his work. Is it, however, sound pathology? Probably not; for, if we were to suppose, in the present instance, the cutaneous exhalants preternaturally relaxed and open, the profuse secretion of perspiration would still require for its explanation an increased action of the cutaneous vessels and glands from which it is derived. The expression, "relaxed fibres," made use of in the text, can be understood as meaning nothing more than a debilitated habit. In this sense, there may be some truth in it; but—if it were to be received in its literal meaning, it would be liable to criticism.—ED.

without any evil : such is the wonderful effect of an established habit. But the moment the general health suffers, or the system becomes seriously weakened by its continuance, the sweat is apt to become colliquative, and to terminate in a decline.*

Tulpius gives a case of its continuing for seven years.—(Lib. iii., cap. 42.) Astringents of all kinds have been tried, but with variable effects. Dr. Percival relied chiefly on bark ; De Haen employed the white agaric (Rat. Med., p. xii., cap. vi., ◊ 6), and in the Journal de Médecine (tom. xlviii.), the same medicine is recommended under the name of *fungus laricis* ; it is the *boletus laricis* of the present day. It was given in the form of troches and pills. Cold sea-bathing, and the mineral acids, with temperate exercise, light animal food, and the use of a hair mattress, instead of a down bed at night, have proved successful on many occasions, and form the best plan.

SPECIES II.
EPHIDROSIS CRUENTA.
BLOODY SWEAT.
CUTANEOUS PERSPIRATION INTERMIXED WITH BLOOD.

THIS species has not been very commonly described by nosologists ; but the cases of idiopathic affection are so numerous and so clearly marked by other writers, that it ought not to be passed over.—(Ploucq. Init., vii., 316.)

We have noticed a sympathetic and vicarious affection of this kind under the genus MISMENSTRUATION, and have there observed, that the cutaneous exhalants, in such instances, become enlarged in their diameter, and suffer red blood, or a fluid of the appearance of red blood, to pass through them. In cases of extreme debility from other causes, as in the last and fatal stage of atonic fevers, or in sea or land scurvy (N. Act. Nat. Cur., vol. iv., obs. 41 ; Bresl.

* Little doubt can be entertained, that what is here stated to be the cause of the decline is the effect of it. In phthisis, hectical symptoms, and among them profuse perspirations, always show themselves in the course of the disease. It is difficult to understand how tuberculated lungs could arise from profuse perspiration. The cause of the profuse sweats into which certain individuals readily fall, though their health seems good, has not hitherto been satisfactorily explained. Convalescents sometimes have similar dispositions, which cease as the strength returns. The effusion of sweat with coldness of the skin, often noticed in dying persons, is quite as familiar as it is inexplicable. As Andral has remarked (Anat. Pathol., tom. i., p. 337), we know nothing about the reason of certain diseases, or stages of them, being attended with perspiration ; why acute rheumatism should be accompanied by frequent and copious sweats ; why sweats should be so constantly an attendant of suppurated pulmonary tubercles ; while, on the contrary, the skin is so remarkably dry in chronic gastritis. Is it that in phthisical subjects the cutaneous exhalation makes up for the suspension of that from the lungs ?—ED.

Samml., 1725, i., p. 183), blood has been known to flow from the cutaneous exhalants in like manner. None of these, however, are idiopathic affections. When the discharge shows itself as a primary disease, the cause has generally been some violent commotion of the nervous system forcing the red particles into the cutaneous excretories, rather than a simple influx from a relaxed state of their fibres. And hence it has taken place occasionally during coition (Paullini, cent. iii., obs. 46 ; Eph. Nat. Cur., dec. ii., ann. vi., Appx., pp. 4, 45, 55) ; sometimes during vehement terror ; and not unfrequently during the agony of hanging or the torture.—(Bartholinus, epist. i., p. 718.) It is said also to have occurred in new-born infants.— (Eph. Nat. Cur., dec. ii., ann. x., obs. 65.)

SPECIES III.
EPHIDROSIS PARTIALIS.*
PARTIAL SWEAT.
CUTANEOUS PERSPIRATION LIMITED TO A PARTICULAR PART OR ORGAN.

THERE are some persons who rarely perspire ; others, who perspire far more freely from one organ than another, as the head, or the feet, or the body. Such abnormities rather predispose to morbid affections, than are morbid affections themselves. Sauvages, in illustration of the present species, quotes a case from Hartmann, of a woman who was never capable of being thrown into a sweat, either by nature or art, in any part of her body, except when she was pregnant, at which time she perspired on the left side alone.—(Hartmanni, De Sudore unius Lateris, 4to., 1740.) Schmidt has noticed a like anomaly.—(Collect. Acad., vol. iii., p. 577.)

In this last case, it is probable that the kidneys became a substitute for the action of the cutaneous exhalants, as we see they do on various occasions, as when their mouths become collapsed from the chilly spasm that shoots over them on plunging into a cold bath, or in a fit of hysterics.

The sweat thus discharged from a partial outlet is frequently fetid, as under the fifth species of the present genus ; and, when it is constitutional, it is often repelled with great danger to some more important organ.

SPECIES IV.
EPHIDROSIS DISCOLOR.
COLOURED SWEAT.
CUTANEOUS PERSPIRATION POSSESSING A DEPRAVED TINGE.

SWEAT is often tinged with a deeper yellow than is natural to it, from a resorption of bile into the bloodvessels ; and, as we have already seen, it is sometimes intermixed with blood, from violence, or a relaxed state of the cutaneous exhalants. And when these, or causes

* E. partialis sometimes accompanies paralytic affections.—D.

like these, co-operate, we can readily account for the various colours it has sometimes exhibited, as green, black, blue, saffron, or ruby (*Swediaur, Nov. Nos. Meth. Syst.*, i., 219) ; in the language of Professor Frank, "color nunc pallidè flavescens, nunc lacteus, vel croceus, sanguineus, ac interdum subviridis, cœruleus, aut ater" (*De Cur. Hom. Morb. Epit.*, tom. v., p. 27, Manuh., 8vo., 1792) ; examples of all which are referred to in the volume of Nosology. We see, indeed, the whole of these hues produced daily under the cuticle from the extravasation of blood, according as the effused fluid is more or less impregnated with the colouring matter of the blood, and the finer and more limpid parts are first absorbed and carried off. It is possible also, that in some of the cases referred to, the stain may have been produced by inhaling a vapour impregnated with metallic corpuscles or some other pigment ; and especially when working in metallurgical trades or quicksilver mines.*

SPECIES V.
EPHIDROSIS OLENS.
SCENTED SWEAT.
CUTANEOUS PERSPIRATION POSSESSING A DEPRAVED SMELL.

THE varieties that have been chiefly noticed are those of a sulphureous scent ; of a sour scent ; of a rank or fetid scent ; of a violet (Id., dec. iii., ann. ix., x., obs. 96), and of a musky scent.—(*Paullini*, cent. i., obs. 21 ; *Eph. Nat. Cur.*, dec. ii., ann. v., Appx., p. 9.) The rank or fetid scent is sometimes partial ; being only evacuated from particular organs, as the feet and axillæ. De Monteaux, however, has found the same thrown off generally (*Maladies de Femmes*, tom. ii.) : and, as a symptom in atonic fevers, it must have been witnessed by most practitioners, as also in several sordid cutaneous eruptions.† In fevers, moreover, we frequently meet with a secretion of sour perspiration, which, in a few instances, has had the pungency of vinegar. When such smells accompany diseases, they usually cease on the cessation of the disease which gives rise to them. When they are habitual, they often depend upon a morbid state of the stomach, or of the cutaneous excretories ; and will often yield to a course of aperients or alterants, a frequent use of the warm, and, when the constitution will allow, of the cold bath, and such exercise, as shall call forth a copious discharge of perspira-

---

* In the London Medical Gazette for 1832-3, p. 211, the reader may find the particulars of a case of green perspiration, which was ascertained to derive its colour from an admixture of the acetate of copper. The patient, a young lady æt. 14, had had the milk which she took for breakfast boiled in a copper vessel, the tin lining of which was worn away, to the extent of one half of it. The case is drawn up by Dr. Prichard of Leamington.—ED.
† The discharge or matter of eruptions cannot be called sweat or perspiration, with any degree of correctness.—ED.

ble matter, and free the cutaneous follicles or orifices of whatever olid materials may lodge in them.

Many of these, however, are often dependant upon the diet or manner of life. Thus, the food of garlic yields a perspiration possessing a garlic smell ; that of peas a leguminous smell, which is the cause of this peculiar odour among the inhabitants of Greenland ; and acids a smell of acidity. Among glass-blowers, from the large quantity of sea-salt that enters into the materials of their manufacture, the sweat is sometimes so highly impregnated that the salt they employ and imbibe by the skin and lungs has been seen to collect in crystals upon their faces. A musky scent is not often thrown forth from the human body ; but it is perhaps the most common of all odours that escape from the skin of other animals. We discover it in many of the ape kind, and especially in the *simia jacchus ;* still more profusely in the opossum, and occasionally in hedgehogs, hares, serpents, and crocodiles. The odour of civet is the production of the civet-cat alone,—the *viverra zibetha* and *viverra civetta* of Linnéus,—though we meet with faint traces of it in some varieties of the domestic cat. Among insects, however, such odours are considerably more common, and by far the greater number of them are of an agreeable kind, and of very high excellence ; for the musk scent of the *cerambix moschatus,* the *apis fragrans,* and the *tipula moschifera,* is much more delicate than that of the musk quadrupeds : while the *cerambix suaveolens,* and several species of the ichneumon, yield the sweetest perfume of the rose ; and the petiolated sphex a balsamic ether highly fragrant, but peculiar to itself.

SPECIES VI.
EPHIDROSIS ARENOSA.
SANDY SWEAT.
CUTANEOUS PERSPIRATION, CONTAINING A DISCHARGE OF SANDY OR OTHER GRANULAR MOLECULES.

As the odorous particles of both animal and vegetable food are sometimes absorbed by the lacteals, and impregnate the matter of perspiration, so at times are the more solid particles of the materials employed in handicraft trades absorbed by the lungs, and equally thrown forth upon the surface. This, as observed under the last species, is particularly the case with glass-blowers, upon whose forehead and arms salt is often seen to collect and crystallize in great abundance, from the quantity of this material which they employ in the manufacture of glass, and its diffusion through the heated atmosphere of the workshop in minute and imperceptible particles.

But a reddish sandy material is occasionally found to concrete on the surface of the body under other circumstances, and which cannot be charged to any material volatilized in the course of business. Bartholin (*Hist. Anat.*, cent. i., 34), Schurig (*Litholog.*, p. 235), Mollenbroek

(*De Vasis*, cap. xiii.), and various other writers, have given instances of this kind of crystallization, which seems to consist in an excess of free uric acid, translated from the kidneys to the skin by an idiopathic sympathy, and forming red sand on the surface, as it probably would otherwise have done in the bladder or the urinal. It is possible, indeed, that a man may hereby escape from the fabrication of a urinary calculus, or stone in the bladder : and were such a transfer at all times in our power, we should gladly avail ourselves of it in many cases of a lithic diathesis, and employ it as a preventive of urinary concretions. When the sand is troublesome from the quantity collected, the alkaline and other medicines recommended under *lithia renalis* will easily remove it.*

GENUS II.

EXANTHESIS.

CUTANEOUS BLUSH.

SIMPLE, CUTANEOUS, ROSE-COLOURED EFFLORESCENCE, IN CIRCUMSCRIBED PLOTS, WITH LITTLE OR NO ELEVATION.

EXANTHESIS is a Greek compound, from ἰξ, "extra," and ἀνθέω, "floreo," superficial or cutaneous efflorescence, in contradistinction to ENANTHESIS, in Class III., Order IV., rash fever, or "efflorescence springing from within."

This genus affords but one known species, the specific name for which is taken from Dr. Willan :—

1. Exanthesis Roseola.　　　Rose-rash.

SPECIES I.

EXANTHESIS ROSEOLA.

ROSE-RASH.

EFFLORESCENCE IN BLUSHING PATCHES, GRADUALLY DEEPENING TO A ROSE-COLOUR, MOSTLY CIRCULAR OR OVAL ; OFTEN ALTERNATELY FADING AND REVIVING ; SOMETIMES WITH A COLOURLESS UMBO ; CHIEFLY ON THE CHEEKS, NECK, OR ARMS.

ROSEOLA was sometimes employed by the older writers, though in a very loose sense, to signify scarlet fever, measles, and one or two other exanthems, that were often confounded ; but, as it is now no longer used for these, it

---

* The cases described in this section require confirmation ; for, in their nature, they approach the marvellous. With respect to the crystallization of salt on the faces and arms of glass-blowers, the very parts on which they are alleged to occur seem to imply, that the salt is not perspired in that abundant manner in consequence of a previous absorption of it ; but, that the atmosphere, being impregnated with its vapour, some of this collects on the brow and arms, and, mixing with moisture really perspired there, becomes crystallized. But, whether this explanation be more probable than what is offered in the text or not, it is certain that the examples cited by our author require the stamp of modern and unprejudiced observation, to give them all the authenticity which is desirable.—ED.

may stand well enough as a name for the present species, which Fuller has described as a flushing all over the body like fine crimson, which is void of danger, and "rather a ludicrous spectacle than an ill symptom."—(*Exanthematologia*, p. 128 ; *Bateman's Synops.*, 95.)

As a symptom, this rash is frequently met with in various maladies. Thus, in the dentition of infancy, it appears on the cheeks ; in the inoculated cowpox, around the vesicle ; in dyspepsy and various fevers, in different parts of the body, constituting varieties, several of which by Dr. Willan are named, according to the disease they accompany, Roseola infantilis, R. variolosa, R. vaccina, and R. miliaris : but which, as mere symptoms of other disorders, are to be sought for in the diseases of which they occasionally form a part.

In the spring and autumn it often appears to be idiopathic, especially in irritable constitutions. The occasional causes are fatigue, sudden alternations of heat and cold, or the drinking of very cold water after violent exercise. Dr. Willan mentions one instance of its occurring after sleeping in a damp bed. It has sometimes been mistaken for an eruption of the measles, and still oftener for that of a mild rosalia or scarlet fever, of which last error the same author gives an example in a child that was extensively affected with it, about midsummer, for several years in succession, and whose attendant physician informed the parents that the scarlet fever had recurred in their child seven times.*

The attack is sometimes preceded, during the heat of summer, by a slight febrile indisposition. It appears first on the face and neck, and, in the course of a day or two, is distributed over the rest of the body. The eruption spreads in small patches of various figures, but usually larger and more irregular than those of measles, often as large as a shilling, at first of a brightish red, but soon settling into the deeper hue of the damask rose. It sometimes assumes an annular form, R. annulata, and appears over the body in rose-coloured rings, with central areas, or umbos, of the usual colour of the skin : the rings being at first small, but gradually dilating to the diameter of half an inch.†

---

* Roseola may be discriminated from the appearances of the skin in scarlet fever, by the redness returning at all points, directly after the pressure of the finger is removed ; whereas, in scarlet fever, if pressure be made on the rash with the finger, the redness, on the discontinuance of such pressure, spreads gradually from the circumference of the part to the centre.—(Traité Théor. et Prat. des Maladies de la Peau, tom. i., p. 47.) When children are said to have had measles and scarlet fever half a dozen times, they have generally experienced frequent attacks of roseola only. It is, indeed, this circumstance which gives to the subject of roseola more interest than it would otherwise possess, and makes the study of its characters very necessary.—ED.

† According to Rayer, when roseola follows gastro-enteritis, it is preceded for a few days by more or less fever. It may present itself over the whole surface of the body, or it may be confined to particular regions ; in which last circumstance it ordinarily first shows itself on the face, neck,

This rash is troublesome, but of little importance otherwise. In the medical treatment of it, the state of the stomach and bowels should be particularly inquired into, and, for the most part, will be found to require correction.* Acidulated drinks, with occasional and gentle laxatives, generally remove the disease, unless it be connected with any constitutional or visceral affection, when it sometimes proves very obstinate, and can only be cured by curing the primary malady.†

GENUS III.
EXORMIA.
PAPULOUS SKIN.

SMALL ACUMINATED ELEVATIONS OF THE CUTICLE; NOT CONTAINING A FLUID, NOR TENDING TO SUPPURATION; COMMONLY TERMINATING IN SCURF.‡

For the acuminated elevation of the cuticle, which the Latins call papula, the Greeks had

---

or lower extremities. The rings in the annular variety are at first one or two lines in diameter, but gradually enlarge, leaving a central space free from redness. On the second day, roseola is of a bright red colour, and attended with slight itching, but no pricking, like that which is felt in urticaria. It never lasts beyond the fourth or fifth day, unless the disease happen to consist of a succession of eruptions.—See Rayer, Mal. de la Peau, tom. i., p. 44.—Ed.

* Alibert remarks, "Apply leeches to the seat of the disease, if it seems necessary."—D.

† In the *infantile rose-rash*, or that attendant on dentition, or other irritations peculiar to infancy, the proper treatment is that called for by the state of the constitution producing the rash; "but purgatives, and occasionally calomel and cretaceous powder, where there is much acidity of the primæ viæ, are requisite." The following prescription is given by Dr. A. T. Thomson :—

℞. Pulv. contrayervæ comp., gr. xii.
Potassæ nitratis, gr. iv. Misce.
Sit pulvis, 4ta quâque hora sumendus.

For the *annular rose-rash*, the warm bath, gentle laxatives, and the mineral acids, are recommended; and, for the chronic form of it, sea bathing. The autumnal rose-rash is benefited by an infusion of cinchona, with diluted sulph. acid and conf. rosæ, or the following mixture:—

℞. Infus. gentianæ radicis, f. ʒvj.
Magn. sulphatis, ʒiv.
Acid sulph. dilut., ℳ xvj. Misce.

Sumantur cochl. ampla, iij. 6ta quâque hora.
(See Thomson's Atlas of Delineations of Cutaneous Diseases, pp. 37, 38.) Roseola is restricted to no age nor sex; but more commonly affects children (R. infantilis). It may occur at any period of the year, but is most frequent in summer (R. æstiva) or autumn (R. autumnalis). It is often accompanied with a slight gastro-intestinal inflammation.—See Rayer, Maladies de la Peau, tom. i., p. 44.—Ed.

‡ Papulous inflammations of the skin, characterized by *papulæ*, that is to say, by solid and resisting elevations, accompanied by more or less acute itching. Papulæ ordinarily terminate in resolution and furfuraceous desquamation, but occasionally in small ulcerations.—(See Rayer, Traité Théorique et Pratique des Maladies de la Peau, tom. i., p. 560.) They are very different

---

two synonymous terms, ecthyma (ἐκθυμα) and exormia (ἐξόρμια). The first was used most frequently in this sense; but as this has by some unaccountable means been employed very generally to import quite a different eruption, a crop of large pustulous, rather than of small solid pimples, forming a species of ECPYESIS, or the sixth genus of the present Order, I have chosen the second term for the present purpose.

The common terminating diminutive (*ula* or *illa*) is probably derived from the Greek ὕλη (ulè or ilè) "materia," "materies"—*of the matter, make, or nature of*; thus, "papula, or papilla," of the matter or nature of pappus; "lupula," of the matter or nature of the lupus; "pustula," of the matter or nature of pus; and so of many others.

Papula and pustula, which by Sauvages are degraded into mere symptoms of diseases, and not allowed to constitute diseases of themselves, are raised to the rank of genera by Celsus, Linnéus, and Sagar, and, under a plural form (papulæ and pustulæ), to that of orders by Willan. In the present system, exormia and ecphlysis, intended to supply their place, are employed as generic terms, and run parallel with those papulæ and pustulæ of Willan which are not essentially connected with internal disease; and are only made use of instead of papula and pustula, first, as being more immediately Greek, and next, in order to prevent confusion from the variety of senses assigned to the latter terms by different writers. Exormia and ecphlysis, therefore, as distinct genera under the present arrangement, import eruptions of pimples and pustules in their simplest state, affecting the cuticle, or, at the utmost, the superficial integument alone, and consequently without fever or other internal complaint, as a necessary or essential symptom; although some part or other of the system may occasionally catenate or sympathize with the efflorescence. It is difficult, indeed, to draw a line of separation, and perhaps impossible to draw it exactly, between efflorescences strictly cutaneous and strictly constitutional, from the numerous examples we meet with of the one description combining with or passing into the other. But a like difficulty belongs to every other branch of physiology, in the widest sense of the term, as well as to nosology; and all we can do in any division of the science is, to lay down the boundary with as much nicety and

---

from exanthematous inflammations, which present spots instead of elevations; and they are equally dissimilar from bullous, vesicular, and pustular inflammations, in which a serous or purulent fluid is deposited between the cuticle and the corpus reticulare. However, in order to distinguish the papulæ of lichen and prurigo from the minute vesicles of the itch and eczema, it is necessary, as Rayer observes, carefully to inspect these different elevations with a magnifying-glass. When papulæ have been injured by scratching, or when they have been replaced by furfuraceous desquamations or excoriations, the diagnosis is sometimes involved in such obscurity that it can only be dispelled by watching the formation of new elevations, whose papular form reveals the nature of the previous ones.—Op. cit., tom. i., p. 562.—Ed.

caution as possible, and to correct it, as corrections may afterward be called for.

The species which belong to this genus, or which, in other words, are characterized by a papulous skin not necessarily connected with an internal affection, are the following:—

1. Exormia Strophulus.　Gum-rash.
2. ――― Lichen.　Lichenous Rash.
3. ――― Prurigo.　Pruriginous Rash.
4. ――― Milium.　Millet-rash.*

SPECIES I.
EXORMIA STROPHULUS.
GUM-RASH.

ERUPTION OF RED PIMPLES IN EARLY INFANCY, CHIEFLY ABOUT THE FACE, NECK, AND ARMS, SURROUNDED BY A REDDISH HALO; OR INTERRUPTED BY IRREGULAR PLOTS OF CUTANEOUS BLUSH.†

Dr. Willan has observed, that the colloquial name of red-gum, applied to the common form of this disease, is a corruption of red-gown, under which the disease was known in former times, and by which it still continues to be called in various districts; as though supposed, from its variegated plots of red upon a pale ground, to resemble a piece of red printed linen. In effect, it is written red-gown in most of the old dictionaries; in Littleton's, as late as 1684: and, I believe, to the present day. The varieties in Willan are the following, whose descriptions are large and somewhat loose. We may extract from them, however, the subjoined distinctions of character:—

a Intertinctus. Pimples bright red; distinct;
　Red-gum.　intermixed with stigmata and red patches; sometimes spreading over the body.

β Albidus.　Pimples minute, hard, whitish;
　White-gum.　surrounded by a reddish halo.

γ Confertus.　Pimples red, of different sizes,
　Tooth-rash.　crowding or in clusters; the larger surrounded by a red halo; occasionally succeeded by a red crop.

δ Volaticus.　Pimples deep-red, in circular
　Wildfire-rash.　patches, or clusters; clus-

---

ters sometimes solitary on each arm or cheek; more generally flying from part to part.

ε Candidus.　Pimples large, glabrous, shi-
　Pallid gum-　ning; of a lighter hue than
　rash.　the skin: without halo or blush.*

Generally speaking, none of these varieties are of serious importance; and all of them, being consistent with a healthy state of the functions of the body, require but little attention from medical practitioners. Several of them are occasionally connected with acidity, or some other morbid symptom of the stomach and bowels, and hence particular attention should be paid to the primæ viæ.† The system, also, suffers generally, in many cases, if the efflorescence be suddenly driven inwards by exposure to currents of cold air, or by the use of cold bathing. Both these, therefore, should be avoided while the efflorescence continues; and if such an accident should occur, the infant should be immediately plunged into a warm bath, which commonly succeeds in reproducing the eruption, when constitutional illness ceases.—(*Bronzet, sur l'Education des Enfans,* p. 187.) In every variety, indeed, the nurse should be directed to keep the child's skin clean, and to promote an equable perspiration by daily ablutions with tepid water, which are useful in most cutaneous disorders; and will be found, in other respects, of material importance to the health of children.‡

---

* The papulæ of strophulus are whiter or redder than the surrounding healthy skin; those of prurigo, when not disturbed, are nearly of the same colour as the skin. Besides, each of the successive eruptions constituting strophulus constantly exhibits the course of an acute disease, while prurigo partakes more of the nature of a chronic one. On the contrary, according to Rayer, a marked line of demarcation between strophulus and lichen is difficult to form. It seems to him that the shades of difference between these two diseases are probably the result of differences in the ages and conditions of the individuals affected with them. The papulæ of lichen are, indeed, sometimes red, inflamed, scattered, or collected in groups, like those of strophulus; but the latter has intermissions and periodical exacerbations more frequently than the former; while, on the other hand, strophulus never terminates in excoriations like those of lichen agrius. Strophulus confertus may be known from marbled or mottled patches of erythema, the latter being smooth, not prominent, and destitute of papulæ.—See Rayer, tom. i., p. 567.—Ed.

† Strophulus is sometimes brought on by direct irritation of the skin from coarse woollen clothes, exposure of the body to too much heat or uncleanliness; but, most commonly, it is symptomatic of gastro-intestinal inflammation, excited by food in too great abundance, or of bad quality, the process of dentition, &c.—See Rayer, Traité Théorique et Pratique des Maladies de la Peau, tom. i., p. 564.—Ed.

‡ When strophulus has arisen from any irritation of the surface of the body, the first and principal indication is to remove this cause. The pruritus may be temporarily relieved by applying

---

* Rayer, in noticing the three kinds of papulous inflammation usually described, namely, strophulus, lichen, and prurigo, expresses his opinion, that their number ought to be reduced to two; strophulus appearing to him to be only a modification of lichen in new-born children and those at the breast.—(Op. cit. vol. cit., p. 560.) Strophulus is a disease of early infancy; lichen affects children and adults; prurigo children and aged persons. None of these diseases is contagious; but individuals who have once had them, almost always have fresh attacks of them at variable intervals, and especially from atmospherical vicissitudes.—Ed.

† Strophulus is a cutaneous inflammation, common in children at the breast, characterized by pruriginous, red, or white papulæ, of variable size, appearing in succession, disappearing and returning sometimes in an intermittent manner, and ending in resolution or a furfuraceous desquamation.—See Rayer, Traité des Maladies de la Peau, tom. i., p. 563.—Ed.

In the tooth-rash, *strophulus confertus*, there is no difficulty in tracing the ordinary cause. Yet this, also, has often been ascribed to a state of indigestion, or some feverish complaint in the mother or nurse. "I have, however," says Dr. Willan, "frequently seen the eruption where no such cause for it was evident. It may, with more propriety, be ranked among the numerous symptoms of irritation arising from the inflamed and painful state of the gums in dentition, since it always occurs during that process, and disappears soon after the first teeth have cut through the gums." It may, however, like the red-gum, *s. intertinctus*, be occasionally connected with a weak and irritable state of the bowels : though the tender and delicate state of the skin, and the strong determination of blood to the surface which evidently takes place in early infancy, and is the common proximate cause of the red-gum, is probably the common remote cause of the tooth-rash.

The tooth-rash is the severest form in which strophulus shows itself. Instead of being confined to the face and breast, it often spreads widely over the body, though it appears chiefly, in a diffused state, on the forearm. Dr. Willan notices a very obstinate and painful modification of this disorder, which sometimes takes place on the lower extremities. " The papulæ spread from the calves of the legs to the thighs, nates, loins, and round the body, as high as the navel : being very numerous and close together, they produce a continuous redness over all the parts above mentioned. The cuticle probably becomes shrivelled, cracks in various places, and finally separates from the skin in large pieces." It has some resemblance to the intertrigo, which however may be distinguished by having a uniform red, shining surface, without papulæ, and being limited to the nates and thighs.

In like manner, those children are most liable to the *strophulus volaticus*, or wildfire-rash, who have a fair and irritable skin, though this also occasionally catenates with the morbid state of the stomach and bowels. It appears sometimes as early as between the third and sixth month, but more frequently later.

This last is the erythema volaticum of Sauvages, the æstus volaticus of many earlier writers : whence the French name of feu volage. All these terms have, however, been often used in a very indefinite sense, and hence, also, applied to one or two species of porrigo, and especially *porrigo crustacea*, or crusta lactea.—(*Astruc, De Morb. Infant.*, p. 44.) And hence, Dr. Armstrong has described this last disease as a strophulus, or tooth-rash.—(*On the Diseases of Children*, p. 34.)

The *strophulus albidus*, and *strophulus candidus*, are the two slightest varieties of this species of indisposition. The first is chiefly limited to the face, neck, and breast, and often continues in the form of numerous hard, whitish specks, for a long time, which on the removal of their tops do not discharge any fluid, though it is probable that they were originally formed by a deposition of fluid, which afterward concreted under the cuticle. The pimples in the strophulus candidus are larger, and diffused over a wider space ; often distributed over the loins, shoulders, and upper part of the arms ; though they rarely descend further.

Several of the varieties occasionally coexist and run into each other, particularly the first two.*

SPECIES II.
EXÒRMIA LICHEN.
LICHENOUS RASH.

ERUPTION DIFFUSE ; PIMPLES RED ; TROUBLESOME SENSE OF TINGLING OR PRICKING.†

LICHEN (λειχὴν-ος) is a term common to the Greek phytologists as well as the Greek pathologists. By the former it is applied to that extensive genus of the algæ, or rather to many of its species, which still retains the name of lichen in the Linnéan system : and it is conjectured by Pliny that the physicians applied the same name to the species of disease before us from the resemblance it produces on the surface of the body to many of the spotty and minutely tubercular lichens, which are found wild upon stones, walls, and the bark of trees or shrubs. Gorræus, however, gives two other origins of the term ; one of which he does not approve, from the eruption being supposed to be cured by

---

cold water, containing a little of the muriate of soda, or vinegar, to the papulæ. These lotions will even be serviceable when strophulus is symptomatic of inflammation of the digestive organs. But, in this case, it is above all things necessary to combat the internal affection by suitable diet, and the daily use of a tepid bath of a decoction of bran. The cold bath will lessen and completely remove this papulous inflammation with great rapidity ; but it exasperates the gastro-intestinal inflammation frequently existing as a complication. Rayer pronounces purgatives to be equally hurtful, and expresses disapprobation of the emetic and tonic treatment recommended by Willan ; for he considers that the digestive organs should not be disturbed and irritated with such medicines.—See Rayer, Traité Théorique et Pratique des Maladies de la Peau, tom. i., p. 568.—ED.

* Underwood, on the Diseases of Children, vol. i., passim. Whatever may be the form of the eruption, strophulus is always attended with a good deal of itching, which is increased by the heat of the bed. Children are thus rendered uneasy, and prevented from sleeping ; and, with the symptoms of strophulus itself, is frequently combined disorder arising from gastro-intestinal inflammation, or dentition.—See Rayer, Traité des Maladies de la Peau, tom. i., p. 566.—ED.

† A cutaneous inflammation, frequent in adults, characterized by a simultaneous or a successive eruption of red pruriginous papulæ, either scattered or arranged in groups in one region, or over the whole surface of the body ; ordinarily terminating in a furfuraceous desquamation, and more rarely in superficial, but particularly obstinate excoriations.—(See Rayer, op. et vol. cit., p. 571.) Under the name of *papular venereal disease*, Mr. Carmichael has published several examples of lichens developed in individuals who had had contagious affections of the genital organs.—Op. et vol. cit., p. 589.—ED.

its being licked with the human tongue ; and the other, to which he inclines, from its creeping in a lambent or tongue-like form, over different parts of the body. The derivation in both these cases being λείχω, "lambo," "lingo."

It is a far more troublesome rash than the preceding ; from the severest modifications of which, however, it chiefly differs by the intolerable tingling or pricking which accompanies and peculiarly characterizes it. The following are its chief varieties :—

α Simplex. Simple lichen.	General irritation; sometimes a few febrile symptoms at the commencement ; tingling aggravated during the night ; pimples scattered over the body ; which fade and desquamate in about a week.
β Pilaris. Hair lichen.	Pimples limited to the roots of the hair; desquamate after ten days ; often alternating with complaints of the head or stomach.
γ Circumscriptus. Clustering lichen.	Pimples in clusters or patches of irregular forms, appearing in succession over the trunk and limbs; sometimes coalescing ; and occasionally reviving in successive crops, and persevering for six or eight weeks.
δ Lividus. Livid lichen.	Pimples dark-red or livid; chiefly scattered over the extremities ; desquamation at uncertain periods, succeeded by fresh crops, often persevering for several months.
ε Tropicus. Summer-rash. Prickly heat.	Pimples bright-red, size of a small pin's head ; heat, itching, and needle-like pricking ; sometimes suddenly disappearing, and producing sickness or other internal affection ; relieved by the return of a fresh crop.
ζ Ferus. Wild lichen.	Pimples in clusters or patches, surrounded by a red halo ; the cuticle growing gradually harsh, thickened, and chappy : often preceded by general irritation.
η Urticosus. Nettle lichen.	Pimples very minute, slightly elevated, reddish : intolerably itching, especially at night ; irregularly subsiding, and reappearing ; chiefly spotting the limbs ;* occa-

sionally spreading over the body,· with gnat-bite shaped wheals : from the violence of the irritation, at times accompanied with vesicles or blisters, and succeeded by an extensive exfoliation of the cuticle.* ˙

Under this species, as under the last, we may observe that all the varieties are in their purest state simple ·affections of the skin, though occasionally, probably, from peculiarity of habit, or some accidental disorder of the digestive function, connected with the state of the constitution or of the stomach or bowels. Dr. Willan, indeed, makes it a· part of his specific character, that lichen is "connected with internal disorder :" but his description is at variance ·with his definition ; for with respect to the first variety, or simple lichen, he expressly asserts (*Willan*, p. 39) that it " sometimes appears suddenly without any manifest disorder of the constitution." While in regard to the tropical lichen or prickly heat, one of the severest modifications under which the disease appears, he states, and with apparent approbation, from Winterbottom, Hillary, Clark, and Cleghorn, that it is considered as salutary; that even "a vivid eruption of the prickly heat is a proof that the person affected with it is in a good state of health ;"—that "its appearance on the skin of persons in a state of convalescence from fevers, &c., is always a favourable sign, indicating the return of health and vigour" (Id., p. 35, from *Winterbottom*); that " it· seldom causes any sickness or disorder, except the troublesome itching and pricking" (Id., p. 59, from *Hillary*) ; that "it is not attended with any febrile commotion while it continues out" (Id., p. 61, from *Clark*); and that "it is looked upon as a sign of health, and, indeed, while it continues fresh on the skin, no inconvenience arises from it except a frequent itching."—(Id., p. 63, from *Cleghorn*.) And, in like manner, Dr. Heberden observes, that some patients have found themselves well on the appearance of the eruption, but troubled with pains of the head and stomach during the time of its spread; but by far the greater number experience no other evil from it besides the intolerable anguish produced by the ·itching, which sometimes makes them fall away by breaking their rest, and·is often so tormenting as to make them almost weary of their lives. Most of these remarks apply equally to the urticose variety, one of its severest forms, as I shall have occasion to observe presently.

The simple lichen shows itself first of all by an appearance of distinct ·red papulæ about

* According to Rayer, it shows itself especially on the neck and sides of the face. The papulæ are of an irregular shape, and inflamed like the elevations produced by the bites of bugs or gnats. While the first papulæ are ending in resolution or a furfuraceous desquamation, others present themselves successively on the trunk and limbs, where they become confluent, and form small patches. Lichen urticatus is rare in young persons and

adults. Rayer has never seen it but in the heat of summer or spring. When it occurs in children, it cannot be distinguished from strophulus candidus, which seems to correspond to this variety of lichen in adults.

* Lichen urticatus (Rayer), first described by Bateman, and added to the species enumerated by Willan, received its name from the analogy which it presents in several respects to urticaria.—Ed.

the cheeks and chin, or. on the arms, with but little inflammation round their base : in the course of three or four days, the eruption spreads diffusely over the neck, body, and lower extremities, attended with an unpleasant sensation of tingling, which is sometimes aggravated during the night. In about a week, the colour of the eruption fades, and the cuticle separates in scurf. All the surface of the body, indeed, remains scurfy for a long time, but particularly the flexures of the joints. The duration of the complaint varies ; and hence, in different cases, a term of from fourteen to thirty days intervenes between the eruption and a renovation of the cuticle. "The eruption sometimes appears suddenly, without any manifest disorder of the constitution" (*Willan*, ut suprà, p. 39); and sometimes there is a febrile state, or rather a state of irritation, at the beginning of the disorder, though "seldom considerable enough to confine the patient to the house" (Id., p. 37) ; and which is relieved by the appearance of the eruption. It has occasionally been mistaken for measles or scarlatina : but its progress, and, indeed, the general nature of its symptoms, from the first, are sufficiently marked to distinguish it from either of these.*

The causes are not distinctly pointed out by any writers, and it is singular that they should have been passed by both by Willan and Bateman. So far as I have seen, this and all the varieties depend upon a peculiar irritability of the skin as its remote cause, and some accidental stimulus as its exciting cause. The irritability of the skin is sometimes constitutional, in which case the patient is subject to frequent returns of the complaint ; but it has occasionally been induced by various internal and external sources of irritation : as, a diet too luxurious or too meager; the debility occasioned by a pro-

tracted chronic disease, or an exacerbated state of the mind; an improper use of mercury, or of other preparations that have disagreed either with the stomach or the chylifacient viscera. Under any of which circumstances, a slight occasional cause is sufficient for the purpose ; as, exposure to the burning rays of a summer sun, a sudden chill on the surface, cold water drunk during great heat or perspiration ; a dose of opium or any other narcotic, or substance that disagrees with the stomach or the idiosyncrasy. Dr. Heberden has suggested another cause, as perhaps operating in various cases, and inquires, whether it may not be produced by some irritant floating in the atmosphere, of so fine a structure as to be invisible to the naked eye, as the down of various plants or insects ; and he particularly alludes to the delicate hairs of the *dolichos pruriens*, or cowhage, as occasioning the disease in the West Indies, from their attacking the skin in this manner imperceptibly. But since general ablutions afford little or no relief, and all medicated lotions are even more ineffectual ; and as we can often trace it to other causes in our own country, and are at no loss for a different cause in the West Indies, the present can hardly be allowed to be the ordinary cause, though it may become an occasional excitement.*

The remedial process should consist in keeping the bowels cool and free by neutral salts ; a mixed diet of vegetables, ripe fruits, especially of the acescent kind, as oranges and lemons, and fresh animal food ; with an abstinence from fermented liquors, a light and cool dress, an open exposure to pure air, and an occasional use of the tepid bath.† The mineral acids have sometimes proved serviceable, but not always ;‡ and the red or black hydrargyri sulphuretum

---

* The lichen simplex, even in an extensive form, cannot be confounded with measles, scarlatina, and other exanthemata, the spots or cutaneous rednesses of which are entirely different from the papulæ of lichen. The only affections which it is liable to be mistaken for, are the itch and prurigo. In the latter, however, which is a papulous disease, as well as lichen itself, the papulæ are more considerable, and of the same colour as the skin ; not red and vivid, like those of lichen. Prurigo is attended with violent pruritus, while lichen usually brings on only a degree of pricking or tickling, the patient not experiencing pruritus except when his body has been exposed to heat, or he has been guilty of some excess in diet, especially with reference to spirituous liquors. As for itch, *vesicles* are its special character ; whereas lichen is an eruption of *papulæ*. The vesicles of itch are almost always situated on the inside of the arm and forearm, on the wrists, and between the fingers ; but the papulæ of lichen usually occupy the outer and posterior surfaces of the limbs. In a few rare cases, simple lichen affects the hands ; but then the papulæ are commonly in groups on the dorsal surface of the hand, while the vesicles of itch are chiefly situated in the interspaces of the fingers. The papulæ of lichen, particularly when confluent, are surrounded by small delicate scales : the vesicles of itch are never encircled by scales, but by small scabs.—See Rayer, op. et vol. cit., p. 581. —ED.

* The following are the remarks on the prognosis, delivered by Rayer :—The duration of simple lichens, occasioned by the heat of summer, differs from one to two or three weeks. When lichen is the effect of unknown causes, or of such as have not acted immediately on the skin, it is sometimes very incontrollable, and may last, whatever may be the disposition of the papulæ, for several months, or even years. In general, lichen is serious and difficult of cure, when it is of long standing, and characterized by successive eruptions, formed in individuals of advanced age and impaired constitutions. The lichen agrius of the face is ordinarily very obstinate, and subject to frequent relapses.—Op. et vol. cit., p. 585.—ED.

† In the summer time, Rayer prefers cold bathing, which he finds often sufficient to remove the complaint, and this without any danger. Warm baths, he says, often increase the inconveniences, and especially in cases of lichen urticatus.—ED.

‡ When the eruption resists cold bathing, Rayer approves of the trial of beverages strongly acidulated with the nitric, muriatic, or sulphuric acid ; and, when the digestive organs are too irritable to bear these acids, lemon-juice or vinegar may be substituted for them. When the papulæ are very numerous, crowded together, and confluent at several points, as in the lichen agrius, he recommends the antiphlogistic treatment to be more energetic, and, in young subjects, general and local bleeding frequently repeated, care being taken, when leeches are used, to place them out

has been thought useful by many ; but the plan proposed by Mr. Wilkinson for the severer kinds of the disease, will here also be often found well worthy of trial ; which consists in a calomel purge twice a week, and the internal use of the subcarbonate of ammonia,.in a dose of five or six grains, four or five times a day.— (*Remarks on Cutaneous Diseases*, 1822.)

When the system is evidently in an empoverished state, from previous sickness, innutritive food, or any mesenteric affection, bark, the mineral acids, or the metallic tonics, afford a reasonable hope of relief, and especially such preparations of iron as may sit easy on the stomach.*

The HAIR LICHEN and CLUSTERING LICHEN differ from the preceding in little more than a difference of station or of form. Their causes or mode of treatment run parallel, and it is not needful to enlarge on them farther.

The LIVID LICHEN is evidently connected with a weak and debilitated habit. Its papulæ are often interspersed with petechiæ, sometimes, indeed, with purple patches or vibices, and manifest a state of constitution bordering on that of scurvy or porphyra. Here the diet, regimen, and medical treatment should be altogether tonic and cordial, and may be taken from the plan already proposed for this last malady.—(Cl. III., Ord. IV., Spe. 10.)

of the circle of the eruption, as otherwise the irritation of their bites would augment the papulous inflammation. Cold lotions, soothing fomentations, and bathing the parts in tepid mucilaginous lotions, are the local means advised by this author. Coarse linen should not be allowed to touch the skin, as it would occasion irritation ; and thick clothes, which would heat the body too much, are to be avoided. These means are to be aided with low diet.—Op. et vol. cit., p. 586.—ED.

* As Rayer has observed, however, the practitioner must not forget to employ likewise such remedies as operate immediately on the skin. When lichen is extensive, and affects the integuments deeply, the complaint will sometimes be benefited by gentle friction with an ointment, containing sulphur, combined with the subcarbonate of potash or soda; the parts being at the same time bathed in cool emollient lotions. If the skin were dry, a few trials of the vapour-bath might do good; but if repeated too often, they might render the papulæ worse. Rayer observes, that sulphureous baths constantly prove pemicious in acute, and are seldom useful in chronic lichen ; never succeeding, indeed, but in the decline of this affection. When the state of the digestive organs does not prohibit the practice, he approves of the diluted mineral acids. In cases of excoriated lichen agrius, they lessen the secretion from the broken papulæ, appease the pruritus, and contribute to the cure. Then, also, gentle purgatives, frequently repeated, are proper ; but care is to be taken not to bring on, by the rash employment of purging remedies, a gastro-intestinal inflammation, as a substitute for that of the cutaneous surface. Rayer only sanctions the exhibition of arsenical medicines in the treatment of chronic lichen with extreme caution and moderation, and never except when the complaint resists all other modes of treatment. Previously to their being prescribed, the state of the digestive organs is to be considered ; any inflammation of them, if existing, previously removed ; and the doses of the liquor arsenicalis increased very

The TROPICAL LICHEN, or PRICKLY HEAT, is a disease of high antiquity, and is equally described by the Greek and Arabian writers. The latter denominate it ESHERA ﺍﺷﻮﻝ, which is the plural of sheri ﺷﻮﻯ, literally *papulæ*, and hence THE PAPULÆ, or PAPULOUS DISORDER, by way of emphasis. And this term, softened or corrupted into essera, has been adopted and employed as the name of the disease by many European writers of great reputation, as Bartholin, Hillary, and Ploucquet. The term, however, has sometimes been used both in the east and among Europeans in a looser sense, so as occasionally, but most improperly, to embrace urticaria, and some other febrile rashes as well.

The symptoms of the disease I shall give in the words of my valued friend Dr. James Johnson, who delineates the disease as he has felt it, and as, in recollection, he seems almost to feel it still ; and hence his description flows " Warm from the heart, and faithful to its fires."

"From moschetoes," says he, " cock-roaches, ants, and the numerous other tribes of depredators on our personal property, we have some defence by night, and in general a respite by day ; but this unwelcome guest assails us at all, and particularly the most unseasonable hours. Many a time have I been forced to spring from table and abandon the repast which I had scarcely touched, to writhe about in the open air for a quarter of an hour ; and often have I returned to the charge, with no better success, against my ignoble opponent ! The night affords no asylum. For some weeks after arriving in India, I seldom could obtain more than an hour's sleep at one time, before I was compelled to quit my couch, with no small precipitation, and if there were any water at hand, to sluice it over me, for the purpose of allaying the inexpressible irritation ! But this was productive of temporary relief only ; and, what was worse, a more violent paroxysm frequently succeeded.

" The sensations arising from prickly heat are perfectly indescribable : being compounded of pricking, itching, tingling, and many other feelings, for which I have no appropriate appellation.

" It is usually, but not invariably, accompanied by an eruption of vivid red pimples, not larger in general than a pin's head, which spread over the breast, arms, thighs, neck, and occasionally along the forehead, close to the hair. This eruption often disappears, in a great measure, when we are sitting quiet, and the skin is cool ; but no sooner do we use any exercise that brings out a perspiration, or swallow any warm or stimulating fluid, such as tea, soup, or wine, than the pimples become elevated, so as to be distinctly seen, and but too sensibly felt !

" Prickly heat being merely a symptom, not a cause, of good health, its disappearance has been erroneously accused of producing much

gradually, and never beyond fifteen or twenty drops in the twenty-four hours.—See Traité Théorique et Pratique des Maladies de la Peau, tom. i., p. 588.—ED.

mischief; hence the early writers on tropical diseases, harping on the old string of 'humoral pathology,' speak very seriously of the danger of *repelling*, and the advantage of 'encouraging the eruption, by taking small warm liquors,' as tea, coffee, wine whey, broth, and nourishing meats.'

"Indeed, I never saw it repelled even by the cold bath: and in my own case, as well as in many others, it rather seemed to aggravate the eruption and disagreeable sensations, especially during the glow which succeeded the immersion. It certainly disappears suddenly sometimes on the *accession* of other diseases, till the onset reason to suppose that its disappearance *occasioned* them. I have tried lime-juice, hair-powder, and a variety of external applications, with little or no benefit. In short, the only means which I ever saw productive of any good effect in mitigating its violence, till the constitution got assimilated to the climate, were—light clothing—temperance in eating and drinking—avoiding all exercise in the heat of the day—open bowels—and last, not least, a determined resolution to resist with stoical apathy its first attacks."*

In this species, as also in the next, it is obvious that the extremities of the nerves which accompany the cutaneous papillæ, are in a peculiar state of irritation. And when we reflect that the organ of the skin possesses the most acute sensibility of any of the structures of the body, and suffers more pain than any other part under amputation; and when to this we add, that the nerves are uniformly most sensible at their extremities, we can be at no loss to account for the maddening distress which is hereby produced.—(*Bostock, Elementary System of Physiol.*, p. 85, 8vo., 1824.).

The wild lichen, or LICHEN FERUS, is particularly noticed by Celsus, under the name of AGRIA, as applied to it by the Greeks, from the violence with which it rages. It occurs in him after a brief description of a variety of papula of a milder kind, which Willan supposes, and with some reason, to be the clustering. "Altera autem est, quam 'Αγρίαν Græci appellant: in qua similiter quidem, sed magis cutis exasperatur, exulceraturque, ac vehementius et roditur, et rubet, et interdum inter pilos remittit. Quæ minus rotunda est, difficilius sanescit: nisi sublata est, in impetiginem vertitur."—(*De Med.*, lib. v., cap. xxviii.) This variety, however, in its general range, its vehemence, and protracted duration, approaches nearer to the nettle lichen than to any other: yet the pimples are larger, more clustered, and more apt to run into a pustular inflammation, so as often to produce cutaneous exulcerations and black scabs; and hence the remark of Celsus, that it is disposed to terminate in an impetigo,† or, as others have it, in psora or lepra.

* See James Johnson, M. D., on the Influence of Tropical Climates on European Constitutions, 8vo., Lond., 1821.

† One disease has often been mistaken for the other. The small pustules of impetigo are sometimes collected in groups, like the papulæ of lichen

The URTICOSE or NETTLE LICHEN is, perhaps, the most distressing form of all the varieties, if we except the tropical: and, like the tropical, notwithstanding its violence, it is often totally independent of any constitutional affection. I can distinctly say, from various cases that have occurred to me, that even when the patient has been worked up to such a degree of madness as to force him against his own will into a perpetual scratching, which greatly exasperates it, still the constitution has remained unaffected, the pulse regular, the appetite good, and the head clear. In most of the cases the author alludes to, however, there was an established or idiopathic irritability of the system, and especially of the skin; and in one or two of them, it was unfortunate that opium, under every form, and in every quantity, always increased the irritability; while no other narcotic was of any avail. I freely confess that I have been more perplexed with this obstinate and intractable variety, which has in some cases irregularly subsided for a few days or weeks, and then reappeared with more violence than ever, than I have been with almost any other complaint that has ever occurred to me. The subcarbonate of ammonia, as just referred to, has sometimes been serviceable, but by no means always. A tepid bath, and especially of seawater, has sometimes also been useful; but I have often found even this fail, and have uniformly observed the bath mischievous when made hot; for the skin will not bear stimulation. The hydrocyanic or prussic acid, in doses of four minims, two or three times a day, has occasionally also subdued the irritability, though in a few instances it has produced more mischief than it has removed.

From the alterant apozems of sarsaparilla, elm-bark, juniper-tops, and snake-root, no benefit has accrued; and as little from sulphur, sulphurated quicksilver, nitre, the mineral acids, and the mineral oxydes and salts. I once tried the arsenic solution, but the stomach would not bear it. Sea-bathing, however, in connexion with sea-air, has rarely failed; and I am hence in the habit of prescribing it to a delicate young lady, who has been several times most grievously afflicted with this distressing malady, as soon as it reappears, as well from the known inefficacy of every other remedy, a long list of which she has tried with great resolution, as from the benefit which this has almost uniformly produced.*

Mr. Wilkinson recommends that the itching parts be frequently moistened with a lotion consisting of a scruple of subcarbonate of ammonia and acetate of lead dissolved in four ounces of rose-water, and be slightly touched every day,

agrius; but, in the latter, there are only minute incrustations, difficult of separation; whereas, in impetigo, the scabs are thick, and easily fall off. The possibility of lichen being transformed into psoriasis or impetigo, though a rare occurrence, is admitted by Rayer.—Op. et vol. cit., p. 579.–ED.

* According to Alibert (Monogr. des Dermatoses, vol. ii.), individuals who suffer from ecthyma should use emollient baths daily. Gelatinous baths also have recently been found very successful.—D.

or every other day, with aromatic vinegar diluted with one third part of water.—(*Remarks on Cutaneous Diseases*, p. 25, 1822.)

I have said that the wild lichen in its severity and duration offers a near resemblance to this. The former, however, is more apt to run into a pustular inflammation, though in the nettle lichen we sometimes find a few of the vesicles* filled with a straw-coloured fluid, but which are not permanent. There is also a greater tendency to some constitutional affection in the wild than in the nettle modification, and particularly to a sickness, or some other disorder of the stomach, upon repulsion by cold. Under the nettle lichen, the patient seldom finds the stomach or any other organ give way, and will endure exposure to a sharp current of air with a full feeling of refreshment, without any danger of subsequent mischief.

There is a singular modification of this disease described in a letter from Dr. Monsey, of Chelsea College, to Dr. Heberden, in which the cause was exposure of the skin to a bright sun in the open air. The patient was a man thirty ears of age, of a thin, spare habit: and his skin, as soon as the solar rays fell upon it, became instantly almost as thick as leather, and as red as vermilion, with an intolerable itching: the whole of which abated about a quarter of an hour after he went into the shade. Dr. Monsey adds, that this was not owing to the heat of the sun, for the sun in winter affected him full as much, if not more, and the heat of the fire had not such an effect. He was in consequence thrown into a state of " confinement for near ten years. It may not be amiss," continues Dr. Monsey, "to mention one particular, which is, that one hot day having a mind to try if he were at all benefited by his immersions" (he seems to have used a salt bath under cover for many weeks), "he undressed himself and went into the sea in the middle of the day; but he paid very dearly for the experiment, the heat diffusing itself so violently over his whole body by the time he had put on his clothes, that his eyesight began to fail, and he was compelled to lie down upon the ground to save himself from falling. The moment he lay down, the faintness went off; upon this he got up, but instantly found himself in the former condition: he therefore lay down, and immediately recovered. He continued alternately getting up and lying down till the disorder began to be exhansted, which was in about half an hour, and so gradually went off. He had frequently been obliged to use the same practice at other times when he was attacked with this disorder."

That this case is to be regarded as a peculiar form of the present species, the extraordinary irritation and intolerable itching of the skin

seem to vouch for sufficiently. It discovers, however, a cutaneous excitement of an idiopathic and most singular kind : and keeping this idea in mind, it is not difficult to account for the tendency to deliquium related in the latter part of the account. The patient, it seems, could endure cold bathing under cover or in the shade, and was not rendered faint by the reactive glow that ensued upon his quitting the water ; but when to this reactive glow was united, in consequence of his bathing in the open air, and in the middle of the day, the pungent heat of the sun, he was incapable of enduring both, till, by a certain length of exposure to this conjoint stimulus, the cutaneous nerves became torpid, which it seems they did in about half an hour, when the affection, we are told, "gradually went off."

A daily exposure to the same exhausting power would, in all probability, soon have rendered the torpitude habitual, or at least have reduced the cutaneous sensibility to its proper balance, which, after all, forms the real cure in the West Indies, and in most of the chronic cases of our own country. This, however, does not seem to have been thought of; but after having tried a long list of different series of medicines in hospital and in private practice to no purpose, the patient was at length fortunate enough, when under the care of Dr. Monsey, to be put as a forlorn hope upon a brisk course of calomel, of which he took five grains every night, with a purge of rhubarb or cathartic extract the ensuing morning, for nearly a fortnight in succession ; and having thus transferred the morbid irritability of the skin to the intestinal canal, the disease left him.

SPECIES III.

EXORMIA PRURIGO.

PRURIGINOUS RASH.

ERUPTION DIFFUSE : PIMPLES NEARLY OF THE COLOUR OF THE CUTICLE ; WHEN ABRADED, EMITTING A FLUID THAT CONCRETES INTO MINUTE BLACK SCABS ; INTOLERABLE ITCHINGS, INCREASED BY SUDDEN EXPOSURE TO HEAT.*

IN the symptoms of a papular eruption and an intolerable itching, this species makes an approach to the preceding ; but it differs from it

---

* This term does not seem correct, as applied to a papulous disease. Rayer observes, that lichen, whether simple or complicated, is seldom transformed to any other modification of inflammation ; though occasionally, wnen the inflammation continues a long while in the same places, it degenerates into psoriasis or impetigo.—See Traité des Maladies de la Peau, tom. i., p. 579.—ED.

* Prurigo, a chronic inflammation of the integuments, characterized by papulæ, which are nearly of the same colour as the skin, and accompanied with acute itching ; they naturally terminate in resolution, and with small black circular scabs, when they have been broken by the nails.—(See Rayer, Traité des Maladies de la Peau, tom. i., p. 601.) The symptoms of itching, or pruritus, in a greater or less degree, is common to most diseases of the skin, and especially to urticaria, the itch, eczema, strophulus, lichen, &c Now, as Rayer correctly remarks, although this sensation has a particular character in prurigo, it cannot be regarded as a pathognomonic symptom of it. The true character of this disease consists in an eruption of papulæ, whose form and colour, like that of the skin, distinguish them from the papulæ of lichen and strophulus.—Op. et vol. cit., p. 610.—ED.

essentially in the colour of the papulæ, and in the nature of the itching, which is often far more simple ; and when combined with a sense of stinging, gives a feeling peculiar to itself, like that of a nest of ants creeping over the body and stinging at the same time.

It offers the three following varieties, the last of which chiefly differs from the second in being more inveterate :—

a Mitis. Mild prurigo.	Pimples soft and smooth : itching at times subsiding ;* chiefly common to the young and in spring time.
β Formicans. Emmet prurigo.	Pimples varying from larger to more obscure than in the last ; itching incessant,† and accompanied with a sense of pricking or stinging, or of the creeping of ants over the body ; duration from two months to two or three years, with occasional but short intermissions : chiefly common to adults.
γ Senilis. Inveterate prurigo.	Pimples mostly larger than in either of the above, sometimes indistinct, giving the surface a shining and granulated appearance ; itching incessant :‡ common to advanced years, and nearly inveterate.

In all the varieties, the itching differs in its extent ; being sometimes limited to a part only of the body, and sometimes spreading over the entire frame.—(*Sitonus*, tract. 34, *Loescher.*) Courmette relates a case in which it alternated from side to side (*Journ. Med.*, tom. lxxxv.): and in many instances it appears periodically. Hence, in Willan, we have not only an account of the three preceding varieties, but of several

---

* The itching is generally most troublesome when the patient is in bed. It is excited or aggravated by the part being touched or rubbed with the clothes, by the body being heated, by the process of digestion, violent exercise, &c. The pruritus sometimes has intermissions of three or four hours, especially at periods when the patient's mind is very much engaged.—See Rayer, Traité des Maladies de la Peau, tom. i., p. 602.—Ed.

† The paler the papulæ, the more violent in general the itching. The papulæ extend over the whole body excepting the face, feet, and palms of the hands ; and particularly form on parts exposed to friction, or subject to have bands round them, as the nape of the neck, the loins, and the thighs. —(See Rayer, tom. i., p. 603.) The apices of most of the papulæ are torn off by the patient scratching the part, and the skin appears studded with small thin black scabs, which are more conspicuous than the unbroken papulæ ; the latter, on account of their diminutive size, and of their colour being like that of the skin, being often difficult to distinguish.—Ed.

‡ The part is generally a good deal injured by scratching, and there is an abundant furfuraceous desquamation.—Rayer, op. et vol. cit., p. 604.—Ed.

others, which chiefly, if not entirely, differ from them in being limited to particular parts; as prurigo podicis, p. præputii, p. urethralis, p. pubis, p. pudendi muliebris.

A common cause of this species in all its varieties, though by no means the only cause, is want of proper cleanliness of the skin and of apparel ; and hence it is found most frequently in the hovels of the poor, the squalid, and the miserable.* Yet as it is not always found under these circumstances, even where there is the grossest uncleanliness, some other cause jointly operating in such situations, some idiopathic condition of the skin, by which the sordes thus collected and obstructing the mouths of the cutaneous exhalants becomes an active irritant, must be admitted.† One of these conditions appears to be a skin peculiarly delicate and sensible, which is mostly to be found in early life ; and another, a skin peculiar dry and scurfy, which is a common condition of old age ; on which account repelled perspiration is correctly set down as a cause by Riedlin. Even in the cleanliest habits, these peculiarities of the skin often become causes of themselves, and of a more intractable kind than mere sordes, as they are far more difficult of removal. A diet of fish alone has sometimes excited such a habit ; and an habitual addiction to spirituous drinks, whether wine, ale, or alcohol, produces also in many persons a like sensibility of the surface, and lays a foundation for the disease in its most obstinate form.

Where the rash continues long, and becomes pertinacious, the papulæ form minute exulcerations, degenerating, in the first variety, into a species of contagious itch, and in the second, into a running scall ; which last, in the third or inveterate variety, sometimes forms nests for various parasitic insects,‡ and especially for

---

* Prurigo is particularly disposed to attack the extremes of life ; it is more common among the poor than the rich, and oftener seen in men than women.—Rayer, op. et vol. cit., p. 609.—Ed.

† According to Rayer, prurigo is often produced by residence in low, damp situations, and especially by uncleanliness.—Ed.

‡ Sommer, Diss. de affectibus pruriginosis Senûm. Loescher, Diss. de pruritu senili totius corporis, Witeb., 1728. Rayer observes, that besides the papulæ characteristic of prurigo, accidental lesions are sometimes noticed, which disappear as soon as the irritation occasioning them itself ceases. When individuals, afflicted with prurigo, neglect cleanliness, pustules, vesicles, and furuncles may originate in the midst of the papulæ ; the skin may have more or less considerable cracks in it, and indeed become of great thickness. When the disease is of long standing, especially in old persons, the epidermis is thrown off in small scales, or a furfuraceous desquamation occurs at different points on the trunk and limbs. Itch and impetigo may accidentally complicate prurigo ; but Rayer deems it incorrect to say, with Willan and Bateman, that they take place as terminations of this disease.—(See Rayer, Traité Théorique, &c. des Maladies de la Peau, tom. i., p. 605.) Independently of these accidental affections of the skin, general prurigo may be complicated with other internal inflammations. In prurigo formicans, the eruption of papulæ is sometimes preceded by headache, uneasiness, and pain in the epigastrium.

several species of the acarus and pediculus, to which Dr. Willan adds the pulex. In treating of intestinal animalcules, we had occasion to observe, that " they appear, from the luxuriance of their haunts and repasts, to be in various instances peculiarly enlarged and altered from the structure they exhibit out of the body ; whence a difficulty in determining, in many cases, the external species to which a larve, worm, or animalcule found within the body, may belong."— (Vol. i., *Helminthia erratica,* p. 178.) This remark applies with peculiar force to the parasites detected in the diseases before us, some of which grow to such an enormous size, and with such altered characters, from rioting on so plentiful a supply of juices, that it is by no means easy to recognise them. Dr. Willan describes an insect of this kind, found in great abundance on the body of a patient suffering under the inveterate prurigo, which he at first took for a pediculus, though from the nimbleness of its motions, as well as from other characters, he at length ascertained it to be a pulex, not described by Linnæus : more probably, from the causes just stated, so altered in its form as not to be easily referred to the species to which it really belongs.

Thorough and regular ablution and cleanliness are here, therefore, peculiarly necessary, and these will often succeed alone, especially in the first variety.* If they should not, sulphur and the sulphureous waters, as that of Harrowgate, taken internally, and applied to the skin itself, have sometimes been found serviceable.† Soda, combined with sulphur, and taken internally, with infusion of sassafras or juniper-tops, is peculiarly recommended by Dr. Willan. Small doses of the blue-pill, as three or four grains every night, combined with a like proportion of the extract of colocynth, is often found serviceable, and especially where the complaint is obstinate and has become chronic. Where it is of fresher origin, washing the parts affected with a diluted solution of ammonia or potash, as, for example, a drachm of liq. ammon. subcarbonatis, or hartshorn, to an ounce of water; or half a drachm of the liquor potassæ to the same proportion of water. This will produce a new excitement or counter-stimulus ; and the specific irritation will be generally lost in the common, which we may rest from as soon as necessary : a remark, which it may be advantageous to bear in mind through most of the cutaneous af-

On the other hand, when individuals, affected with prurigo, are seized with an acute disorder, the papulous eruption is almost always lessened, and sometimes it completely disappears.—Rayer, loco cit.—Ed.
  * Cold or tepid baths are set down by Rayer as the best of all the local remedies for prurigo. Sometimes, however, the patients experience the greatest relief from plunging themselves every day for an hour in a bath of some emollient decoction, like that of bran.—Ed.
  † A cure has occasionally been effected by means of sulphureous fumigations, though the irritation produced by them sometimes makes it necessary to suspend their employment, and to have recourse to simple bathing, vapour-baths, or emollients. —See Rayer, op. et vol. cit., p. 613.—Ed.

fections before us ; as in numerous instances they will yield, if early attended to, under a like treatment, and it is for the same reason that they have often given way to an occasional use of aromatic vinegar, or a diluted solution of nitrate of silver. In a very obstinate and chronic case, Mr. Wilkinson tells us that he derived very great benefit from a free use of an ointment consisting of equal parts of sulphur* and tar, united, by means of lard, with two drachms of hydrosulphuret of ammonia, and four ounces of chalk to every pound and a half. This was liberally applied over the whole extent of the eruption every day, and washed off every other day. The compound calomel pill and the arsenic solution, however, were employed internally in the meanwhile ; and the parts occasionally washed with undiluted aromatic vinegar, or else a solution of nitrate of silver, previous to the application of the ointment.—(*Remarks on Cutaneous Diseases,* p. 30, 1822.) If the constitution have suffered from a meager diet, or be otherwise exhansted, general tonics and a nutritive food must necessarily form a part of the plan.

In many cases, however, of the second variety, and in still more of the third, this pertinacious and distressing complaint bids defiance to all the forms of medicine, or the ingenuity of man : and I cannot adduce a stronger illustration of this remark, than by referring to an attack which it lately made on one of the brightest ornaments of medical science in our own day, whose friendship allows me to give the present reference to himself. It is now something more than four years since he was first visited with this formicative but colourless rash, which affected the entire surface, but chiefly the legs : and he has since tried every means that the resources of his own mind or the skill of his medical friends could suggest, yet for the most part without any thing beyond a palliative or temporary relief. The tepid bath produced more harm than good, though several times repeated : Harrowgate water, internally and externally had recourse to, was of as little avail : acids and alkalis, separate or conjoined, in whatever way made use of, failed equally ; nor did purgatives or diaphoretics, or any of the alterative dietdrinks, or the alterative metallic preparations, answer better. The coldest spring-water employed as a bath or lotion, and free doses of opium as a sedative, were the only medicines from which he at any time derived any decided relief, and these constantly afforded it for a short time. In the middle of the coldest nights of the preceding winter, and the still colder nights of the winter before, he was repeatedly obliged to rise and have recourse to sponging with cold

  * Rayer states, that benefit is seldom derived from mercurial or sulphur ointment, lime-water lotions, or a solution of the sublimate; but he mentions, that the pruritus may be appeased by applying an ointment containing hellebore and hydro-chlorate of ammonia. Mercurial washes may be prescribed with advantage for prurigo formicans, especially when complicated with pediculi. Under other circumstances, ablution with cold or tepid water affords great relief.—Ed.

water, often when on the point of freezing. The opium he took never procured real sleep, nor abated the complaint, but generally threw him into a quiet kind of revery, which produced all the refreshment of sleep ; and to obtain this happy aphelxia, or abstraction of mind, he was compelled to use the opium in large doses, often to an extent of ten grains every twenty-four hours, for weeks together, and rarely in less quantity than five or six grains a day and night for many months in succession. The change operated on the general habit by this peculiar sensibility of the skin was not a little singular ; for first, in the midst of the distraction produced by so perpetual a harassment, and the necessary restlessness of nights, neither his animal spirits nor his appetite in any degree flagged, but, upon the whole, rather increased in energy, and his pulse held true to its proper standard. And next, though opium was wont to disagree with him in various ways antecedently, it proved a cordial to him through the whole of this tedious affection, without a single unkindly concomitant, and never rendered his bowels constipated. From the long-continued excess of action, there was at length an evident deficiency in the restorative power of the skin ; for two excoriations, arising from the eruption, degenerated into sloughing ulcers. At the distance of about nineteen or twenty months from the first attack, he began to recover ; the skin, which had been so long in a state of excitement, lost its morbid sensibility, and became torpid : he had rarely occasion to have recourse to cold ablutions, but dared not trust himself through the day without a dose of opium, as an exhilarant, though the quantity was considerably reduced. For many months, also, he took the bark and soda as a general tonic. Perhaps the most instructive part of this case is, the great advantage and safety of the external application of cold water, as a refrigerant and tonic, in cutaneous eruptions accompanied with intolerable heat and irritation. And it is possible, that half the wells which in times of superstition were dedicated to some favourite saint, and still retain his proper name, derive their virtue from this quality, rather than from any chymical ingredient they contain, which has often as little to do with the cure as the special interposition of the preternatural patron.*

I do not know that the prussic acid† has hitherto been introduced into practice in this

* Of all the general remedies for prurigo, blood-letting and cooling diluent beverages seem to Rayer the most useful; as whey, barley-water, lemonade, &c.—(Tom. i., p. 614.) Bleeding he considers as invariably called for in young plethoric individuals. In women, whose menses are suppressed, he advises leeches to be applied to the vulva. Persons who have indulged too much in high-seasoned dishes and spirituous liquors, he recommends to be kept for some time on a vegetable diet, or asses' or goats' milk.—Ed.

† The editor has frequently employed the following lotion with success :—

　Ŗ Hydrarg. oxymuriatis, gr. iij.
　　Acidi hydrocyanici, f. ʒj.
　　Mist. amygdalæ amaræ, f. ʒviij.
　Ft. lotio partibus affectis subinde applicanda.

kind of rash : but as I have reason to think it has occasionally proved successful in the wild lichen, as well as in various other disorders of the skin accompanied with severe irritation, it may be tried with some hope internally, in doses of three or four minims two or three times a day ; and, perhaps, not without a beneficial effect, in a dilute solution externally : for which, however, the laurel-water itself may form a convenient substitute.

SPECIES IV.

EXORMIA MILIUM.

MILLET-RASH.

PIMPLES VERY MINUTE ; TUBERCULAR ; CONFINED TO THE FACE ; DISTINCT ; MILK-WHITE ; HARD ; GLABROUS ; RESEMBLING MILLET-SEEDS.

This species is taken from Plenck, who denominates it grutum sive milium. It is a very common form of simple pimple or exormia, and must have been seen repeatedly by every one ; though, with the exception of Plenck, I do not know that it has hitherto been described by any nosologist. It has a near resemblance to the white-gum of children, as described by Dr. Underwood, the strophulus albidus of Willan, and the present system. But the pimples in the milium are totally unattended with any kind of inflammatory halo or surrounding redness ; and are wholly insensible. They are sometimes solitary, but more frequently gregarious. It is a blemish of small importance, and rarely requires medical interposition ; but as it proceeds from a torpid state of the cutaneous excretories, or rather of their mouths or extremities, which are obstructed by hardened mucus, stimulant and tonic applications have often been found serviceable, as lotions of brandy, spirit of wine, or tincture of myrrh, or a solution of sulphate of zinc with a little brandy added to it.

When this species becomes inflamed, it lays a foundation for a varus or stonepock, which we have already described under the order of INFLAMMATIONS in the third class of the present system.—(Vol. i., p. 448.)

GENUS IV.

LEPIDOSIS.

SCALE-SKIN.

EFFLORESCENCE OF SCALES OVER DIFFERENT PARTS OF THE BODY, OFTEN THICKENING INTO CRUSTS.*

LEPIDOSIS is a derivative from λεπίς, -δος,

* It is the character of scaly inflammations to make their appearance as elevations, or red spots, on which scales form, consisting of layers of altered cuticle, continually separating from the surface of the skin.—(Rayer, tom. ii., p. 1.) In psoriasis and lepra, these elevations unite, spread, and are soon transformed into scaly layers of various shapes and dimensions. In pityriasis, however, the scales seem to be composed of the cuticle unchanged ; but in lepra and psoriasis, they consist of layers of cuticle thickened, opaque, silky, and very brittle. When these scales are removed or spontaneously thrown off, the subja-

"squamma." The Greek is preferred to the Latin term, in concurrence with the general rule adopted in the present system in regard to the names of the classes, orders, and genera. The genus includes those diseases which consist in an exfoliation of the cuticle in scales or crusts of different thickness, and with a more or less defined outline, in many cases owing to a morbid state or secretion of the rete mucosum or adipose layer of the part immediately beneath, which is sometimes too dry or deficient in quantity; sometimes perhaps absent altogether; sometimes charged with a material that changes its natural colour; and sometimes loaded with an enormous abundance of a glutinous fluid, occasionally combined with calcareous earth. In the severer cases, the true skin participates in the change.

As this colorific substance, forming the intermediate of the three lamellæ that constitute the cutaneous integument, is only a little lighter in hue than the true skin among Europeans, it is not often that we have an opportunity in this part of the world of noticing the changes effected upon it by different diseases: but as among negroes it contains the black pigment by which they are distinguished, such changes are among them very obvious: for the individual is sometimes hereby, as we shall see presently, rendered piebald, or spotted black and white; and there are instances in which the whole of this substance, or rather of its colouring part, being carried off by a fever, a black man has suddenly been transformed into a white.

Changes of this kind often occur without any separation of the cuticle from the cutis; but if the fever be violent, such separation takes place over the entire body, and the cuticle is thrown off in the shape of scurf, or scales, or a continuous sheath. And sometimes the desquamation from a hand has been so perfect that the sheath has formed an entire glove. The same effect has followed occasionally from other causes than fever, as on an improper use of arsenic (*De Haen, Rat. Med.*, part x., cap. ii.) or

cent corpus reticulare is found red and inflamed. Lastly, inveterate scaly inflammations are always accompanied by cracks and a morbid thickening of the skin. These inflammations, as Rayer observes, are sometimes confined to the points where they first commenced; and occasionally get well in these situations, but break out in others. They excite itching, pricking, and heat, which are invariably exasperated by whatever increases the temperature of the surface of the body. These sensations are commonly most acute when the disease is in the axillæ or on the scalp. Cutaneous transpiration is interrupted in the places occupied by the scales; and when they have invaded successively almost the whole surface of the body, the urinary secretion and pulmonary exhalation are usually increased in quantity. According to the same authority, scaly inflammations are often blended together,—a proof of the identity of their nature; and they are more rarely conjoined with other kinds of inflammation. They are more frequent in the lower than the upper classes of society, and in women than men. None of them are contagious; but numerous facts prove that they may be hereditary.—Ed.

other mineral poisons, on being bitten by a viper (*Eph. Nat. Cur.*, dec. i., ann. iv., v., obs. 38), and sometimes on a severe fright.—(*Act. Nat. Cur.*, vol. vii., obs. 43.) There are various instances in which the nails have exfoliated with the cuticle (*Eph. Nat. Cur.*, dec. iii., ann. ii., obs. 124), and others in which the hair has followed the same course. Sometimes, indeed, a habit of recurrence has been established, and the whole has been thrown off and renewed at regular periods (*Gooch, Phil. Trans.*, 1769); in one instance, once a month.—(*Eph. Nat. Cur.*, dec. iii., ann. i., obs. 134.)

In the genus before us, the exfoliations are of a more limited kind, and, in some instances, very minute and comparatively insignificant. In the severer forms, however, the true skin participates in the morbid action, and the result is far more troublesome.

The species it presents to us are the following :—

1. Lepidosis	Pityriasis.	Dandruff.
2. ————	Lepriasis.	Leprosy.
3. ————	Psoriasis.	{ Dry Scall. { Scaly Tetter.
4. ————	Ichthyiasis.	Fish-Skin.*

SPECIES I.
LEPIDOSIS PITYRIASIS.
DANDRUFF.

PATCHES OF FINE BRANNY SCALES, EXFOLIATING WITHOUT CUTICULAR TENDERNESS.†

This species is the slightest of the whole : its varieties are as follow :—

a Capitis. Dandruff of the head.	Scales minute and delicate : confined to the head ; easily separable. Chiefly common to infancy and advanced years.
β Rubra. Red dandruff.	Scaliness common to the body generally ; preceded by redness, roughness, and scurfiness of the surface.
γ Versicolor. Motley dandruff.	Scaliness in diffuse maps of irregular outline, and diverse colours, chiefly brown and yellow ; for the most part confined to the trunk.

Pityriasis is a term common to the Greek physicians, who concur in describing it, to adopt the words of Paulus of Ægina, as "the separation of slight furfuraceous matters (πιτυρώδων σωμάτων) from the surface of the head, or other parts of the body, without ulceration." The

* Rayer considers that Willan, in arranging ichthyiasis with the other three scaly diseases above specified, has attached too great an importance to the scales, which seem to be only secondary productions.—(See Traité des Maladies de la Peau, tom. ii., p. 2.) The scaly eruption of syphilis he also prefers classing with another order of cutaneous diseases.—Ed.

† A chronic superficial inflammation of the skin, characterized by small red spots, often scarcely discernible, and followed by a permanent scurfy desquamation.—Rayer, tom. ii., p. 56.—Ed.

same character is given by the Arabian writers, and especially by Avicenna and Ali Abbas. But several writers, both Greek and Arabian, who have thus described it generally, limit its extent to the head, which is the ordinary seat of the porrigo or scabby scall, characterized by ulceration and a purulent discharge, covered by minute scabs ; and hence in some writers, pityriasis has been confounded with porrigo ; or, in other words, the dry and branny scale with the pustular scab ; which, however, there is no difficulty in accounting for, since the variety, whose seat is also in the head, has a tendency, if neglected, and the minute and scurfy scales grow thicker and broader, and crustaceous, to degenerate into porriginous pustules.

The FIRST VARIETY, or DANDRUFF OF THE HEAD, when it attacks infants, exhibits minute scales; and when it appears in advanced age, scales of larger diameter. It shows itself at the upper edge of the forehead and temples as a slight whitish scurf, set in the form of a horse-shoe ; on other parts of the head there are also cuticular exfoliations, somewhat larger, flat, and semi-pellucid. Sometimes, however, they cover nearly the whole of the hairy scalp, either imbricated, or with an overlap, as in tiling.

Little attention is necessary in this complaint beyond that of cleanliness, and frequent ablution ; when, however, the hairy scalp is attacked, it is better to shave the head, after which the scales may be removed by a careful use of soap and warm water, or by an alkaline lotion.[*] This is the more expedient, because the scales in this situation are often intermixed with sordes, and pustules containing an acrimonious lymph are formed under the incrustations : and in this way pityriasis, as we have already observed, may, and occasionally does, degenerate into porrigo.

The SECOND VARIETY, or RED DANDRUFF, sometimes affects the general health in a perceptible degree, from the suppression which takes place in the perspiration, and the consequent dryness, stiffness, and soreness of the skin ; and the general itching which hence ensues is often productive of much restlessness and languor. This, which is the severest modification of the disease, appears chiefly at an advanced period of life, though it is not limited to old age. A tepid bath of seawater is, perhaps, the most useful application, as serving to soften the skin, and produce a gentle diapnoë. With this external remedy Dr. Willan advises us to unite the compound decoction of sarsaparilla, and antimonials, which operate towards a like effect. The tinctura hellebori nigri in small doses has also sometimes been found useful ; and when the irritability of the skin is not very great, Dr. Bateman was in the habit of using a gently restringent lotion or ointment, consisting of the acetate of lead with a certain proportion of borax or alum.

---

[*] Soapy lotions, or decoctions of poppies, or bran, with or without the addition of acetate of lead, to diminish the itching.—Rayer, tom. ii., p. 59.—ED.

The variegated or MOTLEY DANDRUFF, pityriasis versicolor, often branches out over the arms, back, breast, or abdomen, but rarely in the face, like many foliaceous lichens growing on the bark of trees ; and sometimes, where the discoloration is not continuous, suggests the idea of a map of continents, islands, and peninsulas, distributed over the skin.

We have a more distinct proof of a morbid condition of the rete mucosum, or adipose colorific layer of the skin, in this, than in any other affection belonging to the entire genus. The morbid action, indeed, seems confined to this quarter, and consists in the secretion of a tarnished pigment, though possibly, in some instances, it may be only discoloured, by a mixture with a small portion of extravasated blood. And, were it not for the furfuraceous scales, which determine its real nature, this affection would belong to the genus EPICHROSIS of the present order. There is no elevation ; and the staining rarely extends over the whole body. Dr. Willan tells us that it seldom appears over the sternum or along the spine of the back. I had lately a patient, however, in a gentleman about forty years old, who was suddenly attacked with a discoloration and branny efflorescence of this kind, which extended directly across the spine over the loins, and very nearly girded the body. It continued upon him for about three years without any constitutional indisposition, or even local disquietude, except a slight occasional itching, and then went away as suddenly as it made its appearance. The hue was a fawn-colour : and, as the patient was anxious to lose it, he tried acids, alkalis, and other detergents of various kinds, but without any effect whatever. This variety of dandruff generally continues for many months, and not unfrequently, as in the present case, for several years. Being altogether harmless, it requires no medical treatment.

The pityriasis nigra of Willan, referred to by Bateman, but only glanced at by either of them, so far as I have seen it, is rather a modification of the genus EPICHROSIS, and species *Pœcilia*, under which it will be noticed. It is a cuticular discoloration, but without cuticular exfoliation.

SPECIES II.
LEPIDOSIS LEPRIASIS.
LEPROSY.

PATCHES OF SMOOTH, LAMINATED SCALES ; OF DIFFERENT SIZES, AND A CIRCULAR FORM.[*]

THIS genus constitutes the vitiligo of Celsus. The term LEPRIASIS is a derivative from λιπρὸς, "scaber, vel asper ex squammulis decedentibus ;" with a termination appropriated, by a sort of common consent, to the squamose tribe of diseases.—(See the author's volume of Nosology ; *Prelim. Diss.*, p. 60.) Lepra, which is

---

[*] Rayer adds,—surrounded by a reddish prominent circle, and depressed in their centre, scattered over the surface of the integuments, and their formation has not been preceded by vesicles or pustules.—See Traité Théorique et Pratique des Maladies de la Peau, tom. ii., p. 4.—ED.

the more common term, is derived from the same root: but lepriasis is preferred to lepra, as a more general term, and hence better calculated to comprise the different varieties of this species, so generally described or referred to by the Greek and oriental writers, but whose descriptions, not very definite when first written, at least, with a few exceptions, have been rendered altogether indefinite and incongruous in modern times, from a misunderstanding or confusion of the names under which the descriptions are given. It is to this cause we must ascribe it, that even in the learned epitome of Dr. Frank, lepra is made to include diseases so different, as genuine leprosy in all its forms, ichthyiasis, elephantiasis, and elephantia, which he distinguishes from elephantiasis from its locality, and a few other symptoms.—(*De Cur. Hom. Morb. Epit.*, tom. iv., p. 211, Mannh., 8vo., 1792.)

The embarrassment which Dr. Bateman felt upon this subject, when writing on the genus ELEPHANTIASIS, and which has been noticed already (Cl. III., Ord. IV., Gen. VIII., Spe. 1), he was equally sensible of when he came to LEPRA, and the researches of Dr. Willan gave him little or no assistance. I could not then find time to render him the aid he stood in need of, but I have since directed my attention to the subject, and will now give the reader its results as briefly as possible.

In the admirable and exact description of the cutaneous efflorescences and desquamations to which the Hebrew tribes were subject on their quitting Egypt, and which they seem to have derived from the Egyptians, drawn up by Moses, and forming a part of the Levitical law (*Levit.*, cap. xiii.), there are three that distinctly belong to the present species, all of them distinguished by the name of BERAT (כהרת) or "BRIGHT SPOT;" one called BOAK (בהק), which also imports brightness, but in a subordinate degree, being "a dull-white beras," not contagious, or, in other words, not rendering a person unclean, or making it necessary for him to be confined; and two called TSORAT (צרעת) "venom or malignity:" the one a *berat lebena*, or "bright-white berat" (Id., xiii., 38, 39), and the other a *berat cecha*, "dark or dusky berat" (Id., v., 3), spreading in the skin; both of which are contagious, or, in other words, render the person affected with it unclean, and exclude him from society.—(Id., v., 6, 8.)

The Arabic and Greek writers have in fact taken notice of and described all these, but with so much confusion of terms and symptoms, from causes I will presently point out, that without thus turning back to the primary source, it is difficult to unravel them or understand what they mean.

The boak, or slighter and uncontaminating berat, is still denominated by the same name among the Arabians, BOAK بَهَاق, and is always the λέπρα αλφός, or "dull-white leprosy," of the Greeks: while the bright-white and dusky berats of the Hebrews, which the latter distinguished on account of their malignity by the

name of צרעת (*tsorat*), are still called, among the Arabians, by the Hebrew generic term, with a very slight alteration; for the *berat lebena* (כהרת לבנה) or bright-white berat of the Hebrew tongue, is the *beras bejas* برص بياض of the Arabic, and the *berat cecha* (בהרת כהה), or dusky berat, its *beras asved* برص أسود : the former of these two constituting the λέπρα λευκή, or "bright-white" leprosy of the Greeks, and the latter their λέπρα μέλας, "dusky or nigrescent leprosy."

So far the whole seems to run in perfect harmony: but as many of the Arabians, in process of time, used boak and beras indiscriminately, the different species of the disease, as well as their qualities, became immediately confounded, and we are told sometimes that leprosy is, and at other times that it is not, unclean or contagious. And what increased the confusion is, that the Arabians employed also another term of still wider import than either of these, being قوبا, (*kuba* or *kouba*), which imported scaly eruptions of every kind, running not merely parallel with the entire genus LEPIDOSIS before us, but something beyond, so as to include the humid as well as the dry scall; and consequently diseases of very different qualities and degrees of malignancy, contagious and uncontagious, cuticular and ulcerative. It is a term peculiarly common to the writings of Avicenna and Serapion. And as kouba, or with the article alkouba, was also frequently applied to all the species of beras or leprosy, the real characters of the latter were rendered doubtful and intricate. And hence a very obvious source of confusion upon this subject originating among the Arabians.

But while the Arabian writers borrowed two terms appropriated to the disease before us from the Hebrew tongue, beras and boak, and employed both of them in a loose and indefinite manner, the Greeks themselves borrowed one and employed it still more indeterminately: for from the Hebrew *tsorat* they obtained their ψώρα (*psora*)—as our own language has since the word SORE. Tsorat, as we have already seen, is restrained by the Hebrew legislator to the two forms of beras or leprosy which were contagious or rendered a man unclean: and, as the Greeks introduced this term into their own tongue, it would have been better to have restrained it to the same import, and to have used psora as the translation of tsorat. But the Greeks had the word lepra already by them, as significative of the same disease *generally*, or a synonyme of berat or beras; and hence, instead of psora, they employed lepra, which is the word made use of in the Greek as well as in the Latin versions. As lepra, however, is a generic term, and runs parallel with berat, so as to include the boak or uncontaminating, as well as the contaminating forms of the disease, the clearness, if not the entire sense of the Hebrew, is greatly diminished in the Greek version. When we are told by Moses, in the language of the *Hebrew* Bible, that the priest shall examine the berat, or bright spot, accurately, and if it have the specific marks, it is a TSORAT (which the berat is not necessarily), we readily understand what he means. But when he tells us, in the language of the *Greek* Bible, that the priest shall look at the berat or τηλαυγης (which is itself necessarily a lepra), and if it have the specific marks it is a LEPRA, the meaning, to say the least of it, is obscure and doubtful. It is probable, however, that psora, when first introduced into the Greek tongue, imported the very same idea as in the Hebrew: but it soon gave way to the older term of lepra: and having thus lost its primitive and restricted signification, it seems to have wandered in search of a meaning, and had at different times, and by different persons, various meanings attributed to it; being sometimes used to express scaly eruptions generally, sometimes the scales of leprosy, but at last, and with a pretty common assent, the far slighter efflorescence of scaly tetters or scalls, denominated in the Levitical code saphat (הספחת); and by the Latins scabies, or *impetigo sicca*: constituting the PSORIASIS, or ensuing species, of the present classification. So that while in Hebrew, or under its primitive sense, tsorat or psora denoted the most malignant form of lepidosis, in Greek, or under its secondary sense, it denoted one of the mildest forms of the same. And hence another source of confusion upon the subject before us, originating among the Greek writers, as the preceding originated among the Arabian.

And when to these two sources of perplexity we add that the Greek term lepra was, from a cause I have formerly explained, employed equally to express elephantiasis, we shall easily be able to account for the indefinite and incoherent descriptions of all these diseases which are given by many of the Greek and Arabian writers, and the inaccuracy with which the symptoms of one specific disease are run into another. Actuarius endeavoured to throw something of order into the midst of this confusion, by contemplating all these maladies, in conjunction with lichen, as different forms of a common genus, and dividing them into four separate species:—"A less violent disease," says he, "than elephantiasis, is lepra; lepra is, however, more violent than psora, and psora than the lichenes." But lepra penetrates deep, forms circular eruptions and certain funguses or deliquescences of flesh (τινας σύντηξεις σαρκὸς), and throws off scales, from which also it derives its name: while psora is more superficial, assumes intermediate shapes, and only casts off furfuraceous corpuscles. A roughness and itching of the skin are common to both."—(*Actuar. De Meth. Medend.*, ii., 11.) And to the same effect Paulus of Ægina.—(*Paul. Ægin.*, iv., 2; *Serapion, Breviar.*, tr. v., cap. iv.; *Avicenna*, lib. i., iii., 1.)

The real fact is, that the two last are nearly connected in nature, and in the present work follow in immediate succession, while both are widely remote from the first: and though it is possible they have occasionally terminated in it,

are by no means naturally connected with it, or form a necessary harbinger.

Lepra or lepriasis in Celsus occurs under the name of vitiligo, and, like the berat of the Hebrew legislator, is made to include three modifications; the ordinary forms of it, indeed, that have descended to us, though delineated with much error and incongruity. The description of Celsus is drawn up with peculiar accuracy and concinnity, and makes the nearest approach to that of Moses of any I am acquainted with: and by uniting them, and combining a few well-ascertained symptoms from other authors, we shall be able to obtain a pretty clear insight into the genuine characters of these modifications, freed from the extraneous concomitants that have so often bewildered us.

α Albida. Boak (בהק). Heb. Boak ﺑﻖ. Arab. Alphos. ('Αλφὸς.) Auct. Gr. Cels. Common or dull-white leprosy.	Scales glabrous, dull-white, circular and definite; preceded by reddish and glossy elevations of the skin; surrounded by a dry, red, and slightly elevated border; scattered; sometimes confluent; irregularly exfoliating and reproduced; rarely found on the face: not contagious.
β Nigricans. Berat cecha; (בהרת כהה) Hebr. Beras asved, Arab. نرص اسود Melas. (Μέλας.) Auct. Gr. Cels. Dusky or black leprosy.	Scales glabrous, dusky, or livid, without central depression; patches increasing in size; scattered or confluent. Contagious.
γ Candida. Berat lebena; (בהרת לבנה) Hebr. Beras bejas, Arab. برص بياض Leuce. (Λευκη.) Auct. Gr. Cels. Bright-white leprosy.	Scales on an elevated base, glossy-white, with a deep central depression; encircled with a red border; patches increasing in size; hairs on the patches white or hoary; diffused over the body. Contagious.

All these, at least in their origin, are strictly cutaneous affections: though we shall probably have to observe, that the last two, when they become inveterate, sometimes seem to affect the habit; and it is hence possible that the first may do so in a long course of time, if neglected.

It is on this account that the boak, common or DULL-WHITE LEPROSY, has been regarded as in every instance a constitutional malady by many writers of recent times: but it was not so regarded either by the best Greek and Arabian physicians, who also duly distinguished it from elephantiasis and other complaints, with which it has been confounded by later writers, nor is it so regarded by Dr. Willan, who ascribes it chiefly to cold, moisture, and the accumulation of sordes on the skin, especially in persons of a slow pulse, languid circulation, and a harsh, dry, and impermeable cuticle ; or whose diet is meager and precarious. It is hence found chiefly in this metropolis among bakers and bricklayers' labourers ; coal-heavers, dustmen, laboratory-men, and others who work among dry, powdery substances, and are rarely sufficiently attentive to cleanliness of person.

In the common, and, perhaps, in all the varieties, the scaly patches commence where the bone is nearest to the surface, as along the skin about the elbow, and upon the ulna in the forearm, on the scalp, and along the spine, os ilium, and shoulder-blades. They rarely appear on the calf of the leg, on the fleshy part of the arms, or within the flexures of the joints. Both sides of the body are usually affected at the same time and in the same manner ; but, contrary to the erysipelatous erythema and some other maladies of the skin, the parts first affected do not run through their action and heal as other parts become diseased, but continue with little alteration, till from medical application, or the natural vigour of the constitution, returning health commences ; when all the patches assume a like favourable appearance at the same time,those nearest the extremities, and where the disease, perhaps, first showed itself, going off somewhat later than the rest. The scaly incrustations sometimes extend to the scalp, and a little encroach on the forehead and temples ; but it is very rarely that they spread to the cheeks, chin, nose, or eyebrows. The eruption is seldom attended with pain or uneasiness of any kind, except a slight degree of itching when the patient is warm in bed, or of tingling on a sudden change of temperature in the atmosphere.

We have said that this variety is strictly a cutaneous eruption, and rarely, if ever, affects the constitution. It is in consequence regarded as of but little importance in the Levitical code, which contemplates it as not penetrating below the skin of the flesh, and not demanding a separation from society. " If a man or a woman," says the Jewish law "have in *the skin of their flesh* a berat, a white berat, then the priest (who, after the manner of the Egyptians, united the character of a physician with his own), shall look ; and behold, if the berat in the skin of the flesh be dull, it is a BOAK *growing in the skin :* he is clean."—(*Levit.*, cap. xiii., 38, 39.) Not essentially different Celsus :—" The vitiligo, though it brings no danger, is nevertheless offensive, and springs from a bad habit of body. The dull-white and the dusky forms, in many persons, spring up and disappear at uncertain periods. The bright-white, when it has once made its attack, does not so easily quit its hold. The cure of the two former is not difficult : the last scarcely ever heals."—(*De Medicina*, lib. v., cap. xxviii., sect. 19.)

We may hence distinctly affirm, that the variety of the dull-white or common leprosy is not contagious : and had it been so among the Jews, Moses would have condemned the patient to a quarantine under this form, as well as under the two ensuing. Dr. Willan, indeed, yielding to the general opinion upon this subject,

derived from a proper want of discriminating one form of the disease from another, inclines to believe, that it may occasionally become in time so interwoven with the habit as to be propagable, but still rejects the idea of its being contagious. In reality, although in most countries where leprosy is a common malady, places of separate residence are usually allotted to those who are affected with it, under whatever modification it may appear, this has rather been from an erroneous interpretation of the Jewish law, and in ignorance of the exceptions that are introduced into it. The lepers of Haha, a province in the Barbary states, though banished from the towns, are seen in parties of ten or twenty together, infesting the roads, and approach travellers to beg charity. In Morocco they are confined to a separate quarter, or banished to the outside of the walls. They are, according to Mr. Jackson, but little disfigured by the disease, except in the loss of the eyebrows, which the females endeavour to supply by the use of lead ore ; while they give an additional colour to their complexion by the assistance of al akhen, or rouge.

In like manner, Niebuhr asserts, that one of the species of leprosy to which the Arabs are subject, is by them still called boak ; but that it is neither contagious nor fatal. Upon which remark, his annotator, M. Forskål, adds, " the Arabs call a sort of leprosy, in which various spots are scattered over the body, behaq ; which is without doubt the same as is named בהק (bohak or behaq) in Lev. xiii. They believe it to be so far from contagious, that one may lie with the person affected without danger. On May 15, 1763," says he, " I saw at Mokha a Jew who had the leprosy bohak. The spots are of unequal size ; they do not appear glossy ; they are but little raised above the skin, and do not change the colour of the hair ; the spots are of a dull-white, inclining to red."—(*Reisebeschreibung nach Arabien und andern unliegenden Landern*, Kopenhag., 4to., 1774.)

The NIGRESCENT LEPROSY, forming the second variety, is improperly called *black*, though it was so named by the Greeks. The colour, as repeatedly described by the Jewish legislator, is rather obscure, darkling, or dusky. The term is כהה (cecha), whence the Latin cœcus : and it immediately imports obfuscous, or overcast with shade or smoke. The character in Celsus is in perfect accordance with this, as he explains to us that μέλας, or, " niger," in its application to this variety, imports "umbræ similis," " shadelike," or " shadowed." The hue is tolerably represented in Dr. Willan's plate, but better in Dr. Bateman's, in which it has been retouched. The natural colour of the hair, which in Egypt and Palestine is black, is not changed, as we are repeatedly told in the Hebrew code, nor is there any depression in the dusky spot ; while the patches, instead of keeping stationary to their first size, are perpetually enlarging their boundary. The patient labouring under this form was pronounced unclean by the Hebrew priest or physician, and hereby sentenced to a separation from his family and friends; and hence there is no doubt of its having proved contagious. Though a much severer malady than the common leprosy, it is far less so than the *leuce* or third variety; and on this account is described more briefly than in the Hebrew canon. In our own quarter of the world, the exfoliated surface in the nigrescent or dusky leprosy remains longer without new scales, discharges lymph, often intermixed with blood, and is very sore. When it covers the scalp it is particularly troublesome. With us· it is chiefly found among· soldiers, sailors, sculler-men, stage-coachmen, brewers' labourers, and others whose occupations are·attended with much fatigue, and expose them to cold and damp, and to a precarious or improper mode of diet. For the same reason, women, habituated to poor living and constant hard labour, are also liable to this form of the disease.

In consequence of the increased excitement and irritability of the skin in the hot and sandy regions of Egypt and Palestine, there is, however, a far greater predisposition to leprosy of all kinds, than in the cooler temperature of Europe. And hence, under the next variety, we shall·have occasion to·observe, from the Levitical account, that all of them were apt to follow various cracks or blotches, inflammations, or even contusions of the skin.

The BRIGHT-WHITE LEPROSY is by far the most serious and obstinate of all the forms which the disease assumes. The pathognomonic characters, dwelt upon by the Hebrew legislator in deciding it, are, "a glossy-white and spreading scale, upon an elevated base; the elevation depressed in the middle, but without a change of colour; the black hair on the patches, which is the natural colour of the hair in Palestine, participating in the whiteness, and the patches themselves perpetually widening their outline." Several of these characters taken separately belong to other lesions or blemishes of the skin as well, and therefore none of them were to be taken alone :. and it was only when the whole of them concurred, that the Jewish priest,.in his capacity of physieian, was to pronounce the disease a *tsorat* (צרעת), or malignant leprosy. We have said that in lepriasis, the rete mucosum, or colorific layer of the skin, is peculiarly affected, and we have here a still more distinct proof of this assertion in the change of the hair, the colour of which has a relation to this material. This change is produced by the barter of a black for a white colouring material, probably a phosphate of lime, which gives also the bright glossy colour, not hoary or dull, to the scaly patches; and which, in ichthyiasis, forming the fourth species of the present· genus, we shall find is occasionally deposited on the surface in prodigious abundance.

. Common as this form of leprosy was among the Hebrews,· during and subsequent to their residence in Egypt, we have no reason to believe it was a family complaint, or even known among them antecedently : and there is hence little·doubt, notwithstanding the confident assertions of Manetho to the contrary, that they received the infection from the Egyptians, instead of communicating it to them. Their subjugated and distressed state, however, and the peculiar nature of their employment, must have rendered them very liable to this as well as to various other·blemishes and misaffections of the skin : in the production of which there are no causes more active or powerful than a depressed state of body and mind, hard labour under a burning sun, the body constantly covered with the excoriating dust of brick-fields, and an empoverished diet; to all of which the Israelites were exposed while under the Egyptian bondage.

It appears also from the Mosaic account, that in consequence of these hardships, there was, even after they had left Egypt, a general predisposition to the tsorat or contagious form of leprosy, so that it often occurred as a consequence of various other cutaneous affections; sometimes appearing as a *berat lebena* (בהרת לבנה), or bright-white leprosy, and sometimes as a *berat cecha*, (בהרת כהה), dusky leprosy, according to the peculiar habit or idiosyncrasy. The cutaneous blemishes or blains, which had a tendency to terminate in leprosy, and which were consequently watched with a suspicious eye from the first, are stated by Moses to have been the following :—

1. Shaat (שאת).*   Herpes or tetter, οὐλή, Sept. an irritated cicatrix.

2. Saphat (ספהת).†   Psoriasis, or dry scall.— Dry sahafata ﺷﺤﻔﺔ. Ara.

3. Netek (בתק).‡   Porrigo, or humid scall. Porrigo. Lat. vers. Jun. et Tremel. Moist sahafata ﺷﺤﻔﺔ. Arab.

4. Berat (בהרת).§   Leuce, bright-white scale; the critical ·sign of contagious leprosy.

5. Boak (בהק).‖   Alphos, dull-white scale; the critical sign of uncontagious leprosy.

6. Nega (נגע).¶   Ictus, blow or bruise; ἀφή, Sept.

7. Shechin (שחין).**   Furunculus, or bile, as in Job ii., 7.

8. Mecutash (אש מכות).††   Anthrax, or carbuncle; literally " a fiery inflammation."

On the appearance of any one of these affections upon a person, he was immediately brought before the priest for examination. If the priest perceived that, in connexion with such blemish, there were the distinctive signs of a tsorat or contagious leprosy,‡‡ as a bright, glossy, and

---

* Levit., cap. xiii., 2, 10, 19, 43.
† Id., v, 2, 6, 7, 8.   ‡ Id., v. 30, 31.
§ Id., v. 2, et sæpè alibi.   ‖ Id., v. 39.
¶ Id., v. 29, 42.   ** Id., v. 18.   †† Id., v. 24.
‡‡ Rayer admits, that the etiology is very obscure; but he maintains that 'lepriasis is not. propagated by contact, either mediate or immediate. Husband and wife, he says, may live togeth-

squamous surface, with a depression in the middle, and white hairs, the person was immediately declared unclean, and is supposed to have been sent out of the camp to a lazaretto provided for the purpose. If the priest had any doubt upon the subject, the person was put under domestic confinement for seven days, when he was examined a second time; and if, in the course of the preceding week, the eruption had subsided, and discovered no tendency to the above distinctive characters, he was discharged at once. But if the eruption were stationary, and the result still doubtful, he was put under confinement for seven days more; at the expiration of which, on a third examination, the nature of the disease always sufficiently disclosed itself; and he was either sentenced to a permanent separation from the community, or pronounced clean and set at liberty.

These doubtful cases, as we have just noticed, sometimes superinduced the bright-white and sometimes the dusky leprosy, apparently according to the particular constitution of the skin, or of the habit generally. And we are further told, that there are two ways in which the disease, and particularly the severest or bright-white form of it, terminated;—a favourable and an unfavourable. If it spread over the entire frame without producing any ulceration, it lost its contagious power by degrees; or, in other words, ran through its course and exhausted itself. In which case, there being no longer any fear of further evil either to the individual himself or to the community, the patient was declared clean by the priest, while the dry scales were yet upon him, and restored to society.—(*Levit.*, cap. xiii., v. 12, 13.) If, on the contrary, the patches should ulcerate, and quick or fungous flesh (כשר חי) (Id., v. 10, 14, 15) spring up in them, the priest was at once to pronounce it an inveterate leprosy (Id., v. 11); a temporary confinement was declared to be totally unnecessary, and he was regarded as unclean for life. The accuracy with which this second termination is described, is fully confirmed by the passage quoted already, but for another purpose, from Actuarius; and it is curious to observe how closely they coincide. "The lepra," says the latter, speaking of it in

its worst form, "penetrates deep, forms circular eruptions, and certain funguses or deliquescences of flesh." But we meet with nothing in the Mosaic account that approximates it to elephantiasis: nothing of a thick, rugose, livid, tuberculate, and particularly an insensible skin; nothing of fierce and staring eyes, hoarse and nasal voice, or of a general falling off of the hair. And hence we have additional proof, that these maladies were distinct and unconnected. This malignant state of the disease, however, is still generally called, after the Greek misnomer, elephantiasis: and the two maladies in consequence hereof are to this hour confounded in the Greek islands, and even as far north as Iceland, the *ultima Thule* to which the literature of the Greeks had travelled: but we have sufficient proof in all these cases, from some of the best travellers of the present day, that the disease thus described is not the tubercular or thick-legged elephantiasis, but the above malignant form of genuine leprosy. Thus, Mr. Jowett, in his very interesting "Christian Researches in the Mediterranean," in describing the beautiful, but now, from its political reverses, most pitiable island of Haivali or Kydonia, near Scio :— "A little farther on is the hospital for lepers : it was founded by a leper. Elephantiasis is no uncommon disorder in these parts : its effects are very offensive. I saw poor men and women with their fingers or legs literally *wearing* or *wasting away*" (*Christian Researches in the Mediterranean*, p. 65, 8vo., 1822); forming a character directly opposite to what occurs in proper elephantiasis : where the limbs, though they continue to crack, continue to thicken enormously, even to the moment of separation. Dr. Henderson, on the contrary, while describing the real elephantiasis in Iceland, calls it the Jewish leprosy, and offers a sort of apology for Moses that he "has not noticed the very striking anæsthesia, or insensibility of the skin" (*Iceland; or, the Journal of a Residence in that Island*), which, continues he, "is an inseparable attendant of the genuine elephantiasis." The direct answer is, that Moses delineates a different disorder, and one in which no such symptom exists.*

er without communicating it to each other. All that has been written about the pretended contagiousness of lepriasis he pronounces to be incorrect, and declares that the most false inferences on this point have been drawn from receptacles for lepers, established in the eighth, ninth, and tenth centuries.—(See Traité Théorique, &c. des Maladies de la Peau, tom. ii., p. 12.) The disease appears sometimes to have been excited by stimulating viands, and the abuse of spirituous liquors. It has been known to originate shortly after the introduction of poisonous substances into the digestive organs, as, for instance, salts of copper, or from the abuse of acids. An habitual indulgence in eating game, salt spicy dishes, fish, or shell-fish, has been suspected to be concerned in producing lepriasis, though the disease is not more common on the seacoast than in the interior. Grief and poverty have also been mentioned as causing it; but it has been known to attack the rich and voluptuous.—Rayer.—Ed.

* Lepriasis differs in several respects from other chronic inflammations of the skin, and even from those which, like it, have a scaly form. In psoriasis, it is true, the cuticle, as in lepriasis, is more or less rough and scaly, and red on its adherent surface; but the shape of the scaly layers is irregular, whereas in lepriasis they have a regular orbicular form. In psoriasis, the edges of the scales are neither elevated nor inflamed; and the surface of the subjacent skin has often fissures in it, of greater or less depth, and is generally more tender and irritable than in lepriasis. However, one variety of psoriasis (psoriasis guttata) has so much analogy to lepriasis, that it constitutes a kind of intermediate case between this disease and other varieties of psoriasis, the scales being distinct and isolated, like those of lepriasis, though they are small, seldom more than two or three lines in diameter, and their circumference is less regular. Syphilitic scaly eruptions also resemble lepriasis in their situation and their circular shape. In their size, and copper or livid colour,

As leprosy, except in its less common and contagious modifications, has always been accounted a blemish, rather than a serious disease, in the east, the art of medicine has rarely, in that quarter, been gravely directed towards it, save in the use of the oxyde of arsenic, which is by far the most efficacious of every remedy that has hitherto been tried in any quarter. I have already had occasion to notice the preparation and proportion of this mineral, employed from time immemorial, in treating of elephantiasis, for which disease, also, it is in common use ; and the reader may turn to the passage at his leisure. But, with the exception of arsenic, the remedies proposed by the Asiatics are trifling, and little worthy of notice.

In Europe, the mode of treatment has, indeed, been far more complicated, but I am afraid not much more skilful or successful : consisting, till of late years, of preparations quite as insignificant as any that occur in the Arabian writers, and often highly injurious by their stimulating property. Of the insignificant, the simplicity of modern practice has banished by far the greater number : and it is now, perhaps, hardly known to the general, or even to the medical botanist, that *meadow scabious*, and several other species of the same genus, were so denominated, from their being supposed, when employed as a wash in the form of decoction, to possess an almost specific virtue against leprosy, itch, and almost every other kind of foul and scabious eruption.

Warm-bathing, simple or medicated, and this frequently repeated, is advantageous in all the varieties ; for it tends to remove the scales, soften the skin, and excite perspiration. In the nigrescent leprosy, which proceeds chiefly from poor diet in connexion with sordes, the bath should be of pure fresh water, and the remainder of the cure will generally, in such case, depend upon a better regimen and general tonics. In the other varieties, when they occur among ourselves, the sulphureous waters of Harrowgate, Croft, and Moffat, whether applied externally or internally, seem frequently to prove more efficacious. As external applications, most benefit appears to be derived from the tar ointment, as employed by Dr. Willis, and a dilute solution of sublimate, or the unguentum hydrargyri nitrati, as recommended by Dr. Willan. These medicines should be applied to the skin, and the

---

they are like the lepra nigricans of Willan, and their centre is flat, and covered with a very thin scale ; but they are seldom more than six or eight lines in diameter. Besides, as Rayer adds, not only are the dryness and roughness, which are so remarkable in lepriasis, not observed in syphilitic scaly eruptions, but the latter, when old, are almost as soft and supple as other parts of the skin. Besides, the circles are livid or purple, destitute of scales, and rarely complete. Lastly, syphilitic scaly eruptions fade away, and are cured under the use of mercury, usually healing from the circumference, whereas the orbicular eruption of lepriasis gets well in the contrary direction, from the centre to the margin.—See Rayer, Traité des Maladies de la Peau, tom. ii., p. 14. —ED.

former of them be well rubbed in upon the parts affected, every night, and carefully washed off the next morning with warm water, a slight alkaline lotion, or the aromatic vinegar diluted with a third part of water. *

As internal medicines, the most useful seem to have been the *solanum dulcamara*, and *ledum palustre*, in decoction or infusion. Dr. Crichton strongly recommends the former, and speaks in high terms of its success. I have not been so fortunate in the trials I have given it. The ledum in Sweden,† and, indeed, over most parts of the north of Europe, as high up as Kamtschatka, has long maintained a very popular character, and the form of using it is thus given by Odhelius in the Stockholm Transactions for 1774. Infuse four ounces of the ledum in a quart of hot water ; strain off when cold ; the dose from half a pint to a quart daily.

The bark of the *ulmus campestris*, or elm-tree, has also been warmly recommended by various writers, for this, as well as numerous other cutaneous eruptions ; and, in connexion with more active medicines, appears to have been of some use ; but it is feeble in its effect when trusted to alone. Its form is that of a decoction, two ounces to a quart of water : the dose half a pint, morning and evening.—(*Medical Transactions,* vol. ii., p. 203.)

The *œnanthe crocata*, or hemlock dropwort, is another plant that has been recommended in obstinate and habitual cases of this kind ; and

* When lepriasis is recent and extensive, and the affected parts of the skin are highly inflamed, thickened, vascular, and excessively itchy, and motion of the joints difficult, the disease would certainly be rendered worse by sea-bathing, friction, or sulphureous lotions. Here bleeding, anointing the parts with cream, fresh butter, or lard, afford prompt relief. If the eruptions are large, but not numerous, leeches may be applied near their circumference. The emollient, gelatinous, and vapour-baths are also advantageous. When the case is of some standing, and attended with scarcely any inflammation, the skin is first to be cleaned with lotions, the warm bath, and slight frictions ; and then, if the scales are strongly adherent, or consist of thick strata, stimulating lotions, such as alcohol diluted, or a solution of sulphuret of potash, will promote the falling off of the scales, and advantageously influence the progress of the disease. When the scales have thus been detached, a little tar ointment, or of the ung. hydrarg. nitrat. diluted with ung. plumbi acet., may be applied to the skin in the evening, and the part washed the next day with warm water, or a lotion containing a little soap. It is under such circumstances, also, that sulphureous baths and waters are of service. Brimstone vapour-baths have sometimes effected a cure, but according to Rayer, they more frequently fail. Acid vapour-baths, sea-bathing, alkaline baths, and various natural warm mineral baths, are occasionally successful. When the leprous patches are few and of long standing, they may sometimes be cured by covering them with small blisters, or touching them superficially with a solution of chlorine, or diluted nitrate of mercury.—Rayer, op. et vol. cit., p. 19.—ED.

† Linnæus, Diss. de Ledo Palustri, Upsal, 1775. Abhandl. der Königl. Schwed. Academie der Wissenschaften, band xli., p. 194.

there are unquestionable examples of its having produced a beneficial effect. Dr. Pulteney has especially noticed its success in a letter to Sir William Watson. The herb, however, is one of the most violent poisons we possess in our fields, and when mistaken for wild celery, water parsuip, or various other herbs, has frequently proved fatal a few hours after being swallowed, exciting convulsions, giddiness, locked jaw, violent heat in the throat and stomach, and sometimes sickness and purging : and where the patient has been fortunate enough to recover, it has often been with the loss of his nails and hair. Goats, however, eat it with impunity, though it is injurious to most other quadrupeds. As a medicine, it is given in the form of an infusion of the leaves : though sometimes the juice of the roots has taken the place of the leaves. Three teaspoonfuls of the juice is an ordinary dose, which is repeated every morning.

But by far the most active and salutary medicine for every form of leprosy, in Europe as well as in Asia, is arsenic. I have already adverted to its common use in the latter quarter ; and at home, in the form of the College solution, it has often been found to succeed, when every other medicine has been abandoned in despair. The ordinary dose is five minims twice or even three times a day, increased as the stomach will allow, or till the patient appears to be over-dosed, when he will exhibit several or all of the following symptoms : headache, a pain and often a sense of inflation in the stomach and bowels, cough, restlessness, irritation in the skin generally, redness and stiffening of the palpebræ, soreness of the gums, and ptyalism.*

SPECIES III.
LEPIDOSIS PSORIASIS.
DRY-SCALL.

PATCHES OF ROUGH, AMORPHOUS SCALES ; CONTINUOUS, OR OF INDETERMINATE OUTLINE : SKIN OFTEN CHAPPY.†

PSORIASIS is a derivation of ψώρα, "scabies,

---

* The tincture of cantharides, in doses of five drops, increased sometimes to thirty, will occasionally remove leprous inflammation with rapidity.—See Rayer, Traité des Maladies de la Peau, tom. ii., p. 21.—ED.

† A chronic inflammation of the skin, confined to one region of the body, or extending over its whole surface, characterized by scales of various shapes and sizes, not depressed in the centre, and whose irregular margins are not prominent, like those of lepra or lepriasis.—(See Rayer, Traité Théorique, &c. des Maladies de la Peau, tom. ii., p. 28.) Psoriasis is only liable to be confounded with three other diseases ; namely, lepriasis, pityriasis, and syphilitic scaly patches. As Rayer observes, there is, indeed, a great analogy between lepriasis and psoriasis, especially psoriasis guttata. They both begin with solid, and, as it were, papulous elevations ; both are extremely obstinate ; they soon assume the form of scaly circular patches ; and finally, in the same patient, scaly patches are often seen taking the shape of psoriasis guttata on the trunk, and that of lepriasis on the elbows and knees. The patches of psoriasis guttata, however, are always narrower, and

asperitas," with a terminal ιρις, as in the preceding species. The primary term ψώρα, or psora, was used in very different senses among the Greek writers, from a cause I have already explained under LEPRIASIS, where it has been shown, that the real radical is the Hebrew term צרע (tsora), " to smite malignantly or with a disease," whence צרעת (tsorat) imports the leprosy in a malignant or contagious form, but not in an uncontagious. The lexicographers, not hitting upon the proper origin of ψώρα, have supposed it to be derived from ψάω (psao), which means, however, unfortunately, " tergo, detergo," " to cleanse, purify, or deterge," instead of " to pollute :" but, as one way of cleansing is by scraping, and as persons labouring under psora scrape or scratch the skin on account of its itching, the difficulty is supposed to be hereby solved, and psora is allowed to import derivatively what, upon this explanation, it opposes radically.

The actual origin of the term, however, is of little importance. It was mostly employed by the Greek writers, and has been very generally so in modern times, to import a dry scall or scale ; for the terms are univocal : the Saxon sceala or scala being the origin of the former, and denoting the latter, of a rough surface and indeterminate outline, as expressed in the specific definition.

Psoriasis, as thus interpreted, is the dry Sahafata ڎﻪﻣ of the Arabian writers, the ספחת (Saphat) of the Levitical code, as already explained ; the Arabic being derived from the Hebrew root. It embraces the following varieties :

α Guttata. Guttated dry-scall.	Drop-like, but with irregular margin. In children contagious.	
β Gyrata. Gyrated dry-scall.	Scaly patches in serpentine or tortuous stripes. Found chiefly on the back, sometimes on the face.	

generally more crowded together, than those of lepriasis ; their margins are not raised, and their centre is not depressed, like those of the latter affection : in psoriasis, the inflammation of the corpus reticulare is more acute, giving a redder appearance to the scales, which are more adherent than those of lepriasis. The differences between lepriasis and psoriasis diffusa are still more remarkable. The patches of the latter are irregular, and not depressed in the centre : those of lepriasis are exactly circular, and even when several leprous patches conjoin, their circular arrangement is yet manifest in the segments of circles visible at their circumference. Then psoriasis differs from the scaly eruptions of syphilis, which are encircled by a copper-coloured areola, and have scales of diminutive size, not well marked : there is sometimes a small pustule in their middle, soon followed by a scab. They have a strong disposition to ulcerate, are not accompanied by pruritus, and are often complicated with syphilitic affections of the conjunctiva, pharynx, nodes, &c. They rapidly yield to mercury, and especially to corrosive sublimate. Lastly, they disappear first at their circumference, and then at their centre, where they frequently leave a small white cicatrix.—See Rayer, tom. ii., p. 39.—ED.

γ Diffusa.
Spreading dry-
scall.

Patches diffuse, with a ragged, chapped, irritable surface : sense of burning and
itching when warm : skin
gradually thickened and furrowed, with a powdery scurf
in the fissures. Extends
over the face and scalp.

δ Inveterata.
Inveterate dry-
scall.

Patches continuous over the
whole surface ; readily falling off, and reproducible,
with painful, diffuse excoriations. Extend to the nails
and toes, which become convex and thickened. Found
chiefly in old persons.

ε Localis.
Local dry-scall.

Stationary, and limited to particular organs.

In the FIRST, or GUTTATED VARIETY, the
patches very seldom extend to the size of a sixpence ; and are distinguished from those of leprosy by having neither an elevated margin nor
an elliptic or circular form, often spreading an-
gularly, and sometimes running into small serpentine processes.* The eruption commences
in the spring, mostly on the limbs, and appears
afterward distributed over the body, sometimes
over the face. It subsides by degrees towards
the autumn, and sometimes reappears in the
spring ensuing.†

In children, probably from the greater sensibility of their skin, this variety of scall spreads
often with great rapidity, and is scattered over
the entire body in two or three days.

The SECOND, or GYRATED VARIETY, runs in a
migratory course, and apes the shape of earthworms or leeches when incurvated, with slender vermiform appendages. Not unfrequently
the two ends meet, and give the scall an annu-
lated figure like a ringworm, particularly about
the upper part of the shoulders or on the neck, in
which case they are sometimes confounded with
shingles, or some other modification of herpes.‡

* The scaly patches are small, distinct, irregular, and two or three lines in diameter, each commencing with a little solid red elevation, of the
size of a pin's head, the apex of which soon becomes covered with a diminutive, dry, white
scale. The patches are rounded, prominent, lenticular, and, at first, separated from one another
by considerable interspaces. Their centre is always more raised than their edges ; but, when
they get well, as the cure takes place from the
centre towards the circumference, the middle of
the patches, composed of sound skin, or skin
somewhat altered in colour, then becomes accidentally depressed. As the cure advances further,
the patches are transformed into segments of circles.—See Rayer, Traité des. Mal. de la Peau,
tom. ii., p. 29.—ED.

† Psoriasis guttata most frequently makes its
attack in autumn or spring, and sometimes gets
well of itself in the summer. It may in this manner appear and disappear again, for several years
in succession.—(See Rayer, op. et vol. cit., p. 30.)
It is the most common species of psoriasis, for it
amounts, according to Rayer's calculation (p.
39), to three fifths of the total number of different
examples of the disease.—ED.

‡ Psoriasis gyrata, like all the other varieties

The SPREADING SCALL commences commonly
on the face or temples,* as the first of the preceding does on the extremities, and the second
on the back. It is sometimes confined to a single patch, which, nevertheless, is occasionally
to be seen in some other part, as the wrist, the
elbow-joint, breast, or calf of the leg. It is
often obstinate and of long duration, and has
been known to continue for a series of years :
in which cases, however, there is usually an aggravation or extension of it at the vernal periods. It is at times preceded by some constitutional affection ; and at times seems to produce the same. When limited to the back of
the hand, this, like some other forms of lepidosis, is vulgarly called the Baker's Itch.† On
the hands and arms, and sometimes on the face
and neck, it is peculiarly troublesome to washerwomen ; probably from the irritation of the soap
they are continually making use of.

The inveteracy of the FOURTH VARIETY seems
principally to spring from the general torpitude
and want of power in the class of persons
whom it chiefly attacks, which is those who
are in the decline of life. It is accompanied
with painful excoriations, in many instances occasioned by the pressure of some parts of the
clothing against the sores, or by the attrition of
contiguous surfaces, as of the nates, groins,
thighs, and scrotum. At an advanced period
of the disease, the cuticle is often still more
extensively destroyed ; and the extremities, the
back, and nates, have been seen excoriated at the
same time, with a very profuse discharge of thin
lymph from the surface : after which the discharge itself thickens, from an absorption of the

of psoriasis, undergoes marked remissions during
summer, and almost always grows worse in winter.
—See Rayer, tom. ii., p. 30.—ED.

* According to Rayer, more frequently on the
limbs than the trunk ; the patches sometimes disappearing in one region and appearing in another.
The arrangement of them, either in small circular spots, or within a broader form, makes no difference in the nature of the disease, and often
psoriasis guttata is seen on the trunk, and psoriasis diffusa on the limbs, of the same individual.—
(Op. et vol. cit., p. 31.) The patches, like those
of psoriasis guttata, usually begin as small, solid,
very numerous, and, as it were, papulous elevations, on the summit of which, little dry scales,
of a dead white colour, are formed. The skin inflames, and becomes scaly in the interspaces ; the
scales enlarge and conjoin ; their surfaces are
red, and they are frequently separated by dry,
linear, and painful cracks. On the legs and forearms the united patches sometimes constitute but
a single extensive one, or else represent a broad
band running in the direction of the length of the
affected limb. In these cases, instead of complete
scales, one sometimes perceives on the inflamed
skin only diminutive furfuraceous scaly particles,
resembling powdered mustard in colour ; and
when the scales are removed with the aid of lotions, warm-bathing, steam, &c,, the subjacent
surface appears smooth, glossy, and inflamed.—
See Rayer, op. et vol. cit., p. 31.—ED.

† Grocer's itch, also, is described by Rayer as a
variety of psoriasis diffusa. Indeed, this itch and
baker's itch are considered by him as the same
disease.—ED.

finer parts, and forms a dry, harsh, and almost horny cuticle, which progressively separates in large pieces.* At first this variety intermits in the summer, but at length becomes permanent and intractable.

The LOCAL VARIETY is found chiefly on the lips, eyelids, prepuce, scrotum, and inside of the hands. It is peculiarly common to shoemakers, and artificers in metallic trades, as braziers, tinmen, and silversmiths : probably from filth and the irritation of the substances they make use of.†

The DRY-SCALL, under one or other of the above forms, is one of the most frequent cutaneous diseases in this kingdom ; and the first variety, guttated or drop-scall, psoriasis guttata, is sometimes contagious in irritable skins, and especially among children.‡ Several of these modifications are also found, occasionally, as symptoms or sequels of lues, particularly the first three ; but are in every instance distinguishable by the livid or chocolate hue of the scales.

As cutaneous sordes, in connexion with a peculiarity in the constitution of the skin, and especially in connexion with a meager diet, in-

dolence, and want of exercise,* appears to be the general cause of this as well as of many other, perhaps most other, simple cutaneous eruptions, the first principles of a curative intention must consist in washing and softening the skin by warm-bathing, regularly persevered in ; and in improving the diet, and exciting to a life of more activity. Beyond this, the common treatment of psoriasis should be, with little exception, that of lepriasis' [varied, as in this case, according to the more or less inflamed state of the skin]. Hence the alterant and stimulant ointments of sulphur and tar in equal proportions ; lotions' of diluted aromatic vinegar, or nitrate of silver, and the sulphureous waters of Harrogate, Croft, Sharpmore, Broughton, Wrigglesworth, and other places, used both externally and internally, will succeed better than common spring or river-water, as detergents.† Chalybeate medicines, and particularly chalybeate waters, have been powerfully recommended by Dr. Willan and many others : but, excepting where the disease is combined with a languid circulation, as in the inveterate form, and demands excitement, these do not appear to be of any certain efficacy. Bleeding and the repetition of purgatives are of no avail, though a common practice with many, and founded also on the authority of Dr. Willan.‡

---

* Whether the disease begin in the form of psoriasis guttata, or that of psoriasis diffusa, after it has continued several months or years, and especially when it has occurred in old persons, enfeebled by misery or the abuse of spirituous liquors, the redness of the skin under the scales diminishes ; its tissue becomes indurated and swollen ; the patches are covered with hard, dry, white, thick scales ; the skin, stiffened and tense, yields with difficulty to the movements of the limbs ; and very soon numerous deep fissures intersect it in various directions, emitting blood, and sometimes pus, that dries into linear scabs. A burning itching is experienced in the skin, particularly in the night. This inveterate form of psoriasis may extend over the greater part of the surface of the body. When limited to one region, the skin really undergoes there a species of hypertrophy, rising sometimes a quarter of a line higher than the level of the surrounding healthy skin.— See Rayer, tom. ii., p. 33.—Ed.

† The grocer's itch, as already noticed, is regarded by Rayer as a variety of psoriasis ; it occurs sometimes on the dorsal surface of the hands of grocers, but it is observed likewise in bakers, washerwomen, bleachers, and the higher classes of society. The disease begins with two or three small scaly elevations, which successively spread over all the back of the hand. The inflamed skin is soon pervaded by dry painful fissures, especially about the wrist and the joints between the first phalanges of the fingers and the metacarpal bones. This variety of psoriasis may be known from the confluent and chronic lichen of the back of the hand, because, in the latter, the scaly state of the skin is always preceded by a considerable eruption of small papulæ. When this or any other form of psoriasis invades the whole of the hand, the matrix of the nails itself becomes the seat of chronic inflammation ; then the nails thicken, curve, split, and are ultimately thrown off, being replaced by others, which may undergo similar changes.—See Rayer, tom. ii., p. 37.—Ed.

‡ Rayer does not regard psoriasis as a contagious disease ; but notices its hereditary character, as being often unequivocally exemplified.— Tom. ii., p. 39.—Ed.

* The seasons have a very marked influence on psoriasis diffusa and psoriasis guttata, the attacks of which commonly begin in the commencement of autumn or spring. The influence of employments and trades seems to be restricted to a few local varieties ; in short, whatever directly or indirectly irritates the skin may probably excite psoriasis, which has been known to follow repeated attacks of lichen or prurigo, the application of a blister, or the development of some other acute disease of the skin.—See Rayer, tom. ii., p. 39.—Ed.

† Dr. A. T. Thomson has seen much benefit from the following lotion :—℞ Sulphureti potassæ ʒj ; saponis ʒij ; aq. distillatæ ℥viij ; ft. solutio, partibus affectis ope spongiæ applicanda ;—or from an unchymical lotion, composed of sulphate of zinc, acetate of lead, each twenty grains ; aq. rosæ, ℥v ; mucil. acaciæ ℥j.—See Atlas of Delineations of Cutaneous Diseases, p. 19, 4to.—Ed.

‡ Notwithstanding our author's statement, Willan's practice has high authorities in its favour. When psoriasis guttata is recent, and in an adult subject, Rayer recommends the treatment to commence with one or more general bleedings. Duffin, Wallace, and Graves are also advocates for the same plan. When psoriasis is general, blood is to be taken occasionally from the neighbourhood of the inflamed points, on the neck, the trunk, and limbs, for several weeks, the patient employing at the same time simple baths, or, which Rayer prefers, cool narcotic emollient baths, which powerfully lessen the cutaneous inflammation and excessive itching. In adults, pouring warm water on the parts, and the vapour-bath, are of service in detaching the scales ; and by alternating this practice and that of sulphureous baths, psoriasis diffusa, not attended with much inflammation, may sometimes be cured in three or four months. When, however, psoriasis diffusa is of long standing, the modification of irritation of the skin should be changed by frictions with antimonial ointment, which sometimes prove useful even in inveterate psoriasis, though, in this case, the af-

"Strong mercurial preparations," observes Dr. Willan, "are of no advantage, but eventually rather aggravate the complaint."* Nor do the fresh juices of the alterant plants, scurvy-grass, succory, fumitory, or sharp-pointed dock, appear to be of any material benefit. The solution of arsenic, however, has seemed at times to restore the habit to a healthy reaction.

A gentle purgative should open the course of medical treatment ; to which should succeed an internal use of the fixed alkalis, with precipitated sulphur, and decoctions of elm-root, sarsaparilla, sassafras, mezereon, or dulcamara ; and when the skin is very dry, an antimonial at night, or five grains of Plummer's pill, the compound submuriate mercurial pill of the London College. Yet here, as in the preceding species, the most effectual remedy, in obstinate cases, is the arsenic solution, with an abstinence from fruits, acids, and fermented liquors : under which plan, in conjunction with the above regimen, most of the ordinary cases will be found to disappear in about three weeks or a month.

How far the sulphureous vapour-bath may succeed in any of the varieties of this as well as of the ensuing, and of several other species, has not hitherto been sufficiently determined. M. Galés of Paris, and, in consequence of his recommendation, M. de Carn of Vienna, have tried it upon an extensive scale, and apparently with considerable success.† But, as in most other cases of a new invention, it is represented as being successful in such a multiplicity of diseases, and diseases essentially dissimilar, that its very popularity abroad has operated against a free and decisive trial of its powers among the more cautious practitioners of our own country. A few institutions, however, I am glad to find, are at length founded, both in this metropolis and in Dublin, for the laudable purpose of carrying on a full investigation : so that we shall soon be enabled to draw a correct estimate.‡

---

fection of the skin is so deep, that it is almost always incurable, at least in old persons, Psoriasis inveterata, according to Rayer, is benefited by emollient narcotic baths, employed to bring about the separation of the scales. He advises also occasional local bleeding in the vicinity of the most irritated points. This palliative treatment be prefers to any attempt at a complete cure, when the skin is thickened, fissured, and indurated, in nearly every region of the body.—See Rayer, tom. ii, p. 42.—Ed.

* Dr. A. T. Thomson excepts the more severe cases of P. diffusa, for which small doses of three or five grains of Plummer's pills are sometimes useful, given in conjunction with cinchona and soda :—

℞ Sodæ bicarbonatis ʒij.
Infusi cinchon. lancif. ℥vss.
Tinet. cascarillæ, ʒiv.

Fiat Mist., cujus 4ta pars bis in die sumatur. In the P. guttata he also gives hydrargyrum cum creta, in doses of twelve grains at bedtime, until the gums are slightly affected.—See Atlas of Delineations of Cutaneous Diseases, p. 19, 4to.—Ed.

† Ueber Kraetze, und derem bequemste schnellwirkendeste und sicherste Heilart, &c., von D. Karsten, &c., &c., Hanover, 1818.

‡ Observations on Sulphureous Fumigation as

SPECIES IV.

LEPIDOSIS ICHTHYIASIS.

FISH-SKIN.

THICK, INDURATED INCRUSTATION UPON THE SKIN, TO A GREATER OR LESS EXTENT ; SCALINESS IMPERFECT.*

The specific term is derived from ιχθὺς, "piscis," with the terminal adjunct of the preceding species. The word is commonly written, but less correctly, ichthyosis, since, as I have already observed, the suffix *iasis* is by general consent applied to all species appertaining to the genus or tribe of diseases before us.

In the disease before us, the cutaneous excretories throw forth such an excess of calcareous matter, that it often covers the entire body like a shell; and the cutis, the rete mucosum, and the cuticle, being equally impregnated with it, the order of the tegumental laminæ is destroyed, and the whole forms a common mass of bony or horny corium, generally scaly or imbricate, according as the calcareous earth is deposited with a larger or smaller proportion of gluten, in many instances of enormous thickness, and sometimes giving rise to sprouts or branches of a very grotesque appearance : thus offering to us numerous varieties, of which the following are the chief :—

α Simplex, Simple fish-skin.	The incrustation forming a harsh, papulated, or watery rind ; hue dusky ; subjacent muscles flexible.— Sometimes covering the whole body, except the head and face, palms of the hands, and soles of the feet.
β Cornea. Horny fish-skin.	The incrustation forming a rigid, horny, imbricated rind ; hue brown or yellow ; subjacent muscles inflexible. Sometimes covering the entire body, including the face and tongue.

---

a Remedy in Rheumatism and Diseases of the Skin, by W. Wallace, &c., Dublin, 1820. With reference to psoriasis inveterata, Dr. A. T. Thomson, after noticing the liquor arsenicalis, speaks highly of the liquor potassæ, which, he says, is the most effectual remedy, in doses of ℳ xxx. gradually increased to ℳ cl., given in the bitter almond emulsion, twice a day ; or, if the patient be delicate, in some bitter infusion, and the hydrargyrum cum creta at bedtime. The psoriasis palmaria receives benefit from the steam of warm water, and should then have the ung. hydrarg nitrat. applied to it in a very diluted form.—See Dr. A. T. Thomson's Atlas of Delineations of Cutaneous Diseases, p. 19.—Ed.

* Ichthyasis is characterized by a morbid development of the cuticle, often accompanied by hypertrophy of the cutis. The cuticle forms on the surface of a part, or of nearly the whole of the skin, a thick gray stratum, divided into small irregular compartments, not overlapping, however, like the scales of fish.—Rayer, Traité des Maladies de la Peau, tom. ii., p. 302.—Ep.

γ Cornigera.   The incrustation accompa-
  Cornigerous fish-   nied with horn-like, incur-
  skin.'   vated sproutings; some-
        times periodically shed
        and reproduced.

This indurated incrustation commences with
a change in the papillæ of the cutis, which are
elongated and enlarged into roundish cones or
tubercles, often void of sensation. Some of the
scaly papillæ have a short, narrow neck, and
broad, irregular tops. Sometimes the scales are
flat and large,-and imbricated or placed like
tiling, or the scales on the back of fishes, one
overlapping another.* They also differ considerably in colour in different instances, and are
blackish, brown, or white. The skin, to a very
considerable extent, has sometimes been found
thickened into a stout, tough leather. In a singular enlargement of the lower extremity, produced by a puerperal sparganosis, Mr. Chevalier found the thickness of the corium in some
parts nearly a quarter of an inch; which, on
being cut into, presented the same grained appearance that is observable in a section of the
hides of the larger quadrupeds. Below the coriaceous skin, the adipose membrane exhibited
an equal increase of substance, and, in front of
the tibia, was not less than an inch and a half
thick. And there is a singular case, recorded
by Dr. Baillie, in which the same crassitude
was found in the skin of an infant who died a
few days after birth.—(*Wardrop's edition of his
Works*, vol. i., p. 75.) Mr. Machin gives a very
extraordinary case of ichthyiasis of the same
kind, originating, indeed, from a different and
unknown cause, which covered the whole body,
with the exception of the head and face, the
palms of the hands, and the soles of the feet.†

* Rayer considers the name objectionable, because, according to his observations, the scales do
not lie one upon the other, like the scales of a fish.
The stratum of thickened cuticle, divided into irregular compartments, he thinks, is more analogous to the skin of the claws of a fowl, than to
the very diversified scales of fishes and serpents.
At a certain distance, the skin looks as if it were
soiled with mud, though the appearance of the disease varies according to its degree. Sometimes
the alteration of the cuticle is slight; the skin
being of a dull colour, mealy, and communicating,
when touched, a feel like that of the skin of some
old persons. When ichthyiasis is more developed,
it appears on the limbs in the form of a thick layer
of the cuticle, compared, not without some exaggeration, to the bark of trees, and composed of
small, very irregular compartments, not overlapping, and not exceeding two or three lines in diameter, but wider in proportion as they are thin.
Their colour, which is usually a dull gray or
earthy hue, is in some rare examples shining, and
almost like pearl, but more frequently a dark
brown.—See Rayer, tom. ii., p. 303.—ED.

† In parts of the skin naturally very smooth,
the disease is least disposed to occur. The fur-
row at the side of the spine is stated by Willan
never to be the seat of scales; but in one example,
under Dr. Elliotson, some of them occupied that
situation.—(Clin. Lect. in Lancet, 1830-31, p.
593.) The disease often begins in childhood, and
sometimes in early infancy; and it is more common in males than females; and the girls of the

The entire skin formed a dusky, ragged, thick
case, which did not bleed when cut into or scarified, was callous and insensible, and was shed
annually, like the crust of a lobster, about autumn, at which time it usually acquired the
thickness of three fourths of an inch, and was
thrust off by the sprouting of a new skin beneath.
—(*Phil. Trans.*, No. 424.) This man married,
and had a family of six children, all of whom
possessed the same ragged covering as himself.*
The father was twice salivated for the complaint, and threw off the casing each time, as did
one of the children during the smallpox; but the
disease soon returned on both of them. One
case is recorded in which the face was the only
part exempted from the fish-scale covering.—
(*Trans. Medico-Chir. Soc.*, vol. ix., p. 52.)

There is a remarkable passage in the Lettres
Edifiantes et Curieuses of the Jesuits, which intimates that this disease is by no means uncommon among the inhabitants of Paraguay; the
words, which have been quoted by M. Buffon
and Dr. Willan, are as follow:—"Il règne par-
mi eux une maladie éxtraordinaire: c'est une
espèce de Lèpre qui leur couvre tout le corps, et
y forme une croûte semblable à des écailles de
poisson: cette incommodité ne leur cause aucune douleur, ni même aucun autre dérangement dans la santé."† There is perhaps no part

same parents have sometimes all been affected
with ichthyiasis, while all the boys were free from
it.—(See Rayer, tom. ii., p. 305.) The morbid
development of the cuticle always produces the
greatest thickening of it in situations where the
skin is naturally thickest, and the cuticle itself
coarse, as round the joints, on the anterior and external surface of the lower extremities, on the forepart of the kneepan, at the back of the upper extremities, over the olecranon, &c. In all other
places, the morbid deposite is generally much thinner, and it is usually absent from the prepuce, eyelids, groins, armpits, &c. Neither is it found on
the soles of the feet or the palms of the hands,
doubtless in consequence of the particular texture
of these parts.—See Rayer, tom. ii., p. 302.—ED.

* According to Rayer, ichthyiasis is almost always congenital, and its hereditary character is
the best ascertained cause of it.—(Tom. ii., p. 305.)
Dr. Elliotson had two brothers under his care in
St. Thomas's Hospital, both of whom were affected with ichthyiasis; and he refers to another instance, in which a mother and her female child
were affected. This disease is placed among the
scaly diseases by Dr. Willan, but Rayer separates
it from lepra and psoriasis, and classes many diseases of the skin as inflammatory affections. The
plan is highly approved of by Dr. Elliotson, to
whom it appears that a large number of cutaneous
disorders are merely inflammatory, and will yield to
nothing without antiphlogistic treatment. If, says
he, you take blood from a patient who has lepra or
psoriasis, you will frequently find that it is buffed;
the skin is unnaturally red, hot, and smarting; but
in ichthyiasis there is no mark of inflammation
whatever. The skin is not hot; the skin does not
tingle; and if you take blood away, it is not
buffed. There is no pain in the head, nor thirst:
the case is merely an organic affection of the skin.
—See also Rayer, tom. ii., p. 306.—ED.

† Recueil des Lettres, &c., xxv., p. 122. Rayer
observes, that this statement is only vulgar tradi-
tion, destitute of foundation. Climate, regimen,

of the world where we should sooner expect to meet with this, and indeed various other species of squamose or leprous affections of the skin, considering the sultry heat of the atmosphere, the rankness of the perspiration that issues from the bodies of the natives, and their deficiency in personal cleanliness; yet I do not know that the same account has been given by any other travellers, and have looked in vain over Estella and Dobrizhoffer: nor does this particular incrustation of the skin seem to be prevalent in other inland countries exposed to the same excitements, though most of them exhibit squamose disorders of the surface of some kind or other.

In our own country, it often shows itself locally, and is restricted to a single limb, as an arm, leg, or the soles of the feet;* and it has sometimes fixed on a cheek, an interesting figure of which is given in Dr. Bateman's Delineations.

Examples of the cornigerous variety, or that in which the incrustation is accompanied with a sprouting of horns or horn-shaped projections, are by no means uncommon. Sir Everard Home has given two cases in the Philosophical Transactions that occurred within his own knowledge. The patients were women about the middle of life, or rather later : one had four horns, and the other a single horn. Each of them grew from a cyst, which formed gradually, and at last opened spontaneously, and discharged " a thick gritty fluid."—(*Phil. Trans.*, vol. lxxxi., p. 95.) The foreign journals are full of similar accounts ; in some of which the horns are of considerable length, mostly growing upon the head, though in a few instances on the back.† In the British Museum is shown, as a curiosity, a horn of this kind, eleven inches long, and two and a half in circumference at the base. It is said to have issued from a wen that formed in the head of a woman, and to have reached its full length in four years.

When these are single, they rather, perhaps, belong to the genus ECPHYMA,‡ and particularly the species verruca and clavus ; but they are very frequently connected with a dry, furfuraceous, or scaly skin, often oozing a calcareous material.§ A very singular example of this complex

and kind of constitution, he says, have no particular influence in producing this disease.—(Tom. ii., p. 306.) Women, he admits, are less frequently afflicted than men ; but their being attacked is not very uncommon, and he has seen a dozen instances of it.—Ed.

　. * These parts, as Rayer mentions, are usually exempted.—Ed.
　† Eph. Nat. Cur., dec. i., ann. i., obs. 30. See also Hist. de la Société Royale de la Médecine, 1776, p. 316.
　‡ The arrangement of horny excrescences under ichthyiasis seems hardly allowable : for, whatever may have been the cause of the very curious disease that occurred in the heifer referred to in the text, it is certain that, in the human subject, the horny excrescences usually met with are the productions of the cysts of particular wens, which, after bursting, continue to secrete and protrude the horny substance.—Ed.
　§ A case of this kind occurred in the practice of Dr. Valentine Mott. The part diseased was

modification occurred a few years ago in a Leicestershire heifer, which was publicly exhibited, and of which the author presented a description and a drawing to the Royal Society. The whole of the skin was covered with a thick, dry, chalky scurf, often producing an itching ; and wherever the skin was scratched, a calcareous fluid oozed from it, that soon hardened, and put forth corneous, recurvating excrescences, frequently divaricating, and assuming sometimes a leafy, sometimes a horn-shaped appearance. The back was covered with them ; over the forehead, below the dewlap, they hung in some hundreds ; many as large as natural horns, and rattling together whenever the animal moved. The heifer was otherwise in good health, and secreted the same chalky fluid whatever food she was fed upon.

Medicine has hitherto been found of but little avail under any form of this affection. Dr. Willan recommended immersing the incrusted part in water, and picking off the scales with the finger-nails, while thus soaked. Dr. Bateman recommends that the bath should be of sulphureous waters, and the scales rubbed off with a flannel or rough cloth. But both admit that their methods produce only a partial cure ; that the skin does not recover its proper texture, and that the eruption will probably recur.* Dr. Bateman further recommends, as having been actually serviceable, pills made of pitch, hardened

the scrotum ; and the patient was a wealthy farmer, seventy-three years of age ; he had been affected for two or three years with a disease of the stomach, attended with an ulceration of the scrotum, from which there was also an extremely fetid discharge. "On examination, the scrotum exhibited," says Dr. Mott, "a monstrous, and, to me, a very unique appearance, reaching fully two thirds the length of his thighs, being from twelve to fifteen times its ordinary bulk, and studded, particularly on each edge, it being flattened anteriorly and posteriorly, with several dozen tumours, of a stony hardness, covered with the integuments, from the size of nutmegs to that of a large pea. It resembled an enormous bunch of grapes, or more closely, some morbid conditions of the pancreas and spleen which we have occasionally met with. The tumours had all a very white appearance, and the integuments of two or three of the largest having been ulcerated for upwards of a year, poured forth a constant and very fetid discharge. At these openings white bodies were seen, which, when touched with a probe, felt of a stony hardness. A white substance resembling mortar was discharging from these openings, which resulted from the crumbling away of the calculi, and the combination of this substance with the fluid from the ulcers. This state of the scrotum had continued for upwards of twenty years, and had been gradually increasing, the tumours multiplying as the scrotum augmented in size. The patient knew of no cause to which it could be ascribed." The diseased mass was removed by Dr. Mott, a new scrotum formed, and the man recovered.— (See the Phil. Journal of the Med. and Phys. Sc., vol. xiv.)—D.
　* Rayer observes that ichthyiasis is seldom cured, unless it be slight, and that the long continuance of emollient applications, vapour, alkaline, and tepid baths, will only be of service in freeing the skin from the scales.—Ed.

by flour or any other farinaceous substance, which makes the cuticle crack and fall off, as he tells us, without the aid of external means, and leaves a sound skin underneath.* When there is an evident excess of calcareous earth, the most efficacious remedy is probably to be found in a free use of acids, and especially the mineral acids. The arsenic solution, however, is worth trying, but I have no documents of its effects.†

GENUS V.
ECPHLYSIS.
BLAINS.

ORBICULAR ELEVATIONS OF THE CUTICLE, CONTAINING A WATERY FLUID.

Eᴄᴘʜʟʏsɪs (ἐκφλυσις, from ἐκφλύζω, "ebullio," "efferveo," "to boil or bubble up or over"), imports "vesicular eruption confined in its action to the surface;" as ᴇᴍᴘʜʟʏsɪs, which we have long since described (vol. i., p. 608), is "vesicular eruption essentially connected with internal and febrile affection." The term is intended to include all those utricles, or minute bladders of the cuticle, containing a watery fluid, and not necessarily connected with internal disease, whether *bullæ* or *vesiculæ*, between which Dr. Willan has made but little difference in his definitions, except in respect to size : and which were equally denominated by the Greek physicians phlyctænæ, a term derived from the present source. And hence the species that fairly ap-

pertain to this genus appear to be the following :—

1. Ecphlysis Pompholyx.   Water-blebs.
2. ————— Herpes.   Tetter.
3. ————— Rhypia.   Sordid Blain.
4. ————— Eczema.   Heat-eruption.

SPECIES I.
ECPHLYSIS POMPHOLYX.
WATER-BLEBS.

ᴇʀᴜᴘᴛɪᴏɴ ᴏꜰ ʙʟᴇʙs, ᴄᴏɴᴛᴀɪɴɪɴɢ ᴀ ʀᴇᴅᴅɪsʜ, ᴛʀᴀɴsᴘᴀʀᴇɴᴛ ꜰʟᴜɪᴅ ; ᴍᴏsᴛʟʏ ᴅɪsᴛɪɴᴄᴛ ; ʙʀᴇᴀᴋɪɴɢ ᴀɴᴅ ʜᴇᴀʟɪɴɢ ᴡɪᴛʜᴏᴜᴛ sᴄᴀʟᴇ ᴏʀ ᴄʀᴜsᴛ.*

Pᴏᴍᴘʜᴏʟʏx, or pomphus, was used among the Greek writers in the same sense as ᴘᴇᴍᴘʜɪx, of which we have treated already (vol. i., p. 608, *Emphlysis Pemphigus*), and equally imported a bladdery tumour of the skin, distended with a fluid : the Latins denominated it bulla, of which our own term, ᴡᴀᴛᴇʀ-ʙʟᴇʙ, is an apt and exact representative. Pᴇᴍᴘʜɪx, in the modern use of the term, is necessarily accompanied with fever, and hence, under the present arrangement, is an ᴇᴍᴘʜʟʏsɪs, as ᴘᴏᴍᴘʜᴏʟʏx, being without fever or other constitutional affection necessarily connected with it, is an ᴇᴄᴘʜʟʏsɪs.† The latter is hence denominated Pemphigus apyretos by Plenck, and Pemphigus sine pyrexia by Sauvages. It has, however, been properly separated from Pemphigus by Dr. Willan, who has arranged it as it stands in the present work. It offers the four following varieties :—

α Benignus. Mild water-blebs.	Blebs pea-sized, or filbert-sized ; appearing successively on various parts of the body ; bursting in three or four days, and healing readily.
β Diutinus. Lingering water-blebs.	Blebs gradually growing from small vesicles to the size of walnuts ; yellow-

---

* Dr. Willan recommended pitch as an excellent remedy, in the quantity of half an ounce a day. Rayer asserts that experience has not confirmed its efficacy ; but Dr. Elliotson tried it in conjunction with the hot bath and the application of olive oil to the body every day ; and a perfect cure was effected in about a month, though the disease had existed four years. After the oil had been applied, it was not wiped off, but flannel clothes were put on, and these were continued, without being washed, during the treatment ; so that the patient was continually immersed, as it were, in grease.—(Clin. Lect., op. et. vol. cit., p. 595.) Dr. Elliotson found the bath so harmless, that his patient was able to take an ounce and a quarter of it in the day. The hot bath was soon discontinued ; but the inunction, he thinks, from the rapidity of the cure, must have had some effect, as well as the pitch. In cases of partial ichthyiasis, Rayer suggests the trial of repeated blisters, experience having proved that congenital ichthyiasis has sometimes disappeared for a time on the accession of various cutaneous inflammations, as that of variola.—Tom. ii., p. 307.—Eᴅ.

† Such horny excrescences as are the productions of certain encysted swellings require to be taken away with a scalpel, care being observed to leave none of the cyst behind ; for if this important indication be neglected, the disease will return. The editor was once required to remove, from the nates of an old respectable medical gentleman in town, a complete horn, a similar one to which had been removed on a former occasion by another surgeon, but not effectually, because a portion of the cyst had been left. The second operation was followed by a radical cure ; and the patient is at the present time alive, and quite free from his horny annoyance.—Eᴅ.

* Rayer's definition of pemphigus, which in his classification seems to comprise both pemphigus and pompholyx, is somewhat different from that of Dr. Good ; indeed, pemphigus with him is a bullous disorder ; with our author, a vesicular one. " Pemphigus," says he, " is an inflammation of the skin, principally characterized by one or several large yellowish transparent bullæ, the eruption of which may take place simultaneously or successively. After a few days' duration, each bulla terminates by an effusion of the fluid which it contains, the formation of a scab of greater or less thickness, or superficial ulceration."—See Rayer, Traité des Mal. de la Peau, tom. i., p. 154.—Eᴅ.

† The two fundamental divisions of pemphigus, adopted by Rayer, is into acute and chronic.— (See Traité des Mal. de la Peau, tom. i., p. 155.) The first, a febrile disorder, described by Dr. Good in the first volume of this work, under the name of emphlysis pemphigus, as already mentioned : the second differing from the foregoing in the long duration of the eruption, which usually lasts several months ; in the mode in which the bullæ are developed, which is always successive ; and in the absence of any febrile reaction, at least in the early periods of the disease.—Eᴅ.

ish; often spreading in succession over the whole body and interior of the mouth; occasionally reproduced, and forming an excoriated surface with ulceration. Often preceded by languor or other general indisposition for several weeks. Duration from two to four or five days.

γ Quotidianus.
Quotidian water-blebs.

Blebs with a dark red base, appearing at night and disappearing in the morning, or appearing in the morning and disappearing at night. Found chiefly on the hands and legs.

δ Solitarius.
Solitary water-bleb.

Bleb solitary; but reproductive in an adjoining part; very large, and containing a teacupful of lymph. Preceded by tingling: often accompanied with languor.

The third, or quotidian variety, is here introduced upon the authority of Sauvages, for it does not occur in Willan, who seems to have overlooked it: and hence it is not noticed by Bateman. Sauvages, from the time of its more usual appearance, calls it *epinyctis*; but as Vandermonde has given a case of an opposite kind, in which the bulla showed itself daily and subsided nightly, this name will not properly apply. Frank regards it as a variety of eczema, or hidroa (*De Cur. Hom. Morb.*, tom. iv., p. 159), but his arrangement of eruptive diseases is one of the least masterly parts of his work.

Under whatever form, however, the pompholyx appears, its causes seem to be debility and irritability, either general, or confined to the cutaneous exhalants. The benign variety has hence been found in infancy during teething and bowel complaints, and occasionally immediately after vaccination. The quotidian has evidently succeeded to great anxiety, fatigue, watching, and low diet. It appears also chiefly in persons of advanced age, or who have been unduly addicted to spirituous liquors. It is by far the most severe of all the forms of the disease, as being painful as well as tedious. The other varieties are to be referred to like causes.*

In early or middle life, Peruvian bark, given freely, with an improved diet where necessary,

has formed the most successful remedy. In old age, softening the skin, and gently exciting the cutaneous exhalants, has been equally useful: but, while the bark is less serviceable in old age, warm-bathing has proved rather injurious in earlier life.*

SPECIES II.

ECPHLYSIS HERPES.

TETTER.

ERUPTION OF VESICLES IN SMALL, DISTINCT CLUSTERS; WITH A RED MARGIN; AT FIRST PELLUCID, AFTERWARD OPAQUE; ACCOMPANIED WITH ITCHING OR TINGLING; CONCRETING INTO SCABS: DURATION FROM FOURTEEN TO TWENTY-ONE DAYS.

HERPES, from ἕρπω, "serpo," "repo," has been used in very different senses by different writers: being sometimes restricted to one or two of the modifications of the present classification, and by others extended so widely as to include both the preceding and the ensuing genus; or, in other words, cutaneous eruptions, dry, vesicular, and pustular; and, in this latitudinarian sense of the term, it is employed by Mr. B. Bell, who gives us a herpes farinosus and pustulosus, as well as a herpes miliaris and exedens.

In the present arrangement, the term is limited to minute and clustering *cutaneous vesicular eruptions* alone, which form a clear and distinctive indication. The fluid contained in the vesicles, is for the most part highly acrimonious and excoriating; and hence the terms δάρσις and δαρτός (darsis and dartus), "excoriatio and excoriatus," have been applied to it; from which the French have derived their popular name for it

---

* The chronic pemphigus of Rayer is often preceded and accompanied by chronic inflammation of the gastro-intestinal or the genito-urinary mucous membrane; and in these complicated cases, the functional disorders of the digestive and of the urinary organs are combined with the phenomena produced by the inflammation of the skin. The formation of bullæ is then preceded by languor, lassitude, headache, nausea, dysuria, pains in the limbs, &c. These examples, however, strictly belong to the emphlysis pemphigus of Dr. Good's arrangement.—ED.

* When any degree of febrile excitement is present, bleeding and other depleting measures should precede the employment of bark. Then the infusion of cinchona, with gentle cordials and diuretics, may be prescribed, or the sulphate of quinine, with mineral acids, provided the mucous membranes are unaffected, which rarely happens.— (See Rayer, tom. i., p. 165.) The following formula is recommended by Dr. A. T. Thomson:—

℞. Infusi cinchonæ f. ʒxss.
Spiritus etheris nitrosi f. ʒss.
Tinct. cascarillæ f. ʒj.
Misce; ft. haustus, bis in die sumendus.

In chronic pemphigus, purgatives are found by Rayer to be invariably hurtful.—(Tom. ii., p. 165.) When excoriations occur, they should be dressed with the ung. zinci, or the parts beyond the excoriated surface touched with the nitrate of silver.—(See Dr. A. T. Thomson's Atlas of Delineations of Cutaneous Diseases, p. 47.) The prognosis of chronic pemphigus is always more unfavourable than that of acute, or the emphlysis pemphigus of the present system, which is only a serious disease when complicated with inflammation of the mucous membrane of the alimentary canal, or lungs, cephalitis, or pneumonitis. Chronic pemphigus, especially in old persons, is always followed by extensive and numerous excoriations, occasioning severe pain and continual restlessness. It is often attended with vomiting and a colliquative diarrhœa, which mostly carries the patient off.—See Rayer, tom. i., p. 162.—ED.

of dartre, which, by an easy corruption, has been changed in our own tongue into tetter.* Dr. Frank has made herpes a division of porrigo (*De Cur. Hom. Morb. Epit.*, tom. iv., p. 133), in doing which, instead of simplifying and generalizing cutaneous eruptions, which was obviously his intention, he has rather perplexed and confounded them.

The following are the varieties which seem fairly to belong to it:—

a Miliaris. Miliary tetter.	Vesicles millet-sized; pellucid; clusters commencing at an indeterminate part of the surface, and progressively strewed over the body; succeeded by fresh crops.
β Exedens. Erosive tetter.	Vesicles hard; of the size and origin of the last; clusters thronged; fluid dense, yellow or reddish; hot, acrid, corroding the subjacent skin, and spreading in serpentine trails.
γ Zoster. Shingles.	Vesicles pearl-sized; the clusters spreading round the body like a girdle; at times confluent. Occasionally preceded by general irritation or other constitutional affection.
δ Circinatus. Ringworm.	Vesicles with a reddish base, uniting in rings, the area of the rings slightly discoloured; often followed by fresh crops.
ε Iris. Rainbow-worm.	Vesicles uniting in small rings, surrounded by four concentric rings of different hues; vesicular and prominent. Usually found about the hands or instep.
ζ Localis. Local tetter.	Limited to particular organs; stationary or vicinous.

The FIRST, or MILIARY VARIETY, is the herpes miliaris of Hippocrates and Hoffmann, the H. phlyctenoides of Bateman. The cause of this peculiar irritability of the skin that excites this affection is very obscure.† The lymph con-

---

* Rayer takes a different view of this subject; for though he agrees with Willan and Bateman in considering herpes to comprehend a group of vesicular inflammations of the skin, resembling one another in the form of the inflammatory process, and merely differing in situation (H. labialis, H. præputialis), the disposition of the vesicles in clusters (H. phlyctenoides vel miliaris), or in a ring (H. circinatus); yet, says he, the term herpes, taken in this signification, is not synonymous with the words *dartre* and *tetter*. It denotes, also, affections very different from those which Lorrey, Turner, Alibert, &c., have comprised under the name of herpes; for it has a precision of meaning which would be sought in vain in the nomenclature of these several writers.—Tom. ii., p. 226. —ED.

† According to Rayer, the disease is ordinarily connected with a slight chronic irritation of the digestive organs, indicated after meals by tardiness

tained in the vesicles is sometimes brownish, and for the space of two or three days, other clusters successively arise near the former. The eruption commences in any part of the body.* The enclosed lymph sometimes becomes milky or opaque in the course of ten or twelve days, from an absorption of its finer parts; and, about the fourth day, the inflammation around the vesicles assumes a duller red hue, while the minute utricles break and discharge their fluid; or dry into scales, which fall off, and leave a considerable degree of inflammation below, that still continues to exude fresh matter, which also forms into cakes, and falls off like that which preceded. The itching is always very troublesome: and the matter discharged from the vesicles is so tough and viscid, that every thing applied in the way of dressing adheres very closely, and is removed with great trouble and uneasiness.

To the SECOND, or EROSIVE VARIETY, the Greeks gave the name of ἕρπης ἐσθιόμενος, or "herpes esthiomenos," of which the Latin herpes exedens is a mere translation. The herpes esthiomenos, however, has hitherto been much misunderstood, and been held of a far severer character than it really possesses, in consequence of an error that has long since crept into the text of Celsus, and been propagated in the common editions, in which he is made to say that the livid and fetid ulcer, which the Greeks called θηρίωμα, sometimes degenerates into a herpes

of digestion, thirst, heat in the epigastrium, flatulent tension of the belly, &c. In some cases it is this internal affection which claims the principal attention.—See tom. i., p. 228.—ED.

* This variety of vesicular inflammation, so well described and delineated by Bateman, is sometimes, according to Rayer, developed exclusively on the forehead, cheeks, neck, or still more frequently on the limbs; or else it is successively propagated over several of these regions. A pricking sensation in the parts where the eruption is about to appear, followed by heat, itching, and red spots, precedes, by a few hours, and sometimes by one or two days, the formation of the vesicles. These first contain a colourless or lemon-coloured fluid, and present themselves in the form of irregular clusters, of from twelve to fifty vesicles at most, which clusters are not numerous themselves, though sometimes followed by a succession of others of a similar nature. Between the different clusters the integuments retain their natural colour, though seldom between the vesicles composing the clusters themselves. The formication and pricking are increased by external heat, and by that of the bed at night. Most of the vesicles rapidly increase in size, and some of them even attain considerable dimensions. Scarcely have twenty-four or thirty-six hours elapsed from the formation of each of them, when the fluid in them begins to be turbid. The smaller soon assume a milky look, and the larger become brownish, being filled with a bloody serosity. Between the sixth and tenth days, all of them shrivel and lessen, fresh clusters coming out; when the eruption is successive. The fluid of the smaller ones is often absorbed; that of the larger escapes on their bursting, or is converted into yellowish or dark-coloured scabs, which are usually detached between the fifteenth or twentieth day.—See Rayer, tom. i., p. 227.—ED.

esthiomenos, or exedens, "eating herpes;" as though the herpes exedens formed the worst and most gangrenous stage of this ulcer. In the volume of Nosology I have examined this passage critically, and have shown that for herpes esthiomenos we ought to read φαγίδαινα, "the ulcer called *phagedæna*," as it is properly given in the corrected text of the variorum edition, which settles the dispute at once, and clears Celsus from the absurdity which has been ascribed to him, of converting a cutaneous vesicular affection into a deep-spreading ulcer of a cancerous character. Celsus, therefore, in reality, makes no mention whatever of the herpes exedens or esthiomenos ; and it is to other writers we must turn for its character. Galen has described it very accurately : and in the volume of Nosology I have copied and translated Galen's description, as it occurs in different parts of his writings. The definition given of it above is entirely taken from his representation. The ulcerative ringworm of Dr. Bateman is, perhaps, a modification of this variety : it is of tedious and difficult cure, but is limited to hot climates.

Where this variety is connected, as it is sometimes found to be, with the state of the constitution, and particularly of the stomach, and the patches are accompanied with a sensation of actual burning or scalding, so as to resemble a more papulated form of measles, like the measles of this modification, they are denominated nirles in some parts of Scotland.

The THIRD VARIETY, HERPES ZOSTER, is the zona ignea of many writers, both which terms imply a belt or girdle, and are evidently given to the eruption from its ordinary seat and course as surrounding the body. The Latin word for these is *cingulum*, and from cingulum our own SHINGLES has been derived in a corrupt way.*

A slight constitutional affection sometimes precedes the appearance of this form, as sickness and headache, but by no means generally ; for, in most instances, the first symptoms are those of heat, itching, and tingling in some part of the trunk, which, when examined, is found to be studded with small red patches of an irregular shape, at a little distance from each other, upon each of which numerous minute elevations

* By Rayer termed zona, and arranged with bullæ. The following is his definition of it :—An acute inflammation of the skin, mostly appearing on the trunk in the form of a semicircular band, consisting of inflamed *vesicles* and *bullæ*. The disease in reality constitutes, according to Rayer's view, the intermediate link between bullous and vesicular inflammations.—(See Traité Théorique et Pratique des Maladies de la Peau, tom. i., p. 202.) It rarely comes on in a completely simple form. In the midst of the bullæ and vesicles characterizing it, psydracious pustules may accidentally present themselves. The lymphatic glands of the axilla or thorax are sometimes inflamed in zona of the thorax or abdomen. Among the internal lesions accompanying that of the skin, none is more frequent than that of the stomach or intestines.—(See Rayer, tom. i., p. 206.) The seat of zona is in the corpus reticulare : the inflammation is not so deep as that of erysipelas, and rarely extends to the subcutaneous cellular tissue.—Ibid. —ED.

are seen clustering together. These, when accurately inspected, are found to be distinctly vesicular ;* in the course of twenty-four hours, they enlarge to the size of small pearls, are perfectly transparent, and filled with a limpid fluid. The clusters are of various diameter, from one to two, or even three inches, and are surrounded by a narrow red margin, in consequence of the extension of the inflamed base a little beyond the congregated vesicles. During three or four days, other clusters continue to arise in succession, and with considerable regularity ; that is, nearly in a line with the first, extending always towards the spine at one extremity, and towards the sternum or linea alba at the other ; most commonly passing round the waist like half a sash, but sometimes, like a sword-belt, across the shoulder.† As the patches which first appeared subside, the vesicles become partially confluent, and assume a livid or blackish hue, and terminate in thin dark scabs, the walls of the utricles being thickened by the exsiccation of the grosser parts of the contained fluid. The scabs fall off about the twelfth or fourteenth day,

----

* According to Rayer, they consist of grayish or yellowish transparent bullæ and vesicles, surrounded by a red and inflamed areola. They are full of serosity, some being as small as a lentil-seed, and others as large as an almond. Although usually separated from one another, several are so close together as to be, as it were, in bunches. In a more advanced stage, the latter are confounded together, and become confluent. In five or six days, the fluid of the vesicles assumes an opaline colour, and becomes sero-purulent ; and if the inflammation be more intense, the fluid is converted in topus. Between the second and fourth days some of the vesicles and bullæ spontaneously burst, and discharge a limpid, inodorous, serous fluid. The cuticle is detached, and the corpus reticulare exposed, leaving so many small inflamed surfaces, which, for a few days, secrete pus, just as a part that has been blistered does. Others shrivel up without bursting, and are transformed into small scabs, which turn to a dark colour, and are soon detached. The appearance of vesicles and bullæ is always successive.—See Rayer, tom. i., p. 203. —ED.

† Zona, as Rayer calls it, is most disposed to begin on the trunk, and especially on the abdomen. It extends from some point of the median line outwards, as far as the vicinity of the vertebral column, and thus produces a sort of half girdle, or semicircle. It never makes a complete circle. Pliny, Turner, Russel, and Tulp, it is true, mention such an occurrence ; but they have not detailed the particulars of any cases of it. Sometimes, when it attacks a part whose circumference is not extensive, it forms three quarters of a circle, thus surrounding the neck like a collar, the arm like a bracelet, the knee like a garter, &c. Instances of zona taking a perpendicular direction, or one parallel to the axis of a limb, are very rare. However, Rayer has seen this happen on the thigh, from the trunk down to the knee. In another case, it occurred on the shoulder-joint. When the disease occurs on the face, the inflammation is sometimes propagated into the mouth, only one side of which is affected, and a considerable salivation may thus be excited. In ten cases of zona referred to by Rayer, eight were on the right side of the body.—See Traité des Mal. de la Peau, tom. i., p. 205.—ED.

when the exposed surface of the skin appears red and tender ; and, where the ulceration and discharge have been considerable, is pitted with numerous cicatrices. The complaint is generally of little importance, but is sometimes accompanied, especially on the decline of the eruption, with an intense, deep-seated pain in the chest, which is not easily allayed by medicine. By some authors, as Hoffmann and Platner, it is said to be occasionally malignant and dangerous, and Languis alludes to two cases in noblemen that terminated fatally.—(*Epist. Med.*, p. 110.) The disorder, however, seems in these instances to have been of a different kind from shingles, and to have depended upon a morbid state of the constitution.—(*Plumbe, on Diseases of the Skin,* p. 140, 8vo., 1824.)

This affection is found most frequently in the summer and autumn,* when the skin is most irritable from increased action ; and in persons of a particular diathesis, disposed to herpes, rather than to any other form of scaly eruption. Under these circumstances, slight exciting causes will produce it, as exposure to cold after violent exercise with great heat ; cold cucurbitaceous vegetables, or other substances that disagree with the stomach ; inebriety ; or even a sudden paroxysm of passion, or other strong mental emotion, of which Schwartz tells us that he has seen not less than three cases.—(*Diss. de Zonâ Serpigniosâ,* Hal., 1745.) It is more common to early than to later life, being found principally between twelve and twenty-five years of age. It has sometimes appeared critical in bowel complaints or pulmonic affections.—(*Bateman, on Cutaneous Diseases,* p. 227, 8vo., 1813.) It does not seem to be contagious, though asserted to be so by some writers. " In the course of my attendance," says Dr. Bateman, " at the Public Dispensary during eleven years, between thirty and forty cases of shingles have occurred, none of which were traced to a contagious origin, or occasioned the disease in other individuals."

The RINGWORM is a still slighter variety of herpes than shingles, both with respect to disquieting symptoms and range of the disease. Here the vesicles are restricted to the circumference of the herpetic patch, thus forming an annular outline ; the central area, however, in some degree participating in the inflammation, becomes roughish, and of a dull red colour, and throws off an exfoliation as the vesicles decline, leaving a red and tender surface beneath. The process is completed in about a week ; but a fresh crop of herpetic circles often springs up in the neighbourhood, or in some other part of the body ; and, as such crops are occasionally repeated many times in succession, the course of the disease is not unfrequently protracted through a long period, and migrates over the entire surface from face to foot. Yet no other inconvenience attends it than a disquieting

itching and tingling in the patches. It is found most frequently in children, and, though deemed contagious, affords no real ground for such an opinion. It has, indeed, been traced, in some instances, in several children of the same school or family at the same time ; but, perhaps, only where the same occasional cause, whatever that may be, has been operating upon all of them : while, in most instances, the examples have consisted in single patients who have not been debarred communication, or even sleeping, with their school-fellows, or other branches of a family.

The RAINBOW-WORM, or tetter, is of a rare occurrence, and was by Dr. Willan at first mistaken for an exanthem, in consequence of his having only seen it in its earliest stage : on which account, in the first edition of his Table of Classification, he called it a rainbow rash. The error has been corrected by Dr. Bateman, to whom we are indebted for the first accurate description of it. Its usual seat is on the back of the hands, or the palms and fingers, sometimes on the instep. The patches are very small, and, at their full size, do not exceed that of a sixpence. Its first appearance is that of an efflorescence ; but by degrees the concentric and irridescent rings become distinctly formed and vesiculated, and even the area partakes of the vesication, and becomes an umbo. The utricles are distended in about nine days ; they continue stationary for two days more ; and then gradually decline, and disappear a week afterward. The central vesicle is of a yellowish-white colour ; the innermost ring of a dark or brownish-red ; the second of nearly the central teint ; the third, which is narrower than the rest, is dark-red ; the fourth, or outermost, which does not appear till the seventh, eighth, or ninth day, is of a light-red hue, and is gradually lost in the ordinary colour of the skin.

This variety has only been seen in young persons, and is unconnected with any constitutional affection. Its exciting cause is not known : though it has occasionally followed a severe catarrhal affection, accompanied with hoarseness. It has also occasionally recurred several times in the same person, always occupying the same parts, and going through its course in the same periods of time.

The LOCAL RINGWORM is accompanied with a considerable sense of heat and itching or tingling irritation in the region in which it riginates. That of the lip renders the adjoining parts hard, and tumid, and painful, and especially the angle of the mouth ; the form is usually semicircular ; and though the herpes does not spread to any considerable distance, it is sometimes found at the same time within the mouth, forming imperfect rings on the tonsils and uvula, and producing an herpetic sore throat. It usually appears, however, as a symptom or sequel of some disease of the abdominal viscera, and sometimes proves critical to them. It terminates, as in other cases, in ten or fifteen days, in dark thick scabs, which form over a red and tender new cuticle.

The local ringworm of the prepuce is apt to be mistaken at first for a chancre, and still more

---

* The causes of this disease seem to Rayèr not to be very well made out but he observes that it is most common in hot weather.—Tom. ii., p. 206.—Ed.

so if, under the influence of this mistake, it be treated with irritants ; for the base will then become much more thickened and inflamed, and the natural course of the vesicles will be interrupted. If the eruption be left alone, it will prove itself in about twenty-four hours by the enlargement and distinct form of the vesicles, and their assuming an annular line. They die away after having run their course, as in the other varieties. The exciting cause of this is not known. It has been ascribed, however, by Mr. Pearson, to a previous use of mercury. Like several of the other modifications, it has a tendency to recur after it has once shown itself.

No internal use of medicine is necessary in the treatment of any of the varieties of herpes, except when the constitution becomes affected from the irritation ; and, in such case, a gentle purgative or two should be administered at first,[*] and a plan of tonics[†] be laid down afterward, the diet being simple and plain.[‡]

External applications are almost of as little avail ; for the eruption must have time to run through its course, and, if this be interrupted, we shall certainly prolong the period, and add to the irritation. Stimulating ointments[§] and lotions were in use formerly, but they have

now been judiciously laid aside, as only tending to exacerbate the affection. When, from the viscosity of the discharged fluid, the vesicles are apt to adhere to the clothes or whatever covering they come in contact with, they may be covered with a layer of cetaceous cerate on lint : but keeping the part clean with soap and water, and the application of a layer of lint alone, will be most useful in the local variety of the prepuce, as even oleaginous applications are apt to cause irritation.[*]

SPECIES III.
ECPHLYSIS RHYPIA.
SORDID BLAIN.

ERUPTION OF BROAD, FLATTISH, DISTINCT VESICLES ; BASE SLIGHTLY INFLAMED ; FLUID SANIOUS ; SCABS THIN AND SUPERFICIAL ; EASILY RUBBED OFF AND REPRODUCED.[†]

FOR a distinct arrangement of this species in medical classification we are altogether indebted to Dr. Bateman, who has denominated it *rupia*, from ῥύπος, "sordes," as indicative of the ill smell and sordid condition of the diseased parts : and, in his Delineations, he has given two excellent coloured plates of its appearance under different modifications. Ῥύπος, however, with its aspirate and the ordinary power of the *v*, should be rendered in Latin characters RHYPIA, as now given, and only altered for the sake of greater correctness.

The species offers three varieties, as follow :—

a Simplex.	Scab flat ; livid or blackish ;
Simple sordid blain.	shape circular.
β Prominens.	Scab elevated, conical, and
Limpet-shelled blain.	blackish ; shape, limpet-shelled.
γ Escharotica.	Sanious discharge ; erosive,
Erosive blain.	producing gangrenous eschars.

The vesicles under this species never become confluent : their progress is slow, and leads to an ill-conditioned discharge, which concretes into thin, superficial, and chocolate-coloured scabs, of the distinctive characters noticed

---

* The annexed formula is given by Dr. A. T. Thomson :—

℞ Magnesiæ carbonatis ℨss.
Sodæ bicarbonatis ℨj.
Vini colchici f. ℨj.
Aq. distillatæ f. ℨix.
Syrupi tolutani ℳx.

Fiat haustus, in effervescentiæ impetu ipso, cum succi limonum cochleari amplo uno, bis in die sumendus.—ED.

† ℞ Sodæ bicarbonatis ℨss.
Infusi gentianæ comp. f. ℨix.
Tinct. columbæ f. ℨj.
Syrupi aurantii f. ℨss.

Fiat haustus, in impetu effervescentiæ, cum succi limonum recentis cochleari amplo uno, ter in die sumendus.—(See Dr. A. T. Thomson's Atlas of Delineations of Cutaneous Diseases, p. 80.) In obstinate cases he prescribes the foregoing draughts, or the hydrargyrum cum creta, with decoction of sarsaparilla.—ED.

‡ Repose, the antiphlogistic regimen, cooling beverages, venesection, and, still more commonly, topical bleedings on the epigastrium, and near the verge of the anus, are set down by Rayer as the proper measures for relieving the symptoms which are the forerunners of herpes zoster, or rather, for relieving the gastro-intestinal inflammation that is the cause of them. When the eruption has made its appearance, their intensity may diminish, or it may continue in the same degree for several days, so as to require a repetition of local bleeding and emollient clysters. Rayer is of opinion that general bleeding is only right when herpes zoster covers an extensive surface, or is conjoined with another more or less serious inflammation.—Tom. i., p. 208.—ED.

§ For herpes circinatus (ringworm), and herpes iris (tetter), solutions of sulphate of copper, or zinc, or borax, or alum, are still in common use. When considerable pain and heat are experienced, Dr. A. T. Thomson looks upon one part of tincture of opium, and two parts of water, as the best application for herpes circinatus.—ED.

* In herpes zoster, when the areolæ of the bullæ and vesicles are very red, much inflamed, and painful, Rayer advises leeches to be applied round the part affected, or near the most tender places ; and the patient to be plunged in a tepid emollient narcotic bath. Topical emollients, he says, rarely expedite the cure. Opiate liniments, he admits, are sometimes useful in assuaging the pain and restlessness. The inflamed skin, he thinks, should always be preserved from the contact of the air and from the friction of the clothes, by covering it with silk paper dipped in oil, or an opiate liniment.—See Rayer, Traité des Maladies de la Peau, tom. i., p. 209.—ED.

† Rayer classes rupia, the rhypia of Dr. Good, with bullous inflammations of the skin ; he defines it as characterized by small flattish bullæ, few in number, with inflamed bases, and containing a serous fluid, that very soon thickens, and becomes purulent or bloody, drying into dark-coloured scabs, thin, or elevated.—See Rayer, Traité des Mal. de la Peau, tom. i., p. 196.—ED.

above.* When the ulcers under the scab, in the two first varieties, heal, they still leave the surface of a livid or blackish colour, as if from a pigment in the rete mucosum. The second variety assumes the direct form and swell of a small limpet-shell, with its open part downwards, but its colour is much darker.†

All the modes of this eruption are connected with a debilitated, and hence frequently with a cachectic, state of the system, and the first is sometimes accompanied with symptoms resembling those produced by a morbific poison. They occasionally make a near approach to the ecthymata (see *the ensuing Genus*, Spe. 3, *Ecpyesis Ecthyma*), but differ in the form, shape, and size of the vesicle, and in the colour and consistence of the contained fluid, as consisting of flattened muddy blains, and forming large and more circular scabs.

The escharotic variety affects only infants and young children, when reduced by bad diet and nursing, or some severe disease, as the smallpox. The vesicles are generally found on the loins, thighs, and other parts of the extremities, and appear to contain a corrosive sanies: some of them frequently terminate in gangrenous eschars, which leave deep indentations.

The disease is only to be combated by supporting the system, and restoring it to a state of vigour, by means of good, light, nutritious diet, and the use of alterative and tonic medicines, as the compound pill of the submuriate of mercury, bark, columbo, and sarsaparilla.‡

SPECIES IV.
ECPHLYSIS ECZEMA.
HEAT ERUPTION.

ERUPTION OF MINUTE, ACCUMULATED VESICLES, DISTINCT, BUT CLOSELY CROWDING ON EACH OTHER; PELLUCID OR MILKY; WITH TROUBLESOME ITCHING OR TINGLING; TERMINATING

---

* When the small bullæ of rupia are prematurely broken or torn, the skin becomes excoriated, and not covered with scabs.—See Rayer, tom. i., p. 197.—ED.

† Bateman, ut suprà, p. 237. Rupia mostly occurs on the legs, but sometimes on the loins and thighs. It usually attacks children of delicate constitutions, or enfeebled by previous illnesses. Scrofulous children are deemed particularly subject to it. Winter is the time when it is most disposed to occur, attacking principally such as are badly clothed, badly lodged, or badly fed, and especially after they have been suffering from smallpox, ecthyma, &c. Rayer has known rupia complicated with subcutaneous hemorrhages, or bleeding from the mucous membranes. According to this author, rupia is never itself a dangerous disease, and if the cure is sometimes tedious, this is because the disorder often takes place in individuals afflicted with hemorrhages, chronic inflammation of the digestive organs, &c., or labouring under the debilitating influence of misery.—See Traité Théorique, &c. des Maladies de la Peau, tom. i., p. 198.—ED.

‡ Another indication is, to combat any internal inflammation that may be present. Rayer recommends opening the bullæ, if they contain serosity.—ED.

IN THIN SCALES OR SCABS; OCCASIONALLY SURROUNDED BY A BLUSHING HALO.

ECZEMA, from ἐκζέω, " efferveo," is the hidroa of Sauvages and Vogel : it is common to all countries in the summer, and has been described in all ages. Its proximate cause is irritation in consequence of exposure to the direct rays of the sun, or to air of a high temperature, or to violent exercise. Hence it chiefly affects those parts that are most exposed to this influence, as the face, neck, and forearms in women, but particularly the back of the hands and fingers ; the latter being sometimes so tumefied that the rings cannot be drawn off. The blushing halo by which they are surrounded is popularly called a *heat-spot.* In men of a sanguine temperament, and who use violent exercise in hot weather, these vesicles are intermixed in various places with minute pustules, possessing a hard circular base, the phlyzacium of Willan, or with hard and painful tubercles, which appear in succession, and rise to the size of small biles, and suppurate very slowly, though without a central core. The vesicles are apt to be confounded with two other eruptions of very different kinds ; miliaria, while it spreads widely over the body, and scabies, when fixed chiefly about the wrists, the ball of the thumbs, and the fingers. It is, however, distinguishable from the former, by being unaccompanied with fever, or any other constitutional derangement ; and from the latter by the pellucidity and acumination of the vesicles, the closeness and uniformity of their distribution, and the absence of surrounding inflammation or subsequent ulceration. The sensation, moreover, to which it gives rise, is that of a smarting or tingling, rather than of an itching.

The eruption is irregularly successive, and has no determinate period of decline, which very much depends upon the irritability of the skin itself. Generally, however, it runs its course in two or three weeks, and subsides slowly and almost imperceptibly. But when the skin is highly irritable, it will sometimes continue till the weather grows cool in the autumn, and consequently for two or even three months.

Medicine, external or internal, seems to accomplish but little. In most cases, the reaction of a cold bath increases the irritation : and hence a tepid bath is most serviceable. Astringent lotions add equally to the irritability, as do unguents of all kinds. Washing the parts with mild or Windsor soap and tepid water I have found most effectual—when in a few days the skin will bear a soap of a coarser kind with still more advantage. When the irritability of the skin is connected with that of the general frame, the mineral acids, and other astringent tonics, have proved decidedly beneficial.

The *eczema impetiginodes* of Dr. Bateman is an eczema set down on an impetiginous habit of the skin, and is hence a mixed complaint.*

---

* Whether this statement is correct may admit of doubt : eczema impetiginodes is usually regarded as a local eruption, consisting of separate vesicles, containing a transparent fluid, slightly

His *eczema rubrum*, or *mercuriale*, has already been described as an erythema.

GENUS VI.

ECPYESIS.

HUMID SCALL.

ERUPTION OF SMALL PUSTULES, DISTINCT OR CONFLUENT; HARDENING INTO CRUSTULAR PLATES.

ECPYESIS is a Greek term, from ἐκπυῶ, "suppuro." It is here used in contradistinction to EMPYESIS, already employed to import deep-seated suppurations; and consequently is intended to describe pustular eruptions simply cutaneous, or not necessarily connected with internal affections, as opposed to those which result from an internal cause. The genus, therefore, embraces the pustulæ of Dr. Willan, which he has correctly defined "elevations of the cuticle, with an inflamed base containing pus."

The old English term for ecpyésis or pustula in this sense of the word is *scall*, from the Saxon scala or sccala, not essentially different from the medical sense of scale. The scall was of two kinds, dry and moist: both which are clearly referred to in the Levitical law that governed in the matter of plague. The former is there denominated ספחת (saphat), as we have already observed when treating of lepra, and the latter, or the eruption before us, נתק (netek). —(*Leviticus*, xiii., 30, 31.) The Arabians, like our own ancestors, denominated both these by a common name ﺳﺤﺎﻓﺔ (sahafata) from ﺳﺤﻒ

elevated, attended with pain, heat, smarting, and intense itching, and some degree of swelling. When the vesicles break, the effused lymph irritates and inflames the surrounding skin, which becomes red, and the cuticle thick and rough, like what is observed in impetigo. The diseases termed grocers' itch and bricklayers' itch are by some writers considered as varieties of psoriasis, by some as modifications of impetigo, and by others as specimens of eczema impetiginodes. Thus, Dr. A. T. Thomson observes, that this last species of eczema often arises from local irritants, as blisters; the ointment of tartarized antimony; the acrid powders with which the hands of many artisans are constantly covered; as, for instance, grocers, bricklayers, and filemakers. It may be mistaken for itch when it appears on the wrists and fingers; but in scabies, the itching, which returns in paroxysms, is very different from the stinging sensations of eczema; neither is eczema contagious.—(See Dr. A. T. Thomson's Atlas of Delineations of Cutaneous Diseases, p. 88.) For allaying the pain and tingling of eczema impetiginodes, this author recommends the following lotions :—

R Acidi hydrocyanici f. ℈ij.
　Hydrarg. oxymuriatis gr. iij..
　Mist. Amygdalæ amaræ f. ℥vj.
　Fiat lotio subinde utenda.

Or touching the parts with a solution of nitrate of silver :—

R Argenti nitratis ℈iss.
　Aq. distillatæ f. ℥v.
　Solve : pauxillum, ope pencilli, partibus affectis applicandum.—ED.

(sahaf), squammæ, or rather from the Hebrew ספהת (saphat) : distinguishing the one from the other, like our ancestors also, by the adjuncts dry and humid : so that the sahafata of the Arabians is a direct synonyme of the old English or Saxon scale. In our established version, the Hebrew נתק (netek), which imports the eruption before us, or *humid* scall, is by mistake rendered *dry* scall, which, as remarked above, is a ספחת (saphat). The expletive *dry* does not occur in the original, and that נתק (netek) denotes humid scall rather than dry scall is clear from the explanation contained in the Bible context, in which it is represented as a scall, seated on the hair or beard, and affecting its strength and colour, forming so thick a crust or scab, that its removal by shaving cannot be accomplished, or ought not to be attempted. It is distinctly, therefore, a porrigo or scabby scall, and is thus verbally rendered in the Latin version of Tremellius and Junius, forming one of the species of the present genus; and seems to be one of the two modifications of it which, in our own language, are denominated honey-comb scall, and scalled head. Θραῦσμα, by which *netek* is rendered in the Septuagint, is literally *crust*, a very significant term in common use to express the peculiar nature of the scab that hardens on the porriginous sore. Tetter, a corruption from the French dartre, or the Greek δαρτὸς, has of late years been used synonymously with scall, and has almost supplanted it : but the proper meaning of dartre, or tetter, is herpes, to which in this work it is confined, an excoriating eruption of a vesicular or ichorous kind.

The species that belong to this genus are the following :—

1. Ecpyesis Impetigo.	Running Scall.
2. —— Porrigo.	Scabby Scall.
3. —— Ecthyma.	Papulous Scall.
4. —— Scabies.	Itch.

All these specific terms have been loosely employed, and in very different significations, by most writers. They are here limited to the definite senses assigned them by Dr. Willan; and, with the exception of ecthyma, by Celsus, whom Willan has followed. Ecthyma does not occur in Celsus, though it is found in Galen; but in a sense somewhat different from its use in modern times, as will be further noticed hereafter.

SPECIES I.

ECPYESIS IMPETIGO.*

RUNNING SCALL.

PUSTULES CLUSTERING, YELLOW, ITCHING; TERMINATING IN A YELLOW SCALY CRUST, INTERSECTED WITH CRACKS.

THE specific term is a derivative from impeto,

* A cutaneous inflammation, not essentially attended with fever, nor contagious, characterized by small pustules, agglomerated or discrete, termed by Willan *psydracious*, and the fluids of which, after their bursting, dries in the form of yellow laminated or elevated scabs.—(See Rayer, Traité

"to infest:" it is used in its ordinary and restrained sense, as opposed to the unauthorized latitude assigned to it by Professor Frank, who, as already observed, employs it as the name for an entire class :- and the following are its varieties :—

a Sparsa. Scattered humid scall.	Clusters loose ; irregularly scattered ; chiefly over the extremities ; often succeeded by fresh crops.
β Herpetica. Herpetic scall.	Clusters circular, crowded with pustules, intermixed with vesicles ; often with exterior concentric rings surrounding the interior area as it heals : itching accompanied with heat and smarting. Chiefly in the hands and wrists.
γ Erythematica. Erythematic scall.	Pustules scattered ; preceded by erythematic blush and intumescence ; often by febrile or other constitutional affection. Chiefly in the face, neck, and chest.
δ Laminosa. Laminated scall.	Pustules confluent ; chiefly in the extremities ; the aggregate scabs forming a thick, rough, and rigid casing around the affected limb, so as to impede its motion ; a thin ichor exuding from the numerous cracks.
ε Exedens. Erosive scall.	The purulent discharge corroding the skin and cellular membrane.
ζ Localis. Local humid scall.	Confined to a particular part ; mostly the hands or fingers ; and produced by external stimulants, as sugar or lime.

The differences are sufficiently clear from these definitions. The first variety, or scat-

Théorique et Pratique des Maladies de la Peau, tom. i., p. 471.) The principal forms of impetigo, according to Rayer, are two : sometimes the psydracious pustules are disposed in clusters (the impetigo figurata of Willan), sometimes they are scattered over the parts affected (the impetigo sparsa of Willan). Each of these varieties may be acute or chronic, according as it may consist of one or of several successive eruptions of pustules. The impetigo figurata of Willan most commonly attacks young subjects of a lymphatic temperament. It may come on unpreceded by any admonitory symptoms, or may be ushered in with symptoms of gastro-enteritis, pain in the epigastrium, restlessness, lassitude, &c. It is most frequently noticed on the face, and almost always on the middle of the cheeks. It may cover the whole of these parts, and then extend to the commissure of the lips, and form a circle round the chin. It has also been observed on the neck, trunk, and limbs ; the clusters of psydracious pustules and the scabs following them are usually circular on the forearm and hands, and on the lower extremities are broader than on the upper.— See Rayer, tom. i., p. 474.—Ed.

TEREO HUMID SCALL, has sometimes been confounded with varieties of PORRIGO and SCABIES, constituting two subsequent species of the present genus. It differs from porrigo, however, in having the purulent discharge succeeded by an ichorous humour soon after the eruption has shown itself, and in the possession of a thinner and less extensive scab.* It differs from scabies in its more copious exudation of ichor, when the latter is secreted, in the magnitude and slower progress of the utricles [in the conversion of the discharge into yellow, prominent, or laminated scabs], and in the sensation of heat and smarting, rather than of itching, which accompanies the disease ; and differs from both in being uncontagious.†

The ERYTHEMATIC FORM commences with the ordinary signs of an erysipelas, as a redness and puffy swelling of the upper p of the face, with an œdema of the eyelids, and the irritation is sometimes accompanied with some degree of pyrexy for two or three days. But a critical eye will easily perceive that, instead of the smooth polish of the erysipelas, there is a slight inequality on the surface, as if it were obscurely papulated ; and, in a day or two, the disease will show its true character by the formation of numerous psydracious pustules‡ over the inflamed and humid skin, instead of the large irregular bullæ of erysipelas. The pustules are formed with a sense of heat, smarting,

---

* The small pustules of porrigo favosa are never humid, like those of impetigo, but covered with a yellow dry scab, excavated in the form of a little cup. The diminutive pustules of porrigo scutulata, or circinata, are indeed disposed in clusters, like those of impetigo figurata ; but the fluid which they contain is contagious. Impetigo figurata usually occurs on the face, and in adults ; while porrigo circinata is almost exclusively seen in children, and on the scalp. The porrigo larvalis of Willan is more difficultly discriminated from the impetigo sparsa.—See Rayer, tom. i., p. 479. —Ed.

† Impetigo sparsa, though most frequent on the limbs, may appear on the neck, shoulders, face, and ears. On the lower extremities of old debilitated persons, or in those of sedentary habits, it is always a tedious disease, sometimes spreading over the whole leg, from the knee down to the ankle and instep, and rendering motion of the limb painful. The scabs become large and adherent, and the leg is at length covered with one thick yellowish scab, which, as it dries, becomes rough and grooved, like the bark of a tree. The inflamed parts are the seat of annoying heat and acute itching, and out of the several fissures a yellow matter oozes and dries up, so as to produce additional scabs. Sometimes the disease extends to the toes, and the nails are detached ; and among the frequent consequences of this form of impetigo are œdema and ulcers of the limb ; the impetigo exedens of the present system, it is to be presumed, though Dr. Good describes it as affecting the side of the chest or the trunk. The impetigo sparsa of the upper extremities is mostly situated on the forearm ; it differs from that of the lower in being less severe, while in its chronic state it is more rarely complicated with œdema and ulceration.—See Rayer, tom. i., p. 476.—Ed.

‡ Small, not pointed, and very little raised.— EDITOR.

and itching, and, as they break, they discharge a hot and acrid fluid, which adds to the irritation and excoriation of the surface. In this painful condition, the face or other part remains for ten days or a fortnight, when the discharge begins to diminish, and to concrete into thin yellowish scabs. Fresh pustules, however, arise in the neighbourhood, and the disease runs on from one to two or three months, according to the irritability of the skin, and its tendency to be affected by continuous sympathy. It has sometimes perambulated the entire surface from head to foot : during the whole of which course the constitution is scarcely disturbed, or in any way affected.*

The LAMINATED HUMID SCALL is sometimes conjoined in the lower limbs with cellular dropsy, and produces severe ulceration : and its incrustation occasionally extends to the fingers and toes, and destroys the nails, being succeeded by nails of an imperfect fabrication, thick, notched, and irregular.

The EROSIVE FORM is rare, and highly intractable. It commences on the side of the chest or trunk of the body, and gradually extends itself. The pustules are here intermixed with vesicles, the fluid is peculiarly acrid and erosive, and the skin and cellular texture are slowly, but deeply and extensively, destroyed, with very great pain and irritation : insomuch that the disease is said by some, though with little foundation, to be of a cancerous nature.

The LOCAL FORM is mostly produced by the use of irritant materials, constantly applied to the parts affected, which are chiefly the hands, as sugar among the labourers in grocery warehouses, and lime among bricklayers. Whence this variety has been vulgarly called *Grocers' Itch*,† or *Bricklayers' Itch*. According to the peculiar character of the skin, the eruption is sometimes vesicular, and belongs to the preceding genus, being a modification of eczema ; but more generally pustulous, and appertains to

the genus before us. In neither instance does it seem to be contagious.

Most of the causes enumerated under LEPRIASIS, and many of the species of ECPHLYSIS, operate in the present species ; as general debility or relaxation, with a skin peculiarly irritable ; poor diet, filth, fatigue, and local stimulants.* And hence, when the constitution seems to catenate with the disease, the same general remedies have been found successful ; as the alkalis, sulphur taken freely, Plummer's pill, the alterative decoctions or infusions of dulcamara, ledum palustre, juniper-tops, sarsaparilla, and mezereon, together with frequent warmbathing for the purpose of purifying and softening the skin.† In connexion with these, we should have recourse to such external applications as may best tend to diminish the irritability of the cutaneous vessels, and give tone to their action. The most useful of these are the metallic oxydes, with the exception of those of lead, which are rarely useful, at least if employed alone, and are often found injurious. About ten grains of sublimate dissolved in a pint of distilled water, with a small proportion

* The causes of impetigo seem to Rayer to be very obscure. Young persons of fine delicate complexions are occasionally attacked by it in the face, after exposing themselves to the heat of the sun ; but, according to the same authority, it occurs in adults more frequently than either in children or old subjects. It is capable of being excited by other cutaneous inflammations, especially by repeated attacks of lichen agrius. It is often accompanied with inflammatory affections of the digestive organs ; and this is particularly noticed in children, during the period of the first or second dentition.—See Rayer, tom. i., p. 478.—Ed.

† In the cases under Dr. Elliotson, already quoted, in which a full pulse, heat, thirst, drowsiness, and giddiness, &c., existed, the treatment consisted in bleeding, low diet, and small quantities of mercury. In the commencement of impetigo, and whenever it is attended with redness of the skin, or a considerable eruption of pustules, Rayer advises bleeding. He states 'that general or local tepid bathing in emollient anodyne decoctions, and gentle frictions with the ung. zinci, vel plumbi acetatis, are useful in lessening the inflammation and morbid secretion which are the effect of it. When the disease is no longer acute, the detachment of the scabs is to be promoted by the application of steam ; which, however, will be hurtful, if employed before the inflammation has been removed. If no gastro-intestinal inflammation be present, Rayer sanctions the exhibition of saline purgatives ; but, in the contrary case, he orders leeches to the epigastrium and verge of the anus. In chronic impetigo, he advocates repeated abstractions of blood from the neighbourhood of the inflamed parts, and the employment of emollient sedative lotions, and the steam of hot water, with a purgative occasionally, when the state of the digestive organs will admit of it. In a later stage, when the skin is not tender nor inflamed, sulphureous mineral waters may be employed, or sea-bathing. It is in this state of the disease that the ung. hydrarg. nitrat., or caustics, have sometimes answered. Antimonial, mercurial, and arsenical medicines, Rayer disapproves of, as producing chronic affections of the digestive organs worse than the disease of the skin.—See tom. i., p. 481.—Ed.

* This is not always the case ; in some examples, mentioned by Dr. Elliotson in his Clinical Lectures, (Lancet, 1830–31, p. 489), the patients had headache and a full pulse, with drowsiness, sometimes giddiness, heat, thirst, &c. The blood taken away exhibited a buffy crust and concave surface. In fact, the local symptoms of impetigo may be combined with those of gastro-intestinal inflammation ; the lymphatic glands in the vicinity of the cutaneous affection may inflame and swell; and the excessive itching of the skin may prevent sleep, and disorder various functions. But, according to Rayer, one of the most important complications to be studied is that of the pustules of impetigo with the vesicles of eczema (Eczema impetiginodes). This vesiculo-pustular disease, mentioned by Dr. Good under the name of E. impetigo exedens, is generally very severe, and, when it attacks the arms, usually begins on the wrists, thence spreads to the backs of the hands, phalanges of the fingers, and matrices of the nails, while it is extending itself in an opposite direction up the forearm.—See Rayer, tom. i., p. 477. —Ed.

† Rayer describes this affection as a variety of psoriasis diffusa.—See Traité des Mal. de la Peau, tom. ii., p. 37.—Ed.

of muriated ammonia, will frequently prove a valuable remedy. Or the oxyde of zinc may be applied in the form of an ointment, which I have often found serviceable, prepared in the manner already noticed under the species pru-rigo. Lime-water is also recommended by many writers, and has proved useful as a stim-ulant astringent; as have also solutions of alum, and sulphate of zinc, and sulphuret of potash, the old liver of sulphur: but I have found them less useful than the zinc ointment.

The acrid oil contained in the shell of the cashew-nut, has often been employed with great advantage in some of these varieties, and espe-cially when the disease is decidedly local, and a local change of action is the grand desideratum. In many cases, however, the skin is too irrita-ble for stimulants of any kind, and will only bear warm water, or a decoction of mallows, poppy-heads, or digitalis: after which the exco-riated surface may be smeared with cream, or an emulsion of almonds. In general, neverthe-less, astringent stimulants agree far better with this affection than with herpes. The burning and maddening pain in the erosive scall can rarely be alleviated but by opium. The Har-rowgate waters are generally recommended, and, in many instances, have certainly been found useful.

SPECIES II.
ECPYESIS PORRIGO.*
SCABBY SCALL.

PUSTULES STRAW-COLOURED; CONCRETING INTO SCALES OR YELLOW SCABS.

This is the porrigo of Celsus and Willan, from *porrigo*, "to spread about;" and the tinea of Sauvages and most of the nosologists. It offers the following varieties:—

α Crustacea. Milky scall. — Pustules commencing on the cheeks or forehead in patch-es; scabs often confluent, covering the whole face with a continuous incrustation (porrigo larvalis). Found chiefly in infants, during the period of lactation.

β Galeata. Scalled head. — Pustules commencing on the scalp in distinct, often dis-tant, patches; gradually spreading till the whole head is covered as with a helmet; cuticle below the scabs red, shining, dotted with papillous apertures, oozing fresh matter; roots of the hair destroyed: con-tagious. Found chiefly in children, during dentition.

γ Favosa. Honeycomb scall. — Pustules common to the head, trunk, and extremi-ties;* pea-sized; flatten-ed at the top: in clusters, often uniting; discharge fetid: scabs honeycomb-ed, the cells filled with fluid. Found both in ear-ly and adult age.†

δ Lupinosa. Lupine scall. — Pustules minute, in small patches, mostly commen-cing on the scalp; patch-es terminating in dry, del-ving scabs, resembling lu-pine-seeds; the interstices often covered with a thin, whitish, exfoliating incrus-tation. Found chiefly in early life.

ε Furfuracea. Furfuraceous scall. — Pustules very minute, with little fluid; seated on the scalp; terminating in scur-fy scales. Found chiefly in adults.

ζ Circinata. Ringworm scall. — Clusters of very minute pus-tules, seated on the scalp in circular plots of bald-ness, with a brown or red-dish, and somewhat fur-furaceous base. Found chiefly in children.

The FIRST VARIETY is the *crusta lactea* of nu-merous authors, the *tinea lactea* of Sauvages, so called from the milky or rather the creamy ap-pearance and consistency of the discharge, whence the French name of *croute de lait*, and our own of milky scall. It is almost exclusive-ly a disease of infancy, at which period the skin of the head is peculiarly tender and delicate. It commences ordinarily on the forehead and cheeks, in an eruption of numerous minute and yellowish-white pustules, which are crowded to-

* Rayer, careful not to confound ptyriasis, pso-riasis, lepra, impetigo, chronic eczema, syphilitic eruptions of the scalp, with tinea, or porrigo, ad-mits four species of the latter disease: tinea fa-vosa (porrigo favosa); tinea annularis (porrigo circinata); tinea granulata (porrigo lupinosa); and tinea mucosa (porrigo crustacea). He con-siders, likewise, these four cases as very distinct from one another, and not as varieties of the same affection. Their individual existence is founded upon characters as striking as those of other pustular inflammations of the skin. Some tineæ are contagious, while others are not so; a cir-cumstance which obviates every supposition of the identity of their nature. What renders the consideration of them as varieties of the same in-flammation still less admissible, is, that they are seldom combined together.—See Rayer, Traité des Maladies de la Peau, tom. i., p. 496.—Ed.

* It takes place ordinarily on the scalp, some-times extending to the temples, eyelids, and fore-head; and more rarely to the shoulders, elbows, and forearm. Rayer saw an instance in which it covered all the back of the trunk down to the sacrum, and likewise the knees, and the upper and outer part of the legs. The patient, who was twelve years of age, had none of the disease on the scalp.—Op. cit., tom. i., p. 497.—Ed.

† But not in equal proportions; the majority of cases at the Bureau Central des Hôpitaux being in children of seven, eight, and nine years, and especially seven.—See Rayer, Traité des Mal. de la Peau, tom. i., p. 502.—Ed.

gether upon a red surface, and break and discharge a viscid fluid, that concretes into thin yellowish scabs. As the pustular patches spread, the discharge is renewed, and continues to be thrown forth from beneath the scabs, increasing their thickness and extent, till the forehead, and sometimes the cheeks and entire face, become covered as with a cap : the eyelids and nose alone remaining free from the incrustation. The quantity of the discharge varies considerably, so that in some instances the scabs are nearly dry. As they fall off and cease to be renewed, a red and tender cuticle is exposed to view, like that in impetigo, but without a tendency to crack into fissures. Smaller patches are occasionally formed about the neck and breast, and even on the extremities, and the disease runs on for several weeks, sometimes several months ; during which the constitution suffers but little, except from a troublesome itching, which sometimes interferes with the rest and destroys the digestion. And, when the last takes place, a foundation is immediately laid for general debility, and especially for torpitude and enlargement of the mesenteric glands. In many instances the eruption returns at irregular intervals, after having appeared to take its leave ; apparently reproduced by cutting additional teeth, or some other irritation. Dr. Starck affirms that, when the disease is about to terminate, the urine acquires the smell of that voided by cats ; and that, when there is no tendency to this change of odour, the disease is generally of long continuance.* It is singular that, notwithstanding the extensive disfigurement and sometimes depth of the ulcerations, no permanent scar or deformity is hereby produced.†

The SECOND VARIETY, or SCALLED HEAD, originates generally in the scalp, and consists of

* With regard to this statement, Rayer observes, that he finds it liable to numerous exceptions.—Tom. i., p. 533.—ED.

† Porrigo crustacea, described by Rayer under the name of teigne muqueuse, is set down by him as not contagious. He believes its real frequency to be greater than the register of the Bureau Central des Hôpitaux makes out, where it stands in comparison with porrigo favosa as 71 to 908.—(See Rayer, Traité des Mal. de la Peau, tom. i., p. 532.) In the treatment he almost invariably abstains from the application of zinc and satumine ointments. Mercurial purgatives he considers dangerous. In infants at the breast, he finds tepid, emollient, mucilaginous lotions sufficient to produce a gradual cure. In older children, when the inflammation causes restlessness, he applies from two to six leeches under the ears or jaw. If no amendment take place, he next puts a small blister on the arm, and keeps it open. When the disease is on the scalp, after cutting off the hair, he applies an emollient poultice, bathes the head two or three times a day with a decoction of linseed, and if the child is strong, puts leeches on its temples, or the nape of the neck. In a few days a blister is applied to the arm, and kept open. In very old chronic cases, if the foregoing means are insufficient, he employs sulphureous lotions, or friction with the ung. hydrarg. nitratis. Depletion he only deems necessary in a very few cases, where the hair-follicles themselves are inflamed.—Tom. i., p. 532.—ED.

pustules somewhat larger, and loaded with a still more viscid material, than the first. The pustules are circular in form, with a flattish and irregular edge. They sometimes commence on the cheeks ; but when the face is affected, the ordinary course is from the scalp towards the cheeks by the line of the ears. They are usually accompanied with a considerable degree of itching, and harass children from six months to four or five years of age. The disease is rarely found in adults. From the quantity of the discharge, the hair is matted together, the scabs become considerably thickened, the ulceration spreads into the integuments, and the indurated patches seem, in some cases, to be fixed upon a quagmire of offensive fluid. The lymphatic system, if not in a state of debility before the appearance of the eruption, soon becomes affected, and exhibits marks of irritation ; but whether from general debility, or the absorption of irritating matter, it is difficult to say. The glands on the side of the neck enlarge and harden, exhibiting at first a chain of small tumours lying loose under the skin ; after which some of them inflame, the integuments become discoloured, and a slow and painful suppuration ensues. The ears unite in the inflammation, and from behind them, or even from their interior, a considerable quantity of the same viscous and fetid fluid is poured forth. In some cases, the submaxillary and parotid glands catenate in the inflammatory action. The fluid is peculiarly acrimonious, and consequently, whatever part of the body it accidentally touches, becomes affected by it. Hence the arms and breasts of nurses evince frequently the same complaint, and other domestics receive the disease by contagion. Its duration is uncertain, but it is more manageable than the preceding species ; and if not maintained by the irritation of teething or any other excitement, it may be conquered in a few weeks.

The HONEYCOMB SCALL, or THIRD VARIETY, differs very little from the preceding, except in the seat of the patches, and in an increased size and thickness of the scab, which is often cellular or honeycombed. And as pustules of this form have been called favi, from their resemblance to honeycombs, this variety of the disease, from the time of Ali Abbas to the present, has been distinguished by the name of tinea favosa, scabies favosa, or porrigo favosa. By Dr. Bateman it is united with the preceding variety. The colour of the scab is yellowish or greenish, and semitransparent, its surface highly irregular and indented, and its consistency softish. The pustules are found on the face, trunk, and extremities. The irritation they produce excites the little sufferer to be perpetually picking and scratching them about the edges, by which means the skin is kept sore and the ulceration extended. This is particularly the case about the heels and roots of the toes, the extremities of which last are sometimes ulcerated, while the pustules even creep under the nails. The odour from this and the preceding variety is not only most rank and offensive to the smell, but occasionally inflames the eyes of nurses and others, who are officially surrounded by its vapour.*

The LUPINE VARIETY† is peculiarly characterized by the dryness of its scabs, which are formed upon small clusters of minute pustules, the finer part of whose fluid is rapidly absorbed, so that the part remaining concretes,‡ and shows in the central indentations of its surface a white scaly powder. The size of the scab is that of a sixpence : it is found in the head, and elsewhere ; but when in other parts than' the head, it is often much smaller in diameter, and sometimes does not exceed two lines. It is liable to increase if neglected, and is usually tedious and of long duration.§

The PURFURACEOUS or BRANNY SCALL makes a still nearer approach to the tribe of lepidosis, and is often mistaken for a pityriasis, or lepriasis, particularly when it appears in the scalp, which is its most common seat. It commences, however, if its course be watched, with an eruption of minute pustules, which nevertheless possess

---

* The disease is contagious, and readily propagated among children who employ the same comb or hair-brush. This is particularly the case when any trivial excoriations of the scalp are present : uncleanliness is also known to give a predisposition to the disease. According to Rayer, no other variety of porrigo is characterized by small pustules, scarcely rising above the level of the skin, and not bursting ; no other terminates in dry, slightly-depressed, or excavated scabs, and leaves red lenticular impressions on the skin, after these scabs have separated from it.—Op. cit., tom. i., p. 503.—ED.

† La teigne granulée of Rayer ; who describes it as characterized by small pustules, less deeply implanted than those of porrigo favosa, irregularly scattered over the scalp, and drying into gray or brown scabs, not excavated like a little cup, and sometimes quite loose among the hairs.—Op. cit., tom. i., p. 523.—ED.

‡ Into numerous hard granules, containing, as is alleged, a considerable portion of lime.—(See Lancet for 1831-32, No. ccclxv., p. 513.) "Lorsqu' elles ne sort pas abreuvées par le pus, elles ont une consistance très dure et comme pierreuse, que les cataplasmes ramollissent difficilement."—(Rayer, tom. ii., p. 523.) Porrigo lupinosa is rarely met with in adults, and is remarked by Rayer to be much more frequent in the hospitals of Paris than the porrigo favosa, from which it differs by the humidity of the pustules from their first appearance ; by the ragged and irregular form of its scabs ; and by its not being contagious.—(See Rayer, tom. i., p. 525.) Recent cases are treated by this author on the antiphlogistic plan, followed by blisters on the arms ; while, for those of longer duration, he prefers the depilatory ointments and powders of MM. Mahon, adverted to in a subsequent note, p. 681.—ED.

§ The itching, which is extremely acute, is often much increased by the presence of numerous lice. Porrigo lupinosa is sometimes complicated with sympathetic inflammation of the lymphatic glands of the neck, and also with symptoms of inflammation in the chest or abdomen. It only affects the bulbs of the hair, and occasions baldness when it is of very long duration. We never find more than a few of the pustules perfect ; most of them are dry ; the scabs are but slightly adherent to the skin ; and the corpus reticulare is red and inflamed. —See Rayer, tom. i., p. 524.—ED.

---

a very small quantity of fluid, so that the whole is soon absorbed, and the excoriation or ulceration is but slight. It is apt to be renewed, is attended with a considerable degree of itching, and some soreness of the scalp ; the hair partially falls off, becomes thin, less strong in its texture, and somewhat lighter in its colour ; none of which symptoms occur in any species of the true scaly eruption. The glands of the neck, moreover, are occasionally swelled and painful.

The RINGWORM SCALL* has been known and described under different names, from the Greek writers to our own day. It consists of clusters of very minute pustules, forming circular plots of a brown or reddish hue. There is sometimes only a single plot, and the pustules are so small as to elude all notice, unless very closely examined, though a papular roughness is obvious.† The exudation is small, yet, if neglected, it concretes into thin scabs, sometimes irregularly tipped with green, while the plots expand and become confluent. The hair is injured from the first attack ; appearing thinner and lighter in colour, and breaking off short : in progress of time the roots are affected, and the plots are

---

* The tinea annularis, or teigne annulaire of Rayer, defined by him as a chronic and contagious inflammation, characterized by circular clusters of small pustules, which ordinarily form on the hairy scalp. They dry in the form of thin scabs, but little adherent.—Op. cit., tom. i., p. 518.—ED.

† It commences with circular, red, inflamed spots, on which arise small pustules of a yellowish-white colour, and the centre of each of which is usually perforated by a hair. By degrees this circle enlarges, and becomes from half an inch to an inch and a half in diameter. The fluid of the pustules dries into thin, hard, slightly-adherent scabs, under which the skin is red and inflamed. In the course of two or three weeks, not only do the first clusters extend themselves, but additional ones are produced, either spontaneously or from the successive inoculations caused by the fluid of the pustules, with which the children's fingers become impregnated when they scratch the scalp. If porrigo circinata be left to itself, the patches, after becoming very numerous, may be blended together at their edges, and form more or less irregular surfaces. However, the circular disposition of the original patches is still denoted by the segments of circles, perceptible at the circumference of the disease. In the vicinity of the patches, the skin becomes red and scaly. The inflammation is very often propagated to the hair-follicles, a circumstance which, Rayer conceives, led Underwood and others to ascribe the primitive seat of the disease to the bulbs of the hair. The hairs either break or are detached from the skin, and are replaced by others, which, in their turn, sooner or later, fall off like the former, if the skin continue inflamed, covered with scabs, or a new eruption of pustules should take place. The baldness is permanent only in a few rare examples, where the scalp is deeply ulcerated, or the hair-follicles destroyed. So long as there is redness and a furfuraceous desquamation of the skin, an eruption of fresh pustules is to be apprehended : on the contrary, the cure is not far off when the morbid redness disappears, and the hairs, growing again on the denuded parts, have the same colour and strength as those out of the limits of the disease. —See Rayer, op. cit., tom. i., p. 519.—ED.

quite bald; and, as they spread into each other, the baldness extends over the whole head, and nothing remains but a narrow border of hair, forming the outline of the scalp. It is chiefly confined to children; and since the multiplication of large boarding-schools and manufactories, in which last they are employed with too little attention to their health, it has been strikingly common in our country : and from its contagious property, has been propagated with great rapidity.* It sometimes spreads from the head over the forehead and neck.

Porrigo, therefore, is a disease which appears under different modifications of ulceration, from sores of some depth, emitting a thick fetid pus, and covered with a broad scaly scab, to eruptions so minute as to require the aid of a glass, being covered with fine furfuraceous exfoliations, and discharging a thin purulent ichor, manifested rather by its effects than its presence.

The predisposing cause is in every instance irritability of the cutaneous exhalants; and, as we find this irritability much greater in infancy than in mature life, the different varieties of porrigo are chiefly confined to this season. The exciting causes are filth, or want of cleanliness, bad nursing, innutritious diet, want of pure air, and whatever else has a tendency to weaken the system generally, and irritate the skin locally. And we may hence see why some of the varieties are found occasionally as sequels of lues, or in those who have debilitated their constitutions by high living, and especially by an immoderate use of spirits.

It is hence obvious that many, perhaps all these varieties, may, in some instances, be connected with the general state of the system; and, in such cases, the restorative diet-drinks and alterative tonics enumerated under the genus ecphlysis will often be equally advantageous here. Sulphur and the vegetable alkalis have also been found serviceable, but especially small doses of calomel, or the black or red oxyde of mercury. And, if there be much general irritation, it will be advisable to unite these with the conium or hyoscyamus. The pansy or heart's-ease (*Viola tricolor*) was in high vogue for cutaneous eruptions generally, and particularly for those before us, during the sixteenth and seventeenth centuries. It fell, however, into disrepute, but was revived by Dr. Starck towards the close of the eighteenth century.† He directs that a handful of the fresh, or half a drachm of the dried leaves, be boiled in half a pint of milk, to be strained for use, and form a single dose, which is to be repeated morning and evening. He asserts, that during the first eight days, the eruption usually increases considerably, and that the patient's urine acquires

the cat-like smell we have already alluded to: but that, when the medicine has been taken a fortnight, the scab or scurf begins to fall off in large scales, leaving the skin clear. The remedy is to be persisted in till the skin has resumed its natural appearance, and the urine its natural odour. Dr. Starck also recommends as an internal remedy, which we should little have expected, a decoction of the leaves of the *Tussilago farfara*, or coltsfoot, which I should scarcely have noticed were it not that this medicine is equally well spoken of by Professor Frank (*De Cur. Hom. Morb. Epit.*, tom. iv., p. 204), and was also esteemed useful by Dr. Cullen, as we had formerly occasion to observe, in sores dependant upon a scrofulous habit, many of which, he tells us, he has seen healed under its employment, both in extract and decoction.—(*Mat. Med.*, part ii., chap. xviii.) As to the *Viola tricolor*, Baldinger, who seems also to have tried it, and upon a pretty large scale, asserts that it is of inferior value to sulphur (*Neues Magazin für practische Aerzte*, ix., p. 117), and Selle, that if given in small doses it is useless, and, if in larger, that it does more harm than good.— (*Medicina Clinica*, i., 185.)

There is some difficulty in determining upon the external applications. Generally speaking, the skin, under all the modifications of this species, will bear astringent and even stimulant remedies well, and yield without obstinacy to their use : but, in a few instances, we meet with the contrary, the slightest irritants aggravating the pustules, and extending their range. The most irritable varieties are the honeycomb, where it occurs at the extremities of the joints, as about the toes and heel, and behind the ears, and the furfuraceous. The last, however, will usually bear a lotion of mild soap and water, and afterward equal parts of starch and calamine reduced to a very fine powder, and dusted over the patches. The honeycombed scall often requires, at first, sedative fomentations and cataplasms, but will afterward allow an application of the zinc ointment, or even that of the nitric oxyde of mercury diluted with an equal part of calamine cerate. Dr. Willan was attached to the Cocculus indicus in cases of this sort, which he prescribed in the proportion of two drachms of the powdered berry to an ounce of lard; but the ointment of galls generally succeeds better. In common, however, we may employ a bolder practice, and use rather active alkaline or acid lotions, or solutions of zinc, or warm resinous ointments of tar, pitch, or gum elemi. A dilute solution of nitrate of silver, or equal parts of water and aromatic vinegar, will often be found equally beneficial ; or the less elegant process of Dr. Frank, which is however formed upon the same principle. "Patentia nunc ulcera *cum urinâ recenti ac sanâ* quotidie lavantur, ac mox unguento populeo, vel unguento albo, aut rubro, aut demum citrino mercuriali, obtecta, tali methodo simplicissima ad sanationem perducuntur."—(*De Cur. Hom. Morb. Epit.*, tom. iv., p. 201, Manuh., 8vo., 1792.) All that is wanting is the excitement of a new and healthier action, which the cutaneous vessels for the most

---

* Rayer sets it down as highly contagious, and quotes Willan in support of this statement, who knew this disease in a school spread from one boy to fifty others in the course of a month.—Op. cit., tom. i., p. 519.—Ed.

† De Crustâ Lacteâ Infantûm, Francf., 1779 ; see also Comment. Lips., vol. xxvii., p. 170. Marcard, Beschreibung von Pyrmont. Mezger, Vermischte Schriften, b. ii.

part receive with but little trouble; and this, with a punctilious attention to cleanliness, is in most cases sufficient to ensure a cure.

. With the sulphur ointment, .or, which is better, sulphur and cream, I have ofteh succeeded in curing very virulent attacks of the *porrigo favosa*, that have covered the whole of the face, and matted the beard into a most disgusting spectacle.*

In the external treatment of *porrigo galeata*, or scalled head, one of the most effectual applications is a modification of Banyer's unguentum ad scabiem, for in its original form it is both too irritant and too astringent, as well as very unscientifically compounded. I was first induced to try this preparation from the recommendation of my excellent and learned friend Dr. Parr; it has since been recommended by Professor Hamilton, and more lately by Dr. Bateman. Each has altered its composition in a slight degree, and the following form, which is more simple than any of the rest, is that which I have been in the habit of employing with great success for many years. To a powder consisting of two drachms of calomel and an ounce of exsiccated alum and of cerusse, add six drachms of Venice turpentine and an ounce and a half of spermaceti cerate. The hair is first to be cut off as close as may be, for shaving is often impossible; the scalp is then to be slowly and carefully washed with soap and water; and, when there is very little irritation, with soft soap, as being more stimulant, in preference to hard; the washing to be repeated night and morning, and the scalp to be well dried afterward. The ointment is to be applied after the washing every night, and is to be well rubbed all over the head. It

may be washed off in the morning; and when the scalp is made dry, instead of applying it through the day, the head may be thoroughly powdered with nicely levigated starch, contained in a fine linen or cambric bag. The scabs and incrustations will hereby become desiccated, and often brittle, for the ointment alone will diminish, and at length utterly suppress the morbid secretion. And in this state they should be gently picked or combed off, one after another, as they grow loose and become detached at the edges.

In the last variety, the ringworm porrigo, or *alopecia porriginosa* of Sauvages, though the appearance is far less disgusting, and unaccompanied with smell of any kind, the bulbs of the hair seem more affected than in any of the preceding. And hence this, which is one of the most common modifications of the disease, and, as we have already observed, has been peculiarly frequent of late years, has been found one of the most obstinate. It has ordinarily made its appearance among children at school, but is not confined either to schools or to childhood; for I had not long since a medical friend under my care, troubled with the same complaint, whose age is about forty.

- The disease appears to be seated under the cuticle, in the mouths of the secernents of the rete mucosum, which secrete a material of a different colour from what is natural and healthy, and hence give a brown or reddish hue to the entire patch. This material affords no nutriment to the bulbs of the hair, and seems sometimes to be acrimonious; whence the hair, like the rete mucosum itself, changes its colour; and, with the change of colour, becomes thinner and weak-

---

* Two principal objects have generally been kept in view in the treatment of porrigo favosa; in some methods the cure of the pustular inflammation of the skin, either rationally or empirically, is the main thing aimed at; in others, the evulsion of the hairs constitutes the chief measure. Among the former plans, what Rayer terms the antiphlogistic and derivative, appears to him the best. The abstraction of blood is seldom necessary. Decoction of linseed, and emollient cataplasms, applied to the shaven scalp, loosen the scabs, and diminish the inflammation; but in order to bring about a cure, Rayer assists these means with two blisters on the arms, from which a discharge is to be maintained for two or three months.—(Op. cit., tom. i., p. 504.) But from the moment that the inflammation has extended to the bulbs of the hair, Rayer sets down every treatment that does not aim at producing either the evulsion, or the falling off of the hair, as ineffectual. For this purpose he prefers the depilatory treatment adopted by MM. Mahon, who pay particular attention to the following objects :—1. To that of cleansing the scalp, and keeping it as much so as possible. 2. To that of separating, without pain, the hairs whose bulbs are inflamed. They begin with cutting the hair so as to leave it only two inches in length. They then loosen and remove the scabs with hog's lard, or a linseed poultice; and afterward wash the head with soap and water. This plan is continued for four or five days, at the expiration of which the second part of the treatment begins, and a depilatory pomatum is applied to all the affected points of the scalp

every other day. This practice is persisted in for a month, six weeks, or two months. On the days when the pomatum is not used, a fine comb is passed through the hairs, by which means they are detached without pain. At the end of a fortnight, a depilatory powder is sprinkled among the hairs once a week. The next day the fine comb is used, and the depilatory pomatum employed again. In a month or six weeks the first depilatory pomatum is discontinued, and another substituted for it during a fortnight or month; after which, the inunctions are made only twice a week, till the redness is completely removed. The comb, which is to be used on the days when the pomatum is not applied, is to be smeared with lard or oil, and only lightly to be pressed upon. MM. Mahon's depilatory powder and pomatum seem to owe their activity to their containing lime, with a small quantity of subcarbonate of potash and charcoal.—(See Rayer. tom. i., p. 508.) This depilatory treatment, which was deemed unnecessary by Willan and Bateman, is considered indispensable by Rayer; yet at the Bloomsbury Dispensary we cure all cases without it. The hair is kept short, the head gently washed or fomented every day, and as soon as the inflammation has abated, and the scabs have been removed with a little lard, an ointment is applied, consisting of about 3½ grs. of oxymuriate of mercury, ℨj of white precipitate, and ℨj of lard. A few grains of subcarbonate of soda and rhubarb, with or without a small proportion of hydrargyrum cum creta, according to circumstances, are likewise given once or twice a day.--Eᴅ.

er, and breaks off short at the base of the cuticle, sometimes at the roots below.

The acrimony of the secretion occasionally produces a morbid sensibility in the minute vessels of the part affected, so that the patient can hardly bear the patch to be pressed upon, or the comb to pass over it ; yet this is not a common effect, for irritants may usually be employed from the first.

When this morbid sensibility exists, we must endeavour to shorten its stage ; for it will at length pass off naturally by tepid and sedative fomentations, as of poppy-heads or digitalis : and afterward have recourse to depilatories, without which we can do nothing, for we cannot otherwise penetrate to sufficient depth ; and hence, the more active they are, the more radical will be their effects. Different preparations of mercury have for this purpose been chiefly employed, and mostly a solution of sublimate. The other metallic acids have been tartar-emetic, sulphate of zinc, sulphate of iron, ærugò, or the green oxyde of copper, and even arsenic ; while practitioners of a more timid character have confined themselves to the pitch-plaster, balsam of sulphur, or decoctions of tobacco, hemlock, or the *Viola tricolor*.

In slight cases, most of these applications will be found sufficient ; but, in severe and obstinate cases, none of them. And hence, in every case, I have for many years confined myself to a solution of the nitrate of silver, in the proportion of from six to ten grains to an ounce of distilled water, according to the age of the patient, or the irritability of his cuticle ; and with this application I have never failed. It destroys the hair to its roots, gives tone to the morbid vessels, and changes their action. It often excites a slight vesication or soreness on the surface, and it is in most instances necessary to push it to this point. And when this stimulant astringent has answered its purpose, the decalvate plots should for some weeks afterward be daily washed with the acetated solution of ammonia, or aromatic vinegar.*

When porrigo is of long standing, and has become chronic, the irritation must be lessened gradually ; and a steady use of alterants is absolutely necessary, especially in the varieties accompanied with a considerable discharge ; for many writers of authority, as Pelargus (*Medicinische Jahrgänge*, i., P. 1, p. 50), Sennert (*Paral. ad L. V. Med. Práct.*, 4, 2), Stoll (*Prælect*, p. 48), and Morgagni (*De Sed. et Caus. Morb.*, ep. lv., art. 3), have given examples of epilepsy, apoplexy, and even death itself, from a sudden retrocession of the eruption. In the Berlin Medical Transactions, there is a case or two of amaurosis produced by a metastasis of this disease.—(Dec. i., vol. vii., p. 7 ; ii., vol. vi., p. 28.) One of the best medicines for the present purpose is the arsenical solution.

* Few remedies seem to be more popular with American practitioners than the ung. picis et sulph., for the treatment of various modifications of porrigo. In some instances, a weak lotion of arsenic has caused a salutary change in cases of this character.—D.

The cure is generally protracted by a strumous diathesis.*

SPECIES III.
ECPYESIS ECTHYMA.
PAPULOUS SCALL.

PUSTULES LARGE ; DISTINCT ; DISTANT ; SPARINGLY SCATTERED ; SEATED ON A HARD, ELEVATED, RED BASE ; TERMINATING IN THICK, HARD, GREENISH, OR DARK-COLOURED SCABS.†

ECTHYMA, from ἰκθύειν, "to rage, or break forth with fury," was used by the Greek writers synonymously with exormia, in the sense of papula : to which effect Galen " apertum est ab ἰκθύειν, quod-est ἰξυρμᾶν, id est erumpere, derivatum esse ἰκθύμασι, id est PAPULIS, nomen in iis quæ sponte *extuberant* in cute."—(In *Hippocr.*, lib. iii., sect. 51.) I have observed, however, under EXORMIA (suprà, p. 642), forming Genus III. of the present Order, that ecthyma has of late years been limited by the nosologists, and especially by Willan, Young, and Bateman, to the species before us, probably on account of its more papulated form ; and there seems no reason for deviating from their arrangement.

The following are its chief varieties :—

α Vulgare.	Base bright-red ; eruption completed with a single crop. Duration about fourteen days.
Common papulous scall.	
β Infantile.	Base bright-red ; eruption recurrent in several successive crops, each more extensive than the preceding. Found chiefly in weakly infants du-
Infantile papulous scall.	

---

* My friend Mr. Macilwain considers porrigo to be a constitutional disease, though, as explained in the text, some forms of it are contagious, and accidentally transmitted from one child to another by the use of the same comb, &c. Mr. Macilwain's doctrine naturally leads him to place greater reliance on internal than external remedies ; and he deems a farinaceous diet better in these cases than one of animal food. He allows, however, milk, the yolk of eggs, " which, with rusks, bread in various forms, sago, arrow-root, tapioca, and plain puddings, constitute the diet." —See Clinical Obs. on the Constitutional Origin of the Various Forms of Porrigo, p. 43, 8vo., Lond., 1833.—ED.

† Ecthyma, an inflammation of the skin, not contagious, characterized by large pustules, raised on a hard, circular, bright-red base. They are always discrete, usually make their appearance in succession in several regions of the body, and become covered with brown, thick, adherent scabs, under which a new cuticle or cicatrix forms, and more rarely the pustules terminate in ulceration, or tubercular induration.—(Rayer, tom. i., p. 430.) It attacks all ages and all constitutions, but is most frequent in adults. It may originate from some previous or still existing inflammation of the skin. It often follows variola, confluent scabies, and more rarely measles, scarlatina, leech-bites, &c. It may be connected with gastro-intestinal inflammation, and sometimes with disease of the lungs. In women, ecthyma is most common during pregnancy.—See Rayer, tom. i., p. 435.—ED.

ring the period of lactation.
Duration two or three
months.

γ Luridum.   Base dark-red ; elevated ; pus-
Lurid papulous   tules larger and more free-
scall.   ly scattered, discharging a
bloody or curdly sanies.
—Found chiefly in advan-
ced age. Duration several
weeks, sometimes months.

This last is the melasma of Linnæus, Vogel,
and Plenck. They are all diseases of debility,
local or general ; and hence, whether they occur in infancy, adult life, or age, are to be
cured by general tonics, pure air, and exercise,
tepid bathing, and preparations gently stimulating applied externally in the form of lotions,
ointments, or powders. None of them are contagious, and in this, as well as in their approaching more nearly to a papulous or broad pimply
character, especially that of the smallpox, they
differ essentially from the preceding. Nutritious food alone, with pure air and regular exercise, is often sufficient for a cure.* But as
this species is manifestly dependant upon a debilitated or cachectic state of the constitution, it
is often connected with those other symptoms
which appertain to such a condition, as a tumid
belly, diarrhœa, and general emaciation, in in-
fauts ; and dyspepsy and scirrhous parabysmata,
or enlargements of the abdominal viscera, in
adults. Dr. Bateman has given a very excellent coloured print of what he calls a cachectic,
or fourth variety, in his Delineations, in which
the scabby pustules are thickly scattered over
the limbs, mimicking very closely in size and
number an ordinary appearance of discrete smallpox at the time of its scabbing. It is, however,
distinctly a symptomatic affection, or rather, a
sequel of some long or chronic disease of an exhausting nature, and always disappears in the
train of its cure.†

---

* If acute ecthyma consist of merely a few
scattered pustules, without any complication,
Rayer prescribes diluent beverages, bathing the
parts in cold water, or bran and water, and enjoin-
ing a quiet and regular mode of living. When the
eruption is more extensive, and the patient young
and strong, one bleeding is advised, with cold or
temperate bathing, repeated according to the degree of inflammation in the skin. In chronic ecthyma, Rayer considers the indications to be the
same ; but, as in this case, the health has often
suffered from inattention to cleanliness, and from
unwholesome food, bleeding can only be practised
with great caution, and a good nutritious diet is a
chief object. Here, also, instead of common bathing, a bath of mineral or seawater is sometimes
to be preferred. When chronic ecthyma takes
place in an infant at the breast, the quality of the
nurse's milk is to be considered, a change of whom
is often indispensable. Rayer only sanctions prescribing laxatives and bitters in a few rare cases,
where no symptom of gastric or intestinal inflammation prevails ; and he thinks that Bateman has
recommended too generally chalybeates, quinine,
serpentaria, sarsaparilla, and antimonials.—Op.
cit., tom. i., p. 438.—ED.
† The varieties of ecthyma laid down by Willan
and Bateman appear to Rayer, in a certain degree, well founded, inasmuch as some particular-

---

SPECIES IV.
ECPYESIS SCABIES.
ITCH.

ERUPTION OF MINUTE PIMPLES, PUSTULAR, VESIC-
ULAR, PAPULAR, INTERMIXED OR ALTERNA-
TING ; INTOLERABLE ITCHING ; TERMINATING
IN SCABS ; FOUND CHIEFLY BETWEEN THE
FINGERS OR IN THE FLEXURES OF THE JOINTS ;
CONTAGIOUS.*

THIS disease is peculiarly complex ; but the
ities belong to them ; but he does not adopt them
himself, because he considers their basis not determinate enough ; and he prefers the division into
acute ecthyma and *chronic ecthyma*. The latter
which is the most common, always consists of
several successive eruptions, situated on the neck,
the scalp, the limbs, and even the face, and taking
place at intervals of various lengths. Sometimes
the pustules become very large, with a hard purple circumference (ecthyma luridum of Willan).
When the successive eruptions occur in weakly,
ill-fed children, they constitute the ecthyma infantile of Willan ; and when in old subjects, whose
constitutions are impaired by hard labour and the
abuse of spirituous liquors, this form of chronic ecthyma corresponds to Bateman's ecthyma cachec-
ticum. Whether ecthyma be acute or chronic, or
consist of one or of several successive eruptions,
its broad pustules always retain striking external
characters. They cannot be mistaken for the
small pustules of impetigo, acné, mentagra, and
porrigo. They are not navel-shaped, like those
of smallpox ; nor multilocular, like those of cowpox ; nor are they, like the pustules of these two
diseases, contagious. As for syphilitic pustules,
a mistake can only arise when ecthyma takes
place slowly and successively ; and it is to be remembered, that such pustules are rarely encircled
by so broad an areola as those of ecthyma. They
have also a greater tendency to ulcerate, and in
shape bear a stronger resemblance to little biles.
Farther, the difference in the diagnosis of ecthy-
matous and syphilitic pustules may frequently be
facilitated by our acquaintance with the previous
disorders which the patient has had, by the existence of other syphilitic complaints, and by the beneficial effects of mercury. The itch has no similarity to ecthyma, except when it is complicated
with pustules, or the vesicles characterizing it are
accidentally transformed into pustules. In ecthyma, the pustules are seldom numerous ; their appearance is successive ; the course of each is independent of that of the others ; some being on
the decline, while others are just beginning. On
the contrary, in itch, the accidental pustules form
at the most inflamed points, and are constantly
blended with the small vesicles which characterize this disease. The pustules are more crowded
together than those of ecthyma, and frequently
situated on the back of the hand, between the fingers, and especially between the thumb and forefinger. They are accompanied by pruritis, while
the pustules of ecthyma occasion a lancinating
pain, like that of a bile. The itch is vesicular and
contagious ; ecthyma is pustular, and cannot be
propagated either by mediate or immediate contact. Ecthyma differs from a bile in the extension of the inflammation from within outward ;
and even when it does reach the cellular tissue,
no central slough is produced, as always takes
place in furuncular inflammation.—See Rayer,
Traité des Mal. de la Peau, tom. i., p. 435-437.
—ED.

* This definition does not at all correspond to
that offered by Rayer, according to whom itch is

specific characters now given embrace the modifications which constitute its chief varieties,
and which are as follow :—

a **Papularis.**
  Rank itch.
Eruption of miliary, aggregate
pimples ; with a papular,
slightly-inflamed base, and
vesicular apex ; pustules
scantily interspersed ; tips,
when abraded by scratching,
covered with a minute, globular, brown scab.

β **Vesicularis.**
  Watery itch.
Eruption of larger and more
perfect vesicles, filled with
a transparent fluid, with an
uninflamed base ; intermixed with pustules ; at times
coalescing and forming scabby blotches.

γ **Purulenta.**
  Pocky itch.
Eruption of distinct, prominent,
yellow pustules, with a
slightly-inflamed base ; occasionally coalescing, and
forming irregular blotches,
with a hard, dry, tenacious
scab.

δ **Complicata.**
  Complicated
  itch.
Eruption complicated of pustular, vesicular, and papular
pimples, co-existing ; spreading widely over the body ;
occasionally invading the
face ; sometimes confluent
and blotchy.

ε **Exotica.**
  Mangy itch.
Eruption chiefly of rank, numerous pustules, with a hard
inflamed base, rendering the
skin rough and brownish ;
itching extreme ; abrasion
unlimited, from excessive
scratching. Produced by
handling mangy animals.

That all these affections are not distinct species of a common genus, but mere varieties of a
single species, is manifest from the fact, that in
different individuals, or under different conditions of the skin, every variety, even the mangy
itch itself, will produce every other variety,
while all of them in some instances coexist, and
are destroyed by the same means.* The above

an apyrectic contagious inflammation, characterized by vesicles slightly raised above the level of
the skin, constantly attended with pruritus, transparent at their apex, filled with a viscous and serous
fluid, and capable of forming on all parts of the
body, but particularly in the flexures of the joints,
and in the interspaces of the fingers.—(Op. cit.,
tom. i., p. 254.) Our author, in his definition and
subsequent history of the disease, plainly includes
various other inflammations with which scabies
may be comphcated.—ED.

* Even the varieties spoken of by Dr. Good
would probably be referred by Dr. Rayer to other
affections with which the itch may be complicated. According to the latter, writer, however,
other *vesicular* inflammations seldom take place together with the itch ; and when this becomes complicated with eczema, it is almost always in consequence of the use of stimulating lotions or frictions. Yet he has observed vesicles, like those of
eczema, and true bullæ, like those of a blistered

English names for the first three are those in
common or vulgar use, and it would be difficult
to find names more appropriate. The pocky
itch is so denominated from the resemblance of
the pustules to minute smallpox, and not from
any supposed connexion with syphilis. It gives
the largest pimples of all the modifications, as
well as the most purulent ; but it has never the
hard base of either the smallpox, or the ecthyma, or papulous scall we have just noticed, nor
has it the hard raised border or round imbedded
scab of the last, and hence is easily distinguished
from both. The two former varieties are far
more readily confounded with some varieties of
prurigo and of lichen, and especially in consequence of the black dots on the tips of the papulæ, and the long red lines common to all as produced by scratching. But they are distinguished
by the greater simplicity of the itching sensation, which, however intolerable, is not combined with tingling or formication ; and by their
being highly contagious, which the others are
not. Yet, from their general resemblance, all
these have by many writers been confounded,
and by others, who were fully sensible of their
distinction, been incorrectly described under
scabies or psora as a common name.

As a *primary* disease, itch is, in every instance, the result of personal uncleanliness, and
an accumulation of sordes upon the skin, though
the most cleanly are capable of receiving it by
contact ; and it always appears most readily
where close air, meager diet, and little exercise
are companions of personal filth ; for here, as
we have already had frequent occasions of observing, the skin is more irritable and more
easily acted upon by any morbid cause. Like
many other animal secretions, the fluid hereby
generated is contagious ; and, on close intercourse, but not otherwise, and chiefly in the
warmth of a common bed, or of a bed that has
been slept in before by a person affected with
the disease, is capable of communication.*

surface, on the dorsal and palmar surfaces of the
hands, when they were the seat of a great number
of psoric vesicles. *Papulous* inflammations are
those with which the itch is almost always complicated. When the vesicles of the itch are multiplied over a great many points, they often excite
lichen, the papulæ of which may be scattered
about, or formed in clusters. Prurigo also sometimes presents itself in persons afflicted with inveterate itch ; a circumstance that has led to the
supposition that the itch may degenerate into a
papulous disease. When the irritation of the skin
is exceedingly acute, the pustules of ecthyma, and
even true biles, may be combined with the vesicles of scabies. Lastly, in some rare examples,
the inflammation of the skin arising from the itch,
or some of the affections which complicate it, may
be so extensive and intense as to produce inflammation of the mucous membrane of the lungs or
digestive canal ; and, if this latter disorder attain
a high degree, the vesicles of the itch shrivel, fade,
and disappear.—(See Rayer, tom. i., p. 256.)
These observations will reconcile some of the differences between Dr. Good's account of the present subject, and the history of it delivered by Rayer.—ED.

* M. Mouronval was unable to transmit the dis-

Where the cutaneous irritation hereby produced is general to the surface, and has been suffered to remain without check or with little attention for a long time, a sudden suppression of the irritation by a speedy cure, like the sudden suppression of a long-standing ulcer or issue, is often attended with some severe internal affection;* in one instance, indeed, related by Wontner, it was succeeded by mania. And in camps and prisons, where the constitution has been debilitated by confined air and innutritious diet, the eruption has sometimes been known to assume a malignant character; of which Baldinger gives us an example, the whole surface of the body, in the instance to which he refers, having exhibited a sordid tesselation of crusts, excoriations, and broad livid spots, with an indurated base, accompanied with fever at night and severe headache.

Whenever an organ is weakened in its action, it is extremely apt to become a nidus for worms or insects of some kind or other to burrow in. Hence the numerous varieties of helminthia or invermination in debility of the stomach or other digestive organs; and hence the lodgment, as we have already observed, of the grubs of a minute insect, probably a species of pulex, in one or two of the varieties of prurigo; and hence again, in gangrenous ulcers, and especially in warm climates, the appearance almost every morning of innumerable grubs or maggots. A similar deposite of eggs, apparently of the genus acarus or tick, is sometimes found in itch pustules, or in the immediate vicinity of them. And hence itch has, by Wichmann, Frank, and many other writers of great intelligence, been ascribed solely to this cause:† while others, who have sought for the appearance of the grub hereby produced, but in vain, have peremptorily denied the existence of such a fact in any

ease by inoculation with the serosity of the vesicles, either in the manner of friction or that of insertion.—(Recherches et Obs. sur la Gale, faites à l'Hôpital St. Louis, 8vo., Paris, 1821.) As the itch is known to be readily communicable from one person to another by mediate as well as immediate contact, the result of M. Mouronval's experiments is not what one would have anticipated. When the itch has been impaited from one individual to another, a slight pruritus is experienced a few days afterward in the parts which have been most exposed to the contagion. The pruritus increases at night, from the heat of the bedding, and in the day from the effect of spirituous beverages, acrid food, and every thing that causes a determination of blood to the integuments. Small elevations are soon noticed, scarcely exceeding the level of the skin. In children, the eruption takes place in four or five days after infection; in adults, in a week or fortnight; and in old subjects, or persons labouring under chronic diseases, sometimes not till one or several months have elapsed from the period of catching the disorder. In young, sanguine individuals, the elevations are of a light red colour; but in valetudinarians they are of the same colour as the skin.—See Rayer, tom. i., p. 255.—Ed.

* Rayer's explanation of this part of the subject is given in a foregoing note.—Ed.
† Wichmann, Aetiologie der Krätze, Hanov., 1786. Rochard, Journ. de Méd., tom. xli., p. 26.

case.* Dr. Frank confides, indeed, so implicitly in the acarus as a cause of itch, as to affirm that, where this insect does not exist, the eruption is nothing more than a spurious itch (De Cur. Hom. Morb. Epit., tom. iv., pp. 165, 166); and, as he further affirms that the disease is sometimes epidemic, he endeavours to account for this fact by supposing that the atmosphere, in particular states of constitution, favours the production of the itch acarus, as of earthworms and intestinal worms, far more than in other states. The explanation now given constitutes, however, the actual history, and readily reconciles these conflicting opinions. Such insects are not always to be traced, but they may be seen occasionally: and whenever they appear, they are not a cause, but a consequence of the disease.

There are few complaints that have been treated with so many remedies, and none with so many pretended specifics. Sulphur, zinc, acids of all kinds, bayberries, white hellebore, arsenic, alum, muriate and other preparations of quicksilver, alkali, tobacco, and tar, have all been used externally in the form of lotions or ointments; and sulphur and sulphuric acid have been given internally, and been strongly recommended, both in Germany and in our own country, for their success. Sulphuric acid was first used in the Prussian army in 1756, by Dr. Colthenius, chief physician; after which Professor Schroeder, of Gottingen, employed it very freely, and asserted that he never failed herewith to cure the itch in fourteen days at furthest.—(See Dr. Helonich's Dissertatio de Olei Vitriolis usù, &c., Hal., 1762.)

Dr. Linckius, in the Nova Acta Naturæ Curiosorum, gives an account of an epidemic itch which raged very generally around Nuremburg about the middle of the last century, and resisted all the usual means of sulphur, lead, turpentine, arsenic, mercury, human and animal urine, chalybeate waters, lime-water, and drastic purgatives, and only yielded to diuretics, urged to such an extent as to irritate the urethra with a considerable degree of pain. The medicine he em-

* Sager, Baldinger, N. Magazin, b. xi., p. 484. Hartman, Diss. Quæstiones super Wichmanni Ætiologiâ Scabiei, Fr., 1789. Drs. Galeotti and Chiarurgi, of Florence, and MM. Lugol, Biett, and Mouronval, of Paris, have tried in vain, on a vast number of itchy persons, to detect the acarus scabiei, with the aid of powerful magnifying-glasses and excellent microscopes. Rayer was not more successful in his investigations; for he could never trace on the skins of persons affected with scabies any other insect than pediculi, which were met with in examples of great negligence and uncleanliness. Neither could he or other experimenters with the names discover any white living globules in the fluid of the vesicles, or the subcutaneous perforations of the insect, spoken of by certain authors.—See Traité des Mal. de la Peau, tom. ii., p. 413. The acarus scabiei is said, however, to have been at length unequivocally detected by M. Renucci, who lately received from M. Lugol the sum of 300 francs, the reward offered by the latter for such discovery.—For additional particulars, see Lond. Med. Gaz., Oct. 4, 1834, p. 29.—Ed.

ployed was a subnitrate of potash, obtained by deflagrating common nitre with charcoal. The first hint of this practice he received from a treatise of Mauchart. The urine hereby excreted was very fetid, and threw down a copious sediment.*

It is very possible that all of these have been successful under peculiar degrees and modifications of the complaint. For the itch is not difficult to cure, and seems only to require an application that will excite a new and more healthy action in the cutaneous vessels. The simplest and most certain cure is to be obtained by the sulphur ointment, of which that of the London College gives as good and as simple a form as any. On the continent they usually combine with the sulphur an equal quantity of powdered bayberries and of sulphate of zinc, which is mixed up into an ointment with linseed or olive oil. This form was first proposed by Jasser, and under the name of unguentum Jasserianum, has maintained an unrivalled character for the last half century.† The offensive smell of the sulphur, whether in the simple ointment or Jasser's compound preparation, is very much diminished by adding to the materials a few drops of the essence of burgamot, and as much rosewater as the powders will absorb before they are mixed with the animal or vegetable oil.‡ Perhaps, however, the neatest, as well as the most rapid mode of cure by sulphur, is that of fumigation, as long ago proposed by Professor Frank (Ubi suprà, tom. iv., p. 174), though lately brought forward again as a new discovery. It has been successfully and commodiously applied by M. Gales, of Paris, and since extensively employed in Germany by the advice of Dr. de Carro, of Vienna, and Dr. Karsten, of Hanover.§ The pa-

tient, for this purpose, is enclosed naked in a commodious box, with a neck-opening for his head to rise above it, and a stool to sit upon. The box is numerously perforated at the bottom, and the sulphureous fumes are communicated to the interior of the box, by means of these perforations: the sulphur being placed on a stone hearth below, and volatilized by a fire underneath it. He must remain in this state for half an hour or an hour; and, as he is hereby thrown into a considerable degree of perspiration, it is better for him to be put into a warm bed immediately afterward, till the perspiration has subsided. Other cutaneous complaints have yielded to the same process.*

These are the safest and most effectual applications, and should be employed whenever practicable. But, under other circumstances, the most elegant mode of treatment is to be obtained by a mercurial lotion made by dissolving a drachm of oxymuriated quicksilver in half a pint of water, and adding two drachms of muriate of ammonia, and half an ounce of nitre. The hands are to be washed with this solution night and morning, and a little of it is to be applied with a clean sponge to the pustules in other parts.†

About eight-and-forty hours' steady use of this lotion, or the sulphur ointment, will generally be found sufficient to effect a cure; after which the person should be well cleansed and rinsed with warm water. And it will tend much to expedite and ensure a cure, if the body be in like manner exposed to a warm bath before the curative process is entered upon, as much of the contagious matter and impacted sordes will hereby be removed, and the ointment or lotion will have a chance of taking a greater effect. When the constitution has been influenced, aperient and alterative medicines will also be necessary, and ought not to be neglected.

In India a pleasant and easy cure is said to be effected by wearing linen that has been dipped in juice expressed from the agreeable fruit of the bilimbi-tree (*averrhoa bilimbi*, Linn.), which has also the reputation of being an anti-

---

* Therapeia Scabiei epidemicæ per Diuresin, &c., tom. iv. Yet Rayer says,—" La gale n'est ni épidémique, ni endémique; ce n'est point par des causes climatériques et par des conditions locales qu'elle se propage dans certaines contreés, mais par des habitudes de malpropreté.—See Traité Théorique et Pratique des Maladies de la Peau, tom. i., p. 258.—ED.

† Schmucker, Vermischte-Chir. Schriften, b. iii., p. 183, Franckf., 1783, 8vo.

‡ A proportion of the subcarbonate of potash, or muriate of ammonia, is often blended with the brimstone ointment.
　　　℞ Sulph. (vivi dicti) ʒij.
　　　　Muriatis ammoniæ ʒij.
　　　　Adipis ʒxii.
Tere optime, ut fiat unguentum, quo partes affectæ nocte maneque inungantur.
　Another application is a solution of a scruple of sulphuret of lime in a little olive oil, with which the parts affected are smeared every night and morning. The sulphuric acid ointment is occasionally applied, consisting of ʒss of the diluted acid to an ounce of lard.
　　　℞ Potassæ subcarbonatis ʒiv.
　　　　Aq. rosæ f. ʒj.
　　　　Hydrarg. sulphur. rubri ʒj.
　　　　Olei volatilis burgamotæ f. ʒss.
　　　　Adipis
　　　　Sulphuris sublimati, ā ā ʒix.
Tere, et misce secundum artem, ut fiat unguentum.—See Dr. A. T. Thomson's Atlas of Delineations of Cutaneous Diseases, p. 74.—ED.

§ Ueber Kraetze, und derer bequemste, schnell-

wirkendeste und sicherste, Heilart, &c., Hanov., 1818.
* When scabies is complicated, the pruritus violent, the vesicles exceedingly numerous and crowded, and the disorder of long standing, and accompanied by much inflammation of the skin, Rayer deems it best to let the treatment begin with one or two bleedings from the arm, a few baths, and the employment of antiphlogistic beverages.—Op. cit., tom. i., p. 260.—ED.
† The following lotions are sometimes employed :—
　　　℞ Potassæ sulphureti ʒj ad ʒij.
　　　　Aq. distillatæ ʒxiv.
　　　　Spir. lavandulæ ʒij.
Misce; ft. lotio partibus affectis continue applicanda.
　　　℞ Acidi hydro-chlorici ʒiss ad ʒij.
　　　　Aq. rosæ ℔j.
Misce; ft. lotio ope spongiæ utenda.
Or,　℞ Liq. chlorureti calcis ʒj.
　　　　Aq. distillatæ Oj. Misce.—ED.

dote in many other cutaneous disorders : but I cannot speak of its effects from any personal knowledge.

How far scabies may, under any circumstances, cease naturally, I cannot say : we are informed, however, by Bennet, that a case, which had resisted all remedies, was cured by a phthisical expectoration that continued for a month.*

GENUS VII.
MALIS.
CUTANEOUS VERMINATION.
THE CUTICLE OR SKIN INFESTED WITH ANIMAL-CULES.

MALIS and maliasmus (μάλις, μαλιασμὸς) are Greek nouns importing cutaneous vermination. In the present system, the genus is designed to include both the malis and phthiriasis of Sauvages and several other writers, which are very unnecessarily divided. Common as this disease is to man, it is still more so to animals of perhaps every other class and description, from the monkey to the fish-tribes, and from these to the lowest worms. All of them are infested with parasitic and minute living creatures on their skins, shells, or scales, which afford them an asylum, and for the most part supply them with nutriment. Yet the same affection is still more common to plants, which are not only infested with parasitic plants, but with parasitic animals as well. The volume of Nosology contains many curious examples of this kind, which the reader may turn to at his leisure.

These external parasites, whether animal or vegetable, by our old botanical writers, were significantly called *dodders*, from a term which has lately, but improperly, been restrained to a particular tribe or genus of plants, to which Linnéus has given the name of *cuscusa*, a parasite found very extensively on the nettles and the wild thyme of our own wastes : but which formerly was applied to external parasitic plants of all kinds ; and hence Dryden in his Fables speaks of doddered *oaks*, and in his Æneid of doddered *laurels* :—

> " Near the hearth a laurel grew
> *Dodder'd* with age, whose boughs encompass round
> The household gods, and shade the holy ground."

Dodders are therefore parasites generally, and as strictly apply to those which constitute the present genus, as to any that infest the vegetable world.

Generally speaking, vermination is a proof of weakness, whether in animals or in plants ; and hence, the weaker the plant or the animal, the

more subject is it to be attacked, and the more readily to be infested.

A few instances may possibly be adduced of plants and animals in perfect health being thus haunted, but they do not oppose the general rule. The remote cause of this disease, however, is most commonly filth.

The animalcules that infest mankind are the following, which will constitute so many species :—

1. Malis Pediculi.		Lousiness.
2. —— Pulicis.		Flea-bite.
3. —— Acari.		Tick-bite.
4. —— Filariæ.		Guinea-Worm.
5. —— Œstri.		Gadfly-bite.
6. —— Gordii.		Hair-Worm.

SPECIES I.
MALIS PEDICULI.
LOUSINESS.

CUTICLE INFESTED WITH LICE, DEPOSITING THEIR NITS OR EGGS AT THE ROOTS OF THE HAIR : TROUBLESOME ITCHING.

THE insects of this name that trouble our own race are the two following :—

α Pediculi humani. Common louse.	Infestment of the *common louse,* chiefly inhabiting the head of uncleanly children, where it produces a greasy scurf or other filth ; and sometimes exulceration and porrigo : occasionally migrates over the body.
β Pediculi pubis. Crab-louse.	Infestment of the morpio or *crab-louse ;* found chiefly on the groins, pubes, and eyebrows of uncleanly men : itching extreme, without ulceration.*

The COMMON PEDICULUS is too well known to render any particular description necessary. Leewenhoeck, who cautiously watched it, by way of experiment, on his own person, affirms that the male is furnished at the extremity of the abdomen with a sting, and that it is this sting which produces the usual irritation, the suction of the proboscis hardly seeming to occasion any irksome sensation on the skin of the hand. The male is readily distinguished from the female by having the tail or tip of the abdomen rounded, which in the female is forked or bifid. The animal is produced from a small oval egg, vulgarly called a nit, which is agglutinated by its smaller end to the hair on which it is deposited. From this egg proceeds the insect complete in all its parts, and differing only from the parent animal in its size. To determine the time of pregnancy and proportion of increase, this indefatigable physiologist took two females and placed them in a black silk stocking, which he

---

* Young, on Consumptive Diseases, p. 171. We have already mentioned, on the authority of Rayer, the occasional dying away of itch, in consequence of severe inflammation of the mucous membrane either of the lungs or bowels. Putting this case out of present consideration, he affirms that the itch never terminates spontaneously, and that, in an individual who neglects to employ proper means of cure, it may annoy him during the whole of his life.—Op. cit., tom. i., p. 256.—ED.

* Three species are commonly mentioned as infesting the human body :—1. Pediculus humanus capitis (De Geer). 2. Pediculus humanus corporis (De Geer). 3. Pediculus pubis (Linnéus).

wore day and night, that they might have the full benefit of feeding upon him. He found that in six days each laid fifty eggs without exhausting its store, and that, in twenty-four days, the young were capable of laying eggs themselves: and, carrying on the calculation, he estimates that the two females conjointly might have produced eighteen thousand in two months.

The largest animals of this kind were discovered by Linnéus in the warm caverns of Fahlum in Sweden. It has been observed, however, by many entomologists, that those which conceal themselves in clothes, or the *pediculi vestimentorum*, are, in some respects, a different animal from the lice of the hair, or *p. capitis.* Dr. Willan remarks, that the latter lay single nits on the hairs of the head, and do not spontaneously quit the scalp or its natural covering. The former are large, flat, and whitish, and seldom appear on the head, but reside on the trunk of the body, on the limbs, and on the clothes. The nits are conglomerate, and usually deposited in the folds of linen, or in other articles of dress.

Swediaur once saw a young woman, thirty years of age, in the Westminster Infirmary, who was covered very generally with minute pustules and tubercles produced by an unlimited assault of these animalcules over the whole body ; and supposes that universal phthiriasis was by no means an unfrequent disease among the ancients.—(*Nov. Nosol. Meth. Syst.*, ii., p. 233.)

The PEDICULUS PUBIS is distinguished by the cheliform structure of its legs, whence its name of crab-louse : its antennæ consist of five articulations. Its excrement stains the linen, and appears like diluted blood. It is a frequent cause of local prurigo ; for these animals burrow in the skin, and, being almost unknown among decent persons, may remain a long time unsuspected, since even an examination for the purpose will scarcely detect them. They are chiefly discoverable by their nits, which may be seen attached to the basis of the hairs, the insects themselves appearing only like discolorations of the skin.

All these are bred among the inhabitants of sordid dwellings, jails, and workhouses, or who are habitually uncleanly. Monkeys, the Hottentots, and some tribes of negroes, are said to eat them: The cutaneous secretion is sometimes so changed by disease, that it becomes offensive to them, and they quit the person who is labouring under it : various infectious fevers seem to produce this result.

It is affirmed by some writers, that the *pediculus capitis* or *humanus* has been found useful in epilepsies, diseases of the head, and in scrofula, and that the worst consequences have arisen from drying the little ulcerations they produce. In Russia, and other parts of the continent, where this kind of uncleanliness is, perhaps, less attended to than in our own country, all this may have occurred ; for we have already had occasion to observe, that any cutaneous irritation, whether from scabies, porrigo, or any other excitement, maintained till it has become habitual, should be suppressed gradually, or we shall

endanger a transfer of the morbid action to a part of far more importance. Upon the whole, however, such remarks are only apologies for filth and indolence, as we are in no want of much more effectual cutaneous irritants, where such means are called for, than can be obtained from so disgusting a source.

The most fatal poisons to all these vermin are the mercurial oxydes, staphisacre, menispermum, rue, opium, angelica, and laurel ; saffron, pepper, sedum, lycopodium, pinguicula, tobacco, and the seeds of veratrum. Cleanliness itself, however, is a sufficient antidote, and a sure prophylactic. The *pediculus pubis* is best destroyed by calomel mixed with starch-powder, and applied by means of a down-puff.*

SPECIES II.
MALIS PULICIS.
FLEA-BITE.

CUTICLE INFESTED WITH FLEAS ; OFTEN PENETRATING THE CUTIS WITH THEIR BRISTLY PROBOSCIS, AND EXCITING PUNGENT PAIN ; EGGS DEPOSITED ON OR UNDER THE CUTICLE.

THIS species offers us the two following varieties :—

α Pulex irritans. Common flea.	Infestment of the *common flea,* with a proboscis shorter than the body; eggs deposited on the roots of the hair, and on flannel.
β Pulex penetrans. Chiggre.	Infestment of the *chigoe* or *chiggre,* a West Indian flea, with a proboscis as long as the body ; often penetrating deeply into the skin, and lodging its *eggs* under the cuticle, particularly of the feet ; producing malignant, occasionally fatal ulcers.

The COMMON FLEA infests not mankind only, but quadrupeds and birds of all kinds. It is probable that it has many varieties ; but these have not been ascertained by entomologists. Contrary to the economy of the pediculus, the flea undergoes all the changes of the metamorphosing tribes of insects, being produced from an egg, which gives rise to a minute vermicle

---

* A few frictions on the part with common or camphorated mercurial ointment, or bathing it with a lotion of the oxynuriate of mercury, will generally answer, without any occasion to shave the pubes. As for the pediculi corporis, they may be easily destroyed by means of the sulphur vapour-bath, or frictions with ointments containing sulphur and the alkalis. Rayer mentions as an effectual application, a pomatum composed of three parts of red sulphuret of mercury, one of the hydro-chlorate of ammonia, and thirty-two of lard. The clothes should be fumigated with sulphur or mercury. The ung. nicotianæ, sometimes recommended, has been known to excite convulsions and vomiting.—See Rayer, Traité Théorique et Pratique des Maladies de la Peau, tom. ii., p. 403. —ED.

or larve, that is transformed into a chrysalis, and finishes in a winged animal. The eggs, in the summer months, take six days before they are hatched, the larve the same period before it becomes a chrysalis, the chrysalis twelve days before it assumes its perfect form : so that the entire process is completed in a little more than three weeks in the summer, though a longer period of time is consumed in the colder months. It obtains its nourishment from the juices of the animal it infests, by driving its sharp proboscis under the cuticle.

The CHIGOE or chiggre is thus excellently described by Catesby. "It is a very small flea, found only in warm climates. It is a very troublesome insect, especially to negroes and others that go barefoot and are slovenly. They penetrate the skin, under which they lay a bunch or bag of eggs, which swell to the bigness of a small pea or tare, and give severe pain till taken out; to perform which great care is required, for fear of breaking the bag, which endangers mortification and the loss of a leg, and sometimes life itself. This insect, in its natural size, is not above a fourth part so big as the common flea. The egg is so small as to be scarcely discerned by the naked eye."[*]

As these animalcules are fostered, like the pediculus, by filth and laziness, they are best destroyed by vigilance and cleanliness; and, in the meantime, most of the poisons recommended in the former case will prove effectual in the latter. The cuticular or cutaneous haloes, often accompanied with a slight elevation of the skin, crowned with minute vesicles, or dandruff, produced by the present and various other bites or stings of insects, as that of the gadfly, harvest-bug, or wasp, are called by Frank (*De Cur. Hom. Morb. Epit.*, tom. iv., p. 181, Manuh., 8vo., 1792) and many other writers psydrasia or psydrasiæ. Dr. Willan's definition of the term does not widely differ from this explanation.

SPECIES III.

MALIS ACARI.

TICK-BITE.

CUTICLE INFESTED WITH THE TICK : ITCHING HARASSING ; OFTEN WITH SMARTING PAIN.

The tick insect offers us the following varieties :—

a Acari domestici. "Observed on the head in
Domestic tick. considerable numbers."— This is not a common variety, but Dr. Young has an example, and I have introduced the variety upon his authority and in his words.

β Acari scabiei.† Infestment of the *itch-tick ;*
Itch-tick. burrowing under the cuti-

cle, in or near the pustules or vesicles of the scabs in those affected.

γ Acari autumna- Infestment of the *harvest-*
lis. *bug ;* less in size than the
Harvest-bug. common mite ; inflicting its bite in the autumn, and firmly adhering to the skin ; itching intolerable, succeeded by glossy wheals.

The acarus is a numerous genus of very minute insects, including, besides those enumerated above, a multitude of other species, well known to every one, as *a. ricinus* or dog-tick, *a. siro* or mite, *a. dysenteriæ* or dysentery-tick, of which we have spoken already.—(Vol. i., p. 170.)

The first in the above varieties is probably the *a. leucurus* of Linnéus, with a testaceous exterior, found frequently in the neighbourhood of gangrenous sores and dead bodies. The second *a. scabiei* or *exulcerans,* for though enumerated as two by Linnéus, they are the same animal, white, with reddish legs. It burrows, not in, but near the exulcerations of the itch, as already observed under scabies, as also in the neighbourhood of other exulcerations, and adds considerably to their irritation.[*] The harvest-bug is a globular ovate-red insect, with an abdomen bristly behind. From the glossy wheals which its bite produces, it has sometimes been called WHEAL-WORM.

The wounds inflicted by vermin of this kind are to be avoided by avoiding their haunts ; or, when we have been exposed, a tepid bath is the best means of preventing the ill effects. When the punctures have taken place, they may be relieved by a lotion composed of equal parts of the aromatic spirit of ammonia and water, which I have often found also highly serviceable in the bite of an animal that does not, indeed, harbour in the cuticle or on the skin, though he is as troublesome by his sudden and predacious sallies ; I mean the gnat and the moschето-fly.

SPECIES IV.

MALIS FILARIÆ.

GUINEA-WORM.†

SKIN INFESTED WITH THE GUINEA-WORM ; WINDING AND BURROWING UNDER THE CUTICLE,

insect, made by Lugol, Biett, Galeotti, Chiarurgi, and Rayer, with powerful glasses and microscopes, have been already noticed in a note to the section of this work treating of *ecpyesis scabies.* The authorities in support of the reality of the acarus scabiei are chiefly Hauptmann, Cestoni, Galès, Bonomo, Linnéus, Morgagni, and Renucci, the latter of whom recently obtained a prize for the clear discovery of it from M. Lugol.—ED.

* Rayer's investigations lead him to believe, that the acarus scabiei is only the pediculus corporis in very uncleanly persons affected with itch. —Op. cit., tom. ii., p. 412.—ED.

† Rudlophi, Entozoorum sive Vermium Intestinalium Historia Naturalis, 3 vols., 8vo., Amst., 1808, art. FILARIA. Blainville, art. FILAIRE, Dict. des Sciences Naturelles.—ED.

---

* Pulices penetrantes may be destroyed by washing the parts with a decoction of tobacco.— (See Rayer, Traité des Mal. de la Peau, tom. ii., p. 407.) Of course this statement refers to cases in which they are not lodged in the cutis.—ED.
† The unsuccessful attempts to discover this

FOR THE MOST PART, OF THE NAKED FEET OF WEST INDIAN SLAVES ; SEVERE ITCHING, OFTEN SUCCEEDED BY INFLAMMATION AND PAIN.

THIS worm is found chiefly in both the Indies, most frequently in the morning dew ;[*] often twelve feet long, not thicker than a horsehair. It may be felt under the skin, and traced by the fingers, like the string of a violin : and excites no uneasy sensation, till the skin is perforated by the animal. It should be drawn out with great caution, by means of a piece of silk tied around its head ; for if, by being too much strained, the animal break, the part remaining under the skin will grow with redoubled vigour, and often occasion a fatal inflammation.

This animal is the *irk Medini* مدينى برقا of Avicenna and the Arabians, literally, *vermis Medinensis*, but which has, by some means or other, been by most writers corruptly translated *nervus*, or *vena Medinensis*.

The Guinea-worm was well known to the Greek writers, who, according to Pliny, denominated it δρακοντία (dracontia); whence the name of dracunculus, which is frequently applied to it. Aëtius and Agatharcides have both given an account of this worm, as has also Paulus of Ægina.

The inflammation produced by this animal commences with an itching in the part affected, without acute pain. The part swells and inflames, and at length resembles a furunculus or bile in hardness, and, when on the point of breaking, in vehement pain. Soon after the tumour has burst, the head of the worm may be seen peeping from the bottom of the sore, whence it is to be cautiously laid hold of, as already described. Sir James M'Grigor informs us, that the native practitioners are far more expert in extracting it than Europeans ; and that, after an exact feel with their fingers for the body of the worm, they make an incision, as nearly as they can judge, through its middle, and by nicely tying a piece of silk to each end, curl out both at the same time.[†] Mr. Hutchinson gives an ac-

count of his having extracted one that measured three yards and a half in length.[*] It more usually, however, measures from eighteen inches to six feet. It is elastic, white, transparent ; and contains a gelatinous substance.

Other varieties, or perhaps species, of the filaria are traced under the skin of numerous animals,—mammals, birds, and even insects : and it seems sometimes to infest the aqueous humour of the horse's eye ; and by exciting inflammation, has produced blindness.

SPECIES V.
MALIS ŒSTRI.
GADFLY-BITE.

SKIN INFESTED WITH THE LARVES OF THE GADFLY ; CHIEFLY BURROWING IN THE SCHNEIDERIAN MEMBRANE OF THE NOSTRILS.

THIS complaint is more common to quadrupeds than to mankind ; especially to sheep, horses, and black cattle ; the insect depositing its eggs in different parts of the bodies of these animals, and hence producing painful tumours, occasionally succeeded by death, from the violence of the inflammation. We sometimes, however, and in the West Indies not unfrequently, find the eggs of this insect deposited in the interior membrane of the human nostrils ; accidentally inhaled with the air, or lodged by a sudden ascent of the insect itself. Mr. Kilgour, of Jamaica, gives a striking example of this, though he does not exactly indicate the insect. The patient was reduced almost to a state of madness before the appearance of a single larve denoted the real nature of the disease. The cure was effected by an injection of tobacco decoction. Two hundred were discharged in ten days.—(*History of a Case in which Worms in the Nose were removed*, &c., 8vo., 1782.)

SPECIES VI.
MALIS GORDII.
HAIR-WORM.

SKIN INFESTED WITH THE HAIR-WORM ; CHIEFLY INSINUATING ITSELF UNDER THE CUTICLE OF THE BACK OR LIMBS OF INFANTS ; PRODUCING PRICKING PAINS, EMACIATION, AT TIMES CONVULSIONS.

THIS is the *morbus pilaris* of Horst, the *malis à crinonibus* of Etmuller and Sauvages.

The nature of the disease is still involved in some uncertainty ; the fibrils thrown forth from the surface of the skin, accompanied with the symptoms above described, are by some authors supposed to be a morbid production of real

---

[*] It is now believed that the Guinea-worm is never developed out of the human body. Loefler, who resided many years in Africa, never knew an instance of its having been observed in water. Neither could Lind ever detect it in the waters of that quarter of the globe.—(See Rayer, Traité des Mal. de la Peau, tom. ii., p. 420.) For a refutation of an old opinion, of late revived (see Trans. of the Med. and Physical Society of Calcutta, vol. i.), that the filaria medinensis is not an individual animal, but a dead portion of lymphatic vessel, see a letter by Professor Grant, in the Edin. Med. and Surgical Journ., No. cvi., p. 116.—ED.

[†] Medical Sketches of the Expedition to Egypt from India, 8vo., Lond., 1804. - This worm chiefly gets into the subcutaneous cellular tissue of the lower extremities. Out of 181 cases referred to by Sir James M'Grigor, 124 were in the feet ; 33 in the legs ; 11 in the thighs ; 2 in the scrotum ; and 2 in the hands. Kæmpfer met with this worm in the cellular tissue of the ham and scrotum ; Peret in that of the head, neck, and trunk ; and Bajon asserts, that he saw two instances of it under the mucous membrane of the eyeball.

According to Chardin, the filaria is always single ; but Bajon and Bosmann state, that it is not unusual to meet with several in the same patient. —See Rayer, Traité des Mal. de la Peau, tom. ii., p. 420.—ED.

[*] Edin. Med. Essays, vol. v., part ii., p. 309. Fermin describes one that was eight ells in length.— See also Rayer, Traité des Mal. de la Peau, tom. ii., p. 419.—ED.

hairs; but the greater number, and among the rest Ambrose Paré, ascribe to them a distinct living principle.

The disease is uncommon: but, upon the whole, it seems to be often produced by a species of the gordius or hair-worm; some of which are well known to infest other animals in like manner; and especially the *cyprinus al. burnus*, or bleak, which, at the time, appears to be in great agony.

Hoffmann tells us that the children of Misnia are much infested with worms of this kind, which he describes as resembling black hairs lodged under the skin: and which, by a perpetual irritation, so emaciate them, that they become little more than living skeletons. When the skin is warm, they appear; but, while it is cold, they keep buried under its cover.

A similar disease is said by M. Bassignet to have been peculiar, in 1776, to the town of Seyne and its neighbourhood, and to have made its attack upon almost all the new-born children. In Seyne, it was at that time called cées, a corruption of ceddés, a provincial term for a bristle. It appeared from the first twelve hours till the end of the first month after birth, rarely later than the last period. The symptoms were, a violent itching, and general erethism, so as to prevent sleep; hoarseness, a diminution of the voice, and an inability of sucking. Friction with the hand over the body proved a certain cure, and brought forth a kind of dark rough filaments resembling hair, often not more than the twelfth of an inch in length, in some cases furnished with a minute bulb at the extremity.—(*Hist. de la Société Royale*, &c., an. 1776.)

A decoction of the cocculus indicus is serviceable in most of the preceding species: but, perhaps, the most determinate cure for the whole is to be found in the civadilla, supposed to be a species of the veratrum, which I have already recommended in many cases. No insect nor vermin of any kind is capable of resisting or living under the pungent and acrid aroma of its seeds when reduced to powder, which it is only necessary to sprinkle over the linen or bedclothes that are thus infested. The powder, indeed, is a powerful errhine; and, when tasted, affects the tongue with the pungency of needles, and excites a severe and protracted ptyalism. On account of this acrid and penetrating power, it ought not to be used where the surface of the body is exulcerated. In porrigo,-or scabby scall, it has even proved fatal: and hence it is omitted in Rosenstein's third edition of his work "On the Diseases of Children," though recommended in the two preceding.

GENUS VIII.
ECPHYMA.
CUTANEOUS EXCRESCENCE.
SUPERFICIAL, PERMANENT, INDOLENT EXTUBE-RANCE; MOSTLY CIRCUMSCRIBED.

ECPHYMA is a Greek term, from *ἐκφύω*, "educo, egero," in contradistinction both to *phyma*,

"an inflammatory tumour," and *emphyma*, "a tumour without inflammation," originating below the integuments. Extuberances, similar to those belonging to this genus, are frequently found in the rinds of fruits, as apples and oranges, and form a peculiar character in some species of melon; none of which are produced by insects, nor are we acquainted with the immediate cause.

The species of this genus are the four following:—

1. Ecphyma Caruncula.	Caruncle.
2. ——— Verruca.	Wart.
3. ——— Clavus.	Corn.
4. ——— Callus.	Callus.

SPECIES I.
ECPHYMA CARUNCULA.
CARUNCLE.
SOFT, FLESHY, OFTEN PENDULOUS, EXCRESCENCE OF THE COMMON INTEGUMENT.

THIS species is found over the surface generally, and occasionally, as a sequel of lues, about the anus and sexual organs.

From its shape or position, it often obtains a particular name; as *ficus*, when fig or raisin-shaped; *encanthis*, when seated on the canthus or angle of the eye.

These excrescences, on their first formation, seem to be productions of the cuticle alone;[*] but by gradually thickening, and a fresh vascularity, they come at length to be connected with the skin itself, and, in some instances, even to proceed to the depth of the subjacent muscles. They are of very different degrees of hardness: being in some instances not much firmer than the parts with which they are connected: while, in others, they are found to acquire the obduracy of a rigid scirrhus. Their colour also is very various: in some cases they are of a pale white, and in others of different shades of red. In some instances they are single, and in others gregarious. In many cases, they are not larger than ordinary warts; but, in others, they are much broader and thicker.

Where they are neither painful nor unsightly, there can be no reason for attacking them; but, in other cases, they should be removed. Those of a soft consistency may be often destroyed by rubbing them frequently with a piece of crude sal ammoniac, or washing them with a strong solution of it. Savin powder is a still more effectual escharotic. Pressure alone will also sometimes succeed when it can be fairly applied. But, if none of these answer, recourse must be had to lunar caustic, or the scalpel.

SPECIES II.
ECPHYMA VERRUCA.
WART.
FIRM, HARD, ARID, INSENSIBLE EXTUBERANCE OF

---

[*] No doubt this part of the description is incorrect with reference to the examples specified by the author.—ED.

X x 2

THE COMMON INTEGUMENT: FOUND CHIEFLY ON THE HANDS.

WARTS are small sarcomata that offer the following varieties:—

a Simplex.	Simple and distinct : sessile
Simple Wart.	or pensile.
β. Lobosa.	Full of lobes and fissures.
Lobed Wart.	
γ Confluens.	In coalescing clusters.
Confluent Wart.	

All these rise, like the caruncle, from the cuticle at first, and gradually become connected with the cutis by being supplied with minute arteries, that rarely extend far into the substance, as the surface, when of any bulk, is hard, ragged, and insensible, though the base is endued with extreme sensibility.*

Warts may be destroyed by ligature,† the knife, escharotics, or powerful astringents. Many of our common pungent plants are employed by the vulgar for the same purpose, and, in various instances answer sufficiently. One of the most frequent is the celandine, or *Chelidonium majus*, whose yellow acrid juice is applied to the excrescence daily or occasionally till it disappears. The pyroligneous acid, however obtained, answers the same purpose, as does the *Meloë pro-*

* Rayer describes two kinds of warts, the *common* (verrues vulgaires), and *those with pedicles* (verrues pédiculées). Common warts are usually formed on the hands. When perpendicularly cut through, the thickness of the cuticle is observed to increase progressively as far as the middle of the wart. The cutis, which is thickened as well as the cuticle, sends prolongations into the substance of the latter, which are termed the roots of the wart. Sometimes these, being surrounded by a layer of cuticle, are separated from one another, so as to give the wart a split or lobulated appearance (verrucca lobosa). When warts are cut into, small black points are sometimes perceived ; and Cruveilhier has traced bloodvessels in them in the form of red streaks, following the prolongations of the cutis. Warts with pedicles are represented by Rayer to be small appendages of the skin, shaped like the finger of a glove, and with a smooth polished surface, often of the same colour as the nipple of the breast. He states, that they consist of two very fine reddish layers of skin, connected together by means of a delicate cellular tissue. They are mostly situated on the neck, back, or limbs, and are sometimes flattish, with a broad base (verrues charnues).—(See Rayer, Traité des Mal. de la Peau, tom. ii., p. 296,) Common verrucæ are well known to form much more frequently in children and young subjects than in old persons. Habitual irritation seems to promote their formation on the hands, and hence their frequency on individuals who are in the custom of handling hard bodies, or whose hands are much exposed to great variations of atmospheric temperature, or remain in an uncleanly state. Warts differ from syphilitic excrescences, inasmuch as the latter are attended or have been preceded by other venereal complaints, occur on or near the genitals, or on the chin and face; and often yield to mercury, or the deutochlorure of gold or soda. Syphilitic excrescences are also red, and, when wounded, bleed more freely than warts.—Op. cit., loco cit.—ED.

† When the pedicle is narrow, horsehair or silk is often used for this purpose.—ED.

scarabæus, the liquor potassæ or ammoniæ, mineral acids, muriated ammonia. In Sweden, they are destroyed by the *Gryllus verrucivorus,* or wart-eating grasshopper, with green wings spotted with brown. The common people catch it for this purpose ; and it is said to operate by biting off the excrescence, and discharging a corrosive liquor on the wound. They often disappear spontaneously, and hence are sometimes supposed to be charmed away.*

SPECIES III.
ECPHYMA CLAVUS;
CORNS.†

ROUNDISH, HORNY, CUTANEOUS EXTUBERANCE, WITH A CENTRAL NUCLEUS, SENSIBLE AT ITS BASE : FOUND CHIEFLY ON THE TOES, FROM THE PRESSURE OF TIGHT SHOES.

CORNS originate in the same manner as caruncles and warts. They are sometimes spontaneous and gregarious, spreading over the whole head and body ; and sometimes rise to a considerable height, and assume a horny appearance. In the last case the tuber makes a near approach to some of the species of the genus LEPIDOSIS, especially *L. ichthyiasis cornea,* and *cornigera.* In the ninth volume of the Transactions of Natural Curiosities, is a case of an annual fall by a spontaneous suppuration.

The cure consists in cutting or paring the excrescence down nearly to its roots ; and then applying some warm resinous or other stimulating preparation, as the juice of squills, houseleek, or purslane, or the compound galbanum or ammoniac emplaster.‡

* Rubbing warts with muriate of ammonia will remove them in the course of time, without any inflammation or pain, unless they happen to be of a peculiarly hard description. Rayer prefers touching them with nitric acid, as a more expeditious and certain means of cure. In this metropolis, a strong solution of the nitrate of silver, the concentrated acetic acid, and the tinctura ferri muriatis, are favourite applications.—ED.

† Small accidental rounded productions of the cuticle, very hard, circumscribed, ordinarily formed on the upper surface or sides of the toes, and sometimes on the sole of the foot, near the anterior extremities of the metatarsal bones. They compress, irritate, inflame, and sometimes penetrate the cutis, or even affect the bones and subjacent articulations. The cuticle of which corns are composed is so thickened, that several layers of it may be successively removed with a cutting instrument, and in their centre a point of horny appearance, whiter, and extending more deeply than them, may be distinguished. Pressure on a corn occasions acute pain. The induration is sometimes surrounded by a slight ecchymosis, situated between the cutis and the semitransparent layers of the corn, and commonly increasing in proportion to the thickness and consistence of the small central induration. The thickened cuticle was found, on maceration of a corn, to have depressed and thinned the cutis underneath it; but Rayer was not able to detect any vessels in the substance of the corn itself, as some anatomists pretend to have done.—See op. cit., p. 321-323.—ED.

‡ The nitrate of silver and kreosote will be found useful in removing corns.—D.

SPECIES IV.
ECPHYMA CALLUS.
CALLUS.

CALLOUS, EXTUBERANT THICKENING OF THE CU-
TICLE ; INSENSIBLE TO THE TOUCH.*

THIS species is found chiefly on the palms of
the hands and soles of the feet, as a consequence of hard labour. Among those who accustom themselves to long journeys over the
burning sands of Egypt, some have had their
feet as indurated with a thick callus as an ox's
hoof, so as to bear shoeing with iron ; and, in
Siam, such persons have been known to walk
with their naked feet on redhot iron bars.

This species is produced also by a frequent
exposure of the hands or feet to hot water or
to mineral acids. The cuticle of the feet has
been rendered so thick and insensible by the
use of sulphuric acid as to endure fire without
pain. This acid is hence commonly employed
by professed fire-walkers and fire-eaters, the interior of the mouth being hardened and seared in
the same way as the soles of the feet.

In the Medical Museum is a singular case of
this complaint, as it occurred in a young man,
the cuticle of whose hands was so thickened and
indurated as to render them of no use. He was
by trade a dier ; and the disease was gradually
brought on by cleaning brass wire, with a fluid
consisting of sulphuric acid, tartar, and alum.
His fingers were so rigid from the callosity of
the cuticle, that on a forcible endeavour to
straighten them, blood started from every pore.
As the disease was chiefly ascribed to the use
of the acid, the patient was ordered to apply to
his hands an emollient liniment, consisting of
equal parts of olive-oil and liquor potassæ. After two days, one-half the alkali was omitted,
and the yolk of two eggs added. By means
of this application, the hardened cuticle began to
peal off, and a new flexible one to appear beneath ; he acquired the use of his fingers by degrees, and in about two months the cure was
perfected.

GENUS IX.
TRICHOSIS.
MORBID HAIR. ●

MORBID ORGANIZATION OR DEFICIENCY OF HAIR.

TRICHOSIS (τρίχωσις), "pilare malum," is a
term of Actuarius and other Greek writers,
from θρίξ, "pilus." TRICHIASIS is the more
common appellation ; but it has often been used
in a somewhat different and more limited sense.
The terms athrix and distrix, which express two
of the species under this genus, are evidently
from the same root.

Hair may be regarded as a vegetation from
the surface of the body ; it rises from a bulbous
root, of an oval form, which is situated within

the cutis. The separate hairs are spiral and
hollow, filled with a pulp, furnished with vessels,
and knotted at certain distances, like some sorts
of grass, and in some cases, send out branches
at their knots. Their roots or bulbs are found
over the whole surface of the body, though they
only vegetate in particular parts, for which it is
not easy to assign a reason. [According to
Professor Macartney, all true hairs, whatever
may be their figure, agree in certain circumstances. Thus, they all grow upon vascular
pulps, which, with the tubular roots that surround them, are enclosed in bulb-shaped capsules, or investments situated within the skin.*
The minute parts which are concerned in the
production of small hairs, such as those which
grow on the human head, or the bodies of quadrupeds in general, cannot be easily distinguished. In these instances, the bulbs appear to be
short transparent membranous tubes, which permit the root of the hair to be seen through them.
They usually contain a clear gelatinous fluid,
and sometimes a particle of blood. These capsules have but a slight adherence to the subcutaneous substance, or to the skin ; as frequently, on pulling out a hair, the bulb comes
along with it. The bulbs are larger in proportion as the hair is young. The pulp on which
the hair is formed passes through the bottom
of the capsule, in order to enter the tube of the
hair, into which it penetrates for a short distance, but never, in common hairs, reaching to
the external surface of the skin. The pulp is
supplied by one artery, which, when injected,
renders the whole perfectly red.† The pulp secretes the matter of which the hair is composed,
and it is found only to extend to that portion of
the hair which is in a state of growth ; and in
those which are deciduous, or which are cast at
particular seasons of the year, such as the hairs
of quadrupeds, the pulp becomes entirely obliterated before the period of shedding the hair, and
its root is converted into a solid pointed mass.]—
(*Macartney, in Rees's Cyclopædia*, art. HAIR.)

As hairs, at least in a state of health, have no
more nerves than the filaments of vegetables, it
is probable that the circulation is carried on in
them in the same manner as in plants. By
combing, we free the fluid from those obstruc-

---

* A callus, or callosity, as it is more commonly
called, when the term is employed in the sense assigned to it by Dr. Good, differs from a corn in
having no central white cone that penetrates more
deeply than the rest of it.—ED.

* Most of the changes to which the hairs are
liable arise, like those of the nails, from an affection of the bulbs, or the organs by which they are
produced. The hair-follicles inflame in several
inflammatory diseases of the scalp, as in porrigo
favosa and porrigo lupinata, and in certain cases
of impetigo, &c.—(See Rayer, tom. ii., p. 358.)
The growth of hairs is considerably influenced by
the state of the organs of generation. Thus Mo-
reau presented to the Faculty of Medicine at Paris
a child only six years old, the precocious development of whose testicles had so forced the growth
of hair on its body, that its breast was as shaggy
as that of an adult. On the other hand, the beards
of eunuchs are known frequently to cease in a
great measure to grow.—See Rayer, tom. ii., p.
385.—ED.

† M. Frederick Cuvier is alleged to have seen
the bulbs of feathers of various birds very much
injected with blood, and highly inflamed.—See
Rayer, op. cit., tom. ii., p. 359.—ED.

tions which must necessarily be produced by their being bent in all directions ; and hereby promote a circulation through the bulb, and relieve the head from accumulations ; for, though the vessels of the bulb are small, they are numerous.* And we are hence enabled to account for the relief and refreshment which are often felt by a patient after the operation of combing. : Long hair has been in all ages esteemed an ornament. There is no question, however, that it requires more nutriment for its support than short hair ; and some physiologists have gone so far as to doubt whether it may not hereby be injurious to the general health, as productive of debility. But there seems no real ground for such a belief ; as a healthy system, like the roots or trunk of a healthy tree, will always be able without inconvenience to furnish sustenance enough for its branchy foliage. Dr. Parr, however, affirms, that suddenly cutting off long hair has to his knowledge been injurious, and attended with every appearance of plethora :† while very thick hair may occasionally weaken by the undue warmth and perspiration it occasison.

Next to the bones, hair appears to be the most indestructible of the constituents of the body ;‡ and there are accounts of its having been found in old tombs, after all the soft parts had entirely disappeared. The hair of different individuals differs considerably in thickness, in the proportion of 1-300 to 1-700 of an inch in diameter : and it is no less variable in its other physical qualities, some kinds being much more dense and elastic than others, which Mr. Hatchett ascribes to the different proportion of jelly contained in it.—(*Bostock's Elementary System of Physiology*, p. 91, 8vo., 1824.)

* This passage requires some little explanation. By circulation, Dr. Good could not mean a circulation of blood in the hairs themselves, but only in their pulps, which, we find, do not extend into their tubes beyond the level of the skin, at least in the healthy common hair of the human subject. Dr. Good, by circulation, however, may possibly refer also to the oily and other secretions which pervade the hair, and are no doubt produced from the vessels either of the bulb or pulp. Bichat supposes that there is a species of circulation in the interior of the hair, by which he explains the changes of colour, and the sympathy which is well known to exist between the hair and many important organs of the body. If, however, these effects are produced by any vital action, it must go on likewise, as Dr. Macartney justly observes, in the horny substance of the hair, which is the seat of many of those effects. The fibrous structure of the hair seems calculated to admit that sort of movement, or circulation of the juices, which takes place in plants ; and an organic action in the substance of hairs, Dr. Macartney conceives, must be admitted to exist, in order to account for the changes to which it is subject.—ED.

† See also Lanoix, Observations sur le Danger de couper les Cheveux dans quelques Maladies aiguës.—Mém. Soc. Méd. d'Émulation, Paris, tom. i., 8vo.—ED.

‡ We have examined hair taken, together with sculls, from the tumuli which exist on the western coast of South America, and which contain the relics of nations of whom no other records exist : it was apparently unchanged.—D.

According to the experiments of Vauquelin, read to the Institute in 1808, human hair is not soluble in boiling water ; but when exposed to a greater temperature in Papin's digester, it dissolves readily. From a solution of black hair, a black matter was deposited, which proved to be an oil of the consistence of bitumen, together with iron and sulphur. And as the hair of some persons has a smell approaching to that of sulphur, and especially those who have red hair, we are no longer at a loss to account for this.

. The same excellent chymist found that alcohol extracts from black hair a whitish and a grayish-green oil, the last of which separates as the alcohol evaporates. It is probable, therefore, that the black matter is gummy or albuminous ; the white, we are told, resembles cetaceum in appearance, though it differs in chymical affinity. Red hair affords the white matter, and, instead of the grayish-green oil, an oil as red as blood. White hair contains phosphate of magnesia, and its oil is nearly colourless. When hair becomes suddenly white from terror, Vauquelin thinks it may be owing to a sudden extrication of some acid, as the oxymuriatic acid is found to whiten black hair ; but it is suggested by Parr, that this may more probably be owing to an absorption of the oil of the hair by its sulphur, as in the operation of whitening woollen cloths. Dr. Bostock has more plausibly conceived, that the effect depends upon the sudden stagnation in the vessels which secrete the colouring matter, while the absorbents continue to act, and remove that which already exists.— (*Elementary System of Physiology*, p. 92. For additional remarks on gray hair, see Trichosis poliosis.)

These remarks will assist us in comprehending something of the nature of the following species of diseases, which are included in the genus before us :—

1. Trichosis Setosa.	Bristly Hair.
2. ——— Plica.	Matted Hair.
3. ——— Hirsuties.	Extraneous Hair.
4. ——— Distrix.	Forky Hair.
5. ——— Poliosis.	Gray Hair.
6. ——— Athrix.	Baldness.
7. ——— Area.	Areated Hair.
8. ——— Decolor.	Discoloured Hair.
9. ——— Sensitiva.	Sensitive Hair.

SPECIES I.

TRICHOSIS SETOSA.

BRISTLY HAIR.

HAIRS OF THE BODY THICK, RIGID, AND BRISTLY.

THIS is the hystriacis or porcupine hair of Plenck. It is, in fact, a stiff corpulence of hair produced by a gross or exuberant nutriment, and has been sometimes limited to the head, sometimes to other organs, and sometimes common to the body.* The remarks already offered will sufficiently account for its production.

* Bichat saw an unfortunate individual at Paris, whose face was covered from his birth with hairs as rigid as the bristles of a wild boar.—(Anatomic Gen., tom. iv., p. 827.) M. Villermé like-

In the fifth volume of the Philosophical Transactions, we have an extraordinary example of hair of this kind being thrown off and renewed every autumn, like the horns of the deer and various other quadrupeds. The affection was also hereditary ; for five sons exhibited the same morbid state of the hair.—(See also *Samml. Med. Wahrnehmung.*, band iv., p. 249.)

SPECIES II.
TRICHOSIS PLICA.
MATTED HAIR.

HAIRS VASCULARLY THICKENED; INEXTRICABLY ENTANGLED AND MATTED BY THE SECRETION OF A GLUTINOUS FLUID FROM THEIR ROOTS.*

This disease affords a sufficient proof by itself, if other proofs were wanting, of the vascularity of the hairs. Vauquelin ascribes it to a superfluous excretion of the fluid that nourishes them ; but there must be something more than this :† there must be also an intumescence or dilatation of the vascular tunic of the hairs, since their capacity is always augmented, and in some cases so much so as to permit the ascent of red blood ; in consequence of which they bleed when divided by the scissors.‡

wise, in 1808, met with a child, about six or eight years old, at Poictiers, with a great number of brown prominent patches of different sizes dispersed over the whole body, excepting the hands and feet, and which were covered with hairs shorter and less coarse than those of a wild boar, yet somewhat analogous to them. The hairs, and spots on which they grew, occupied about one fifth of the surface of the body.—See Rayer, Traité des Mal. de la Peau, tom. ii., p. 384.—ED.

* "By plica," says Rayer, "I understand, with J. F. A. Schlegel (Ueber die Ursachen des Weichselzopfes der Menschen und Thieren, &c., Jena, 1806, 8vo.), a particular inflammation of the bulbs of the hair, ordinarily accompanied by an anormal development and entanglement of it. The disease is sometimes complicated with chronic inflammation of the matrix of the nails."—(See Traité des Mal. de la Peau, tom. ii., p. 359.) The nails, he observes, both of the fingers and toes, usually become long, yellowish, livid, black, and sometimes crooked (p. 361). Notwithstanding Rayer's adoption of the foregoing definition, he afterward confesses, that more precise and minute anatomical researches than those hitherto made, are requisite to dispel the doubts which may be entertained about plica consisting of a particular inflammation of the bulbs of the hairs.—(Tom. ii., p. 361.) Indeed, in another part of his treatise, he admits, that the circumstance of porrigo and some other inflammations of the scalp making the hair fall off, instead of accelerating its growth, is adverse to the doctrine. The exact source of the exudation that takes place on the skin where plica exists, seems also, to Rayer, a point that has not been duly examined.—ED.

† Dr. Otto remarks, that the chymical composition of the hair is so changed in this disease that it dissolves in boiling.—D.

‡ The reality of any disease, corresponding to plica polonica, as described by writers, is sometimes doubted ; but, if there be such a case, agreeing with the particulars ascribed to it in books, it

Most authors ascribe it to uncleanliness, which is no doubt the ordinary exciting cause, though there seem to be others of equal efficiency. It is also very generally affirmed to be contagious ; and I had hence added this character to the disease in the volume of Nosology. But as Dr. Kerckhoffs strenuously maintains the contrary, after a very minute attention to the complaint in Poland itself, and more especially after having in vain endeavoured to inoculate first himself, and then two children, from the matter issuing from the bulbs of hair pulled for this purpose from a boy who was suffering from it in the most loathsome manner, I have here withdrawn the symptom.

Dr. Kerckhoffs reduces plica to a much simpler principle than it has hitherto been described under, and strips it of many of the most formidahle features by which it has been characterized ; particularly its connexion with hectic fever, or any idiopathic affection of the brain.— (*Observations Médicales, par Jos. Rom. Louis Kerckhoffs, Médecin de l'Armée,* &c. ; see *Med. Trans.,* vol. vi., art. iii.) He regards it as a mere result of the custom common among the lowest classes of the Polonese, of letting the hair grow to an immense length,* of never combing, or in any other way cleaning it, and of constantly covering the head with a thick woollen bonnet or leathern cap. And hence, says he, while the rich are in general exempt from the disease, it is commonly to be met with among the poor alone, who wallow in filth and misery, and particularly among the Jews, who are proverbially negligent of their persons. He contends, in consequence, that it is more endemic to Poland than to any other country ; and that nothing more is necessary to effect a cure than general cleanliness, and excision of the matted hair.

The first person he saw labouring under this disease, and he gives the case as a general specimen, was a boy from fifteen to eighteen years old, in a miserably poor village in the neighbourhood of Posen : most offensively filthy, lying in a dark hole, and stinking (*puant*) beside the beasts. He had black hair, very long, very coarse, and braided into thick plaits of a twelvemonth's standing. His head was covered with grease, his brain was greatly affected, and he was complaining of terrible headaches. The medical practitioner that attended him opposed a removal of the hair, from a vulgar belief, that the common outlet of morbid humours being thus cut off, such humours would flow rapidly to the brain, and produce apoplexy or some other cerebral affection. At length, he consented

certainly shows an inordinate action of the blood-vessels of the pulp, which probably passes further than usual into the tube of the hair.—ED.

* On the etiology of plica, we find nothing but unsatisfactory and even contradictory matter : thus, it is alleged by some writers, that the way to prevent this disease is to avoid the protracted impression of cold and damp, and the *custom of most of the Poles, to shave their heads on assuming the national costume.*—See Rayer, op. cit., vol. ii., p. 362, —ED.

that after a brisk purge the process of cutting the hair should commence ; but only to be proceeded in by degrees. The length of two fingers was therefore first removed ; and this producing no mischief, it was again shortened to the same extent two days afterward ; and in this manner the whole was cut off in about twenty days. After this the patient was allowed to comb his head a little, and wash it with milk : a few bitters and other tonics were prescribed for him, and he was very shortly restored to perfect health.

Admitting Dr. Kerckhoffs' explanation of this disease to be correct, it is somewhat singular, that the same explanation has never hitherto been given by the most intelligent and most celebrated Polish or even German physicians ; as it is also that the disease should be unknown in other countries, where the hair is, in like manner, suffered to grow without cutting, and where as little attention is paid to cleanliness. Hence Sinapius (*Paradoxa Med.*), and numerous other writers, deny uncleanliness to be the only, or even the ordinary cause. They contend for a predisposition in the habit, and affirm that under such predisposition any local accident, and a variety of affections in remote organs, may become exciting causes. In the Ephemera of Natural Curiosities is a case, in which it seems to have been produced by a wound in the head.—(Dec ii., ann. ii., obs. 1.) Vehr relates another, in which a suppression of catamenia for three months was followed by it and a jaundice.—(*Diss. Icterus fuscus cum Plicâ Polonicâ*, &c., Fr., 1708.) It is also occasionally a sequel of several of the varieties of psoriasis. Swediaur relates a case, in which the removal of the hair was accompanied with severe pain, though the scissors were applied at a considerable distance from the head : but he seems to have credited report upon this subject too readily ; for he tells us of another case in which the patient, then residing in one of the hospitals at Paris, suffered acute headache on the abscission of her matted hair, and died not long after.— (*Nov. Nos. Meth. Syst.*, ii., 231.) In one instance it appears to have followed gout in the head, and to have kept pace periodically with its paroxysms. The patient was about fifty years of age, and whenever attacked with this podagral affection, his hair began to curl and become hard ; insomuch that often in a single night, instead of hanging down straight, it formed a complicated wreathy mass, which no combing could reduce to order. As soon, however, as the paroxysm of gout subsided, the hair lost its tendency to twist, and was easily disentangled.*

Cutting off the hair, however, though generally supposed to exasperate the disease, or to lead to some secondary evil, does not appear to produce these effects ; and hence Vicat recommends the use of the scissors whenever the hairs bleed.—(*Mémoire sur la Plique Polonoise*, Lausanne, 1775.) It is far better, with Dr. Kerckhoffs, to use them beforehand.*

Though the disease has been usually confined to the hair of the scalp, it has occasionally appeared in other quarters, as in the beard, the armpits, and even the pudendum : authorities for which are quoted in the volume of Nosology.

From the great afflux of fluids, and even of blood, to the head, during this disease, it is often accompanied with hemicrania, or some other cephalalgic affection.

SPECIES III.
TRICHOSIS HIRSUTIES.
EXTRANEOUS HAIR.

GROWTH OF HAIR IN EXTRANEOUS PARTS, OR SUPERFLUOUS GROWTH IN PARTS COMMON.

THE most frequent example of this misaffection is that of bearded women. In a few instances, the female beard has even been bristly, thus uniting the present with a preceding species. Hippocrates ascribed hirsuties under this form to a deficient menstruation (*Epidem.*, lib. vi., sect. vii. ; *Schurig, Parthenologia*, p. 185, Dresd., 1729, 4to.), whence it is occasionally met with in young women. This cause is admitted generally in modern practice ; but one of the most striking cases in a young woman that has ever occurred to the present author, was accompanied with an habitual *paramenia superflua*, under which the patient at length sunk at about forty years of age.†

---

* Journ. of Foreign Med., No. xvii. The previous or simultaneous existence of the other diseases mentioned in the text might have been accidental, without any essential connexion with the origin of plica. At all events, such connexion cannot be explained. According to Rayer, the scalp is painful when touched. The bulbs of the hair are swollen, and contain a greater quantity of fluid than usual ; they are also so sensitive, that the slightest motion communicated to the hairs occasions acute pain at their roots ; a morbid se-

cretion oozes from the inflamed bulbs, and glues the hairs together, sometimes without their being mixed together and entangled. The hairs may stick together in separate locks of greater or less thickness, lengths, and degrees of flexibility, like so many cords (the plique multiforme of Alibert) ; or else, besides adhering together, they may acquire an immoderate length, so as to resemble a horse's tail (the plique à queue of Alibert) ; or, lastly, they may be agglutinated and mixed together, without ever separating, making a misshapen mass of greater or less size (the plique en masse of Alibert).—See Rayer, tom. ii., p. 360. —ED.

* The use of the warm bath, or pediluvium, residence in a mild temperature, the application of tepid lotions to the head or other parts, where the bulbs of the hair are liable to be affected, cutting off the hair, and an habitual attention to cleanliness, are the means specified by Rayer as most generally proper in the treatment of plica. The more or less serious affections which precede, accompany, or follow it, present likewise particular indications, the comprehension and fulfilment of which can only be taught by experience.—See Rayer, tom. ii., p. 362.—ED.

† Women are well known to be disposed to acquire a beard at the change of their constitutions, between forty and fifty, when the menses permanently stop. In the section on trichosis setosa,

In like manner, a beard has sometimes been found on boys (*Paullini*, cent. iii., obs. 64), and, in a few instances, on infants.—(*Eph. Nat. Cur.*, dec. ii., ann. iv., obs. 163, ap. 203.)

Hair has often also sprouted forth from organs whence it does not grow naturally ; which, however, in most examples, can be accounted for without any great difficulty, by bearing in mind a remark offered in the opening of the present genus ; I mean, that " the roots or bulbs of hairs are found over the entire surface of the body, though they only vegetate in particular parts." Yet Amatus Lusitanus has given us an example to which this explanation will not apply ; for, in this, the exotic hairs grew on the tongue (cent. vi., cur. 65), as the feathers of the toucan grow naturally. Criniti and Bose found the heart covered in the same manner.— (*Pr. Hist. de Anitomenis Messenii hirsuto corde*, Paris, 1525 ; *Pr. Sistens historiam cordis villosi*, Leips., 1771.)

Of organized animal substances, however, hair seems to originate most easily : and this, too, without having, at least in many cases, any apparent bulb or root to shoot from. We had lately occasion, when treating of PARURIA STILLATITIA, to notice their discharge from the bladder as constituting one of the causes of this complaint. So in MALIS GORDII (suprà, p. 690) they have been apparently solicited by friction from different parts of the body of an infant, with seeming relief to his distress. And under the genus ECCYESIS (suprà, p. 508, et passim), numerous examples have been given of their formation in various internal organs. It is on this account the hair and beard are said by wri-

some facts are quoted, equally illustrative of the present subject. Rayer, in 1806, saw a young woman in the Hôpital de la Pitié, twenty-six years of age, whose shoulders were covered with black hairs, the bulbs of which made the skin form so many little brownish prominences. Various morbid conditions seem to be conducive to extraneous hair. Boyer used to mention in his lectures a case, in which an inflammatory tumour of the thigh was followed by a rapid growth of numerous long hairs on the part. All surgeons know that certain kinds of nævi usually have hairs upon them. The following case is recorded by M. Bricheteau :—A young woman of fair complexion, dark hair, and delicate constitution, after being reduced to a complete state of marasmus by a painful pregnancy, a miscarriage, and an extraordinary difficulty of swallowing, at length recovered her health in the summer of 1826. Scarcely had she begun to take food and gain strength, when her skin, which had been parched, and agglutinated, as it were, to her bones, became covered with a multitude of small elevated points, like those produced by the impression of cold. They were particularly observed on the back, loins, chest, and abdomen ; and, in a few days, they assumed a brownish colour, and very soon each of them put forth from its apex a hair, which was at first very short, light-coloured, and silky, but grew so rapidly, that in a month the whole surface of the body and limbs, with the exception of the hands and face, was perfectly shaggy. In another few months the hairs dropped off spontaneously, and were not reproduced.—See Rayer, tom. ii., p. 383.—ED.

ters of grave authority occasionally to grow for some time after the death of every other part of the body ; of which examples may be found in Heister (*Heist. Compend. Anat.*) and Camerarius.—(*Camerar. Memorab.*, cent. vi., p. 47.)

SPECIES IV.
TRICHOSIS DISTRIX.
FORKY HAIR.
HAIRS OF THE SCALP WEAK, SLENDER, AND SPLITTING AT THEIR EXTREMITIES.

THIS is a common affection, and depends upon a deficiency in the supply of proper nutriment from the bulb or root of the hair, in consequence of which the upper part of the tube becomes arid and brittle, and splits into minute filaments, as already explained in the introductory remarks to the present genus.[*] Its cure is to be accomplished by cutting the hair short, and stimulating the roots by irritant pomatums, unguents, or oils.

SPECIES V.
TRICHOSIS POLIOSIS.
GRAY HAIR.[†]
HAIRS PREMATURELY GRAY OR HOARY.

THE SPECIFIC term POLIOSIS is a Greek derivative from πολὸς, " candidus," " canus,"— " white or hoary."

The general principle of this diseased appearance has been explained in the introductory remarks to the present genus. The colour of the hair is derived from the rete mucosum, which secretes a very compound material for this purpose, a part of the occasional ingredients of which are iron, sulphur, lime, a grayish-green and a blood-red oil. In the silvery white and glossy hair of young persons, the nutritive mat-

* Rayer, in speaking of compound hairs (poils composés), which are often split at their extremities, and consist of hairs of different colours, remarks, that they are produced from follicles which are united, but have only a single external opening, common to both of them. See Traité des Mal. de la Peau, tom. ii., p. 385.—ED.

† The *canities* of many writers, which, as Rayer observes, may be congenital, the effect of advanced age, or an accidental occurrence. It may also be partial or general. The hairs of the head, and especially of the temples, are those usually the first which undergo this change in old persons. When gray hairs fall off, others are seldom formed, and baldness is therefore usually a consequence of a person becoming gray-headed. Naturally light hair is said by Rayer seldom to become white, which is undoubtedly a mistake (see op. cit., tom. ii., p. 360) ; but his observation, that it generally falls off at a comparatively early period of life, may be more correct. The hairs commonly become gray in a slow, gradual manner ; though authentic examples of the change taking place suddenly, as, for instance, in the course of one night, are upon record.—(See Bichat, Anat. Gén., tom. iv., p. 815 ; Cassan, in Archives Gén. de Méd., Janvier, 1827.) These facts prove, as Rayer observes, that phenomena take place within the hair which are dependant upon vitality.—ED.

ter is, perhaps, the rete mucosum in its purest and most uncoloured state. Gray hair is produced in two ways. In one there is no colouring material whatever, except apparently a small portion of the sulphur: and in this case the hair is directly hoary, or of a yellowish or rusty white. In other circumstances, the rete mucosum or nutriment of the hair, from causes already explained under the genus PAROSTIA, is loaded with calcareous matter, but deficient in its proper oil; and hence the hair is somewhat whiter, but of a dead hue, harsher, and coarser, very brittle, and apt to fall off from the roots.

White hair, probably produced by the former of these means, has been found occasionally in every stage of life; and Schenck gives a case in which it appeared on birth.* It has sometimes been transmitted hereditarily (*Eph. Nat. Cur.,* dec. ii., ann. i., obs. 69): and, in some instances, seems to have taken place from terror,† the spasm of the capillaries of the skin extending to the bulbs of the hair, which no longer communicated a supply of the ordinary pigment. It has for the same reason followed an obstinate cephalæa (*Journ. des Sçavans,* 1684), and is said to have occurred after death.‡

* Lib. i., obs. 3, ex Stuckio. The occurrence of gray hairs in young persons not more than eighteen or twenty years of age is so frequent, that few individuals have not had opportunities of noticing it.—ED.

† Camerar. Memor., cent. ii., N. 14. Doute, Ergo Canities à timore? Paris, 657. J. P. Frank, De Cur. Hom. Morb., tom. v., p. 123. Also from anger, from unexpected afflicting news, from diseases of the scalp, as porrigo, deep wounds, leaving scars destitute of pigment, &c., profuse hemorrhage, immoderate indulgence in venery, the employment of mercury too often repeated, violent emotions of the mind, &c.—(See Rayer, tom. ii., p. 366.) Canities is sometimes partial. The editor has known more than one instance of a tuft of gray hair being situated on one of the temples, while all the rest of the hair was of its original brown colour. Rayer refers to similar cases (tom. ii., p. 366).—ED.

‡ Eph. Nat. Cur., dec. ii., ann. i., obs. 69. It does not appear to be proved, that the colour of the hair is derived, as our author states, from the rete mucosum; but every fact tends to show, that it is secreted by the vascular pulp or root of the hair itself. With respect to the manner in which the hairs are turned gray, the subject is one of difficulty, in whatever light it is viewed. We have adverted to Dr. Macartney's conclusion, that an organic action in the substance of hairs must be admitted to exist, in order to account for the changes to which it is subject. If this were not the case, he deems it impossible to explain, in particular, the alterations in the colour of the hair. He tried to trace the progression of the colour in the hair, and the change of organization accompanying the process; but without being able to satisfy himself on some points. "In almost all the specimens we have examined of human hair, during the process of becoming gray, *we have found the loss of colour to commence at the point, and gradually to advance towards the root.* In a few instances we have observed *short portions of the hair gray in the middle;* and we have seen the hairs of the mane and tail of horses becoming white at their roots. Some hairdressers also as-

SPECIES VI.
TRICHOSIS ATHRIX.
BALDNESS.

DECAY AND FALL OF THE HAIR.

THE general principle of this defect has been so fully detailed under the preceding species, and in the introductory remarks to the present genus, that it is not necessary to add any thing farther.

This affection of the hair is the alopecia of Sauvages and other modern nosologists, but not that of Celsus and Galen, which is a variety of the next species. Alopecia is a Greek term, derived from ἀλωπήξ, "vulpes," *a fox,* this animal being supposed to lose its hair and become bald sooner than any other quadruped. The Arabian writers named it from the same source

sert, that the hairs of the human head occasionally first change to gray next the roots.* The term *gray* is not so proper as *transparent* would be, since it consists not in an alteration of colour, but a total disappearance of it; and which is not in the interior substance, as supposed by Bichat, but in the horny or external part of the hair." Dr. Macartney inclines to the suspicion, that *the colouring matter is carried back into the system by absorption.*—(See Rees's Cyclopædia, art. HAIR.) If a hair become gray by the desiccation or evaporation of any of its parts, he conceives, that the change would not be confined to particular portions of it, and the whole would afterward appear withered or shrunk. Weak hairs, and those whose pulp is obliterated, would likewise be most apt to lose their colour. The contrary of this, however, takes place. None but permanent hairs ever become gray. The strongest and darkest hairs are most liable to the change, and afterward appear to be stronger and thicker than before, and are longer in being shed than others which have preserved their colour. It may be added, that no means will have the effect of turning hairs gray, after they have been removed from the body. This observation, by Dr. Macartney, we see is directly repugnant to a statement made in the text, and is also at variance with the alleged effect of oxymuriatic acid in whitening the hair. The whole of the subject seems to call for further researches.—ED.

* The following are Rayer's remarks on this point:—"The hairs always begin to turn white at their loose end." He adds, however, they are sometimes observed to be white at the part near the skin, and dark-coloured throughout the rest of their extent. This disposition, the reverse of the first, he says, depends upon the hairs being first secreted of a dark colour, and then white in consequence of an affection of their bulbs.—(Op. cit, tom. ii., p. 365.) Dying gray hair with nitrate of silver is found to render it hard and rigid. Nothing useful can be done for obviating the gray hair of old age: when plucked out, or removed with depilatories, if it grow again, it returns with the same silvery appearance. But, when canities is partial, or consequent to chronic inflammation of the scalp, implicating the bulbs, the hair, after falling off or being plucked, will sometimes grow again with its natural primitive colour. It is likewise noticed by Rayer, that a part of a hair secreted white, is followed by another part furnished with colouring matter. In situations where the bulbs have been destroyed by deep wounds or ulcers, the hair cannot be regenerated. See Rayer, tom. ii., p. 368.—ED.

دَآءُ ٱلثَّعْلَى, *daussaleb*, literally " morbus vulpis." The species admits of the following varieties :—

α Simplex.	Hairs of the scalp of a natural hue ; gradually dying at the bulbs, or loosened by a relaxation of the cutaneous texture.
Bald head.	
β Calvities.	Hairs gray or hoary ; baldness chiefly on the crown of the head ; and confined to the head. Mostly common to advanced age.
Bald crown.	
γ Barbæ.	Decay and fall of the beard.
Bald beard.	

The FIRST VARIETY is the defluvium capillorum of Sennert. Whatever tends to give an established relaxation and want of tone to the cutaneous vessels, becomes a cause of this affection :*—and it is hence a frequent sequel of fevers of various kinds. It is also found as a symptom in tabes, phthisis, porrigo favosa, chronic eczema, and impetigo [in which three last affections the fall of the hair appears to be a consequence of an inflammation of the hair-follicles.]

When it is an indiopathic affection, general tonics and cold bathing form the most promising treatment ; and when it is a secondary complaint, it must follow the fortune of the disorder that gives rise to it.†

The SECOND VARIETY proceeds from a cause precisely opposite to the preceding. Here the cutaneous secernents, instead of being too loose and relaxed, are too dry and rigid ; there is little nutriment afforded to the roots or bulbs of the hair, whence they become arid and brittle, particularly at the extreme point of the head or crown, and are perpetually breaking off at their origin.‡ The cause of the whiteness or hoari-

---

* It has been stated in a previous note, that most of the changes to which the hair is liable, depend upon some affection of its bulbs, or the hair-follicles, as they are often called ; the organs by which it is produced.—ED.

† According to Rayer, the examples which happen during the convalescence from acute diseases, frequently seem to be preceded by a slight erythema, or ptyriasis of the scalp. They are accompanied by an exceedingly copious furfuraceous desquamation. A great quantity of cuticular pellicles are detached by the comb, which are quickly reproduced, and under them the skin is usually erythematous. In other instances, the fall of the hair is accompanied with a morbid secretion from sebaceous follicles. But it must be allowed, that the most curious specimen of baldness is what has been erroneously named porrigo decalvans ; a case treated of by Dr. Good in the ensuing section under the denomination of trichosis area, in which neither vesicles, pustules, nor any inflammatory process, can be detected.—See Rayer, tom. ii., p. 372.—ED.

‡ The baldness of age comes on slowly and progressively, without any perceptible change in the scalp. In men, it frequently extends to all the upper and anterior part of the head, so that merely a semicircle of hair is left, reaching from one temple to the other. The hair of women turns gray ; but it is not generally so much disposed to

---

ness of the hair has been explained under the preceding species. Other causes than that of old age are noticed by pathologists, and have no doubt a foundation ; as terror, which has sometimes operated very rapidly, insolation or exposure of the head to the rays of the sun, unlimited sexual indulgence (*Gilbert, Adversus Pract. Prin. ; Merlet, Diss. Ergo à Salacitate Calvities?* Paris, 1662), cephalæa, and worms.—(*Paullini Lanx Sat.,* dec. iv., obs. 9.)

This affection is far more common to males than to females ; it is asserted by many writers that it never occurs in eunuchs (*De Moor, Dis. in Hipp.,* App. vi., 28, L. B., 1736 ; *Schenck,* l. i., obs. 10), and by Schenck, that it never takes place in any person before the use of sexual copulation, and hence ought not to exist in bachelors ; and, provided the remark be well founded, on which I cannot speak from my own knowledge, might be employed as a test of their continence.

The most promising remedies are to be sought for in an external application of warm animal oils, and oily aromatic essences, as lavender-water.*

Baldness of the chin, or want of beard, is not a common defect ; but examples of it are referred to in the volume of Nosology.† And a few rare instances are to be met with of the baldness extending over every part of the body. Professor Frank has given us a striking example of

---

* The cause of the loss of hair, and the nature of the affection of the hair-follicles, ought manifestly to be considered. When the detachment of the hair depends upon inflammation of the latter organs, the treatment should be different from what is called for by other states, which likewise bring on baldness. The calvities of old age is incurable. Loss of hair occasioned by eczema, impetigo, and porrigo, requires no other treatment than what these complaints respectively demand. If the skin be dry, tense, and furfuraceous, the parts should be shaved, and smeared with oils or ointments. In porrigo decalvans, and other cases not attended with inflammation of the skin or hair-follicles, Rayer recommends stimulating the parts by the application of a decoction of walnut-leaves, morel, lesser centaury, or mustard-powder, with aromatic spirituous lotions, or with embrocations of oil of lavender, juniper, chamomile, &c.—See Rayer, Traité des Mal. de la Peau, tom. ii., pp. 374, 375.—ED.

† The chin is liable to all the varieties of alopecia, and even to porrigo decalvans, or trichosis area.—ED.

---

fall off as that of men. According to Bichat, before the hair of old persons falls off, its bulbs gradually diminish, and the small tubes that contain its roots finally disappear. There is also a destruction of the hair-follicles in certain cases of partial alopecia occasioned by subcutaneous tumours. This alteration of the hair-follicles does not occur in accidental baldness. In the body of a man rendered almost completely bald by an attack of fever, Bichat found all the tubes of the hair perfect, and young hair beginning to grow at the bottom of them. Hence, as Rayer observes, there is a difference between the fall of the hair of aged individuals, and the loss of it induced by certain disorders : in the first cases, all perishes ; in the second, only the stalk of the hair becomes detached.—ED.

this in a young man, who, about two months before he saw him, had suffered a sudden falling off of the hair from the chin, head, eyelashes, and pubes, while his fingers appeared dead, as though destroyed by a dry gangrene ; his voice, meanwhile, was unchanged, the full power of procreation continued, and, with the exception of a slight debility which he had felt, for a few days, he was free from complaint. There was no perceptible cause, though thirteen years before he had laboured under syphilis.[*]

SPECIES VII.
TRICHOSIS AREA.
AREATED HAIR.

PATCHES OF BALDNESS WITHOUT DECAY OR CHANGE OF COLOUR IN THE SURROUNDING HAIR ; EXPOSED PLOTS OF THE SCALP GLABROUS, WHITE, AND SHINING ; SOMETIMES SPREADING AND COALESCING, RENDERING THE BALDNESS EXTENSIVE.

THIS species is taken entirely from Celsus, who gives two varieties of it almost in the following words :—

a Diffluens. Diffluent areated hair.	Bald plots of an indeterminate figure ; existing in the beard as well as in the scalp ; obstinate of cure. Common to all ages.
β Serpens. Serpentine areated hair.	Baldness commencing at the occiput, and winding in a line, not exceeding two fingers' breadth, to each ear, sometimes to the forehead : often terminating spontaneously. Chiefly limited to children.

The FIRST-VARIETY forms the true alopecia of the Greeks, of which I have spoken already, and is so denominated by Celsus, Galen, and other Greek and Roman writers. The second is called by them ophiasis, from ὄφις, " a serpent," in consequence of the serpentine direction in which the disease trails round the head.

Dr. Bateman has described this species under the name of *porrigo decalvans*, while he admits that the surface of the scalp offers no porriginous or other eruption whatever, but " within these areæ is smooth, shining, and remarkably white. It is probable, however," he adds, " *though not ascertained*, that there may be an eruption of minute achores about the roots of the hair, in the first instance, which are not permanent, and do not discharge any fluid." It must be obvious that this fall of the hair has no connexion whatever with porrigo ;[†] depending upon a partial

operation of the causes that we have already noticed as giving rise to the two preceding species of poliosis and athrix.

A frequent shaving of the entire scalp, with affusion of cold water, and the use of stimulant liniments, as aromatic vinegar, or a solution of two drachms of the oil of mace in three or four ounces of alcohol, will sometimes be found to produce a fresh crop of hair : though, in most instances, all applications are equally unavailing ; and, even in successful cases, it is usually many weeks or even months, and has been years, before the patches are duly supplied with hair.[*]

SPECIES VIII.
TRICHOSIS DECOLOR.
MISCOLOURED HAIR.

HAIR OF THE HEAD OF A PRETERNATURAL HUE.

As the hair receives its tint from the pigment communicated to the bulbs by the rete mucosum,[†] whatever varies the character or colour of this material, will vary also the colour of the hair. Some of the causes of such variation we shall have to notice under the ensuing genus ; but there are others which are not so easily explained. Hair contains iron and sulphur. The blood-red oil, which is procured by digestion from the red hair, forms a third constituent. The grayish-green oil, which M. Vauquelin has been also able to extract from black and other dark kinds of hair, is another distinct principle : and, from an excess or deficiency, or a peculiar combination of the colorific constituents, we are able to account for some of the extraordinary hues which the hair is occasionally found to exhibit, though others seem to preclude all explanation.[‡] The chief varieties they display are the following :—

a Cærulea.	Of a blue colour.§
β Denigrata.	Changed from another colour to a black.‖

---

* De Cur. Hom. Morh. Epit., tom. iv., p. 124. A singular instance of a baldness, restricted to one side of the body, is related by Ravaton ; it followed a violent commotion, and was accompanied by amaurosis in the eye of the same side. The hairs of the head, those of the eyebrow, and the eyelashes, underwent a change of colour, and were then detached.—ED.

† On this point, as explained in the previous section, Rayer coincides with Dr. Good. Porrigo,

too, is a contagious disease, which trichosis diffluens is not.—ED.

- *. The editor has had several cases of this curious disease under his care ; but he has never seen any benefit result from the stimulating applications in ordinary use.—ED.

† The derivation of the colouring matter of the hair from the rete mucosum is not the hypothesis generally entertained by the latest physiologists. Indeed, it is rather contrary to anatomy, which teaches us that the bulbs of the hair are frequently in the cutis, and deeper than the rete mucosum ; and there is every reason to conclude, that the colouring matter, as well as the substance of the hair, is secreted by the pulp, or the vascular part of the bulb. This is the view adopted by M. Rayer, as appears from the following quotation :—" Les poils peuvent éprouver divers changemens de couleur, liés sans doute à quelques modifications de la partie du bulbe, qui fournit leur matière colorante."—Traité des Mal. de la Peau, tom. ii., p. 386.—ED.

‡ Otto remarks, that in persons with light hair, who work in metals, it is found green or blue.—D.

§ Paullini, cent. i., obs. 93.

‖ Id., cent. iii., obs. 59.

γ Viridis.　　Of a green colour. Of which we have had very numerous examples.*

δ Variegata.　Spotted like the hair of a leopard.† Of this the examples are more common than of any of the preceding varieties.

Many of these singular hues are said to have followed some natural colour of the hair: and, in some instances, suddenly. This is particularly the case with the second variety; or that in which the hair has abruptly become black, which seems to have occurred as a result of fever, of exsiccation, and of terror. Schurig gives a case in which the beard, as well as the hair, was transformed from a white to a black.‡

We have observed, under the fifth species, that one of the causes of white or rather hoary hair, is a dry, shrivelled, or obstructed state of its bulbs, by which the colorific matter is no longer communicated. And it is possible, that as both terror and fevers, and many other violent commotions, have sometimes proved a cure for palsy, they may occasionally produce a like sudden effect upon the minute vessels of the bulbs of the hair, remove their obstruction, or arm them with new power, and thus re-enable them to throw up into the tubes of the colourless hair the proper pigment.

SPECIES IX.
TRICHOSIS SENSITIVA.
SENSITIVE HAIR.
HAIR OF THE HEAD PAINFULLY SENSITIVE.

This species is added in consequence of a singular case that has occurred since the publication of the first edition, and on the special recommendation of the learned and indefatigable editor of the Edinburgh Medical and Surgical Journal, to whom the author is also indebted for suggesting the specific name. It shows us that, under a morbid condition of the scalp, not only bloodvessels, but nerves, will sometimes shoot forth into the tubes of the hair, and convey a very high and acute degree of sensibility.

In the hospital of the Royal Guard at Paris was a private soldier, who had received a violent kick on the occiput from a horse. The cerebral excitement produced was extreme, and could only be kept under by almost innumerable bleedings, both local and general. Among a series of phenomena produced by this state of preternatural excitation, the sensibility acquired by the hairs of the head was not the least remarkable. The slightest touch was felt instantly; and cutting them gave exquisite pain, so that the patient would seldom allow any one to come near his head. Baron Larrey, on one occasion, to put him to the test, gave a hint to an assistant, who was standing behind the patient, to clip one of his hairs without his perceiving it. This was done with dexterity, but the soldier broke out into a sally of oaths, succeeded by complaints; and it was some time before he could be appeased.*

GENUS X.
EPICHROSIS.
MACULAR SKIN.
SIMPLE DISCOLORATION OF THE SURFACE.

Epichrosis (ἐπίχρωσις) is a term common to the Greek writers, and employed to express a

. *. Bartholin, Hist. Anat.; Paullini, cent. i., obs.93.
† Eph. Nat. Cur., dec. iii., ann. 3, obs. 184.
‡ Schurig. Spermatos. M. Alibert relates the case of a lady who, in a fever brought on by a difficult labour, lost a fine head of light-coloured hair, while every part of the scalp was inundated with a viscous fluid; but that, after her recovery, the hair returned, and assumed a very black colour. The same writer likewise mentions another example, in which a person, during an attack of illness, lost all his hair, which was naturally brown, and afterward, when the hair grew again, it was of a fiery red colour. It is even alleged, that the gray hair of a woman sixty-six years of age turned black a few days before her death, the bulbs presenting an extraordinary state, and seeming as if they were gorged with the matter from which the hair derived its colour; while the gray hair had only a dry shrivelled root, much smaller than that of the black.—(Journ. Gén. de Méd., tom. iv., p. 290.) A curious instance is recorded of a woman, whose naturally light-coloured hair used always to become of a reddish-yellow colour whenever she was attacked by fever, but returned to its natural hue as soon as the febrile disturbance ceased.—(Journ. Complém. des Sciences Méd., tom. v., p. 59.) Lastly, M. Villermé recites the particulars of a young lady, sixteen years of age, who, after some trivial headaches, perceived, in the course of the winter of 1817 and 1818, that several parts of her head were entirely bald; and six months after this period, she had not a hair on her scalp. In the beginning of January, 1819, her head became covered with a sort of black wool at the points from which the hair was first detached, and with brown hair elsewhere. Some of the hairs fell off when they had attained the length of three or four inches; the colour of others altered at a greater or less distance from their extremities, while the other parts of them, towards their roots, put on a chestnut hue.—(Dict. des Sciences Méd., tom. xliii., p. 302.) These curious accounts are inserted by M. Rayer, in his important publication on Diseases of the Skin, tom. ii., p. 387. There is a person in York, the colour of whose hair is continually changing. At present, it is a mixture of white, brown, and red; sometimes it is all white; at others, dark brown and red, and frequently red and white. His hair has been subject to these changes for many years. —See Morning Herald, Oct. 11, 1834.—ED.

* Edin. Med. Journ., July, 1823, p. 481. From Journ. of For. Med., No. xvii. In a case of this description, much care would be necessary not to confound the morbid sensibility of the scalp with that alleged to be actually in the hairs themselves. When the scalp is exquisitely tender, the slightest handling or disturbance of the hair will sometimes give pain; and perhaps the present species ought to have received further confirmation previously to its introduction into a nosological system. It is curious, however, that considerable branches of the fifth nerve should be distributed to the whiskers of animals. In a cat, which lived after the division of the fifth nerve in the cavity of the scull, the whiskers of the mutilated side became thin and crooked.—See Mayo's Outlines of Human Physiology, p. 502, 2d edit.—ED.

coloured or spotted surface of any kind. The genus is new, but it seems called for. Like the last, it consists of blemishes, many of which cannot always either be cured or even palliated; but, as all these are morbid affections, the nosological system that suffers them to pass without notice is imperfect Many of them, however, are not of serious consequence, and have been arranged by Professor Frank under EPHELIS, employed as a genus, and with a latitude beyond its ordinary use.—(*De Cur. Hom. Morb.*, tom. iv., p. 77, Mannh., 8vo., 1792.)

The following are the species that belong to it:—

1. Epichrosis Leucasmus.   Veal Skin.
2. ——— Spilus.   Mole.
3. ——— Lenticula.   Freckles.
4. ——— Ephelis.   Sunburn.
5. ——— Aurigo.   Orange Skin.
6. ——— Pœcilia.   Piebald Skin.
7. ——— Alphosis.   Albino Skin.

SPECIES I.
EPICHROSIS LEUCASMUS.
VEAL SKIN.

WHITE, GLABROUS, SHINING, PERMANENT SPOTS, PRECEDED BY WHITE TRANSITORY ELEVATIONS OR TUBERCLES OF THE SAME SIZE; OFTEN COALESCING AND CREEPING IN A SERPENTINE DIRECTION; THE SUPERINCUMBENT HAIRS FALLING OFF AND NEVER RESPROUTING.

THIS is the vitiligo, or veal skin of Willan, so called from the veal-like appearance which these spots produce on the general colour of the surface. It is common to the different parts of the body, but chiefly found about the face, neck, and ears. The term leucasmus (λευκασμὸς), importing whiteness, is merely employed instead of vitiligo to avoid confusion, as Dr. Willan has used vitiligo in a sense somewhat different from that of Celsus, or of any one who preceded him; though Professor Frank has made an approach to it by giving it the meaning of Celsus, importing a variety of leprosy, and afterward confounding it with numerous other affections of the skin that have no possible connexion with it, of which the present forms one instance.—(*De Cur. Hom. Morb. Epit.*, tom. iv., p. 119.)

The size of these spots varies considerably, from that of a large pin's head to that of a shilling or half a crown. The blank and morbid whiteness remains through life, and seems to show that the patches are no longer possessed of red bloodvessels, and that the white hue of the rete mucosum alone is visible in their respective areas, exhibiting a pure white, only differing from that of death in being glossy from the action of a living principle.

SPECIES II.
EPICHROSIS SPILUS.
MOLE.

BROWN, PERMANENT, CIRCULAR PATCH; SOLITARY; SOMETIMES SLIGHTLY ELEVATED, AND CRESTED WITH A TUFT OF HAIR.

THE specific term, from σπίλὸς, "macula," has

been long in use. The blemish is common, but unimportant.

We have already remarked, that the rete mucosum is a substance which forms the second or middle of three laminæ that constitute the external integument. It is improperly called either *rete* or *mucosum*, for it is neither a network nor a mucous material, being in effect nothing more than an adipose secretion of a peculiar kind, which, when black, has a considerable resemblance to the grease that is interposed between the axles and wheels of our carriages.

Its existence was first noticed by Malpighi, who gave it the name of rete, as thinking that, through the structure of soft and uniform matter, he could trace certain fibres, crossing each other in various directions, but which have not been ascertained since, not even in the skin of the negro, in whom this layer is most conspicuous. In many animals, indeed, there is no rete mucosum whatever, and Bichat has expressed his doubts whether it has a distinct existence in any species, and conceives Malpighi was mistaken. But Cruickshank appears to have confirmed satisfactorily the assertion of Malpighi in the human form, and even to have traced it in some of the internal parts of the body, as well as in the skin (*On Insens. Persp.*, passim): and Dr. Gordon (*Anat.*, p. 244), after a scrutinous examination, has added his testimony to the same fact.—(*Bostock, Syst. of Physiol.*, p. 79; see also *Edin. Med. Journ.*, vol. xviii., p. 247.)

It is in truth the common pigment or colouring principle of the skin, and hence differs very considerably in hue, as is sufficiently obvious in the respective individuals of the same country, but still more so in those of remote regions; giving a white or fair hue to the inhabitants of the south side of the Caucasus, and their probable descendants, the great body of Europeans; a black to the negroes of Africa; an olive hue to the Mongo-Tartar race; a brown to the islanders of Australasia; and a red to the native tribes of North America.

In temperate climates, and in its purest state, it is a clear glossy white; and when reddened under a delicate cuticle, by the minute and innumerable arteries that are distributed over the surface of the body, it gives that rich but dainty tone of colour which constitutes beauty of complexion.

It sometimes happens, however, that persons who are perfectly fair in their general complexion, from an equal diffusion of this substance in its utmost purity, have a few small spots of a lighter or deeper brown in the face, limbs, or body, from an occasional dash of brown in the rete mucosum, produced by causes which it is impossible to unravel; and which, as we shall show presently, in other persons extends over the entire surface, and is consequently intermixed with the whole of the secretion: and it is this occasional dash that constitutes a spilus or mole. Possibly, the rete mucosum possesses a certain portion of iron, a concentration of which in the coloured part may constitute the colorific material. Be this as it may, we perceive, wherever these coloured spots exist, there is a greater tendency to increased action than elsewhere : and hence we often find a slight elevation, and additional closeness of structure, and not unfrequently an enlargement of the natural down into a tuft of hairs.

If this reasoning be correct, alkaline lotions (and all soaps are of this character, though not sufficiently strong for the present purpose) should form the best cosmetics. But the spots are rarely removable by any means ; and the less they are tampered with the better.

These differ essentially from nævi, or genuine mother-marks, inasmuch as the latter are produced by a distention of the minute bloodvessels of the skin, so that those which should contain only colourless blood, admit the red particles, and hereby exhibit stains of different shapes and ranges, and of different shades of crimson or purple, according to the quantity of red blood that is hereby suffered to enter, or the nature of the vessels that are distended.

SPECIES III.
·EPICHROSIS LENTICULA.
FRECKLES.

CUTICLE STIGMATIZED WITH YELLOWISH-BROWN DOTS, RESEMBLING MINUTE LENTIL-SEEDS ; GREGARIOUS ; OFTEN TRANSITORY.

LENTICULA is more generally written in modern times *lentigo* ; it is here given as it occurs in Celsus. The root is the Latin term *lens*, a lentil-seed.; the Greek word for which is φάκια : and this, without a diminutive termination, was also applied to the same blemish when the spots were of a larger size.

Its causes are various ; most commonly it is produced by an exposure to the rays of the sun ; but it frequently arises without any such exposure, and is sometimes transmitted hereditarily. The mode by which the colorific rays of the sun operate in the production of this effect, we shall explain under EPHELIS, or sunburn, forming the next species. Where the remote cause is constitutional, it is probably a result of the same colorific material as that to which we have just referred spilus or mole, existing in the rete mucosum, and operating more diffusely, though in much smaller patches. How it comes to pass that this middle layer of the exterior integument should at any time be thus interruptedly charged with a coloured pigment, so as to form the freckled appearance which constitutes the present cuticular blemish, it is not easy to say ; but that it has a remarkable tendency to do so is obvious, not only from the present and preceding species, but still more so from the very striking and singular patchwork which constitutes EPICHROSIS PŒCILIA, or the sixth species of the genus before us ; where we shall be again under the necessity of touching upon the subject.

Freckles are most frequently found on persons of fair complexions and red hair ; and, as we have already observed, this hue of the hair is produced by a peculiar pigment, or a blood-red oil, by which the substance of the hair-tubes is stained.

Freckles are often transitory. They occur

in many instances in great abundance in pregnant women, and disappear after lying-in, sometimes, indeed, in the latter months of pregnancy.[*] Riedlin affirms, but upon what authority I know not, that they are a foresign of a female offspring.[†]

It is well observed by Frank, that the more tender leaves of plants and the cuticle of fruits have a tendency to the same affection, and particularly after a descent of very gentle rains which the burning ray of the sun does not suddenly disperse ; in which case we often meet with as many dots as there have been drops of rain.—(*De Cur. Hom. Morb. Epit.*, tom. IV., p. 79, Mannh., 8vo., 1792.) Similar marks are likewise sometimes produced by the defedation of insects.

Cosmetics are of less avail in this than in the ensuing species ; but those we shall have there occasion to notice may be tried under the species before us.[‡]

SPECIES IV.
EPICHROSIS EPHELIS.
SUNBURN.

CUTICLE TAWNY BY EXPOSURE TO THE SUN : OFTEN SPOTTED WITH DARK FRECKLES, CONFLUENT OR CORYMBOSE : DISAPPEARING IN THE WINTER.

EPHELIS (ἔφηλις) is a term of Celsus, as well

---

* The chloasma gravidarum of several pathologists.—ED.

† Lin. Med., 1695, p. 393. In some women the spots here alluded to make their appearance only for a few days, at the period of menstruation. They are also observed in patients afflicted with chronic disease of the stomach or lungs.—See Rayer, Traité des Maladies de la Peau, tom. ii., p. 210.—ED.

‡ The following is the advice given by M. Rayer, respecting the best manner of removing the spots of chloasma :—" When they occur," says he, " in women a few days after conception, they sometimes disappear on the expiration of the first month of pregnancy, together with the symptoms indicating that event ; but they have been known to continue throughout the whole term of pregnancy, and even after parturition. In the latter case, and always when the spots take place independently of any other affection, they should be treated with sulphur-baths, which, in the space of a month or six weeks, will frequently disperse them. This means is preferable to acid lotions, or to frictions of the parts affected with emulsions, liniments containing camphire or the borate of soda, or pomatums medicated with the lauro-cerasus." When chloasma originates from the influence of some other organic disease, or when it is accompanied with chronic diseases of the stomach, bowels, uterus, &c., Rayer very properly recommends the appropriate remedies for these original disorders to be first administered.—(See Rayer, Traité des Mal. de la Peau, tom. ii., p. 211.) For the removal of freckles, the hands and face are sometimes bathed with a solution of albumen, or gum, cream, skim-milk, distilled aromatic waters, or even with more active spirituous applications. But, as Rayer observes, these means rarely answer the purpose of taking away freckles, which ordinarily fade of themselves on the approach of winter.—Op. et vol. cit., p. 207.—ED.

as the name appropriated to the preceding species: and its real meaning is "sunburn," or "sunspot"—"vitium faciei solis ustione." In Celsus, however, the term is used in a much wider sense, and applied to blemishes which have no connexion with sunburning. It is here restrained to its proper signification.

The sun in hot climates, or very hot summer-seasons, has a tendency to affect the colour of the skin in a twofold manner. First, by a direct affinity of its colorific rays, or those of light, with the oxygen of the animal surface, and particularly with that of the rete mucosum, in consequence of which a considerable part of the oxygen is detached and flies off, and the carbon and hydrogen with which it was united, being freed from its constraint, enter into a new combination, and form a more or less perfect charcoal, according to the proportion in which they combine. And secondly, by the indirect influence which the calorific rays of the sun, or those of heat, produce upon the liver, and excite it to a more abundant secretion of bile, possessing a deeper hue, and which is more copiously resorbed into the system. That a certain proportion of bile is resorbed at all times, is clear from the colour of the urine, and the stain which the perspirable fluid gives to clean linen: and that this proportion is greater in hot summers than in cold winters, and particularly in intertropical climates, is well known to every one who has attended to the subject.

These, then, are the ordinary causes of that effusive brown stain of the skin which we denominate sunburn. But whether the deeper spots or freckles which so often accompany a sunburnt skin be owing to an equal action of either of these causes, and particularly of the first, upon the rete mucosum, or to an extrication of any colouring matter, as of iron, for example, existing in the rete mucosum itself, and unequally distributed, is beyond our power to determine. Either cause is sufficient to produce such an effect, though perhaps the real cause is the latter: and we have already seen, that in the distribution of this adipose layer over the surface, and its connexion with the cuticle and the cutis, there is a frequent obstruction to a free flow of whatever colouring material may exist in it, which is in consequence accumulated in spots or patches, instead of being equally diffused.

As sunburn is chiefly occasioned by an inordinate separation of oxygen from the other constituent principles of the rete mucosum with which it was united, the most rational cosmetics in this case are those which have a tendency to bleach the skin, by containing a considerable proportion of some vegetable or mineral acid. Homberg's cosmetic, which has long been in vogue on the continent, is a dilute solution of oxymuriate of mercury, with a mixture of oxgall. Hartmann's, which has also been in high estimation, consists of a simple distillation of arum-root in water. This forms a very pungent lotion, and its object is to dilute or wash out the brown pigment by exciting an increased flow of perspirable fluid towards the surface, and to carry off a part of it by an increased action of the cutaneous absorbents. Spirit of lavender, or any of the essential oils dissolved in alcohol, may be employed for the same purpose; and some have used a diluted eau de luce, which is also useful as an alkaline irritant. In Schroeder's Pharmacopœia there is a preparation for the same purpose which we should little expect, and the virtues of which are not very likely to be tried in the present day: it is entitled aqua stercoris humani: but in former times, dung of all kinds was a standard article in almost every Materia Medica, and there are few diseases for which it was not recommended by some practitioners; occasionally, indeed, internally as well as externally. The general intention was that of obtaining a very pungent ammonia; but this we are able to do at present by far less offensive means.

When the hands are deeply discoloured, they may often be bleached by exposing them to the fumes of sulphur.

In drupaceous fruits, and especially those of a fine cuticle, as apples, we sometimes meet with spots and miscolorations of the same character as moles, freckles, and sunburn; the causes of which we do not always know, though we can sometimes trace them to small punctures in the cutis by birds and insects.

SPECIES V.
EPICHROSIS AURIGO.
ORANGE SKIN.

CUTICLE SAFFRON-COLOURED, WITHOUT APPARENT AFFECTION OF THE LIVER OR ITS APPENDAGES; COLOUR DIFFUSED OVER THE ENTIRE SURFACE: TRANSIENT; CHIEFLY IN NEW-BORN INFANTS.

THIS orange hue of infants, and which is occasionally to be met with in later periods, appears, as Dr. Cullen observes, to depend either on bile, not as in the usual manner excreted, but received into the bloodvessels and effused under the cuticle, or on a peculiar yellowness of the serum of the blood distinct from any connexion with bile.—(Synops. Nosol. Med. Gen., xci., 5.) Sauvages has rightly distinguished between this disease as a mere cutaneous affection and proper jaundice. In him it occurs under the name of ephelis lutea, an improper name, however, as the affection is not an ephelis or sunburn; while the jaundice of infancy he calls aurigo neophytorum, which ought rather to be icterus neophytorum.—(Nosol. Method. in rebus.)

It may in general be remarked, that while the sclerotic tunic of the eyes, as well as the skin, is tinged with yellow in the genuine jaundice of infants, the former retains its proper whiteness in aurigo. Whence the serum derives the yellow hue it so strikingly evinces on some occasions, except from the bile, it is difficult to determine. That a certain proportion of bile exists constantly in the blood in a healthy state is manifest, as we have already observed, from the colour of the urine, and the tinge given to linen by the matter of insensible perspiration:

and that this proportion varies in different climates, and different seasons of the year, without producing genuine jaundice, we have also observed. And hence infants, under particular circumstances, may be subject to a like increase, with a like absence of icteritious symptoms. But what those circumstances are, does not seem to be clearly known. We see, nevertheless, that whatever rouses the system generally, and the excretories peculiarly, readily takes off the saffron die : and hence it often yields to a few brisk purges, and still more rapidly to an emetic.

SPECIES VI.
EPICHROSIS PŒCILIA.
PIEBALD SKIN.

CUTICLE MARBLED GENERALLY, WITH ALTERNATE PLOTS OR PATCHES OF BLACK AND WHITE.

PŒCILIA (ποικιλία) is a term of Isocrates, from ποικιλὸς, "versicolor," "pictus diversis coloribus ;" whence *pœcile*, the porch or picture-gallery of the Stoics at Athens. The species is new to the nosological classification ; but the morbid affection has been long known to physiologists, and ought to have had a niche in the catalogue of diseases before now.

This affection is chiefly found among negroes, from an irregular secretion or distribution of the pigment which gives the black hue to the rete mucosum. In albinoes, as we shall have occasion to observe presently, this pigment is entirely withheld, and the matter of the rete mucosum seems to be otherwise affected ; in the species before us, it is only irregularly or interruptedly distributed.

What the cause of this interrupted distribution consists in, we know not ; but in several of the preceding species of the present genus, and particularly in moles and freckles, we perceive a striking tendency to such an effect ; and, if we turn our attention to the animal and vegetable world around us, we shall observe it springing up before us in a thousand different ways, and giving rise to an infinite diversity of the nicest and most elegant cutaneous tapestry. It is, in truth, as the author has already remarked in the volume of Nosology, to the partial secretion or distribution of this natural pigment, that we are indebted for all the variegated and beautiful hues evinced by different kinds of animals and plants. It is this which gives us the fine red or violet hue that tinges the nose and hindquarters of some baboons, and the exquisite silver that whitens the belly of the dolphin and other cetaceous fishes. In the toes and tarsal membrane of ravens and turkeys, it is frequently black ; in common hens and peacocks, gray ; blue in the titmouse ; green in the waterhen ; yellow in the eagle ; orange in the stork ; and red in some species of the scolopax. It affords that sprightly intermixture of colours which besprinkle the skin of the frog and salamander. But it is for the gay and glittering scales of fishes, the splendid metallic shells of beetles, the gaudy eye-spots that bedrop the wings of the butterfly, and the infinitely diversified hues of the flower-

VOL. II.—Y y

garden, that nature reserves the utmost force of this ever-varying pigment, and sports with it in her happiest caprices.

While I am writing, says Dr. Swediaur, I have before me a friend who, after residing abroad for many years, at first in the East Indies, and then in the West, returned to Europe with a skin variegated with white spots like those of a tiger. In other respects he is well.—(*Nov. Nosol. Meth. Syst.*, vol. ii., p. 204.)

In some cases, a diversified colour of the skin appears to be hereditary among mankind. Blumenbach gives an example of a Tartar tribe whose skin was generally spotted like the leopard's.—(*De Generis Hum. Varietate Nativâ.*) Individuals thus motley-coloured are commonly called piebald negroes, or are said to have piebald skins.

The Medico-Physical Society of New-York has lately published a case, communicated by Dr. Emery Bissel, in which a man of the Brotherton tribe of Indians, ninety years of age, had been gradually becoming white for the last thirty years of his life. The first appearance of this change was a small white patch near the pit of the stomach, soon after an attack of acute rheumatism ; which was shortly accompanied with other white spots in the vicinity, that enlarged, and at length intermixed. And the spread of the white hue continuing to range over the whole body, the original colour was only visible at the time of writing on the forehead and forepart of the face and neck, with a few small patches on the arm. The skin, as it became white, was of a fine clear teint, and had nothing of the dull earthy appearance or the livid hue observed in albinoes. Whence it should seem, that not merely the black or dark-coloured pigment had been absorbed and carried off, but that a fair, whitish, and glossy rete mucosum, like that secreted under the cuticle in white men, had taken its place.—(*Journ. of Science and Arts*, No. xii., p. 379.)

This extraordinary change, however, is sometimes produced far more rapidly ; for, in the American States, a black man has, in a few instances, had the whole of the colouring pigment carried off in the course of a severe fever, and has risen from his bed completely transformed into a white man. And in the famous American trial of Alexander Whistelo, the supposed father of a white bastard child, a variety of cases are given of a like kind, the black pigment being in some of them more generally removed, and in others less so.—(*The Commis. of the Almshouse v. Alexander Whistelo*, &c., New-York, 8vo., 1808.) Buchner, on the contrary, relates the case of a white man, who, on recovering from a like disorder, had his face tinged with a black hue, doubtless from a morbid secretion of a pigment the skin had never before elaborated.

A course of nitrate of silver, continued internally for some weeks, has often produced a deep tawny and uniform discoloration of the skin, approaching to a black, being deepest in the parts most exposed to the light. Fourcroy, Butini, Alberti, Reimarus, and many other writers, have given cases of this change ; and Dr.

Roget has lately published another instance, in which the discoloration preserved its intensity of hue six years after a discontinuance of the medicine, the general health not being interfered with.—(*Med. Chir. Trans.*, vol. vii., p. 290.) In some instances, the upper half of the body only has been discoloured, and more rarely, the pigment has appeared, like that of piebald negroes, in patches. Vesper relates the case of an old man, afflicted with hemiplegia, who presented the singular phenomenon of one half of the body, that which was paralyzed, completely yellow, while the other retained its natural colour; the distinction prevailed so accurately in the face, that the two hues ran through the nose, and were only separated by an imaginary line. In this instance, however, jaundice was the cause.—(*Dict. des Sciences Médicales*, art. CAS RARES.)

Plenck asserts that he once saw a man with a green face, the right side of his body black, and the left yellow, produced by a previous disease: and Dr. Bateman informs us, "that subsequent to the period of his publication, Dr. Willan had observed a variety of ptyriasis in children born in India and brought to this country, which commenced in a partially papulated state of the skin, and terminated in a black discoloration, with slightly furfuraceous exfoliations. It sometimes affected half a limb, as the arm or leg; sometimes the fingers or toes."—(*Cutaneous Diseases*, p. 48.)

SPECIES VII.
EPICHROSIS ALPHOSIS.
*ALBINO SKIN.**

CUTICLE DULL WHITE: PUPILS ROSY: SIGHT WEAK, AND STRONGEST IN THE SHADE.

THIS species occurs not among negroes only, as commonly supposed, but among the inhabi-

---

* A doubt may be entertained whether the state of an albino should be regarded as one of disease. Blumenbach and some other writers consider that the peculiarities of an albino proceed from a disease nearly allied to leprosy.—(De Gen. Hum. Varietate Nat., cap. iii., sec. 77, and Winterbottom on the Native Africans, vol. ii.) On the other hand, it is argued by Mr. Lawrence, that albinoes do not exhibit a single character of disease. All their functions are executed as in other persons. They are born of healthy parents, occur among the robust and hardy members of savage tribes, and a similar deviation takes place in many wild animals. He quotes two writers of very different characters, both of whom had seen African albinoes, and were convinced that the notion of disease was quite unfounded. "Prétendre que ce sont des nègres nains, dont une espèce de lèpre a blanchi la peau, c'est comme si l'on disoit que les noirs eux-mêmes sont des blancs que la lèpre a noircis."—(Voltaire, Essai sur les Mœurs, Introd.) Pallas writes,—"Cæterum hasce varietates Æthiopum albas non magis morbo sane naturam (quod Blumenbachio placuit) appellari posse puto, quam ipsa Æthiopum nigredo morbus est."—(Novæ Species Quadrupedum, p. 11.) Rayer, however, in his valuable work on the Diseases of the Skin, includes among them what he terms *albinism* or *leucopathia*, which he divides into *congenital* and

---

tants of Europe as well. [Experience proves, that the essential peculiarities which constitute an albino are not restricted to certain individuals of hot climates, but are occasionally noticed in natives of almost every country; and that the singular constitution of an albino is in fact not indicated merely by its effects on the surface of the body, but by equally remarkable characters in the eyes and hair. Certainly this deviation of human nature from its ordinary type was first observed in Africa, as might naturally be expected, because the contrast which a negro thus affected formed to the rest of the sable natives of that country, would be more striking than what resulted from the analogous condition of a European viewed among other Europeans, possessing their ordinary complexion. Hence, also, the individuals who thus deviated from the general black colour of their parents, were at first termed *leucæthiopes*, or *white negroes*. Afterward, however, similar varieties of the human species attracted remark in other parts of the globe, where sundry names were applied to them. Thus, in consequence of the annoyance which they suffered from the light, and their habit of avoiding it, such as were met with in the island of Java received from the Dutch the contemptuous appellation of *kakkerlakken*, *cockroaches*, insects that run about in the dark. Hence also the French term *chacrelas*. Of epichrosis alphosis, regarded by our author as a species of disease, he notices the two following varieties:]—

α Æthiopica. Negro albino.	Hair white and woolly: irids white. Found among negroes.	
β Europæa. European albino.	Hair flaxen and silky. Found among Europeans and other white nations.*	

The FIRST of these varieties is by far the most striking, on account of the greater change in the colour of the skin, and the peculiar contrast it forms with the general cast of the negro features.†

---

accidental, general or partial, proceeding from the absence of the pigment of the skin, and the colouring matter of the hair. A general accidental leucopathia, he observes, has hitherto only been noticed in negroes; though white persons, after a long residence in dark places, become blanched, so as to make an approach to albinism.—(See Traité des Mal. de la Peau, tom. ii., p. 194.) The subject of partial leucopathia, which may be either congenital or accidental, has been already considered under the sixth species of epichrosis. The forms of albinism termed by Rayer accidental, and occurring subsequently to birth, must undoubtedly be regarded as morbid conditions, whatever may be decided, in this respect, concerning albinoes, born as such.—ED.

* As albinoes occur in Java and Ceylon, and among the yellow or copper-coloured Indians of the Isthmus of Darien (see Lionel Wafer's New Voyage and Description of the Isthmus of America, 8vo., Lond., 1699), the African and European varieties will not comprehend all which have been noticed in various other parts of the world.—ED.

† See Jefferson's account of three albino negro women in the same family, in Cox's Philadelphia Museum, vol. i., p. 151.—D.

The name of albino was first employed by the Portuguese, and applied to such Moors as were born white, or rather who continued so from the time of birth ; for the children of negroes have little discoloration on birth, nor for several weeks afterward (see *Whistelo's Trial, as referred to in* p. 705) ; and who, on account of this morbid hue, were regarded as monsters ; and the term has since passed into our own and most other languages of the world. In these persons, however, there were other peculiarities observed besides the hue of the skin ; for their hair, in all its natural regions, was equally white, the iris of the eyes white, and the pupil rose-coloured. This whiteness of the surface, however, is not the clear and glossy teint of the uncoloured parts of the European frame in a healthy state, but of a dead or pallid cast, something like that of leprous scales. The eyes, in consequence of the deficiency of their natural pigment, are so weak that the individuals can hardly see any object in the day, or bear the rays of the sun ; though under the milder light of the moon they see with great accuracy, and run through the deepest shades of their forests with as much ease and activity as other persons do in the brightest daylight. They are also said to be less robust than other men ; and to sleep through the day and go abroad at night; both which last facts are easily accounted for, from the weakness of their sight and the discomfort of the sunbeams to their eyes.

It was at one time a subject of inquiry, whether these persons were a distinct variety of the human race, or merely instances of an occasional aberration from the ordinary laws that govern the human fabric : and the former opinion derived some support from its being found that male and female albinoes, who not unfrequently intermarried, being rejected by the rest of the world, produced an offspring with the same imperfections as their own.*

The question, however, has long been sufficiently set at rest, since albino children have been found produced in most parts of the world, and from parents of all tribes and colours, black and olive-hued, and red and tawny ; and since the subject has been more closely attended to, from white parents or inhabitants of Europe, as well as black or copper-coloured Africans. Nor does the anomaly appear to be confined to recent times ; for Pliny seems distinctly to allude to it in the following passage, as existing in his

day :—In Albaniâ gigni quosdam *glaucâ* oculorum *acie à pueritie* statim *canos,* qui *noctû plusquam interdiu cernunt.*—(*Nat. Hist.,* lib. vii., cap. 2.)

It is the appearance of the characteristic albino signs in European children, that constitutes the sᴇᴄᴏɴᴅ of the two varieties before us. These signs are, a dull or unglossy white diffused over the body, with white or flaxen hair, white irids and red pupils. The disease is rare, but we have had at least eleven examples* described by different authorities to the present time. Two by De Saussure, four by Buzzi, one by Helvetius, one by Maupertuis, and three by Dr. Traill. It is singular that all these are males ;[†] and still more so that the female offspring of the same families were, without an exception, destitute of the albino degeneracy. The three described by Dr. Traill were part of a family of six, the daughters of which were in every respect unaffected.[‡] How far this disorder is in Europe capable of being produced hereditarily, as abroad, is not known ; nor indeed does there yet appear to have been an opportunity of forming an intermarriage between a male and female of this kind, as not a single female has yet been discovered possessing the imperfect formation.

<hr>

* See further, Cox's account of an albino in the Phil. Med. Museum, vol. i., and J. Vaughan's description of two, in the second volume of the same work.—D.

† According to M. Saussure, female albinoes are more rare than male ones.—Voyages dans les Alpes, &c.

‡ In the year 1809, Rayer saw at Paris two examples of universal congenital albinism. The subjects of them were a brother and a sister, the one aged twenty, the other nineteen, both natives of France. Rayer is also acquainted with two children, one eight years old, the other ten, who have the same affection: their parents are healthy, and their brothers do not participate in their peculiarity. In March, 1827, Rayer tells us, he went to the Bicêtre, to see a person named Roche, an albino by birth, but better known in that place by the appellation of *lapin blanc* (white rabbit). He was then forty-three years of age, and, at first sight, presented the aspect of an old man. The hairs of his head and eyebrows, his eyelashes, beard, and the hairs of his limbs, were of a milk-white colour. The uvea was but slightly coloured, and pervaded by little red and gray streaks. The pupil was of blood-red colour. The skin looked very nearly like that of a person who has a fine complexion ; but it did not exhibit the dead white usually seen in albinoes. The mucous membranes of the eyelids, tongue, and genitals, presented the natural red colour seen in Europeans. The nails were of proper size and form. The eyes could not bear the light, the eyelids being commonly nearly closed, and subject to an incessant winking motion. The muscles of the trunk and limbs were well developed. The intellects weak ; and his power of articulation imperfect, as if he had a cleft in his palate. The genital organs were well formed. He appears to have had no brothers nor sisters. His father was a native of Picardy; his mother, who was a brunett, was born in Auvergne ; she ascribed the peculiarities in her son's conformation to her having experienced, during her pregnancy, a fright at the sight of a large white cat.—(See Rayer, op. cit., tom. ii., p. 198.)—Eᴅ.

<hr>

* In the natural history of our own species, Mr. Lawrence remarks, the albinoes have not met with much better treatment than the negroes ; for some have doubted whether they, as well as the latter, belong to the same species with us.—(See Voltaire, Essai sur les Mœurs, Introd. and chap. 143.) The negroes were too black, the albinoes too white. They have been supposed incapable of propagation. They are, in truth, not numerous enough to breed together, and thus form a permanent variety ; but that they can both beget and conceive is most abundantly proved. Mr. Lawrence knows of no instance of two being matched together ; but when they are paired with common negroes, the offspring is generally black, sometimes white.—Eᴅ.

The same delicacy of constitution that distinguishes the foreign or negro albino, distinguishes the European, of which we may form an estimate from Dr. Traill's account of one of the three we have already alluded to. "The oldest of these albinoes," says he, "is nine years of age, of a delicate constitution, slender, but well formed both in person and in features: his appetite has always been bad: he frequently complains of a dull pain in his forehead: his skin is exceedingly fair; his hair flaxen and soft; his cheeks have very little of the rose in them. The iris and *pupil* of his eyes are of a bright red colour, reflecting in some situations an opaline tinge. He cannot endure the strong light of the sun. When desired to look up, his eyelids are in constant motion, and he is incapable of fixing his eye steadily on any object, as is observed in those labouring under some kinds of slight ophthalmia, but in him is unaccompanied by tears. His mother says that his tears never flow in the coldest weather; but when he is vexed, they are shed abundantly. He goes to school, but generally retires to the darkest part of it to read his lesson. His disposition is very gentle; he is not deficient in intellect. His whole appearance is so remarkable, that some years ago a person attempted to steal him, and would have succeeded in dragging him away, had not his cries brought him assistance."[*]

The disease consists altogether in a defective secretion of the rete mucosum; which is not only without the colouring constituent principles that naturally belong to it, and particularly its power of affording a black pigment, but seems to be also untempered and imperfectly elaborated

___

[*] Nicholson's Journ. Nat. Phil., Feb., 1808. An account of an albino that was living near Vienna, is contained in Voigt's Magazin für das Neuste der Naturkunde, b. iii., p. 178. An albino boy of this country is briefly mentioned by Mr. Hunter. "Those of the human species," says he, "who have the pigmentum of a light colour, see much better with a less degree of light than those who have it dark; and this in proportion to their fairness; for, when the hair is quite white, they cannot see at all in open day, without knitting their eyebrows, and keeping the eyelids almost shut. In many of these instances, there is a universal glare of light from the pupil, tinged with a share of red, which colour most probably arises from the blood in the vessels of the choroid coat. I have likewise observed that the pigmentum is thinnest when it is light, so that some of the light which is reflected from the point of vision would seem to be thrown all over the inner surface of the eye, which, being white, or rather a reddish white, the light appears to be again reflected from side to side. This seemed to be the case in a boy at Shepperton, when about three years of age; of whom I have a portrait to show that appearance. He is now (1786) about thirteen years of age. The common light of the day is still too much for him; the twilight is less offensive. When in a room, he turns his eyes from the window; and when made to expose his face to the light, or when out in the open air, he knits his eyebrows, half shuts his eyelids, and bends his head forwards, or a little down; yet the light seems to be less obnoxious to him now than formerly, probably from habit."—(On Animal Economy, p. 250, 2d edit.)—ED.

in other respects, judging from the dulness or deadness of the white hue it gives to the surface of the body, instead of the life and glossiness it diffuses in a state of perfect health. That this cutaneous layer is not altogether wanting is clear, since in such case the red vascularity of the cutis would be conspicuous through the delicate transparent cuticle, in albinoes peculiarly delicate, and tinge the surface with a red, instead of a white colour.[*]

That the flaxen hue of the hair and the whiteness of the irids were derived from an imperfection in the secretion or elaboration of the rete mucosum, admits of no doubt; and the opinion long ago expressed by Professor Blumenbach (*Med. Bibl.*, ii., 537), that the red colour of the pupils in the two adult albinoes whom he had examined at Chamoun was equally owing to the want of the usual black pigment, has since been confirmed by M. Buzzi, of Milan, who has had an opportunity of dissecting an albino, and has proved that the pigmentum nigrum of the choroid coat, and also that portion of it which lies behind the iris, and is called uvea, were totally wanting.[†]

___

[*] Naturalists have soared into the regions of conjecture, in order to account for the origin of albinoes. Thus Buffon ascribes them to an effort of the constitution to resume, what he calls, the primitive colour of nature, which he fancies is white, and degenerates, in consequence of various circumstances, into the different shades now observed. All this, however, is merely fancy, unsupported by facts. Mr. Hunter's reasoning even inclined him to consider the opposite conclusion as most probable. "Animals," says he, "living in a free and natural state, are subject to few deviations from their specific character; but nature is less uniform in its operations when influenced by culture. *These changes are always*, I believe, *from the dark to the lighter teints*; and the alteration very gradual in certain species, requiring in the canary-bird several generations, while in the crow, mouse, &c., it is completed in one. But this change is not always to white, though still approaching nearer to it in the young than in the parent, &c. This alteration in colour being constantly from dark to lighter, may we not reasonably infer, that in all animals subject to such variation, the darkest of the species should be reckoned nearest to the original? and that where there are specimens of a particular kind entirely black, the whole have been originally black? Without this supposition, it will be impossible, on the principle I have stated, to account for individuals of any class being black."—(See Hunter on the Animal Economy, p. 244, 2d edit.)—ED.

[†] Dissertazione storico-anatomica sopra una varietà particolare de uomini bianchi, &c., Milan, 1784; Le Cat, Traité de la Couleur de la Peau humaine. The facts stated in the text do not amount to proof, that the colour of the hair and iris depends upon an imperfect secretion of the rete mucosum itself; for those parts have undoubtedly, in the natural state, a distinct colouring matter of their own. The following is, perhaps, a more correct representation of the subject:—The characters of the albino are found to depend upon a deficiency of the colouring principle of the skin, hair, and eyes. Thus, the former has the hue which its cellular and vascular contexture produces; the hair is reduced to its simple organic groundwork; and in the eyes, which are entirely

. We have observed, under the preceding species, that other animals are as richly supplied with a rete mucosum as mankind, and that they are indebted to it for their respective colours; and as there can be no reason why they may not at times endure a like deficiency, we have reason to expect, à priori, that they may occasionally exhibit proofs of the same complaint. In accordance with this reasoning, Blumenbach has traced this affection in many tribes, and especially in white dogs, owls, and rabbits [but, what is curious, only in warm-blooded animals]: and Dr. Traill has lately observed a case of the same disease in a young sparrow which he accidentally shot. This seems to have been a perfeet albino, with red eyes, pale reddish beak and neck, snow-white plumage, of a satin gloss on the head, neck, wing-coverts, and back. The nest from which it issued contained another young sparrow of the common colour; and when the albino-bird quitted the nest, which it was seen to do a few days before it was shot, it was instantly attacked by fifty or sixty common swallows, and obliged to take refuge in a tree.— (*Edinburgh Philosophical Journal*, No. 4, p. 390.)

·lestitute of pigmentum, the colour of the iris depends on the fine vessels which are so numerous in its composition, and that of the pupil in the still greater number of capillaries which almost entirely form the choroid membrane.—(See Hunter on Animal Economy, p. 250, 2d edit.) The close connexion of these parts, in respect to their colour, is evinced by the fact, that neither is ever separately affected.—(See Lawrence's Lect. on Physiology, &c., p. 281.) In piebald horses, however, as is well known, the iris is white, though most of their hair may be of another hue; and it is a curious fact, first pointed out by Mr. Hunter, that in variegated animals, the colour of the pigmentum of the eye is regulated by that of the eyelashes. "The magpie, for instance, is nearly one third or fourth part white; and the two colours, if blended, would make the compound gray; but, the eyelashes being black, the pigmentum is black also. We sometimes meet with people whose skin and hair are very white, and yet the iris is dark, which is a sign of a dark pigmentum; but if we examine more carefully, we shall also find that the eyelashes are dark, although the eyebrows may be of the colour of the common hair."—(On Animal Economy, p. 247, 2d edit.) It is alleged that the moral character of albinoes is in relation to the feebleness of their organization. Their intelligence, like that of negroes, is also stated to be of a limited description, though some instances to the contrary have been cited.—(See Rayer, Traité des Mal. de la Peau, tom. ii., p. 194.)—ED.

*The following memorandum and prayer, having been found among the late **Dr.**
Good's papers, are annexed to this work, in compliance with the directions which he
left upon the subject.*

JULY 27, 1823.

FORM OF PRAYER,

Which I purpose to use, among others, every morning, so long as it may please God that I shall
continue in the exercise of my profession; and which is here copied out, not so much to assist
my own memory, as to give a hint to many who may, perhaps, feel thankful for it when I am
removed to a state where personal vanity can have no access, and the opinion of the world can
be no longer of any importance. I should wish it to close the subsequent editions of my
STUDY OF MEDICINE.

O THOU great Bestower of health, strength, and comfort! grant thy blessing
upon the professional duties in which I may this day engage. Give me judgment to discern disease, and skill to treat it; and crown with thy favour the
means that may be devised for recovery: for, with thine assistance, the hum-
blest instrument may succeed; as, without it, the ablest must prove unavailing.

Save me from all sordid motives; and endow me with a spirit of pity and
liberality towards the poor; and of tenderness and sympathy towards all: that
I may enter into the various feelings by which they are respectively tried; may
weep with those that weep, and rejoice with those that rejoice.

And sanctify thou their souls, as well as heal their bodies. Let faith and patience, and every Christian virtue they are called upon to exercise, have their
perfect work: so that, in the gracious dealings of thy Spirit and of thy Providence, they may find in the end, whatever that end may be, that it has been
good for them to have been afflicted.

Grant this, O Heavenly Father, for the love of that adorable Redeemer who,
while on earth, went about doing good, and now ever liveth to make intercession
for us in Heaven. Amen.

GENERAL INDEX.

A.

Abortion, ii. 482.
Abscess, how distinguished from Aposteme, i. 428.
  of the abdomen, i. 429.
  of the loins, i. 434.
  of the liver, i. 435.
  of the chest, i. 437.
  of the breast, i. 443.
  of the eye, i. 527.
Absence of mind, ii. 208.
Absorbent system, physiology of, ii. 518.
  whether veins are absorbents, ii. 525.
  general effects from the union of this
    and the secement system, ii. 526.
Absorption in cataract, ii. 238.
Abstraction of mind, ii. 209.
Acari malis, ii. 689.
Acarus dysenteriæ, i. 548.
  scabiei, ii. 685.
  cutaneous, ib.
Acid bath, i. 205.
  uric, produced more copiously from animal
    than vegetable food, ii. 621.
  oxalic, predominant principle in diabetic
    urine, ib.
Acidum abietis, i. 266.
ACROTICA, ii. 637.
Acrotism, ii. 311.
Acrotismus, ib.
Acupunctura, in neuralgia, ii. 264.
Ædoptosis, ii. 471.
  uteri, ib.
    vaginæ, ii. 473.
    vesicæ, ib.
    complicata, ib.
    polyposa, ii. 474.
Ægophonism, ii. 52.
ÆSTHETICA, ii. 221.
Æstus volaticus, ii. 644.
Æthusa cynapium, or fool's parsley, i. 122.
After-pains in labour, ii. 507.
Agenesia, ii. 464.
  impotens, ii. 465.
  dysspermia, ii. 466.
  incongrua, ii. 468.
Agria, ii. 648.
Agrypnia, ii. 338.
  excitata, ib.
  pertæsa, ii. 339.
Ague, i. 350.
  quotidian, i. 353.
  tertian, i. 354.
  quartan, i. 355.
  irregular, ib.
  complicated, ib.
  has raged in high grounds, while low have
    escaped, i. 357.
  treatment of, i. 358.
Ague-cake, i. 356.

Air, average of inspired in a minute, i. 240, 243.
  vesicles or cells, i. 237.
  expired, i. 240.
  whether secreted by organs, ii. 593.
Albinism, ii. 706.
Albino-skin, ib.
Albugo, ii. 230.
Albumen, i. 320.
Algor, ii. 258.
Al-gridi (Arab.), i. 625.
Al-jedder (Arab.), ib.
Alimentary canal or cavity, i. 24.
  in some animals imperforate, ib.
  comparative length of, ib.
  extent in relation to kind of food,
    ib.
    DISEASES OF, i. 38.
Alopecia, ii. 681, 698, 700.
Alphabets, why they differ in different languages,
  i. 259.
  mostly derived from the Phœnician, i.
    260.
  Devanagari, and some others not, ib.
Alphos, ii. 655.
Alphosis, ii. 706.
Alternating calculus in the bladder, ii. 627.
Alusia, ii. 200.
  elatio, ib.
  hypochondrias, ii. 203.
Alveoli, absorbed in old age, i. 41.
Alvine worms, i. 174.
Alysmus, ii. 341.
Alyssum, ii. 306.
Amaurosis, ii. 238.
  varieties, ii. 239.
Ambition, ungovernable, ii. 195.
Amblyaphia, ii. 258.
Amblyopia senilis, ii. 240.
Amenorrhœa, ii. 431.
Ammoniaco-magnesian phosphate of the bladder,
  ii. 627.
Amnesia, ii. 217.
Anacatharsis, i. 263.
Anal hemorrhage, ii. 12.
  worms, i. 177.
Anaphrodisia, ii. 465.
Anaptysis, i. 263.
Anasarca, ii. 563.
Anas cygnus, i. 235.
  olor, ib.
Anetus, i. 350.
  quotidianus, i. 353.
  tertianus, i. 354.
  quartanus, i. 355.
  erraticus, ib.
  complicatus, ib.
  treatment of, i. 357.
Aneurisma, ii. 122.
  varieties, ii. 123.

THE END.

NATURAL HISTORY.

THE BOOK OF NATURE. By JOHN MASON GOOD, M.D., F.R.S. To which is now prefixed, a Sketch of the Author's Life. Complete in one volume, 8vo.

"This work is certainly the best philosophical digest of the kind which we have seen."—*Monthly Review.*

NATURAL HISTORY ; or, Uncle Philip's Conversations with the Children about Tools and Trades among the Inferior Animals. 18mo. With numerous Engravings.

THE NATURAL HISTORY OF INSECTS. With numerous Engravings. 18mo.

The study of Natural History is at all times, and to almost every person, eminently pleasing and instructive: the object in this admirable volume has been to render it doubly captivating by the plain and simple style in which it is treated, and by the numerous engravings with which the text is illustrated. There is no branch of this delightful science more pleasing than that which exhibits the wonderful goodness and wisdom of the Creator, as they are displayed in the endless varieties of insect life— their forms, habits, capacities and works—and which investigates the nature and peculiarities of these diminutive tribes of animated existence.

A POPULAR GUIDE TO THE OBSERVATION OF NA- TURE. By ROBERT MUDIE, Esq. 18mo. With Engravings.

AN OUTLINE OF THE NATURAL HISTORY OF EGYPT. By Rev. MICHAEL RUSSELL, LL.D. [No. 23 of the Family Library.] 18mo.

AN OUTLINE OF THE NATURAL HISTORY OF PALES- TINE. By Rev. M. RUSSELL, LL.D. [No. 27 Fam. Lib.] 18mo.

AN OUTLINE OF THE NATURAL HISTORY OF NU- BIA AND ABYSSINIA. By Rev. M. RUSSELL, LL.D. 18mo. No. 61 of the Family Library.] Engravings.

DESCRIPTIVE SKETCHES OF THE NATURAL HIS- TORY OF THE NORTH AMERICAN REGIONS. By JAMES WILSON, Esq. 18mo. [No. 53 of the Family Library.] Engravings.

ILLUSTRATIONS OF THE CLIMATE, GEOLOGY, AND NATURAL HISTORY OF THE POLAR SEAS AND REGIONS ; with an Account of the Whale-Fishery. By Professors LESLIE and JAMESON. With Engravings. [No. 14 of the Family Library.] 18mo.

ILLUSTRATIONS OF THE ZOOLOGY, BOTANY, CLI- MATE, GEOLOGY, AND MINERALOGY OF BRITISH INDIA. By JAMES WILSON, Esq. R. K. GREVILLE, LL.D. and Professor JAMESON. 18mo. [Nos. 47, 48, & 49 of the Family Library.] Engravings.

ILLUSTRATIONS OF THE GEOLOGY, MINERALOGY, AND ZOOLOGY OF AFRICA. By Professor JAMESON and JAMES WILSON, Esq. [No. 16 of the Family Library.] 18mo.

CLASSICAL WORKS.

XENOPHON. The Anabasis: Translated by EDWARD SPEL-
MAN, Esq. The Cyropædia: Translated by the Hon. MAURICE ASHLY COO-
PER. In 2 vols. 18mo. With a Portrait.

SALLUST. Translated by WILLIAM ROSE, M.D. With Notes.
18mo. Portrait.

CÆSAR. With Hirtius's Continuation. Translated by WIL-
LIAM DUNCAN. 2 vols. 18mo. Portrait.

CICERO. The Orations Translated by Duncan, the Offices by
Cockman, and the Cato and Lælius by Melmoth. In 3 vols. 18mo. With a
Portrait.

THE WORKS OF HORACE, translated literally into English
Prose. By C. SMART, A.M. In 2 vols. 18mo.

THE ORATIONS OF DEMOSTHENES. Translated by
THOMAS LELAND, D.D. In 2 vols. 18mo. Portrait.

MEDICINE AND SURGERY.

LEXICON MEDICUM; OR, MEDICAL DICTIONARY;
Containing an Explanation of the Terms in Anatomy, Botany, Chemistry, Materia Medica, Midwifery, Mineralogy, Pharmacy, Physiology, Practice of Physic,
Surgery, and the Various Branches of Natural Philosophy connected with Medicine. By ROBERT HOOPER, M.D. With Additions from American Authors,
by SAMUEL AKERLY, M.D. Two volumes in one, 8vo.

A DICTIONARY OF PRACTICAL SURGERY: compre-
hending all the most Interesting Improvements, from the earliest Times down
to the Present Period; an Account of the Instruments and Remedies employed
in Surgery; the Etymology and Signification of the Principal Terms; and
Numerous References to Ancient and Modern Works. By SAMUEL COOPER,
M.D. With numerous Notes and Additions, embracing all the Principal Improvements and Greater Operations introduced and performed by American
Surgeons. By DAVID MEREDITH REESE, M.D. In 2 vols. 8vo.

THE STUDY OF MEDICINE. By JOHN MASON GOOD, M.D.
New and Improved Edition. *In press.*

DIRECTIONS FOR INVIGORATING AND PROLONGING
LIFE; OR, THE INVALID'S ORACLE. Containing Peptic Precepts,
pointing out agreeable and effectual Methods to prevent and relieve Indigestion,
and to regulate and strengthen the Action of the Stomach and Bowels. By
WILLIAM KITCHENER, M.D. Revised and Improved, by THOMAS S. BARRETT,
M.D. 18mo.

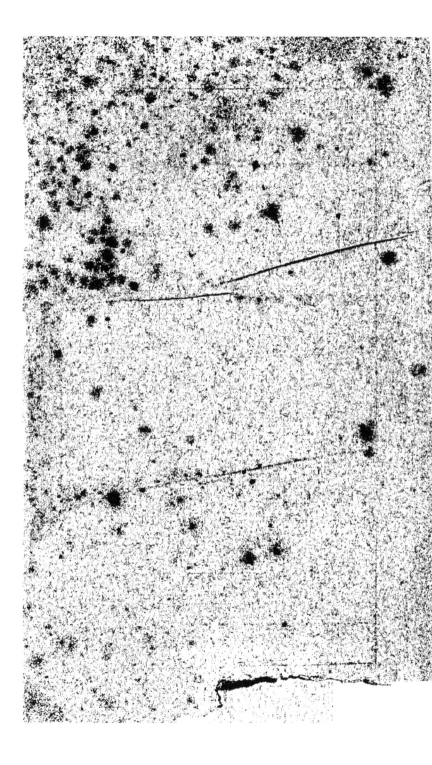

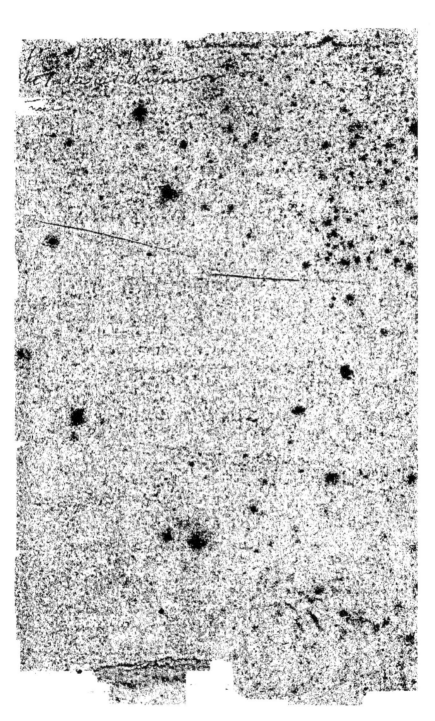

Lightning Source UK Ltd.
Milton Keynes UK
UKHW042146220219
337760UK00014B/1537/P